NURSING INTERVENTIONS & CLINICAL SKILLS

ANNE GRIFFIN PERRY, EdD, RN, FAAN
Professor Emerita
Former Interim Dean
School of Nursing
Southern Illinois University—Edwardsville
Edwardsville, Illinois

PATRICIA A. POTTER, PhD, RN, FAAN
Director of Research
Patient Care Services
Barnes-Jewish Hospital
St. Louis, Missouri

WENDY R. OSTENDORF, RN, MS, EdD, CNE
Professor of Nursing
Neumann University
Aston, Pennsylvania

ELSEVIER

ELSEVIER

3251 Riverport Lane
St. Louis, Missouri 63043

NURSING INTERVENTIONS AND CLINICAL SKILLS, SIXTH EDITION   ISBN: 978-0-323-18794-7

Notices

Knowledge and best practice in this field are constantly changing. As new research and experience broaden our understanding, changes in research methods, professional practices, or medical treatment may become necessary.

Practitioners and researchers must always rely on their own experience and knowledge in evaluating and using any information, methods, compounds, or experiments described herein. In using such information or methods they should be mindful of their own safety and the safety of others, including parties for whom they have a professional responsibility.

With respect to any drug or pharmaceutical products identified, readers are advised to check the most current information provided (i) on procedures featured or (ii) by the manufacturer of each product to be administered, to verify the recommended dose or formula, the method and duration of administration, and contraindications. It is the responsibility of practitioners, relying on their own experience and knowledge of their patients, to make diagnoses, to determine dosages and the best treatment for each individual patient, and to take all appropriate safety precautions.

To the fullest extent of the law, neither the Publisher nor the authors, contributors, or editors, assume any liability for any injury and/or damage to persons or property as a matter of products liability, negligence or otherwise, or from any use or operation of any methods, products, instructions, or ideas contained in the material herein.

Previous editions copyrighted 2012, 2007, 2004, 2000, 1996

International Standard Book Number: 978-0-323-18794-7

Executive Content Strategist: Tamara A. Myers
Traditional Content Development Manager: Jean Sims Fornango
Publishing Services Manager: Deborah L. Vogel
Senior Project Manager: Jodi M. Willard
Design Direction: Brian Salisbury

Printed in United States of America
KV

Last digit is the print number: 9   8   7   6   5   4   3   2   1

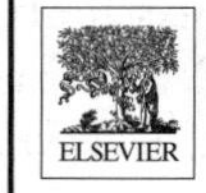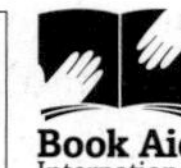

QUICK REFERENCE FOR STANDARD PROTOCOL FOR ALL NURSING INTERVENTIONS

All nursing skills must include certain basic steps for the safety and well being of the patient and the nurse. To prevent repetition, these steps are referred to at the beginning of and the end of each skill as standard protocols. The complete Standard Protocol includes the essential steps that must be done consistently with each patient contact in order to deliver responsible and safe nursing care.

BEFORE THE SKILL

1. **Verify health care provider's orders if the skill is a dependent or collaborative nursing intervention.** Independent nursing interventions are verified with the nursing care plan or primary nurse. *Dependent and collaborative interventions include invasive procedures and medically determined therapies, such as medication administration, wound care applications, and urinary catheterization.*
2. **Gather equipment/supplies and complete necessary charges according to agency policy.** Some equipment is reusable and is kept at the bedside. Some equipment is disposable and charged to the patient as used. *Check agency policy.*
   SUPPLIES for all nursing interventions:
   - Armband (or picture) for patient identification
   - Consent Form if required by facility policy
   - Clean disposable gloves if contact with mucous membranes, nonintact skin, or moist body substances is anticipated. (Consider latex allergies in choice of gloves.)
3. **Perform hand hygiene for at least 15 seconds following the Hand Hygiene guidelines in Chapter 5.** For hand rub solutions, check manufacturers' label for directions on use. *The CDC recommends rubbing for 15 seconds.*
4. **Introduce yourself to patient (and family),** including both your name and title or role. In this text "family" is used in an expanded sense to include husband/wife, domestic partner, or significant others. *Patients have the right to know the credentials of the persons providing their care.*
5. **Explain the procedure and describe what the patient can expect in simple terms.** *Understanding what is being done relieves patient's level of anxiety and enhances ability to cooperate.*
6. **Adjust the bed to appropriate height and lower side rail on the side nearest you.** Check locks on the bed wheel. *Minimizes caregiver's muscle strain and prevents injury. Prevents bed from moving.*
7. **Provide adequate lighting for procedure** *Ensures adequate illumination of patient's body and equipment.*
8. **Provide privacy for patient. Position and drape patient as needed.**

DURING THE SKILL

9. **Promote patient independence, decision making, and involvement if possible.** *A patient-centered approach to care enhances patient motivation and cooperation.*
10. **Assess patient tolerance, being alert for signs of discomfort, shortness of breath, and fatigue.** *Ability to tolerate interventions varies depending on severity of illness or pain. Use nursing judgment to provide rest and comfort measures.*

COMPLETION PROTOCOL (END OF SKILL)

11. **Assist patient to a position of comfort, and organize needed toiletry or personal items within reach.**
12. **Be certain patient has a way to call for help with call-light or alarm in easy reach and patient knows how to use it.** *Minimizes risk of falls.*
13. **Raise the appropriate number of side rails and lower the bed to the lowest position. Side rails are considered a restraint and cannot be used to prevent a patient from getting into and out of bed.** *Nursing judgment may allow alert, cooperative patients to have side rails down.*
14. **Dispose of used supplies and equipment.** Leave patient room tidy. *(See CDC Guidelines, Chapter 5)*
15. **Remove and dispose of gloves, if used. Perform hand hygiene for at least 15 seconds.** *Wearing gloves does not eliminate the need for hand hygiene.,*
16. **Document and report patient's response and expected or unexpected outcomes.** *Enhances continuity of nursing care.*

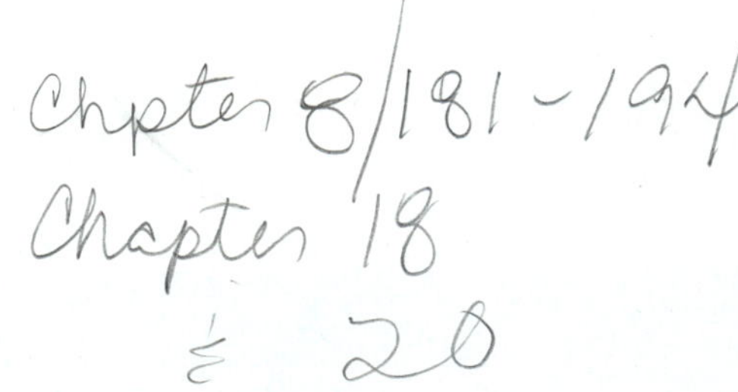

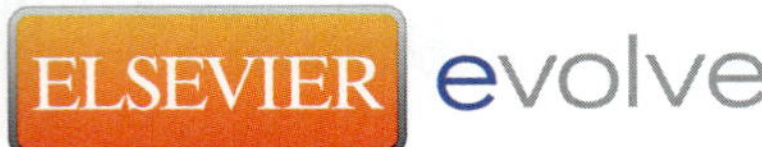

YOU'VE JUST PURCHASED
MORE THAN
A TEXTBOOK!

Evolve Student Resources for *Perry: Nursing Interventions & Clinical Skills, 6th,* include the following:

- Additional Review Questions
- Audio Glossary
- Skills Performance Checklists

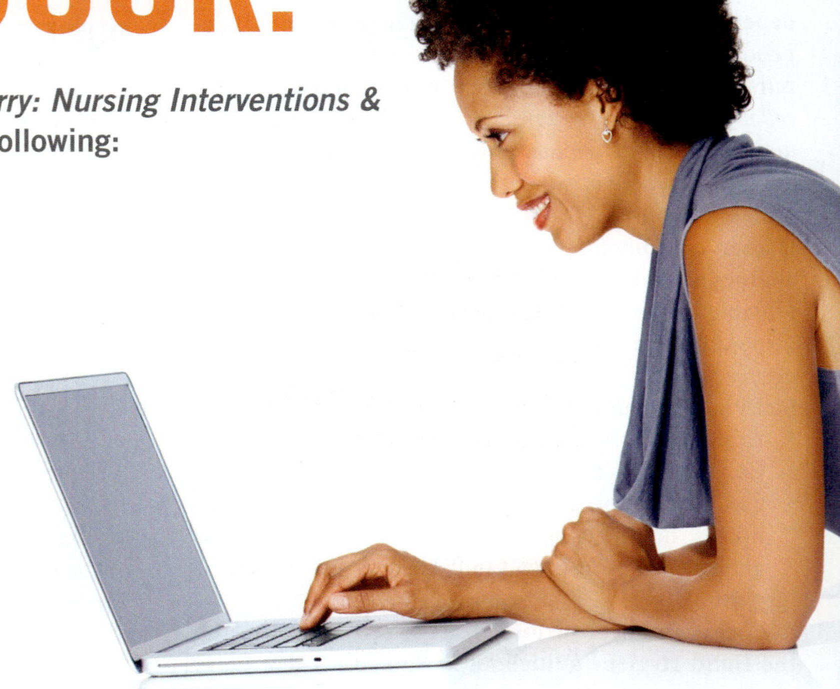

Activate the complete learning experience that comes with each *NEW* textbook purchase by registering at

http://evolve.elsevier.com/Perry/

REGISTER TODAY!

ANNE GRIFFIN PERRY, RN, EDD, FAAN

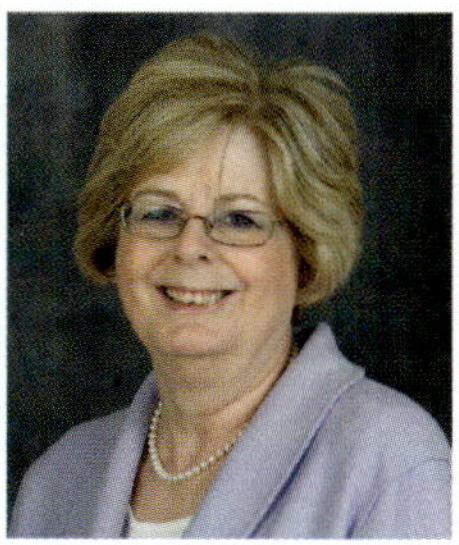

Dr. Anne G. Perry, Professor Emerita and Former Interim Dean and Associate Dean of Nursing at Southern Illinois University Edwardsville, is a Fellow in the American Academy of Nursing. She received her BSN from the University of Michigan, her MSN from Saint Louis University, and her EdD from Southern Illinois University at Edwardsville. Dr. Perry is a prolific and influential author and speaker. Her work includes four major textbooks (*Basic Nursing, Fundamentals of Nursing, Nursing Interventions and Clinical Skills,* and *Clinical Nursing Skills and Techniques*), 24 journal articles, 10 abstracts, and 12 nursing research and education grants. She has presented over 50 papers at conferences across the United States. She has acted as an editorial board member of numerous journals (*Journal of Nursing Measurement, Intensive Care Medicine, AACN Clinical Issues,* and *Perspectives in Respiratory Nursing*), and she was one of a few key consultants on *Mosby's Nursing Skills Videos* and *Mosby's Nursing Skills Online.* Dr. Perry currently serves on the NANDA board of directors and was formerly on the Advisory Board for Lewis and Clark Community College, School of Nursing.

Dr. Perry has been involved in the front lines of nursing education since 1973 at Saint Louis University, first as an instructor. She then advanced to full professor and held various leadership positions. As a clinician and researcher, Dr. Perry's contributions to pulmonary nursing and nursing language development involve both research and policy-making. She has investigated and published findings regarding topics that include weaning from mechanical ventilation, uses of the therapeutic intervention scoring system, critical care, and validation of nursing diagnoses.

PATRICIA A. POTTER, RN, MSN, PhD, FAAN

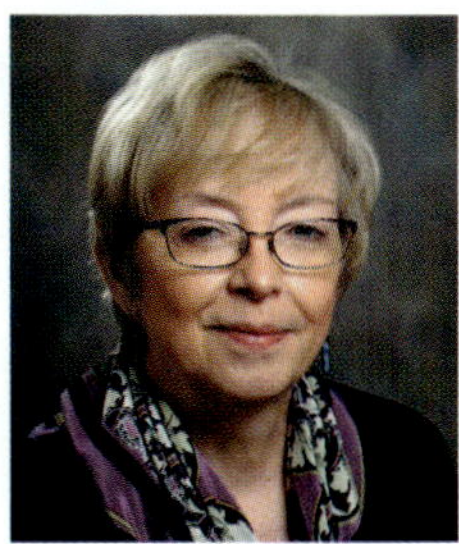

Dr. Patricia Potter received her diploma in nursing from Barnes School of Nursing, her BSN at the University of Washington in Seattle, Washington, and her MSN and PhD at Saint Louis University in St. Louis, Missouri. A ground-breaking author for more than 25 years, her work includes four major textbooks (*Basic Nursing, Fundamentals of Nursing, Nursing Interventions and Clinical Skills,* and *Clinical Nursing Skills and Techniques)* and over 20 journal articles. She has been an unceasing advocate of evidence-based practice and quality improvement in her roles as administrator, educator, and researcher.

Dr. Potter has devoted a lifetime to nursing education, practice, and research. She spent a decade teaching at Barnes Hospital School of Nursing and Saint Louis University. She entered into a variety of managerial and administrative roles, ultimately becoming the director of nursing practice for Barnes-Jewish Hospital. In that capacity she sharpened her interest in the development of nursing practice standards and measurement of patient outcomes in defining nursing practice. Her most recent passion has been in the area of nursing research, specifically cancer family caregiving, the effects of compassion fatigue on nurses and, more recently, fall prevention. Dr. Potter is currently the Director of Research for Patient Care Services at Barnes-Jewish Hospital in St. Louis, Missouri.

WENDY R. OSTENDORF, RN, MS, EdD, CNE

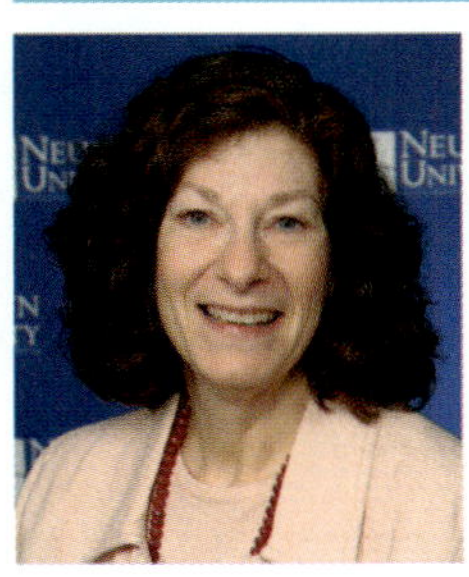

Dr. Wendy R. Ostendorf received her BSN from Villanova University, her MS from the University of Delaware, and her EdD from the University of Sarasota. She currently serves as a full professor of nursing in the Division of Nursing and Health Sciences at Neumann University in Aston, Pennsylvania. She has contributed over 26 chapters to multiple nursing textbooks and has served as co-author for *Clinical Nursing Skills and Techniques.* She has presented over 25 papers at conferences at the local, national, and international levels.

Professionally, Dr. Ostendorf has a diverse background in pediatric and adult critical care. She has taught at the undergraduate and graduate level for 30 years. With decades of practice as a clinician, her educational experiences have influenced her teaching philosophy and perceptions of the nursing profession. Dr. Ostendorf's current interests include the history and image of nursing as it has been represented in film, as well as the use of dedicated units and preceptors on students' transition to practice.

CONSULTANTS AND CONTRIBUTORS

CLINICAL CONSULTANTS

Nancy Laplante, PhD, RN,AHN-BC
Associate Professor
Widener University
Chester, Pennsylvania

Rita Wunderlich, PhD, RN, CNE
Associate Professor
Goldfarb School of Nursing
Barnes-Jewish College
St. Louis, Missouri

CONTRIBUTORS TO THE SIXTH EDITION

Janice C. Colwell, RN, MSN, CWOCN, FAAN
Advanced Practice Nurse
University of Chicago, Department of Surgery
Chicago, Illinois

Kelly Jo Cone, RN, PhD, CNE
Professor, Graduate Program
Saint Francis Medical Center College of Nursing
Peoria, Illinois

Patricia Conley, RN, MSN, PCCN
Staff Nurse
Research Medical Center
Kansas City, Missouri

Jane Fellows, MSN, RN, CWOCN
Wound/Ostomy CNS
Duke University Health System
Durham, North Carolina

Susan Fetzer, RN, GSWN, MSN, MBA, PhD
Associate Professor
College of Health and Human Services
University of New Hampshire
Durham, New Hampshire

Roberta L. Harrison, PhD, RN, CRRN
Assistant Professor
School of Nursing
Southern Illinois University—Edwardsville
Edwardsville, Illinois

Diane M. Heizer, MSN, RN
Practice Specialist
Barnes-Jewish Hospital
St. Louis, Missouri

Anne Marie Herlihey, DNP, RN, CNOR
Administrative Director for Perioperative, Endoscopy, and
    Ambulatory Services
Alexian Brothers Medical Center
Elk Grove Village, Illinois

Nancy Laplante, PhD, RN,AHN-BC
Associate Professor
Widener University
Chester, Pennsylvania

Nelda K. Martin, RN, CCNS, ANP-BC
Clinical Nurse Specialist / Adult Nurse Practitioner
Barnes-Jewish Hospital, Heart and Vascular Program
St. Louis, Missouri

Angela McConachie, DNP, FNP-C
Instructor
Goldfarb School of Nursing at Barnes-Jewish College
St. Louis, Missouri

Theresa Pietsch, Ph.D, RN, CRRN, CNE
Assistant Professor
Neumann University
Aston, Pennsylvania

Elizabeth S. Pratt, DNP, RN, ACNS-BC
Research Scientist, Clinical Nurse Specialist
Barnes-Jewish Hospital
St. Louis, Missouri

Jacqueline Raybuck Saleeby, PhD, RN, BCCS
Associate Professor, Nursing
School of Health Professions
Maryville University
St. Louis, Missouri

Amy Spencer, MSN, RN-BC
Staff Development Specialist
Christiana Care Health Systems
Newark, Delaware

E. Bradley Strecker, PhD, RN, CRRN
Associate Professor
Program Director, Accelerated BSN Program
Mid America Nazarene University
Olathe, Kansas

Virginia Strootman, RN, MS, CRNI
Vice President of Clinical Services
Specialty Pharmacy Nursing Network, Inc.
Sarasota, Florida

Donna L. Thompson, MSN, CRNP, FNP-BC, CCCN
Nurse Practitioner—Continence Specialist
Urology Health Specialist
Drexel Hills, Pennsylvania

Rita Wunderlich
Associate Professor
Goldfarb School of Nursing
Barnes-Jewish College
St. Louis, Missouri

Valerie J. Yancey, PhD, RN, HNC, CHPN
Associate Professor
Southern Illinois University—Edwardsville
Edwardsville, Illinois

CONTRIBUTORS TO PREVIOUS EDITIONS

Elizabeth A. Ayello, RN, BSN, MS, PhD, CS, CETN

Margaret R. Benz, RN, MSN(R), BC, APN

Barbara J. Berger, MSN, RN

V. Christine Champagne, APRN, BC

Janice C. Colwell, Rn, MS, CWOCN

Kelly Jo Cone, PhD, RN, CNE

Karen S. Conners, RNC, MSN

Eileen Costantinou, MSN, RN

Deborah Crump, RN, MS, CHPN

Sheila A. Cunningham, BSN, MSN

Wanda Cleveland Dubuisson, PhD, RN

Julie Eddins, RN, BSN, MSN, CRNI

Deborah Oldenburg Erickson, RN, BSN, MSN

Joan O. Ervin, RN, BSN, MN, CCRN

Sue Fetzer, BA, BSN, MSN, MBA, PhD

Melba J. Figgins, MSN, BSN

Janet B. Fox-Moatz, RN, BSN, MSN

Lynn C. Hadaway, MEd, RNC, CRNI

Amy Hall, RN, PhD

Susan A. Hauser, RN, BSN, BA, MS

Mimi Hirshberg, RN, MSN

Carolyn Chaney Hoskins, RN, BSN, MSN

Maureen B. Huhmann, MS, RD

Meredith Hunt, MSN, RNC, NP

Nancy Jackson, RN, BSN, MSN(R), CCRN

Linda L. Kerby, RN-C-R, BSN, MA, BA

Marilee Kuhrik, BSN, MSN, PhD

Nancy Kuhrik, BSN, MSN, PhD

Amy Lawn, BSN, MS, CIC

Kristine M. L'Ecuyer, RN, MSN, CCNS

Antoinette Kanne Ledbetter, RN, BSN, MS, TNS

Mary MacDonald, RN, MSN

Mary Kay Knight Macheca, MSN(R), RN, CS, ANP, CDE

Cynthia L. Maskey, RN, MS

Constance C. Maxey, RN-BC, MSN

Barbara McGeever, RN, RSM, BSN, MSN, DNS(c)

Mary "Dee" Miller, RN, BSN, MS, CIC

Peter R. Miller, RN, MSN, ONC

Rose M. Miller, RN, BSN, MSN, MPA, ACLS

Karen Montalto, RN, DNSc

Kathleen Mulryan, RN, BSN, MSN

Elaine K. Neel, RN, BSN, MSN

Kim Campbell Oliveri, RN, MS, CS

Marsha Evans Orr, RN, MS

Wendy R. Ostendorf, RN, MS, EdD, CNE

Shirley E. Otto, MSN, RN, AOCN

Deborah Paul-Cheadle, RN

Roberta J. Richmond, MSN, RN, CCRN

Paulette D. Rollant, RN, BSN, MSN, PhD, CCRN

Jacqueline Raybuck Salleby, PhD, RN, MSN

Linette M. Sarti, RN, BSN, CNOR

Lynn Schallom, RN, MSN, CCRN, CCNS

Kelly Schwartz, RN, BSN

Julie Snyder, RN, MSN, BC

Phyllis G. Stallard, BSN, MSN, ACCE

Victoria Steelman, PhD, RN, CNOR

Patricia A. Stockert, RN, PhD

Sue G. Thacker, RNC, BSN, MS, PhD

Donna L. Thompson, MSN, CRNP, FNP-BC, CCCN

Nancy Tomaselli, RN, MSN, CS, CRNP, CWOCN, CLNC

Stephanie Trinkl, BSN, MSN

Kathryn Tripp, BSN

Paula Vehlow, RN, MS

Pamela Becker Weilitz, MSN(R), RN, CN, ANP

Jana L. Weindel-Dees, RN, BSN, MSN

Joan Domigan Wentz, MSN, RN

Trudie Wierda, RN, MSN

Laurel A. Wiersema-Bryant, MSN, RN, CS

Terry L. Wood, PhD, RN, CNE

Rita Wunderlich, MSN, PhD

Rhonda Yancey, BSN, RN

Valerie J. Yancey, PhD, RN, HNC, CHPN

Shannon Patton, RN, MSN
Instructor of Clinical Nursing
School of Nursing
The University of Texas at Austin
Austin, Texas

Patricia L. Pence, EdD, MSN, RN
Nursing Professor
Illinois Valley Community College
Oglesby, Illinois

**Susan Porterfield, PhD, MSN, MS, BSN,
    BS, FNP-C**
NP Coordinator/Assistant Professor
Florida State University
Tallahassee, Florida

Jill Reed, MSN, APRN-C
Nursing Instructor
College of Nursing
University of Nebraska Medical Center
Kearney, Nebraska

Erin K. Rodgers, MSN, RN, CPN
Assistant Professor
School of Nursing
Vanderbilt University
Nashville, Tennessee

Diane Rudolphi, MSN, RN
CNTT Faculty
School of Nursing
University of Delaware
Newark, Delaware

Gale P. Sewell, PhD(c), MSN, RN, CNE
Associate Professor
Department of Nursing
University of Northwestern St. Paul
St. Paul, Minnesota

**Mary Ann Shinnick, PhD, RN,
    ACNP-BC, CCNS**
Director Simulation Lab
School of Nursing
University of California—Los Angeles
Los Angeles, California

**Benjamin A. Smallheer, PhD, RN,
    ACNP-BC, CCRN**
Assistant Professor
Acute Care Nurse Practitioner
School of Nursing
Vanderbilt University

Sarah A. Smith, Ph.D, RNC-OB
Nursing Laboratory and Simulation
    Coordinator
School of Nursing
University of Hawaii—Hilo
Hilo, Hawaii

Lanette E. Tanaka, MSN, RN
Assistant Teaching Professor
College of Nursing
University of Missouri—St. Louis
St. Louis, Missouri

Lynne L. Tier, MSN, RN, LNC
Associate Professor of Nursing
Adventist University of Health Sciences
Orlando, Florida

Jodi VanKleef, MS, RNC-OB
Instructor
School of Nursing
Southern Illinois University at Edwardsville
Edwardsville, Illinois

Susan A. Wheaton, MSN, RN
LRC Director/Lecturer/Clinical Instructor
School of Nursing
University of Maine

**Paige D. Wimberley, PhD, APRN,
    CNS, CNE**
Associate Professor of Nursing
Arkansas State University
Jonesboro, Arkansas

Aimee Woda, PhD, RN, BC
Assistant Clinical Professor
Marquette University
Milwaukee, Wisconsin

Thanks to the talented and dedicated professionals at Elsevier: Tamara Myers, Executive Editor, who provided support, leadership, enthusiasm, and a healthy sense of humor during the revision process; Jean Sims Fornango, Managing Editor, who spent countless hours tracking the progress of this text. Her organizational skills, commitment to accuracy, and dedication to quality kept the project on target; Jodi Willard, Senior Project Manager, whose organization, careful editing, and guidance of the project through the production process helped to ensure an accurate, consistent book; and Brian Salisbury, whose creativity provides an attractive and unique visual appeal to the text. These contributions significantly enhance the learning process.

Notes from the Authors

I wish to acknowledge the nurse educators at Saint Louis University and Southern Illinois University—Edwardsville Schools of Nursing. Their knowledge of the discipline and commitment to nursing education help to shape the practice of nursing in the region. These educators skillfully integrate the science and the art of nursing into their classes and clinical experiences. These faculty, together with the expert nursing staff in the clinical settings, provide the initial foundation for caring clinical practice.

Anne Griffin Perry

As I continue to enjoy a nursing career enriched by knowing so many outstanding nurse professionals, I wish to acknowledge the nurses at Barnes-Jewish Hospital. They practice excellence each day by always seeking ways to improve their practices. They are also deeply caring individuals who strive to bring comfort and healing for their patients.

Patricia A. Potter

It is an ongoing honor to contribute to a book that will support the education of so many future nurses. I would like to thank my husband, who has endless patience and offers me so much love, as I take so much time to work on my career.

Wendy R. Ostendorf

PREFACE TO THE STUDENT

Numerous features are built into this textbook to develop your skills as a highly qualified nurse. Look for these elements to focus your study time for more efficient effort:

- **Quick Reference for Standard Protocol for All Nursing Interventions** in the front of the text reminds you of steps to be consistently taken before, during, and after every care interaction with a patient. Each skill and procedure will remind you to review these steps.
- **Clean glove logo** reminds you when it is essential to apply clean gloves to protect yourself and your patient from transmission of microorganisms.

- **Safe Patient Care** boxes help you identify important safety issues for each skill and procedure.
- **Additional review questions, checklists, and an audio glossary** are available for your use on the companion Evolve site: http://evolve.elsevier.com/perry/nursinginterventions

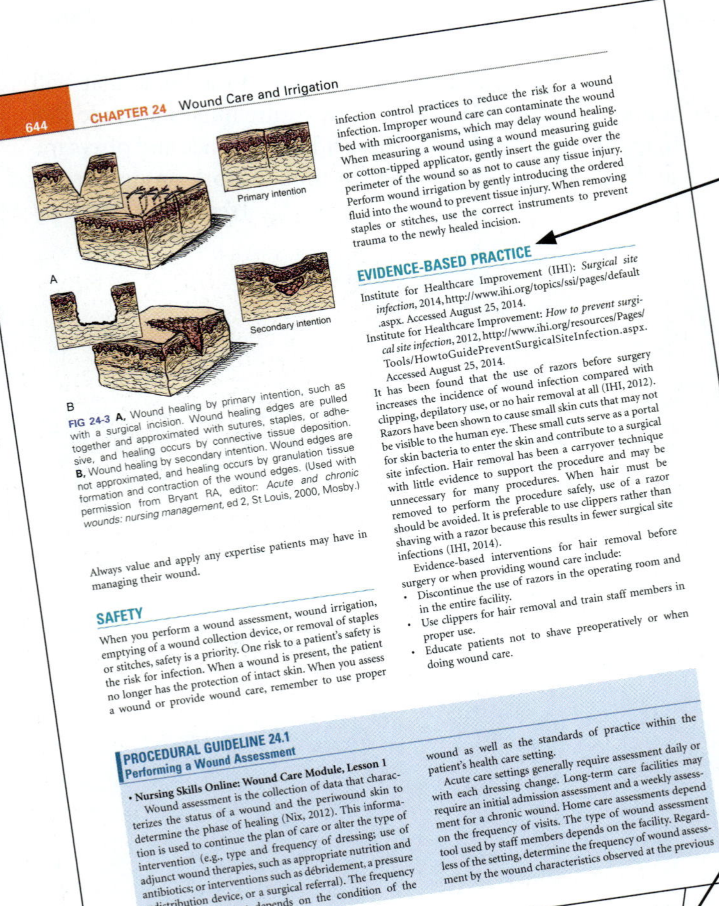

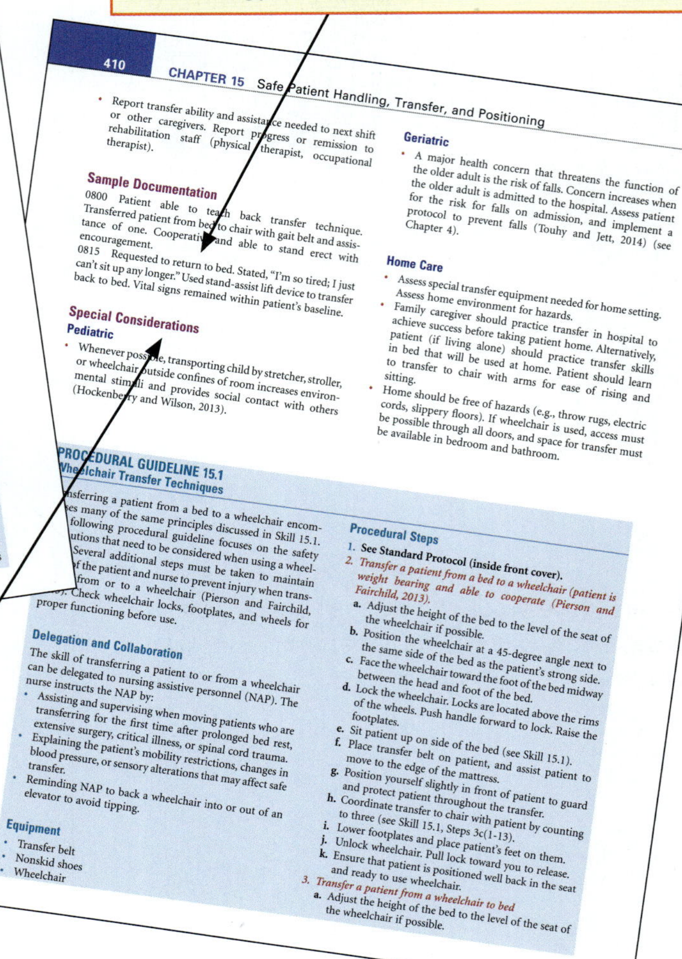

Every chapter has an Evidence-Based Practice section to help you understand how research outcomes inform evidence-based nursing practice.

Sample Documentation shows you how to record a nurse's narrative note with proper terminology and phrasing.

Special Considerations indicate modifications needed for pediatric, geriatric, or home care performance of a skill.

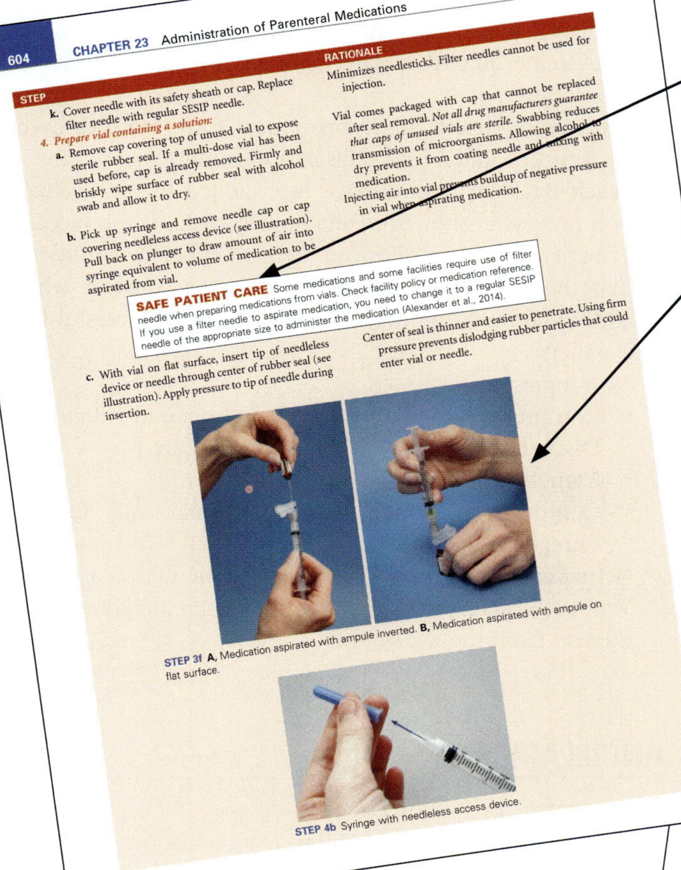

STEP	RATIONALE
k. Cover needle with its safety sheath or cap. Replace filter needle with regular SESIP needle.	Minimizes needlesticks. Filter needles cannot be used for injection.
4. *Prepare vial containing a solution:*	
a. Remove cap covering top of unused vial to expose sterile rubber seal. If a multi-dose vial has been used before, cap is already removed. Firmly and briskly wipe surface of rubber seal with alcohol swab and allow it to dry.	Vial comes packaged with cap that cannot be replaced after seal removal. *Not all drug manufacturers guarantee that caps of unused vials are sterile.* Swabbing reduces transmission of microorganisms. Allowing alcohol to dry prevents it from coating needle and mixing with medication.
b. Pick up syringe and remove needle cap or cap covering needleless access device (see illustration). Pull back on plunger to draw amount of air into syringe equivalent to volume of medication to be aspirated from vial.	Injecting air into vial prevents buildup of negative pressure in vial when aspirating medication.

SAFE PATIENT CARE Some medications and some facilities require use of filter needle when preparing medications from vials. Check facility policy or medication reference. If you use a filter needle to aspirate medication, you need to change it to a regular SESIP needle of the appropriate size to administer the medication (Alexander et al., 2014).

STEP	RATIONALE
c. With vial on flat surface, insert tip of needleless device or needle through center of rubber seal (see illustration). Apply pressure to tip of needle during insertion.	Center of seal is thinner and easier to penetrate. Using firm pressure prevents dislodging rubber particles that could enter vial or needle.

STEP 3f **A,** Medication aspirated with ampule inverted. **B,** Medication aspirated with ampule on flat surface.

STEP 4b Syringe with needleless access device.

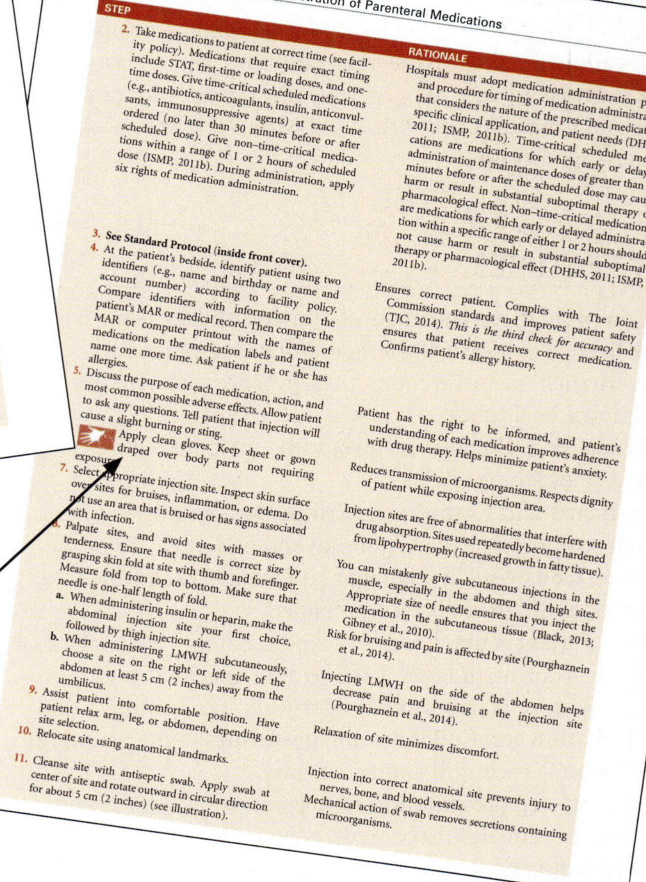

STEP	RATIONALE
2. Take medications to patient at correct time (see facility policy). Medications that require exact timing include STAT, first-time or loading doses, and one-time doses. Give time-critical scheduled medications (e.g., antibiotics, anticoagulants, insulin, anticonvulsants, immunosuppressive agents) at exact time ordered (no later than 30 minutes before or after scheduled dose). Give non–time-critical medications within a range of 1 or 2 hours of scheduled dose (ISMP, 2011b). During administration, apply six rights of medication administration.	Hospitals must adopt medication administration policy and procedure for timing of medication administration that considers the nature of the prescribed medication, specific clinical application, and patient needs (DHHS, 2011; ISMP, 2011b). Time-critical scheduled medications are medications for which early or delayed administration of maintenance doses of greater than 30 minutes before or after the scheduled dose may cause harm or result in substantial suboptimal therapy or pharmacological effect. Non–time-critical medications are medications for which early or delayed administration within a specific range of either 1 or 2 hours should not cause harm or result in substantial suboptimal therapy or pharmacological effect (DHHS, 2011; ISMP, 2011b).
3. See Standard Protocol (inside front cover).	
4. At the patient's bedside, identify patient using two identifiers (e.g., name and birthday or name and account number) according to facility policy. Compare identifiers with information on the patient's MAR or medical record. Then compare the MAR or computer printout with the names of medications on the medication labels and patient name one more time. Ask patient if he or she has allergies.	Ensures correct patient. Complies with The Joint Commission standards and improves patient safety (TJC, 2014). *This is the third check for accuracy and* ensures that patient receives correct medication. Confirms patient's allergy history.
5. Discuss the purpose of each medication, action, and most common possible adverse effects. Allow patient to ask any questions. Tell patient that injection will cause a slight burning or sting.	Patient has the right to be informed, and patient's understanding of each medication improves adherence with drug therapy. Helps minimize patient's anxiety.
6. Apply clean gloves. Keep sheet or gown draped over body parts not requiring exposure.	Reduces transmission of microorganisms. Respects dignity of patient while exposing injection area.
7. Select appropriate injection site. Inspect skin surface over sites for bruises, inflammation, or edema. Do not use an area that is bruised or has signs associated with infection.	Injection sites are free of abnormalities that interfere with drug absorption. Sites used repeatedly become hardened from lipohypertrophy (increased growth in fatty tissue).
8. Palpate sites, and avoid sites with masses or tenderness. Ensure that needle is correct size by grasping skin fold at site with thumb and forefinger. Measure fold from top to bottom. Make sure that needle is one-half length of fold.	You can mistakenly give subcutaneous injections in the muscle, especially in the abdomen and thigh sites. Appropriate size of needle ensures that you inject medication in the subcutaneous tissue (Black, 2013; Gibney et al., 2010).
a. When administering insulin or heparin, make the abdominal injection site your first choice, followed by thigh injection site.	Risk for bruising and pain is affected by site (Pourghaznein et al., 2014).
b. When administering LMWH subcutaneously, choose a site on the right or left side of the abdomen at least 5 cm (2 inches) away from the umbilicus.	Injecting LMWH on the side of the abdomen helps decrease pain and bruising at the injection site (Pourghaznein et al., 2014).
9. Assist patient into comfortable position. Have patient relax arm, leg, or abdomen, depending on site selection.	Relaxation of site minimizes discomfort.
10. Relocate site using anatomical landmarks.	
11. Cleanse site with antiseptic swab. Apply swab at center of site and rotate outward in circular direction for about 5 cm (2 inches) (see illustration).	Injection into correct anatomical site prevents injury to nerves, bone, and blood vessels. Mechanical action of swab removes secretions containing microorganisms.

Safe Patient Care alerts help you promote patient safety.

Extensive illustrations demonstrate key step-by-step procedures.

Glove logo reminds you when to apply clean gloves during the course of performing a skill or procedure.

The evolution of knowledge and technology influences the way we teach clinical skills to nursing students. The foundation for success in performing nursing skills remains a competent and well-informed nurse who thinks critically and asks the right questions at the right time to provide appropriate, high-quality nursing care. This edition of *Nursing Interventions & Clinical Skills* retains the successful elements of previous editions but incorporates material key to this shift in how nurses practice.

Emphasis on QSEN Competencies may be easily found throughout the text. You will find sections on *Patient-Centered Care*, *Safety*, and *Evidence-Based Practice* at the beginning of each chapter. Information on *Delegation and Collaboration*, *Safe Patient Care*, and *Documentation* appear in each skill and procedure as needed. We have retained the concise format, clear language, and streamlined approach that were hallmarks of previous editions. New photos and line drawings update the generous illustration program. All skills and procedures are presented within the framework of the nursing process.

KEY FEATURES

- **Comprehensive coverage** of nursing skills—from basic skills such as measuring temperature to complex advanced skills such as intravenous therapy and management of endotracheal tubes
- **Extensive full-color art program**, including dozens of new photographs
- **Standard and Completion Protocols**—simplifying basic steps common to the beginning and end of each skill
- **Glove icons** visually highlight circumstances in which the use of clean gloves is recommended
- **Safe Patient Care boxes** incorporated into skill alerts, which inform students when to take special precautions and the specific risks to consider when performing a skill
- **Delegation and Collaboration guidelines** in the planning section for each skill and procedure
- **Step-by-step presentation of steps** of each skill, with supporting rationales that are often evidence based
- **Recording and Reporting** sections provide a concise, bulleted list of information to be documented and reported
- **Sample Documentation** sections provide examples of clear variance notes or narrative documentation
- **Special Considerations** sections provide information on how to adapt skills in specific circumstances, such as in the home care setting or when caring for a child or older adult

NEW TO THIS EDITION

- Introduction of the concept of **HCAHPS** (Hospital Consumer Assessment of Healthcare Providers and Systems), which is a patient survey now widely used to evaluate quality of care delivered by hospitals across the country.
- Institute of Healthcare Improvement **Care-bundles** have been incorporated into skills as appropriate.
- **Teach-Back** techniques have been added to the Evaluation process to show students how to evaluate the success of patient teaching, allowing them to either be confident that the patient has mastered a task or consider what additional teaching methods may be more successful for a patient.
- New topics:
  - Communication with Cognitively Impaired Patients
  - Discharge Planning and Transitional Care
  - Catheterizing a Urinary Diversion
  - Compassion Fatigue for Professional and Family Caregivers
- **Returned to the text:** Care of a Patient with a Central Venous Access Device. This skill has been reintegrated into the text from the Evolve site.

ANCILLARIES

Evolve Instructor Resources:
- *TEACH for RN* provides objectives, lesson plans, teaching strategies, clinical activities, additional case studies, integration guides for media, nursing curriculum standards correlation (including concepts based), and PowerPoint sets for each chapter
- *Test Bank* includes 750 completely updated testing items in a variety of testing formats
- *PowerPoint* slide sets for each chapter

Evolve Student Resources:
- Audio glossary
- Interactive review questions
- Skills Performance Checklists for every skill and procedure in interactive PDF format

Also available:
- **Nursing Skills Online 3.0** contains 18 modules rich with animations, videos clips, interactive activities, and exercises to help students prepare for their clinical lab experience. The instructionally designed lessons focus on topics that are difficult to master and pose a high

risk to the patient if done incorrectly. Lesson quizzes allow students to check their learning curve and review as needed, and the module exams feed out to an instructor grade book. Available alone or packaged with the text.

- **Mosby's Nursing Video Skills: Basic, Intermediate, Advanced, 4th edition,** provides 128 skills with overview information covering skill purpose, safety, and delegation guides; equipment lists; preparation steps ; procedure videos with printable step-by-step guidelines; appropriate follow-up care; documentation guidelines; and interactive review questions. Available online or as a student DVD, either of which may be packaged with the text. The online version feeds unit exams to an instructor grade book.

CONTENTS

APPENDIXES

Using Evidence in Nursing Practice

EVOLVE WEBSITE/RESOURCES LIST

http://evolve.elsevier.com/Perry/nursinginterventions
Audio Glossary • Checklists • Review Questions

Nurses have a critical role in health care delivery. As health care facilities in the United States continue to optimize care delivery systems, the Institute of Medicine (IOM) emphasizes six aims to achieve quality: Care must be safe, effective, efficient, timely, patient-centered, and equitable (IOM, 2001). Nurses are at the forefront of health care, providing direct care to patients and their family caregivers. Nurses must understand the implications of providing care using evidence-based practice (EBP) to achieve the six aims noted by the IOM. The IOM report, along with initiatives from groups such as The Joint Commission (TJC) and the National Quality Forum (NQF), has led to greater scrutiny as to why certain health care approaches are used. As a result, EBP became a response to the broad societal forces that nurses and other health care professionals face. The Quality and Safety Education for Nurses (QSEN) Institute recognizes that EBP is an essential tool for nursing graduates, who must be able to integrate EBP to deliver optimal health care (QSEN Institute, 2014).

The IOM published *The Future of Nursing* (2010), which stressed that EBP should be a core competency in nursing education. As a nurse, you must employ best practices for your patients. EBP is the method that incorporates current research evidence, clinical expertise, health care resources, and patient and family values and preferences to determine safe care practices. The application of research findings is just one piece of EBP. In contrast, research utilization is the process by which only scientifically produced knowledge (e.g., research study findings) is transferred to practice. "Evidence-based practice is broader than research utilization because clinicians are encouraged to consider a number of dimensions in clinical-decision making, one of which is evidence" (Melnyk and Fineout-Overholt, 2011).

The American Nurses Association (ANA) highlights EBP in *Nursing: Scope and Standards of Practice* (2010). Standard 9 states that "the registered nurse integrates evidence and research findings into practice" (ANA, 2010) to promote positive patient outcomes (Fig. 1-1). All health care professionals should use EBP in their clinical practice. For example, a nursing student reviews the most current literature on the proper implementation of a new skill. A nurse educator applies current evidence to improve a simulated laboratory teaching technique for nursing students. A group of staff nurses studies the evidence and works with an interdisciplinary team on the unit to find ways to improve communication among the team and the patients. In each case, nurses and other health care professionals use a problem-solving approach that integrates use of the best available scientific evidence rather than making decisions on intuition, past policy, or experience alone.

New evidence in the research literature is reported every day. The rapid growth in health care and technology requires

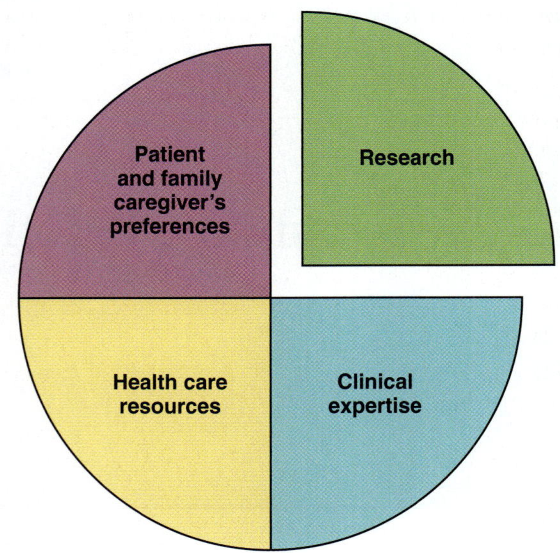

FIG 1-1 Evidence-based practice. (Melnyk and Fineout-Overholt, 2011; Newhouse et al., 2007.)

nurses to have up-to-date knowledge to provide the most effective care for patients (Poe and White, 2010). Relying only on experience or previous knowledge gained in schooling can limit care and possibly harm patients. Maintaining up-to-date knowledge on best practices is essential for you to provide the best care to your patients (Box 1-1). The challenge is to obtain the very best, most current information when you need it in your practice.

COMPARING EVIDENCE-BASED PRACTICE WITH RESEARCH AND PERFORMANCE IMPROVEMENT

Health care providers frequently confuse the similarities and differences between EBP, research, and performance or quality improvement (Fig. 1-2). Table 1-1 compares the three related processes. Performance improvement processes are designed to bring about immediate improvement in health care delivery settings. Change in processes can occur quickly. Often when members of a performance improvement team review their internal monitoring data (e.g., fall rates, falls with injuries), they might decide to change their processes by applying EBP (applying fall prevention evidence). When a quality improvement process is completed, there may be unanswered questions (e.g., what is the best approach to reduce falls in cancer patients) that may lead to the need for a research study.

Applying EBP optimizes clinical care and improves patient outcomes by applying the most current and relevant evidence that pertains to a clinical problem (e.g., inpatient falls). Using EBP, incorporating patient's and family's preferences in conjunction with clinical expertise and health care resources, allows a health care team to use research and other sources

<table>
<tr><td>BOX 1-1</td><td>EVIDENCE-BASED PRACTICE CASE STUDY</td></tr>
</table>

A health care provider orders penicillin G benzathine intramuscular (IM) injection for a bacterial infection. A new nurse has given influenza vaccines to his adult patients but has not given any other medication intramuscularly. He asks his clinical nurse specialist (CNS) about the best sites for IM injections. A search of the literature results in several articles. The CNS and nurse discuss the findings relative to the medication orders. The Z-track method for giving an injection (see Chapter 23) is the best technique to prevent medication leakage (Cocoman and Murray, 2010). Nurses may be most comfortable using the deltoid muscle (upper arm) for an injection because it is most often used in adult vaccinations. The deltoid is the preferred site for adult vaccines because the medication is low volume, and the site is easy to access (Centers for Disease Control and Prevention, 2014). In contrast, the literature highlights that the ventrogluteal (lateral hip) and vastus lateralis (lateral quadriceps) are the best sites for larger volume IM injections (Hopkins and Arias, 2013). These sites have no nerves or blood vessels, preventing injury with larger volume medications, such as the antibiotic ordered. The CNS assists the new nurse in administering a ventrogluteal IM injection to give the antibiotic because it was his first time using a new site. The patient experiences little discomfort and has no side effects from the vaccination.

The best evidence comes from well-designed, systematically conducted research studies found in scientific journals. The journals come from nursing and all related health care disciplines. However, there are other sources of evidence that do not originate from research. They include quality or performance improvement data, risk management and infection control information, medical record audits, and clinicians' expertise. Non–research-based data offer valuable information about practice trends and the nature of problems in a specific setting. For example, expert clinicians are an invaluable resource because of their experience and their familiarity with the current literature. However, it is important not to rely solely on non–research-based information. Research-based evidence is more likely to be timely and relevant to current practice conditions. When you face a practice problem, always seek the best sources of evidence that help you find the best solution in caring for your patients.

of evidence in a dynamic and ever-changing environment. Sometimes a health care team undertakes an EBP project (e.g., best approach to reduce falls in cancer patients) and finds that there is no conclusive, reliable evidence available. A gap exists. When that happens, a research project is necessary to provide the evidence needed.

Investigating a problem or area of interest by way of research takes time and commitment. A problem might be identified following the performance improvement or EBP process or from the researcher's personal interests. Research can be lengthy because the researcher must review evidence that does exist, demonstrate why the problem of interest has

TABLE 1-1	COMPARISON OF THREE EVIDENCE-BASED PROCESSES		
PROCESS	**AIM**	**SOURCE OF EVIDENCE**	**TIME FRAME**
Evidence-based practice	Apply existing evidence to change a practice (clinical, educational, or managerial)	Current research evidence, clinical expertise, health care resources, and patient and family values and preferences	Rigorous review and critique of literature regarding current evidence-based practices Pilot test practice changes
Research	Generate *new* scientific knowledge that is generalizable to other patient populations or health care settings	Researcher reviews current literature, identifies a gap or area that has been unanswered, and designs a study to offer new evidence	Systematic investigation takes time—observing or testing something that is new, unanswered
Performance improvement	Improve systems or processes so as to improve outcomes within a work unit or health care setting	Systematic process that evaluates work flow and outcomes of specific processes (e.g., fall rates, patient readmissions). May use benchmark data from other health care settings to evaluate results	Rapid cycle—makes process actionable Results do not provide new knowledge that is generalizable but may raise unanswered questions

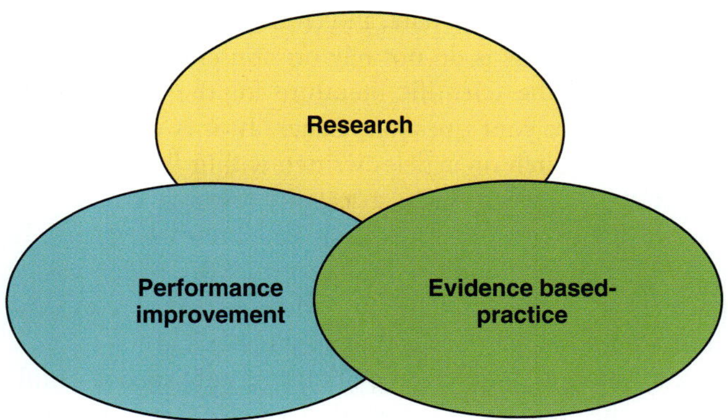

FIG 1-2 The interrelated processes of evidence-based practice, performance improvement, and research.

not been clearly answered, design a proper study that will explain the problem of interest, conduct that study, and evaluate the results. If the results of a research study explain the problem, new knowledge has been developed.

STEPS OF EVIDENCE-BASED PRACTICE

EBP is a problem-solving approach to clinical practice that integrates the conscientious use of best evidence along with a clinician's expertise and patient's preferences and values in making decisions about patient care (Melnyk and Fineout-Overholt, 2011). Using a step-by-step approach ensures that you will obtain the strongest available evidence to apply in a patient care situation. There are six steps of EBP:

1. Ask a clinical question.
2. Collect the most relevant and best evidence.
3. Critically appraise the evidence you gather.
4. Integrate all the evidence along with your clinical expertise, patient preferences, and values in making a practice decision or change.
5. Evaluate the practice change or decision.
6. Share or communicate the outcomes with others.

Ask a Clinical Question

EBP begins with forming a relevant and meaningful clinical question. Nurses and other health care providers face questions in their practice each day. Make it a habit always to question what does not make sense to you, such as a recurring problem in the care of patients or a problem or area of interest that is time-consuming, costly, or not logical. Titler et al. (2001) suggest using either problem-focused or knowledge-focused triggers to identify clinical questions.

Problem-Focused Trigger

A problem-focused trigger is a question faced while caring for a patient or a trend seen in a practice setting.
Examples:
- "How can we reduce the rate of pressure ulcers since it has been increasing over the last 3 months on our surgical unit?"
- "What approaches can be used to reduce the fall rate on the neurology floor?"

Knowledge-Focused Trigger

A knowledge-focused trigger is a question regarding new information about a topic.
Examples:
- "What is the current evidence for reducing phlebitis in peripheral intravenous (IV) catheters?"
- "What is known about ways to enhance learning in older adults?"

Typically, practice questions begin to form as health care professionals talk more about patient care. EBP becomes an easier process when you and your colleagues agree on a relevant clinical question. The clinical question may be either a background question, asking a general or broad range question, or a foreground question, asking a focused question that is well defined (Newhouse et al., 2007). An example of a background question is as follows: "What are the best practices for glucose control in a hospital?" A foreground question is more specific, such as the following: "In hospitalized patients, does obtaining a blood glucose and giving the insulin within 30 minutes of a meal improve blood glucose levels compared with giving insulin within 60 minutes?"

When you ask a focused foreground question, the next step is to search for evidence. Melnyk and Fineout-Overholt (2011) suggest using a PICO format to state foreground questions. Box 1-2 summarizes the four elements of a PICO question. Let's use the following example: You are a staff nurse working on a medical oncology unit. You are meeting with colleagues on the EBP committee to review monthly performance measures for the unit. One measure is reducing hospital-acquired infection (HAI) rates. As your colleagues discuss the issue, one nurse mentions that the critical care units are using chlorhexidine instead of bar soap for bathing (Ritz at al., 2012). Infection rates, most notably for methicillin-resistant *Staphylococcus aureus*, decreased within 60 days in these units after the use of chlorhexidine for daily bathing. Your colleagues wonder if chlorhexidine bathing is a good option for all hospitalized patients. As a result, you ask this PICO question, "In hospitalized patients (*P*), does chlorhexidine soap (*I*) compared with bar soap (*C*) reduce the rate of hospital-acquired infections (*O*)?"

A clearly stated PICO question leads you to the most relevant research and clinical articles from the literature that applies to your clinical situation. The question should identify knowledge gaps and reveal the type of evidence that you lack for your clinical practice. A well-designed PICO question does not have to include all four elements. However, the goal is to ask a question that contains as many of the PICO

elements as possible in a logically framed question. Sometimes nurses ask meaningful questions that do not require all four elements. For example, "How do oncology nurses (*P*) cope with the death of a cancer patient (*I*)?"

Incomplete PICO questions do not lead you to a well-defined set of scientific articles. For example, background questions such as "What are the best practices for pain management?" and "What approaches can be used to assess health literacy?" would lead you to the scientific literature, but the articles would be too numerous and diverse. You want to state a foreground question in a PICO format and then gather a few very good, current scientific articles.

Collect the Best Evidence

After you identify a clear and concise PICO question, the next step is to search for the available evidence, both external and internal. External evidence consists of the scientific literature (computerized bibliographical databases), national guidelines, and national benchmarking. Internal evidence includes facility policy and procedure (P&P) manuals, quality or performance improvement data, and clinical practice guidelines. One rule to follow is do not rely on nonscientific evidence. Always go to the scientific literature for the most current evidence about your question. Generally, it is wise to focus your article search on articles written within the last 5 years unless your search includes a "classic" research article (e.g., one written by a well-known, established researcher).

When searching the scientific literature for evidence, seek the help of a medical librarian when possible. A medical librarian knows the relevant databases (Box 1-3).

A database is an electronic library of published scientific studies, including peer-reviewed research. A peer-reviewed article has been evaluated by a panel of experts familiar with the topic of the article. The medical librarian helps translate elements of your PICO question into the language or key words that yield the most relevant articles you want to read. For example, consider the PICO question, "In hospitalized patients (*P*), does chlorhexidine soap (*I*) compared with bar soap (*C*) reduce the rate of hospital-acquired infections (*O*)?" The key words in the question are *hospitalized patients*, *chlorhexidine*, (bar) *soap*, and (hospital-acquired) *infections*. When conducting a search, it is necessary to enter and manipulate the different key words until you get the combination that gives you the articles you want to read about your topic. Sometimes when you enter a key word to search, you get results for articles that seem unrelated to your topic. The word you select sometimes has one meaning to one author and a different meaning to another. For example, you might choose a key word *oncology* when use of the key word *cancer* might be more successful. Another example is using two separate terms such as *infection* and *incidence* instead of the term *infection rate*. A medical librarian helps you learn how to choose alternative words or terms that identify your PICO question.

MEDLINE, CINAHL, and PubMed are among the most comprehensive databases and represent the scientific knowledge base of health care (Melnyk and Fineout-Overholt, 2011). PubMed is a free resource on the Internet. MEDLINE

<table>
<tr><td colspan="2" style="background:#2e6b3e;color:white">BOX 1-2   DEVELOPING A PICO QUESTION</td></tr>
</table>

P = Population

Identify your population (e.g., patients, families, staff) by age, gender, ethnicity, or disease or type of health problem (as appropriate).

I = Intervention or Area of Interest

Identify the intervention that you want to use in practice and that you believe is worthwhile (e.g., a treatment, a diagnostic test, an educational approach).

C = Comparison Intervention or Area of Interest

What is the usual standard of care or current intervention that you want to compare against the intervention of interest?

O = Outcome

What result do you wish to achieve or observe as a result of an intervention (e.g., change in patient's behavior, physical status, or perception)?

<table>
<tr><td>

BOX 1-3   SEARCHABLE SCIENTIFIC LITERATURE DATABASES AND SOURCES

- **CINAHL:** Cumulative Index of Nursing and Allied Health Literature; studies in nursing, allied health, and biomedicine (http://www.cinahl.com)
- **MEDLINE:** Studies in medicine, nursing, dentistry, psychiatry, veterinary medicine, and allied health (http://www.ncbi.nim.nih.gov)
- **EMBASE:** Biomedical and pharmaceutical studies (http://www.embase.com)
- **PsycINFO:** Psychology and related health care disciplines (http://www.apa.org/psycinfo)
- **Cochrane Reviews:** Full text of regularly updated systematic reviews prepared by the Cochrane Collaboration; completed reviews and protocols (http://www.cochrane.org/reviews)
- **National Guidelines Clearinghouse:** Repository for structured abstracts (summaries) about clinical guidelines and their development; also includes condensed version of guidelines for viewing (http://www.guideline.gov)
- **PubMed:** Health science library at the National Library of Medicine; offers free access to journal articles (http://www.nlm.nih.gov)
- **On-Line Journal of Knowledge Synthesis for Nursing:** Electronic journal containing articles that provide a synthesis of research and an annotated bibliography for selected references (http://nursingsociety.org/publications/journals)
- **Interagency Council on Information Resources in Nursing:** Offers the Essential Nursing Resources, 26th Edition (2012); includes a list of print, electronic, and web sources to support nursing practice, education, administration, and research activities (http://www.icirn.org)

</td></tr>
</table>

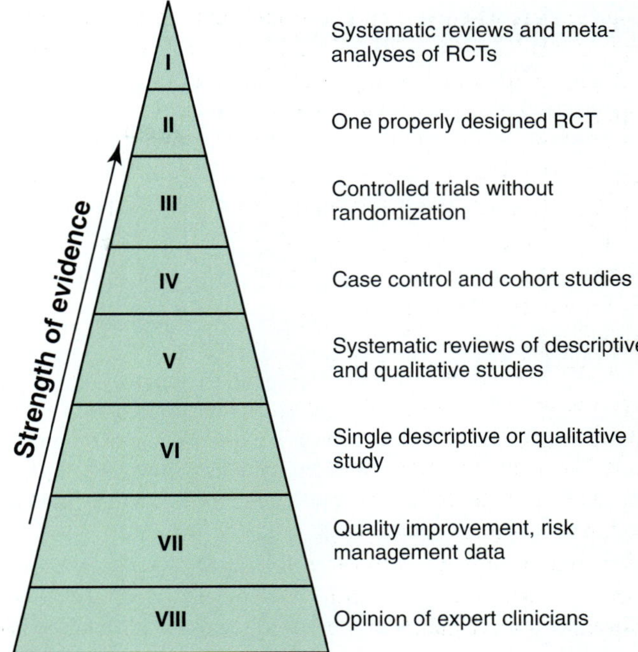

FIG 1-3 The evidence hierarchy pyramid. *RCT,* Randomized controlled trials. (Modified from Guyatt G, Rennie D: *User's guide to the medical literature,* Chicago, 2002, American Medical Association: AMA Press; Harris RP et al: Current methods of the U.S. Preventive Services Task Force: a review of the process, *Am J Prev Med* 20[3 Suppl]:21, 2001.)

Table 1-2 describes types of studies in the evidence hierarchy.

If your PICO question yields an article on your topic that is a systematic review, celebrate! This type of article provides an excellent summary of the evidence available. In a systematic review, a researcher has asked the same PICO question that you asked and then examined all of the well-designed experimental research studies on that topic. The review determines whether the evidence for which you are searching exists and whether it is strong enough for you to change practice.

An individual randomized controlled trial (RCT) is an experimental study that aims to establish cause and effect and is the best way for testing a therapy or intervention. Historically, there have been few RCTs conducted in nursing. The nature of nursing makes RCTs difficult to conduct in a clinical setting. Nurses care for patients' responses to health problems in busy clinical settings. For example, a nurse might be interested in studying a new approach for managing a patient symptom such as pain. The nurse wants to try the use of massage and analgesics compared with analgesics alone. To conduct an RCT, the nurse would have to refrain from offering the new approach (massage and analgesia) to a subgroup of patients (control group). In busy clinical settings, there are often barriers that make conducting RCTs difficult. Nurse researchers often rely on quasiexperimental, descriptive, and qualitative studies to conduct their research.

The use of clinical experts is at the bottom of the evidence pyramid, but do not consider clinical experts a poor source

and CINAHL can be accessed only through vendors, which are usually available through academic institutions by subscription. The Cochrane Reviews is a valuable source of synthesized or preappraised evidence. The database includes the full text of regularly updated systematic reviews and protocols for reviews currently in progress. The National Guidelines Clearinghouse (NGC) is a database supported by the Agency for Healthcare Research and Quality (AHRQ) that contains clinical guidelines, which are systematically developed statements about a plan of care for a specific set of clinical circumstances involving a specific patient population. The NGC is valuable when you are developing a plan of care for a patient.

When you search the literature, you get a list of many different types of scientific articles. You might ask, "Which articles are the best to read?" The pyramid in Fig. 1-3 is one example of a hierarchy for ordering the strength of available evidence. At the top of the pyramid are systematic reviews, the strongest source of scientific evidence. At the bottom is the opinion of expert clinicians. At this point in your nursing career, you are probably not an expert on the different types of scientific studies. However, you can learn enough about the types of studies to help you decide which articles to read.

TABLE 1-2   TYPES OF STUDIES IN THE EVIDENCE HIERARCHY

STUDY TYPE	DESCRIPTION	EXAMPLE
Systematic review or meta-analysis	A panel of experts reviews the evidence from all randomized controlled trials about a specific clinical question. The review summarizes all findings and describes the state of the science. In a meta-analysis there is the addition of a statistical analysis that combines data from all studies.	Experts examined 19 randomized trials comparing the use of small-bowel feeding with gastric feeding and ICU patient outcomes. Meta-analysis revealed that small-bowel feeding, compared with gastric feedings, reduced the risk of pneumonia in critically ill patients without affecting mortality, length of ICU stay, or duration of mechanical ventilation (Alhazzani et al., 2013).
Randomized controlled trial	A researcher tests an intervention against the usual standard of care. Participants are randomly assigned to either a control group (receives standard care) or a treatment group (receives experimental intervention), with both measured based on the same outcomes to see if there is a difference.	Researchers randomly assigned 60 adults to either web-based training or use of educational pamphlets before surgery. Both groups had face-to-face education after surgery. There was no difference in pain ratings, but the experimental group reported less pain interference with coughing, had fewer pain-related barriers, and consumed more opioids. This pilot study shows that web-based training can be beneficial for postoperative pain management and increase accessibility to education without adding more costs (Martorella, Cote, and Racine, 2012).
Case control study	Researchers study one group of subjects with a certain condition (e.g., obesity) at the same time as another group of subjects who do not have the condition to determine if there is an association between the condition and predictor variables (e.g., exercise pattern, family history, history of depression).	Swedish researchers evaluated 702 participants, all same-sex twins, 80 years or older, from a longitudinal population-based study. Individuals with CHF (n = 138) had a higher prevalence of vascular dementia (16% versus 6%) and all types of dementia (40% versus 30%) than individuals without a diagnosis of CHF. Subjects with dementia had a higher prevalence of depression, hypertension, and diabetes (Hjelm et al., 2014).
Descriptive study	A researcher gathers data from subjects to describe a concept under study (e.g., the prevalence or magnitude of a condition or problem) or characteristics of a concept.	Researchers explored nurses' and nursing students' experiences of journal clubs implemented as learning methods for collaborative learning. Journal clubs support competencies and discussion required for producing evidence-based care (Laaksonen et al., 2013).
Qualitative study	Studies explore phenomena such as individuals' experiences with health problems and the contexts in which the experiences occur. Typically, a qualitative study involves interviewing, observations, or spending time with the subjects under study.	Researchers in Sweden interviewed 10 patients to understand their experiences after undergoing gastric bypass surgery. Themes from the interviews included feeling inferior with the body as an obstacle, waiting for surgery, waking up and feeling both vulnerable and safe, and coming home with expectations about a changed body. This study focused on the value of understanding patients' presurgical inferiority with their bodies and the importance of strengthening the new motivation after surgery (Forsberg, Engstrom, and Soderberg, 2014).
Quality improvement data, risk management information	Data collected within a health care facility offers important trending information about clinical conditions and problems. Staff in the facility review the data periodically to identify problem areas and seek solutions.	A research scientist and two staff nurses performed a quality improvement project to evaluate nurse bedside rounding as a strategy to reduce hospital-acquired pressure ulcers. Rates of ulcers reduced from 27% to 0% for three quarters after nurse-focused rounding was implemented (Kelleher, Moorer, and Makic, 2012).
Clinical experts	Accessing clinical experts on a nursing unit is an excellent way to learn about current evidence. Clinical experts often write clinical articles on topics that require application of evidence in the literature.	A clinical leader wrote an article describing the evidence supporting bedside shift report using the SBAR (Situation-Background-Assessment-Recommendation) framework for enhanced patient and family outcomes on pediatric hospital units (Novak and Fairchild, 2012).

CHF, Congestive heart failure; *ICU,* intensive care unit.

of evidence. Expert clinicians often use evidence as they build their practice, and they are rich sources of information for clinical problems. The use of experts coupled with scientific literature provides a strong source of evidence.

Critique the Evidence

After you have conducted a literature search and gathered any data you might have related to your question, it is time to critique the evidence. A critique tells you if there is sufficient evidence to answer your PICO question and to change practice. In most settings, nurses and other health care providers collaborate in critiquing the evidence. For example, each member of an EBP committee shares in reading articles and using specific criteria for each article review.

The critique of evidence determines the value, feasibility, and use of evidence for making a practice change. During the critique, you evaluate the scientific merit and clinical applicability of each of the studies from the literature. You then review findings from the group of studies and determine if there is a strong enough basis for use of the evidence in practice. In the example of the PICO question described earlier on use of chlorhexidine, a critique answers if there is strong evidence to use chlorhexidine soap instead of bar soap to reduce the rate of HAIs.

It takes time to acquire the skills to critique evidence from the literature. Ideally, a member of an EBP committee has experience in this area. When you read an article, do not let the statistics or technical wording cause you to put it down and walk away. Know the elements of an article, and use a careful approach when reviewing each one. Evidence-based articles include the following elements:

- *Abstract:* An abstract is a brief summary of the article that quickly tells you if it is research or clinically based. It summarizes the purpose of the study or clinical topic, the major themes or findings, and the implications for nursing practice.
- *Introduction:* The introduction contains information about the purpose of the article and brief supporting evidence as to why the topic is important from the author's point of view.

Together, the abstract and introduction determine if you want to continue to read an entire article. You will know if the topic of the article is similar to your PICO question or related closely enough to provide you with useful information. If so, continue reading the next elements of the article.

- *Literature review or background:* A good author offers a detailed background of the level of scientific or clinical information that exists about the article topic. The background is a discussion about what led the author to conduct a study or report on a clinical topic. Perhaps the article does not address your PICO question the way you hope, but possibly it leads you to other, more useful articles. The literature review of a research article usually gives you a good idea of how past research led to the researcher's question.
- *Narrative:* The "middle section" or narrative of an article differs according to the type of evidence-based article it is,

either clinical or research (Melnyk and Fineout-Overholt, 2011). A clinical article describes a clinical topic, which often includes a description of a patient population, the nature of a certain disease or health problem, how it affects patients, and the appropriate nursing therapies. Clinical articles often describe how to use a therapy or new technology. A research article describes the research study, including its purpose, the study methods or design, results or conclusions, and clinical implications. The narrative of a research article includes the following subsections:

- *Purpose statement:* This section explains the focus or intent of a study. It identifies what concepts will be researched (including research questions or hypotheses). The purpose statement makes predictions about the relationship or expected differences between study variables (a concept or characteristic that varies within subjects in the study.)
- *Methods or design:* This section explains how a research study is organized and conducted to answer the research question or test hypotheses. This is where you learn about the type of study (e.g., RCT, case control) that was performed (see Table 1-2). You also learn how many subjects or participants were in the study. In health care studies, subjects sometimes include patients, family members, or health care staff. The language in the methods section is sometimes confusing if it explains details about how the researcher designed the study to minimize bias to obtain the most accurate results possible. It is important to understand how a study was conducted to help determine if the results are relevant to your situation. For example, did the study involve patients similar to the types you care for? Was it conducted in a setting similar to yours? Was the way an intervention was tested feasible in your setting?
- *Results or conclusions:* Clinical and research articles have a summary section. In a clinical article, the author explains the clinical implications for the topic presented. In a research article, the author describes the results of the study and explains whether a hypothesis is supported or how a research question is answered. A qualitative study presents a thorough summary of the descriptive themes and ideas that arise from the researcher's analysis of data.

A quantitative study includes a statistical analysis section. It is important to learn common statistical terms, especially in clinical trial studies. Statistics reveal if a tested intervention had a significant effect or if the effect size was large enough to adopt the intervention in practice. When reading statistical analyses, ask these questions: Does the researcher describe the results related to the study's purpose? What was the sample size? Were the results statistically significant? What was the size of the effect of the intervention? A good author discusses any limitations or weaknesses to a study in the results section. The information on limitations further helps you to decide if you want to use the evidence with your patients.

- *Clinical implications:* A research article includes a section that explains if the findings from the study have clinical implications. The researcher explains how the findings are relevant to clinical practice for the type of subjects studied.

After you critique each article, synthesize or combine the findings from all of the articles to determine the strength of evidence. Depending on the type of articles you read, evidence will range from rigorous or strong to weak. It is a challenge for members of an EBP committee to weigh each article and collectively judge the level of evidence available. Are findings from the studies valid, reliable, and relevant to the patient population or area of interest? Use critical thinking to consider the accuracy of the evidence and how well the evidence addresses the PICO question. Also consider the evidence in light of the concerns, values, and preferences of your patient population. Ethically, it is important to consider evidence that would benefit patients and do no harm. You decide to use the evidence in your practice when it is relevant, is easily applicable in your setting of practice (e.g., resources and support are available), and has the potential for improving patient outcomes.

Apply the Evidence

When you determine that the evidence is strong and applicable to your question, you decide how to incorporate it into practice. One way you may choose to use evidence is by directly applying it in the care of a patient. For example, you may find evidence in the literature for the use of an alternative pain therapy (e.g., music therapy) for patients with cancer. You then try the therapy the next time you care for a patient who is receptive to its use.

Most practice changes involve a group such as the members of an EBP committee. In this case, it is always wise to pilot a practice change, which means implementing the change for a small group of patients over a limited time frame (e.g., 3 months). Piloting a practice change allows you to identify any issues with implementation and determine if the change resulted in beneficial patient outcomes. When a pilot is successful, it becomes easier to make a change on a larger scale and evaluate the outcome.

In the example of the medical-oncology staff nurses who are exploring the use of chlorhexidine soap compared with bar soap in hospitalized patients, the evidence shows that chlorhexidine is more effective in reducing the rate of HAIs. The staff now must decide how to gain support to offer chlorhexidine soap instead of bar soap for daily bathing. In this step of EBP, it becomes important to know your resources and understand how change is made in your organization and how to gain consensus for a practice change. It is important to involve all of the health care disciplines that the change would affect. For example, physicians, the infection prevention department, and skin care team should be involved in the practice change. Also, health care professionals who assisted in the critical care areas, who initially used chlorhexidine in your hospital, would be helpful in understanding how bathing practices may change with the change from using bar soap to using liquid chlorhexidine soap.

There are various options for integrating evidence, such as through a new Policy and Procedure, a clinical practice guideline, or new assessment and teaching tools. When choosing a way to integrate evidence, always consider how the staff who would be affected by the change would most likely accept it. For example, the nurses reviewing evidence on chlorhexidine soap choose to meet with the nurses and physicians in the infection control department. They present the results of their literature critique in a professional manner and emphasize how the evidence shows that hospitalized patients may benefit from daily chlorhexidine bathing to reduce HAIs. The infection prevention department is excited to hear about the evidence and will collaborate with the nurses to implement the practice. The physician agrees to speak with the physician leadership in the hospital and gain support from them. The pilot on a nursing unit is scheduled for 1 month with a plan to offer chlorhexidine bathing to all patients the following month.

Evaluate the Practice Change

When nurses apply evidence in clinical practice, it is important to evaluate the effect or outcome. An outcome is an observable effect of an intervention, such as a clinical procedure, care delivery model, or educational approach. Measuring outcomes reveals if an intervention is effective and can determine if patients progress, if students learn, or if staff benefit. Collecting initial baseline data and identifying the outcomes you choose to measure before implementing a change gives you a basis for evaluating the effects of any change. This approach is often called a predata and postdata collection method.

It is essential to be precise in identifying the outcomes you want to measure before you begin implementation. This outcome identification allows you to know what specific data to collect to measure the outcome before you begin and then collect during implementation.

Sometimes evaluation is as simple as determining if the expected outcomes you set for an intervention are met. For example, after using a new transparent intravenous (IV) dressing, does the IV line dislodge, or does the patient develop the complication of phlebitis? When using a new approach to preoperative teaching, does the patient learn what to expect after surgery?

Selecting appropriate outcomes requires careful thinking. Box 1-4 outlines the features of a desirable outcome. The medical-oncology nurses collaborate with infection prevention staff to identify the outcomes for their project. The staff decide to measure infection rates, which are already collected by the infection prevention department. They will also work with the clinical supplies department to track the number of bottles of chlorhexidine used per day. The nurses will compare it with the number of patients per day, a report their nurse manager has available. This information will allow the team to track the use of chlorhexidine for bathing (adherence) and decide if units with high usage have low rates of HAIs.

<table>
<tr><td>

BOX 1-4   FEATURES OF OUTCOME MEASURES

- Reliable
- Valid
- Measurable
- Suited to population
- Not overly costly to collect
- Sensitive to change in the individual
- Nondirectional—defined as the desired behavior or response

</td></tr>
</table>

Data from Melnyk BM, Fineout-Overholt E: *Evidence-based practice in nursing & healthcare: a guide to best practice*, ed 2, Philadelphia, 2011, Lippincott Williams & Wilkins.

When selecting outcomes, consider how you will measure them. Observations, physical measurements, surveys, and questionnaires are examples of how you can measure outcomes. For example, if your outcome is a change in weight, the obvious measurement approach is use of a scale. If your outcome is a patient's adherence to a treatment plan, you might choose to use self-report or have the patient complete a daily diary.

When an EBP change occurs on a large scale, an evaluation is more formal. For example, after the team implements chlorhexidine soap for daily bathing, nurses on the medical-oncology unit (the pilot unit) collect information about infection rates, usage of chlorhexidine bottles, and the patient census. The nurses are able to take this information and compute rates of infection and track trends before and after chlorhexidine bathing. The nurses can track the expected usage of chlorhexidine bottles and compare it with the daily patient census to determine if all patients are given a daily bath with chlorhexidine. Also, the nurses can collect feedback from nurses and patients about their experiences using the new soap. With the analysis, the nurses can present data to the nursing leadership to determine if using chlorhexidine versus bar soap is effective in reducing HAIs for all nursing units. In this example, the intensive care units already demonstrated a reduction in HAIs. After the pilot on the medical-oncology unit, the nurses demonstrated that chlorhexidine soap reduced infection rates in their population and shared the nurses' and patients' comments about the ease of change to the new product and the satisfaction that they knew that this change would help protect patients while in the hospital. Outcome data tell you if the practice change was beneficial.

Sometimes evaluation data show the need to modify a practice change or discontinue it.

Share the Outcomes with Others

After applying evidence, it is important to share outcomes from the change in practice to nursing and other health care colleagues. Sharing of outcomes is important whether the results are successful or unsuccessful. There are many ways to communicate the outcomes of EBP, including talking with a colleague, sharing results in staff meetings or a committee, presenting in workshops or seminars, submitting an abstract for a poster presentation, and publishing an article. In the case example, the lead nurse on the EBP medical-oncology committee and an infection prevention physician decide to make a joint presentation at a nursing grand rounds session.

As a professional, you are responsible for communicating important information about nursing practice. Sharing evidence and the effects of any practice change motivates others and makes them excited about practice improvements.

EVIDENCE IN NURSING SKILLS

Nurses who work in clinical settings must use the current best evidence to guide their practice and improve patient outcomes. One way is through the use of P&Ps that provide direction for implementing procedures such as the skills in this text. Nurses rely on P&Ps to contain the most current information regarding safe and effective practices.

An increasing number of nursing organizations have adopted an approach for ensuring evidence-based P&Ps (Becker et al., 2012). As P&Ps are reviewed or developed, nursing should include the evidence that supports clinical practice (Poe and White, 2010). Documentation that P&Ps include evidence strengthens the reason for the process and demonstrates that nursing is using the best research available to lead clinical practice.

It is common for nurses to raise questions about day-to-day clinical issues such as why procedures are performed the way they are. Implementing EBP into P&P development makes sense. Nurses on P&P committees are adopting formal processes for the routine review of P&Ps to ensure that new evidence is integrated into organizational policy. An EBP approach to P&P review and development demonstrates how an organization integrates EBP into practice, an important consideration for TJC and Magnet hospital review (Oman et al., 2008).

▌CRITICAL THINKING EXERCISES

Case Study

The nurses on a medical-surgical unit are discussing problems in providing their diabetic patients education about insulin injections before discharge. One nurse has just attended a 1-day workshop on the Teach Back method of education. The nurse shares with the group that after providing teaching, you have to ask the patient to explain what you just taught them. Based on the patient's reply and demonstration of the skill, you can determine what the patient learned. If the patient has difficulty sharing or demonstrating what he or she has learned, you need to repeat the training. This process may need to be repeated several times for the patient to understand the education you are providing. The staff nurses express interest in this method of teaching and ask the nurse manager to assist in developing a Teach Back tool for the nurses to use for training patients about insulin injections with needle safety. The nurse manager contacts a certified diabetes educator, who has a tool she uses for her outpatient diabetes classes. At the next meeting, the nurses talk about how they will educate their peers about using the Teach Back tool. One of the nurses asks, "How will we know if the patients learn more with the Teach Back method compared with the verbal education and handout we currently provide?"

1. Write a PICO question for the clinical case study.
2. What would be an outcome that the nurses would measure in a study designed to educate their patients, and how would they measure it?

Review Questions

1. When you conduct a scientific literature review, your aim is to gather articles about studies that involved scientific rigor. Order the following sources of scientific evidence, beginning with the most rigorous and ending with least rigorous.
   1. Single descriptive study
   2. Controlled trial without randomization
   3. Systematic review
   4. Case control study
   5. One randomized controlled trial
   6. Systematic review of qualitative study
2. A committee of nurses has collected a set of six articles about approaches for preventing pressure ulcers. They have read each article, reviewed the relevance of the articles to their practice, and discussed the strength of evidence available. This is an example of which step of EBP?
   1. Ask a clinical question.
   2. Collect the most relevant and best evidence.
   3. Critically appraise the evidence.
   4. Apply the evidence along with your clinical expertise, patient preferences, and values.
3. Staff nurses are meeting to discuss EBP issues. Which of the following clinical questions is an example of a knowledge-focused trigger?
   1. The unit has seen an increased rate of falls, and the staff nurses wonder if it is related to patients receiving opioid analgesics.
   2. The nurses on the unit have seen an increase in wound infections.
   3. The nurses anticipate that physicians will be using more local anesthesia for surgical procedures.
   4. The unit has had more medication errors during the last 3 months.
4. When attempting to identify a PICO question, what are the limitations of asking a background question? Select all that apply.
   1. The background question will lead you to too many articles to read.
   2. The background question will limit your search to only systematic review articles.
   3. The background question will lead you to a set of articles on diverse topics.
   4. The background question limits the focus of your search.

5. Nurses on an EBP committee find an article that describes a research study that measured nurses' perceptions of communication during handoffs with other staff members. This is an example of which of the following types of studies?
   1. Descriptive study
   2. Case control study
   3. Randomized controlled trial
   4. Systematic review
6. Which of the following are characteristics of a randomized controlled trial research study? Select all that apply.
   1. The study examines the subjective context in which persons' experiences occur.
   2. The study includes two groups, both measured on the same outcomes, to see if there are differences.
   3. The study tests a new intervention against the usual standard of care.
   4. The study examines subjects with a certain condition at the same time as another group of subjects who do not have the condition.
7. When reading a scientific article, what information will the nurse find in the literature review or background section?
   1. A discussion about what led the author to conduct a study or report on a clinical topic
   2. Information about the purpose of the article and the importance of the topic for the audience who reads it
   3. Identification of the concepts that will be researched
   4. Explanation of whether a hypothesis is correct or how a research question is answered
8. In the following PICO question, identify the four elements: Does the use of hourly rounds compared with standard observations reduce the number of falls in medical inpatients? Fill in the elements.
   P:
   I:
   C:
   O:
9. Which question contains the primary components of a PICOT question?
   1. Are oral steroids effective for female adults with adult-onset asthma?
   2. Which steroid preparations are best for male teenagers with activity-induced asthma who play sports?
   3. Does the use of inhalers improve bronchial air flow?
   4. Does the use of medication via an inhaler versus a nebulizer affect oxygen saturation in asthmatic children?
10. A UPC is planning to adopt a new type of pulse oximeter to improve accuracy of measurement and reduce patient discomfort while wearing the device. Which resources should the committee consider before beginning a pilot evaluation of the oximeter? Select all that apply.
    1. The accuracy of the device
    2. Cost of the device
    3. Support from doctors for the change
    4. The patients' satisfaction with the device

REFERENCES

Alhazzani W, et al: Small bowel feeding and risk of pneumonia in adult critically ill patients: a systematic review and meta-analysis of randomized trials, *Crit Care* 17(4):R127, 2013.

American Nurses Association: *Nursing: scope and standards of practice*, ed 2, Silver Spring, MD, 2010, American Nurses Association.

Becker E, et al: Clinical nurse specialists shaping policies and procedures via an evidence-based clinical practice council, *Clin Nurs Spec* 26(2):74, 2012.

Centers for Disease Control and Prevention: Vaccinations: dose, route, site, and needle size, http://www.immunize.org/catg.d/p3085.pdf. Accessed January 19, 2014.

Cocoman A, Murray J: Recognizing the evidence and changing practice on injection sites, *Br J Nurs* 19(18):1170, 2010.

Forsberg A, Engstrom A, Soderberg S: From reaching the end of the road to a new lighter life—people's experiences of undergoing gastric bypass surgery, *Intensive Crit Care Nurs* 30(2):93, 2014.

Hjelm C, et al: Factors associated with increased risk for dementia in individuals age 80 years or older with congestive heart failure, *J Cardiovasc Nurs* 29(1):82, 2014.

Hopkins U, Arias C: Large-volume IM injections: a review of best practices, *Oncology Nurse Advisor* 2013. http://media.oncologynurseadvisor.com/documents/44/ona_feature0213_injections_10767.pdf. Accessed January 31, 2014.

Institute of Medicine: *Crossing the quality chasm: a new health system for the 21st century*, Washington, DC, 2001, National Academy Press.

Institute of Medicine (IOM): The future of nursing: Leading change, advancing health, 2010. Retrieved from http://books.nap.edu/openbook.php?record_id=12956&page=R1.

Kelleher A, Moorer A, Makic MF: Peer-to-peer nursing rounds and hospital acquired pressure ulcer prevalence in a surgical intensive care unit, *J Wound Ostomy Continence Nurs* 39(2):152, 2012.

Laaksonen C, et al: Journal club as a method for nurses and nursing students' collaborative learning: a descriptive study, *Health Sci J* 7(3):285, 2013.

Martorella G, Cote J, Racine M: Web-based nursing intervention for self-management of pain after cardiac surgery: pilot randomized controlled trial, *J Med Internet Res* 14(6):e177, 2012.

Melnyk BM, Fineout-Overholt E: *Evidence-based practice in nursing & healthcare: a guide to best practice*, ed 2, Philadelphia, 2011, Lippincott Williams & Wilkins.

Newhouse R, et al: *Johns Hopkins evidence-based practice model and guidelines*, Indianapolis, IN, 2007, Sigma Theta Tau International.

Novak K, Fairchild R: Bedside reporting and SBAR: improving patient communication and satisfaction, *J Pediatr Nurs* 27(6):760, 2012.

Oman K, et al: Evidence-based policy and procedures: an algorithm for success, *J Nurs Adm* 38(1):47, 2008.

Poe S, White K: *Johns Hopkins nursing evidence-based practice: implementation and translation*, Indianapolis, IN, 2010, Sigma Theta Tau International.

QSEN Institute: http://qsen.org/. Accessed January 19, 2014.

Ritz J, et al: Effectiveness of 2 methods of CHG bathing, *J Nurs Care Qual* 27(2):171, 2012.

Titler MG, et al: The Iowa model of evidence-based practice to promote quality care, *Crit Care Clin North Am* 13(4):497, 2001.

Communication and Collaboration

 **EVOLVE WEBSITE/RESOURCES LIST**

http://evolve.elsevier.com/Perry/nursinginterventions
Audio Glossary • Checklists • Review Questions

Communication is a basic human need and the foundation for establishing a caring relationship between a nurse and patient. It involves the expression of emotions, ideas, and thoughts through verbal (words or written language) and nonverbal (e.g., behaviors) exchanges. Verbal communication includes both the spoken and the written word. Nonverbal communication includes body movement, physical appearance, personal space, touch, and facial expression. The interaction between a skilled nurse and a patient progresses to a therapeutic level in which the nurse offers goal-directed activities to help the patient share thoughts and feelings. With time and practice, you develop therapeutic communication skills and maintain a congenial and warm style that helps patients feel comfortable in sharing their feelings.

Multiple interpersonal skills are essential to communicate therapeutically with patients. These skills include having empathy and a nonjudgmental attitude, being aware of both verbal and nonverbal communication, using appropriate body language, being patient and sensitive to patients' cues, and giving feedback appropriately. Many factors influence the complex process of communication (Box 2-1).

Communication is an interaction between two or more people that involves an exchange of information between a sender and a receiver. The basic elements of communication include a message, a sender, a receiver, and feedback (Fig. 2-1). The message is the information expressed and can be motivated by experience, emotions, ideas, or actions. The message may be sent through different channels, including visual, auditory, and tactile senses. For communication to be effective, the receiver must be aware of the sender's message. The message received is understood as filtered through perceptions shaped from previous experiences. People tend to interpret life experiences through general assumptions and values they hold; in essence, this is the concept of filtering. The more aware people are of how these assumptions influence how they perceive the world and others, the more open they can be when interacting with others. Feedback, verbal or nonverbal, is a response to the sender that indicates if the meaning of the message sent was received. Because communication is a two-way process, you give feedback to and seek feedback from patients to validate patients' understanding of the messages sent.

<table>
<tr><td>

BOX 2-1 FACTORS THAT INFLUENCE COMMUNICATION

Perceptions: Personal views based on past experiences.
Values: Beliefs that a person considers important in life.
Emotions: Subjective feelings about a situation (e.g., anger, fear, frustration, pain, anxiety, personal appearance).
Sociocultural background: Language, gestures, and attitudes common for a specific group of people relating to family origin, occupation, or lifestyle.
Knowledge level: Level of education and experience influences a person's knowledge base.
Roles and relationships: Conversation between two nurses differs from conversation between the nurse and a patient.
Environment: Noise, lack of privacy, and distractions influence effectiveness.
Space and territoriality: A distance of 18 inches to 4 feet is ideal for sitting with a patient for an interaction. Patients from different cultures often have different needs for personal space.

</td><td>

BOX 2-2 INEFFECTIVE RESPONSES AND BEHAVIORS

- Not listening
- Talking too much
- Appearing too busy
- Using clichés
- Seeming uncomfortable with silence
- Laughing nervously
- Not paying attention
- Smiling inappropriately
- Being opinionated
- Showing disapproval
- Avoiding sensitive topics
- Belittling feelings
- Arguing
- Minimizing problems
- Being superficial
- Being defensive
- Changing the subject
- Focusing on personal problems of the nurse
- Having a closed posture
- Making flippant remarks
- Ignoring the patient
- Lying or being insincere
- Making false promises
- Making sarcastic remarks

From Keltner N et al: *Psychiatric nursing: a psychotherapeutic management approach*, ed 6, St Louis, 2011, Mosby.

</td></tr>
</table>

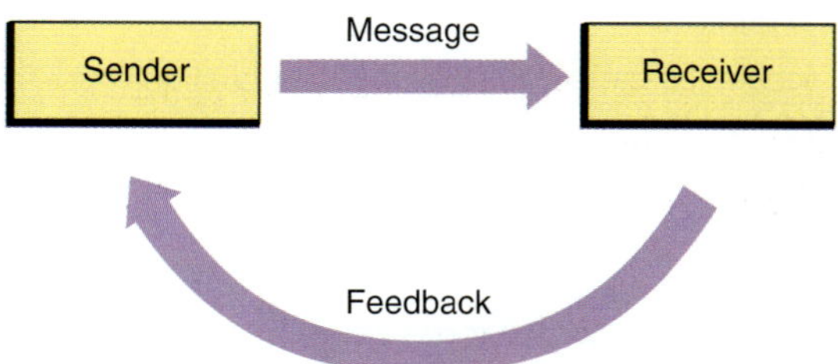

FIG 2-1 Communication is a two-way process.

Silence is a therapeutic technique, and it gives a nurse and patient time to think. It is important for you to be aware of a patient's inner feelings and nonverbal behavior that provides cues to the patient's feelings. Reflecting your impressions can validate what the patient is experiencing. If silence lasts too long or becomes uncomfortable for the patient, it can be helpful to say, "You seem very quiet," or "Could you tell me what you need right now?" or "How are you feeling?"

Barriers to effective therapeutic communication techniques exist in the form of ineffective responses and behaviors (Box 2-2). The use of these nontherapeutic techniques hinders the therapeutic relationship between the patient and the nurse.

Effective communication requires practice similar to any other skill. An attitude of acceptance is helpful to promote open communication. To listen effectively, face the patient, maintain eye contact, pay attention to what the patient is conveying, and give feedback to verify accurate understanding. Although you may not agree with a patient response, it is important to accept the patient's right to an opinion. Avoid arguing with patients; instead, simply reflect understanding of what they are communicating without agreeing or disagreeing.

Preoccupation with the techniques of communication can interfere with rather than enhance the communication process. Ineffective communication may not halt conversation, but it often tends to inhibit patients' willingness to express concerns openly. Find an appropriate environment, allow for sufficient time, and facilitate communication according to patients' circumstances and needs. Be aware of techniques that facilitate or inhibit communication (Table 2-1).

PATIENT-CENTERED CARE

Patient-centered care involves an awareness and respect for patient's needs, preferences, and values. High-quality communication between the nurse and the patient and family facilitates patient-centered care. You need to address the patient as a person and listen to the patient, encouraging questions and concerns (Slatore et al., 2012). Providing privacy is important; ideally, communication between you and your patient should occur in a quiet place with minimal external distraction. It is important to minimize any hospital noises because excessive noise hinders communication and negatively affects a patient's health (Eggertson, 2012).

It is important to recognize cultural diversity and demonstrate respect for people as unique individuals. Culture is just one factor that influences communication between two people. Awareness of cultural norms or values enhances understanding of nonverbal cues. Be aware of your own cultural values and expectations and how they may "filter" or direct your care. Consider any potential communication barriers with people from other cultures, including cultural perspective, heritage, and health traditions of both the patient and the nurse. Examples of questions to consider include: Who is the nurse from a cultural perspective? Who is the patient from a cultural perspective? What is the nurse's heritage? What is the patient's heritage? What are the health

TABLE 2-1   FACILITATING AND INHIBITING COMMUNICATION

TECHNIQUE	EXAMPLES	RATIONALE
Initiating and Encouraging Interaction		
Giving information	"It is time for me to ...." "I will be here until ...."	Informs patient of facts needed to understand situation Provides a means to build trust and develop a knowledge base for patients to make decisions
Stating observations	"You're smiling." "I see you're up already."	By calling patient's attention to what is observed, nurse encourages patient to be aware of behavior
Open questions/ comments	"What is your biggest concern?" "Tell me about your health."	Allows patient to choose the topic of discussion according to circumstances and needs
General leads	"And then?" "Go on ...." "Tell me more ...."	Encourages patient to continue talking
Focused questions/ comments	"Tell me about your pain or comfort." "What did your doctor say?" "How has your family reacted?" "What is your biggest fear?"	Encourages patient to give more information about specific topic of concern
Helping Patient Identify and Express Feelings		
Sharing observations	"You look tense." "You seem uncomfortable when ...."	Promotes patient's awareness of nonverbal behavior and feelings underlying behavior; helps clarify meaning of behavior
Paraphrasing	Patient: "I couldn't sleep last night." Nurse: "You've had trouble sleeping?"	Encourages patient to describe the situation more fully; demonstrates that nurse is listening and concerned
Reflecting feelings	"You were angry when that happened?" "You seem upset ...."	Focuses patient on identified feelings based on verbal or nonverbal cues
Focused comments	"That seems worth talking about more." "Tell me more about ...."	Encourages patient to think about and describe a particular concern in more detail
Ensuring Mutual Understanding		
Seeking clarification	"I don't quite follow you ...." "Do you mean ...?" "Are you saying that ...?"	Encourages patient to expand on a topic that is not yet clear or that seems contradictory
Summarizing	"So there are three things that you're upset about: your family being too busy, your diet, and being in the hospital so long."	Reduces the interaction to three or four points identified by nurse as significant; allows patient to agree or add other concerns
Validation	"Did I understand you correctly that ...?" "What made you decide to eat that when you know it gives you stomach pain?"	Allows clarification of ideas that nurse may have interpreted differently than intended by patient
Inhibiting Communication		
"Why" questions	"Why did you go back to bed?"	Asks patient to justify reasons; implies criticism and makes patient feel defensive; better to state what happened and encourage telling the whole story (e.g., "I noticed you went back to bed.")
Sidestepping or changing subject	Patient: "I'm having a hard time with my family." Nurse: "Do you have any grandchildren?"	Eases nurse's own discomfort and avoids exploring topic identified by patient
False reassurance	"Everything will be okay." "Surgery is no big deal."	Vague and simplistic and tends to belittle patient's concerns; does not invite a response
Giving advice	"You really should exercise more." "You shouldn't eat fast food every day."	Keeps patient from actively engaging in finding a solution; often patient knows what should or should not be done and needs to explore alternative ways of dealing with issue
Stereotyped responses	"You have the best doctor in town." "All patients with cancer worry about that."	Does not invite patient to respond
Defensiveness	"The nurses here work very hard." "Your doctor is extremely busy."	Moves focus away from patient's feelings without acknowledging concerns

traditions of the nurse's heritage? What are the health traditions of the patient's heritage? Transcultural communication is most effective when each person attempts to understand the point of view of the other from that person's cultural heritage. Adopt an attitude of flexibility, respect, and interest to bridge any communication barriers imposed by cultural differences.

- *Use of language, gestures, and vocal emphasis of words:* Taking care to determine if understanding was achieved is important. Avoid overly technical jargon or terms unique to a culture.
- *Eye contact:* Direct eye contact is valued in some cultures, whereas other cultures find it improper and intrusive (e.g., it may be improper to make eye contact with an authority figure).
- *Use of touch and personal space:* Some cultures are "noncontact" cultures and have needs for clear boundaries; other cultures value close contact, handshakes, and embracing (Fig. 2-2).
- *Time orientation:* Many cultures are oriented to the present; some cultures value planning for the future.
- *Nonverbal behaviors:* Use gestures with shared meaning.

The United States is culturally and ethnically diverse, reflecting a mixture of health care beliefs and practices. As society becomes more diverse, it is essential for health care providers to learn about cultural and ethnic differences. This process begins with self-awareness and involves getting to know oneself: one's personality, values, beliefs, and ethics when caring for patients who are different from oneself (Purnell, 2013). Race encompasses one's skin, eye, and hair color. Ethnicity is not just a person's race; rather, it is about embracing the tradition and customs from one's country of origin. Race remains constant because it does not have customs, whereas one can identify with another ethnic group. Culture is the knowledge and values shared by a society. Using culturally competent communication begins with addressing these differences.

Patients with limited English proficiency may not possess adequate vocabulary skills to communicate effectively. A translator or interpreter often is needed when a patient does not speak the nurse's language (Giger, 2013). It is important in health care settings and in home care to use professional interpreters. Health care language is often complex, and interpreters decode the patient's words and provide meaning behind the message, whereas translators just restate the words from one language to another. Often the patient speaks the same language with limited ability or uses language with a meaning different from the nurse's meaning. For example, the patient may know customary greetings such as "How are you?" and not understand "pain" or "nausea." When communication fails, avoid the tendency to speak louder, stop talking, concentrate on the tasks, or begin doing things for rather than with the patient. Inappropriate responses may result in painful isolation, anger, or misunderstanding for the patient and his or her inability to cooperate. The use of professional interpreters is associated with decreased errors and increased quality of care; consequently, health care providers should not rely on family members as translators when caring for patients with limited English proficiency. Box 2-3 describes special approaches to communicate to patients who speak different languages; these approaches are useful even when an interpreter is available.

Patients with sensory losses require communication techniques that maximize existing sensory and motor functions. Some patients are unable to speak because of physical or neurological alterations, such as paralysis; a tube in the trachea to facilitate breathing (Fig. 2-3); or a stroke resulting in aphasia, difficulty understanding, or verbalizing. A patient with receptive aphasia has impaired comprehension of both written and spoken language. Expressive aphasia affects the motor function of speech so that the patient has difficulty speaking and writing but is able to hear and understand. Speech pathologists are helpful for patients with speech difficulties.

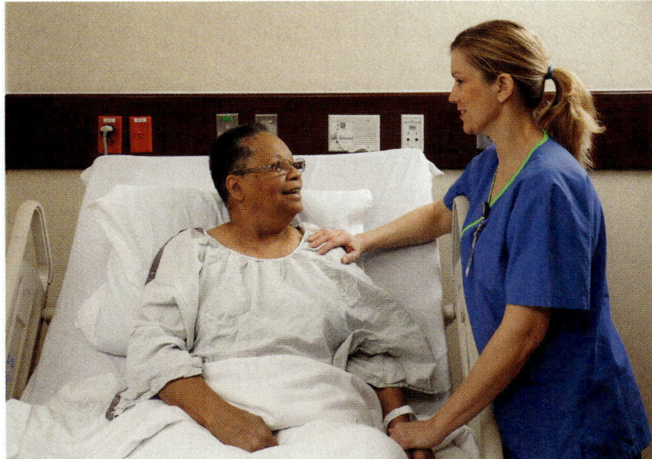

FIG 2-2 Therapeutic use of touch needs to take cultural factors into consideration.

BOX 2-3   SPECIAL APPROACHES FOR A PATIENT WHO SPEAKS A DIFFERENT LANGUAGE

- Use a caring tone of voice and facial expression to help alleviate the patient's fears.
- Speak slowly and distinctly but not loudly.
- Use gestures, pictures, and role playing to help the patient understand.
- Repeat the message in different ways if necessary.
- Be alert to words the patient seems to understand and use them frequently.
- Keep messages simple and repeat them frequently.
- Avoid using medical terms that the patient may not understand.
- Use an appropriate language dictionary or have a medical interpreter make flash cards to communicate key phrases.

Modified from Giger J: *Transcultural nursing: assessment and intervention*, ed 6, St Louis, 2013, Mosby.

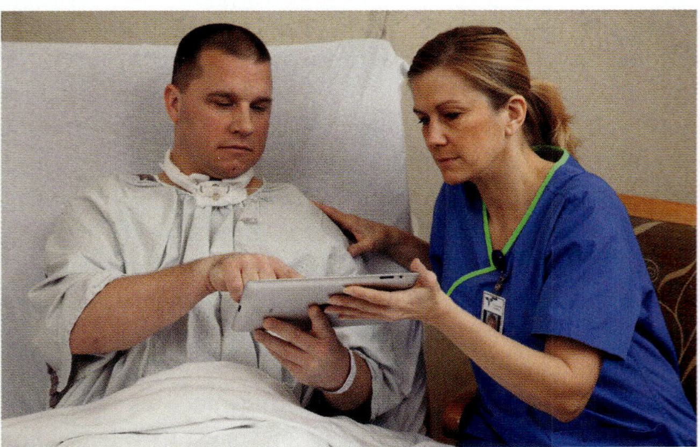

FIG 2-3 Communication tools are available for patients who cannot speak because of a tracheostomy.

BOX 2-4	COMMUNICATION AIDS

- Pad and felt-tipped pen or magic slate
- Board with words, letters, or pictures denoting basic needs (e.g., water, bedpan, pain medication)
- Call bells or alarms
- Sign language
- Use of eye blinks or movement of fingers for simple responses (e.g., "yes" or "no")
- Flash cards with pictures rather than words
- Computer or electronic devices

Hearing impairment affects one's quality of life and may be easily overlooked by health care providers. Communication is impaired when a message is lost or misinterpreted because the patient did not hear correctly. Aids such as pictures, electronic communication, two-way text messaging, and communication software can be used to communicate with patients successfully (Box 2-4).

SAFETY

Miscommunication, between health care providers and between provider and patient, can adversely affect patient safety. Consider your personal safety when interacting with patients who are potentially violent. Patients who are angry and frustrated and believe that no one is listening may be more likely to behave in a violent manner.

The illness experience is a stressor, and some patients have trouble coping. Do not be offended by challenging and difficult patients; approach them with patience, acknowledging their distress. Ineffective communication between the nurse and patient or family can lead to low satisfaction and negative health outcomes. It is important to express genuine concern and acknowledge the patient's beliefs and fears (Delbanco et al., 2013).

EVIDENCE-BASED PRACTICE

Dinh T et al. The effectiveness of health education using the teach-back method on adherence and self-management in chronic disease: a systematic review protocol, *JBI Datab System Rev Implement Rep* 11(10):30-41, 2013.

Sarkar U et al. Literacy and patient care, *UpToDate*, 2014, http://www.uptodate.com.ezproxy.neumann.edu/contents/literacy-and-patient-care?source=machineLearning&search=Teach+Back&selectedTitle=1%7E150§ionRank=1&anchor=H12#H12. Accessed May 12, 2014.

There is evidence that when there is improved communication of health-related information, there can be improved patient outcomes, especially for individuals identified as having low or limited literacy skills (Sarkar et al., 2014). Evidence suggests that using an approach to communication that seeks to teach to a goal until identified learning outcomes have been met has been an effective patient teaching strategy.

Teach Back is a technique used by health care providers to allow patients or caregivers to use their own words to explain recently taught information (Dinh, 2013). Teach Back allows for immediate identification and correction of misunderstood or misinterpreted information, with the ultimate goal of preventing adverse events related to inadequate understanding. This technique has been validated as a strategy for teaching new skills. Several strategies have been shown to improve communication using Teach Back:

- Use plain language.
- Use concrete and specific phrases.
- Question until patient understanding has been assessed.
- If a gap in knowledge is assessed or an incorrect explanation provided, repeat the information.
- Develop an educational strategy that can be understood by the patient.
- Encourage questions from the patients.
- Confirm patient comprehension.

SKILL 2.1	ESTABLISHING THE NURSE-PATIENT RELATIONSHIP AND INTERVIEWING

A therapeutic nurse-patient relationship is the foundation of nursing care and involves patient-centered, goal-directed interactions using therapeutic communication skills.

Therapeutic communication empowers patients to make decisions. Factors that influence communication include a patient's perceptions, values, sociocultural background, and knowledge level. Therapeutic communication differs from social communication because it is patient-centered and goal-directed with limited disclosure from the professional. However, an important aspect of therapeutic communication is the nurse's ability to demonstrate caring for patients. Caring establishes trust and openness and facilitates patient communication.

Nurses usually avoid sharing details of their personal lives with patients. Sometimes personal self-disclosure is effective if it helps a patient to focus on key issues. However, social communication that involves equal opportunity for personal disclosure and in which both participants seek to have personal needs met is inappropriate between nurses and patients (Keltner et al., 2011). An appropriate example is sharing personal thoughts and life experiences with a patient and family to show that you understand what the patient might be experiencing.

The nurse-patient relationship is characterized by three overlapping phases: orientation, working, and termination. The *orientation phase* involves learning about the patient and any initial concerns and needs. During the orientation phase, clarify your role and the roles of other health care professionals, collect information, establish goals, correct misunderstandings, and establish rapport between yourself and the patient. It is quite common to encounter a patient who needs comfort and support while experiencing threatening situations. A newly diagnosed illness, separation from family and friends, the discomfort of surgery or diagnostic and treatment procedures, grief, and loss are a few examples of health-related situations that require the skill of comforting.

Various communication techniques facilitate or inhibit communication during the *working phase* (see Table 2-1). Active listening and empathy are two of the most effective ways to facilitate communication. Active listening conveys interest in a patient's needs, concerns, and problems and requires complete attention to understand the entire verbal and nonverbal message. Listening techniques are learned behaviors. At first they seem awkward and time-consuming. However, as with any skill, they become more comfortable with practice. It is essential that you appear natural, relaxed, and at ease while listening.

Empathy is the act of effectively communicating to other people that their feelings are understood. After they know that their feelings are accepted, people do not have to struggle to explain or justify their reactions (Fortinash and Holoday-Worret, 2012).

During the working phase, you may be conducting a patient interview. The interview involves communication initiated for a specific purpose and focused on a specific content area, such as the initial assessment of newly admitted patients or obtaining a health history in a health care provider's office. The interviewer obtains information about the patient's health state, lifestyle, support systems, patterns of illness, patterns of adaptation, strengths and limitations, and resources. This information is used for an admission database or health

BOX 2-5   INTERVIEW DATABASE

- Health-related concerns
- Perception of health status
- Past health problems, all current medications, and therapies
- Effect of health status on role; influence on relationship with members of household
- Influence on occupation
- Ability to complete activities of daily living

history and provides data for identifying the patient's expectations and for responding appropriately to individualized patient needs.

The interview facilitates a positive nurse-patient relationship, which makes it easier for patients to ask questions about the health care environment and expectations regarding daily routines and procedures. Schedule the interview at a time when there are minimal interruptions and visitors are not present. Sometimes it is beneficial to include family members in the interview, with the focus clearly kept on identifying the patient's needs. Before beginning, tell the patient about the purpose of the interview and the types of data to be obtained. Let the patient know that it is important to ask questions at any time and that he or she has the right not to answer questions. Spend time becoming acquainted with the patient. Establish a time frame for the interview, and honor this commitment to the patient. Ask questions to form a database from which you can develop a care plan (Box 2-5). Carefully observe for evidence of discomfort and be willing to stop the interview when appropriate.

The direct question technique is a structured format requiring one-word or two-word answers and is frequently used to clarify previous information or obtain basic routine information (e.g., allergies, marital status). The open-ended question technique promotes a more complete description of identified areas of concern. Examples of open-ended questions and comments include "What are your health concerns?" "How have you been feeling?" and "Tell me about your problem."

Prepare for the *termination phase* at the beginning of the interaction by indicating the purpose of the communication session and the amount of time available. The termination phase consists of evaluation and summary of progress toward identified goals.

ASSESSMENT

1. The first contact a nurse has with a patient occurs during the orientation phase. Address the patient by name and introduce yourself and your role on the health care team ("Hello, my name is Sally Regan, and

I am the registered nurse assigned to take care of you today ….”). Use clear, specific communication (verbal and nonverbal) to provide information and clarify concerns. *Rationale: Clear, specific communication decreases confusion and anxiety and improves the quality of health care.*

2. Assess the following behaviors: patient's needs, coping strategies, defenses, and adaptation styles. *Rationale: Assessing for individualized behaviors helps to identify patient needs.*

3. Determine patient's need to communicate (e.g., patient who constantly uses call light, is crying, does not understand an illness, has just been admitted to the hospital or nursing home). *Rationale: Patients in need of support, comfort, knowledge, or encouragement benefit from meaningful communication.*

4. Assess the reason patient needs health care.

5. Assess factors about yourself and the patient that influence communication, including perceptions, values and beliefs, emotions, sociocultural background, severity of illness, knowledge, age, verbal ability, roles and relationships, environmental setting, physical comfort, and discomfort. *Rationale: Attention to factors that influence communication facilitates accurate assessment of the experiences of the patient.*

6. Assess personal barriers to communicating with the patient (e.g., bias toward patient's condition, anxiety from inexperience). *Rationale: Barriers prevent you from conveying empathy and caring and obtaining relevant assessment information.*

7. Assess patient's language and ability to speak. Does the patient have difficulty finding words or associating ideas with accurate word symbols? Does the patient have difficulty with expression of language or reception of messages? *Rationale: This assessment identifies the appropriate communication aids to be used (e.g., use of an interpreter, use of communication board).*

8. Assess patient's health literacy level. Does the patient skip over uncommon or hard words, avoid asking questions, or have difficulty discussing concepts related to illness or treatments? *Rationale: Health literacy has a direct effect on health outcomes. Assessing the patient's level of health literacy allows you to design more effective communication and teaching approaches.*

9. Assess patient's ability to hear. Be sure the patient's ears are free of cerumen, and determine that hearing aids are functional (see Chapter 11).

10. Assess resources available in selecting communication methods: review information from medical records, and consult with family, health care providers, and other members of the health care team. *Rationale: Collaboration with health care team members facilitates your response to patient based on integration of knowledge. Seek information from family after obtaining the patient's approval. Patient privacy must be maintained.*

11. Before initiating the working phase of the nurse-patient relationship, assess the patient's readiness to work toward goal attainment. *Rationale: Patient's goals are identified and agreed on by effective communication skills such as restating and clarifying.*

12. Consider when patient is due to be discharged or transferred from the health care facility. *Rationale: This allows you to anticipate the amount of time available to work with the patient and when termination of the relationship is to occur.*

PLANNING

Expected Outcomes focus on using therapeutic communication skills to develop a therapeutic relationship with the patient and obtain information about the patient's ideas, needs, and concerns, and focus on gathering information through the interview process for a database to develop an appropriate plan of care.

1. Patient expresses ideas, fears, and concerns clearly and openly without anxiety.
2. Patient's health care goals are identified and achieved.
3. Patient verbalizes understanding of information communicated by health care providers.

Orientation Phase

1. Prepare by providing a warm and accepting environment, establishing trust, formulating individualized treatment goals, considering time allocation, formulating initial questions, and mentally preparing to keep your mind clear of other concerns or distractions.
2. Prepare patient and environment physically; provide a quiet environment, maintain privacy, reduce distractions or interruptions, and take care of the patient's physical needs before beginning the discussion.
3. If others are present, ask patient if they should stay.

Working Phase

1. Use open-ended questions to identify strategies to develop a realistic plan to meet identified goals of patients.

Termination Phase

1. Prepare by identifying methods of summarizing and synthesizing information pertinent for aftercare.

Delegation and Collaboration

All health care providers must practice effective communication. Establishing a therapeutic nurse-patient relationship and interviewing are professional nursing skills and may not be delegated. Nursing assistive personnel (NAP) may observe and receive a lot of important information because of the length of time they are with the patient. The nurse instructs the NAP about:

- The proper way to interact verbally and nonverbally with patients.
- Special ways to communicate with patients who are cognitively impaired, anxious, angry, children, or older adults.
- Communicating to the nurse patient concerns, including anger and anxiety, to determine if additional nursing interventions are needed.

IMPLEMENTATION *for* ESTABLISHING THE NURSE-PATIENT RELATIONSHIP AND INTERVIEWING

STEPS	RATIONALE
1. Orientation Phase	
a. Create a climate of warmth and acceptance. Be aware of nonverbal cues, both sent and received. Provide comfort and support to patient.	This facilitates open exchange without fear or anxiety.
b. Use appropriate nonverbal behaviors (e.g., good eye contact, open relaxed posture, sitting eye level with patient).	Appropriate nonverbal behaviors facilitate communication by providing a nonverbal message that shows interest in what the patient has to say.
c. Observe patient's nonverbal behaviors, including body language. If verbal behaviors do not match nonverbal behaviors, seek clarification from patient.	Congruence between patient's verbal and nonverbal behaviors ensures that you receive the correct message.
d. Explain purpose of interaction when information is to be shared.	Information and explanation can decrease anxiety about the unknown.
e. Use active listening.	Active listening conveys interest in patient's needs, concerns, and problems and conveys empathy.
f. Identify patient's expectations in seeking health care.	Identifying expectations conveys a level of interest in patient's needs.
g. Encourage patient to ask for clarification at any time during the communication.	This gives patient a sense of control and keeps channels of communication open.
2. Working Phase	
a. Use therapeutic communication skills (see Table 2-1), such as restating, reflecting, and paraphrasing, to identify and clarify strategies for attainment of mutually agreed-on goals.	These techniques establish a greater understanding of messages sent and received.
b. Discuss and prioritize problem areas.	Patients' misinterpretations need to be clarified because patients experiencing emotionally charged situations may not comprehend the message (Keltner et al., 2011).
c. Provide information to patient, and help patient express needs and feelings.	A patient, nonjudgmental, supportive approach minimizes patient anxiety.
d. Use questions carefully and appropriately. Ask one question as a time, and allow sufficient time for patient to answer. Use direct questions. Use open-ended statements as much as possible, such as, "Tell me about how you are feeling today."	Patient is able to respond to help, develop workable solutions based on goals, and participate fully in a realistic plan for his or her well-being. This helps patient to express himself or herself and allows you to obtain thorough information about patient's needs and concerns.
e. Avoid communication barriers (see Table 2-1).	Barriers result in a message not being received, being distorted, or not being understood.
f. If a patient interview is necessary (e.g., health history), tell the patient the reason for the interview and how long it is expected to take. Assure patient that all information obtained during the interaction is confidential.	This assurance relieves anxiety about giving information to a stranger and encourages participation.
1) Interview patient about health status, lifestyle, support systems, patterns of health and illness, and strengths and limitations.	Interview facilitates a positive nurse-patient relationship and the development of trust, putting patients at ease.
2) If patient is alert enough to state name, where he or she is, and what day it is, proceed with the interview. Confirm information obtained from patient with other caregivers or family members if patient is disoriented or confused or seems unreliable.	An alert and oriented patient is a reliable source of information.

Continued

STEPS

3) Ask what led patient to seek health care. Attempt to obtain a descriptive account of all the events in the order in which they occurred. Ask open-ended questions and listen to patient's story.

4) For each symptom that patient reports, determine when, where, and under what circumstances it occurred. Also determine location; quality; quantity; duration; and aggravating, alleviating, and associated factors and related symptoms (Table 2-2).

5) Identify past hospitalizations, past surgical procedures and complications, and previous major health problems.

6) Determine whether patient regularly takes medications and, if so, for what period of time. Ask the name, reason for taking, dosage, and frequency of medication. Specifically ask about dietary supplements or over-the-counter (OTC) medications such as aspirin, acetaminophen, ibuprofen, laxatives, sleeping pills, diet pills, herbal supplements or remedies, or other types of alternative therapies.

7) Clarify if patient takes narcotics, insulin, digitalis, contraceptives, steroids, or hormone replacements.

8) Identify risk factors related to lifestyle that influence the patient's health, knowledge level, and awareness of the risk.

9) Continue with additional areas of interest or concern according to the focus of the interview. As appropriate, indicate when you are nearly finished with the interview.

3. **Termination Phase** (see illustration)

   a. Continue to use therapeutic communication skills to discuss discharge or termination issues and guide discussion related to specific patient changes in thoughts and behaviors.

RATIONALE

Active listening encourages exchange of information. Conducting an interview by asking questions only may make patient feel like a subject of interrogation.

This refines and clusters assessment data associated with each symptom.

Patients may not think of dietary supplements or OTC medications because these do not require prescriptions. However, both of these classifications of medications may have interactive effects with current or future prescribed medications.

Patients may not mention these if such drugs seem unrelated to the reason for admission or when they think that the health care provider would have previously conveyed this information.

Risk factors include smoking, alcohol use, drug abuse, lack of exercise, stress, nutritional factors (e.g., fluids, cholesterol, carbohydrates, fiber, salt), exposure to violence, and unprotected sexual activity.

This conveys empathy and keeps focus of interview on patient. This offers patient a chance to ask final questions.

Communication skills reinforce knowledge and skills learned during working phase of relationship.

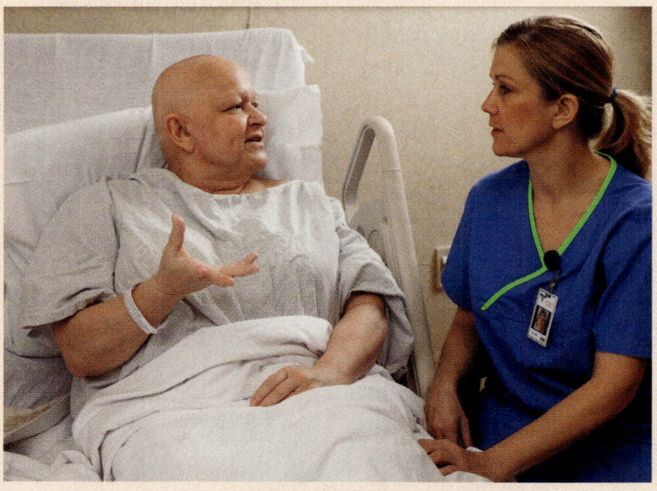

STEP 3 Sitting facing the patient may facilitate communication.

STEPS	RATIONALE
b. Summarize with patient what you have discussed during interaction or interview, including goal and achievement. Summarize your understanding of patient's health concerns.	This summary provides a sense of closure and mutual understanding and provides a method to verify that the nurse's information is correct and complete. It also enables the patient to correct misconceptions or clarify data.
c. Provide information that tells the patient you are nearly finished.	This offers a chance to ask final questions.

EVALUATION

1. Observe patient's verbal and nonverbal responses (e.g., body language, verbal statements) after discussion of feelings and circumstances that were identified.
2. During working phase, ask patient for feedback regarding the message communicated. Was communication accurately interpreted? Verify if information obtained from the patient regarding his or her thoughts, needs, and concerns is accurate.
3. During termination phase, summarize and restate. Ask if patient or significant other has had an adequate opportunity to describe health concerns.

Unexpected Outcomes and Related Interventions

1. Patient continues to express verbally and nonverbally feelings of anxiety, fear, anger, confusion, distrust, and helplessness.
   a. Reassess patient's level of anxiety, fear, and distrust.
   b. Come back at another time to repeat the message.
   c. Determine influences affecting clear communication (e.g., cultural issues, literacy issues, physical limits).
2. Feedback between nurse and patient reveals a lack of understanding.
   a. Assess for and remove barriers to communication.
   b. Repeat the message using another approach if possible.

3. Nurse is unable to acquire information about patient's ideas, fears, and concerns.
   a. Try alternative communication techniques to promote the patient's willingness to communicate openly.
   b. Rephrase question after there has been time for understanding and response.
   c. Offer the patient the opportunity to talk with another professional to obtain the necessary information.
4. Family member or significant other answers for patient, even when patient is capable of answering.
   a. Direct the question to patient, using patient's name.
   b. Acknowledge the answer given by a family member, then state that you are interested specifically in what the patient has to say about it.
   c. Conclude the interview and resume again after the family members are gone. If necessary, you may suggest that family take a break for a while, get coffee or a meal, or walk outside briefly for some fresh air.
5. Patient is unable to communicate, and family members are present.
   a. Interview a family member as you would the patient.
   b. Explore the needs of family and patient.

Recording and Reporting

- Record information-related interventions and patient responses.

TABLE 2-2	DIMENSIONS OF A SYMPTOM
DIMENSIONS	**QUESTIONS TO ASK**
Location	"Where do you feel it?" "Does it move around?" "Show me where."
Quality or character	"What is it like? Sharp, dull, stabbing, aching?"
Severity	"On a scale of 0 to 10, with 10 the worst, how would you rate what you feel right now?" "What is the worst it has been?" "In what ways does this interfere with your usual activities?"
Timing	"When did you first notice it?" "How long does it last?" "How often does it happen?"
Setting	"Does it occur in a particular place or under certain circumstances?"
Aggravating or alleviating factors	"What makes it better?" "What makes it worse?" "When does it change?" "Have you noticed other changes associated with this?"

- Report pertinent information, subjective data, and nonverbal cues, including response to illness, response to therapy, and questions or concerns.
- Complete the information included in the admission profile: reason for admission; medical-surgical history; family history; allergies; health habits, including cultural beliefs about health, current prescribed therapies (include all OTC medications and supplements), and any current nonprescribed therapies or alternative treatments.

Sample Documentation

Complete standardized assessment form according to facility policy. Document evaluation of patient learning.

1345   Patient expresses anxiety about current hospitalization. Is fidgeting in the bed, wringing his hands. Expresses much concern about fears of cancer with recent diagnostic tests. Knows friends diagnosed with cancer. Encouraged to talk with his wife and the health care provider about concerns and questions.

Special Considerations

Pediatric

- Use vocabulary that is familiar to the child based on level of understanding and usual patterns of communication.
- Consider the child's developmental level to select the most appropriate communication techniques (e.g., storytelling and drawing) (Hockenberry and Wilson, 2013).
- Evaluate the child's usual pattern of communication, including use of age-appropriate language.

- Include parents in the interviewing process when appropriate.

Geriatric

- Be aware of any cognitive or sensory impairment.
- Avoid stereotyping older adults as having cognitive or sensory impairments.
- Speak face-to-face with a patient who has a hearing impairment, articulate clearly in a moderate tone of voice, and assess whether the patient hears and understands the words.
- Ensure that older patients with visual impairments have any necessary assistive devices such as eyeglasses and large-print reading material.
- Encourage patients with auditory or visual impairments to use assistive devices to aid in communication.

Home Care

- Identify a primary caregiver for patient and include in the interview. This individual may be a family member, friend, or neighbor.
- Assess the level of understanding of patient and primary caregiver regarding the patient's condition.
- Incorporate the patient's usual daily habits and routines into the communication event (e.g., bathing and dressing patient).
- Assess for the presence of any cognitive or physical impairments that may hinder communication.
- Identify patient's primary caregiver and include that person in the interviewing process.

SKILL 2.2   COMMUNICATING WITH PATIENTS WHO HAVE DIFFICULTY COPING

Anxiety results from many factors. A newly diagnosed illness, separation from loved ones, the threat of pending diagnostic tests or surgical procedures, a language barrier, and expectations of life changes are just a few factors that cause anxiety. How successfully a patient copes with anxiety depends in part on previous experiences, the presence of other stressors, the significance of the event causing anxiety, and the availability of supportive resources. Effective communication helps to decrease anxiety. Communication methods reviewed in this skill may help an anxious patient clarify factors causing anxiety and cope more effectively. There are stages of anxiety with corresponding behavioral manifestations: mild, moderate, severe, and panic (Box 2-6).

The degree and frequency of anger range from everyday mild annoyance to anger related to feelings of helplessness and powerlessness. It is important to understand that in many cases a patient's ability to express anger is sometimes necessary for recovery. When a patient experiences a significant loss, anger becomes a means to help cope with grief. A patient may express anger toward a health care professional, but often the anger hides a specific problem or concern. A patient with a new diagnosis of cancer may voice anger with the nurse's care instead of expressing a fear of dying.

It is stressful to deal with an angry patient. Anger can represent rejection or disapproval of nursing care. Satisfying the needs of one angry patient often results in a failure to meet the priorities of other patients. Create a safe and private environment for patients to express anger and frustration.

However, anger is the common underlying factor associated with a potential for violence. In the health care setting, health care professionals may become the target of a patient's anger when the patient cannot express it toward a significant other. De-escalation skills are useful techniques for managing a potentially violent patient. These skills range from using nonthreatening verbal and nonverbal messages to safely disengaging and controlling the aggressor physically (Fortinash and Holoday-Worret, 2012).

Depression is more than just sadness; it is a mood disorder with many causes. People with mild depression describe themselves as feeling sad, blue, downcast, and

---

BOX 2-6 BEHAVIORAL MANIFESTATIONS OF STAGES OF ANXIETY

Mild Anxiety
- Increased auditory and visual perception
- Increased awareness of relationships
- Increased alertness
- Able to problem solve

Moderate Anxiety
- Selective inattention
- Decreased perceptual field
- Focus only on relevant information
- Muscle tension; diaphoresis

Severe Anxiety
- Focus on fragmented details
- Headache, nausea, dizziness
- Unable to see connections between details
- Poor recall and problem solvling

Panic State of Anxiety
- Does not notice surroundings
- Feeling of terror
- Unable to cope with any problem

---

tearful. They commonly feel apathetic, hopeless, helpless, worthless, guilty, and angry. Other symptoms include difficulty sleeping or sleeping too much, irritability, weight loss or gain, headaches, and feelings of fatigue regardless of the amount of sleep. In some cases, there is a high level of anxiety, physical complaints, and social isolation. Thoughts of death and decreased libido may also occur (Keltner et al., 2011). Many patients in acute care settings who have either acute or chronic health conditions have symptoms of depression. Some patients with a diagnosis of depression are receiving treatment with medication or psychotherapy or both. Other depressed patients may not be receiving any treatment.

As a result of their illness, patients in the health care setting often experience various emotions including depression, anxiety, or anger. These emotions may have a negative impact on their coping skills, requiring specific nursing interventions, including therapeutic communication strategies, to manage their behaviors.

ASSESSMENT

1. Observe for physical, behavioral, and verbal cues of anxiety, such as dry mouth, sweaty palms, tone of voice, frequent use of call light, difficulty concentrating, wringing of hands, and statements such as "I'm scared." *Rationale: Certain behaviors indicate anxiety.*
2. Assess for possible factors causing patient anxiety (e.g., hospitalization, fatigue, fear, pain).
3. Assess factors influencing communication with the patient (e.g., environment, timing, presence of others, values, experiences, need for personal space because of heightened anxiety).

4. Assess your own level of anxiety as a nurse and make a conscious effort to remain calm. *Rationale: Anxiety is highly contagious, and one's own anxiety can worsen the patient's anxiety.*
5. Observe for behaviors that indicate the patient is angry (e.g., pacing, clenched fists, loud voice, throwing objects) or expressions by patient that indicate anger (e.g., repeated questioning of the nurse, irrational complaints about care, no adherence to requests, belligerent outbursts, threats).
6. Assess factors that influence the angry patient's communication, such as refusal to comply with treatment goals, use of sarcasm or hostile behavior, having a low frustration level, or being emotionally immature.
7. Consider resources available to assist in communicating with the potentially violent patient, such as other members of the health care team and family members.
8. Assess for physical, behavioral, and verbal cues that indicate the patient is depressed, such as feelings of sadness, tearfulness, difficulty concentrating, increase in reports of physical complaints, and statements such as "I'm sad/depressed."
9. Assess for possible factors causing patient's depression (e.g., acute or chronic illness, personal vulnerability, past history).
10. You may need to confer with family members about possible causes of the patient's depression, including past history of the illness.

PLANNING

Expected Outcomes focus on reducing the patient's anxiety or depression through the use of effective communication techniques; focus on promoting effective and socially appropriate verbal and nonverbal expressions of anger.
1. Patient discusses or describes factors causing anxiety, anger, or depression.
2. Patient is able to discuss methods to cope with anxiety, anger, or depression.
3. Patient's anxiety, anger, or depression is mitigated, and problem solving is initiated.
4. Patient states that coping strategies improve well-being.

Delegation and Collaboration

Communicating effectively with an anxious, angry, or depressed patient cannot be delegated to nursing assistive personnel (NAP). The nurse instructs the NAP about:
- Basic skills needed to interact verbally with an anxious, angry, or depressed patient.
- Their role as the nurse uses de-escalation techniques.
- Appropriate safety measures for themselves and other patients.

IMPLEMENTATION *for* COMMUNICATING WITH PATIENTS WHO HAVE DIFFICULTY COPING

STEPS	RATIONALE
1. Provide brief, simple introduction; introduce self; and explain purpose of interaction.	Brief reintroductions help to orient patient continually.
2. Use appropriate nonverbal behaviors (e.g., relaxed posture, eye contact). Stay with patient at the bedside.	Patients experiencing emotionally charged situations may not comprehend the verbally delivered message. Focus on understanding patient, providing feedback, assisting in problem solving, and providing an atmosphere of warmth and acceptance.
3. Use appropriate responses that are clear and concise.	This promotes effective communication so that patient can explore causes of anxiety and steps to alleviate anxious feelings. It conveys empathy.
4. Help patient acquire alternative coping strategies, such as progressive relaxation, slow deep-breathing exercises, and visual imagery.	Stress-reduction techniques are nonpharmacological strategies that patient can use to reduce anxiety.
5. Minimize noise in physical setting.	Decreasing environmental stimuli may reduce patient's anxiety.
6. Adjust the amount and quality of time for communicating depending on patient's needs.	Flexibility and adaptation of techniques may be necessary based on patient's ability to communicate, level of anxiety, and need for more time to establish trust.
7. Create a climate of patient acceptance. Maintain a nonthreatening verbal approach using a calm tone of voice. Try to determine the source of the anger. Use open body language with a concerned nonthreatening facial expression, open arms (not folded), hands not in pockets, relaxed posture, and a safe distance (e.g., not invading the patient's personal space).	A relaxed atmosphere may prevent further escalation.
8. Respond to potentially violent patient with therapeutic silence, and allow patient to ventilate feelings. Use active listening for understanding. Do not argue with patient. Avoid defensiveness with patient.	These techniques often de-escalate anger because anger expends emotional and physical energy; patient runs out of momentum and energy to maintain anger at a high level. Arguing escalates anger.
9. Answer questions calmly and honestly. If patient presents a power-struggle type of question (e.g., "Who said you were in charge; I don't have to listen to you"), set limits using clear, concise language. Inform patient of potential consequences, and follow through with consequences if behaviors are not altered.	Setting limits on power-struggle questions provides structure and diffuses anger (Fortinash and Holoday-Worret, 2012).
10. Maintain personal space. It may be necessary to have someone with you and to keep the door open. Position yourself between patient and the exit.	These steps promote your safety when patient becomes violent.
11. If patient is making verbal threats to harm others, remain calm yet professional and continue to set limits with inappropriate behavior. If a distinct likelihood of imminent harm to others is present, notify proper authorities (e.g., nurse manager, security).	Angry patients lose the ability to process information rationally and may impulsively express themselves through intimidation.

> **SAFE PATIENT CARE** A potentially violent patient can be impulsive and explosive; it is imperative that you keep personal safety skills in mind. In this case avoid touch.

STEPS	RATIONALE
12. Encourage safe coping behaviors (e.g., physical exercise, writing about negative thoughts).	These measures are examples of methods of directing energy in an acceptable way.
13. Use open-ended questions or statements such as, "Tell me about how you are feeling."	An open-ended question or statement encourages the patient to continue talking, facilitating a discussion of symptoms and circumstances.

STEPS	RATIONALE
14. Encourage small decisions and independent actions. When necessary, make decisions that patients are not ready to make.	Depressed patients may be overly dependent and indecisive.
15. Spend time with patient who is withdrawn and provide honest affirmation.	This behavior communicates patient's worth.
16. Ask, "Are you having thoughts of suicide?" If the answer is yes, ask, "Have you thought about how you would do it?" (plan); "Do you have what you need?" (means); "Have you thought about when you would do it?" (time set).	Depressed patients are at increased risk for suicide. Of all suicide hotline callers, 95% answer no at some point in this series of questions or indicate that the time is set for some date in the future. The more developed the plan, the greater the risk of suicide (Keltner et al., 2011). Referral is needed.

EVALUATION

1. Have patient discuss ways to cope with anxiety, anger, or depression in the future and make decisions about the current situation.
2. Observe for continuing presence of physical signs and symptoms or behaviors reflecting anxiety or depression.
3. Ask patient to discuss factors causing or increasing anxiety, anger, or depression.
4. Ask patient if feelings of anxiety, anger, or depression have subsided.
5. Determine patient's ability to answer questions and solve problems.
6. Use **Teach Back:** State to the patient "I want to be sure I explained clearly different ways you can better cope. Can you tell me some of those ways?" Evaluates what the patient is able to explain or demonstrate. Revise your instruction now or develop plan for revised patient teaching to be implemented at an appropriate time if patient is not able to teach back correctly.

Unexpected Outcomes and Related Interventions

1. Physical signs and symptoms of anxiety, anger, or depression continue.
   a. Use refocusing or distraction skills such as relaxation and imagery to reduce anxiety.
   b. Be direct and clear when communicating with patient to avoid misunderstanding.
   c. Touch, when used appropriately, may help control feelings of panic or confusion.
   d. Administering medication for behavior as prescribed may be necessary.
   e. Provide security measures (see facility protocol).
   f. Evaluate support system.
   g. Refer patient to a mental health professional for consultation.
   h. Use distraction techniques or redirection with patients with cognitive impairment.

Recording and Reporting

- Record factors and actions that cause the patient's anxiety, anger, or depression.
- Document nonverbal behaviors; methods used to relieve anxiety, anger, or depression (pharmacological and non-pharmacological methods); and patient response (verbal and nonverbal).
- Document your evaluation of patient learning.
- Record and report threats of violence made and who was notified.

Sample Documentation

1800   Patient expressed extreme anger toward staff related to food served cold and no-smoking policy. Stated, "I just can't take this abuse any more. I have to get out of here now." Threatened to leave the hospital against medical advice. Nurse manager and patient's health care provider were notified. Encouraged to write about his feelings; family plans to stay with patient until he is calmer.

Special Considerations
Pediatric

- Evaluate the child's usual pattern of communication, including use of age-appropriate language.
- Anxiety or depression may be expressed through restless behavior, physical complaints, or behavioral regression.
- Children tend to have less internal control over their behaviors; immediately setting limits for inappropriate behaviors exhibited by the child is effective (Hockenberry and Wilson, 2013).

Geriatric

- Anxiety is often the result of change in usual patterns and environment.
- Depression among older adults is a major health concern; suicide risk is increased in older adults (Keltner et al., 2011).

Home Care Considerations

- Personal safety for the nurse against potentially violent patients or family members extends to all health care settings, including the patient's home. The nurse may be in a potentially dangerous situation while giving care to the patient at home.

- Be aware of physical surroundings, including possible exits. Maintain a nonthreatening position, including body language, body position, and rate of speech, when interacting with an angry or potentially violent patient. Whenever possible, attempt to de-escalate the patient. If de-escalation does not occur and you think that safety may be threatened, call for assistance.
- Have numbers for emergency use posted near phone (e.g., mental health provider, emergency response units, and neighbors).

SKILL 2.3   COMMUNICATING WITH COGNITIVELY IMPAIRED PATIENTS

Patients can have short-term or long-term cognitive impairment. Patients with cognitive impairment pose a challenge for all caregivers. Often patients cannot think, speak, or understand what they were told. Memory loss and confusion may be present in patients who have some form of dementia or brain injury. People with mental illness or developmental disabilities may have some degree of cognitive impairment. Other causes of cognitive impairment include fatigue and effects of medications. Use a normal tone of voice and simple words and speak slowly when communicating with patients with cognitive impairment.

ASSESSMENT

1. Assess for physical, behavioral, and verbal cues that indicate a patient has cognitive impairment. Assess orientation status of the patient (person, place, and time), and perform a mini-mental examination (see Chapter 7). *Rationale: If the patient is unable to think, speak, or understand, communication strategies need to be adjusted to communicate effectively.*
2. Assess for possible factors causing patient's cognitive impairment (e.g., illness, medication, fever, electrolyte imbalances). *Rationale: Causes of cognitive change may be attributed to health status or medications. It is important that these factors be part of an assessment.*
3. Assess factors influencing communication with patient (e.g., environment, timing, presence of others, values, experiences, need for personal space because of cognitive impairments).

4. Assess the level of cognitive impairment and influencing factors. *Rationale: Understanding the cause of mental decline, such as a stroke, fever, or electrolyte imbalance, assists in supporting and communicating with the patient.*
5. Ascertain the most effective means of communicating with the patient with cognitive impairment (i.e., verbal or written communication or nonverbal communication). *Rationale: Understanding factors that influence communication helps to identify effective communication strategies.*

PLANNING

Expected Outcomes focus on recognizing symptoms of cognitive impairment in patients and effectively communicating with patients.
1. Patient's physical and emotional discomforts are acknowledged.
2. Patient is able to communicate needs to the nurse.

Delegation and Collaboration

The skill of communicating effectively with a patient with cognitive impairment cannot be delegated to nursing assistive personnel (NAP). The nurse instructs the NAP about:
- The proper communication skills needed to interact verbally and nonverbally with a patient with cognitive impairment.
- The possible causes and signs and symptoms of the patient's cognitive impairment.

IMPLEMENTATION *for* COMMUNICATING WITH COGNITIVELY IMPAIRED PATIENTS

STEPS	RATIONALE
1. Approach patient from the front and provide brief, simple introduction; introduce yourself; and explain purpose of interaction.	Brief reintroductions help to orient patient continually.
2. Use appropriate nonverbal behaviors (e.g., relaxed posture, eye contact). Stay with the patient at the bedside.	Patients experiencing emotionally charged situations may not comprehend the verbally delivered message. Focus on understanding patient, providing feedback, assisting in problem solving, and providing an atmosphere of warmth and acceptance.
3. Use clear and concise verbal techniques to respond to patient. Use simple language, and speak slowly; use short, simple sentences. Ask "yes" or "no" questions.	This promotes effective communication so the patient can explore causes of anxiety and steps to alleviate anxious feelings. It conveys empathy.

STEPS	RATIONALE
4. Ask one question at a time, and allow time for response. Avoid rushing patient.	This gives patient time to process the information and respond.
5. Repeat sentences using a steady voice, and avoid being too quick to guess what patient is trying to express.	Repetition allows time for patient to respond; it can be frustrating for patient if you misinterpret his or her message or pressure him or her to respond.
6. Use ACC devices to facilitate communication (e.g., pictogram grid, talking mats, objects).	Talking mats are communication aids that use picture symbols so the patient can place relevant images below a visual scale to indicate feelings (McGhee, 2011).
7. Provide assistive devices such as eyeglasses or hearing aids to help with communication.	Use of such devices facilitates clarity of communication experiences.
8. Do not argue with patient or correct patient if mistakes are made.	Arguing can lead to increased frustration and agitation.
9. Maintain meaningful interactions with patient, and use creative methods of communication based on patient's comfort level and ability.	Superficial, brief contact may lead to a sense of isolation and detachment.
10. Help patient acquire alternative coping strategies, such as progressive relaxation, slow deep-breathing exercises, and visual imagery. Minimize noise in physical setting.	Stress-reduction techniques are nonpharmacological strategies that patient can use to reduce anxiety that results from difficulty to communicate because of confusion.

EVALUATION

1. Observe for clarity and patient's understanding of information.
2. Observe verbal and nonverbal behaviors.

Unexpected Outcomes and Related Interventions

1. Patient remains disoriented and cannot communicate effectively.
   a. Be direct and clear when communicating with patient to avoid misunderstanding.
   b. Evaluate patient's support system.
   c. Refer patient to a mental health professional for consultation.
   d. Use distraction techniques or redirection with patient with cognitive impairment.

Recording and Reporting

- Record communication strategies used to interact successfully with the patient with cognitive impairment.
- Report verbal and nonverbal responses by patient.

Sample Documentation

2200 Patient is observed attempting to get out of bed without assistance. Patient does not respond to verbal commands/questions. Showed picture of bathroom to patient, and patient nods head. Assisted patient to ambulate to bathroom.

Special Considerations
Pediatric

- Use vocabulary that is familiar to the child based on child's level of understanding and usual patterns of communication.
- When interviewing the child with cognitive impairment, consider the child's developmental level.
- Include parents in the interviewing process when appropriate.

Geriatric

- Be aware of any cognitive or sensory impairment; patients who have cognitive impairments may exhibit tantrum-like behaviors in response to real or perceived frustration.

Home Care Considerations

- Identify patient's primary caregiver and include in interactions. This individual may be a family member, friend, or neighbor.
- Assess the level of understanding of the patient and primary caregiver regarding the patient's condition.
- Incorporate the patient's usual daily habits and routines into the communication event (e.g., bathing and dressing patient).
- Assess caregiver for the presence of any cognitive or physical impairments that may hinder communication.

IMPROVING INTERPROFESSIONAL COMMUNICATION

Skillful communication between nurses and nurses and other health care professionals improves the continuity of care, contributes to a culture of safety, prevents or resolves conflict, increases collaboration between health care professionals, and helps increase patient satisfaction (Fernandez et al., 2010). When critical information is not communicated clearly, the patient is adversely affected. According to research, a lack of interprofessional cooperation and collaboration and poor communication contribute to fragmented care and negative patient outcomes (Churchman and Doherty, 2010). In recent years, The Joint Commission (TJC) published the *National Patient Safety Goals* and identified as one of its goals to improve the effectiveness of communication among caregivers (TJC, 2014). Hand-off communications (see Procedural Guideline 2.1) and *Situation, Background, Assessment, and Recommendation* (SBAR) communication (see Procedural Guideline 2.2) are two techniques to improve interprofessional communication in health care settings.

PROCEDURAL GUIDELINE 2.1
Hand-Off Communications

The quality of patient care is improved when transferring information from one health care provider to another, called a *hand-off*. This commonly occurs when patient moves to a new unit or facility or at change of shift. Hand-off communication uses clear language and effective communication techniques. These hand-offs are interactive, providing the opportunity for all health care personnel involved to ask questions or seek clarification about the patient's treatment regimen. Hand-offs at the patient's bedside can enhance patient-centered care by involving the patient in the decision-making process. Consequently, inadequate hand-offs can be hazardous to patients and staff (Liu et al., 2012; Novak and Fairchild, 2012).

Delegation and Collaboration

The skill of hand-off communications cannot be delegated to nursing assistive personnel (NAP). The nurse instructs the NAP about:
- Patient information received during the transfer of care.
- Pertinent information or change in clinical status to report to the nurse, such as changes in the patient's vital signs, level of comfort, or clinical condition.

Equipment

- Worksheets; patient care summary; nursing care plan, critical pathway, multidisciplinary treatment plan
- Tape recorder (according to facility policy)

Procedural Steps

1. Develop an organized format for delivering hand-off that provides a description of patient needs and problems.
2. Gather information from documentation sources, NAP report, or other relevant documents.
3. Prioritize information based on patient needs and problems for each patient.
4. For each patient, include the following:
   a. *Background information:* Patient's name, gender, age, current primary reason for hospitalization, and brief history. Also include any known allergies, emergency code status (i.e., do not resuscitate [DNR]), and special needs in regard to any physical challenges (e.g., blind, hearing-impaired)
   b. *Assessment data:* Provide objective observations and measurements made by you during the shift. Describe patient's condition, and emphasize any recent changes. Include any relevant information reported by patient, family, or health care team members, such as laboratory data and diagnostic test results.
   c. *Nursing diagnoses or patient problems:* State the nursing diagnoses or patient problem appropriate for patient. (Some agencies do not include nursing diagnoses in report.)
   d. *Interventions, outcomes, and evaluation* (steps can be combined in a report):
      (1) Describe therapies or treatments administered during shift and expected outcomes (e.g., medication changes, use of oxygen, referral visits). Specify how you implemented interventions uniquely for this patient. Report on evaluation by explaining patient's response and whether outcomes are met. Do not explain basic steps of a procedure.
      (2) Describe instructions or education given in the teaching plan and patient's/family's ability to demonstrate learning.
   e. *Family information:* Report on family visitation or involvement, specifically as it influenced patient. Explain if you included family members in care procedures or instruction.
   f. *Discharge plan:* Review patient's progress toward discharge during each change-of-shift report. Discuss education progress, communication with referral agencies, and family preparation for discharge. This plan also identifies roles and responsibilities of the multidisciplinary team and their follow-up visits.
   g. *Current priorities:* Clearly explain the priorities to which oncoming nurse must attend.
      (1) Report significant clinical changes.
      (2) Report on immediate treatment planned for any new admission.
      (3) Explain status of activities for patients preparing for procedures and treatments.
      (4) Describe current physical status of patients returning from diagnostic or operative procedures.
5. Ask staff from oncoming shift if they have any questions regarding information provided.
6. If using a tape recorder, periodically evaluate for clarity, organization, rate of speaking, and volume level.

PROCEDURAL GUIDELINE 2.2
SBAR Communication

The *Situation, Background, Assessment,* and *Recommendation* (SBAR) communication technique provides a predictable structure for communication of data about a patient's condition among all health care personnel. This communication model includes four components: *Situation*—state what is happening at the present time; *Background*—explain circumstances leading up to situation; *Assessment*—what you think the problem is; and *Recommendation*—what to do to correct the problem. SBAR can be used in hand-off situations and to communicate when a patient's condition changes and applies to both written and verbal communication. It is standardized communication and improves the effectiveness of information delivery. You can use the SBAR tool as a checklist to improve patient safety and help streamline information exchanges from one health care provider to another (Novak and Fairchild, 2012).

Delegation and Collaboration

The skill of SBAR communications cannot be delegated to nursing assistive personnel (NAP). The nurse instructs the NAP about:

- Patient information received during the transfer of care.
- Pertinent information or change in clinical status to report to the nurse, such as changes in the patient's vital signs, level of comfort, or clinical condition.

Procedural Steps

1. *Situation*—Identify self, unit, and patient's name and room number. State what is happening at the present time, including patient's condition and severity.
2. *Background*—Provide background information related to situation. Include admitting diagnosis, reason for admission, allergies, and current medications, laboratory/test results, vital signs, and code status relevant to the situation. Have medical record available when reporting.
3. *Assessment*—Give assessment of the situation.
4. *Recommendation*—Give any care recommendations regarding the patient; explain what you need. Be clear and specific. Explain how you would correct the problem. Read back any verbal or telephone orders received during the recommendation phase.

SKILL 2.4 DISCHARGE PLANNING AND TRANSITIONAL CARE

Discharge planning is an important part of patient care during hospitalization. The discharge process is complex and can be hazardous to the patient, most likely owing to inadequate communication, which can lead to patient errors and other negative outcomes. It is important to involve patients in the discharge process because patient involvement leads to improved health outcomes and greater satisfaction (Shoeb et al., 2012). Developing an agreed-on discharge plan based on the needs and preferences of a patient and family is essential to the discharge process (Graham et al., 2013).

Transitional care refers to the actions of the health care team to ensure the coordination and continuity of care as patients move between various health locations and settings, depending on their health status. Elderly patients and patients with a chronic illness are examples of the types of patients who require transitional care. Examples of health care settings include hospitals, nursing homes, long-term care facilities, and patients' homes. Transitional care may reduce unnecessary use of health care services and improve patient outcomes, while providing cost-effective care in the most appropriate setting (Ornstein et al., 2011; Peikes et al., 2012). Use of clear verbal and written communication is essential to the patient-centered discharge planning process, providing a safe transition from one setting to another. To prevent misunderstandings, have the patient and family members review discharge information. Ask the patient and family members to repeat the information using their own words.

ASSESSMENT

1. Determine patient's appropriateness for discharge. Use patient's plan of care to assess continually patient education and needs after discharge. *Rationale: Premature discharge may result in hospital readmission. Discharge planning begins with admission, and ongoing assessment of patient education and discharge needs enhances patient readiness for discharge.*
2. Assess the health literacy level of patient and family. *Rationale: Because health literacy influences patient care and health outcomes, the nurse must consider the health literacy level of the patient and family when planning patient care, including discharge planning (Dickens and Piano, 2013).*
3. Assess for barriers to learning (e.g., fatigue, pain, lack of motivation). *Rationale: This assessment determines the timing and approach to discharge instruction.*

4. Assess for environmental factors within the home that interfere with self-care (e.g., size of rooms, doorway clearances, steps, bathroom facilities). (A home care nurse is usually available on referral to assist with assessment.) *Rationale: Environmental factors within the patient's home can pose safety risks or problems for self-care. For example, throw rugs are a fall hazard for a patient discharged with crutches or a walker (see Chapter 32).*

5. Collaborate with health care provider and interprofessional team (e.g., physical therapy) in assessing the need for referral for skilled home care services or an extended care facility. *Rationale: Patients eligible for home care must be confined to home as a result of illness, are under a health care provider's care, and require skilled nursing care on an intermittent basis.*

6. Assess patient's and family's perceptions of continued health care needs outside the hospital. Include an assessment of the perceived ability of family caregivers to provide care to patient, including the ability to adjust to demands of patient care, the impact of care demands on their lives (e.g., providing hands-on care, preparing special diets), and the potential ongoing nature of patient's needs. *Rationale: Patients and family members often disagree on health care needs after discharge. Identifying discrepancies early helps in developing the discharge plan more accurately. Being a family caregiver is a highly stressful experience. Family members who are not properly prepared for caregiving are frequently overwhelmed by the patient's needs, which can lead to hospital readmissions (Sobolewski, 2011).*

7. Assess patient's acceptance of health problems and related restrictions. *Rationale: The patient's acceptance affects his or her willingness to follow therapies and restrictions.*

8. Consult other health care team members (e.g., dietitian, social worker) about anticipated needs of the patient after discharge. Make appropriate referrals in a timely manner. *Rationale: Members of all health care disciplines collaborate to determine the patient's needs and functional abilities.*

Expected Outcomes focus on using written and verbal information to develop an individualized discharge plan for the patient and family.
1. Patient or family caregiver explains how health care is to continue at home (or at another facility), which treatments or medications the patient needs, and when to seek medical attention for problems.
2. Patient and family are able to demonstrate self-care activities.
3. Barriers to self-care activities are removed from or modified in patient's home environment.

Delegation and Collaboration

The skill of implementing discharge planning is a professional nursing skill and may not be delegated. Nursing assistive personnel (NAP) may observe and receive a lot of important information because of the length of time they are with the patient. The nurse instructs the NAP to:
- Gather and secure the patient's personal items and home care supplies.
- Transport the patient to the discharge transport vehicle.

IMPLEMENTATION *for* DISCHARGE PLANNING AND TRANSITIONAL CARE

STEPS	RATIONALE
1. Preparation before day of discharge.	
a. Suggest ways to change physical arrangement of home to meet patient's needs (see Chapter 32).	Maintains patient's level of independence and ability to retain function within safe environment.
b. Provide patient and family with information about community health care resources (e.g., medical equipment companies, Meals on Wheels, adult day care). Referrals are usually made while patient is in hospital.	Community resources offer services that patient or family cannot provide.
c. Conduct teaching sessions with patient and family as soon as possible during hospitalization (e.g., signs and symptoms of complications, information regarding medications, use of medical equipment, follow-up care, diet, exercise, restrictions imposed by illness or surgery). Review and give patient discharge materials such as pamphlets, books, or multimedia resources. Refer patient to reliable and current resources on the Internet.	Gives patient opportunities to practice new skills, ask questions, and obtain necessary feedback to ensure learning. A combination of written and verbal information is effective in improving patient satisfaction and knowledge (TJC, 2014).
d. Communicate response of patient and family to teaching and proposed discharge plan to other health care team members.	Facilitates development of individualized discharge plan.

STEPS	RATIONALE

2. Procedure on day of discharge.

a. Let patient and family ask questions or discuss issues related to home care. A final opportunity to demonstrate learned skills is helpful.

Allows for final clarification of information previously discussed. Helps relieve anxiety.

b. Check health care provider's discharge orders for prescriptions, change in treatments, or need for special medical equipment. (Make sure that orders are written as early as possible.) Arrange for delivery and setup of equipment (e.g., hospital bed, oxygen) before patient arrives home.

Only a health care provider is able to authorize a discharge. Early check of orders permits nurse to attend to any last-minute treatments or procedures well before discharge.

c. Determine whether patient or family has arranged for transportation.

Patient's condition at discharge determines method of transport.

d. Provide privacy and assistance as patient dresses and packs all personal belongings. Check all closets and drawers for belongings. Obtain copy of valuables list signed by patient and have security or appropriate administrator deliver valuables to patient.

Prevents loss of personal items. Patient's signature verifies receipt of items and relieves nursing department of liability for losses.

e. Complete medication reconciliation per facility policy. Check discharge medication orders against the medication administration record and home medication list. Provide patient with prescriptions or pharmacy-dispensed medications ordered by health care provider. Offer a final review of information needed to facilitate safe medication self-administration.

Medication reconciliation decreases risk of medication errors and ensures that patient is receiving correct medication at home (TJC, 2014). Review of drug information provides feedback to determine patient's success in learning about medications.

f. Provide information on follow-up appointments to health care provider's office. Provide phone number of unit.

Provides patient with contact for questions that arise after discharge. Ensures continuity of care to prevent rehospitalization.

g. Contact facility business office to determine whether patient needs to finalize arrangements for payment of bill. Arrange for patient or family to visit business office.

Source of concern for many patients is whether facility has accepted insurance or other payment forms.

h. Acquire utility cart to move patient's belongings. Obtain wheelchair for patient. Transport patients leaving by ambulance on ambulance stretchers.

Provides for safe transport.

i. Assist patient to wheelchair or stretcher using safe patient handling and transfer techniques (see Chapter 15). Escort patient to entrance of facility where source of transportation is waiting (see facility policy). Lock wheelchair wheels. Assist patient in transferring into transport vehicle. Help place personal belongings in vehicle.

Prevents injury to nurse and patient. Facility policy requires escort to ensure patient's safe exit. Facility's liability ends when patient is safely in vehicle.

j. Return to division. Notify admitting or appropriate department of time of discharge. Notify housekeeping of need to clean patient's room.

Allows facility to prepare for admission of next patient.

▌EVALUATION

1. Determine patient's ability to understand discharge instructions.

2. Use *Teach Back:* State to the patient, "I want to be sure you correctly understand how to take the medicines you will be taking at home. Can you tell me your daily medications?" Evaluates what the patient is able to explain or demonstrate. Revise your instruction now or develop plan for revised patient teaching to be implemented at an appropriate time if patient is not able to teach back correctly.

Unexpected Outcomes and Related Interventions

1. Patient is unable to understand discharge instructions.
   a. Be direct and clear when communicating with patient to avoid misunderstanding.

b. Evaluate patient's support system.

c. Assess factors that may hinder understanding (i.e., cognitive status; literacy level; presence of anxiety, fear, pain; readiness for discharge).

Recording and Reporting

- Record strategies used to provide discharge teaching with the patient.
- Report verbal and nonverbal responses by the patient.
- Document your evaluation of patient learning.

Sample Documentation

1200   Patient had left hip replacement 5 days ago. Because she lives at home with her husband who has mild dementia, it was determined that the patient be transferred to a skilled nursing facility for several weeks to participate in physical therapy. Discharge checklist reviewed with patient, daughter, and care coordinator from skilled nursing facility. Patient and daughter verbalized understanding of her transitional plan of care and expressed relief that she will not be a burden on her husband. Patient left the hospital in a wheelchair escorted by care coordinator.

Special Considerations
Pediatric

- Use vocabulary that is familiar to the child based on child's level of understanding and usual patterns of communication.
- Consider the child's developmental level when interacting with the child.

- Include parents in the discharge or transfer of care process when appropriate.

Geriatric

- Be aware of any cognitive or sensory impairment.
- Avoid stereotyping older adults as having cognitive or sensory impairments.
- Speak face-to-face with the patient with hearing impairment, articulate clearly in a moderate tone of voice, and assess whether the patient hears and understands the words.
- Ensure that older patients with visual impairments have any necessary assistive devices such as eyeglasses and large-print reading material.
- Encourage patients with auditory or visual impairments to use assistive devices to aid in communication.

Home Care Considerations

- Identify a primary caregiver for the patient. This individual may be a family member, friend, or neighbor.
- Assess the level of understanding of patient and primary caregiver regarding the patient's condition.
- Incorporate the patient's usual daily habits and routines into the communication event (e.g., bathing and dressing patient).
- Assess for the presence of any cognitive or physical impairments that may hinder communication.

CRITICAL THINKING QUESTIONS

Case Study

An 84-year-old patient with a cognitive impairment was transferred from a nursing home to an acute care facility. The patient has a history of vascular dementia from a series of strokes. According to the nursing home staff, the patient has been increasingly agitated and combative in the last few days, and this behavior is unusual for the patient. Laboratory tests revealed a urinary tract infection. The patient began receiving antibiotics for the infection.

1. You are the nurse caring for this patient. Which of the following is an example of an ineffective communication technique to use with this patient with cognitive impairment?
   1. Address patient by name.
   2. Challenge patient if patient is confused.
   3. Ask one question at a time.
   4. Speak slowly and use simple words.

2. The patient's condition is improving, and the patient's daughter wants to move the patient to a different facility. The nurse listens to the daughter's concerns and gives her a list of other appropriate long-term facilities, given the patient's abilities and needs. The nurse should intervene further if the daughter makes which of the following statements? Select all that apply.
   1. "I have a lot to think about before I make a decision that is best for my mother."
   2. "I think I could manage my mother at home with some professional assistance."
   3. "I am afraid of making a bad decision; then again, I can also relocate mother if the facility doesn't work out."
   4. "I will have someone else make the decision, so mother cannot get mad at me."

3. At 2230, the patient is found walking down the hallway of the unit, trying to get off the floor. The patient tries to open the locked door for the stairs. The nurse is busy caring for another patient, so the nurse tells the NAP to check on the patient. The NAP asks the patient what is going on, and the patient states that she needs to leave to get to her hair appointment on time. Which of the following is the most appropriate statement made by the NAP?
   1. "Please come away from the door, and I will show you back to your room."
   2. "Mrs. P, it is Monday evening and you are in the hospital. I work here, and I can help you."
   3. "This door is locked to keep you from getting off the unit."
   4. "I want to you to get dressed before you go to your hair appointment."

Review Questions

1. The nurse is completing the patient assessment and is asking sensitive questions regarding sexuality. The patient tells the nurse, "I don't want to answer these questions; they are personal and private." Which nursing response reflects empathy?
   1. "I know some of these questions are difficult for you."
   2. "Yes, I know just how you feel."
   3. "I understand that this is difficult for you to talk about, but I have to answer these assessment questions."
   4. "I am a professional nurse, and I know what I am doing."

2. What should the nurse know when observing and interpreting a patient's nonverbal communication?
   1. Patients are usually very aware of their nonverbal cues.
   2. Verbal responses are more important than nonverbal cues.
   3. Nonverbal cues have obvious meaning and are easily interpreted.
   4. Nonverbal cues provide significant information and need to be validated.

3. A patient has been withdrawn, suspicious, and explosive since admission. He is wary of staff and other patients. Which approach by the nurse is most appropriate?
   1. Refraining from touch
   2. Patting his arm when he seems frightened
   3. Reaching out to shake his hand as an initial greeting
   4. Placing an arm around his shoulders while walking down the hall

4. The nurse in the mental health unit reviews therapeutic and nontherapeutic communication techniques with a nursing student. Which of the following are therapeutic communication techniques? Select all that apply.
   1. Restating
   2. Listening
   3. Asking the patient "Why?"
   4. Maintaining neutral responses
   5. Giving advice or approval or disapproval
   6. Providing acknowledgment

5. The nonverbal communication that best expresses emotion is:
   1. Cultural artifacts
   2. Body positioning
   3. Facial expressions
   4. Eye contact

6. During a nurse-patient interaction, which nursing statement may belittle the patient's feelings and concerns?
   1. "Don't worry, everything will be alright."
   2. "You seem really uptight."
   3. "I notice you have been biting your fingernails."
   4. "You are jumping to conclusions."

7. Which of the following techniques are examples of nontherapeutic communication? Select all that apply.
   1. Paraphrasing
   2. Challenging
   3. Asking "what" questions
   4. Asking "why" questions

8. Which of the following factors has documented negative effects on patient outcomes?
   1. Interprofessional conflict
   2. Ineffective communication between health care personnel
   3. Stressful working environment for nurses
   4. All of the above

9. Which of the following methods would you use when communicating with an angry patient: (a) maintain personal space, (b) encourage safe coping behaviors, (c) use therapeutic silence, (d) use touch as a therapeutic technique.
   1. a, b, d
   2. a, c, d
   3. a, b, c
   4. b, c, d

10. The nurse is beginning discharge planning for a patient with left-sided weakness. All of the following actions are important, but which one is the most important to ensure that the discharge plan is successful?
    1. Start the discharge plan on admission
    2. Involve family members in discharge planning
    3. Involve the patient in discharge planning
    4. Involve all members of the health care team

REFERENCES

Churchman J, Doherty C: Nurses' views on challenging doctors' practices in an acute care hospital, *Nurs Stand* 24(40):42, 2010.

Delbanco T, et al: A patient-centered view of the clinician-patient relationship, *UpToDate* 2013. http://www.uptodate.com/contents/a-patient-centered-view-of-the-clinician-patient-relationship.

Dickens C, Piano MR: Health literacy and nursing: an update, *Am J Nurs* 113(6):52, 2013.

Eggertson L: Hospital noise, *Can Nurs* 108(4):29, 2012.

Fernandez R, et al: Interdisciplinary communication in general medical and surgical wards using two different models of nursing care delivery, *J Nurs Manag* 18(3):265, 2010.

Fortinash K, Holoday-Worret P: *Psychiatric-mental health nursing*, ed 5, St Louis, 2012, Mosby.

Giger J: *Transcultural nursing: assessment and intervention*, ed 6, St Louis, 2013, Mosby.

Graham J, et al: Nurses' discharge planning and risk assessment: behaviours, understanding and barriers, *J Clin Nurs* 22(15–16):2338, 2013.

Hockenberry MJ, Wilson D: *Wong's essentials of pediatric nursing*, ed 9, St Louis, 2013, Mosby.

Keltner N, et al: *Psychiatric nursing: a psychotherapeutic management approach*, ed 6, St Louis, 2011, Mosby.

Liu W, et al: Medication communication between nurses and patients during nursing handovers on medical wards: a critical ethnographic study, *Int J Nurs Stud* 49(8):941, 2012.

McGhee J: Effective communication with people who have dementia, *Nurs Stand* 25(25):40, 2011.

Novak K, Fairchild R: Bedside reporting and SBAR: improving patient communication and satisfaction, *J Pediatr Nurs* 27(6):760, 2012.

Ornstein K, et al: To the hospital and back home again: a nurse practitioner-based transitional care program for hospitalized homebound people, *J Am Geriatr Soc* 59(3):544, 2011.

Peikes D, et al: The effects of transitional care models on re-admissions: a review of the current evidence, *J Am Soc Aging* 36(4):44, 2012.

Purnell L: *Transcultural health care: a culturally competent approach*, ed 4, Philadelphia, 2013, FA Davis.

Shoeb M, et al: "Can we just stop and talk?" Patients value verbal communication about discharge care plans, *J Hosp Med* 7(6):504, 2012.

Slatore CG, et al: Communication nurses in the intensive care unit: qualitative analysis of domains of patient-centered care, *Am J Crit Care* 21(6):410, 2012.

Sobolewski S: The challenge of improving transitional care, *Home Healthc Nurse* 29(1):640, 2011.

The Joint Commission (TJC): *National Patient Safety Goals*, Oakbrook Terrace, IL, 2014, The Commission. Available at: http://www.jointcommission.org/standards_information/npsgs.aspx. Accessed March 14, 2014.

Documentation and Informatics

Health care documentation is anything entered in written or electronic format into a patient's medical record. Documentation is an essential component of health care delivery because when it is done correctly and appropriately, it ensures better continuity of care to patients, increases communication among care providers, and improves patient safety (Wharvell and Sheldon, 2013). Although some health care facilities still use printed records, electronic documentation is becoming the desired standard. An electronic record is intended to integrate all relevant patient information into one record that is accessible each time a patient enters a health care system. The design of any documentation system is to maintain health care standards, improve care coordination, and increase efficiencies (HealthIT.gov, 2012). The Joint Commission (TJC) (2014) sets standards for documentation of health care.

Informatics refers to the property and structure of information or data. It is important that nurses know how to record and report data and apply the information for patient care. Nursing informatics is a specialty that integrates nursing science, computer science, and information science to manage and communicate data, information, and knowledge in nursing practice. The application of informatics results in an effective nursing information system that better manages and communicates data to improve patient outcomes (Carrington and Tiase, 2013).

PATIENT-CENTERED CARE

Patient-centered care involves nurses individualizing care delivered to patients and being responsive in meeting patient needs (Warren, 2012). Thorough documentation is central to patient-centered care. A nurse is responsible for documenting detailed information about the care that is provided to patients, including aspects of care that are individualized. When you provide a level of detail, the medical record becomes a valuable resource for all health care providers. Communication among members of the health care team through documentation is essential for accurate and timely delivery of therapies. When you record an entry into a patient record, it must convey information about the patient's status, the specific type of interventions delivered, patient responses to care, and critical information that allows all care providers to deliver an organized and comprehensive plan of care.

SAFETY

A patient's medical record is a legal document that reflects all aspects of the patient's care while in a health care setting. As a result, there are standards that all health care agencies integrate into a documentation system (e.g., allergy entries, fall risk information, IV fluid rates) to ensure that the care delivered represents safe practices.

Information entered into the medical record must be accurate, thorough, and current because all care providers rely on the information to deliver and coordinate patient care. Inaccurate or incomplete documentation or falsification of information can result in medical or nursing therapies that are unnecessary, inappropriate, and delayed, all potentially resulting in negative patient outcomes.

ELECTRONIC HEALTH RECORD

The traditional paper medical record is episode oriented, with a separate record for each patient visit to a health care facility. Key information, such as patient allergies, current medications, and complications from treatment, may be lost from one episode of care to the next. The electronic health record (EHR) is a longitudinal electronic record of patient health information generated by one or more encounters in any care delivery setting (Healthcare Information and Management Systems Society, 2012). It automates and streamlines the care provider's workflow. The EHR has the ability to generate a complete record of a clinical patient encounter and support other care-related activities directly or indirectly via interface, including evidence-based decision support, quality management, and outcomes reporting. For example, if a patient develops hypoglycemia, the blood sugar level entered into the EHR may trigger an automatic alert that informs nurses of the need to follow a treatment protocol. Electronic forms and flow sheets are designed by nursing and other health care providers. Professional nursing standards, regulatory requirements, and evidence-based practice are incorporated into the content of many forms. Designing forms that collect pertinent information ensures improved communication among health care providers and ultimately safer patient care.

You must obtain patient consent before information in the EHR is transferred or shared with another facility. Use precautions to protect the patient's information. Facilities need to develop guidelines and policies to ensure privacy and confidentiality of the information consistent with federal and state regulations such as the Health Insurance Portability and Accountability Act of 1996 (HIPAA).

EVIDENCE-BASED PRACTICE

Nwulu U et al: Adoption of an electronic observation chart with an integrated early warning scoring system on pilot wards: a descriptive report, *Comput Inform Nurs* 30(7):371, 2012.

Sidebottom A et al: Reactions of nurses to the use of electronic health record alert features in an inpatient setting, *Comput Inform Nurs* 30(4):218, 2012.

Documentation system designs challenge nurses to know when and how to enter information correctly and use the information to support nursing decisions. Electronic systems can be organized to alert a nurse about important patient changes. A study by Sidebottom et al. (2012) discussed nurses' reactions to EHR alerts notifying nurses of critical changes in data. Nwulu et al. (2012) examined how electronic documentation systems can be used to monitor vital sign changes through preset alerts. Research suggests alerts in electronic documentation systems can benefit nurses in prioritizing their workflow and support their nursing decisions. However, while nurses reported positive reactions to certain alerts, they also reported occasional distrust of the data included in alerts. Regardless of printed or electronic documentation design, good standards of practice in documentation are essential.

- EHRs can alert nurses about important patient changes.
- Nurses may choose to confirm data in alerts to ensure safe practices
- Pop-ups and dashboards are examples of EHR alerts.
- Nurses should have input into the format and upper and lower limits for EHR alerts.
- When EHR alerts are used in the nurse's practice, patient outcomes can be improved.

CONFIDENTIALITY

Nurses are legally and ethically obligated to keep information about patients confidential. Do not disclose information about a patient's status to other patients, family members (unless the patient grants permission), or health care staff not involved in the patient's care. In 1996, HIPAA, legislation to protect patient privacy for health information, was proposed; HIPAA was finalized in 2003 with specific guidelines for communication of patients' personal health information (U.S. Department of Health and Human Services, 2003). Under HIPAA, patients have access to their medical records, and providers must obtain patient consent before information is released for health-related purposes. HIPAA requires the U.S. Department of Health and Human Services to establish national standards for electronic health care transactions and national identifiers for providers, health plans, and employers. These standards are designed to improve the efficiency and effectiveness of the U.S. health care system by encouraging the widespread use of electronic data interchange in health care. HIPAA also addresses the security and privacy of health data.

Only health care providers directly involved in a specific patient's care have legitimate access to the medical record. Other professionals may use records for data gathering, research, or education only with permission and according to established facility, state, and federal guidelines. Many states require reporting of certain infectious or communicable diseases through the public health department, which must be done through proper channels.

Computerized documentation poses risks to patient confidentiality. Most security mechanisms for information systems use a combination of passwords and physical restrictions such as firewalls and antivirus spyware to protect information. However, there are also guidelines for care providers to use to protect patient information, such as proper use of passwords and ensuring a computer terminal is never left unattended when patient information is still displayed (see Procedural Guideline 3.2). It is important to follow a facility's policy if backup files are accidentally deleted. Confidentiality procedures also should be followed for documenting sensitive patient information.

LEGAL GUIDELINES IN DOCUMENTATION

Accurate documentation is one of the best defenses for legal claims associated with nursing care. To limit nursing liability, documentation must clearly indicate that individualized, goal-directed nursing care was provided to a patient based on a nursing assessment. The record needs to describe exactly what happens to a patient. This is best achieved by charting immediately after providing care to a patient. Although nursing care may have been excellent, in a court of law, "care not documented is care not provided." Know your facility policies for documenting, either in paper format or electronically.

The Nurses Service Organization (a medical malpractice, professional liability, and risk management company) (2013) identified common charting mistakes that may result in malpractice, including failure to record pertinent health information, drug information, nursing interventions, and acuity changes. Another documentation problem, unreadable handwriting, has been reduced with EHRs (Austin, 2011). Although EHRs can minimize documentation problems, the nurse is still responsible to adhere to documentation standards for care delivered.

STANDARDS

Current TJC (2014) standards require that all patients who are admitted to a health care facility have an assessment of physical, psychosocial, environmental, self-care, patient education, and discharge planning needs. Documentation within the context of the nursing process provides structure. The nursing process shapes your approach and direction of care and how you document:

- Record assessments that offer a database from which health care team members can draw conclusions about the patient's health problems.
- Record information about the patient's concerns or condition to assist caregivers in problem identification, planning, and setting priorities.
- Describe care activities in detail to reflect the implementation of the plan of care.
- Evaluate patient responses to nursing care to show the patient's progress in achieving expected outcomes of care.

GUIDELINES FOR QUALITY DOCUMENTATION

Nurses practice in a variety of settings and use various forms and formats to communicate specific information about a patient's health care. The use of standard documentation guidelines ensures more efficient, safe, individualized patient care. Ideally, forms are designed to make data easy to enter, find, and interpret and to avoid unnecessary duplication. For example, most nursing forms have a place for patient identification, date and times, and a key to indicate the meaning of abbreviations or entries used and the type of information required. Because of legal requirements, you must follow facility documentation standards. Regardless of the documentation method, all nurses must follow certain basic guidelines.

Factual

A factual record or report contains descriptive and objective information about what a health care provider sees, hears, feels, or smells. An example of an objective description is "pulse 54 beats/minute, strong, and irregular." Avoid using words such as *good, adequate, fair,* or *poor* that are subject to interpretation. Inferences are conclusions based on factual data. An example of an inference is "The patient has a poor appetite," which would be based on factual data, including the amount of food the patient ate during a meal and his or her fluid intake. For example, "The patient ate only two bites of toast for breakfast, with 180 mL of apple juice." The recording of factual data leads to appropriate inferences from which clinical decisions are made.

The only subjective data included in a record or report is what a patient actually verbalizes. Document subjective information using the patient's words in quotes; for example, "Patient states, 'I feel sick to my stomach'" or "Patient states, 'I do not like the food choices here.'" In both cases, document the actual food intake and the patient's subjective report.

Accurate

The use of exact, precise measurements is a means to make comparisons and determine when a patient's condition has changed. Charting that an "abdominal wound is 5 cm in length, without redness, edema, or discharge" is more accurate than the statement "large abdominal wound is healing well." Accurate charting requires you to use only approved health care facility abbreviations and write out all terms that may be confusing. Correct spelling is essential because terms are easy to misinterpret (e.g., *accept* or *except, dysphagia* or *dysphasia*). The Institute for Safe Medicine Practice (2013) publishes a list of abbreviations, symbols, and words that are prone to misinterpretation.

Records need to reflect your accountability during the time frame that you care for a patient. You must chart your own observations and actions. Your signature holds you accountable for any information recorded. When you report observations to another caregiver and interventions are performed by someone else, that fact must be clearly indicated (e.g., "Surgical drain removed by Dr. Jones. Pulse 110, BP 132/78 reported to J. Kemp, RN"). Each written entry must end with your first name or first initial, last name, and title. Electronic entries document your name and title. Nursing students sign off using the approved abbreviation for the school and the program level on any signature.

Complete

The information within a recorded entry must be complete, containing appropriate and essential information. There are criteria for thorough communication for certain health situations. For example, when recording discharge planning, measurable patient goals or expected outcomes, progress toward goals, and need for referrals are always included. When documenting patient behavior, onset, behaviors exhibited, and precipitating factors are included. The following is an example of what may occur when a note has not been recorded completely.

A nurse explains and demonstrates a teaching session about giving insulin injections. The patient eagerly expresses a desire to give the next injection when it is due. Documentation is as follows: "Discussed learning about insulin injection technique." During the next shift, another nurse spends time demonstrating the injection technique and assessing the patient's readiness to give the injection because the previous teaching was not completely communicated. As a result, time is wasted repeating information that the patient learned previously instead of coaching the patient through a self-injection.

Another example of following criteria for complete documentation involves hourly rounding. Recently many hospitals have adopted intentional hourly rounding to decrease patient falls and improve patient satisfaction (Olrich, Kalman, and Nigolian, 2012). Documentation of a patient visit during rounding includes the 4 Ps of care: pain, position, possession, and potty (Institute for Healthcare Improvements, 2012) (Box 3-1).

Concise

Concise documentation facilitates efficient retrieval of pertinent information. EHRs reduce narrative writing and improve accuracy (Kutney-Lee and Kelly, 2011). When you learn to write concisely, less time is needed for documentation. A comparison of a concise and lengthy note follows.

Concise, Factual Entry	Lengthy Entry Using Vague Terms
1900 Left toes cool and pale, without inflammation, capillary return >5 sec; left pedal pulse 1+; right pedal pulse 4+. Patient responds to tactile stimulation and is able to wiggle toes on left foot. Describes pain in left foot as dull, aching 5 (scale 0-10).	1900 The patient's left toes are cool, with pale color. There is no inflammation. There is slow capillary return present greater than 5 seconds. Dorsalis pedis pulse in left foot is weak, and the patient complains of some discomfort. The pain in left foot is described as throbbing without any relief.

Current

Making timely entries in a patient's record avoids omissions and delays in patient care. Many health care facilities keep records and computers near the patient's bedside to facilitate immediate documentation of care activities. Document the following activities or findings at the time of occurrence:

- Acute change in medical condition
- Pain assessment

<table>
<tr><td colspan="2">BOX 3-1   DOCUMENTING THE FOUR Ps OF CARE</td></tr>
<tr><td>Focus of Care</td><td>Documentation</td></tr>
<tr><td>Pain</td><td>Level of pain using a pain scale of 0 to 10. Include interventions to reduce pain.</td></tr>
<tr><td>Position</td><td>Change in the patient's position and interventions to improve comfort.</td></tr>
<tr><td>Possessions</td><td>Possessions are within reach. Include call light, bedside table, and adaptive devices (e.g., eyeglasses).</td></tr>
<tr><td>Potty</td><td>Assistance to use the toilet or bedpan. Record output.</td></tr>
</table>

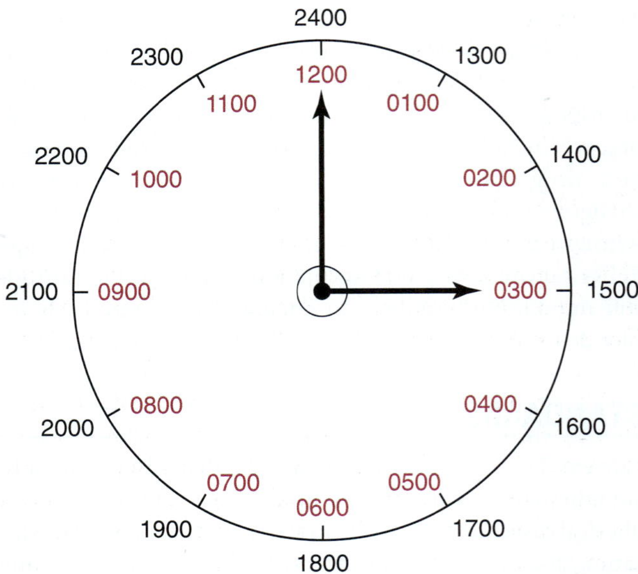

FIG 3-1 Comparison of military time and standard time.

- Administration of medications and treatments
- Preparation for diagnostic tests or surgery
- Change in patient status and who was notified
- Patient response to an intervention
- Admission, transfer, discharge, or death of a patient

Writing notes on a work pad at the time of an event helps to ensure accuracy when you later complete your formal documentation. Often nurses on a care unit design worksheets that incorporate their standards of care.

Many facilities use military time, a 24-hour time system, to avoid misinterpretation of AM and PM times. The military clock ends with midnight at 2400 and begins at l minute after midnight at 0001. The following examples compare standard with military time: 10:22 AM is 1022 military time; 3:15 PM is 1515 military time (Fig. 3-1).

Organized

Organized notes are written in a logical order. For example, an organized note follows the nursing process to describe the assessment, interventions, and patient's response in a sequence. Communication is also more effective when it is organized. When making a record entry, make a list of what to include before beginning to write in the permanent legal record. Identifying relevant content is helpful in deleting unnecessary words. The following compares a well-organized note with a disorganized note:

Organized Note	Disorganized Note
7/17 0630 Patient reports sharp pain 9 (scale 0-10) in left lower quadrant of abdomen, worsened by turning onto right side. Positioning on left side decreases pain to 8 (scale 0-10). Abdomen is tender to touch and rigid. Bowel sounds absent in all 4 quadrants. Dr. Phillips notified. To x-ray for CT scan of abdomen. T. Reis, RN	7/17 0630 Patient experiencing sharp pain in lower quadrant of abdomen. MD notified. Abdomen tender to touch, rigid, with bowel sounds absent. Positioning on left side offers minimal relief of pain. CT scan ordered of the abdomen. J. Adams, RN

Methods of Recording

The method of recording selected by a nursing administration often reflects the philosophy of the department. Staffs use the same method of recording throughout a facility. There are several acceptable methods for recording health care data.

The problem-oriented medical record (POMR) is a structured method of documentation that emphasizes and organizes data by a patient's problems or diagnoses. Any notes about a patient's care are organized using the nursing process. Ideally, each member of the health care team contributes to a single list of identified patient problems. Each recording includes a database, problem list, care plan, and progress notes.

A source record is a way to organize chart information by each discipline instead of by patient problems. The advantage of a source record is that caregivers can easily locate the section of the chart to make entries. Members of each discipline can go to sections such as nurse's notes, physician or health care provider's notes, or laboratory results. A

disadvantage of the source record is fragmented data. Source records are becoming less common.

Charting by exception (CBE) is a method of recording that eliminates redundancy and makes documentation of routine care more concise. The emphasis is on recording abnormal findings and trends in clinical care. It is a shorthand method for documenting based on defined standards for normal nursing assessments and interventions. CBE simply involves completing a flow sheet that incorporates these standards, minimizing the need for lengthy narrative notes. However, the CBE system can be used inappropriately when nurses fail to enter notes that describe abnormal findings or unexpected changes in a patient's condition.

Structured communication using the SBAR approach is a popular technique that provides a framework for communication among members of the health care team. The SBAR approach offers an easy to remember mechanism that you can use to frame conversations, especially critical ones that require a clinician's immediate attention and action. SBAR is a mnemonic for the following:

S: Situation (state what is happening at the present time)

> **Example:** Dr. Sullivan, this is Ed Cashmere, RN on 7200. I am assigned to Mrs. Denise Thomas and she is having a drop in her blood pressure

B: Background (explain the circumstances leading up to the situation)

> **Example:** Mrs. Thomas is 1 day postop and her BP before surgery was 132-144/80. She had a colectomy performed. She is receiving IV fluids of D5½ NS at 80 mL/hr.

A: Assessment (what you think the problem is)

> **Example:** Her BP was 120/78 at 5 AM, now at 6 AM it is 100/60. She is also more restless than before. Her heart rate is 90 and regular. I am concerned she might be bleeding. There is no increase in drainage from her wound.

R: Recommendation (what you would do to correct the problem)

> **Example:** I would like to increase her IV rate and ask that you come take a look at her.

SBAR promotes the provision of safe, efficient, timely, and patient-centered communication (Wentworth et al., 2012).

PROCEDURAL GUIDELINE 3.1
Documenting Nurses' Progress Notes

Nurses practice in a variety of settings and use various forms and formats to communicate information about a patient's health care. Ideally, forms are designed to make data easy to find and interpret and reduce duplication. Medical record forms that nurses traditionally have used for documentation include nursing admission history, physical assessment and vital signs graphic, medication administration records, nurses' notes, and nursing care flow sheets

(Box 3-2). Many facilities have various worksheets that are useful for routine patient care and are not a permanent part of the record.

Progress notes are a format for documenting a record of a patient's progress. Various formats for progress notes, including SOAP (*Subjective* data, *Objective* data, *Assessment* or *Analysis*, and *Plan*), SOAPE (SOAP plus *Evaluation*), PIE (*Problem*, *Intervention*, and *Evaluation*), APIE

Continued

(*Assessment*, *Plan*, *Intervention*, and *Evaluation*), and DAR (*Data*, *Action*, and patient *Response*), are used in focus charting. Any caregiver needs to be able to read a progress note and understand what type of problem a patient has, the level of care provided, and the results of the interventions. The nurse who is responsible for providing care to the patient signs each entry.

Delegation and Collaboration

The skill of documenting nurse progress notes can be delegated to nursing assistive personnel (NAP) (see facility policy). The nurse instructs the NAP about:

- What care activities to document on flow sheets, such as intake and output.
- What information to report to the nurse (e.g., increased pain) so he or she can reassess.

Equipment

- Patient care profile
- Progress note form (written or electronic)

Procedural Steps

1. Review assessment data, problems identified (nursing diagnoses), goals and expected outcomes, interventions, and patient responses during contact with each patient before documentation.
2. After each patient contact, identify information that needs to be documented to ensure quality, accuracy, timeliness, and continuity of information. Consider abnormal findings, changes in patient's status, and new problem identification.
3. Obtain necessary forms or access appropriate computer screens for documentation.
4. Record date and time for each entry, and do not leave open spaces between notes.
5. Use facility format and document in chronological order the following:
   a. Pertinent, factual objective data
   b. Selected subjective data that validate and clarify
   c. Nursing actions taken
   d. Evaluation of patient responses to nursing actions
   e. Any additional nursing actions
   f. To whom information has been reported, including name and status
6. Make progress note entries:
   a. **SOAP format**: *Subjective data*, *Objective data*, *Assessment* or *Analysis*, and *Plan*. Usually based on a numbered list of problems or nursing diagnoses such as "Anxiety related to preparation for surgery":
      S: *Subjective data*—The patient's statements regarding the problem (e.g., Patient stated, "I am dreading this surgery because last time I had a terrible reaction to the anesthesia and such terrible pain.")

O: *Objective data*—Observations that support or are related to subjective data (e.g., frequent turning in bed and loud, agitated voice)

A: *Assessment/Analysis*—Conclusions reached based on data (e.g., fear related to pain/anesthesia)

P: *Plan*—The plan for dealing with the situation (e.g., "Notified anesthesiologist, Dr. Moore, of patient's experience. Discussed with patient alternatives for anesthesia and pain-control options. Stressed importance of activity for circulation and healing. Encouraged patient to keep nurses informed of pain level and need for medication and told patient that pain usually is present but manageable.")

   b. **PIE format**: *Problem*, *Intervention*, and *Evaluation*. Problem-oriented system in which progress notes are written based on a list of numbered or labeled patient problems, such as "Anxiety related to preparation for surgery":
      P: *Problem*—Preoperative anxiety (e.g., Patient stated, "I am dreading this surgery because last time I had a terrible reaction to the anesthesia and such terrible pain when they made me get out of bed."). Observed frequent turning in bed and loud, agitated voice.
      I: *Intervention*—Notified anesthesiologist, Dr. Moore, of patient's experience. Discussed with patient alternatives for anesthesia and pain-control options. Stressed importance of activity for circulation and healing. Told patient to keep nurses informed of pain level and need for medication. Told patient that pain usually is present but manageable.
      E: *Evaluation*—Patient stated that she was "very relieved." Stated she would tell the nurses about pain.

   c. **DAR format**: *Data*, *Action*, and patient *Response*. Used in focus charting; a way to organize progress notes to make them clearer and more organized:
      D: *Data*—Patient states, "I am dreading this surgery because last time I had a terrible reaction to the anesthesia and such terrible pain when they made me get out of bed." Observed frequent turning in bed and loud, agitated voice.
      A: *Action*—Notified anesthesiologist, Dr. Moore, of patient's experience. Discussed alternatives for anesthesia and pain-control options. Stressed importance of activity for circulation and healing. Encouraged patient to keep nurses informed of pain level and need for medication and told patient that pain usually is present but manageable.
      R: *Response*—Patient stated that she was "very relieved." Stated she would tell the nurses about pain.

PROCEDURAL GUIDELINE 3.1
Documenting Nurses' Progress Notes—cont'd

d. Basic narrative note format. Usually not based on a problem list but commonly used when an exception to care occurs, requiring a detailed note:

Patient states, "I am dreading this surgery because last time I had a terrible reaction to the anesthesia and such terrible pain when they made me get out of bed." Observed frequent turning in bed and loud, agitated voice. Notified anesthesiologist, Dr. Moore, of patient's experience. Discussed with patient alternatives for anesthesia and pain-control options. Stressed importance of activity for circulation and healing. Encouraged patient to keep nurses informed of pain level and need for medication and told patient that pain usually is present but manageable. Patient stated, "I feel very relieved after talking with you" and agreed to let nurses know when pain increases.

e. CBE: Charting by Exception system. A progress note describes deviations from the patient's normal assessment findings; nurse uses standardized flow sheets and assessment forms to document normal findings. An exception note is a narrative that describes differences to the norm:

"Patient reports sharp pain in right great toe, rated as a 10 on pain scale of 0 to 10. States the pain began 30 minutes ago. Right great toe is red, warm to touch. Pedal pulses are +3. Unable to assess capillary refill of right great toe because of patient's complaint of pain in toe."

7. Sign progress note with full name or first initial and last name and status according to facility policy. Students are usually required to indicate their level of education and school affiliation.

8. Review previously documented entries with those that you enter, noting if there is significant change in the patient's status. Report any changes to the patient's health care provider.

BOX 3-2   NURSING DOCUMENTATION FORMS AND WORKSHEETS

Nursing History Forms
Complete an assessment for each patient at the time of admission to a health care facility. The history includes basic biographical data (e.g., age, method of admission, health care provider), admitting medical diagnosis or chief complaint, and a brief medical-surgical history (e.g., previous surgeries or illnesses, allergies, medication history, patient's perceptions about illness or hospitalization, physical assessment of all body systems). The nursing history form provides for a systematic and complete patient assessment and the identification of relevant nursing diagnoses. The nursing history provides baseline data to compare with changes in the patient's condition throughout the hospitalization.

Graphic Sheets and Flow Sheets
Forms include routine observations made on a repeated basis using a check mark (e.g., when bath is given, patient is turned) or by entering data (e.g., vital signs and input and output). When completing a flow sheet, review previous entries to identify changes.

Computerized Patient Care Summary
Includes pertinent information about patients and their ongoing care plans, such as basic demographic data (e.g., age, religion), health care provider's name, primary medical diagnosis, current health care provider's orders, nursing orders or interventions, scheduled tests or procedures, safety precautions to use in a patient's care, and factors related to activities of daily living (ADLs).

Nursing Kardex (Worksheet)
The Kardex includes information needed for daily care on a flip card or in a notebook and is usually kept at the nurses' station. Information can be used for change-of-shift report and facilitates access to information without referring to the patient record. The worksheet includes demographic data, tests ordered, therapies, and information related to ADLs. It may include standardized or individualized nursing care plans.

PROCEDURAL GUIDELINE 3.2
Use of Electronic Health Records

EHRs organize data in a standardized format, with screens designed for easy access. The presence of computerized health records in patient rooms allow health care team members to document patient care assessments and interventions immediately and track the patient's progress. Policies and procedures to ensure confidentiality of the patient's information must be maintained at all times.

Delegation and Collaboration

Authorized members of the health care team have access to all parts of the patient's EHR. The skill of charting patient information may be delegated to nursing assistive personnel (NAP) for certain aspects of care, such as vital signs, intake and output, or other content areas as defined by the facility.

Continued

PROCEDURAL GUIDELINE 3.2
Use of Electronic Health Records—cont'd

Equipment

- Computer
- EHR

Procedural Steps

1. Sign on to the EHR using only your user identification and password.
2. Never share passwords, and keep your password private.
3. Do not leave patient information on the monitor where others can view it.
4. Review assessment data, problems identified (nursing diagnoses), goals and expected outcomes, and interventions and patient responses during contact with each patient before data entry.
5. Follow procedures for entering information in all appropriate program functions.
6. Review previously documented entries with those you enter, noting if there is significant change in the patient's status. Report changes to the patient's health care provider.
7. Know and implement procedures to correct documentation errors.
8. Save information as documentation is completed.
9. Sign off when you leave the computer.

PROCEDURAL GUIDELINE 3.3
Documenting an Incident Occurrence

Health care errors do occur. There is no national reporting of such occurrences, but individual health care facilities have their staff complete occurrence reports when deviations in standards of care and adverse events occur. The National Quality Forum (2013) identified a standardized list of preventable, serious adverse events that facilitate the reporting of such events (Box 3-3). An incident or occurrence report is a risk management tool that enables health care providers to identify risks within a facility, analyze them, act to reduce the risks, and evaluate the results. The incident report is completed by any member of the health care or hospital staff when a patient experiences an adverse event while in the hospital. The incident report alerts hospital administration of the event and provides an opportunity to monitor trends and patterns in care and identify ways to improve existing care.

Delegation and Collaboration

The nurse instructs nursing assistive personnel (NAP) to report any incident in which they are involved and complete the document in a timely manner (see policy). An incident report should be completed by the person (or persons) who was involved or witnessed the event.

Equipment

- An incident or occurrence report form or screen
- Black pen for paper report or computer for electronic report

Procedural Steps

1. When you witness an adverse event or find a patient who has just experienced an adverse event, assess the patient's condition and observe the environmental setting.
2. Protect the patient from further injury by calling for assistance immediately or taking action to create a safe environment (e.g., if patient is having an allergic reaction to blood, stop infusion and instill normal saline intravenously; if patient has fallen, call for assistance and ensure that patient is in safe alignment).
3. Take action to be sure the patient is stable.
4. Obtain facility reporting form.
5. Objectively and accurately document what you observed or heard related to the incident.
6. If someone witnessed the event with you, record their information. Identify them as the source of information.
7. Record details of event in chronological order.
8. When a patient is involved, document events in the medical record. However, do not document in the medical record "incident report filed." The incident report is a facility report and not part of the medical record. Document instead your assessment findings of the patient's condition.
9. File the report properly with the risk management department or designated person.

BOX 3-3 EXAMPLES OF SERIOUS REPORTABLE EVENTS OCCURRING WITHIN A HEALTH CARE FACILITY

According to the National Quality Forum (2013), serious reportable events include:

- Surgical procedure or invasive procedure performed on the wrong site or wrong patient
- Patient death or serious injury associated with the nonapproved use of a device or equipment
- Unintended foreign object remained in a patient after surgery or an invasive procedure
- Patient death or serious injury associated with an elopement (unplanned discharge)
- Patient death or serious injury associated with a medication error
- Patient death or serious injury associated with a fall
- Patient death or serious injury associated with unsafe administration of blood products
- Stage 3, stage 4, or unstageable pressure ulcer that occurred after admission to a health care facility
- Patient death or injury associated with physical restraints

CRITICAL THINKING EXERCISES

Case Study

The nurse and NAP are caring for a group of patients on a medical-surgical unit. During the shift, one patient is discharged to a skilled nursing facility, and another patient is sent to surgery. Elements of care for the discharge patient include a physical assessment and discharge teaching. Elements of care for the surgical patient include monitoring vital signs every 2 hours, preoperative teaching, and securing the patient's personal possessions.

1. While the NAP and nurse move the surgical patient from the bed to the stretcher, the patient falls and sustains a hip fracture. Where should the nurse document the patient's fall? Select all that apply.
   1. Medical record
   2. Incident or occurrence report
   3. Personal notes of the nurse
   4. Medication administration record
   5. Discharge teaching record
2. Before sending a patient to the operating room, the nurse notifies the surgeon of the patient's blood pressure of 88/52 mm Hg and a temperature of 38.5° C. The nurse communicates directly to the surgeon using which of the following approaches?
   1. SOAP
   2. PIE
   3. DAR
   4. SBAR
3. Which element of care can a nurse delegate to NAP?
   1. Assessment of the patient who is discharged
   2. Preoperative teaching about surgery
   3. Vital signs when the patient is stable
   4. Evaluation of the patient's response to teaching

Review Questions

1. A nurse manager reviews the nurses' notes in a patient's medical record and finds the following entry, "Patient is uncooperative and refuses to go to therapy." Which of the following directions should the manager give to the staff nurse who entered the note?
   1. Identify which therapy was missed.
   2. Write only your full name in the note with black pen.
   3. Enter only objective and factual information about the patient.
   4. Remove the note from the medical record by eliminating the page.
2. The nurse observes the patient crying in the room and asks the patient what is wrong. The patient states, "I am so scared I will not be able to inject myself. What do you think I should do?" How does the nurse document this interaction with the patient?
   1. "Patient observed to be tearful and confused."
   2. "The patient needs to contact the physician and discuss other medications."
   3. "The patient is upset and does not want to learn how to self-inject."
   4. "The patient stated, 'I am so scared I will not be able to inject myself.'"
3. The nurse is caring for a patient over a 12-hour shift. She conducts her routine assessment at the beginning of the shift and assists the patient to bathe. The nurse administers medications at 0800 and at 1200. At 1300, the patient reports abdominal pain at a level of 7 on a pain scale of 0 to 10 and receives pain medication. At 1330, the dietitian visits the patient to review food preferences. Which of the activities performed by the nurse should be recorded immediately? Select all that apply.
   1. Visit by the dietitian
   2. Medication administration
   3. Assistance in bathing
   4. Food preferences
   5. Pain assessment

4. Charting by exception is a method of recording that:
   1. Includes a factual narrative of all care provided
   2. Streamlines documentation using the acronym DAR
   3. Aims to reduce redundancy and document routine care concisely
   4. Is primarily used to describe psychosocial data
5. The nurse maintains confidentiality of patient data when using an EHR by:
   1. Sharing his or her password with the nurse manager
   2. Logging into the EHR every 4th hour
   3. Not leaving patient data in public view
   4. Disposing of worksheets in trash cans
6. Which of the following are guidelines for quality documentation?
   1. Use descriptive and objective data to describe findings
   2. Include terms such as good and fair to describe ambulation
   3. Use common abbreviations such as *u* or *cc* to minimize space
   4. Include your opinion of how the incident could have been prevented
7. Under HIPAA and quality standards, the nurse must:
   1. Provide the family access to the medical record
   2. Allow NAP to access all medical records in the facility
   3. Protect information by maintaining confidentiality of patient data
   4. Refuse patients access to their personal data while hospitalized

8. A patient was ambulated in the hall at 8:45 PM. What time would it be if documented according to military time?
   1. 0845
   2. 1845
   3. 2045
   4. 1945
9. Which of the following is the correct sequencing of information entered into nurses' progress notes?
   1. Objective, subjective, assessment, and plan
   2. Plan, intervention, assessment, and evaluation
   3. Data, action, and patient response
   4. Problem, evaluation, and intervention
10. After receiving a prn medication for anxiety, a patient's blood pressure decreases from 130/90 to 90/60 mm Hg. What documentation statement best reflects the situation?
    1. "Patient reacts badly to the antianxiety medication; monitoring for safety."
    2. "Assessment of vital signs; monitoring for further changes. Will notify house physician if no improvement"
    3. "No complaints from patient; blood pressure is stable, and patient instructed to lie down."
    4. 0830 Lorazepam 2 mg PO administered. 0915 patient states "I feel dizzy, like I am going to faint. BP 90/60 mm Hg, pulse 110 beats/min and regular.

REFERENCES

Austin S: Stay out of court with proper documentation, *Nursing* 41(4):24, quiz 29, 2011.

Carrington J, Tiase V: Nursing informatics year in review, *Nurs Admin Q* 37(2):136, 2013.

Healthcare Information and Management Systems Society: Electronic health record, 2012, http://www.himss.org/library/ehr/?navItemNumber=13261. Accessed April 22, 2014.

HealthIT.gov: Learn EHR basics, 2012, http://www.healthit.gov/providers-professionals/learn-ehr-basics. Accessed April 22, 2014.

Institute for Healthcare Improvements: Falls prevention, 2012, http://www.ihi.org/offerings/MembershipsNetworks/MentorHospitalRegistry/Pages/FallsPrevention.aspx. Accessed July 19, 2013.

Institute for Safe Medicine Practice: ISMP's list of error-prone abbreviations, symbols, and dose designations, 2013, https://www.ismp.org/tools/errorproneabbreviations.pdf. Accessed April 24, 2014.

Kutney-Lee A, Kelly D: The effect of hospital electronic health record adoption on nurse-assessed quality of care and patient safety, *J Nurs Adm* 41(11):470, 2011.

National Quality Forum: List of SRES, 2013, http://www.qualityforum.org/Topics/SREs/List_of_SREs.aspx. Accessed November 7, 2013.

Nurses Service Organization: 8 Common charting mistakes to avoid, 2013, http://www.nso.com/nursing-resources/article/16.jsp. Accessed April 22, 2014.

Olrich T, Kalman M, Nigolian C: Hourly rounding: a replication study, *Medsurg Nurs* 21(1):25, 2012.

The Joint Commission: *2014 Comprehensive accreditation manual for hospitals: the official handbook*, Oakbrook Terrace, IL, 2014, The Commission.

U.S. Department of Health and Human Services: Standards for privacy of individually identifiable health information, Health Insurance Portability and Accountability Act of 1996, *Fed Reg* 64:60053, 1999, revised 2003, http://www.hhs.gov/ocr/privacy/hipaa/administrative/privacyrule/index.html. Accessed June 18, 2013.

Warren N: Involving patient and family advisors in the patient and family-centered care model, *Medsurg Nurs* 21(4):233, 2012.

Wentworth L, et al: SBAR: electronic handoff tool for noncomplicated procedural patients, *J Nurs Care Qual* 27(2):125, 2012.

Wharvell T, Sheldon J: Record keeping: an accurate reflection of support provided, *Nursing & Residential Care* 15(2):105, 2013.

Patient Safety and Quality Improvement

http://evolve.elsevier.com/Perry/nursinginterventions
Audio Glossary • Checklists • Review Questions

Safety and quality care are the two priorities of all health care facilities. The Institute for Healthcare Improvement (2014a) defines safety as freedom from accidental injury. Innovative health care facilities are making important breakthroughs in the design and performance of safer systems by standardizing approaches and incorporating current evidence into practices. The Institute of Medicine (2013) defines quality as "The degree to which health services for individuals and populations increase the likelihood of desired health outcomes and are consistent with current professional knowledge."

Patient safety is defined as the prevention of physical and psychological harm to patients. Patient safety requires effective communication, teamwork, critical thinking, and timely clinical decisions. Communication failures have been the number one root cause of all sentinel events reported to The Joint Commission (TJC) (Rossi, 2009). TJC annually lists National Patient Safety Goals to reduce risks for medical errors and the potentially serious consequences known as sentinel events (TJC, 2014). This list changes each year to focus on the most challenging problems (Box 4-1).

The National Quality Forum (NQF) and the Centers for Medicaid and Medicare Services (CMS) develop and monitor key health care safety initiatives and provide information to health care facilities and the public to promote patient safety. The NQF (2013) published "Safe Practices for Better Healthcare—2/2013 Update," which includes 34 safe practices that have been demonstrated to be effective in reducing the occurrence of adverse events. Another approach that facilities are adopting to improve safe practices is the incorporation of care bundles. A care bundle is a structured way of improving care processes and patient outcomes (Institute for Healthcare Improvement, 2014b). A bundle is a limited set (usually three to five) of evidence-based practices that, when performed collectively and reliably, have been shown to improve patient outcomes. Examples of care bundles include central intravenous (IV) line care (see Chapter 27) and ventilator care.

Health care facilities foster a patient-centered safety culture by continually focusing on performance-improvement efforts and risk-management findings and safety reports. For example, the ongoing monitoring of the occurrence of falls within a health care facility allows health care providers to identify problem trends and adopt quality/performance improvement processes to change practices aimed at improving patient outcomes (see Chapter 1). Through quality/performance improvement efforts, clinicians integrate evidence-based practices, design safer work environments, adopt current reliable technology, and educate staff on safety issues.

As part of the health care team, a professional nurse is responsible to engage in all activities that support a patient-centered safety culture. Patient-centered is defined as recognizing the patient as the source of control and full partner in providing compassionate and coordinated care based on

---

BOX 4-1   THE JOINT COMMISSION 2014: HOSPITAL NATIONAL PATIENT SAFETY GOALS

- Identify patients correctly
  - Use at least two ways to identify patients
  - Make sure the correct patient gets the correct blood when receiving a blood transfusion
- Improve staff communication
  - Get important test results to the right staff person on time
- Use medicines safely
  - Before a procedure, label medicines that are not labeled. Do this in the area where medicines and supplies are set up.
  - Take extra care with patients who take medicines to thin their blood.
  - Record and pass along correct information about a patient's medicines. Find out what medicines a patient is taking. Compare those medicines with new medicines given to the patient. Make sure the patient knows which medicines to take when at home. Tell the patient it is important to bring an up-to-date list of medicines every time the patient visits a physician.
- Prevent infection
  - Use the hand cleaning guidelines from the Centers for Disease Control and Prevention
  - Use proven guidelines to prevent infections that are difficult to treat
  - Use proven guidelines to prevent infection of the blood from central lines
  - Use proven guidelines to prevent infection after surgery
  - Use proven guidelines to prevent urinary tract infections from catheters
- Prevent mistakes in surgery
  - Make sure the correct surgery is done on the correct patient and at the correct place on the patient's body
  - Mark the correct place on the patient's body where the surgery is to be done
  - Pause before the surgery to make sure that a mistake is not being made.

---

respect for the patient's preferences, values, and needs (QSEN, 2011). There is an emphasis on improving the education of student nurses so that they become more competent in promoting safe health care practices. The QSEN project meets the challenge of preparing future nurses who will have the knowledge, skills, and attitudes needed to improve continuously the quality and safety of the health care facilities within which they work (QSEN, 2011). The QSEN safety competency is stated as "Minimizes risk of harm to patients and providers through both system effectiveness and individual performance." The QSEN skills for safety competency include the following:

- Demonstrate effective use of technology and standardized practices that support quality and safety.
- Demonstrate effective use of strategies to reduce risk of harm to self or others.
- Use appropriate strategies to reduce reliance on memory.

- Communicate observations or concerns related to hazards and errors to patients, families, and the health care team.

Be responsible for incorporating critical thinking skills when using the nursing process. Assess each patient and his or her environment for hazards that threaten safety, and plan and intervene appropriately to maintain a safe environment.

A sentinel event is an unexpected occurrence involving death, serious physical or psychological injury, or risk thereof (TJC, 2013b). These events include any process variation (e.g., medication administration, restraint application) for which a recurrence would carry a significant chance of a serious adverse outcome. They are "sentinel" because they signal the need for immediate investigation and response.

When a sentinel event involving a patient occurs, most facilities initiate a root cause analysis (RCA). The Joint Commission has policies and procedures to report and investigate sentinel events (TJC, 2013a). An RCA is a process of responding to sentinel events with the purpose of discovering the causes of the event and developing an effective plan for preventing future events. TJC (2014) requires an RCA of a sentinel event with a resultant action plan. The RCA needs to be thorough and credible. The RCA is not about placing blame or relieving accountability; it is about looking at all the details that may have contributed to an error. Most facilities have a dedicated safety department that includes a specially trained team to lead all RCAs. The people closest to the error and people close to any system processes that may have contributed to the error must participate. This participation enables the RCA to lead to genuine practice improvement and the prevention of similar events in the future. Refer to facility policy for the RCA process in your facility.

PATIENT-CENTERED CARE

Being hospitalized puts patients at risk for injury partly as a result of unfamiliar environments. Normal life cues, such as a bed without side rails and the direction one usually takes to the bathroom, are absent. Thought processes and coping mechanisms are affected by illness and its accompanying emotions. Patients are more vulnerable to injury. For patients of diverse backgrounds, this vulnerability may be intensified. It is a nurse's responsibility to provide diligent protection of all patients regardless of their socioeconomic status; racial or ethnic group; religion; gender; age; mental health; cognitive, sensory, or physical disability; or sexual orientation or gender identity.

Most untoward events are related to failures of communication. Health care providers must be attentive to communication during assessment. Nurses must use approaches that recognize patients' cultural backgrounds so that appropriate questions can be raised to reveal health behaviors and risks clearly. You enhance a patient's safety by considering the patient in light of the whole person and seeing each care situation through "the patient's eyes" and not just your own perspective. Review the following examples of patient-centered safety guidelines:

- Although a physical restraint is used rarely, when one is needed, clarify the purpose and the monitoring that will occur to the patient and the patient's family caregiver. Listen to their concerns. For example, many families view restraining of older adults as disrespectful.
- When restraints are used, collaborate with family caregivers in accommodating a patient's cultural perspectives. When it is time to remove a restraint, have a family member present to show respect and caring for the patient. (Note: Do not rely on the family member to protect a patient from injury.)
- When seizure precautions are necessary, explain and demonstrate the therapeutic regimen to the patient and family caregiver. Some cultures show different caring practices for people who are having seizures.

SAFETY

All health care facilities strive to achieve a culture of safety among their employees. It is a challenge to minimize adverse events while carrying out complex and hazardous work. The Agency for Healthcare Research and Quality (2012) has outlined key features for a culture of safety:

- Acknowledgment of the high-risk nature of a facility's activities and the determination to achieve consistently safe operations
- A blame-free environment where individuals are able to report errors or near misses without fear of reprimand or punishment
- Encouragement of collaboration across ranks and disciplines to seek solutions to patient safety problems
- Organizational commitment of resources to address safety concerns

Safety begins with proper patient identification. TJC has clear guidelines for using at least two identifiers (e.g., patient name, date of birth, an assigned identifier such as a hospital number) to confirm a patient's identity before administering any medications or treatment and to match the treatment or service to that individual (TJC, 2014). A patient's room number is not an acceptable identifier. For patients with armbands, it is acceptable to use the patient name and ID number on the armband and to compare it with a treatment order in the medical record or medication administration record.

A patient's immediate environment poses many safety hazards. Nurses are responsible for making bedside areas safe for patients. Fig. 4-1 shows environmental interventions for patient safety. The call light/bed control system allows patients to adjust the position of their bed and to signal caregivers when they need assistance. Explain to patients and visiting family members how to operate a call system correctly. A full set of side rails (two or four to a bed) is a physical restraint. Raising only one of two, or three of four, side rails gives patients room to exit a bed safely and move around within the bed. It is also important to keep a bed in low position with wheels locked when stationary. *Always check* a bed for structural risks (e.g., wobbly or damaged rails or soft mattresses). Electronic bed and chair alarms are available to warn a nurse when a patient who needs assistance tries to leave a bed or chair on his or her own. One example of an alarm is pressure-sensitive strips placed beneath a patient on a bed or

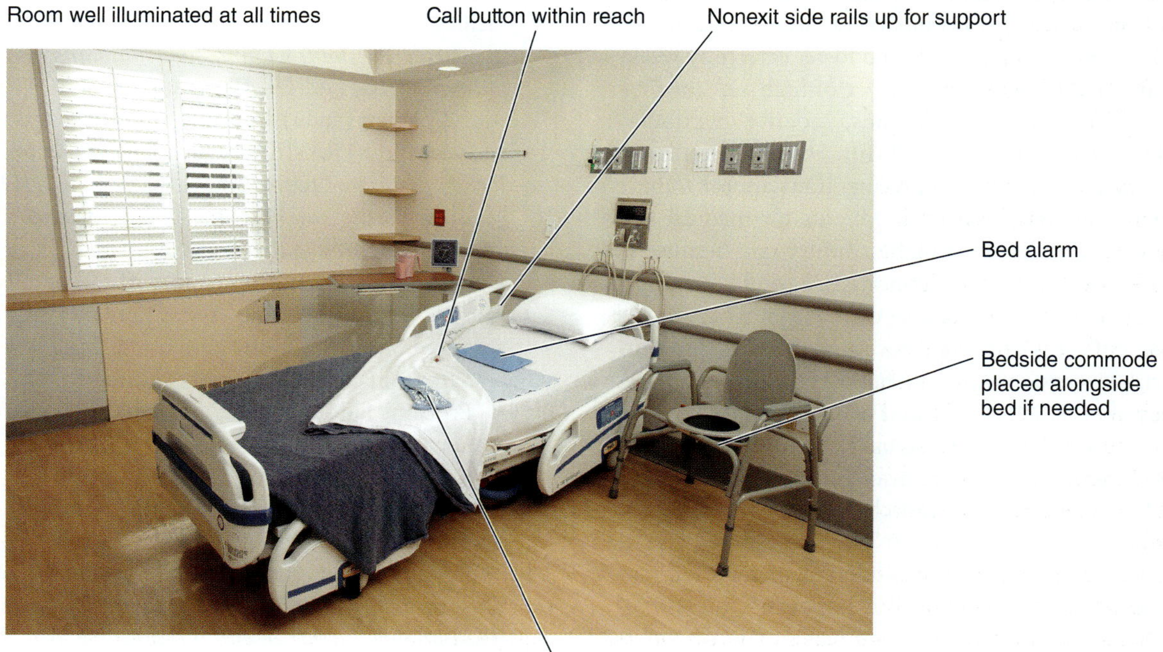

FIG 4-1 Safe patient room environment with bed in low position, bed alarm activated, nonskid footwear (or mat) and call light available, and bedside commode positioned alongside bed.

chair. Additional devices to use at a patient's bedside are a bedside commode, a nonskid floor mat, and an overhead trapeze. Always be alert to conditions within a patient's environment that pose risk for falls and injury (e.g., hazards along walking paths, liquid spilled on floors, poorly functioning equipment).

Strategies for patient safety include encouraging patients to be active participants in their care by making decisions about their treatment and improving communication between caregivers and patients (TJC, 2012a). TJC requires hospitals to have a process for patients and their families to report concerns about safety, such as caregivers not washing their hands. A health care facility must support a "culture of safety" in which a safety concern can be voiced by anyone without fear. For example, if a patient observes a health care provider not washing hands before a dressing change, the patient should be encouraged to point out such omissions. The same applies to health care staff when they witness a colleague not performing hand hygiene.

EVIDENCE-BASED PRACTICE

Hempel S et al: Hospital fall prevention: a systematic review of implementation, components, adherence, and effectiveness, *J Am Geriatr Soc* 61(4):483, 2013.

Krumholz HM: Post-hospital syndrome—an acquired, transient condition of generalized risk, *N Engl J Med* 368(2):100, 2013.

The use of current evidence in practice is essential for achieving safety and quality initiatives. Fall prevention is an ongoing challenge within health care facilities because of the multiple factors that contribute to patient falls (e.g., a patient's disease; the effects of medications and treatments; sensory deficits; cognitive function; physical strength, balance, and coordination). In addition, patients become deconditioned during hospitalization by bed rest or inactivity and are more vulnerable to falling (Krumholz, 2013). A review of studies designed to test interventions for reducing falls in hospitals found promising approaches. However, research studies have not identified any single fall prevention intervention or group interventions to be routinely successful (Hempel et al., 2013). A combination of interventions may be useful in fall prevention, such as the following:

- Hourly bedside rounds
- Use of bed-exit alarms
- Visual risk alert signage
- Patient education about fall risks
- Earlier referral to physical rehabilitation during hospitalization and referral for balance and core-strength training after discharge

• Nursing Skills Online: Safety Module, Lesson 1

Patient falls are one of the most common inpatient adverse events (Department of Health and Human Services, 2010; Oliver et al., 2010). Falls are multifactorial. Risk factors for falls among inpatients include a history of falling, agitation and confusion, urinary incontinence or urgency, decreased vision and hearing, impaired gait and lower extremity weakness, postural hypotension, and the use of high-risk medications (e.g., benzodiazepines, opioids, sedative hypnotics) (Chang et al., 2011; Oliver et al., 2010). Disease also plays a role. For example, patients on oncology units appear to have a higher fall rate compared with patients on medical and neurology units and have the highest injury rate because of disease-related factors (e.g., osteoporosis, coagulation disorders) (Allan-Gibbs, 2010). Because various factors create fall risks for patients, it is important for nurses to perform thorough fall risk assessments and use fall prevention techniques individualized to patients' risks and behaviors.

A consistent approach to assess fall risk is needed. Numerous fall risk assessment tools are available, such as the Morse Fall Scale, STRATIFY scale, Hendrich II Fall Risk Model, and Johns Hopkins Fall Risk Assessment Tool. Most tools generate a score that aims to predict low, moderate, or high fall risk. When a patient's risk is assessed, it is important to communicate the risk for a fall clearly to all health care providers with whom the patient will interact. Assessment findings associated with an increased risk for fall and injury direct your selection of fall prevention interventions.

ASSESSMENT

1. Identify patient using two identifiers (e.g., name and birthday or name and account number, according to facility policy). *Rationale: Ensures correct patient. Complies with The Joint Commission standards and improves patient safety (TJC, 2014).*
2. Assess patient's fall risks using a fall risk assessment tool, such as the STRATIFY. *Rationale: Various physiological factors predispose patients to fall. The STRATIFY tool has good diagnostic validity (accurate in detecting fall risk) (Aranda-Gallardo et al., 2013).*
3. Determine if patient has a history of recent falls or other injuries within the home. Assess previous falls using the acronym *SPLATT* (Touhy and Jett, 2014).
   - **S**ymptoms at time of fall
   - **P**revious fall
   - **L**ocation of fall
   - **A**ctivity at time of fall
   - **T**ime of fall
   - **T**rauma after fall
   Rationale: Key symptoms are helpful in identifying cause for falls. Onset, location, and activity associated with a fall provide further details on causative factors and how to prevent future falls.
4. Review patient's medications (including over-the-counter [OTC] medications and herbal products) for use of

antidepressants, anticonvulsants, antipsychotics, hypnotics (especially benzodiazepines), anxiolytics, diuretics, antihypertensives, antihistamines, anti-Parkinson drugs, hypoglycemics, muscle relaxants, analgesics, and laxatives. *Rationale: Certain medications may increase risk for falls and injury (Chang et al., 2011; Gribbin et al., 2010; Kojima et al., 2011). Use of multiple medications (polypharmacy) is also associated with falls, especially in older adults (Beer et al., 2011).*

5. Assess patient's gait by performing the timed "get up and go" (TGUG) test if patient is able to ambulate:
   - Have patient rise from sitting position without using arms for support.
   - Instruct patient to walk 10 feet (3 m), turn around, and walk back to chair.
   - Have patient return to chair and sit down without using arms for support.
   - Look for unsteadiness in patient's gait.
   Rationale: Reduced gait speed and stability create risk for falls.

6. Assess patient for osteoporosis, current anticoagulant use, history of previous fracture, cancer, and recent chest or abdominal surgery. *Rationale: These factors increase the likelihood of injury from a fall.*

7. Assess risk factors for falls in the health care facility (e.g., being attached to equipment such as sequential compression hose, IV line, or oxygen tubing; improperly lighted room; clutter; obstructed walkway to bathroom; and proximity of frequently needed items such as a urinal or eyeglasses). *Rationale: Environmental barriers pose a risk for falls.*

8. Assess condition of equipment. *Rationale: Equipment in poor repair (e.g., uneven legs on a bedside commode) increases the risk for fall.*

9. Assess patient's fear of falling: consider age older than 75, female sex, lower income or single, perception of poor general health, poor balance, depression, and history of falling in last 3 months. *Rationale: These factors correlate with fear of falling, increasing risk for falls (BMJ, 2010).*

10. Use a patient-centered approach and determine what patient knows about risks for falling and steps that he or she can take to prevent falls. *Rationale: Knowledge of fall risks influences the patient's ability to take needed precautions in reducing falling.*

PLANNING

Expected Outcomes focus on fall and injury prevention and appropriate use of safety equipment.
1. Patient's environment is as free of hazards as possible.
2. Patient or family caregiver is able to identify safety risks.
3. Patient or family caregiver verbalizes understanding of fall prevention interventions.
4. Patient does not sustain a fall or injury.

Delegation and Collaboration

The skill of assessing and communicating a patient's risk for falling cannot be delegated to nursing assistive personnel (NAP). Skills used to prevent falls can be delegated. The nurse instructs NAP to:
- Use fall prevention measures that match a patient's mobility limitations.
- Use specific environmental safety precautions (e.g., bed locked in low position, call light within reach, nonskid footwear).
- Report to the nurse any patient behaviors (e.g., disorientation, wandering) that are precursors to falls.

Equipment
- Fall risk assessment tool
- Hospital bed with side rails
- Wedge cushion
- Call light/intercom system
- Seat belt
- Gait belt
- Wheelchair
- Bed alarm

IMPLEMENTATION *for* FALL PREVENTION IN A HEALTH CARE SETTING

STEPS	RATIONALE
1. **See Standard Protocol (inside front cover).**	

> **SAFE PATIENT CARE** Before using any equipment for the first time, know the safety features and proper method of operation.

STEPS	RATIONALE
2. Explain plan of care. Specifically discuss reasons that patient is at risk for falling. Include family caregivers (as appropriate) in discussion.	This promotes patient cooperation and results in fall prevention measures that are patient-centered and not just routine. Younger patients are very independent and often believe they are not likely to fall.

> **SAFE PATIENT CARE** If patient is taking multiple medications, confer with the health care provider on the possibility of reducing or adjusting the medications.

Continued

STEPS	RATIONALE

3. Adjust bed to low position with wheels locked (see illustration). Place nonslip padded floor mats at exit side of bed.

Height of bed allows ambulatory patient to get in and out of bed easily and safely. Pads provide nonslippery surface on which to stand.

4. Encourage the use of properly fitted skid-proof footwear. Option: Place nonslip padded floor mat on exit side of bed.

Skid-proof footwear or floor mat prevents falls from slipping on floor.

5. Orient patient to surroundings and call light/bed control system.

Orientation to room and call system familiarizes patient with environment and the ability to call readily for assistance.

a. Provide patient's hearing aid and glasses. Be sure each assistive device is functioning and clean.

These assistive devices enable patient to remain alert to conditions in environment.

b. Explain and demonstrate how to turn call light/intercom system on and off at bedside and in bathroom (see illustration). Have patient perform a return demonstration.

Knowledge of location and use of call light is essential for patient to be able to call for assistance quickly.

c. Explain to patient or family caregiver when and why to use call system (e.g., report pain, get out of bed, go to bathroom). Provide clear instructions to patient or family caregiver regarding mobility restrictions.

This instruction increases the likelihood of nurse being able to respond to patient's needs in a timely way.

d. Consistently secure call light/bed control system to an accessible location within patient's reach.

This ensures that patient is able to reach device immediately when needed.

6. Use side rails safely.

a. Explain to patient and family members the reason for using side rails: moving and turning self in bed.

This explanation promotes cooperation.

b. Check facility policy regarding use of side rails.

Side rails are restraint devices if they immobilize or reduce the ability of a patient to move the arms, legs, body, or head freely.

(1) Dependent patients; less mobile patients: In a two–side rail bed, keep both rails up. (Note: Rails on newer hospital beds allow for room at foot of bed for patient to exit bed safely.) In a four–side rail bed, leave only two upper rails up.

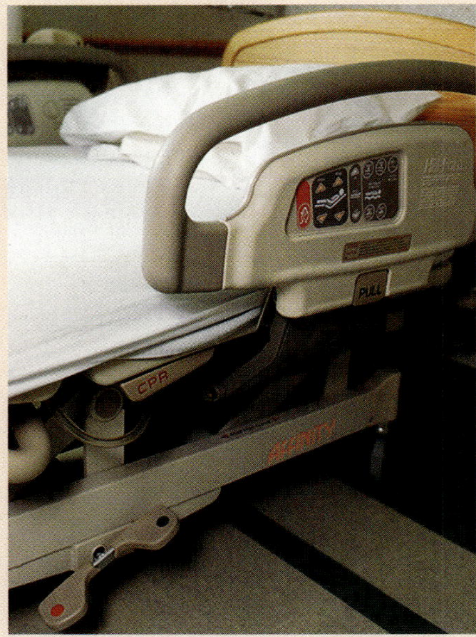

STEP 3 Hospital bed should be kept in the lowest position with wheels locked and side rails up (as appropriate.)

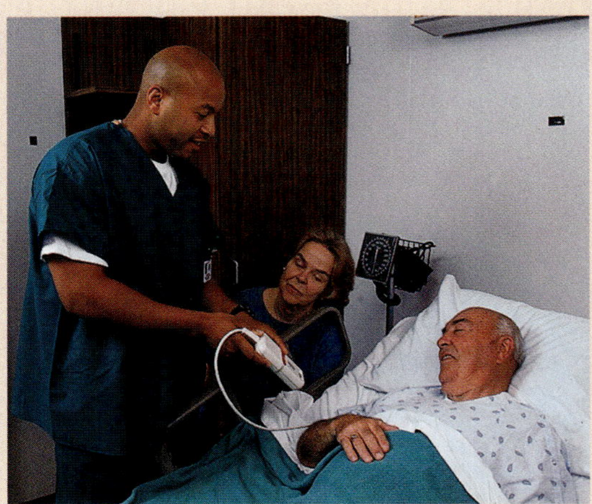

STEP 5b Nurse demonstrates use of call light to patient.

STEPS	RATIONALE

    (2) Patient able to get out of bed independently: In a four–side rail bed, leave only one upper side rail up. In a two–side rail, keep only one rail up.

This allows for safe exit from bed.

7. Make the patient's environment safe.

  a. Remove excess equipment, supplies, and furniture from rooms and halls.

This reduces likelihood of falling or tripping over objects.

  b. Keep floors free of clutter and obstacles, particularly the path to the bathroom.

This reduces likelihood of falling or tripping over objects.

  c. Coil and secure excess electrical, telephone, and any other cords or tubing.

This reduces the risk of entanglement.

  d. Clean all spills promptly. Post a sign indicating a wet floor. Remove the sign when the floor is dry (usually done by housekeeping).

This reduces the risk of falling on slippery, wet surfaces.

  e. Ensure adequate glare-free lighting; use a night-light at night.

Glare may be a problem for older adults because of vision changes.

  f. Have assistive devices (e.g., cane, walker, bedside commode) on exit side of bed.

Availability of assistive devices provides added support when transferring out of bed.

  g. Arrange necessary items (e.g., water pitcher, telephone, reading materials, dentures) within patient's easy reach and in a logical way.

This facilitates independence and self-care and prevents falls related to reaching for hard-to-reach items.

  h. Secure locks on beds, stretchers, and wheelchairs.

This prevents accidental movement of devices during patient transfer.

8. Additional interventions for patients at moderate to high risk for falling (based on fall risk assessment).

  a. Institute facility-specific flagging system (e.g., yellow sign on door indicating risk for fall, yellow sticker on chart, yellow dot on assignment board). Apply yellow Fall Risk armband on patient (see illustration).

Such a system communicates patients at highest risk for fall to all health care team members. A national effort aimed at standardizing the patient wristband color of yellow for fall risk has gained support in several U.S. states.

  b. Prioritize call light responses to patients at high risk, using a team approach

This ensures rapid response by a health care provider when patient calls for assistance.

  c. Establish elimination schedule, using bedside commode when appropriate.

Proactive toileting keeps patients from being unattended with sudden urge to use toilet.

> **SAFE PATIENT CARE** Getting out of bed for toileting is a common event leading to a patient's fall (Tzeng, 2010), especially during evening or night hours when a room is darkened.

  d. Stay with patient during toileting.

Patients often try to get up to stand and walk back to their bed from the bathroom without assistance.

  e. Place patient in a geri chair or wheelchair with wedge cushion. Use wheelchair only for transport, not for sitting an extended time.

A wedge cushion maintains alignment and comfort and makes it difficult to exit chair.

  f. Use a low bed that has low height above floor, and apply floor mats.

This reduces fall-related injuries.

  g. Activate bed alarm for patient.

Alarm activates when patient rises off a sensor and sounds an alert to staff.

  h. Confer with a physical therapist on feasibility of gait training, weight-bearing activities, balance exercise, and strengthening exercises.

Exercise can reduce falls, fall-related fractures, and several risk factors for falls in individuals with low bone density and in older adults (de Kam et al., 2009; Schubert, 2011).

Continued

STEPS	RATIONALE

i. Accompany patient during transport. Alert receiving area to patient's risk for fall.

Safety is provided during transport and transfer.

j. Use sitters or restraints only when alternatives are exhausted (see Skill 4.3).

A sitter is typically a nonprofessional staff member or volunteer who stays in a patient room to provide close observation of patients who are at risk for falling. Use of sitters can be costly. Restraints should be used only as a final option.

9. When ambulating a patient, have patient wear a gait belt and walk along patient's side (see Chapter 16).

A gait belt gives you a secure hold on patient during ambulation.

10. *Safe transport using a wheelchair*

a. Determine level of assistance needed to transfer patient to wheelchair. Position wheelchair on same side of bed as patient's strong or unaffected side (see Chapter 15).

Patient's condition may require more than a one-person assist. Positioning of chair facilitates patient's ability to assist in transfer.

b. Place wedge cushion in chair (see illustration).

A wedge cushion prevents patient from slipping out of chair.

c. Securely lock brakes on both wheels when transferring patient into or out of wheelchair.

Locking the brakes keeps chair steady and secure.

d. Raise footplates before transfer to chair; then lower footplates, placing patient's feet on them after the patient is seated.

This prevents patient from tripping over footplate.

e. Have patient sit with buttocks well back in seat. Option: Apply a quick-release seat belt.

This prevents patient from sliding out of chair.

f. Back wheelchair into and out of elevator or door, leading with large rear wheels first (see illustration).

This prevents smaller front wheels from catching in crack between elevator and floor, causing chair to tip.

11. **See Completion Protocol (inside front cover).**

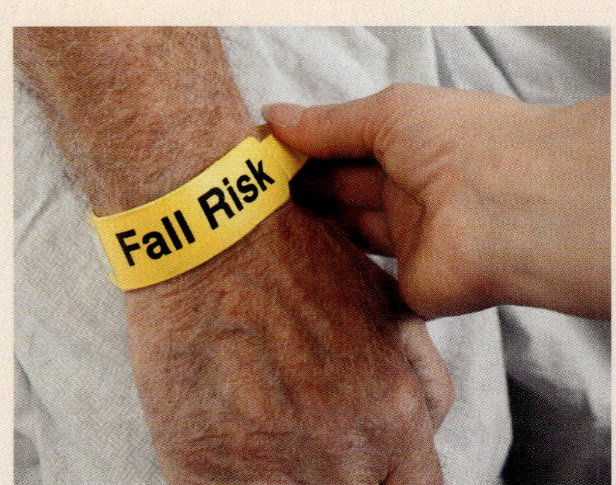

STEP 8a Arm band alerts nursing staff to patient's risk of falling.

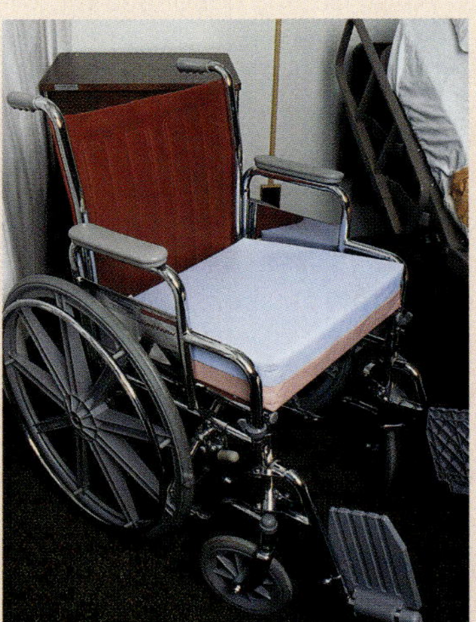

STEP 10b Wheelchair with footplates raised and wedge cushion in place.

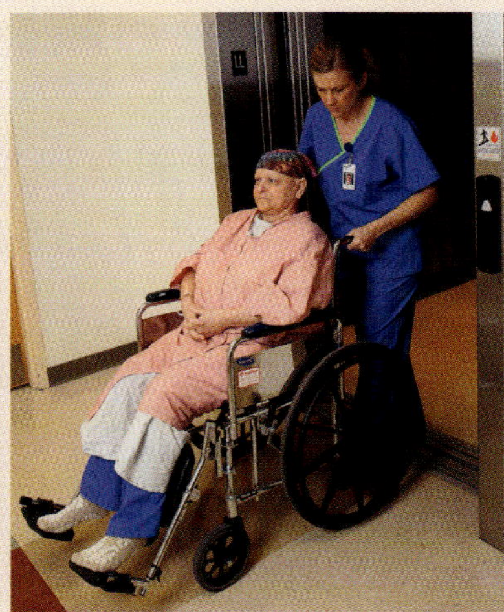

STEP 10f Nurse backing wheelchair into elevator.

EVALUATION

1. Conduct hourly rounds.
2. Observe patient's immediate environment for the presence of hazards.
3. Evaluate patient's ability to use assistive devices such as a walker or bedside commode.
4. Evaluate patient's motor, sensory, and cognitive status, and review if any falls or injuries have occurred.
5. Determine patient's response to safety modifications and that no falls or injuries have occurred.
6. Use *Teach Back:* State to patient and family caregiver, "I want to be sure I explained clearly to you the reasons why you are more likely to fall than other patients. Can you tell me some of those reasons?" Evaluates whether patient or family caregiver is able to explain fall risks. Revise your instruction now or develop plan for revised patient teaching to be implemented at an appropriate time if the patient or family caregiver is not able to teach back correctly.

Unexpected Outcomes and Related Interventions

1. Patient starts to fall while ambulating with a nurse.
   a. Put both arms around patient's waist or grasp gait belt.
   b. Stand with feet apart to provide a broad base of support.
   c. Extend one leg and let patient slide against it to the floor (Fig. 4-2)
   d. Bend knees and lower body as patient slides to the floor (Fig. 4-3)
2. Patient sustains a fall.
   a. Call for assistance.
   b. Assess patient for injury, and stay with the patient until assistance arrives to help lift the patient to the bed or wheelchair.

   c. Notify health care provider and family member.
   d. Note pertinent events related to the fall and treatment provided in the medical record.
   e. Follow sentinel event reporting policy of the health care facility.
   f. Evaluate patient and environment to determine whether the fall could have been prevented.
   g. Reinforce explanation of identified risks with patient, and review safety measures needed to prevent a fall.
   h. Monitor patient closely after the fall because injuries are not always immediately apparent.
3. Patient or family caregiver is unable to explain fall risks.
   a. Offer a reexplanation using plain language, and consider use of printed materials if available.

Recording and Reporting

- Record in the plan of care specific interventions to prevent falls and promote safety.
- Document what patient is able to explain or not explain about fall risks.
- Report patient's fall risks and measures taken to reduce risks to all health care personnel.
- Report immediately to the physician or health care provider if patient sustains a fall or an injury.
- Complete a facility safety event or incident report noting objective details of fall (time, location, patient's condition, treatment, treatment response). Do not place the report in patient's medical record.

Sample Documentation

0900 Fall risk assessment completed. Patient placed on high-risk fall precautions because of history of falls, weakness, and urinary frequency. Call light within reach, top side rails up, hourly room checks completed, night-light on at all times, bedside commode in place. Instructed patient to call for help to ambulate. Patient voiced understanding. Patient demonstrated correct use of call light.

1615 Found patient on floor in bathroom after responding to emergency call light. Patient stated, "I slipped on the wet floor." Patient denies hitting head; alert and oriented × 3; PERRLA. No apparent injury from fall. Blood pressure

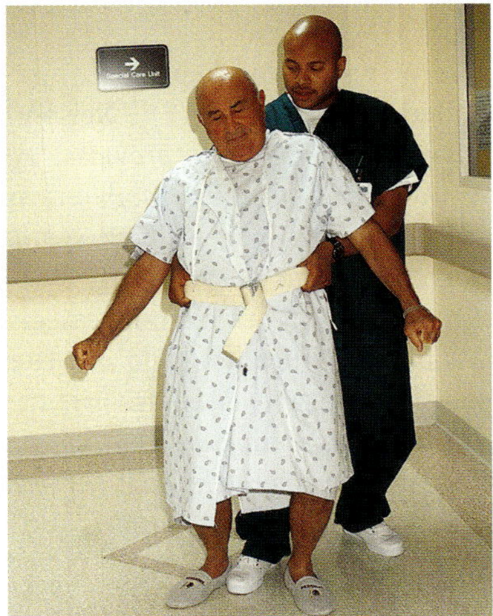

FIG 4-2 Stand with feet apart to provide broad base of support; extend one leg against which patient can slide to floor.

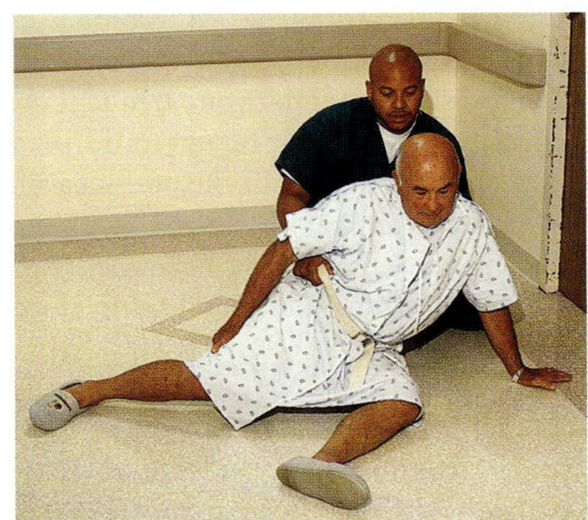

FIG 4-3 Bend knees and lower body as patient slides to floor.

110/74, pulse 82 and regular, respirations 20 per minute. Assisted patient to bed and instructed to call for help before getting out of bed. Patient voiced understanding. Call light placed within patient's reach and patient able to return demonstrate its use. Side rails up × 2. Dr. Justine and patient's wife notified of fall.

Special Considerations
Pediatric

- Children's activity levels and curiosity increase the risk for falls. Eliminate places for a child to climb. Consider using a crib hood if a child is hospitalized.
- Keep side rails of hospital beds down to allow toddlers and preschoolers easy exit and to decrease the need to crawl over the rails (Hockenberry and Wilson, 2011).
- When caring for an infant, keep a hand on the infant when you turn away from the bedside.

Geriatric

- Older patients with short-term memory loss or cognitive dysfunction may be unable to follow directions and may attempt to climb out of bed or get up from a chair unassisted.
- Physical therapy for improving balance, lower body strength, and gait can be beneficial to older patients (Touhy and Jett, 2014).

Home Care

- Assess patient's home environment for hazards, and institute safety measures as appropriate (see Chapter 32).
- Items should be kept in their familiar positions and within easy reach in rooms frequently used.
- If patient has a history of falls and lives alone, recommend that he or she wear an electronic Safe Patient Care device. The device is turned on by the wearer to alert a monitoring site to call emergency services for help.

SKILL 4.2   DESIGNING A RESTRAINT-FREE ENVIRONMENT

Physical and chemical restraints restrict a patient's physical activity or normal access to the body and are not a usual part of treatment indicated by a patient's condition or symptoms. Serious and often fatal complications can develop from the use of restraints. Because of the risks associated with the use of restraints, current legislation emphasizes reducing this use. The CMS set the standard that restraint or seclusion may be imposed only to ensure the immediate physical safety of a patient and must be discontinued at the earliest possible time (Department of Health and Human Services, CMS, 2008). A restraint-free environment is a goal of care for all patients.

When trying to create a restraint-free environment, patients at risk for falling or wandering present special safety challenges. Wandering is meandering, aimless, or repetitive locomotion that exposes a patient to harm and is frequently in conflict with boundaries, limits, or obstacles (NANDA, 2012). Wandering is a common problem in patients who are confused or disoriented or have dementia. Interrupting a wandering patient can increase the patient's distress. The Department of Veteran Affairs has many suggestions for managing a wandering patient, most of which are environmental adaptations. Some of these include hobbies, social interaction, and regular routines (VA National Center for Patient Safety, 2010). Modifications of the environment are effective alternatives to restraints. More frequent observation of patients, involvement of family caregivers during visitation, and frequent reorientation are also helpful measures. Introduction of meaningful and familiar stimuli within a patient's environment can reduce the types of behaviors (e.g., wandering, restlessness, confusion) that may lead to restraint use.

3. Assess patient's behavior (e.g., orientation, level of consciousness, ability to understand and follow directions, combative behaviors, restlessness, agitation), balance, gait, vision, hearing, bowel and bladder routine, level of pain, electrolyte and blood count values, and presence of orthostatic hypotension. *Rationale: Accurate assessment identifies patients with safety risks and the physiological causes for patient behaviors that prompt caregivers to use restraints. Assessment ensures the proper selection of nonrestraint interventions.*
4. Review OTC and prescribed medications for interactions and untoward effects. *Rationale: Medication interactions or side effects often contribute to falling or altered mental status.*
5. For patients who wander or have known dementia, assess for cognitive decline by using the Mini-Mental State Examination (MMSE) (see Chapter 7). *Rationale: Findings of the MMSE assist in selection of effective restraint-free interventions.*
6. Assess degree of wandering behavior using the Revised Algase Wandering Scale (RAWS) (Nelson and Algase, 2007). *Rationale: The RAWS provides a quantitative measure for wandering in several domains as reported by caregivers, including persistent walking, spatial disorientation, and eloping behavior (Futrell et al., 2010).*
7. If a patient has dementia, ask a family caregiver about the patient's usual communication style and cues to indicate pain, fatigue, hunger, and need to urinate or defecate (Touhy and Jett, 2014). *Rationale: This information enables you to determine more accurately a patient's needs. Wandering often occurs if these needs are unmet.*

ASSESSMENT

1. Assess patient's risk for falling (see Skill 4.1).
2. Assess patient's medical history for cognitive deficit, depression, and hyperactivity. *Rationale: Wandering is associated with these common conditions.*

PLANNING

Expected Outcomes focus on providing patient safety while avoiding the need for physical restraints.

1. Patient is injury-free or does not inflict injury on others.

2. Patient displays cooperative behavior toward staff, visitors, and other patients.

Delegation and Collaboration

The skills of assessing a patient's behavior, orientation to the environment, and the decision for safety measures cannot be delegated. Actions for promoting a safe environment can be delegated to nursing assistive personnel (NAP). The nurse instructs the NAP to:

- Use specific diversional or activity measures for making the environment safe.
- Apply appropriate alarm devices.

- Report patient behaviors and actions that suggest wandering (e.g., confusion, combativeness, getting out of bed unassisted) to the nurse.

Equipment

- Visual or auditory stimuli (e.g., calendar, clock, photos, MP3 player, radio, television)
- Diversional activities (e.g., puzzles, games, audio books)
- Wedge cushion
- Ambularm, pressure-sensitive bed, or chair alarm
- Bed enclosure system

IMPLEMENTATION *for* DESIGNING A RESTRAINT-FREE ENVIRONMENT

STEPS	RATIONALE
1. See Standard Protocol (inside front cover).	
2. Orient patient and family members to surroundings, introduce to staff, and explain all treatments and procedures. Frequent reorientation in a calm manner may be needed. Be sure patient is able to read your name badge.	This promotes patient understanding and cooperation.
3. Assign same staff to care for patient as often as possible. Encourage family and friends to stay with patient. In some facilities, sitters are available to stay with a patient as constant observers and in some cases to provide active interaction (Nadler-Moodie et al., 2009).	When one person provides care, patient anxiety is reduced, and safety is increased. Use of sitters is designed to offer constant patient supervision.

> **SAFE PATIENT CARE** There is no research at the present time to suggest the use of sitters to provide constant observation reduces the risk of patient harm related to risk for falling (Harding, 2010).

STEPS	RATIONALE
4. Place patient in a room that is easily accessible to health care staff. Another option is to cohort similar patients in proximity for staff to attend to them frequently if not constantly (Nadler-Moodie et al., 2009).	This facilitates close observation. Watching the activities on a unit distracts a patient (VA National Center for Patient Safety, 2010).
5. Be sure that patient has glasses, hearing aid, or other sensory-aid devices on and functioning.	Sensory deficit increases risk of confusion and disorientation.
6. Provide visual and auditory stimuli meaningful to specific patient (e.g., calendar, radio or MP3 player [patient's choice of music], and family pictures).	Meaningful stimuli orient patient to day, time, and physical surroundings.
7. Anticipate patient's basic needs (e.g., hunger, thirst, toileting, relief of pain) as quickly as possible.	Meeting basic needs in a timely fashion decreases patient's discomfort, anxiety, and risk for fall and injury, by reducing urgency to get out of bed on own.
8. Provide scheduled ambulation, chair activity, and toileting (e.g., ask patient every hour about toileting needs). Organize treatments so that patient has some uninterrupted periods throughout the day.	Regular voiding decreases risk of patient trying to reach bathroom alone. Provide time for sleep and rest. Constant activity may overstimulate patient.
9. Position IV catheters, urinary catheters, and tubes or drains out of patient view. Camouflage by wrapping IV site with bandage or stockinette; place undergarments on patient with urinary catheter or cover abdominal feeding tubes or drains with loose abdominal binder.	Continuous medical treatment can be maintained by reducing visibility of and access to tubes and lines, which patients may want to remove.

Continued

STEPS	RATIONALE
10. Use stress-reduction techniques such as back rub, massage, relaxation, and guided imagery (see Chapter 13).	Reducing anxiety may reduce the urge to wander.
11. Use diversional activities such as puzzles, games, books, folding towels, drawing, or offering an object to hold. Be sure that it is an activity in which patient expresses interest.	Meaningful diversional activities provide distraction, help to reduce boredom, provide tactile stimulation, and minimize wandering.
12. Decrease wandering by eliminating stressors from patient's environment such as cold at night, changes in daily routines, extra or unfamiliar visitors (Futrell et al., 2010). Also remove trigger items, such as keys, coats, shoes, and purses, out of sight.	Reduced stress allows patient's energy to be channeled more appropriately. Triggers cause the person to want to wander.
13. Position patient on a wedge cushion and apply a wrap-around belt. (Note: This is not a restraint if patient is able to self-release.)	A wedge cushion prevents slipping out of a chair and makes it difficult for patient to get out of chair without assistance. A wrap-around belt reminds patient to call for help and allows patient to lift flap for self-release (see illustration).

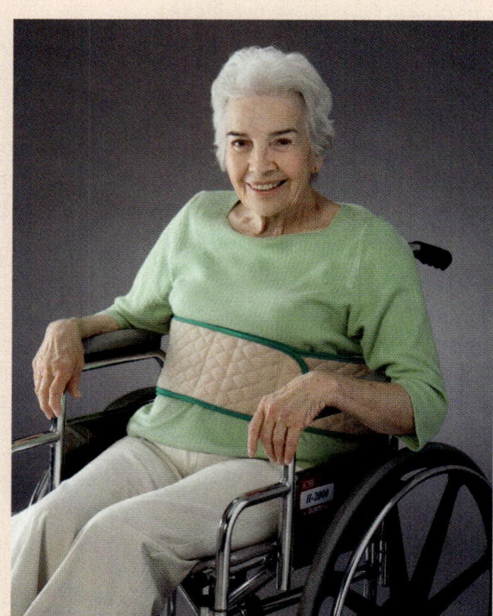

STEP 13 Wrap-around belt. (Courtesy Posey Company, Arcadia, California.)

STEPS	RATIONALE
14. Use pressure-sensitive bed or chair pad with alarms.	
a. Explain use of device to patient and family caregiver.	Alarm alerts staff to patient who is standing or rising up without assistance.
b. When in bed, position device so that it is under the patient's mid-to-low back or under buttocks.	Alarm activates sooner if placed under back. By the time buttocks are off the sensor, patient may almost be out of bed.
c. Test alarm by applying and releasing pressure.	Testing ensures that alarm is audible through call light system.
15. Use an Ambularm monitoring device.	
a. Explain use of device to patient and family caregiver.	This reinforces to patient his or her risk for falling.
b. Measure patient's thigh circumference just above knee to determine appropriate size: leg circumference less than 18 inches (45 cm) requires regular size; 18 inches or greater requires large size.	Band that is too loose slips off; one that is too tight irritates the skin or interferes with circulation.

STEPS	RATIONALE

c. Test battery and alarm by touching snaps to corresponding snaps on leg band.

This ensures device is functional.

d. Apply leg band just above knee and snap battery securely in place (see illustration).

e. Instruct patient that alarm will sound unless leg is kept in horizontal position (see illustration).

f. To assist patient to ambulate, deactivate alarm by unsnapping device from leg band.

Deactivating the alarm prevents false alarm that can be heard by other staff members.

> **SAFE PATIENT CARE** Use of an Ambularm is contraindicated in the presence of impaired circulation, swelling, skin irritation, or breaks in the skin.

16. Place patient in a bed enclosure system (see illustration).

This restraint alternative allows a patient freedom of movement within a protected environment.

17. Consult with family caregiver and physical, speech, and occupational therapists for appropriate activities to provide stimulation and exercise.

Involvement in meaningful and purposeful activities reduces tendency to wander. Exercise improves balance and coordination.

18. Minimize invasive treatments as much as possible (e.g., tube feedings, blood sampling).

Stimuli increase patient's restlessness.

19. See Completion Protocol (inside front cover).

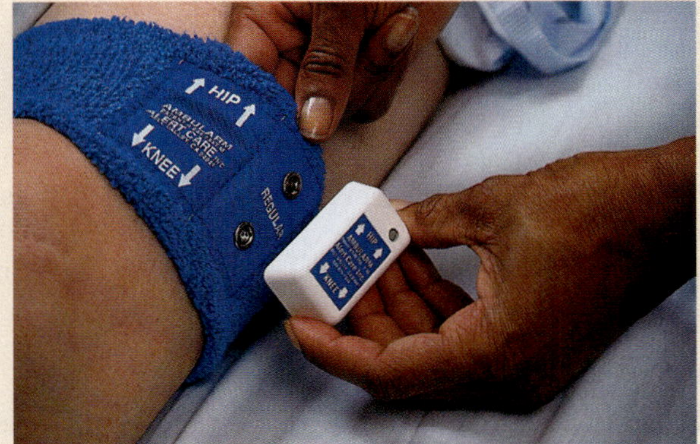

STEP 15d Snap battery in place to activate alarm. (Courtesy Alert Care, Tiburon, California.)

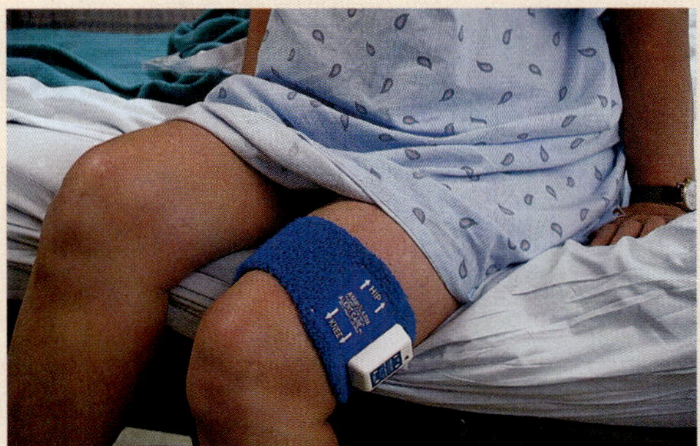

STEP 15e Audio alarm sounds when patient approaches near-vertical position when getting out of bed. (Courtesy Alert Care, Tiburon, California.)

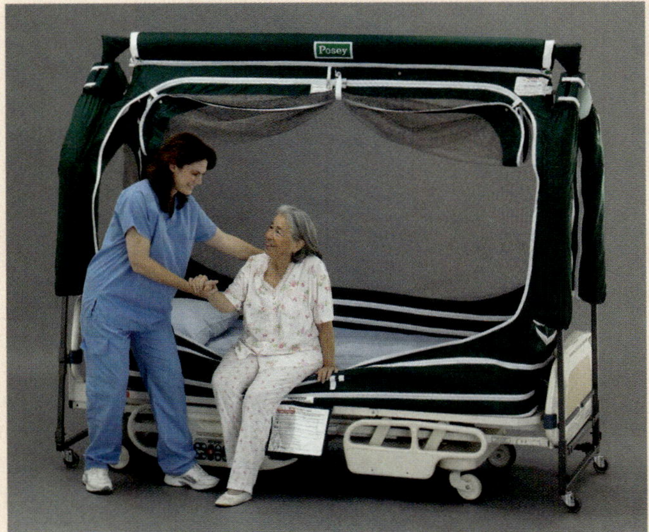

STEP 16 Bed enclosure system. (Courtesy Posey Company, Arcadia, California.)

EVALUATION

1. Observe patient for any injuries.
2. Observe patient's behavior toward staff, visitors, and other patients.
3. Use **Teach Back:** State to the patient, "I want to be sure I explained clearly to you about why you have an Ambu-larm. Can you tell me the reasons?" Evaluates what the patient is able to explain or demonstrate. Revise your instruction now or develop plan for revised patient teaching to be implemented at an appropriate time if patient is not able to teach back correctly.

Unexpected Outcomes and Related Interventions

1. Patient displays behaviors that increase risk for injury to self or others.
   a. Review episodes for a pattern (e.g., activity, time of day) that indicates alternatives that could eliminate the behavior.
   b. Discuss with all health care providers and family care-givers alternative interventions to promote safe, consistent care.
2. Patient sustains an injury or is out of control, placing others at risk for injury.
   a. Notify health care provider and complete a safety event or occurrence report according to facility policy.
   b. Identify alternative measures to promote safety or control behaviors.
   c. As a last resort, identify appropriate restraint to use (see Skill 4.3).

Recording and Reporting

- Record all behaviors that relate to cognitive status and ability to maintain safety: orientation to time, place, and person; ability to follow directions; mood and emotional status; understanding of condition and treatment plan; medication effects related to behaviors; restraint alternatives used; and patient response.
- Document your evaluation of patient learning.
- Report to other health care providers any occurrences of wandering or other behavior that places the patient at risk for injury.

Sample Documentation

0900   Up and dressed; oriented to person but not time or place. Patient became tearful when unable to reach wife by telephone. Pacing in room. Reoriented to place. Explained to patient wife is due to visit later in afternoon. Set radio to favorite talk show.

1000   Participated for 15 minutes with ball toss to music at occupational therapy; then resting in rocking chair, smiling, and interacting socially with roommate.

Special Considerations
Pediatric

- Distraction techniques can decrease the need for restraints. Examples include having a child hold a stuffed animal while an IV line is being inserted or blowing bubbles while a drain is being removed.

Geriatric

- A sudden onset of confusion, weakness, and functional decline in a previously oriented older adult patient may indicate the presence of an underlying illness (e.g., an infection).
- Assess for physical causes of behavior changes, such as urinary or respiratory infection, hypoxia, fever, fluid and electrolyte imbalance, side effects of multiple drug administration, depression, anemia, hypothyroidism, or fecal impaction.
- Reminiscence helps older adults remain oriented (Touhy and Jett, 2014).

Home Care

- Patients at risk for self-injury or violence toward others need intensive supervision. The family caregiver must recognize this need and be able to provide necessary supervision.
- Have the family caregiver set up an area in the home where it is safe for an older adult to wander.

SKILL 4.3   APPLYING PHYSICAL RESTRAINTS

• Nursing Skills Online: Safety Module, Lesson 2

Any form of restraint is discouraged because of the risk of patient injury. There are patient care situations where the use of restraints is allowed. A physical restraint is any manual method or physical or mechanical device, material, or equipment that immobilizes or reduces the ability of a person to move the extremities, torso, or head freely (CMS, 2008). Physical restraints are sometimes used to reduce treatment interference (e.g., preventing patient from removing endotracheal tube or IV catheter), prevent falls, maintain patient position, and protect a patient from harming self or others. Traditionally, the concept of a chemical restraint refers to the use of medications to control delirium, agitation, or violent behaviors or for unplanned endotracheal extubation. However, some behavioral experts argue that medications used to treat specific psychiatric diagnoses should be considered treatment measures rather than restraints (Health

Services Advisory Group, 2012). Typical chemical restraints include sedatives and analgesics, antipsychotics, or a combination of both. Physical or chemical restraints should be the last resort and used only when all other reasonable alternatives fail.

Restraints are most commonly used in hospitals to prevent the disruption of therapy, such as patients pulling out IV, feeding, or urinary catheter tubes. Restraint use is more common in critical care settings, where nurses are concerned that disruption of therapy can significantly injure patients (McCabe, 2011). Protection from physical abuse and patient combativeness is another reason restraints are used in emergency departments (McCabe, 2011). The use of physical restraints is not a safety strategy. Research has shown that patients sustain fewer injuries if left unrestrained (Park and Tang, 2007).

The CMS (2008, 2011) and TJC (2009, 2012b) have set standards for reducing the use of restraints in health care settings and using them only with extreme caution. Hospitals must report to the CMS (2011) any deaths that occur while a patient is in a restraint (exception is soft wrist restraints). Reports must include any deaths directly related to restraint use, deaths that occur within 24 hours after restraint removal, and deaths occurring within 1 week after restraint where it is reasonable to assume that use of the restraint contributed directly or indirectly to a patient's death regardless of the type of restraint used (CMS, 2011). In 2011, the NQF released its National Voluntary Consensus Standards for Public Reporting of Patient Safety Events. The NQF has endorsed a select list of serious reportable events, one of which is patient death or serious disability associated with the use of restraints or bedrails while being cared for in a health care facility.

The CMS standards (2008) for the safe use of restraints in hospitals require that a restraint be used only under the following circumstances:

- To ensure the immediate physical safety of a patient, a staff member, or others.
- When less restrictive interventions have been ineffective.
- In accordance with a written modification to a patient's plan of care.
- When it is the least restrictive intervention that will be effective to protect a patient, staff member, or others from harm.
- In accordance with safe and appropriate restraint techniques as determined by hospital policies.
- It is discontinued at the earliest possible time.

The use of restraints is associated with serious complications, including pressure ulcers, hypostatic pneumonia, constipation, urinary and fecal incontinence, urinary retention, and functional deficits. In some cases, restricted breathing (strangulation) or circulation has resulted in death. Loss of self-esteem, humiliation, fear, and anger are additional serious concerns. The U.S. Food and Drug Administration, which regulates restraints as medical devices, requires manufacturers to label restraints as "prescription only." Many patients do not easily accept use of restraints. Cultural values affect how patients and family members perceive their use. Before using restraints, assess the meaning of restraints for both the patient and the family. Culturally sensitive care may include removing restraints when family members are present.

ASSESSMENT

1. Identify patient using two identifiers (e.g., name and birthday or name and account number, according to facility policy). *Rationale: Ensures correct patient. Complies with The Joint Commission standards and improves patient safety (TJC, 2014).*

2. Assess patient's behavior (e.g., confusion, disorientation, agitation, restlessness, combativeness, or inability to follow directions), and note repeated removal of tubing or other therapeutic devices and inability to follow directions. *Rationale: If patient's behavior continues despite the use of restraint alternative, the use of physical restraint may be necessary.*

3. Review facility policies and state laws regarding restraints. Check for a current health care provider's order. The physician or licensed independent practitioner assesses the patient in person within 1 hour of the initiation of restraints (TJC, 2009). The health care provider's order must include the purpose, type, location, and time or duration of restraint. Long-term care settings require informed consent from a family member before use. Orders may be renewed according to the time limits for a maximum of 24 consecutive hours (TJC, 2009). *Rationale: A health care provider's order for the least restrictive type of restraint is required. Each original restraint order is limited to 4 hours for adults 18 years old and older, 2 hours for children 9 through 17 years old, and 1 hour for children younger than 9 years (TJC, 2009).*

SAFE PATIENT CARE If a nurse or qualified health care provider (see facility policy) restrains a patient in an emergency situation because of violence or aggressive behavior that presents an immediate danger, a face-to-face health care provider assessment within 1 hour is necessary (TJC, 2012a).

1. Determine the most appropriate size restraint following manufacturer's instructions. *Rationale: Applying a restraint that is too small can cause patient injury. A restraint that is too large is easy for a patient to remove.*
2. Inspect the area where the restraint is to be placed. Note any nearby tubing or devices. Assess condition of the skin; sensation, including color; adequacy of circulation; and range of joint motion. *Rationale: This provides a baseline assessment to monitor the patient's response to restraint.*

PLANNING

Expected Outcomes focus on protecting a patient from injury and maintaining prescribed therapy.

1. Patient maintains intact skin integrity; pulses; and skin temperature, color, and sensation of restrained body part.
2. Patient is free of injury.
3. Patient's therapies are uninterrupted.
4. Restraint is discontinued as soon as possible.
5. Patient's self-esteem and dignity are maintained.

Delegation and Collaboration

The skills of assessing a patient's behavior, orientation to the environment, need for restraints, and appropriate use cannot be delegated. Patient and family caregiver education cannot be delegated. The application and routine checking of a restraint can be delegated to nursing assistive personnel (NAP). TJC (2009) requires training on first aid for anyone who monitors patients in restraints. The nurse instructs the NAP about:

- The appropriate type of restraint to use.
- How to check the patient's circulation, skin integrity, and breathing routinely.
- When and how to change the patient's position and provide range-of-motion (ROM) exercises, toileting, and skin care.
- When to report signs and symptoms of the patient not tolerating restraint (e.g., increased agitation, constricted circulation, change in skin integrity or breathing) and what to do.

Equipment
- Proper restraint (e.g., belt, wrist, mitten)
- Padding (if needed)

IMPLEMENTATION *for* APPLYING PHYSICAL RESTRAINTS

STEPS	RATIONALE
1. **See Standard Protocol (inside front cover).**	
2. Educate patient and family caregiver about need for restraint. Talk with patient in a calm, confident manner and explain what you are going to do.	This reduces anxiety and may promote cooperation.
3. Adjust bed to proper height and lower side rail on side of patient contact.	Use of proper body mechanics during restraint application prevents injury.
4. Be sure that patient is comfortable and in proper body alignment.	This promotes comfort, prevents contractures, and prevents neurovascular injury while restraint is in place.
5. If necessary, pad skin and bony prominences that will be covered by the restraint.	Padding protects skin from friction and irritation.
6. Apply restraint; *follow manufacturer's directions.*	A restraint that is applied incorrectly can cause injury by constricting a body part.
a. Belt or body restraint Have patient in a sitting position in bed. Apply belt over clothes, gown, or pajamas. Be sure to place restraint at the waist, not the chest or abdomen. The slot in belt may be positioned in the front for limited movement or rear for increased movement of patient. Remove wrinkles or creases in clothing. Bring ties through slots in belt. Help patient lie down in bed. Have patient roll to side and avoid applying belt too tightly (see illustrations). Ensure that straps secured to bed frame are snug so that belt does not slide to sides of bed.	This type of restraint restrains center of gravity and prevents patient from rolling off stretcher, sitting up while on stretcher, or falling out of bed. Tight application or misplacement can interfere with breathing. This type of restraint may be contraindicated in patients who have had abdominal surgery.
b. Limb (ankle or wrist) restraint Limb restraints are made of a soft quilted material or sheepskin with foam padding. Wrap limb restraint around wrist or ankle with soft part toward skin and secured snugly (but not tightly) in place by a quick-release buckle or tie (see illustration). Insert two fingers under secured restraint (see illustration).	This type of restraint immobilizes one or all extremities to protect patient from fall or accidental removal of device (e.g., IV line, nasogastric tube, or Foley catheter). Tight restraint constricts circulation and causes neurovascular injury or causes occlusion of therapeutic devices. Checking for constriction prevents neurovascular injury.

> **SAFE PATIENT CARE** A patient with extremity restraint is at risk for aspiration if positioned supine. Place the patient in lateral position or with head of bed elevated rather than supine.

STEPS	RATIONALE
c. Mitten restraint A thumbless mitten device restrains patient's hands. Place hand in mitten, being sure that Velcro straps are around wrist rather than forearm (see illustration).	Mitten restraint prevents patient from dislodging invasive equipment, removing dressings, or scratching. This type of restraint allows greater movement than wrist restraint. It is considered a restraint alternative if untethered and patient is physically and cognitively able to remove the mitten.

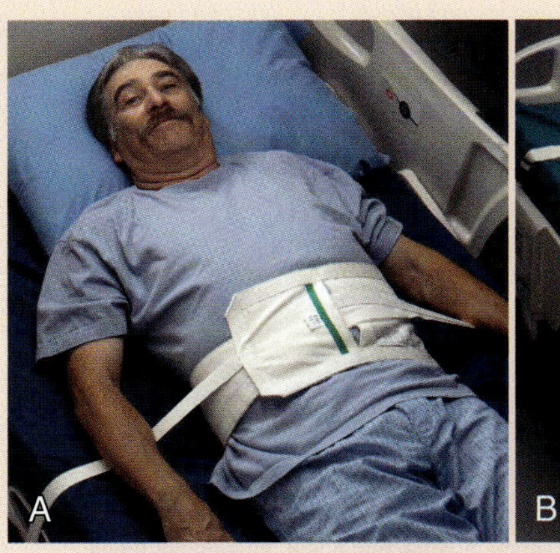

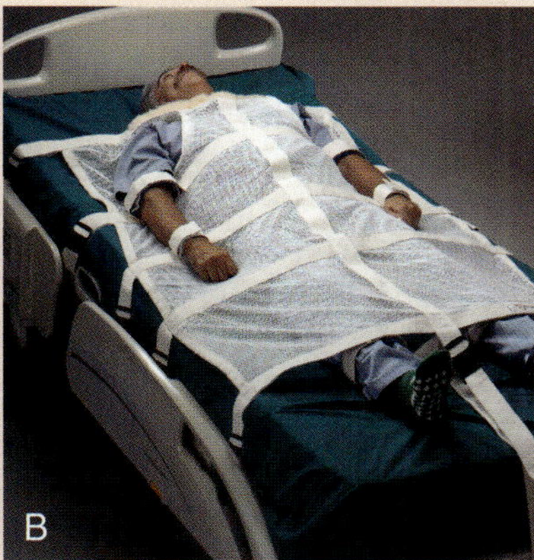

STEP 6a A, Properly applied belt restraint allows patient to turn in bed. **B,** Restraint net limits patient's ability to turn.

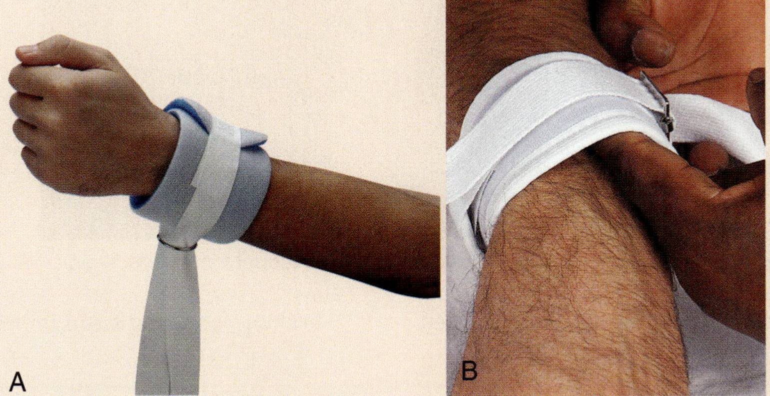

STEP 6b A, Quick-release buckle on extremity restraint. **B,** Check restraint for constriction by inserting two fingers under restraint. (Courtesy Posey Company, Arcadia, California.)

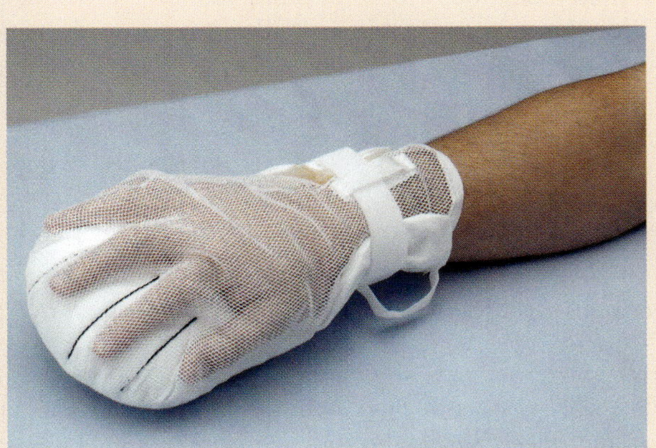

STEP 6c Mitten restraint. (Courtesy Posey Company, Arcadia, California.)

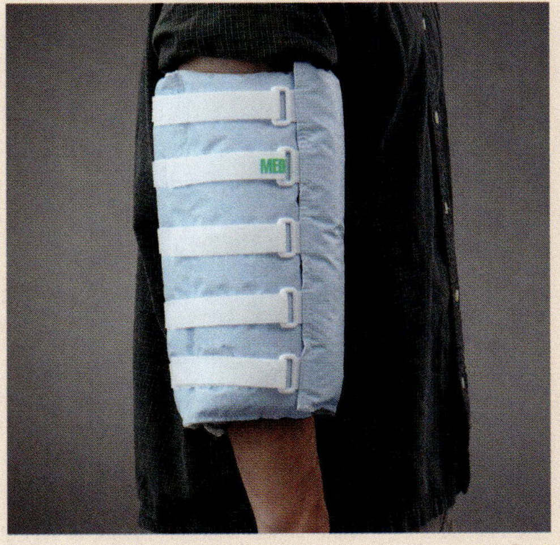

STEP 6d Elbow restraint. (Courtesy Posey Company, Arcadia, California.)

Continued

STEPS	RATIONALE

d. Elbow restraint

Restraint consists of rigidly padded fabric that wraps around the arm. It is closed with Velcro. The upper end has a clamp that hooks to the sleeve of a patient's gown or shirt (see illustration). Insert patient's arm so that elbow joint rests against padded area, keeping joint rigid.

This type of restraint is commonly used with infants and children to prevent elbow flexion (e.g., with IV lines). It may also be used for adults. The restraint keeps elbow joint rigid.

7. Attach restraint straps to portion of bed frame that moves when raising or lowering head of bed. Be sure straps are secure. *Do not attach to side rails.* Restraint can also be attached to chair frame for patient in chair or wheelchair.

Properly positioned strap does not tighten and restrict circulation when bed is raised or lowered.

8. Secure restraint with a quick-release buckle (see illustration) or an adjustable seat belt–like locking device. *Do not tie strap in a knot.*

Quick release is possible in an emergency.

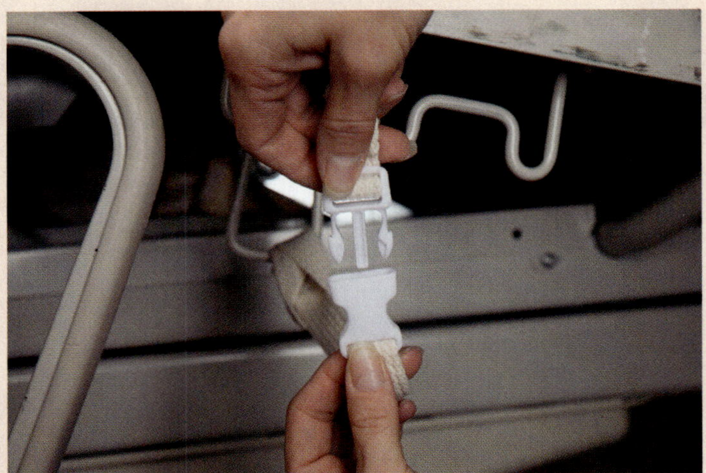

STEP 8 Quick-release buckles make it easier to evacuate patients in an emergency.

9. Double check and insert two fingers under secured restraint.

Checking for constriction prevents neurovascular injury.

> **SAFE PATIENT CARE** Restraints should not interfere with functioning of equipment such as IV tubes. Restraints are not placed over access devices such as an arteriovenous dialysis shunt.

10. Assess proper placement of restraint, including skin integrity, pulses, skin temperature and color, and sensation of the restrained body part. Remove restraints at least every 2 hours (TJC, 2012a) or according to facility policy; reposition patient, provide comfort measures, and evaluate patient each time. If patient is violent or noncompliant, remove one restraint at a time or have staff assist while removing the restraints.

This assessment provides a baseline to determine later if injury develops from restraint. Removal provides an opportunity to change patient's position; perform full ROM, toileting, and exercise; and provide food or fluids.

> **SAFE PATIENT CARE** Do not leave violent or aggressive patients unattended while restraints are off.

11. Secure call light or intercom system within reach.

This allows patient or family to obtain assistance quickly.

12. Leave bed or chair with wheels locked. Keep bed in lowest position.

Locked wheels prevent bed or chair from moving if patient tries to get out. If patient falls when bed is in lowest position, this reduces chance of injury.

13. **See Completion Protocol (inside front cover).**

EVALUATION

1. After restraint application, evaluate patient for signs of injury every 15 minutes (e.g., circulation, vital signs, ROM, physical and psychological status, and readiness for discontinuation). Perform visual checks if patient is too agitated to approach (TJC, 2012a).
2. Evaluate patient's need for toileting, nutrition and fluids, hygiene, and elimination and release restraint at least every 2 hours to provide ROM when an extremity is restrained (see facility policy).
3. Evaluate patient for any complications of immobility (e.g., pressure ulcer).
4. Assess IV catheters, urinary catheters, and drainage tubes routinely to determine that they are positioned correctly and that therapy remains uninterrupted.
5. Evaluate patient's need for restraint use on an ongoing basis (see facility policy). When a restraint is used for violent or self-destructive behavior, a physician or licensed independent practitioner must evaluate the patient in person within 1 hour of the initiation of the restraint.
6. Observe patient's behavior and reaction to the presence of restraint.
7. Use **Teach Back:** Before restraint application, ask patient or family caregiver, "I want to be sure I explained clearly to you the reasons why we are applying a restraint around your wrists at this time. Can you tell me the reason? Can you tell me how we will check on you?" Evaluates what the patient or family caregiver is able to explain or demonstrate. Revise your instruction now or develop plan for revised patient teaching to be implemented at an appropriate time if patient is not able to teach back correctly.

Unexpected Outcomes and Related Interventions

1. Skin underlying restraint becomes reddened or damaged.
   a. Provide appropriate skin care (see Chapter 25).
   b. Notify health care provider, and reassess the need for continued use of restraint and whether you can use alternative measures.
   c. Readjust restraint, use a different type of restraint, or provide additional padding.
   d. Remove restraints more frequently. Change wet or soiled restraints.
2. Patient has altered neurovascular status to an extremity (cyanosis; pallor; coldness of the skin; or complaints of tingling, pain, or numbness).
   a. Remove restraint immediately; stay with patient.
   b. Notify health care provider.
3. Patient becomes confused, disoriented, or agitated.
   a. Identify reason for change in behavior, and attempt to eliminate cause.
   b. Use restraint alternatives (see Skill 4-2), and consider involving family in care.
   c. Determine the need for more or less sensory stimulation, and reorient as needed.
4. Patient becomes physically deconditioned related to restraint use.
   a. Remove restraint if possible.
   b. Notify health care provider.
   c. Implement strict schedule of ROM exercises (see Chapter 16), and consider seeking a physical therapy consultation to begin an exercise regimen.

Recording and Reporting

- Record nursing interventions, including restraint alternatives tried, in nurses' notes.
- Record patient's behavior before restraints were applied, level of orientation, and patient or family member's statement of understanding of the purpose of restraint and consent for application (if required by facility).
- Document your evaluation of patient learning.
- Record purpose for restraint, type and location of restraint, time applied, time restraint ended, and all routine assessments made every 15 minutes in nurses' notes and flow sheet.
- Record patient's behavior after restraint application. Record times patient was assessed, attempts to use alternatives to restraint and patient's response, times restraint was released (temporarily and permanently), and patient's response when restraint was removed.

Sample Documentation

2020 Patient has repeatedly attempted to get out of bed. Remains disoriented to name, date, and location. Provided sitter and attempted to reorient repeatedly without success. Conferred with Dr. Lynch. Patient must remain on bed rest after spinal surgery. Dr. Lynch here to assess patient; ordered belt restraint for next 24 hours.

2030 Belt restraint applied around waist. Patient able to breathe deeply without restriction. Skin under restraint is intact, without redness. Patient able to move extremities. Initiating observations of patient q 15 min. Instructed patient and spouse on purpose of device. Family members at bedside.

Special Considerations
Pediatric

- Limit the use of restraints to clinically appropriate and adequately justified situations (e.g., examination or treatment involving head and neck).
- When a child needs to be restrained for a procedure, it is best that the person applying the restraint not be the child's parent or guardian.
- When an infant or small child requires a short-term restraint for treatment or examination, a papoose board with straps or a mummy wrap using a blanket or sheet effectively controls movements (Hockenberry and Wilson, 2012).
- Stay with a restrained infant and remove the restraint immediately after treatment is complete.

Geriatric

- Restrained older adults often respond with anger, fear, depression, humiliation, demoralization, discomfort, and resignation.

- Consider the risks associated with restraints (e.g., pressure ulcers, impaired strength) for older adults (Touhy and Jett, 2014). Complications of immobility are amplified, leading to greater chance for functional decline.

SKILL 4.4   SEIZURE PRECAUTIONS

A seizure is a sudden, electrical discharge in the brain causing alterations in behavior, sensation, or consciousness. Seizures that appear to begin everywhere in the brain at once are classified as generalized seizures, whereas seizures beginning in one location of the brain are classified as partial seizures (Johns Hopkins Medicine, 2013). There are three phases to a seizure:

- **Aura**—the start of a partial seizure. If the aura is the only phase a patient experiences, the patient has had a simple partial seizure. If the seizure spreads and affects consciousness, it is known as a complex partial seizure. If the seizure spreads to the rest of the brain, it is classified as a generalized seizure.
- **Ictus**—meaning *attack*, ictus is another word for the physical seizure involving a series of muscle contractions, called tonic and clonic contractions.
- **Postictal**—meaning *after the attack*, postictal refers to the aftereffects of the seizure (e.g., arm numbness, loss of consciousness, partial paralysis).

Status epilepticus involves 5 minutes or more of either continuous clinical or electrographic (shown on an electroencephalogram [EEG]) seizure activity or recurrent seizure activity without recovery between seizures (Brophy et al., 2012). It is a medical emergency. Status epilepticus can be convulsive (shown by rhythmic jerking of the extremities) or nonconvulsive (seizure activity shown on an EEG).

Seizure precautions are guidelines that health care providers follow to minimize injury to a patient during any type of seizure. Observation during a seizure is critical. Observe a patient carefully before, during, and after a seizure so that the episode can be documented accurately. Careful observation may help to determine the type of seizure. Your role as a nurse is to protect a patient from harm, assess cardiopulmonary effects, assist with airway management if indicated, and administer antiseizure medications as ordered.

Traditionally, patients who have a partial or mild generalized seizure are immediately placed in the side-lying position to prevent aspiration of oral secretions; this is still a standard of practice. However, more recent findings suggest that in the case of patients who go into status epilepticus, the side-lying position may cause more harm than good (Cherian and Thomas, 2009). Patients who have been rolled onto their side during a major motor seizure are at greater risk for self-injury, such as a dislocated shoulder. Because patients do not breathe during a generalized tonic-clonic seizure, they are not at high risk for aspiration until the event ends. Patients usually take a deep breath immediately after such a seizure and should be rolled over onto their side immediately after the motor activity ceases (Cherian and Thomas, 2009). Refer to your facility policy for positioning guidelines.

The Neurocritical Care Society released practice guidelines for patients with status epilepticus. Within the first 2 minutes, establishing and protecting the airway when a patient loses consciousness is a priority. Noninvasive airway protection and gas exchange with head positioning should be done immediately, keeping the airway patent and administering oxygen. When the seizure begins to subside, intubation (insertion of an artificial airway) should be attempted only if gas exchange is compromised or if the patient is believed to have increased intracranial pressure (Brophy et al., 2012).

ASSESSMENT

1. Assess patient's seizure history, knowledge of precipitating factors (e.g., emotional stress, sleep deprivation, tiredness), frequency of seizures, presence of aura (e.g., metallic taste, perception of breeze blowing on face, noxious odor), body parts affected, and sequence of events if known. Confer with family caregiver. *Rationale: Information about seizure enables nurse to anticipate onset of seizure activity.*

2. Assess for medical and surgical conditions, including history of head trauma, electrolyte disturbances (e.g., hypoglycemia, hyperkalemia), and heart disease; excessive fatigue; and alcohol or caffeine use. *Rationale: These factors are common conditions that precipitate seizures.*

3. Assess medication history (e.g., antidepressants and antipsychotics). Assess the patient's adherence to anticonvulsants, and note the therapeutic drug levels if test results are available. *Rationale: Seizure medications must be taken as prescribed and not stopped suddenly. Stopping or changing doses may precipitate a seizure.*

4. Assess patient's environment for potential safety hazards (e.g., extra furniture). Keep bed in low position, with side rails up at head of bed.

5. Assess patient's cultural perspective about the meaning of seizures and their treatment. *Rationale: Some cultures follow different caring practices for a person with seizures.*

PLANNING

Expected Outcomes focus on maintenance of self-esteem and prevention of injury, airway obstruction, and aspiration.

1. Patient does not sustain traumatic physical injury during a seizure.

2. Patient's airway is patent during seizure activity.

3. Patient verbalizes positive self-feelings after a seizure episode.

Delegation and Collaboration

Assessment of patient's risk for seizures cannot be delegated. However, the skills for making a patient's environment safe and care of patients on seizure precautions can be delegated to nursing assistive personnel (NAP). The nurse instructs the NAP about:

- The patient's prior seizure history and factors that may trigger a seizure.
- Taking immediate action in the event of a seizure by protecting the patient from falling or injury, not attempting to restrain the patient, and not placing anything in the patient's mouth.
- Informing the registered nurse immediately when seizure activity develops.
- Observing the patient's seizure pattern.

Equipment

- Seizure pads for side rails and headboard
- Suction machine and Yankauer suction catheter
- Oral airway
- Oxygen via nasal cannula or face mask
- IV insertion equipment: 0.9% normal saline infusion
- Emergency antiepileptic medications: For emergent condition, IV lorazepam, midazolam for intramuscular administration (also can be given nasally or bucally), diazepam for rectal administration. For urgent treatment, oral valproate sodium or phenytoin; IV midazolam (Brophy et al., 2012)
- Clean gloves
- Equipment for vital signs, pulse oximetry, and blood glucose testing

IMPLEMENTATION *for* SEIZURE PRECAUTIONS

STEPS	RATIONALE
1. **See Standard Protocol (inside front cover).**	
2. For patient with a history of seizures, keep bed in lowest position with side rails up (see facility policy). Have side rails padded. Have oral suction and oxygen equipment ready at bedside.	Modifications to the environment minimize risk of injury during seizure activity. Oral suctioning may be required after a seizure to prevent aspiration of secretions.
3. Patient with a history of seizures should be in hospital room close to nurse's station or room with video monitor.	This improves the likelihood of quick response in an emergency.
4. *Partial or general seizure response*	
a. Position patient safely.	This position protects patient from aspiration and traumatic injury, especially head injury.
(1) If patient is standing or sitting, guide patient to floor and protect head by cradling in your lap or placing pillow under head. Position patient so as to keep head tilted to maximize breathing (if able). Try to position patient on side, but do not force.	
(2) If patient is in bed, turn patient to side and raise side rails.	

> **SAFE PATIENT CARE** Patients who experience status epilepticus and who have been rolled onto their side may be at greater risk for self-injury. A patient should be rolled over onto his or her side immediately after the motor activity ceases (Cherian and Thomas, 2009).

STEPS	RATIONALE
b. Note time seizure began and call for help. Track duration of seizure. Have health care provider notified immediately. Have staff members bring emergency cart to bedside and clear area of furniture and unneeded equipment. Stay with patient.	The aim is to reduce exposure of patient to injury. Description of the seizure may help in ultimate identification of seizure type.
c. If possible, provide privacy. Have staff control flow of visitors in area.	
d. Keep patient in side-lying position, supporting head and keeping it flexed slightly forward.	This position prevents tongue from blocking airway and promotes drainage of secretions, reducing risk of aspiration.

Continued

STEPS	RATIONALE
e. Do not restrain. If patient is flailing limbs, hold them loosely. Loosen restrictive clothing or hospital gown.	This prevents musculoskeletal injury and airway obstruction.
f. *Do not force any objects into patient's mouth*, such as fingers, medicine, tongue depressor, or airway, when teeth are clenched.	This prevents injury to mouth and your hands.

> **SAFE PATIENT CARE** Injury can result from forcible insertion of a hard object into the mouth. **Never insert a tongue blade into a patient's mouth.** Soft objects break and become aspirated. Insert a bite-block or oral airway in advance if you recognize the onset of a generalized seizure, or insert an oral airway when the seizure has terminated to prevent airway obstruction.

STEPS	RATIONALE
g. Maintain patient's airway; suction orally as needed (using oral airway only). Otherwise, suction immediately after seizure. Provide oxygen if ordered. Check level of consciousness and oxygen saturation and perform a fingerstick to check blood glucose.	This prevents hypoxia during seizure activity. Seizures are often the result of severe hypoglycemia (Brophy et al., 2012).
h. Observe sequence and timing of seizure activity. Note type of seizure activity (tonic, clonic, staring, blinking), whether more than one type of seizure occurs, sequence of seizure progression, level of consciousness, character of breathing, presence of incontinence, and presence of autonomic signs (e.g., lip smacking, grimacing).	These observations assist in accurate documentation, diagnosis, and eventual treatment of seizure.
5. *Status epilepticus is a medical emergency.*	
a. Call health care provider and rapid response team immediately.	Rapid response teams are prepared for emergencies.
b. Establish noninvasive airway protection and gas exchange with head positioning. Protect patient as much as possible from injury (supporting head and neck).	Patients do not breathe during a generalized tonic-clonic seizure. It is most important to have a patent airway after convulsions (postictal).
c. Assist health care provider with intubation (introduction of endotracheal tube or oral airway) if oxygen saturation is compromised or elevated intracranial pressure is suspected (see Chapter 29) (**Note:** Apply clean gloves if timing allows) (Brophy et al., 2012). Administer oxygen as ordered.	

> **SAFE PATIENT CARE** Do not place your fingers in the patient's mouth. The patient may accidentally bite your fingers during the seizure. Do not force any type of airway into the patient's mouth.

STEPS	RATIONALE
d. Access oxygen and suction equipment, continuing to keep airway patent.	The aim is to maintain oxygenation.
e. Be sure someone from nursing staff or emergency response team is measuring patient's blood pressure, heart rate, and oxygen saturation and has performed a fingerstick.	It is important to establish and support baseline vital signs and determine if patient is hypoglycemic (common cause of seizure) (Brophy and others, 2012).
f. Perform hand hygiene and apply clean gloves. Prepare for insertion of IV line if saline lock or catheter is not in place. Patient usually receives 0.9% sodium chloride. Assist health care provider in administration of any antiepileptic IV medications either as a bolus or loading dose (see Chapter 23).	IV line establishes route for medications to stop or control seizure activity and to provide hydration.

STEPS	RATIONALE
g. After seizure, suction the patient's airway if secretions have accumulated. If oral airway was inserted, be sure it remains in correct position. Continue oxygen administration.	This maintains oxygenation.
h. Keep patient in side-lying position of comfort in bed with side rails up and bed in lowest position. Place call light in reach.	This position provides for continued safety to reduce risk of aspiration of secretions as patient regains consciousness.
6. As patient regains consciousness, reorient and reassure. Explain what happened and provide a quiet, nonstimulating environment. Foster an atmosphere of acceptance, and give time for patient to express feelings.	Patient may awaken confused and drowsy. Patients who accept the reality of a disease and integrate this into their own self-concept have higher levels of self-esteem.
7. Apply side rail pads or safety bumpers to bed side rails or head of bed or both.	Padding may reduce risk for traumatic injury from future seizures. Do not use pillows to pad side rails because they pose a suffocation risk.
8. See Completion Protocol (inside front cover).	

EVALUATION

1. Check vital signs and oxygen saturation every 15 minutes after convulsion phase. It may also be necessary to check blood glucose (per physician order).
2. Examine patient for injury, including oral cavity (broken teeth, laceration of tongue or mucosa) and extremities.

> **SAFE PATIENT CARE** If onset of the seizure was not witnessed and you suspect that the patient fell and struck his or her head, treat as a closed head injury or spinal injury. Apply a cervical collar before turning or repositioning the patient.

3. Evaluate patient's mental status and orientation after seizure.
4. Ask patient to verbalize his or her feelings after the seizure.

Unexpected Outcomes and Related Interventions

1. Patient sustains a traumatic injury.
   a. Continue to protect patient from further injury.
   b. Notify health care provider immediately.
   c. Administer treatment for injury.
   d. Ensure that the environment is free of additional safety hazards.
2. Patient aspirates oral secretions.
   a. Turn patient onto his or her side, insert oral airway (if possible), and apply suction to remove material in oral pharynx. Maintain a patent airway.
   b. Administer oxygen as needed.

Recording and Reporting

- Record timing of seizure activity, sequence of events, presence of aura (if any), level of consciousness, posture, color, movements of extremities, incontinence, and patient's status (physical and emotional) immediately after seizure.
- Report to health care provider immediately as seizure begins. Status epilepticus is an emergency.

Sample Documentation

1000   Observed patient sitting in chair in room. Cry heard; patient observed sliding to floor, not responding to verbal stimuli. Patient assisted to floor with head supported. Pillow placed under head. Tonic and clonic movements of all four extremities noted, lasting 2 minutes. No cyanosis noted; respiratory pattern slightly irregular. No incontinence noted. At conclusion of tonic and clonic movements, positioned patient on side, airway clear. Blood pressure 142/90, heart rate 96, respirations 20 per minute and regular, oxygen saturation 95%, blood glucose 108.

1020   Patient slept for 20 minutes; now awake and alert; oriented to name, date, and place. Requested nurse describe sequence of events. Stated that this was his "usual type of seizure."

Special Considerations
Pediatric

- Teach parents what to observe for in their child's seizures.
- Child should wear a medical alert bracelet.
- Encourage children with severe atonic seizures (seizures that produce an abrupt loss of muscle tone, also called a drop attack) to wear helmets.

Geriatric

- Older adults may have symptoms such as confusion lasting several days, receptive and expressive speech problems, and unusual behaviors that may make it difficult to recognize a seizure.
- Older adults metabolize anticonvulsants more slowly; drugs accumulate and cause toxicity. Monitor therapeutic blood levels of drugs closely (Meiner, 2011).
- Do not try to remove dentures during a seizure. If dentures loosen, tilt head slightly forward and remove after seizure.

Home Care

- See Box 4-2 for seizure precautions in the home setting.

PROCEDURAL GUIDELINE 4.1
Fire, Electrical, and Chemical Safety

Fires in health care settings are typically electrical or anesthetic related. Although smoking is not allowed in health care facilities, smoking-related fires continue to pose a significant risk because of unauthorized smoking in beds or bathrooms. Prevention is the key to fire safety. Nursing measures include complying with facility smoking policies, using equipment correctly, and keeping combustible materials away from heat sources. If a fire occurs, report the exact location of the fire, contain it, and extinguish it only if it is safe to do so. All personnel help to evacuate patients when needed. Most facilities have fire doors that are held open by magnets and close automatically when a fire alarm sounds. Fire doors should never be blocked.

Health care facilities routinely check and maintain all electrical devices. Every biomedical device (e.g., suction machine, infusion pump, cardiac monitor) must have a safety inspection sticker with an expiration date applied to it. Electrical equipment in good working order requires a three-prong electrical plug for proper grounding. Generally, patients are discouraged from bringing electrical devices to a health care facility. If a patient brings a device, it must be inspected for safe wiring and function before use through the process established by the facility. Many patients with disabilities use battery charges for mobility equipment. These devices also need to be inspected by hospital engineers.

Chemicals in medications (e.g., chemotherapy drugs), anesthetic gases, disinfectants, and cleaning solutions are potentially toxic. They injure the body after skin or mucous membrane contact, after ingestion, or when vapors are inhaled. Health care facilities provide employees access to material safety data sheets (MSDSs) for each hazardous chemical in the workplace (OSHA, 2012). An MSDS form contains information about properties of the chemical (e.g., melting point, boiling point, flash point), toxicity, health effects, first aid, reactivity, safe handling, storage, disposal, protective equipment to use, and procedure for handling a spill.

Delegation and Collaboration

The skill of fire, electrical, radiation, and chemical safety can be delegated to nursing assistive personnel (NAP). A nurse leads the health care team in an emergency response. In the event of fire, the nurse works in collaboration with the fire department. In the event of a radioactive or chemical event, the nurse works in collaboration with the appropriate safety officer.

Equipment

Fire
- Appropriate fire extinguisher for fire: type A, B, C, or ABC

Chemical
- Appropriate personal protective equipment (e.g., clean gloves, gown, mask)
- MSDS form

Procedural Steps

1. Review facility policies regularly for rapid response to fire, electrical, and chemical emergency. Know your responsibilities, such as initiating fire alarm and patient evacuation.
2. Know the location of fire alarms, emergency equipment (e.g., fire extinguishers), MSDS forms, emergency eyewash stations, and exit routes.
3. Assess patient's mental status and ability to ambulate, transfer, or move to anticipate procedure that will be needed to evacuate patient.
4. Be alert to situations that increase the risk for fire. For example, a patient on oxygen is charging his cell phone in the bed. Regularly check room for fire or electrical hazards.
5. Know which patients are on oxygen. Oxygen delivery is shut off in the event of a severe fire.
6. Know the location of current patients on the unit and list of patients who are off the unit.
7. Inspect equipment for current maintenance sticker. Check electrical equipment for basic safety features (e.g., intact cords and plugs, intact casing). Know facility process for tagging and reporting broken or unsafe equipment.
8. *Fire safety (follow the acronym RACE):*
   a. *R*escue the patient from immediate injury by removing from area or shielding from fire to avoid burns.
   b. *A*ctivate the fire alarm immediately. Follow facility policy for alerting staff to respond. (In many situations, perform Steps a and b simultaneously by using the call system to alert staff while you help patients at risk.)
   c. *C*ontain the fire by (1) closing all doors and windows, (2) turning off oxygen and electrical equipment, and (3) placing wet towels along base of doors.
   d. *E*vacuate patients.
      (1) Direct ambulatory patients to walk by themselves to a safe area. Know the fire exits and emergency evacuation route.
      (2) Move bedridden patients by stretcher, bed, or wheelchair.
      (3) If patient is on life support, maintain respiratory status manually (Ambu bag) until he or she is removed from fire area.
      (4) For patients who cannot walk or ambulate, use the following options:
         (a) Place on blanket and drag out of area.

PROCEDURAL GUIDELINE 4.1
Fire, Electrical, and Chemical Safety—cont'd

(b) Use two-person swing: Place patient in sitting position and have two staff members form a seat by clasping forearms together (see illustration). Lift patient into "seat" and carry out of area of danger (see illustration).

> **SAFE PATIENT CARE** Consider the patient's weight and size when choosing an evacuation carry. Use safe patient-handling techniques. Have a staff member assist to avoid injury.

(c) Extinguish fire using appropriate fire extinguisher: type A for ordinary combustibles (e.g., wood, cloth, paper, most plastics), type B for flammable liquids (e.g., gasoline, grease, anesthetic gas); type C for electrical equipment, and type ABC for any type of fire.
(1) To use extinguisher, follow the acronym *PASS*:
  (a) *P*ull the pin (see illustration *A*).
  (b) *A*im nozzle at base of fire.
  (c) *S*queeze extinguisher handles (see illustration *B*).
  (d) *S*weep from side to side to coat area evenly (see illustration *C*).
9. *Electrical safety*
  a. If a person receives an electrical shock, immediately turn off power to electrical source and assess for presence of a pulse. Caution: When disengaging electrical source, check for presence of water on the floor.

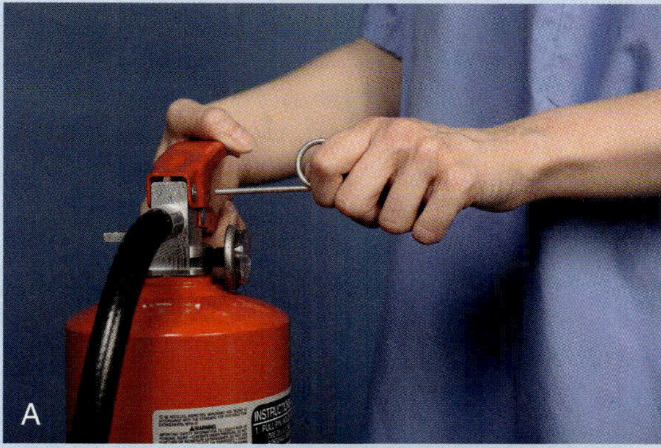

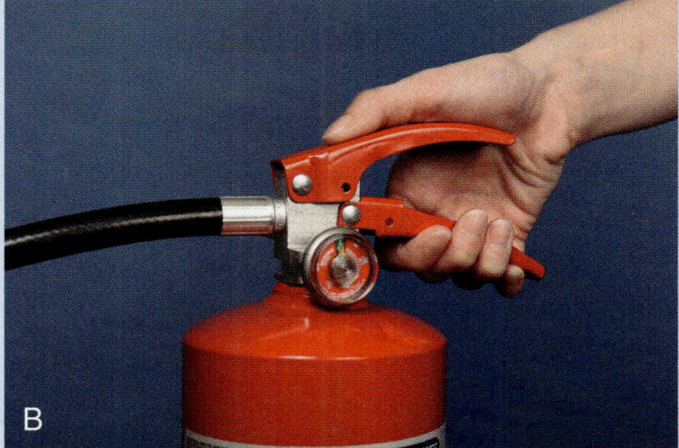

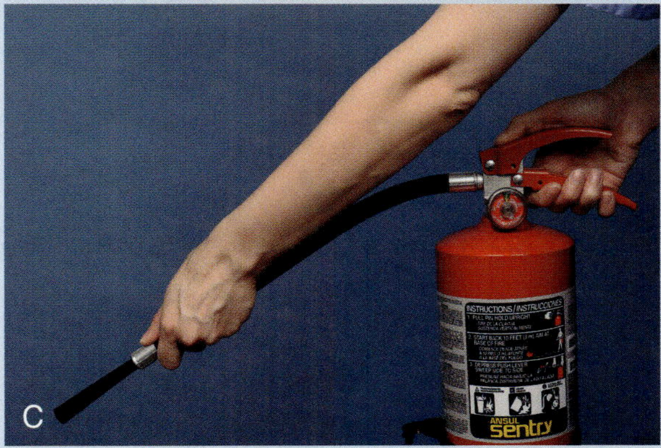

STEP 8d(4)(c)(1) A, Pull safety pin from fire extinguisher. **B,** Aim nozzle of hose at base of fire. **C,** Squeeze handle while sweeping side to side with nozzle.

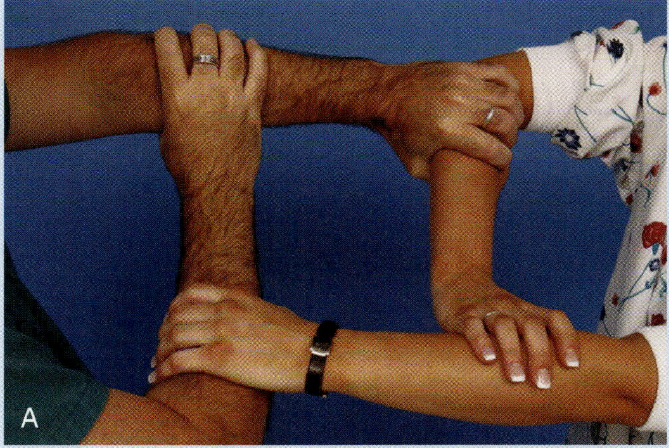

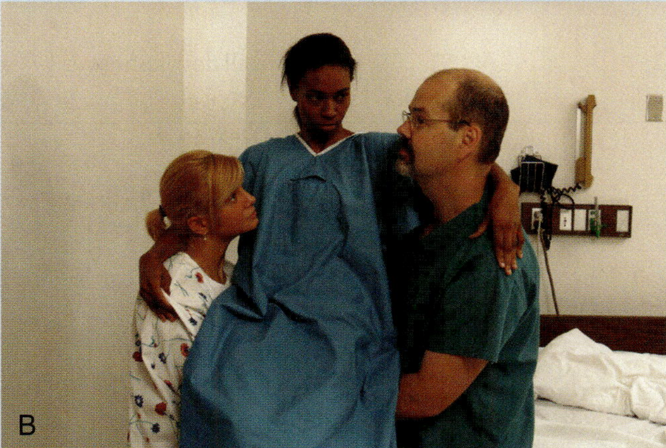

STEP 8d(4)b A, Hands positioned to form two-person evacuation swing. **B,** Patient seated firmly on swing and holding shoulders of nurses for evacuation.

Continued

PROCEDURAL GUIDELINE 4.1
Fire, Electrical, and Chemical Safety—cont'd

SAFE PATIENT CARE Do not touch a person who is being shocked while he or she is still engaged with the source of electricity. If unable to disconnect source, call emergency number for assistance.

b. Once the source of electricity is disconnected, intervene on the person's behalf. If the patient is pulseless, institute emergency resuscitation (see Chapter 29).

c. Notify emergency personnel and the patient's health care provider.

d. If patient has a pulse and remains alert and oriented, obtain vital signs and assess the skin for signs of thermal injury.

10. *Chemical safety*

a. Attend to any person exposed to a chemical. Treat chemical splashes to eyes immediately; flush eyes with water using clean, lukewarm tap water for 15 to 20 minutes; stand under a shower or place head under running faucet. Remove contact lenses if flushing does not remove them (see Chapter 11).

b. Notify persons in the immediate spill area, and evacuate all nonessential personnel from area.

c. Refer to MSDS, and if spilled material is flammable, turn off electrical and heat sources.

d. Avoid breathing vapors of spilled material; apply appropriate respirator.

e. Use appropriate personal protective equipment (refer to MSDS) to clean up spill.

f. Dispose of any materials used in cleanup as hazardous waste.

11. Follow facility policy for reporting a sentinel event. Documentation would likely be made as a sentinel event report and not in nurses' notes.

Box 4-2 HOME SAFETY

Bathroom Safety

A person who has seizures may want to shower instead of bathe to avoid accidental drowning.

- If falls usually occur during a seizure, use a shower seat, preferably one with a safety strap.
- Use nonskid strips in the shower or tub.
- Never use electrical equipment near water to prevent accidental electrocution.
- Consider changing glass in shower doors to shatterproof glass.

Kitchen Safety

A seizure that occurs when a person is cooking could cause injury from a burn or infliction of sharp objects.

- If possible, cook when someone else is nearby.
- Use the back burners of the stove to prevent accidental burns.
- Use shatterproof containers as much as possible. For instance, sauces can be transferred from glass bottles to plastic containers for use.
- Limit time that is required using knives or other sharp objects. If possible, buy foods that are already cut, or ask someone to help in meal preparation.

General Safety

The home environment can be made safer for a person who has seizures.

- Wear a bracelet or carry an identification card noting existing seizure disorder and medications taken.
- Do not smoke or light fires in the fireplace unless someone else is present.
- When alone, avoid using step stools or ladders, and do not clean rooftop gutters.
- Use power tools and motorized lawn equipment that have a safety switch that stops the machine if you release the handle (a "dead man's" switch).

Adapted from Columbia Comprehensive Epilepsy Center, Columbia University (2012).

▮ CRITICAL THINKING EXERCISES

Case Study

A nurse is making rounds on her patients. She walks into a room to find there is a fire in the patient's wastebasket. The patient had surgery the previous day and has been up only once to ambulate. The other patient in the room is scheduled for discharge and is currently in the bathroom.

1. Given this situation, what is the first step the nurse should take?
   1. Activate the fire alarm in the outside hallway.
   2. Contain the fire by placing a wet towel over the waste basket.
   3. Transfer the patient who has not ambulated regularly to a wheelchair quickly and remove the patient from the room.
   4. Evacuate all patients from the patient care unit.

2. The nurse returns to the room after being sure the patient in the wheelchair and the patient in the bathroom have been safely moved to an area down the hall near the floor exit. The nurse returns to the room to try to contain the fire. What is the first step for containing a fire?
   1. Close all doors and windows in the room.
   2. Turn off any oxygen.
   3. Place wet towels along base of doors.
   4. Turn off electrical IV pump.

Review Questions

1. A nurse's co-worker is standing in some spilled water holding the refrigerator door. He is being electrocuted. What is the first thing the nurse should do?
   1. Take his vital signs.
   2. Call the rapid response team.
   3. Unplug the refrigerator.
   4. Wipe up the water from the floor.

2. A nurse is assessing a patient who is just entering the hospital. The patient is 70 years old and reports that she fell a month ago at home but did not sustain an injury. Which of the following would the nurse assess about the previous fall? Select all that apply.
   1. The medications the patient is currently taking
   2. The location of the fall in the home
   3. The patient's medical conditions
   4. The activity the patient was engaged in just before the fall
   5. Whether the patient had dizziness or a sense of weakness just before falling

3. The nurse enters a patient's room. The patient is standing at the sink and begins to actively seize. The patient is having a partial seizure. Which of the following should the nurse initiate first?
   1. Observe sequence and timing of seizure.
   2. Call for help.
   3. Guide the patient to the floor and protect the head.
   4. Suction the mouth of any secretions.
   5. Insert an oral airway into the patient's mouth.

4. Place the following steps for performing the timed "get up and go" (TGUG) test in the correct order.
   1. Look for unsteadiness in patient's gait.
   2. Instruct patient to walk 10 feet, turn around, and walk back to chair.
   3. Have patient rise from sitting position without using chair arms for support.
   4. Have patient return to chair and sit down.

5. The nurse is making rounds on a patient with wrist restraints. It has been 2 hours since the last rounds for this patient. Which of the following will the nurse do? Select all that apply.
   1. Release the restraints for ROM exercises.
   2. Assess the extremity for perfusion and skin integrity.
   3. Offer toileting.
   4. Offer a drink of water.

6. Which of the following describes how a culture of safety is practiced on a nursing unit?
   1. A nurse uses a standardized checklist to observe a patient care technician performing skills.
   2. A nurse completes an annual continuing education requirement on how to report a sentinel event.
   3. A nurse observes another nurse not performing hand hygiene before starting to insert an IV catheter and points out the omission.
   4. A nurse reviews the policy and procedure manual for how to administer a tube feeding.

7. A patient on a medical unit tends to wander. Sometimes the patient forgets where she is. She likes to go down the stairs and outside. What can the nurse do to avoid restraining her? Select all that apply.
   1. Schedule walks throughout her day.
   2. Offer a diversional activity.
   3. Move her to a room close to the nurses' station.
   4. Notify the police that she may be found wandering outside.

8. A nurse working in a home health facility is collaborating with other nurses to develop a fall prevention program for patients in the community. Using evidence from the literature on fall prevention, the nurses would likely include which of the following strategies?
   1. Developing a recommended set of diversional activities for patients to use in the home
   2. Conducting a standard vision assessment when visiting patients the first time
   3. Developing guidelines for using restraints for persons with dementia
   4. Instituting the use of the Revised Algase Wandering Scale (RAWS)

9. A nurse enters a patient's room, finds the patient asleep, and notices sparks and fire coming from an electrical outlet. The patient is in traction for fractures to the legs. Place the following steps for the nurse's response to the fire in their correct order.
   _____ 1. Contain the fire by turning off all oxygen in the room.
   _____ 2. Rescue the patient by moving the bed away from the outlet.
   _____ 3. Alert a staff member to activate the fire alarm.
   _____ 4. Evacuate the patient from the room.

10. Which of the following behaviors demonstrates Quality and Safety Education for Nurses (QSEN) skills for safety competency? Select all that apply.
    1. During rounds on three different patients, you use your memory to recall which patient needs to get an analgesic in the next 30 minutes.
    2. You place a patient on a new bed alarm system without having attended an in-service on the system.
    3. You follow evidence guidelines in your assessment of a patient's fall risk.
    4. During a change of shift report you include a fall occurrence involving a patient for whom you cared.

REFERENCES

Agency for Healthcare Research and Quality: *Patient safety primers: safety culture*, 2012, http://psnet.ahrq.gov/primer.aspx?primerID=5. Accessed May 12, 2014.

Allan-Gibbs R: Falls and hospitalized patients with cancer: a review of the literature, *Clin J Oncol Nurs* 14(6):784, 2010.

Aranda-Gallardo M, et al: Instruments for assessing the risk of falls in acute hospitalized patients: a systematic review and meta-analysis, *BMC Health Serv Rev* 13(1):122, 2013.

Beer C, et al: Quality use of medicines and health outcomes among a cohort of community dwelling older men: an observational study, *Br J Clin Pharmacol* 71(4):592, 2011.

BMJ-British Medical Journal: Fear of falling linked to future falls in older people, *ScienceDaily* 2010. http://www.sciencedaily.com. Accessed October 20, 2013.

Brophy GM, et al: Guidelines for the evaluation and management of status epilepticus, *Neurocrit Care* 17(1):3, 2012.

Centers for Medicare and Medicaid Services (CMS), Department of Health and Human Services: *Revisions to Medicare conditions of participation, 37*, Bethesda, MD, 2008, U.S. Department of Health and Human Services.

Centers for Medicare and Medicaid Services (CMS), Department of Health and Human Services: Medicare and Medicaid programs; reform of hospital and critical access hospital conditions of participation, *Fed Reg* 76(205):2011.

Chang CM, et al: Medical conditions and medications as risk factors of falls in inpatient older people: a case-controlled study, *Int J Geriatr Psychiatry* 26(6):602, 2011.

Cherian A, Thomas SV: Status epilepticus, *Ann Indian Acad Neurol* 12(3):140, 2009.

Columbia Comprehensive Epilepsy Center: *Seizure precautions*, New York, 2012, Columbia University Medical Center. Available at: http://www.columbiaepilepsy.org/patient-education/seizure-precautions.html. Accessed May 12, 2014.

de Kam D, et al: Exercise interventions to reduce fall-related fractures and their risk factors in individuals with low bone density: a systematic review of randomized controlled trials, *Osteoporos Int* 20(12):2111, 2009.

Department of Health and Human Services: *Adverse events in hospitals: methods for identifying events*, 2010, http://oig.hhs.gov/oei/reports/oei-06-08-00221.pdf. Accessed May 12, 2014.

Department of Health and Human Services, Centers for Medicaid and Medicare Services: *Interpretive guidelines for hospitals, 482.13(e) Standard: restraint or seclusion*, 2008, Available at http://www.cms.gov/Regulations-and-Guidance/Guidance/Transmittals/downloads/R37SOMA.pdf. Accessed May 12, 2014.

Futrell M, et al: Evidence-based guideline: wandering, *J Gerontol Nurs* 36(6):40, 2010.

Gribbin J, et al: Risk of falls associated with antihypertensive medication: population-based case-control study, *Age Ageing* 39(5):592, 2010.

Harding A: Observation assistants: sitter effectiveness and industry measures, *Nurs Econ* 28(5):330, 2010.

Health Services Advisory Group: *White Paper on chemical restraint use*, Phoenix, AZ, 2012, Health Services Advisory Group. Available at: http://www.cdph.ca.gov/programs/LnC/Documents/CAHPS-HSAG-White-Paper-Chemical-Restraint-Use-Final.pdf. Accessed May 12, 2014.

Hockenberry MJ, Wilson D: *Wong's nursing care of infants and children*, ed 9, St Louis, 2011, Mosby.

Hockenberry MJ, Wilson D: *Wong's essentials of pediatric nursing*, ed 9, St Louis, 2012, Mosby.

Institute for Healthcare Improvement: *Patient safety*, 2014a, http://www.ihi.org/explore/patientsafety/Pages/default.aspx. Accessed May 12, 2014.

Institute for Healthcare Improvement: *Evidence-based care bundles*, 2014b. http://www.ihi.org/explore/bundles/Pages/default.aspx. Accessed May 12, 2014.

Institute of Medicine: *Announcement: crossing the quality chasm: The IOM Health Care Quality Initiative*, 2013, http://www.iom.edu/Global/News%20Announcements/Crossing-the-Quality-Chasm-The-IOM-Health-Care-Quality-Initiative.aspx. Accessed May 12, 2014.

Johns Hopkins Medicine: *Neurology and neurosurgery: seizures*, 2013, http://www.hopkinsmedicine.org/neurology_neurosurgery/specialty_areas/epilepsy/seizures/index.html. Accessed May 12, 2014.

Kojima T, et al: Association of polypharmacy with fall risk among geriatric outpatients, *Geriatr Gerontol Int* 11(4):438, 2011.

McCabe DE, et al: Perceptions of physical restraints use in the elderly among registered nurses and nurse assistants in a single acute care hospital, *Geriatr Nurs* 32(1):39, 2011.

Meiner SE: *Gerontologic nursing*, ed 4, St Louis, 2011, Mosby.

Nadler-Moodie M, et al: A S.A.F.E. alternative to sitters, *Nurs Manage* 40(8):43, 2009.

National Quality Forum (NQF): *National voluntary consensus standards for public reporting of patient safety events*, 2011, http://www.qualityforum.org/Publications/2011/02/National_Voluntary_Consensus_Standards_for_Public_Reporting_of_Patient_Safety_Event_Information.aspx. Accessed May 9, 2014.

National Quality Forum (NQF): *Safe practices for better healthcare—2/2013 Update, Healthcare Facilities Accreditation Program*, 2013, http://www.hfap.org/pdf/patient_safety.pdf. Accessed May 12, 2014.

Nelson AL, Algase DL: *Evidence-based protocols for managing wandering behavior*, New York, 2007, Springer Publishing.

North American Nursing Diagnosis Association (NANDA) International: *Nursing diagnoses: definitions and classification 2012-2014*, Oxford, 2012, Wiley-Blackwell.

Occupational Safety and Health Administration (OSHA): *Recommended format for Material Safety Data Sheets (MSDSs)*, 2012, https://www.osha.gov/Publications/OSHA3514.pdf Accessed May 9, 2014.

Oliver D, Healey F, Haines TP: Preventing falls and fall-related injuries in hospitals, *Clin Geriatr Med* 26(4):645, 2010.

Park M, Tang J: Changing the practice of physical restraint use in acute care, *J Gerontol Nurs* 33(2):9, 2007.

Quality and Safety Education for Nurses (QSEN), 2011, http://www.qsen.org. Accessed May 12, 2014.

Rossi SM: Tips for improving manager hand-off communication, *Nurs Manage* 40(12):50, 2009.

Schubert TE: Evidence-based exercise prescription for balance and falls prevention: a current review of the literature, *J Geriatr Phys Ther* 34(3):100, 2011.

The Joint Commission (TJC): *Provision of care, treatment, and services: restraint/seclusion for hospitals that use TJC for deemed status purposes*, Chicago, 2009, TJC.

The Joint Commission (TJC): *Comprehensive accreditation manual for hospitals: the official handbook*, Oakbrook Terrace, IL, 2012a, The Commission.

The Joint Commission (TJC): *Revisions to deeming requirements for hospitals*, 2012b, http://www.jointcommission.org/assets/1/18/PREPUB-08-27-2012-HAP-deeming.pdf. Accessed October 20, 2013.

The Joint Commission (TJC): *Sentinel Event Policy and Procedures*, 2013a, http://www.jointcommission.org/Sentinel_Event_Policy_and_Procedures/. Accessed May 9, 2014.

The Joint Commission (TJC): *Sentinel event*, Oakbrook Terrace, IL, 2013b, The Commission. Available at: http://www.jointcommission.org/sentinel_event.aspx. Accessed May 9, 2014.

The Joint Commission (TJC): *National Patient Safety Goals*, Oakbrook Terrace, IL, 2014, The Commission. Available at: http://www.jointcommission.org/standards_information/npsgs.aspx.

Touhy T, Jett K: *Ebersole and Hess' gerontological nursing and health care*, ed 4, St Louis, 2014, Mosby.

Tzeng HM: Understanding the prevalence of inpatient falls associated with toileting in adult acute care settings, *J Nurs Care Qual* 25(1):22, 2010.

VA National Center for Patient Safety: *VHA NCPS escape and elopement management*, 2010, http://www4.va.gov/ncps/CogAids/EscapeElope/index.html#page=page-13. Accessed February 11, 2010.

Infection Control

Infection prevention practices reduce or eliminate sources and transmission of infection that help to protect patients and health care providers from disease. A nurse's role is vital in the prevention and control of infection. Patients in all health care settings are at risk of becoming colonized or infected as a result of an impaired immune response, exposure to an increased number of pathogenic organisms, and performance of invasive procedures (Fardo, 2011). As a nurse, you are responsible for teaching patients and their families about the signs and symptoms of infections, modes of transmission, and methods of prevention.

Health care–associated infections (HAIs), formerly called *nosocomial infections,* are localized or systemic infections that were not present during admission to the facility (CDC, 2013c). HAIs account for an estimated 2 million infections, 99,000 deaths, and a direct medical cost to hospitals greater than $33 billion annually. Such infections are present in 1 of every 20 hospitalized patients (CDC, 2013b).

The presence of a pathogen does not mean that an infection will begin. An infection develops in a cyclical process called the *chain of infection,* which includes six elements: (1) an infectious agent or pathogen, (2) a reservoir or source for pathogen growth, (3) a portal of exit from the reservoir, (4) a method or mode of transmission, (5) a portal of entrance into the host, and (6) a susceptible host. An infection develops if the chain remains intact (Fig. 5-1). Nurses use infection control practices to break an element of the chain so infection will not be transmitted. A nurse's efforts to minimize the onset and spread of infection are based on asepsis and the principles of aseptic technique. The two types of aseptic techniques that a nurse practices are medical and surgical asepsis. The goals of these techniques are to create and maintain an environment that reduces or is absent of disease-producing organisms and to prevent the transfer of these organisms (Linton, 2012).

Medical asepsis, or clean technique, includes procedures used to reduce the number of and prevent the spread of microorganisms (Box 5-1). Hand hygiene, barrier techniques (e.g., use of gloves, mask and gown), and routine environmental cleaning are examples of medical asepsis. Surgical asepsis, or sterile technique, includes procedures used to eliminate all microorganisms from an area (Box 5-2). Nurses in the operating room, labor and delivery, and procedural areas practice sterile asepsis. Nurses also use surgical aseptic techniques at the patient's bedside in the following three situations:

1. During procedures that require intentional perforation of a patient's skin, such as insertion of an intravenous (IV) catheter
2. When the integrity of the skin is broken, such as applying a dressing over a surgical incision or burn
3. During procedures that involve insertion of devices or surgical instruments into normally sterile body cavities, such as insertion of a urinary catheter.

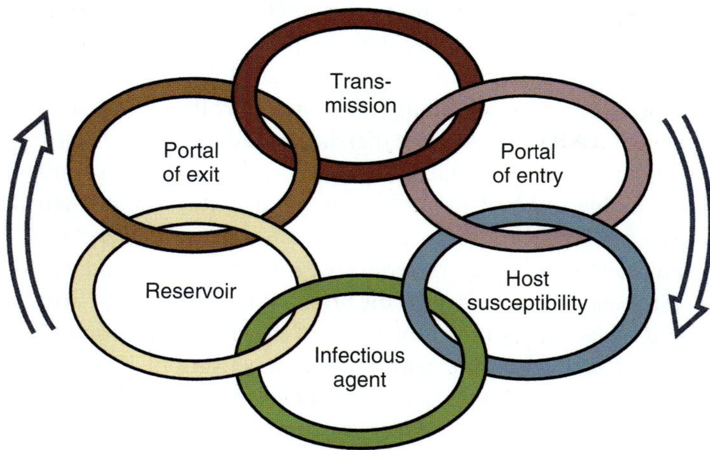

FIG 5-1 Chain of infection.

BOX 5-1	MEDICAL ASEPSIS PRINCIPLES

- Before and after patient contact perform hand hygiene with an appropriate hand antiseptic (e.g., chlorhexidine) or soap and water as an essential part of patient care and infection prevention.
- Always know a patient's susceptibility to infection. Age, nutritional status, stress, disease processes, and forms of medical therapy place patients at risk.
- Recognize the elements of the chain of infection, and initiate measures to prevent the onset and spread of infection.
- Consistently incorporate the basic principles of asepsis into patient care.
- Protect fellow health care workers from exposure to infectious agents through proper use and cleaning or disposal of equipment.
- Be aware of body sites where nosocomial infections are most likely to develop (e.g., urinary or respiratory tract); this enables you to direct preventive measures.

BOX 5-2	SURGICAL ASEPSIS PRINCIPLES

- All items used within a sterile field must be sterile.
- A sterile barrier that has been permeated by punctures, tears, or moisture must be considered contaminated.
- When a sterile package is opened, a 2.5-cm (1-inch) border around the edges is considered unsterile.
- Tables draped as part of a sterile field are considered sterile only at table level.
- If there is any question or doubt about the sterility of an item, the item is considered unsterile.
- Sterile persons or items contact only sterile items; unsterile persons or items contact only unsterile items.
- Movement around and in the sterile field must not compromise or contaminate the sterile field.
- A sterile object or field out of the range of vision or an object held below a person's waist is contaminated.
- A sterile object or field becomes contaminated by prolonged exposure to air; stay organized and complete any procedure as soon as possible.

PATIENT-CENTERED CARE

You are responsible for educating patients about why they are at risk for infection and ways to prevent infection. Patient and family teaching needs to include information concerning signs and symptoms of infection and modes of transmission (especially those in the home). Make your teaching relevant by explaining ways the patient and family caregiver can become involved in preventing infection. Your knowledge of the infectious process, disease transmission, and critical thinking skills associated with use of aseptic techniques and barrier protection is essential to be an effective educator.

When a patient requires isolation in a private room, loneliness can easily develop. Isolation disrupts normal social relationships with visitors and caregivers. Patient safety may be an additional risk for a patient on isolation precautions. Some patients who have an infectious disease also experience self-concept or body image changes. Be aware of the effects of isolation when you plan the time you spend in a patient's room. Give them and their family the opportunity to ask questions and express their concerns. Also be sensitive to a patient's perspective of what isolation means. For some, isolation of a loved one can be considered disrespectful and uncaring. Explain the purpose of isolation thoroughly and the implications when not followed.

In addition, know the cultural views and preferences of your patients. Many may choose to use herbs or other alternative therapies for treating illness and optimizing health (University of Minnesota, 2011).

SAFETY

The U.S. Centers for Disease Control and Prevention (CDC) have guidelines for the set of precautions known as *Standard Precautions* (CDC, 2010b). Part of the rationale for the development of Standard Precautions is that any patient may be a source for infection. Most microorganisms causing infections or disease are in colonized body substances of patients, regardless of whether a culture confirmed an infection and a diagnosis was made.

Body substances such as feces, urine, mucus, and wound drainage can contain potentially infectious organisms. All patients are at risk for carrying an infection, which requires health care workers to use Standard Precautions to prevent exposure. Fundamental to Standard Precautions is the use of barrier protection, which includes the use of personal protective equipment (PPE). Examples of PPE are gloves, masks, eyewear, and gowns to prevent contact of the skin and mucous membranes with blood and body substances (Phillips, 2013).

Barrier protection protects health care workers from patients' blood and body fluids and helps prevent the transfer of organisms to other patients, health care workers, and the environment. It is also an important technique for protecting patients who are immunosuppressed (e.g., patients receiving chemotherapy). The use of some form of PPE is indicated for all patients who potentially have an infection that can be transmitted to others, such as hepatitis B, acquired immuno-deficiency syndrome (AIDS), and tuberculosis (TB).

As a nurse, you help to ensure that all health care providers (e.g., respiratory therapists, physicians, other nurses) working with patients and support staff (e.g., housekeepers) maintain infection-prevention practices at all times; this applies to family members as well. When a hospitalized patient has an infection, a nurse decides on the optimal room placement to minimize the chances of infection spreading to other patients. In addition, two patients with "like" infections can be placed in the same room; this is called *cohorting*. Knowledgeable and judicious use of infection-prevention practices can make a difference as to whether a patient recovers from an illness or develops serious or fatal complications.

EVIDENCE-BASED PRACTICE

Centers for Disease Control and Prevention (CDC): Hand hygiene in health care settings, 2011, http://www.cdc.gov/handhygiene/Guidelines.html. Accessed September 17, 2014.

Centers for Disease Control and Prevention (CDC): Health-care associated infections: *Clostridium difficile,* 2013, http://www.cdc.gov/hai/organisms/cdiff/cdiff_infect. html. Accessed May 6, 2014.

Dubberke ER and Gerding DN: Rationale for hand hygiene recommendations after caring for a patient with *Clostridium difficile* infection, 2011, The Society for Healthcare Epidemiology of America, http://www.shea-online.org/Portals/0/CDI%20hand%20hygiene%20Update.pdf. Accessed May 6, 2014.

Edmonds S et al: Effectiveness of hand hygiene for removal of *Clostridium difficile* spores from hands, *Infect Control Hosp Epidemiol* 34(3):302, 2013.

Jabbar U et al: Effectiveness of alcohol-based hand rubs for removal of *Clostridium difficile* spores from hands, *Infect Control Hosp Epidemiol* 31(5):565, 2010.

A health care–associated infection caused by the germ C. difficile (C. diff) causes severe diarrhea linked to 14,000 American deaths each year (CDC, 2013). *Clostridium difficile* spores are highly resistant to antibiotics and disinfectants and can live for months in the environment. Several disinfectant products were tested to reduce *C. diff* and were compared with soap and tap water. Of the products tested, peracetic acid and surfactant formulation achieved significant reduction of *C. diff* through spore removal and deactivation. However, these results continue to be inferior to the use of soap and water for removing *C. diff* spores from the hands of health care workers working in an area where there has been an outbreak of *C. diff* (Edmonds et al., 2013; Jabbar et al., 2010; CDC, 2011). Hand hygiene with soap and water is not recommended for preventing *C. diff* in non-outbreak settings because no studies have found an increase in *C. diff* with the use of alcohol-based hand hygiene products or a decrease in *C. diff* with the use of soap and water.

- Soap and water is the most effective at removing *C. difficile* spores after caring for a patient with known *C. diff* (Dubberke and Gerding, 2011; Edmonds et al., 2013).
- Apply gloves before entering a room of a patient with *C. diff,* and remove gloves promptly after care.
- Use alcohol-based hand hygiene products for patient care in non-outbreak settings.
- Always perform hand hygiene before and after removing gloves.
- Proper hand hygiene techniques helps to protect other patients and health care workers.

SKILL 5.1   HAND HYGIENE

• **Nursing Skills Online: Infection Control, Lesson 2**

Hand hygiene is a general term that applies to four techniques: handwashing, antiseptic hand wash, antiseptic hand rub, and surgical hand antisepsis. Handwashing is the vigorous, brief rubbing together of all surfaces of the hands lathered in soap and water, followed by rinsing under a stream of water (CDC, 2011). An antiseptic hand wash involves washing hands with warm water and soap or a detergent containing an antiseptic agent. The use of antimicrobial soap (antiseptic) is recommended in certain health care settings. Antimicrobials effectively reduce bacterial counts on the hands and often have residual antimicrobial effects that last for several hours.

An antiseptic hand rub is an alcohol-based waterless product that, when applied to all surfaces of the hands, reduces the number of microorganisms on the hands. These alcohol-based foams or gels contain cosmetic emollients to prevent skin dryness. Alcohol-based hand antiseptics are not effective on visibly soiled hands (CDC, 2013a). Surgical hand antisepsis is an antiseptic hand wash or antiseptic hand rub that surgical personnel use before performing a surgical procedure (see Chapter 28).

The decision to perform hand hygiene depends on four factors: (1) the intensity or degree of contact with patients or contaminated objects, (2) the amount of contamination that may occur with the contact, (3) the patient's or health care worker's susceptibility to infection, and (4) the procedure or activity to be performed (Haas, 2011). *Hand hygiene is not an option.* It is a crucial responsibility of all health care workers. Follow these guidelines for hand hygiene (TJC, 2014; WHO, 2009; CDC, 2011):

1. When hands are visibly dirty, when soiled with blood or other body fluids, before eating, and after using the toilet, wash hands with either plain soap and water or an antimicrobial soap and water.
2. Wash hands with soap and water if exposed to spore-forming organisms such as *C. difficile* or *Bacillus anthracis.*
3. If hands are not visibly soiled, use an alcohol-based hand rub for routinely decontaminating hands in the following clinical situations:
   a. Before and after having direct contact with patients

b. Before applying sterile gloves and inserting an invasive device, such as an indwelling urinary catheter or peripheral vascular catheter

c. After contact with body fluids or excretions, mucous membranes, or nonintact skin

d. After contact with wound dressings (if hands are not visibly soiled)

e. When moving from a contaminated body site to a clean body site during patient care

f. After contact with inanimate objects (e.g., medical equipment) in the immediate vicinity of a patient

g. After removing gloves

ASSESSMENT

1. Inspect the surface of the hands for breaks or cuts in the skin or cuticles. Cover any skin lesions with a dressing before providing patient care. If lesions are too large to cover, you may be restricted from direct patient care. *Rationale: Open cuts or wounds can harbor high concentrations of microorganisms. Facility policy often prevents nurses from caring for high-risk patients if open lesions are present on hands.*

2. Note condition of your nails. Avoid artificial nails, extenders, and long or unkempt nails. Natural nail tips should be less than $\frac{1}{4}$ inch long. See facility policy. *Rationale: Subungual areas of the hand harbor high concentrations of bacteria. Long nails and chipped or old nail polish increase the number of bacteria residing on nails, requiring more vigorous hand hygiene. Artificial nails are not to be worn because they have shown high rates of infectious agents (Felembam, 2012).*

3. Inspect your hands for visible soiling. *Rationale: Visible soiling requires handwashing with soap and water.*

4. Consider the type of nursing activity being performed. The decision whether or not to use an antiseptic depends on the procedure that you will perform and the patient's immune status. *Rationale: The type of nursing activity determines the hand hygiene technique to use.*

PLANNING

Expected Outcomes focus on preventing the transmission of infection.

1. Hands and areas under fingernails are clean and free of debris.

Delegation and Collaboration

The skill of hand hygiene is performed by all caregivers. **Hand hygiene is not optional.**

Equipment

Handwashing

- Easy-to-reach sink with warm running water
- Antimicrobial or nonantimicrobial soap
- Paper towels or air dryer
- Disposable nail cleaner (optional)

Antiseptic Hand Rub

- Alcohol-based waterless antiseptic-containing emollient

IMPLEMENTATION *for* HAND HYGIENE

STEPS	RATIONALE
1. Be sure fingernails are short, filed, and smooth.	Many microorganisms on hands come from beneath the fingernails.
2. Push wristwatch and long uniform sleeves above wrists. Avoid wearing rings during surgical scrubs.	Provides best access to fingers, hands, and wrists. Wearing rings increases the number of microorganisms on hands (Longtin et al., 2011)
3. *Antiseptic hand rub* **a.** Following manufacturer's directions, dispense ample amount of product into palm of one hand (see illustration).	Use enough product to cover hands thoroughly.
b. Rub hands together, covering all surfaces of hands and fingers with antiseptic (see illustration).	Provides enough time for antimicrobial solution to work.
c. Rub hands together until antiseptic is dry. Allow hands to dry completely before applying gloves.	Removes transient organisms. Drying ensures complete antimicrobial action.
4. *Handwashing using regular or antimicrobial soap and water* **a.** Stand in front of sink, keeping hands and uniform away from sink surface. (If hands touch sink during handwashing, repeat steps.)	Inside of sink is a contaminated area. Reaching over sink increases risk of touching the edge, which is contaminated.
b. Turn on water. Turn faucet on or push knee pedals laterally to regulate flow and temperature.	Knee pedals within the operating room and treatment areas are preferred to prevent hand contact with a possibly contaminated faucet.
c. Avoid splashing water against uniform.	Microorganisms travel and grow in moisture.

Continued

STEPS	RATIONALE

d. Regulate flow of water so that temperature is warm.

Warm water removes less of the protective skin oils.

e. Wet hands and wrists thoroughly under running water. Keep hands and forearms lower than elbows during washing.

Hands are the most contaminated parts to be washed. Water flows from least to most contaminated area, rinsing microorganisms into the sink.

f. Apply 3 to 5 mL of soap and rub hands together vigorously, lathering thoroughly (see illustration). Soap granules and leaflet preparations may be used.

Necessary to ensure that all surfaces of hands and fingers are covered and cleansed.

> **SAFE PATIENT CARE** The decision whether to use an antiseptic soap or alcohol-based hand sanitizer depends on whether the hands are visibly soiled, the procedure you will perform, and the patient's immune status.

g. Perform hand hygiene using plenty of lather and friction *for at least 15 seconds*. Interlace fingers and rub palms and backs of hands with circular motion at least five times each. Keep fingertips down to facilitate removal of microorganisms.

Soap cleanses by emulsifying fat and oil and lowering surface tension. Friction and rubbing mechanically loosen and remove dirt and transient bacteria. Interlacing fingers and thumbs ensures that you cleanse all surfaces.

h. Areas underlying fingernails are often soiled. Clean with fingernails of other hand and additional soap or with an orangewood stick *(optional)*.

Area under the nails can be highly contaminated, which increases risk for transmission of infection from nurse to patient.

> **SAFE PATIENT CARE** Do not tear or cut skin under or around nail.

i. Rinse hands and wrists thoroughly, keeping hands down and elbows up (see illustration).

Rinsing with hands down, washes away dirt and microorganisms.

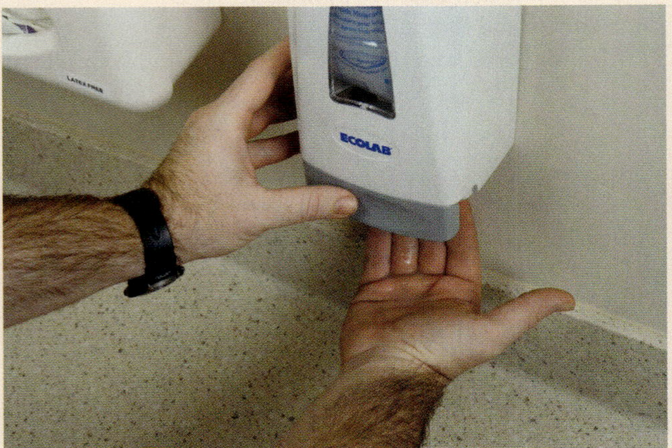

STEP 3a Apply waterless antiseptic to hands.

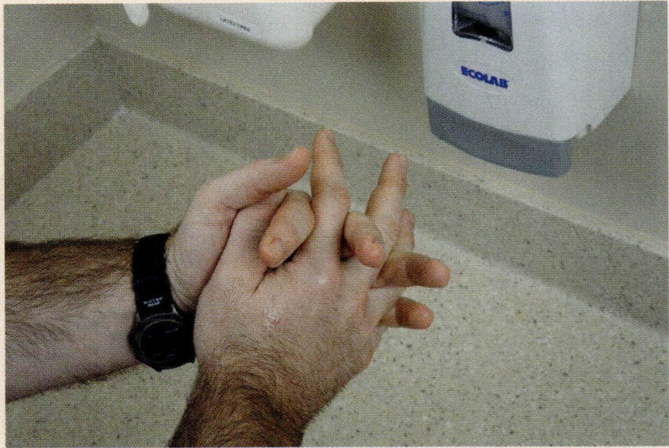

STEP 3b Rub hands thoroughly.

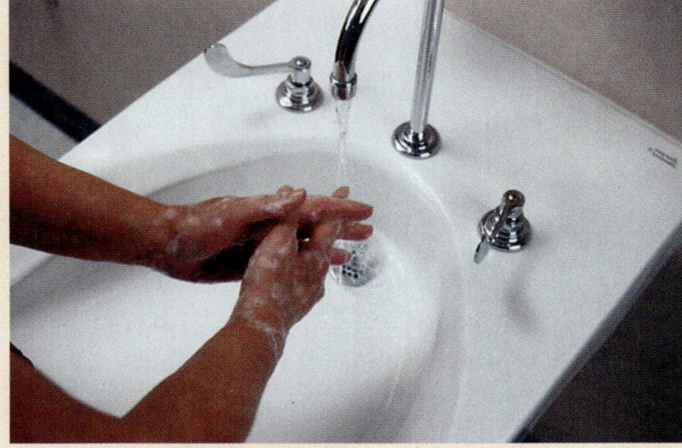

STEP 4f Lather hands thoroughly.

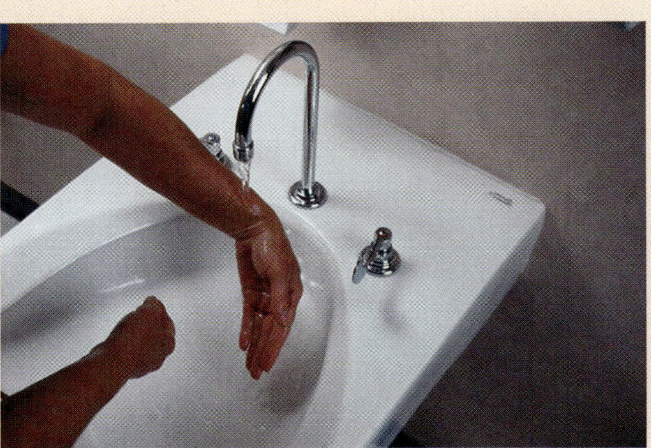

STEP 4i Rinse hands.

STEPS	**RATIONALE**
j. Dry hands thoroughly from fingers to wrists and then forearms with paper towel or warm air dryer.	Drying from cleanest (fingertips) to least clean (forearms) area avoids contamination. Drying prevents chapping and roughened skin.
k. If used, discard paper towel in proper container.	Prevents transfer of microorganisms.
l. Use clean, dry paper towel to turn off hand faucet (see illustration). Avoiding touching handles with hands. Turn off water with knee pedals (if applicable).	Prevents transfer of pathogens from faucet to hands (Haas, 2011).

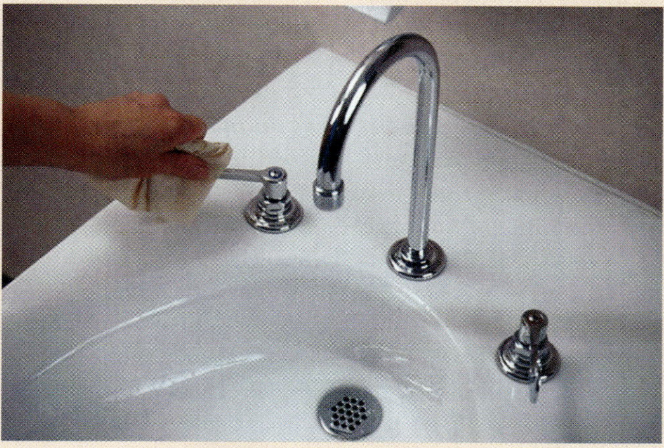

STEP 4l Turn off faucet.

m. If hands are dry or chapped at end of shift, use a small amount of lotion or barrier cream dispensed from an individual-use container.	Large, refillable containers of lotion have been associated with HAIs and should not be used because of the risk of organism growth in lotion.

EVALUATION

1. Inspect surfaces of hands for obvious signs of soil or other contaminants.
2. Inspect hands for dermatitis or cracked skin.

Unexpected Outcomes and Related Interventions

1. Hands or areas under fingernails remain soiled.
   a. Repeat hand hygiene.
2. Repeated use of soaps or antiseptics cause dermatitis or cracked skin.
   a. Rinse and dry hands thoroughly; avoid excessive amounts of soap; try various products; use hand lotions or barrier creams. Small containers are preferred because large containers have been found to harbor pathogens.

Recording and Reporting

- It is unnecessary to document handwashing.
- Report dermatitis, psoriasis, and cuts to facility employee health or infection control department.

Special Considerations
Geriatric

- Older adults are at greater risk for infection.
- The impact of infection is greater for older adults. Hand hygiene by staff is essential.

Certain procedures performed at a patient's bedside require the application of PPE such as a mask, cap, eyewear, gown, or gloves. Standard Precautions require nurses to wear clean gloves before coming in contact with mucous membranes, nonintact skin, blood, body fluids, or other potentially infectious material. Nurses wear gloves routinely when performing various procedures (e.g., nasogastric tube insertion, perineal care, enema administration). Masks are worn when nurses work over sterile areas or with equipment, such as changing a central line dressing. Protective eyewear is important when there is a risk of exposure of the eyes to splattering of blood or other body fluids.

Always assess a patient's potential for acquiring an infection before applying a mask or other PPE (e.g., does the patient have a large open wound, or do you, as the nurse, have a respiratory infection?). If you wear a mask, change it when it becomes moist or soiled (e.g., splattered with blood). Consider wearing a surgical cap to secure loose hair that might contaminate a sterile field. Follow Standard Precautions whenever using PPE.

ASSESSMENT

1. Review the type of procedure to be performed and consult facility policy regarding use of PPE. *Rationale: Not all procedures require PPE. PPE ensures that you and patient are properly protected.*
2. If you have symptoms of a respiratory infection, either avoid performing the procedure or apply a mask. *Rationale: A greater number of pathogenic microorganisms reside within the respiratory tract when infection is present.*
3. Assess the patient's risk for infection (e.g., older adult, neonate, patient with open wound, or immunocompromised patient). *Rationale: Some patients are at greater risk for acquiring an infection; you must use additional protective barriers.*

PLANNING

Expected Outcomes focus on prevention of localized or systemic infection.

1. Patient remains afebrile 24 to 48 hours after a procedure or during the course of repeated procedures.
2. Patient does not develop signs of localized infection (e.g., redness, tenderness, edema, drainage) or systemic infection (e.g., fever, change in white blood cell [WBC] count) 24 hours after the procedure.

Delegation and Collaboration

All health care providers use clean gloves. The skill of applying PPE can be delegated to nursing assistive personnel (NAP). The nurse instructs the NAP to:

- Be available to hand off equipment or assist with patient positioning during a sterile procedure.
- Perform hand hygiene after glove removal.

Equipment

- Clean gloves
- Gown (may be either disposable or reusable depending on facility protocol)
- Mask
- Surgical cap (Note: Use if required by facility policy or to secure hair to prevent contamination of sterile field.)
- Hairpins, rubber bands, or both
- Protective eyewear (e.g., goggles or glasses with appropriate side shields)

IMPLEMENTATION *for* APPLYING PERSONAL PROTECTIVE EQUIPMENT

STEPS	RATIONALE
1. **See Standard Protocol (inside front cover).**	
2. **Apply gown** with opening to the back. Be sure that it covers all outer garments. Pull sleeves down to wrist. Tie securely at neck and waist.	Prevents transmission of infection when patient has excessive drainage or discharges.
3. **Apply a cap.**	
a. If hair is long, comb back behind ears and secure.	Cap must cover all hair entirely.
b. Secure hair in place with pins.	Long hair should not fall down or cause cap to slip and expose hair.
c. Apply cap over head as you would apply a hair net. Be sure that all hair fits under edges of cap.	Loose hair hanging over sterile field contaminates objects on sterile field.
4. **Apply a mask.**	
a. Find top edge of mask, which usually has a thin metal strip along the edge.	Pliable metal fits snugly against bridge of nose.
b. Hold mask by top two strings or loops, keeping top edge above bridge of nose.	Prevents contact of hands with clean facial portion of mask. Mask covers all of nose.
c. Tie two top strings in a bow at top of back of head over cap (if worn) with strings above ears (see illustration).	Position of ties at top of head provides a tight fit. Strings over ears may cause irritation.
d. Tie two lower ties in a bow snugly around neck, with mask well under chin (see illustration).	Prevents escape of microorganisms through sides of mask as nurse talks and breathes.
e. Gently pinch upper metal band around bridge of nose.	Prevents microorganisms from escaping around nose.
f. *Option:* In some cases you will be required to wear a fitted respirator mask. Type of mask and fit-testing depend on type of precautions and facility policy.	

STEPS	RATIONALE

5. Apply protective eyewear.

a. Apply protective glasses, goggles, or face shield comfortably over eyes and check that vision is clear.

Positioning can affect clarity of vision.

b. Be sure that eyewear fits snugly around forehead and face.

Ensures that eyes are fully protected.

6. Apply clean gloves. Pull up gloves to cover each wrist (see illustration). (Note: Provide a latex-free environment if the patient or the health care worker has a latex allergy.)

Prevents transmission of microorganisms.

7. Removal of PPE:

a. Remove gloves. Remove one glove by grasping cuff and pulling glove inside out over hand. Hold removed glove in gloved hand. Slide fingers of ungloved hand under remaining glove at the wrist (see illustration). Peel glove off over first glove. Discard gloves in proper container.

Prevents contamination of hair, neck, and facial area.

b. Remove eyewear. Avoid placing hands over soiled lens. *If wearing a face shield, remove it before removal of mask.*

Reduces transmission of microorganisms.

c. Remove gown by unfastening neck ties and pulling away from neck and shoulders. Touching only the inside of the gown, turn gown inside out, roll or fold into a bundle, and discard.

Front and sleeves of gown are contaminated. This prevents transmission of microorganisms.

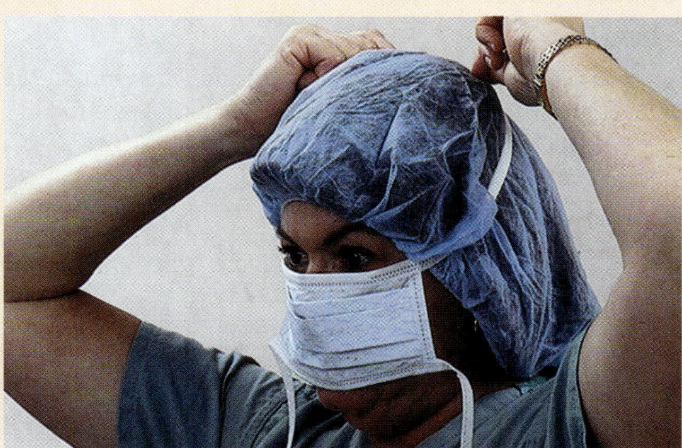

STEP 4c Tie top strings of mask.

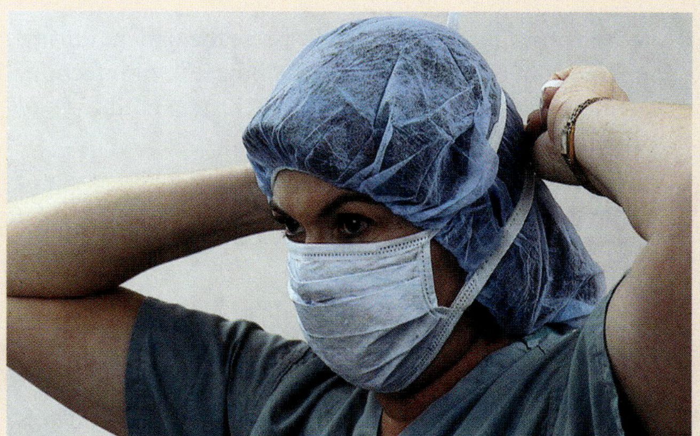

STEP 4d Tie lower strings of mask.

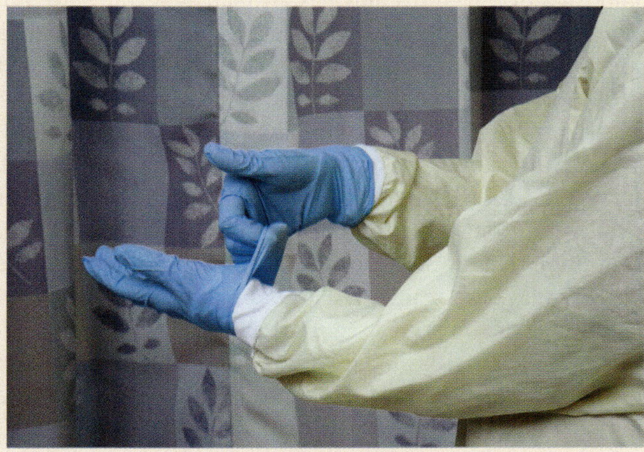

STEP 6 Applying gloves over gown sleeves.

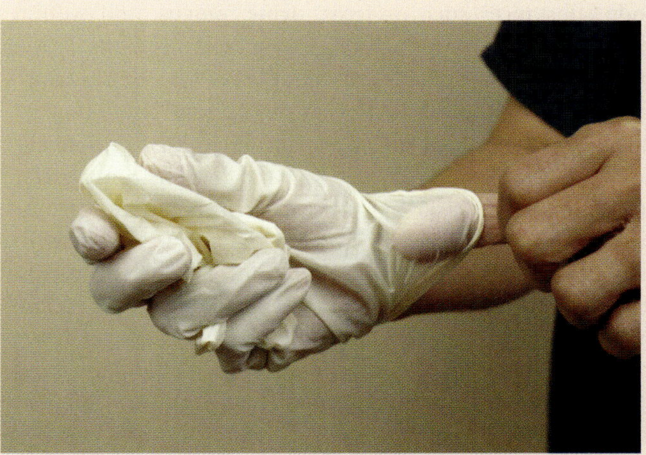

STEP 7a Remove second glove while holding soiled glove.

Continued

STEPS	RATIONALE

d. Untie bottom strings of mask first, hold strings, untie top strings, and pull mask away from face while holding strings. Remove mask from face (see illustrations).

Prevents top part of mask from falling down over your uniform. Contaminated surface of mask could then contaminate uniform.

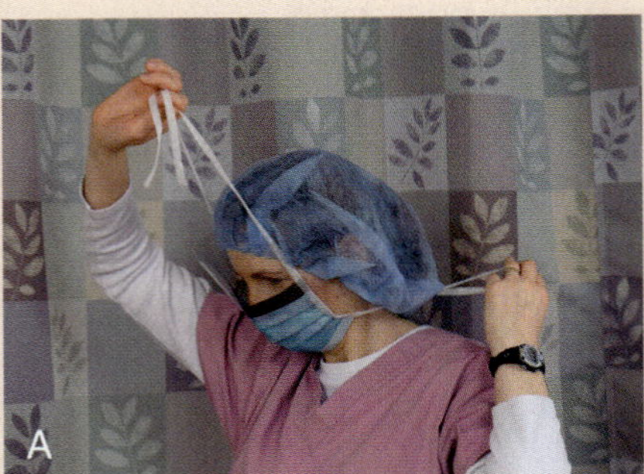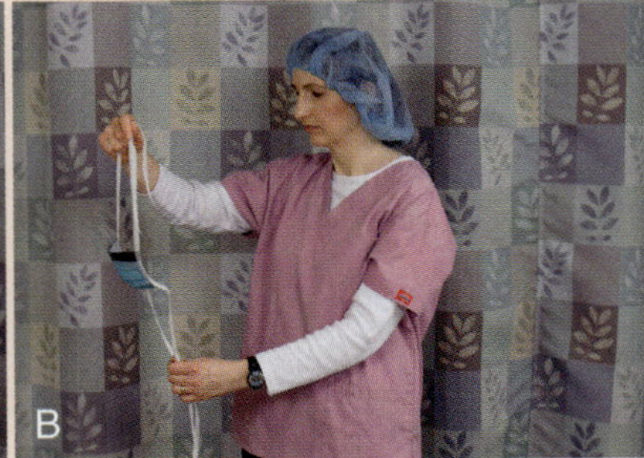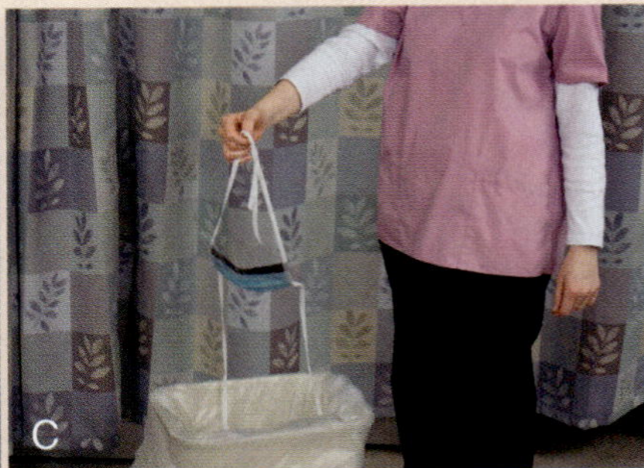

STEP 7d **A,** Untie top strings of mask. **B,** Remove mask from face. **C,** Drop mask in trash.

e. Do not touch outside surface of mask. Discard in plastic-lined receptacle.

Prevents contamination of hands.

f. Grasp outer surface of cap and lift from hair.

Minimizes contact of hands with hair.

g. Discard cap in proper receptacle and perform hand hygiene.

Reduces transmission of microorganisms.

8. **See Completion Protocol (inside front cover).**

EVALUATION

1. After the procedure is completed, assess the patient during your course of care for any changes indicative of infection. Depending on what the PPE equipment was used for, the evaluation will vary.

Recording and Reporting

- It is unnecessary to document use of PPE.

Special Considerations

Home Care

- Instruct a family caregiver on how and when to use PPE.
- Determine ability of family caregiver to observe for signs of infection.

SKILL 5.3   CARING FOR PATIENTS UNDER ISOLATION PRECAUTIONS

When a patient has a source of infection, health care workers follow specific infection prevention and control practices to reduce the risk of cross-contamination to other patients. Body substances such as feces, urine, mucus, and wound drainage contain potentially infectious organisms. Isolation or barrier precautions include the use of PPE (see Skill 5.2). In 2012, the CDC published a National Action Plan to Prevent Healthcare-Associated Infections and included frontline clinicians to improve adherence to hand hygiene and barrier precautions (CDC, 2012a). The guidelines contain recommendations for respiratory hygiene and etiquette as part of Standard Precautions. Standard Precautions, or tier one precautions, are part of care for all patients (Table 5-1). Tier two precautions (see Table 5-1) include precautions for patients with known or suspected infection. A special set of guidelines must be followed if you care for patients with tuberculosis (Box 5-3).

Multidrug-resistant organisms (MDROs) have become increasingly common as a cause of colonization and HAIs.

Three examples of MDROs are methicillin-resistant *Staphylococcus aureus* (MRSA), vancomycin-resistant *Enterococcus* (VRE), and *C. difficile*. MRSA is commonly associated with bloodstream infections and has an increased mortality rate (Becker and Kahl, 2011). Immunocompromised and debilitated patients are at greater risk of acquiring VRE (Archibald, 2011), and patients who have been treated with antibiotics are more likely to test positive for *C. diff*. Gerding (2011) stated that *C. diff* is not only one of the most common HAIs but also is costly. The most common mode of transmission for MDROs is through the health care worker, maximizing the importance of Standard Precautions and hand hygiene. Patients who harbor these MDROs are put on isolation; PPE equipment is frequently used. Patients may also be cohorted, putting patients with similar pathogens together, especially in an outbreak situation (Makamure et al., 2013). MDRO pathogens can survive for days or weeks (even months for *C. difficile* spores) on various environmental surfaces such as patients' overbed tables and side rails (Otter, Yezli, and French,

TABLE 5-1 CENTERS FOR DISEASE CONTROL AND PREVENTION ISOLATION GUIDELINES

Standard Precautions (Tier One) for Use with All Patients

- Standard Precautions apply to blood, blood products, all body fluids, secretions, excretions (except sweat), nonintact skin, and mucous membranes.
- Perform hand hygiene before direct contact with patients; between patient contacts; after contact with blood, body fluids, secretions, and excretions and with equipment or articles contaminated by them; and immediately after gloves are removed.
- When hands are visibly soiled or contaminated with blood or body fluids, wash them with either a nonantimicrobial soap or an antimicrobial soap and water.
- When hands are not visibly soiled or contaminated with blood or body fluids, use an alcohol-based hand rub to perform hand hygiene.
- Wash hands with nonantimicrobial soap and water if contact with spores (e.g., *Clostridium difficile*) is likely to have occurred.
- Do not wear artificial fingernails or extenders if duties include direct contact with patients at high risk for infection and associated adverse outcomes.
- Wear gloves when touching blood, body fluids, secretions, excretions, nonintact skin, mucous membranes, or contaminated items or surfaces. Remove gloves and perform hand hygiene between patient care encounters and when going from a contaminated to a clean body site.
- Wear PPE when your anticipated patient interaction will likely involve contact with blood or body fluids.
- A private room is unnecessary unless the patient's hygiene is unacceptable. Check with the infection prevention and control professional of your facility.
- Discard all contaminated sharp instruments and needles in a puncture-resistant container. Health care facilities must make needleless devices available. Any needles should be disposed of uncapped or a mechanical safety device is activated for recapping.
- Respiratory hygiene and cough etiquette: Have patients cover the nose or mouth when sneezing or coughing; use tissues to contain respiratory secretions, and dispose in nearest waste container; perform hand hygiene after contacting respiratory secretions and contaminated objects or materials; contain respiratory secretions with procedure or surgical mask; sit at least 3 feet away from others if coughing.

Transmission-Based Precautions (Tier Two) for Use with Specific Types of Patients

CATEGORY	DISEASE	BARRIER PROTECTION
Airborne Precautions	Droplet nuclei <5 µm, measles, chickenpox (varicella), disseminated varicella zoster, pulmonary or laryngeal tuberculosis	Private room, negative-pressure airflow of at least 6-12 exchanges per hour via HEPA filtration, mask or respiratory protection device, N95 respirator
Droplet Precautions	Droplets >5 µm; being within 3 feet of the patient; diphtheria (pharyngeal), rubella, streptococcal pharyngitis, pneumonia or scarlet fever in infants and young children, pertussis, mumps, mycoplasmal pneumonia, meningococcal pneumonia or sepsis, pneumonic plague	Private room or cohort patients, mask or respirator (refer to facility policy)
Contact Precautions	Direct patient or environmental contact, colonization or infection with multidrug-resistant organisms such as VRE and MRSA, *Clostridium difficile*, respiratory syncytial virus, shigella and other enteric pathogens, major wound infections, herpes simplex, scabies, varicella zoster (disseminated)	Private room or cohort patients (see facility policy), gloves, gowns
Protective Environment	Allogeneic hematopoietic stem cell transplants	Private room; positive airflow with ≥12 air exchanges per hour; HEPA filtration for incoming air; mask, gloves, gowns

HEPA, High-efficiency particulate air; *MRSA,* methicillin-resistant *Staphylococcus aureus*; VRE, vancomycin-resistant *Enterococcus.*
Modified from Centers for Disease Control and Prevention (CDC), Hospital Infection Control Practice Advisory Committee: Guidelines for isolation precautions in hospitals, *MMWR Morb Mortal Wkly Rep* 57(RR16):39, 2007.

BOX 5-3   SPECIAL TUBERCULOSIS PRECAUTIONS

In 1994, an increase in cases of TB resulted in the CDC publishing guidelines for preventing TB transmission in health care settings. The increase in TB was due to human immunodeficiency virus (HIV) infection, transmission in health care settings, and increase in immigrants from countries with a high rate of TB (CDC, 2011). The current CDC guidelines for preventing and controlling TB focus on early detection of TB infection, protecting close contacts of patients with active TB disease, and applying effective infection control measures in health care settings.

A patient who has respiratory symptoms lasting longer than 3 weeks, unexplained weight loss, night sweats, fever, or a productive cough (might be streaked with blood) should be suspected to have TB. Isolation for patients with suspected or confirmed TB includes placing the patient on airborne infection precautions in a single-patient airborne infection isolation room with negative pressure.

Occupational Safety and Health Administration (OSHA) and CDC guidelines require health care workers who care for patients with suspected or confirmed TB to wear special respirators (e.g., N95 or P100). These respirators are high-efficiency particulate masks that filter particles at a 95% or better efficiency. Health care workers who use these respirators must be fit tested, a procedure to determine adequate fit to minimize leakage into the face piece and provide better protection (CDC, 2012a). OSHA requires employers to provide training concerning transmission of TB, especially in areas where the risk of exposure is high. In addition, the CDC now recommends the use of the QuantiFERON-TB Gold (QFT-G) test (CDC, 2013b), a blood test, in place of the traditional Mantoux TB skin test. The advantages of the QFT-G test are that it does not boost responses measured by subsequent tests, and the results are not subject to reader bias.

There are a few additional things to be aware of while taking care of a patient in isolation for TB. Keep the room door closed at all times in a negative pressure isolation room. Provide instruction to the patient and family on how TB is transmitted and how to prevent infection of others.

2011). Health care workers can contaminate their hands or gloves by touching these contaminated surfaces and then transfer infection to other patients. When a patient with a MDRO is discharged, special cleaning precautions are taken to prepare the room for the next patient. Area decontamination methods such as aerosolized hydrogen peroxide and UV radiation do not rely on housekeeping to ensure distribution and contact time and are generally more efficacious than conventional terminal disinfection (Otter et al., 2011; Rutala and Weber, 2013).

When patients are infected or colonized with specific microorganisms, the CDC recommends transmission-based precautions in addition to Standard Precautions (CDC, 2010b). Health care facilities modify these guidelines according to need and as dictated by state or local regulations.

Isolation precautions are based on the assumption that microorganisms are transmitted by several routes: contact, droplet, air, common vehicle, and vector. The guidelines recommend the use of barrier precautions to interrupt the mode of transmission (see Skill 5.2). Isolation or barrier precautions prescribe the specific use of PPE when a patient is infected or colonized with specific organisms.

The three types of transmission-based precautions may be combined for diseases that have multiple routes of transmission. Whether used singularly or in combination, they are to be used in addition to Standard Precautions. When a patient is found to be infected and requires isolation, determine the reason and mode of transmission. Consult with your infection control professionals and the facility's policy and procedure manual to determine the barrier equipment needed for specific tasks. For example, a patient on Airborne Precautions for measles has an organism that can be carried by the airborne route. A mask is necessary when entering the room for any reason.

One important aspect of care for a patient in isolation is compliance with hand hygiene and the changing of gloves between exposures to body sites and patient equipment. Inadequate glove changes and hand hygiene between exposures to body sites can lead to contamination of previously uncolonized sites (Haas, 2011). For example, do not allow microorganisms in a patient's respiratory secretions to spread to the hub of a central line catheter on your gloved hands. In such a situation, remove gloves after the patient expectorates, perform hand hygiene, and reapply gloves. Noncompliance with glove changing and hand hygiene increases the risk of HAIs.

ASSESSMENT

1. Assess patient's medical history and possible indications for isolation (e.g., purulent productive cough, major draining wound). Review the precautions necessary for the specific isolation category. *Rationale: Ensures that you use appropriate PPE.*
2. Review laboratory test results (e.g., wound culture, acid-fast bacillus [AFB] smears, changes in WBC count). *Rationale: Reveals the type of organism infecting a patient.*
3. Review facility policies and isolation precautions necessary for the type of isolation ordered, and consider types of care measures to be performed while in patient's room. *Rationale: Allows you to organize all equipment needed in the room.*
4. Review nursing care plan notes or confer with nursing colleagues and family members regarding the patient's emotional state and reaction to isolation. Also assess patient's understanding of the purpose of isolation. *Rationale: Allows planning for appropriate social support and education.*
5. Assess whether patient has a known latex allergy. If an allergy is present, refer to facility policy and resources available to provide full latex-free care. *Rationale: Protects patient from a serious allergic response.*

PLANNING

Expected Outcomes focus on preventing transmission of infection to nurse and other patients and improving patient's knowledge of the purpose of isolation.

1. Patient and family verbalize purpose of isolation and treatment plan.
2. Infection does not develop in neighboring patients.

Delegation and Collaboration

The skill of caring for patients under isolation precautions can be delegated to nursing assistive personnel (NAP). The nurse instructs the NAP to:

- Use the correct PPE for the specific isolation.
- Report abnormal findings and any high risk factors (e.g., patient does not adhere to secretion control when coughing) for infection transmission that pertain to the patient.

Equipment

- Barrier protections determined by the type of isolation required: Clean gloves, appropriate mask, eyewear, protective goggles or glasses, face shield, and gown (gown may be disposable or reusable, depending on facility policy)
- Other patient care equipment (as appropriate): Vital signs equipment, sharps container, hygiene items, medication, dressing change items
- Soiled linen bag and trash receptacle
- Sign for door indicating type of isolation in use or for visitors to come to the nurses' station before entering the room
- TB isolation
  - Room with negative airflow
  - N95 or P100 respirator

IMPLEMENTATION *for* CARING FOR PATIENTS UNDER ISOLATION PRECAUTIONS

STEPS	RATIONALE
1. **See Standard Protocol (inside front cover).**	
2. Prepare all equipment to be taken into patient's room. In many cases, dedicated equipment, such as stethoscopes, blood pressure equipment, and thermometers, should remain in room until patient is discharged. Many facilities use disposable single-use equipment. If patient is infected or colonized with a resistant organism (e.g., VRE, MRSA), equipment remains in room and is thoroughly disinfected before removal from room (see facility policy).	CDC recommends use of dedicated noncritical patient care equipment (CDC, 2012b).
3. Prepare for entrance into isolation room.	
a. Apply clean gloves and other PPE following the sequence in Skill 5.2. **NOTE:** A cap is not worn in an isolation room. **NOTE:** Wear unpowdered latex-free gloves if patient or health care worker has a latex allergy.	Prevents transmission of infection by exposure to wound drainage, splashing of body fluids, and airborne microorganisms. Gloves are applied last so they can be placed over the cuffs of the gown.
b. Be sure N95 or P100 mask for TB precautions fits snugly.	
c. When you wear gloves with the gown, bring glove cuffs over edge of gown sleeves.	
4. Enter patient's room. Arrange supplies and equipment. (If equipment will be removed from room for reuse, place on clean paper towel.)	Minimizes contamination of care items.
5. Explain the purpose of isolation and precautions for patient and family to take. Offer opportunity to ask questions. If patient is on TB precautions, instruct to cover mouth with tissue when coughing and to wear disposable surgical mask when leaving room.	Improves patient's and family's ability to participate in care and minimizes anxiety. Identifies opportunities for planning social and diversional activities. Reduces TB microorganism transmission.
6. Assess vital signs (see Chapter 6).	
a. If patient is infected or colonized with a resistant organism (e.g., VRE, MRSA), equipment remains in room including stethoscope and blood pressure cuff (CDC, 2010a)	Decreases the risk of infection being transmitted to another patient.

Continued

STEPS	RATIONALE

b. If stethoscope is to be reused, clean diaphragm or bell and ear tips with alcohol. Set aside on clean surface.

Stethoscopes are a common vehicle for transmission of infection. This action decreases the presence of microorganisms (CDC, 2012a).

c. Use an individual electronic or disposable thermometer.

Prevents cross-contamination.

> **SAFE PATIENT CARE** If a disposable thermometer indicates a fever, assess for other signs and symptoms. Confirm fever using an alternative thermometer. Do not use an electronic thermometer if the patient is suspected or confirmed to have *C. difficile* (Cohen et al., 2010). Infection can be spread to another patient.

7. Administer medications (see Chapters 21, 22, and 23).
   a. Give oral medication in wrapper or cup.
   b. Dispose of wrapper or cup in room.
   c. Wear gloves to administer injection.
   d. Discard needleless syringe or safety sheathed needle into designated sharps container.

Reduces risk of exposure to blood.

Needleless devices should be used to reduce the risk of needlesticks and sharps injuries to health care workers.

8. Administer hygiene, encouraging patient to discuss questions or concerns about isolation.
   a. Avoid allowing isolation gown to become wet. Carry wash basin outward away from gown; avoid leaning against wet tabletop.

   Moisture allows organisms to travel through gown to uniform.

   b. Remove linen from bed; avoid contact with isolation gown. Place in leak-proof linen bag.

   Linen soiled by patient's body fluids is handled so as to prevent contact with clean gown.

   c. Provide clean bed linen and set of towels.
   d. Change gloves and perform hand hygiene if hands become excessively soiled and further care is necessary.

9. Collect specimens (see Chapter 8).
   a. Place specimen container on clean paper towel in patient's bathroom and follow procedure for collecting specimen of body fluids.

   Container will be taken out of patient's room, so outer surface must not be contaminated.

   b. Transfer specimen to properly labeled container without soiling outside of container. After gloves are removed, place container in plastic biohazard bag. Complete and apply biohazard label to outside of bag, and transport to laboratory. Perform hand hygiene and reglove if further procedures are to be performed (see illustration).

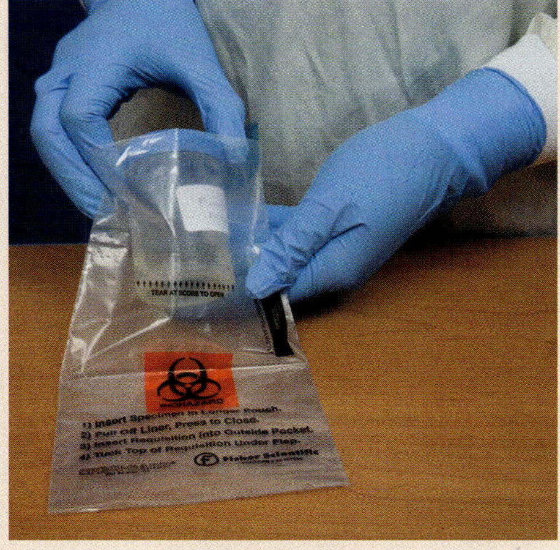

STEP 9b Specimen container placed in biohazard bag and sealed.

10. Dispose of linen, trash, and disposable items.

    Linen or refuse should be contained completely to prevent exposure of personnel to infective material.

    a. Use sturdy moisture-impervious single bags to contain soiled articles. Use double bag if outer bag is torn or contaminated (see illustration).

    Heavy soiling can cause outer side of first bag to become contaminated.

    b. Tie bags securely at top in knot.

11. Remove all reusable pieces of equipment. Clean any contaminated surfaces with disinfectant and allow to dry according to product guidelines (see facility policy).

    Items must be properly cleaned, disinfected, or sterilized for reuse.

12. Resupply room as needed. Have staff hand new supplies to you.

    Limiting trips into and out of room reduces nurse and patient exposure to microorganisms.

13. Leave isolation room. Order for removing PPE depends on what is worn in room. The following sequence describes steps to take if all barriers were worn (CDC, 2010b).

    a. Remove gloves. See Skill 5-2, Step 7a

    Prevents nurse from contacting outer surface of contaminated glove.

    b. Remove eyewear or goggles.

    c. Untie waist and neck strings of gown. Allow gown to fall from shoulders (see illustration). Remove hands from sleeves without touching outside of gown. Hold gown inside at shoulder seams and fold inside out. Discard disposable gown in trash bag.

    Hands do not come in contact with soiled front of gown and have not been soiled.

    d. Remove mask.

    Ungloved hands are not contaminated by touching only mask strings.

    (1) If mask secures over ears, remove elastic from ears and pull mask away from face. For a tie-on mask, while holding onto strings, untie *top* mask strings. Then hold strings while untying bottom strings. Pull mask away from face and drop into trash container. (Do not touch outer surface of mask.) If body fluids splash onto mask, dispose in biohazard waste container.

    (2) If patient is on TB precautions, place reusable mask in labeled paper bag for storage, being careful not to crush mask (check facility policy for number of times it can be used).

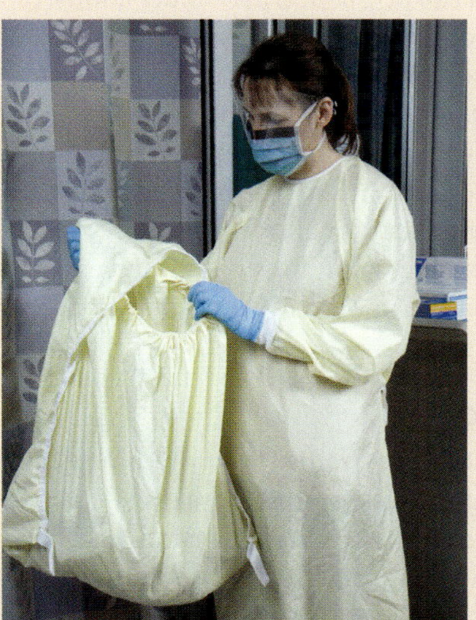

STEP 10a Tie trash bag securely.

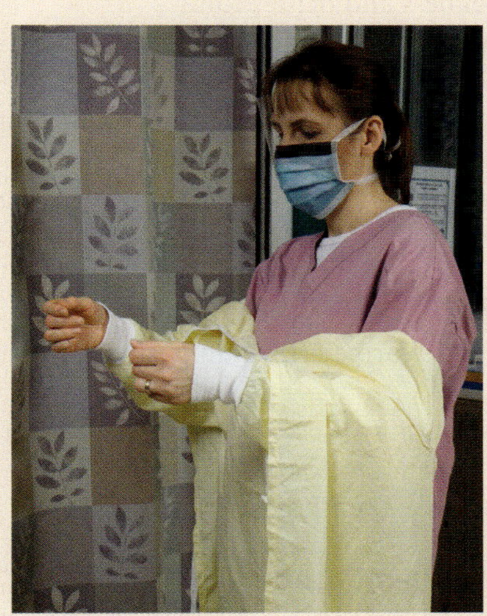

STEP 13c Nurse removes gown.

Continued

STEPS	RATIONALE

e. Perform hand hygiene.

> **SAFE PATIENT CARE** If patient is being treated for *C. difficile* infection, wash hands with soap and water. Alcohol-based hand rubs are not effective against *C. diff* spores

f. Retrieve wristwatch and stethoscope (unless it remains in room) and record vital signs on notepaper or clean paper towel.	Clean hands can contact clean items.
g. Explain to patient when you plan to return to room. Ask if patient requires anything such as personal care items or books or has any requests or needs.	
h. Leave room and close door if necessary. (Close door if patient is on Airborne Precautions.)	Keeping door open too long equalizes pressure in room and allows organisms to flow out.
14. See **Completion Protocol (inside front cover).**	

EVALUATION

1. Observe patient and family members' use of isolation precautions when visiting.
2. Ask patient and family members to explain purpose of isolation in relation to diagnosed condition.
3. Use *Teach Back:* State to the patient, "I want to be sure I explained about the isolation equipment. Can you explain to me why your family needs to apply a gown, mask, and gloves? Evaluates what the patient is able to explain or demonstrate. Revise your instruction now or develop plan for revised patient teaching to be implemented at an appropriate time if patient is not able to teach back correctly.

Unexpected Outcomes and Related Interventions

1. Patient avoids social and therapeutic discussions.
   a. Confer with patient, family, or significant other and determine the best approach to reduce patient's feeling of loneliness and depression.
   b. Use therapeutic listening.
2. Infectious organism spreads to other patients.
   a. Confer with the provider, who may recommend an infectious disease consultation.
   b. Determine appropriate isolation precautions to take with other affected patients.

Recording and Reporting

- Procedures performed (including education) and patient's response
- Type of isolation in use and the microorganism (if known)
- Patient's response to social isolation
- Evaluation of patient learning

Sample Documentation

1320 Contact isolation in place for *Salmonella* in stool. Patient incontinent of liquid stool. Wife at bedside, asking questions about barrier equipment. Discussed method by which *Salmonella* is transmitted and explained purpose of handwashing and use of gown and gloves. Wife verbalized understanding when she requested gloves and gown to assist in cleanup.

Special Considerations
Pediatric

- Isolation creates a sense of separation from family and loss of control. The strange environment confuses a child. Preschoolers are unable to understand the cause-effect relationship for isolation.
- All barriers to be used must be shown to the child. Involve parents in any explanations. Nurses let children see their faces before applying masks so that children do not become frightened (Hockenberry and Wilson, 2013).

Geriatric

- Isolation can be a concern for older adults, especially those who have signs and symptoms of confusion or depression. Patients often become more confused when confronted by a nurse using barrier precautions or when they are left in a room with the door closed. Assess the need for closing door (negative airflow room) along with safety of the patient and additional safety measures required.
- Assess an older adult for signs of depression: loss of appetite, decrease in verbal communications, or inability to sleep.

Home Care

- If patient returns home with a draining wound or productive cough, educate family caregivers on potential sources of contamination in the home and techniques for disposing of biological wastes in accordance with state laws.
- Encourage patients and family to use vigilant hand hygiene and to avoid sharing personal care items with other family members.

SKILL 5.4 PREPARING A STERILE FIELD

• **Nursing Skills Online: Infection Control, Lesson 3**

Performing sterile aseptic procedures requires a work area in which objects can be handled with minimal risk of contamination. A sterile field is an area free of microorganisms and provides a sterile surface for placement of sterile equipment. A field may consist of the inside of a sterile commercial kit or tray, the surface of an opened sterile linen-wrapped package, or the surface of a large sterile drape. Sterile drapes establish a sterile field around a treatment site such as a surgical incision, venipuncture site, or site for introduction of an indwelling urinary catheter. Drapes also provide a work surface for placing sterile supplies and manipulating items with sterile gloves. Drapes are available in cloth, paper, and plastic. They may be wrapped in individual sterile packages or included within sterile kits or trays. These kits or trays contain external and internal sterile (chemical) indicators that indicate that the item has completed a sterilization process. After a kit is opened, the inside surface of the cover can be used as a sterile field. Most drapes are fluid resistant. There are various styles, shapes, and sizes of drapes. For example, bladder catheterization and tracheal suction kits contain sterile items that can be moved with the tray and containers into which sterile solutions can be poured. After you create a sterile field, you are responsible for performing the procedure and making sure that the field is not contaminated.

ASSESSMENT

1. Verify in facility policy and procedure manual that the procedure requires surgical aseptic technique.
2. Assess patient's comfort, oxygen requirements, and elimination needs before the procedure. *Rationale: Certain sterile procedures may last a long time. Anticipate patient's needs so that patient can relax and avoid any unnecessary movement that might disrupt the procedure.*
3. Instruct patient not to touch the work surface or equipment during the procedure and to remain still.
4. Assess for latex allergies. *Rationale: A focused review may reveal latex allergies even when no known allergies are indicated during the chart review.*

5. Check integrity of sterile package for punctures, tears, discoloration, expiration date, and moisture. If using commercially packaged supplies or supplies prepared by the facility, check sterilization indicator as well. *Rationale: Inspection of packaging ensures that only sterile supplies are placed on the sterile field (AORN, 2011).*
6. Anticipate number and variety of supplies needed for the procedure. *Rationale: This ensures that the procedure is organized to prevent break in technique.*

PLANNING

Expected Outcomes focus on prevention of localized or systemic infection.

1. Patient is not exposed to organisms and remains afebrile 24 to 48 hours after a procedure or during the course of repeated procedures.
2. Sterile field is not contaminated.
3. Patient displays no signs of localized infection (e.g., redness, tenderness, edema, drainage) or systemic infection (e.g., fever, change in WBC count) 24 hours after the procedure.

Delegation and Collaboration

The skill of preparing a sterile field cannot be delegated to nursing assistive personnel (NAP). Surgical technicians may prepare a sterile field (see facility policy). The nurse instructs the NAP to:

• Assist in positioning patients and obtaining necessary supplies.

Equipment

• Sterile pack (commercially prepared or prepared by facility)
• Sterile gloves
• Sterile drape or kit that is to be used as a sterile field
• Sterile equipment and solutions specific to the procedure
• Waist-high table or countertop surface
• Appropriate PPE: gown, mask, protective eyewear (see facility policy)

IMPLEMENTATION *for* PREPARING A STERILE FIELD

STEPS	RATIONALE
1. Complete all priority care tasks (e.g., medication administration) before beginning procedure.	Prepare sterile fields as close as possible to time of use to reduce potential for contamination (AORN, 2011).
2. Ask visitors to step out of room briefly during procedure. Discourage movement by staff assisting with procedure.	Traffic and movement increase potential for contamination through spread of microorganisms by air currents.

Continued

 |

3. Prepare equipment at bedside. Position patient comfortably for specific procedure to be performed. If a body part is to be treated, position patient so area is accessible. Have NAP assist with positioning as needed.

Ensures availability before procedure and prevents break in sterile technique (Torch, 2011). (NOTE: Povidone-iodine and chlorhexidine are not considered sterile solutions and require separate work surfaces for prepping.) Patient should be able to lie in one position comfortably without moving during procedure.

4. Apply PPE as needed (consult facility policy) (see Skill 5.2).

5. Select a clean, flat, dry work surface above waist level.

A sterile object below a person's waist is considered contaminated.

6. Check expiration dates on all kits, packs, and supplies to be sure they are sterile.

7. Perform hand hygiene.

Reduces transmission of microorganisms.

8. Prepare sterile work surface.

   a. Sterile commercial kit or tray containing sterile items:

     (1) Place sterile kit or package containing sterile items on work surface above waist level

Once created, sterile field is sterile only at table level. Items placed below waist are considered contaminated.

     (2) Open outside cover and remove kit from dust cover. Place on work surface.

Inner kit remains sterile.

     (3) Grasp outer edge of tip of outermost flap.

Outer surface of package is considered unsterile. A 2.5-cm (1-inch) border around any sterile drape or wrap is considered contaminated.

     (4) Open outermost flap away from body, keeping arm outstretched and away from sterile field (see illustration).

Reaching over sterile field contaminates it.

     (5) Grasp outside surface of edge of first side flap.

Outer border is considered unsterile.

     (6) Open side flap, pulling to side and allowing it to lie flat on table surface. Keep arm to the side and not extended over the sterile surface (see illustration).

Drape or flap should lie flat so it does not rise up accidentally and contaminate inner surface or the sterile items placed on its surface.

     (7) Repeat Step 8a(6) for opening second side flap (see illustration).

     (8) Grasp outside border of last and innermost flap.

     (9) Stand away from sterile package and pull flap back, allowing it to fall flat on work surface (see illustration).

Reaching over sterile field contaminates it.

   b. Sterile linen-wrapped package

     (1) Place package on work surface above waist level.

Items placed below waist level are considered contaminated.

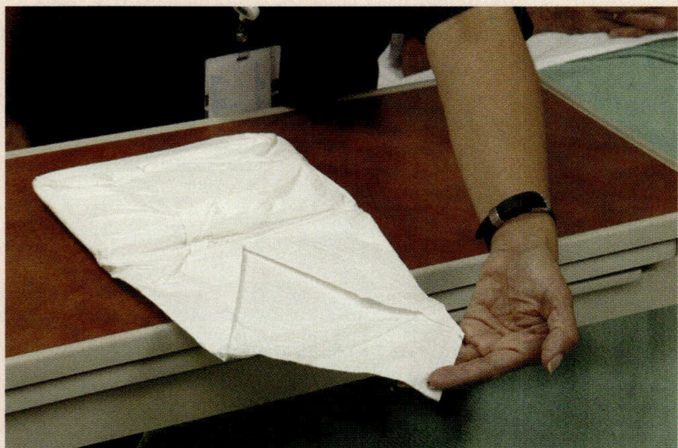

STEP 8a(4) Open outermost flap of sterile kit away from body.

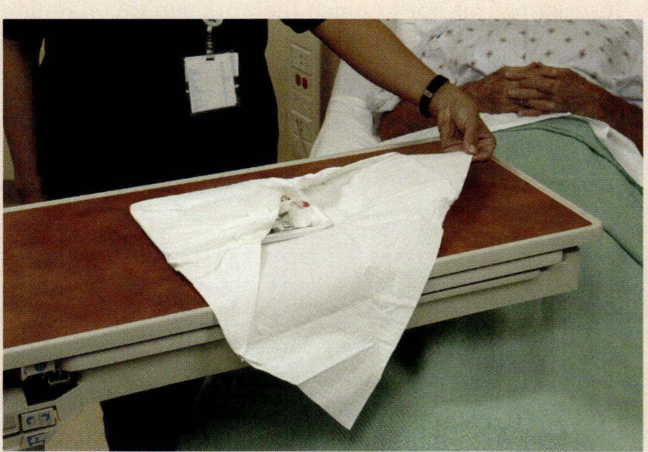

STEP 8a(6) Open first side flap, pulling to side.

<table>
<tr><td>STEPS</td><td>RATIONALE</td></tr>
</table>

(2) Remove sterilization tape seal and unwrap both layers, following Steps 8a(2) through 8a(9) as with sterile kit.

(3) Use opened linen wrapper as sterile field.

Inner surface of wrapper is considered sterile.

c. Sterile drape

(1) Place pack containing sterile drape on work surface and open as described in Steps 8a(2) through 8a(9) for sterile package.

Ensures sterility of packaged drape.

(2) **Apply sterile gloves.** (**NOTE:** This is an option, depending on facility policy.) You may touch outer 2.5-cm (1-inch) border of drape without wearing gloves.

(3) With finger tips of one hand, pick up folded top edge of drape along 1-inch border. Gently lift drape up from its outer wrapper without touching any object. Keep above waist. Discard wrapper with other hand.

If a sterile object touches any nonsterile object, it becomes contaminated.

(4) With other hand, grasp an adjacent corner of drape and hold it straight up and away from body. Allow drape to unfold, keeping it above waist and work surface and away from body (see illustration).

An object held below person's waist or above chest is contaminated. Drape can now be properly placed with two hands.

(5) Holding drape, first position and lay the bottom half over top half of intended work surface.

Prevents you from reaching over sterile field.

(6) Allow top half of drape to be placed over bottom half of work surface (see illustration).

Creates a flat sterile surface for placement of sterile items.

9. Add sterile items to sterile field.

a. Open sterile item (following package directions) while holding outside wrapper in nondominant hand.

Frees dominant hand for unwrapping outer wrapper.

b. Carefully peel wrapper over nondominant hand.

Item remains sterile. Inner surface of wrapper covers hand, making it sterile.

c. Being sure that wrapper does not fall down on sterile field, place item onto field at an angle. *Do not hold arm over sterile field (see illustration).*

Secured wrapper edges prevent flipping wrapper and contaminating sterile field (AORN, 2011).

d. Dispose of outer wrapper.

Prevents accidental contamination of sterile field.

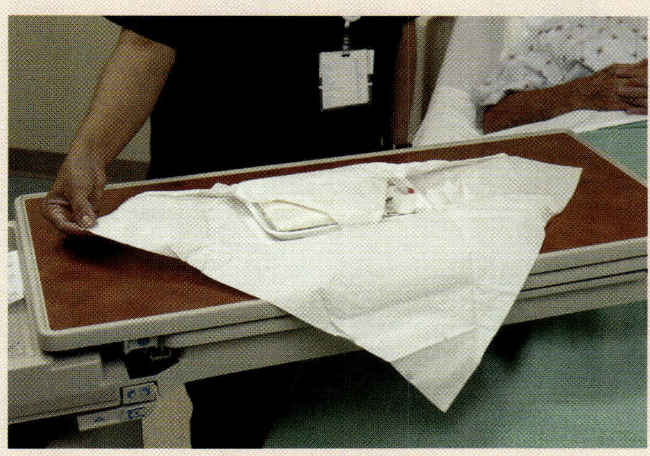

STEP 8a(7) Open second side flap, pulling to side.

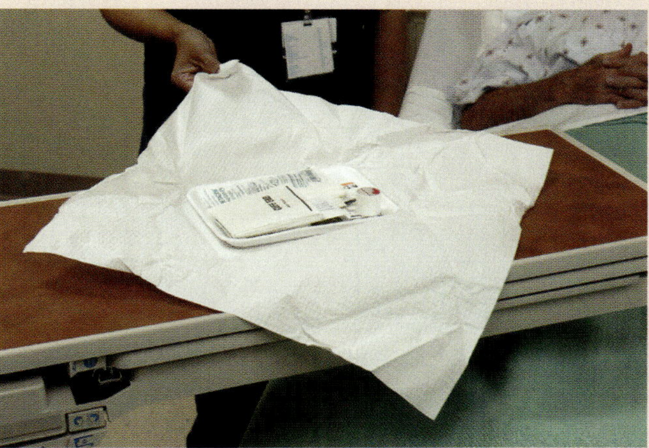

STEP 8a(9) Open last and innermost flap, standing away from sterile field.

Continued

STEPS	RATIONALE

10. *Pour sterile solutions.*

   a. Verify contents and expiration date of solution. — Ensures proper solution and sterility of contents.

   b. Be sure that receptacle for solution is located near or on sterile work surface edge. Sterile kits have cups or plastic molded sections into which fluids can be poured. — Prevents reaching over sterile field.

   c. Remove sterile seal and cap from bottle in an upward motion. — Prevents contamination of bottle lip and maintains sterility of inside of cap.

   d. With solution bottle held away from sterile field, with the label facing up and bottle lip 2.5 to 5 cm (1 to 2 inches) above inside of sterile receiving container, slowly pour contents of solution container (see illustration). Avoid splashing. — Edge and outside of bottle are considered contaminated. Slow pouring prevents splashing liquids, which causes fluid permeation of the sterile barrier, called *strike through*, resulting in contamination. Sterility of contents cannot be ensured if cap is replaced.

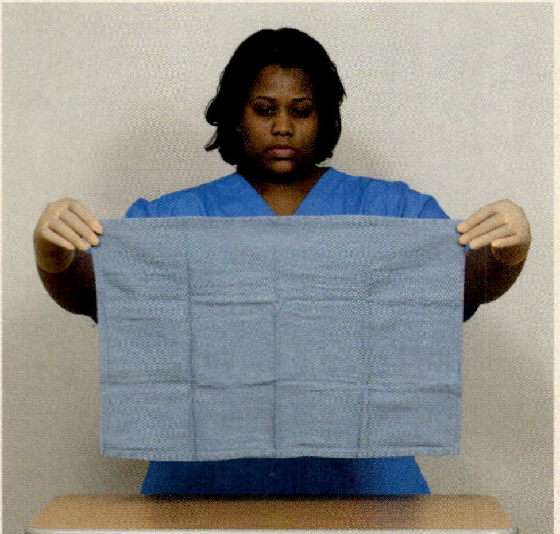

STEP 8c(4) Hold corners of sterile drape up and away from body.

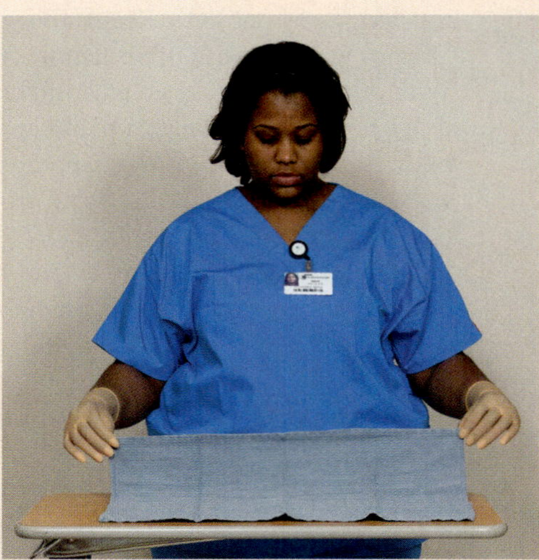

STEP 8c(6) Allow top half of drape to be placed over bottom half of work surface.

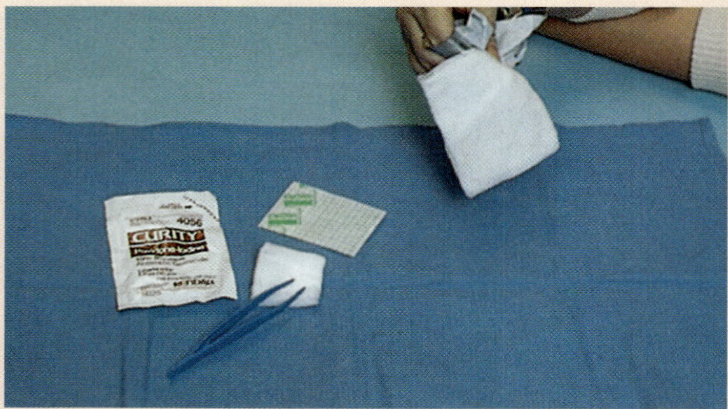

STEP 9c Adding item to sterile field.

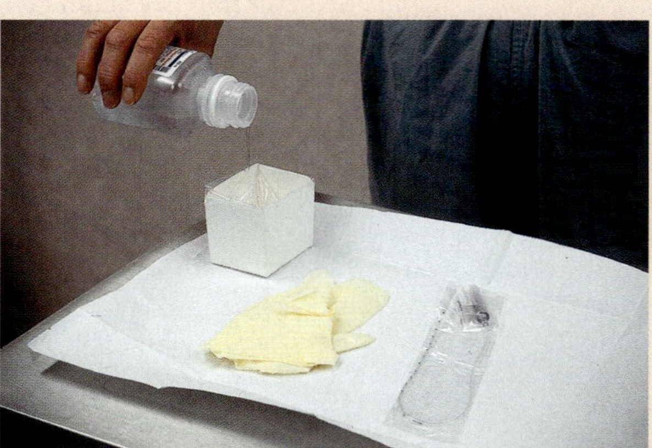

STEP 10d Pour solution into receiving container on sterile field.

EVALUATION

1. Observe for break in sterile technique.

Unexpected Outcomes and Related Interventions

1. Sterile item falls off sterile field.
   a. Add a new sterile item to the field, unless the field becomes contaminated; in the event of contamination, discontinue sterile field preparation and begin again.
2. Sterile field comes in contact with contaminated object, or liquid splatters onto drape, causing strike through.
   a. Discontinue field preparation and start over with new equipment.

Recording and Reporting

No recording or reporting is required for setting up sterile field, but

- Record the sterile procedure performed in the nurses' notes.

Special Considerations
Pediatric

- Children may be unable to cooperate during a sterile procedure, depending on their level of developmental maturity.
- Instruct family members about how they may assist so that the child does not contaminate the sterile field (Hockenberry and Wilson, 2013).

Geriatric

- Memory and sensory deficits may impair an older patient's ability to understand and cooperate with a procedure.

Home Care

- Adaptations may be made for some procedures, such as self-catheterization and home tracheostomy care. In some cases, patients use medical asepsis rather than surgical technique.
- If possible, teach patient and family caregiver to perform sterile procedures well before discharge from acute care so skills can be learned with professional assistance.

SKILL 5.5   STERILE GLOVING

- **Nursing Skills Online: Infection Control, Lesson 4**

Sterile gloves act as a barrier against the transmission of pathogenic microorganisms. You will apply sterile gloves before performing sterile procedures, such as a sterile dressing change or urinary catheter insertion. Sterile gloves do not replace hand hygiene.

You use the open-glove application method for most sterile procedures not requiring a sterile gown. Be careful not to contaminate the gloved hands by touching clean, contaminated, or possibly contaminated items or areas. If a glove becomes contaminated or torn, change it immediately. Once gloved, keep your hands clasped about 30.5 cm (12 inches) in front of your body, above waist level and below the shoulders, until you are ready to perform a procedure.

It is important to choose not only the right glove size but also the correct material. Many patients and health care workers have known latex allergies because of repeat exposure. Box 5-4 lists risk factors for latex allergy. A true latex allergy is a response to the natural rubber latex proteins, and sometimes symptoms can be seen within minutes of contact (Rothrock, 2015). The latex can be inhaled or settle on clothing, skin, or mucous membranes. Reaction to latex can be mild to severe (Box 5-5). Choose latex-free or synthetic gloves when caring for individuals at high risk or with suspected latex sensitivity. Facilities have latex-free procedure kits available for use.

When choosing gloves, be sure that they are tight enough for objects to be picked up easily but that they do not stretch so tightly over the fingers that they can tear easily. Sterile gloves are available in various sizes (e.g., 6, 6½, 7). Sterile gloves are also available in a "one-size-fits-all" style or in "small," "medium," and "large."

ASSESSMENT

1. Consider the type of procedure to be performed and consult facility policy on use of sterile gloves.
2. Consider patient's risk for infection (e.g., preexisting condition, size or extent of area being treated). *Rationale: Directs you to follow added precautions (e.g., use of additional PPE) if necessary.*

BOX 5-4   RISK FACTORS FOR LATEX ALLERGY

- Spina bifida
- Congenital or urogenital defects
- History of indwelling catheters or repeated catheterization
- History of using condom catheters
- High latex exposure (e.g., health care workers, housekeepers, food handlers, tire manufacturers, workers in industries that use gloves routinely)
- History of multiple childhood surgeries
- People with a family history of allergies such as hay fever or hives
- History of food allergies, especially banana, avocado, chestnut, kiwi, apple, carrot, celery, papaya, potato, tomato, melons

Modified from Molinari J, Harte J: Dental services. In Carrrico R, editor: APIC text of infection control and epidemiology, Washington DC, ed 3, 2011, Association for Professionals in Infection Control and Epidemiology (APIC); Mayo Clinic Staff: Latex allergy, November 2011, http://www.mayoclinic.com/health/latex-allergy/DS00621/DSECTION=risk-factor. Accessed May 11, 2014.

BOX 5-5   LEVELS OF LATEX REACTIONS

The three levels of symptoms are mild, more-severe, and anaphylactic shock symptoms. Symptoms are listed in order of increasing severity.

1. *Mild symptoms:* Itching, skin redness, hives or rash.
2. *More-severe symptoms:* Sneezing, runny nose, itchy or watery eyes, scratchy throat, difficulty breathing, wheezing and coughing.
3. *Anaphylactic shock symptoms:* Difficulty breathing, wheezing, decrease in blood pressure, dizziness, loss of consciousness, confusion, rapid or weak pulse. A true latex allergy can be life-threatening, and emergency care is recommended.

Modified from Mayo Clinic Staff: *Latex allergy,* November 2011, http://www.mayoclinic.com/health/latex-allergy/DS00621/DSECTION=symptoms. Accessed March 18, 2014.

3. Select the correct size and type of gloves, and examine the glove package to determine if it is dry and intact. *Rationale: A torn or wet package is considered contaminated. Signs of water stains on the package indicate previous contamination by water.*
4. Inspect the condition of your hands for cuts, open lesions, or abrasions. According to facility policy, a lesion may be able to be covered with an impervious transparent dressing, or it may prevent you from participating in the procedure. *Rationale: Lesions harbor microorganisms. Breaks in the skin integrity may permit microorganisms to enter and increase the risk for infection for both the patient and the nurse (AORN, 2011).*
5. Assess patient for the following risk factors before applying latex gloves (see Box 5-4):
   a. Previous reaction to the following items within hours of exposure: adhesive tape, dental or face mask, golf club grip, ostomy bag, rubber band, balloon, bandage, elastic underwear, IV tubing, rubber gloves, or condom. *Rationale: These items are known to lead to latex allergy.*
   b. Personal history of asthma, contact dermatitis, eczema, urticaria, or rhinitis.
   c. History of food allergies, especially avocado, banana, peach, chestnut, raw potato, kiwi, tomato, or papaya.
   d. Previous history of adverse reactions during surgery or dental procedures. *Rationale: A previous history of adverse reactions is suggestive of an allergic response.*
   e. Previous reaction to latex product. *Rationale: A previous reaction is suggestive of an allergic response.*
6. If patient is expected to be at risk, check facility procedure for obtaining a latex allergy cart. *Rationale: Cart contains nonlatex patient care items.*

PLANNING

Expected Outcomes focus on prevention of localized or systemic infection and latex reaction.
1. Patient remains afebrile with no signs of localized infection 24 to 72 hours after the procedure or during the course of repeated procedures.
2. Patient does not develop signs of latex sensitivity or allergic reaction.

Delegation and Collaboration

The skill of sterile gloving can be delegated to nursing assistive personnel (NAP). However, many procedures that require the use of sterile gloves cannot be delegated (see facility policy). The nurse instructs the NAP to:
- Stop and reapply gloves if they become contaminated.

Equipment

- Package of correct-size sterile gloves: latex or synthetic nonlatex. (Note: Hypoallergenic, low-powder, or low-protein latex gloves may still contain enough latex protein to cause an allergic reaction [Molinari and Harte, 2011].)

IMPLEMENTATION *for* STERILE GLOVING

STEPS	RATIONALE
1. **See Standard Protocol (inside front cover).**	
2. **Apply sterile gloves.**	
a. Perform hand hygiene.	Reduces transmission of microorganisms.
b. Place glove package near work area.	Ensures availability before procedure.
c. Remove outer glove package wrapper by carefully separating and peeling apart sides.	Prevents inner glove package from accidentally opening and touching contaminated objects.
d. Grasp inner glove package and lay it on a clean, dry, flat surface at waist level. Open package, keeping gloves on wrappers inside surface (see illustration).	Inner surface of glove package is sterile. A sterile object held below waist level is contaminated.
e. Identify right and left glove. Each glove has a cuff approximately 5 cm (2 inches) wide. Glove your dominant hand first.	Proper identification of gloves prevents contamination by improper fit. Gloving of dominant hand first improves dexterity.

STEPS	**RATIONALE**

f. With thumb and first two fingers of nondominant hand, grasp edge of cuff of glove for dominant hand. Touch only inside surface of glove.

Inner edge of cuff touches skin and is no longer considered sterile.

g. Carefully pull glove over dominant hand, leaving cuff and ensuring cuff does not roll up wrist (see illustration). Be careful in working thumb and fingers into correct spaces.

h. With gloved dominant hand, slip fingers underneath cuff of second glove (see illustration).

Cuff protects gloved fingers; abducting thumb prevents contamination from contact with unsterile surface.

i. Carefully pull second glove over fingers of nondominant hand (see illustration). Do not allow fingers and thumb of gloved hand to touch any part of exposed nondominant hand. Keep thumb of dominant hand abducted.

Prevents ungloved hand from contaminating sterile glove.

j. After second glove is applied, interlock fingers of gloved hands and hold away from body, above waist level, until beginning procedure (see illustration).

Prevents accidental contamination from hand movement.

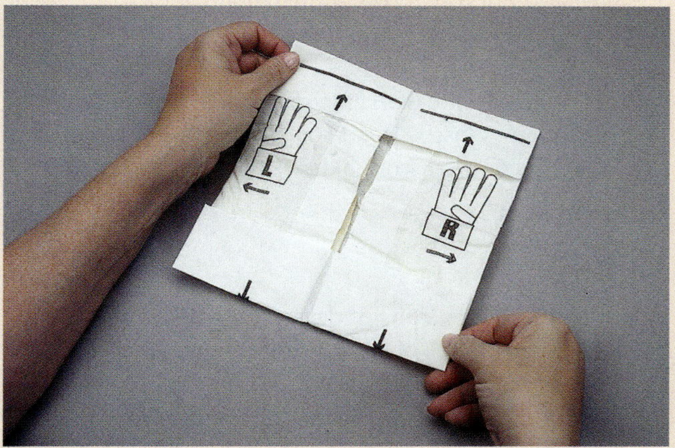

STEP 2d Open inner glove package on work surface.

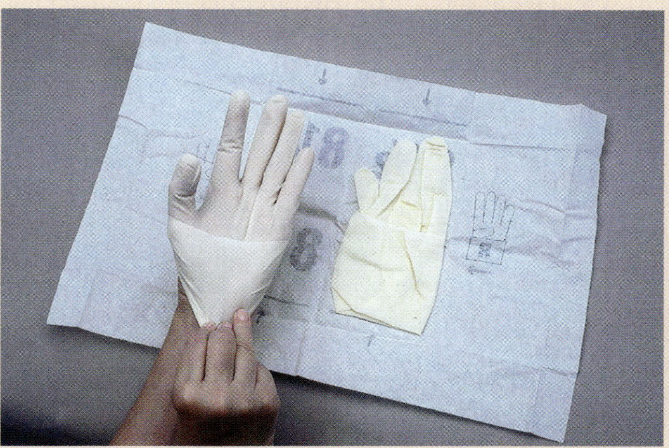

STEP 2g Pick up glove for dominant hand and insert fingers.

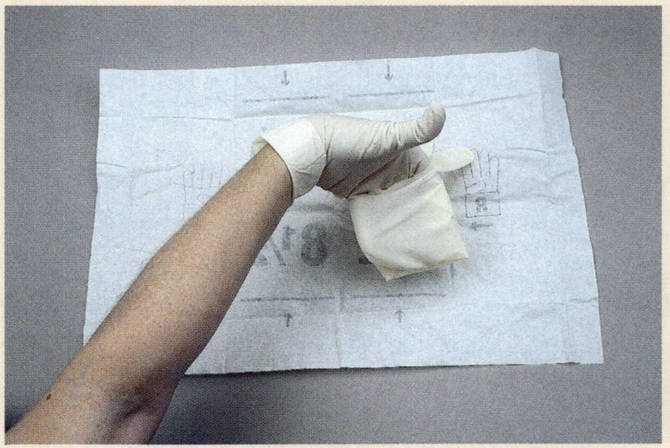

STEP 2h Pick up glove for nondominant hand.

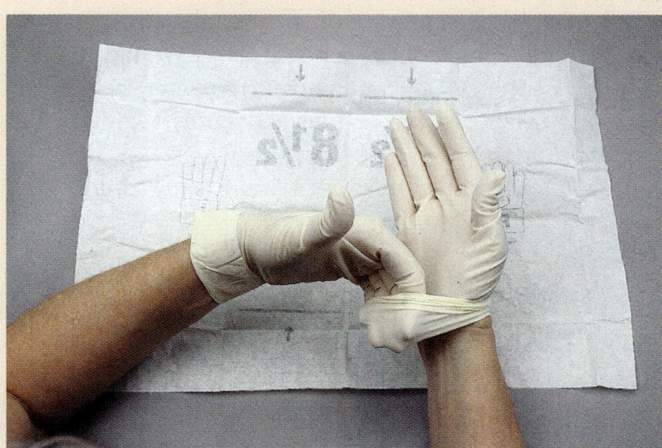

STEP 2i Pull second glove over nondominant hand.

Continued

STEPS	RATIONALE

STEP 2j Interlock gloved hands.

3. Proceed with procedure.
4. **Remove sterile gloves.**
   a. Grasp outside of one cuff with other gloved hand; avoid touching wrist. Pull glove off, turning it inside out. Discard in proper receptacle.

   Outside of glove should not touch skin surface.

   b. Take fingers of bare hand and tuck inside remaining glove cuff. Peel glove off inside out. Discard in trash receptacle.

   Fingers do not touch contaminated glove surface.

   c. Perform thorough hand hygiene.

   Protects health care workers from contamination resulting from any unseen tears or pinholes in gloves; also removes powder from hands to prevent skin irritation.

5. **See Completion Protocol (inside front cover).**

▌EVALUATION

1. Evaluate patient for signs and symptoms of infection (e.g., fever, development of wound drainage) for 48 hours after the procedure.
2. Evaluate patient for signs of latex reaction.

Unexpected Outcomes and Related Interventions

1. Patient develops signs of local or systemic infection.
   a. Notify health care provider of findings. Wound cultures (see Chapter 8) and antibiotic therapy may be needed.
   b. Apply Standard Precautions and sterile technique (as appropriate).
   c. Monitor temperature every 4 hours or per orders.

2. Patient develops signs of dermatitis or latex sensitivity.
   a. Remove source of latex. Bring emergency equipment to bedside.
   b. Notify health care provider of findings.
   c. Have dose of epinephrine and methylprednisolone sodium succinate (Solu-Medrol) available, which may be needed for allergic reaction, and be prepared to initiate IV fluids and oxygen.

Recording and Reporting

- No recording or reporting is required for sterile gloving.
- Record the procedure performed.

▌CRITICAL THINKING EXERCISES

Case Study

A patient is admitted to the emergency department with a productive cough and a history of night sweats. After obtaining further history, it is determined that this patient is at risk for pulmonary TB. Until pulmonary TB is ruled out, this patient is placed on isolation precautions.

1. What type of transmission-based precautions are necessary for this patient? ____________.

2. What kind of mask does the nurse need to wear when she enters the room to care for this patient? ____________.

3. A NAP is caring for this patient. A new nurse informs the NAP that she can decide which mask to wear. What do you tell the nurse and NAP? ____________.

Review Questions

1. A nurse enters the room of a patient who has been given a diagnosis of pneumonia. The nurse instructs the patient to cover the mouth when coughing. This reduces transmission of infection by:
   1. Contact
   2. Small droplet nuclei
   3. Vector
   4. Splashing

2. After the nurse leaves an isolation room, the removal of the PPE should occur in what order? Place steps in the correct order.
   1. Untie bottom mask strings.
   2. Untie waist and neck strings of gown. Allow gown to fall from shoulders.
   3. Remove gloves.
   4. Remove eyewear or goggles.
   5. Untie top mask strings.
   6. Remove hands from gown sleeves without touching outside of gown; hold gown inside at shoulder seams, fold inside out, and discard.
   7. Pull mask away from face and drop into container.

3. Which of the following would be classified as a case of HAI? Select all that apply.
   1. An infected bedsore on a patient just admitted from home
   2. A urinary tract infection that develops after an order is followed for placement of a Foley catheter
   3. A patient tested as HIV positive
   4. The development of purulent drainage exiting from a central venous catheter insertion site
   5. A *Staphylococcus* infection that develops in an incisional wound

4. When a nurse applies clean gloves to collect a urine specimen, how does this technique break the chain of infection?
   1. Blocks the portal of entry of a microorganism
   2. Reduces susceptibility of the host
   3. Controls a reservoir source of organism growth
   4. Blocks the portal of exit

5. Which of the following breaks the chain of infection by controlling the reservoir source of microorganism growth?
   1. Changing a soiled dressing
   2. Washing hands
   3. Avoiding sneezing
   4. Disposing of used needles in a puncture-proof container

6. Identify the procedures that require the use of sterile (aseptic) technique. Select all that apply.
   1. Urinary catheterization
   2. Tracheal suctioning
   3. Insertion of rectal suppository
   4. Insertion of a feeding tube
   5. Lumbar puncture
   6. Sitz bath

7. The nurse has applied the first sterile glove on her right hand (dominant) without touching the sterile outer surface. She takes her gloved right hand and picks up the remaining glove at the top of the cuff and slips it over her left hand. Which of the following statements is correct?
   1. The first glove is applied correctly but is contaminated while applying the second glove.
   2. The first glove is applied incorrectly, but the second glove is applied correctly.
   3. The first glove is applied correctly, and the second glove becomes contaminated.
   4. Both gloves have been applied correctly.

8. When opening a sterile pack, which of the following compromises the sterility of the contents?
   1. Keeping the contents of the pack away from the table edge
   2. Holding or moving the object below the waist
   3. Opening the pack just before the procedure
   4. Movement of sterile products within the sterile field.

9. Which of the following people are at risk for a latex allergy?
   1. A patient who has had a surgical procedure
   2. A health care worker who works in the operating room
   3. A patient who develops pneumonia after hip surgery
   4. A patient with multiple intravenous catheters

10. A health care worker who comes to work with coughing and respiratory congestion is setting up a sterile field. Which of the following actions would require intervention?
    1. The first flap of the sterile package is opened toward the nurse.
    2. The glove for the dominant hand is pulled on first.
    3. The sterile drape is allowed to unfold, keeping it above the waist.
    4. The bottle of solution is poured with the label in the palm of the hand.

REFERENCES

Archibald L: Enterococci. In Carrico R, et al, editors: *APIC text of infection control and epidemiology*, ed 3, Washington, DC, 2011, Association for Professionals in Infection Control and Epidemiology (APIC).

Association of Operating Room Nurses (AORN): *Standards, recommended practices, and guidelines*, Denver, 2011, The Association.

Becker K, Kahl B: Staphylococci. In Carrico R, et al, editors: *APIC text of infection control and epidemiology*, ed 3, Washington, DC, 2011, Association for Professionals in Infection Control and Epidemiology (APIC).

Centers for Disease Control and Prevention (CDC): Hand hygiene in health care settings, 2011, http://www.cdc.gov/handhygiene/Guidelines.html. Accessed September 17, 2014.

Centers for Disease Control and Prevention (CDC): *Healthcare-associated infections (HAIs) elimination: methicillin-resistant Staphylococcus aureus (MRSA) infections*, 2010a, http://www.cdc.gov/HAI/pdfs/toolkits/MRSA_toolkit_white_020910_v2.pdf. Accessed January 10, 2014.

Centers for Disease Control and Prevention (CDC), Hospital Infection Control Practice Advisory Committee: *Guidelines for isolation precautions in healthcare settings 2007*, 2010b, http://www.cdc.gov/hicpac/2007ip/2007isolationprecautions.html. Accessed January 10, 2014.

Centers for Disease Control and Prevention (CDC): *TB: fact sheets*, 2011, http://www.cdc.gov/tb/publications/factsheets/general/tb.htm. Accessed January 10, 2014.

Centers for Disease Control and Prevention (CDC): *National action plan to prevent healthcare-associated infections: roadmap to elimination*, 2012a, http://www.hhs.gov/ash/initiatives/hai/executive_summary.pdf. Accessed January 10, 2014.

Centers for Disease Control and Prevention (CDC): *Respirator trusted-source information*, 2012b, http://www.cdc.gov/niosh/npptl/topics/respirators/disp_part/RespSource3fittest.html#fitb. Accessed January 10, 2014.

Centers for Disease Control and Prevention (CDC): *Wash your hands*, 2013a, http://www.cdc.gov/Features/HandWashing/. Accessed March 18, 2014.

Centers for Disease Control and Prevention (CDC), Division of Tuberculosis Elimination: *Fact sheets: QuantiFERON-TB Gold Test*, 2013b, http://www.cdc.gov/nchstp/tb/pubs/tbfactsheets/250103.htm. Accessed January 10, 2014.

Centers for Disease Control and Prevention (CDC): *Healthcare-associated infections (HAIs)*, 2013c, http://www.cdc.gov/hai/. Accessed January 10, 2014.

Cohen SH, et al: Clinical practice guidelines for *Clostridium difficile* infection in adults: update by the Society for Healthcare Epidemiology of America (SHEA) and the Infectious Diseases Society of America (IDSA), *Infect Control Hosp Epidemiol* 31(5):431, 2010.

Fardo R: Geriatrics. In Carrico R, et al, editors: *APIC text of infection control and epidemiology*, ed 3, Washington, DC, 2011, Association for Professionals in Infection Control and Epidemiology (APIC).

Felembam O, et al: Hand hygiene practices of home visiting community nurses: perceptions, compliance, techniques, and contextual factors of practice using the World Health Organization's five moments for hand hygiene, *Home Healthc Nurse* 30(3):152, 2012.

Gerding D: *Clostridium difficile* infection and pseudomembranous colitis. In Carrico R, et al, editors: *APIC text of infection control and epidemiology*, ed 3, Washington, DC, 2011, Association for Professionals in Infection Control and Epidemiology (APIC).

Haas J: Hand hygiene. In Carrico R, et al, editors: *APIC text of infection control and epidemiology*, ed 3, Washington, DC, 2011, Association for Professionals in Infection Control and Epidemiology (APIC).

Hockenberry MJ, Wilson D: *Wong's essentials of pediatric nursing*, ed 9, St Louis, 2013, Mosby.

Kramer A, Schwebke I, Kampf G: How long do nosocomial pathogens persist on inanimate surfaces? *BMC Infect Dis* 6:130, 2006.

Linton A: *Introduction to medical-surgical nursing*, ed 5, St Louis, 2012, Saunders.

Longtin T, et al: Hand hygiene, *N Engl J Med* 364(13):e24, 2011.

Makamure M, et al: A review of critical care nursing and disease outbreak preparedness, *Dimens Crit Care Nurs* 32(4):157, 2013.

Molinari J, Harte J: Dental services. In Carrico R, et al, editors: *APIC text of infection control and epidemiology*, ed 3, Washington, DC, 2011, Association for Professionals in Infection Control and Epidemiology (APIC).

Otter JA, Yezli S, French GL: The role played by contaminated surfaces in the transmission of nosocomial pathogens, *Infect Control Hosp Epidemiol* 32(7):687–699, 2011.

Phillips N: *Berry & Kohn's operating room technique*, ed 12, St Louis, 2013, Mosby.

Rothrock J: *Alexander's care of the patient in surgery*, ed 15, St Louis, 2015, Mosby.

Rutala W, Weber D: Current principles and practices; new research; and new technologies in disinfection, sterilization and antisepsis, *Am J Infect Control* 41(5 Suppl):S1, 2013.

The Joint Commission (TJC): *National Patient Safety Goals*, Oakbrook Terrace, IL, 2014, The Commission. Available at: http://www.jointcommission.org/standards_information/npsgs.aspx.

Torch J: Raising the red flag, *Prev Strategist* 4(3):44, 2011.

University of Minnesota: *How does culture affect healthcare? Taking charge of your health*, 2011, www.takingcharge.csh.umn.edu. Accessed January 10, 2014.

World Health Organization (WHO): *WHO guidelines on hand hygiene in health care*, Geneva, 2009, WHO Press.

CHAPTER

6

Vital Signs

EVOLVE WEBSITE/EVOLVE RESOURCES LIST

http://evolve.elsevier.com/Perry/nursinginterventions
Audio Glossary • Checklists • Review Questions

Vital signs include temperature, pulse, respirations, and blood pressure. These are indicators of the ability of the body to regulate body temperature, oxygenate body tissues, and maintain blood flow. Pain assessment is considered a fifth vital sign (see Chapter 13). Pain frequently is the symptom that leads patients to seek health care.

PATIENT-CENTERED CARE

Changes in vital signs indicate a patient's response to physical, environmental, and psychological stressors. These changes may reveal sudden alterations in a patient's condition. As a nurse, use clinical judgment to determine which vital signs to measure, when to take measurements (Box 6-1), and when measurements can be delegated safely. A change in one vital sign (e.g., pulse) can reflect changes in the other vital signs (temperature, respirations, and blood pressure). A review of vital sign values helps to determine whether it is necessary to assess specific body systems more thoroughly. For some patients, vital sign assessment may be limited to measuring a single vital sign to monitor a specific aspect of a patient's condition. For example, before and after administering an antihypertensive medication, you measure a patient's blood pressure to evaluate the effect of the drug.

A nurse learns to measure vital signs correctly, understands and interprets the values, begins interventions as needed, and reports findings appropriately. Keeping patients informed of their vital signs promotes understanding of their health status.

SAFETY

Assessing vital signs requires equipment that is clean and in working order. Carefully clean stethoscopes, thermometers, and blood pressure cuffs before and after use with each patient to avoid contamination by microorganisms. The biomedical department of a hospital routinely inspects electronic blood pressure machines for electrical safety. Know how to use each device; if you are unsure, ask for instructions. It is important that each device be used correctly and appropriately to ensure patient safety and to obtain correct, complete patient information.

EVIDENCE-BASED PRACTICE

Zheng D, Giovannini R, Murray A: Effect of respiration, talking and small body movements on blood pressure measurement, *J Human Hyper* 26(7):458, 2012.

BOX 6-1   WHEN TO TAKE VITAL SIGNS

- On admission to a health care facility
- When assessing a patient during home health visits
- In a hospital or care facility on a routine schedule according to the health care provider's order or standards of practice of the facility
- Before, during, and after a surgical procedure or invasive diagnostic procedure
- Before, during, and after a transfusion of any type of blood product
- Before, during, and after administration of medications or application of therapies that affect cardiovascular, respiratory, and temperature-control functions
- When a patient's general physical condition changes (e.g., loss of consciousness, increased severity of pain)
- Before and after nursing interventions influencing a vital sign (e.g., before and after a patient previously on bed rest ambulates, before and after patient performs range-of-motion exercises)
- When a patient reports specific symptoms of physical distress (e.g., feeling "funny" or "different")

TABLE 6-1   VITAL SIGNS: ACCEPTABLE RANGES

VITAL SIGNS	ACCEPTABLE RANGE
Temperature	36-38°C (96.8-100.4°F)
Oral/tympanic	37.0°C (98.6°F)
Rectal	37.5°C (99.5°F)
Axillary	36.5°C (97.7°F)
Pulse	Adult: 60-100 beats/min, strong and regular
Respirations	Adult: 12-20 breaths/min, deep and regular
Blood pressure*	
Systolic	<120 mm Hg
Diastolic	<80 mm Hg
Pulse pressure	30-50 mm Hg
Pulse oximetry	Normal SpO_2: 95%-100%

*In some patients, blood pressure is measured consecutively with the patient lying, sitting, and standing or in both arms. In normal individuals, the change from lying to standing causes a decrease in systolic blood pressure of <15 mm Hg. Record the position and extremity, and compare the measurements for significant differences.

The accuracy of blood pressure readings is affected by measurement conditions. Patient movement and talking are two potential sources of error when blood pressure is measured. In a study by Zheng and colleagues (2012), blood pressures were obtained on healthy adult volunteers three times: at rest, while counting out loud, and while moving the nonmeasurement arm forward and backward. The systolic and diastolic pressure increased during talking by 5 mm Hg and 6 mm Hg compared with the resting measurement. A smaller increase occurred during arm movements. Nurses must carefully control conditions before and during blood pressure measurement using the following strategies:

- Discouraging the patient from talking or moving their arms and legs during manual or electronic blood pressure measurements.
- Asking the patient to remain quiet while the blood pressure is measured.
- Keeping the room cool (12°C [54°F]) during blood pressure measurement.

TEMPERATURE

The measurement of body temperature provides an average of the core temperature of body tissues. Body tissues and cell processes function best within a relatively narrow temperature range of 36° to 38° C (96.8° to 100.4°F). The temperature range of an adult depends on age; physical activity; status of hydration; and state of health, including the presence of infection (Table 6-1). A patient can adjust body temperature by avoiding temperature extremes, adding or removing external clothing or coverings, and ingesting fluids and drugs. Average body temperature varies depending on the measurement site used. Each site and type of

thermometer has unique techniques, contraindications, or limitations and norms (Table 6-2). Several types of thermometers are commonly available to measure body temperature (Box 6-2). You can measure temperature on a Celsius or Fahrenheit scale. Although some electronic thermometers can display both Celsius and Fahrenheit readings, conversion charts are also available to convert from one scale to the other.

PULSE

The pulse is a palpable bounding of blood flow caused by pressure wave transmission from the left ventricle of the heart to the peripheral arteries. Assessing the pulse provides indications of heart function and tissue perfusion (circulation). In adults, the radial pulse is the site for routine pulse assessment. The brachial or apical pulse is the site for routine pulse assessment in infants.

Normally, the pulse is easily palpable, regular in rhythm, and ranges from 60 to 100 beats per minute in adults. When palpated, a normal pulse does not fade in and out and is not easily obliterated by pressure. Pulse abnormalities include bradycardia (pulse <60 beats/min), tachycardia (pulse >100 beats/min), and arrhythmia (irregular pulse rate). *Weak, feeble,* and *thready* are descriptive words for a pulse of low volume that is difficult to palpate. *Bounding* describes a pulse that is very strong. If you identify abnormalities such as an irregular rhythm or an inability to palpate the radial pulse, you must obtain an apical pulse. The apical pulse is the most accurate noninvasive measure of heart rate; you obtain it by

TABLE 6-2 ADVANTAGES AND LIMITATIONS OF SELECTED TEMPERATURE MEASUREMENT SITES

SITE ADVANTAGES	SITE LIMITATIONS
Oral • Easily accessible—requires no position change • Comfortable for patient • Provides accurate surface temperature reading • Reflects rapid change in core temperature • Reliable route to measure temperature for intubated patients	• Causes delay in measurement if patient recently ingested hot or cold fluids or foods, smoked, or chewed gum • Not used with patients who have had oral surgery; are unable to position thermometer in mouth; or have trauma, shaking or chills, or history of epilepsy • Not used with infants; small children; or confused, unconscious, or uncooperative patients • Risk of body fluid exposure
Tympanic Membrane • Easily accessible site • Minimal patient repositioning required • Obtained without disturbing, waking, or repositioning patient • Used for patients with tachypnea without affecting breathing • Sensitive to core temperature changes • Very rapid measurement (2-5 seconds) • Unaffected by oral intake of food or fluids or smoking • Used in newborns to reduce infant handling and heat loss	• More variability of measurement than with other core temperature devices • Requires removal of hearing aids at least 2 minutes before measurement • Requires disposable sensor cover with only one size available • Readings distorted by otitis media and cerumen impaction • Not used with patients who have had surgery of the ear or tympanic membrane; ear drainage; or blood, cerebrospinal fluid, or foreign bodies in the ear canal • Does not accurately measure core temperature changes during and after exercise • Affected by ambient temperature devices such as incubators, radiant warmers, and facial fans • Difficult to position correctly in neonates, infants, and children <3 years old because of anatomy of ear canal • Inaccuracies reported caused by incorrect positioning of handheld unit
Rectal • Argued to be more reliable when oral temperature is difficult or impossible to obtain	• Lags behind core temperature during rapid temperature changes • Not used for patients with diarrhea or patients who have had rectal surgery, rectal disorders, bleeding tendencies, or neutropenia • Requires positioning and is a source of patient embarrassment and anxiety • Risk of body fluid exposure • Requires lubrication • Not used for routine vital signs in newborns • Readings sometimes influenced by impacted stool
Axilla • Safe and inexpensive • Used with newborns and unconscious patients	• Long measurement time • Requires continuous positioning • Measurement lags behind core temperature during rapid temperature changes • Not recommended for detecting fever in infants and young children • Requires exposure of thorax, which results in temperature loss, especially in newborns • Affected by exposure to the environment, including time to place thermometer • Underestimates core temperature

TABLE 6-2	ADVANTAGES AND LIMITATIONS OF SELECTED TEMPERATURE MEASUREMENT SITES—cont'd	
SITE ADVANTAGES		**SITE LIMITATIONS**
Skin		
• Inexpensive • Provides continuous reading • Safe and noninvasive • Used for neonates		• Measurement lags behind other sites during temperature changes, especially during hyperthermia • Adhesion impaired by diaphoresis or sweat • Affected by environmental temperature • Cannot be used on patients with allergy to adhesives
Temporal Artery		
• Easy to access without position change • Very rapid measurement • Eliminates need to disrobe or unbundle • Comfortable for patient with no risk of injury • Used in premature infants, newborns, and children • Reflects rapid change in core temperature • Sensor cover not required		• Inaccurate with head covering or hair on forehead • Affected by skin moisture such as diaphoresis or sweating

using a stethoscope (Box 6-3). A stethoscope magnifies heart sounds as they are transmitted from the chest wall through the tubing to the listener. In adults, you auscultate the apical pulse (heard with a stethoscope) by placing the diaphragm over the point of maximal impulse at the fifth intercostal space on the left midclavicular line (Fig. 6-1).

RESPIRATIONS

Assessing respiration involves evaluating the exchange of oxygen and carbon dioxide between the environment, the blood, and the cells. Obtain the respiratory rate by observing the rate, depth, and rhythm of respiratory movements. Rate refers to the number of times a person breathes in and out in 1 minute. Estimate the depth of respirations by observing the movement of the chest during inspiration. Respiration can be described as deep or shallow. The rhythm of respirations is normally regular; however, irregular respiration patterns may occur (Table 6-3).

Determine breathing patterns by observing a patient's chest or the abdomen. Diaphragmatic breathing results from the contraction and relaxation of the diaphragm and is most visible in the abdomen (Fig. 6-2). Healthy men usually demonstrate diaphragmatic breathing, whereas women breathe more with the thorax, most apparent in the upper chest. In contrast, labored respirations usually involve the accessory muscles of respiration in the neck. A breathing cycle consists of a period of inspiration followed by a period of expiration. When something such as a foreign body (e.g., inhaled peanut) interferes with the movement of air into the lungs, the intercostal spaces retract during inspiration. A longer expiration phase is evident when the outward flow of air is obstructed (e.g., asthma). Auscultate lung sounds if a patient is experiencing dyspnea, a subjective report of inadequate or difficult breathing. Dyspnea is associated with increased effort to inhale

and exhale and may include active use of intercostal and accessory muscles. Orthopnea is difficulty breathing while lying flat and is relieved by sitting or standing. Assess lung sounds when a patient has excessive secretions, complains of chest pain, or has sustained trauma to the chest (see Chapter 7).

BLOOD PRESSURE

Blood pressure is the force exerted by the blood against the arterial walls. The systolic blood pressure is the peak pressure occurring during cardiac contraction when blood is forced from the left ventricle. The diastolic blood pressure is the pressure present in the arteries when the heart is relaxed. The pulse pressure is the difference between the systolic and diastolic pressure; for a blood pressure of 114/72 mm Hg, the pulse pressure is 42 mm Hg.

Many factors influence blood pressure. A single measurement does not adequately reflect a patient's blood pressure. Blood pressure trends, not individual measurements, guide nursing interventions. The most common alteration in blood pressure is *hypertension,* an often asymptomatic disorder characterized by persistently elevated blood pressure. The classification of hypertension is based on the average of at least three seated blood pressure measurements, properly measured with well-maintained equipment and spaced over a period of 1 week apart or more in an office or clinic (Kaplan et al, 2014). A diagnosis of prehypertension in nonpregnant adults is confirmed with a diastolic pressure of 80 to 89 mm Hg *or* systolic readings of 120 to 139 mm Hg (James et al., 2014).

Adoption of healthy lifestyles early in life reduces prehypertension and the risk for hypertension. Factors that increase the risk for hypertension include obesity, increased sodium intake, smoking, and lack of exercise. Hypertension and an elevated pulse pressure (>60 mm Hg) increase the risk for

BOX 6-2 TYPES OF THERMOMETERS

Electronic Thermometers

- Rechargeable battery-powered display unit with a thin wire cord and a temperature-processing probe covered by a disposable cover
- Within 1 minute after placement thermometer displays a digital temperature reading
- Separate probes available for oral and axillary temperature measurement (blue tip) and rectal temperature measurement (red tip) (see illustration *A*)

Tympanic Thermometers

- Probe consists of an otoscope-like speculum with an infrared sensor tip that detects heat radiated from the tympanic membrane of the ear (see illustration *B*)
- Within seconds after placement in the ear canal and depressing the scan button, digital reading appears on display unit; a sound signals when the peak temperature has been measured

Temporal Artery Thermometers

- Infrared scanner displays a digital reading within seconds after scanning while sweeping across the forehead and just behind the ear (see illustration *C*)

Chemical Dot Single-Use or Reusable Thermometers

- Thermometer consists of thin strip of plastic with a temperature sensor at one end that contains chemically impregnated dots formulated to change color to reflect temperature reading usually within 60 seconds (see illustration *D*)
- Useful for screening temperatures, especially in infants; during invasive procedures; and in orally intubated patients in the critical care unit; not appropriate for monitoring fever in acutely ill patients or monitoring temperature therapies
- May underestimate oral temperature by 0.4°C (32.7°F) or more in 50% of adults
- Disposable, easy to store, and can be used for patients requiring isolation
- Reusable thermometer can be used at axillary or rectal site if covered by a plastic sheath with a placement time of 3 minutes

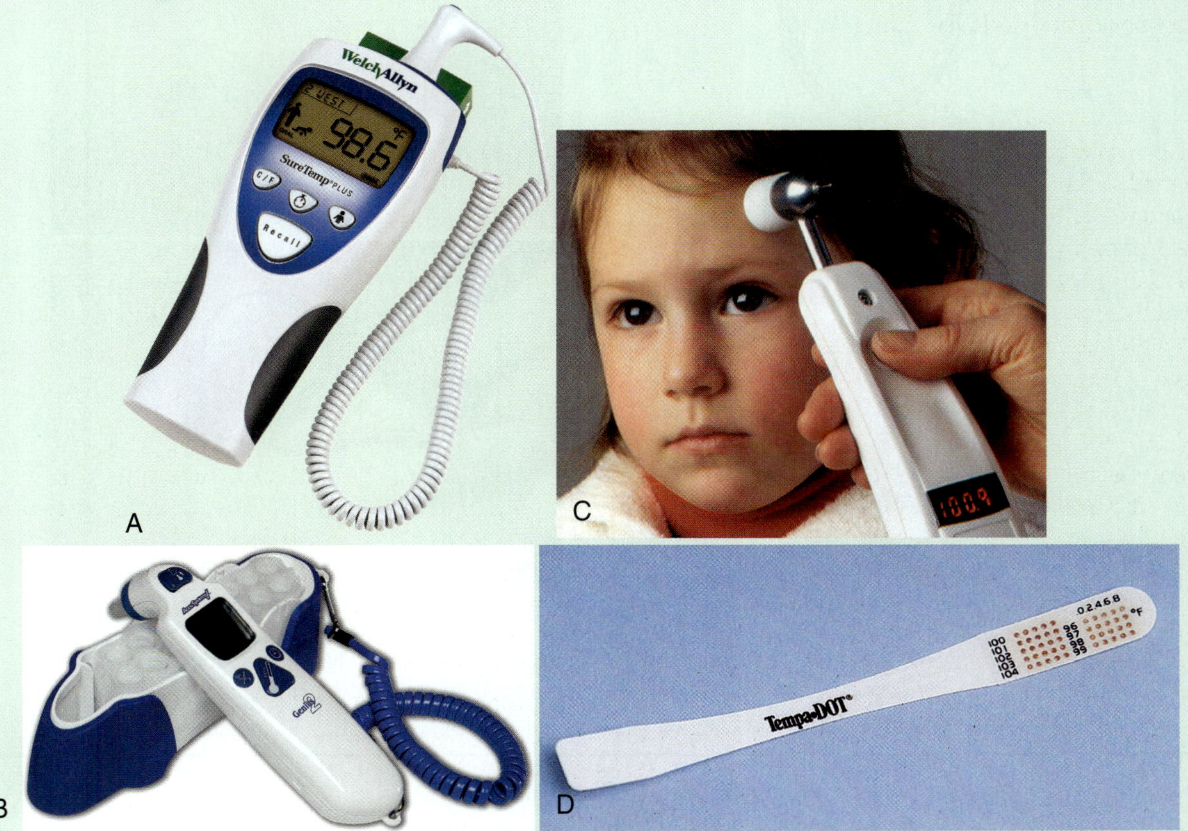

A, Electronic thermometer with oral (blue tip) and rectal (red tip) probes and disposable plastic sheath. **B,** Electronic tympanic membrane thermometer (Genius 2 Thermometer). **C,** Temporal artery thermometer measures heat from blood flowing through the superficial temporal artery. **D,** Chemical dot disposable single-use thermometer. (**B,** Genius 2 Thermometer used with permission of Covidien. All rights reserved. **C,** Photo courtesy Exergen.)

BOX 6-3   EXERCISES FOR LEARNING TO USE A STETHOSCOPE

1. Place earpieces in both ears with tips of earpieces turned toward the face. Lightly blow against the diaphragm (flat side of chest piece). Next, place earpieces in both ears with the tips turned toward the back of the head and again blow against the diaphragm. Compare comfort in the ears and amplification of sounds with earpieces in both directions. Earpieces pointing toward the face should fit snugly and comfortably.

2. If the stethoscope has both a diaphragm (flat side) and a bell (bowl-shaped with a rubber ring) (see illustration *A*), put earpieces in ears and lightly blow against the diaphragm to learn the difference in sound transmission. The chest piece can be turned to allow sound to be carried through either side (bell or diaphragm) of the chest piece. If sound is faint, lightly blow into the bell. Next, turn the chest piece and blow again against both the diaphragm and the bell. The diaphragm is used for higher pitched heart sounds, bowel sounds, and lung sounds (see illustration *B*). The bell is used for lower pitched heart sounds and vascular sounds (see illustration *C*).

3. With earpieces in place and using the diaphragm, move the diaphragm lightly over the hair on your arm. The bristling sound mimics a sound heard in the lungs. When listening for significant sounds, hold the diaphragm still and firmly make a tight seal against the skin to eliminate extraneous sounds.

4. Place the diaphragm over the front of your chest directly on your skin and listen to your own breathing, comparing the bell and the diaphragm. Repeat the process while listening to your heartbeat. Ask someone to speak in a conversational tone and note how the speech detracts from hearing clearly. When using a stethoscope, both the patient and the examiner should remain quiet.

5. With the earpieces in your ears, gently tap the tubing. Tapping also generates extraneous sounds. When listening to a patient, maintain a position that allows tubing to extend straight and hang free. Tubing that rubs or bumps objects creates extraneous sounds. Kinked tubing muffles sounds.

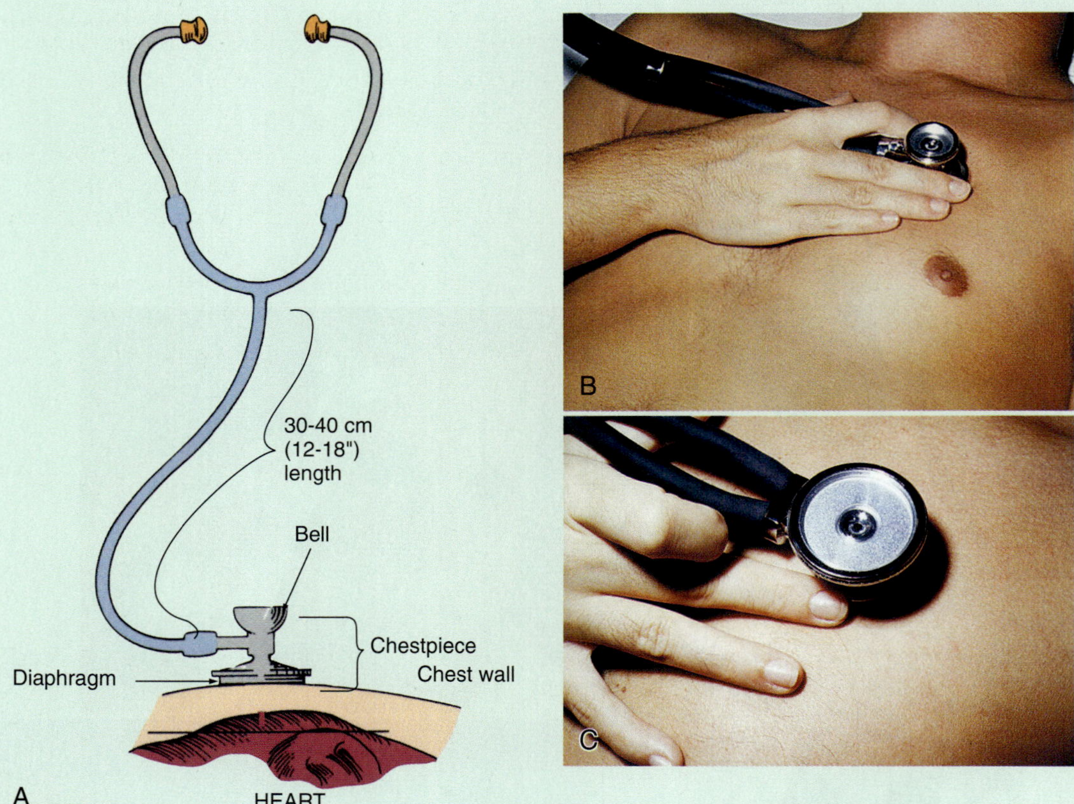

A, Parts of a stethoscope. **B,** The diaphragm is placed firmly and securely when auscultating high-pitched lung and bowel sounds. **C,** The bell must be placed lightly on the skin to hear low-pitched vascular and heart sounds.

stroke, myocardial infarction, and sudden death (Frese, Fick, and Sadowsky, 2011).

Measuring blood pressure using the auscultatory method requires detecting the sounds of the rush of blood (Korotkoff phases) as blood resumes its flow through an artery. The auscultatory method is performed manually with the use of a sphygmomanometer and a stethoscope or electronically with an auscultatory blood pressure machine. An electronic auscultatory blood pressure machine uses a microphone to detect the Korotkoff phases.

A sphygmomanometer includes a pressure manometer, an occlusive cloth or vinyl cuff that contains an inflatable rubber

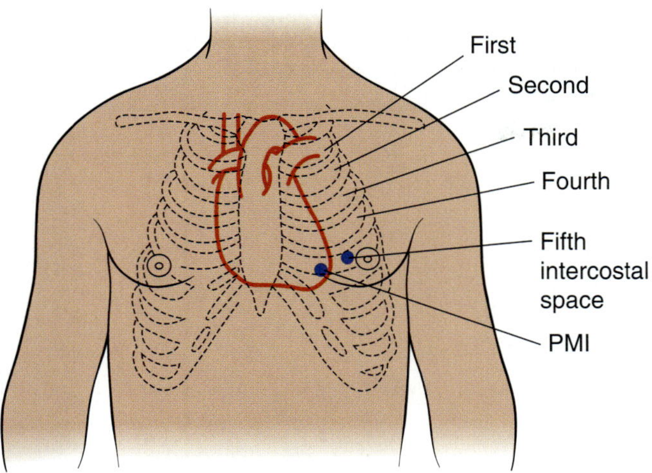

FIG 6-1 Point of maximal impulse (PMI) is at fifth intercostal space.

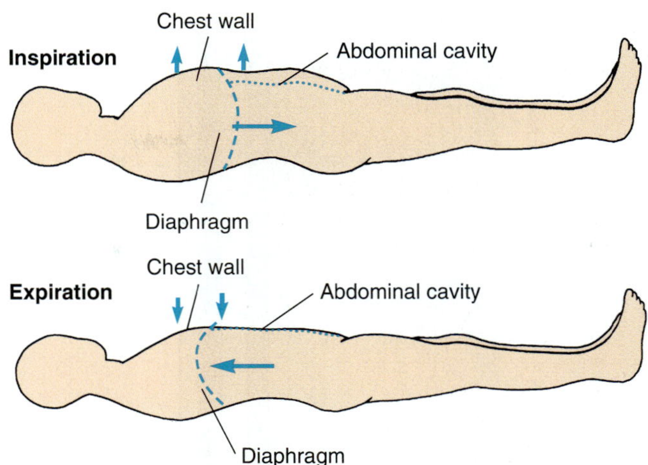

FIG 6-2 Diaphragmatic and chest wall movement during inspiration and expiration.

TABLE 6-3	ALTERATIONS IN BREATHING PATTERN
ALTERATION	**DESCRIPTION**
Apnea	Respirations cease for several seconds. Persistent cessation results in respiratory arrest.
Biot's respiration	Respirations are abnormally shallow for two to three breaths, followed by irregular period of apnea.
Bradypnea	Rate of breathing is regular but abnormally slow (<12 breaths/min).
Cheyne-Stokes respiration	Respiratory rate and depth are irregular, characterized by alternating periods of apnea and hyperventilation. Respiratory cycle begins with slow, shallow breaths that gradually increase to abnormal rate and depth. The pattern reverses; breathing slows and becomes shallow, concluding in apnea before respiration resumes.
Hyperpnea	Respirations are increased in depth. Hyperpnea occurs normally during exercise.
Hyperventilation	Rate and depth of respirations increase. Hypocarbia may occur.
Hypoventilation	Respiratory rate is abnormally low, and depth of ventilation may be depressed. Hypercarbia may occur.
Kussmaul's respiration	Respirations are abnormally deep but regular.
Tachypnea	Rate of breathing is regular but abnormally rapid (>20 breaths/min).

bladder, and a pressure bulb with a release valve that inflates the bladder. It can be portable or wall mounted. The manometer has a glass-enclosed circular gauge containing a needle that registers millimeter calibrations. The needle of the gauge should point to zero when not in use and move freely when the cuff pressure is released.

Place the occlusive cuff of the sphygmomanometer around the arm or thigh. Cuffs come in several different sizes, and the blood pressure measurement is not accurate unless you use the correct-size cuff (Fig. 6-3). Many adults require a large cuff. The inflatable bladder, enclosed by the cuff, should encircle at least 80% of the arm of an adult; the cuff width should be at least 40% greater than the arm circumference. Quickly inflate the cuff until blood flow ceases, and slowly deflate the cuff while the needle begins to fall. Auscultate Korotkoff phases by placing the stethoscope over the artery distal to the blood pressure cuff as the cuff is deflated. In some patients, the sounds are clear and distinct, whereas only the

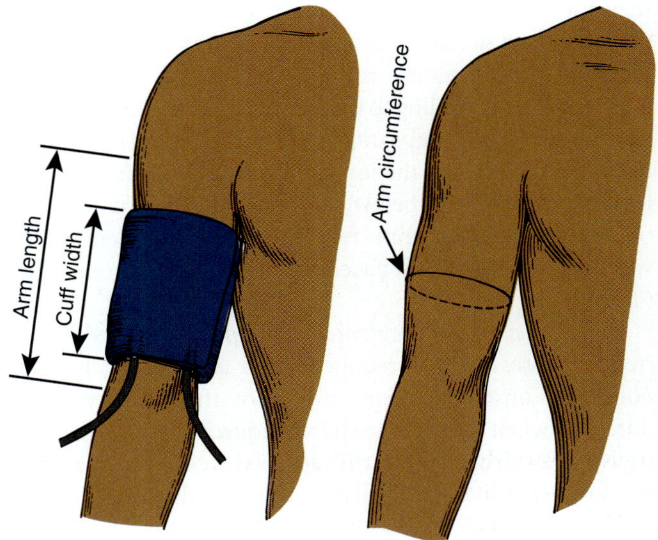

FIG 6-3 Proper cuff size. Length of bladder is 80% of arm circumference; cuff width is at least 40% larger than arm diameter.

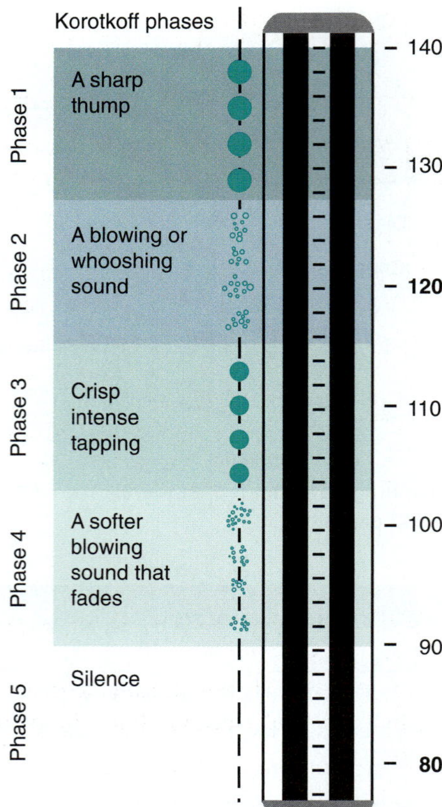

FIG 6-4 Sounds auscultated during blood pressure measurement can be differentiated into five Korotkoff phases. In this example, the blood pressure is 140/90 mm Hg.

beginning and ending sounds are audible in others (Fig. 6-4). You record the blood pressure with the systolic and diastolic numbers written as a fraction. The systolic pressure is the first sound heard as the cuff is deflating. Before the sounds cease, they may become distinctly muffled. The diastolic pressure is the last sound heard. In adults, you identify the systolic and diastolic blood pressure readings and record them by the pressures corresponding to the first of two consecutive sounds heard and the disappearance of sounds (not muffling), respectively. Confirm the last sounds by continuing to listen for 10 to 20 mm Hg below the last sound heard. You will obtain the most accurate readings by being aware of the various factors that influence accurate blood pressure values (Table 6-4).

Electronic blood pressure machines are used when frequent assessment is required, such as in critically ill or potentially unstable patients, during or after invasive procedures, or when therapies require frequent monitoring (e.g., trials of new drugs). Many different styles of electronic blood pressure machines are available; you can also find them in public areas such as shopping malls or patient's homes. Although electronic blood pressure machines are fast and give a nurse time to perform other activities, they do have disadvantages (Box 6-4).

TABLE 6-4   COMMON MISTAKES IN BLOOD PRESSURE ASSESSMENT

ERROR	EFFECT
Bladder or cuff too wide	False-low reading
Bladder or cuff too narrow or too short	False-high reading
Cuff wrapped too loosely or unevenly	False-high reading
Deflating cuff too slowly	False-high diastolic reading
Deflating cuff too quickly	False-low systolic and false-high diastolic reading
Arm below heart level	False-high reading
Arm above heart level	False-low reading
Arm not supported	False-high reading
Stethoscope that fits poorly or impairment of examiner's hearing, causing sounds to be muffled	False-low systolic and false-high diastolic reading
Stethoscope applied too firmly against antecubital fossa	False-low diastolic reading
Inflating too slowly	False-high diastolic reading
Repeating assessments too quickly	False-high systolic reading
Inadequate inflation level	False-low systolic reading
Multiple examiners using different Korotkoff sounds for diastolic readings	False-high systolic and false-low diastolic reading

---

BOX 6-4   ADVANTAGES AND LIMITATIONS OF ASSESSING BLOOD PRESSURE ELECTRONICALLY

Advantages
- Ease of use
- Ability to use a stethoscope not required
- Efficient when frequent repeated measurements are indicated
- Allows blood pressure to be measured frequently, as often as every 15 seconds, with accuracy

Limitations
- Expensive
- Requires source of electricity and space to position machine
- Sensitive to outside motion interference and cannot be used in patients with seizures, tremors, or shivers
- Inaccurate for patients with irregular heart rate or hypotension (blood pressure <90 mm Hg systolic) or in situations of reduced blood flow
- Accuracy standards for electronic blood pressure manufacturers vary
- Vulnerable to error among older-adult and obese patients

• **Nursing Skills Online: Vital Signs, Lesson 2**

Assessment of temperature requires making judgments about the site for temperature measurement, type of thermometer, and frequency of measurement. This skill includes temperature measurement with an electronic thermometer using the oral, tympanic, temporal, rectal, or axillary sites.

ASSESSMENT

1. Consider normal daily fluctuations in temperature. *Rationale: Body temperature tends to be lowest in early morning, peak in late afternoon, and gradually decline during the night. Fever is more accurately identified if you take a temperature between 5 PM and 7 PM.*

2. Identify medications or treatments that may influence temperature. *Rationale: Antiinflammatory drugs, steroids, warming or cooling blankets, and being in a room with fans affect body temperature.*

3. Identify if patient has exercised within the past 30 minutes. *Rationale: Exercise increases metabolism and heat production, resulting in increased temperature (Kaplan et al., 2014).*

4. Identify factors likely to interfere with accuracy of temperature measurement. *Rationale: Smoking, chewing gum, and hot or cold substances cause false temperature readings in the oral cavity for up to 15 minutes. The presence of stool in the rectum decreases accuracy of rectal temperature. Cerumen in the ear canal decreases accuracy of tympanic temperature. Diaphoresis decreases reliability of temporal temperature.*

5. Assess for signs and symptoms that accompany temperature alterations, as follows: for hyperthermia, decreased skin turgor, tachycardia, hypotension, concentrated urine; for heatstroke, hot dry skin, tachycardia, hypotension, excessive thirst, muscle cramps, visual disturbances, confusion or delirium; for hypothermia, pale skin, skin cool or cold to touch, bradycardia and dysrhythmias, uncontrollable shivering, reduced level of consciousness, shallow respirations. *Rationale: Physical signs and symptoms indicate abnormal temperature.*

6. Assess pertinent laboratory values, including complete blood count. *Rationale: A white blood cell count greater than $12,000/mm^3$ in a nonpregnant adult suggests the presence of infection, which can lead to hyperthermia; a white blood cell count less than $5000/mm^3$ suggests that the ability of the body to fight infection is compromised, which can lead to ineffective thermoregulation.*

7. Determine a previous baseline temperature from patient's record. *Rationale: A baseline value allows you to assess for change in condition by comparing vital sign measurements.*

8. Determine an appropriate temperature site and measurement device for patient, considering the advantages and disadvantages of each site (see Table 6-2).

PLANNING

Expected Outcomes focus on identifying abnormalities and restoring homeostasis.
1. Patient's temperature is within acceptable range.
2. Patient identifies the factors that influence body temperature.

Delegation and Collaboration
The skill of temperature measurement may be delegated to nursing assistive personnel (NAP). The nurse instructs the NAP about:
- Appropriate route, device, and frequency for a patient's temperature measurement.
- Precautions needed in positioning the patient for rectal temperature measurement.
- Need to report any significant changes or abnormalities to the nurse.

Equipment
- Thermometer (selected based on site used; see Table 6-2)
- Soft tissue or wipe
- Alcohol swab
- Lubricant (for rectal measurements only)
- Pen and vital sign flow sheet or record or patient's electronic medical record
- Clean gloves, plastic thermometer sleeve, disposable probe or sensor cover
- Towel

IMPLEMENTATION *for* MEASURING BODY TEMPERATURE

STEPS	RATIONALE
1. **See Standard Protocol (inside front cover).**	
2. Explain route by which you will take temperature and importance of maintaining proper position until reading is complete.	Patients are often curious about such measurements and prematurely remove thermometer to read results.
3. *Assess oral temperature (electronic).*	

Continued

STEPS	RATIONALE

a. *Optional:* Apply clean gloves when there are respiratory secretions or facial or mouth wound drainage.

Use of an oral probe cover, which is removable without physical contact, minimizes the need to wear gloves.

b. Remove thermometer pack from charging unit. Attach oral thermometer probe stem (blue tip) to thermometer unit. Grasp top of probe stem, being careful not to apply pressure on the ejection button.

Charging provides battery power. Ejection button releases plastic cover from probe stem.

c. Slide disposable plastic probe cover over thermometer probe stem until cover locks in place (see illustration).

Soft plastic cover will not break in patient's mouth and prevents transmission of microorganisms between patients.

d. Ask patient to open mouth; then gently place thermometer probe under tongue in posterior sublingual pocket lateral to center of lower jaw (see illustration).

Heat from superficial blood vessels in sublingual pocket produces temperature reading. With an electronic thermometer, temperatures in right and left posterior sublingual pockets are significantly higher than in the area under the front of tongue.

e. Ask patient to hold thermometer probe with lips closed.

Maintains proper position of thermometer during recording.

f. Leave thermometer probe in place until audible signal indicates completion and patient's temperature appears on digital display; remove thermometer probe from under patient's tongue.

Ensures that probe stays in place until signal sounds to ensure accurate reading.

g. Push ejection button on thermometer probe stem to discard plastic probe cover into appropriate receptacle.

Reduces transmission of microorganisms.

h. Return thermometer probe stem to storage position/charger of recording unit.

Returning probe stem automatically causes digital reading to disappear. Storage position protects stem.

4. *Assess rectal temperature (electronic).*

a. Draw curtain around bed or close room door. Assist patient to side-lying or Sims' position with upper leg flexed. Move aside bed linen to expose only anal area. Keep patient's upper body and lower extremities covered with sheet or blanket.

Maintains patient's privacy, minimizes embarrassment, and promotes comfort.

b. Apply clean gloves. Cleanse anal region when feces or secretions are present. Remove soiled gloves and reapply clean gloves.

Maintains Standard Precautions when there is exposure to items soiled with body fluids (e.g., feces).

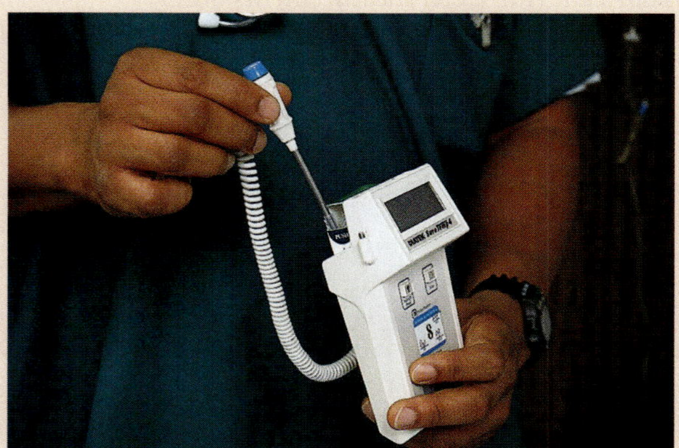

STEP 3c Disposable plastic cover is placed over probe stem and snaps in place.

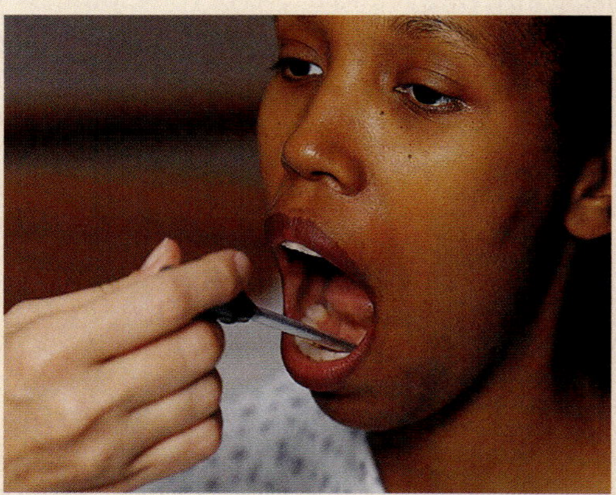

STEP 3d Probe under tongue in posterior sublingual pocket.

STEPS	RATIONALE

c. Remove thermometer pack from charging unit. Attach rectal thermometer probe stem (red tip) to thermometer unit. Grasp top of probe stem, being careful not to apply pressure on the ejection button.

Charging provides battery power. Ejection button releases plastic cover from probe stem.

d. Slide disposable plastic probe cover over thermometer probe stem until cover locks in place.

Probe cover prevents transmission of microorganisms between patients.

e. Squeeze liberal portion of lubricant onto tissue. Dip thermometer probe cover, blunt end, into lubricant, covering 2.5 to 3.5 cm (1 to 1½ inches) for adult.

Lubrication minimizes trauma to rectal mucosa during insertion. Using a tissue avoids contamination of remaining lubricant in container.

f. With nondominant hand, separate patient's buttocks to expose anus. Ask patient to breathe slowly and relax.

Fully exposes anus for thermometer insertion and relaxes anal sphincter for easier thermometer insertion.

g. Gently insert thermometer probe into anus in direction of umbilicus 3.5 cm (1½ inches) for adult. If you feel resistance during insertion, withdraw immediately. Do not force thermometer.

Ensures adequate exposure against blood vessels in rectal wall.

> **SAFE PATIENT CARE**   If you cannot insert the thermometer into the rectum adequately, remove it and consider an alternative method for obtaining temperature.

h. Once positioned, hold thermometer probe in place until audible signal indicates completion and patient's temperature appears on digital display; remove thermometer probe from anus (see illustration).

Probe needs to stay in place until signal sounds to ensure accurate reading.

i. Push ejection button on thermometer stem to discard plastic probe cover into an appropriate receptacle. Wipe probe stem with alcohol swab, paying particular attention to ridges where probe stem connects to probe.

Reduces transmission of microorganisms.

j. Return thermometer stem to storage position/charger of recording unit.

Automatically causes digital reading to disappear. Storage position protects stem.

k. Wipe patient's anal area with tissue or soft wipe to remove lubricant or feces, and discard tissue. Assist patient in assuming a comfortable position.

Provides for comfort and hygiene.

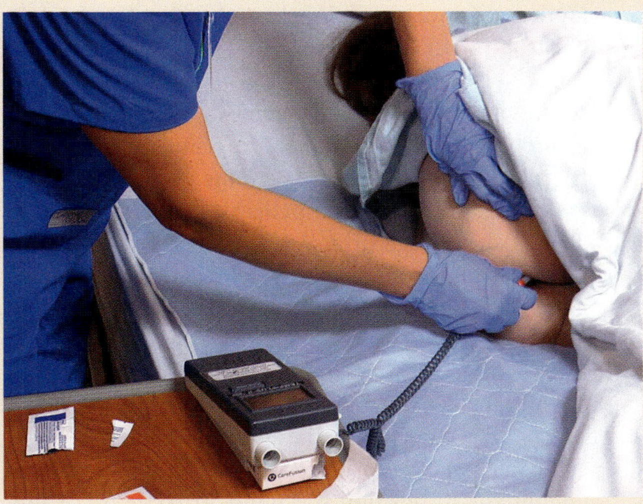

STEP 4h Remove probe inserted into anus.

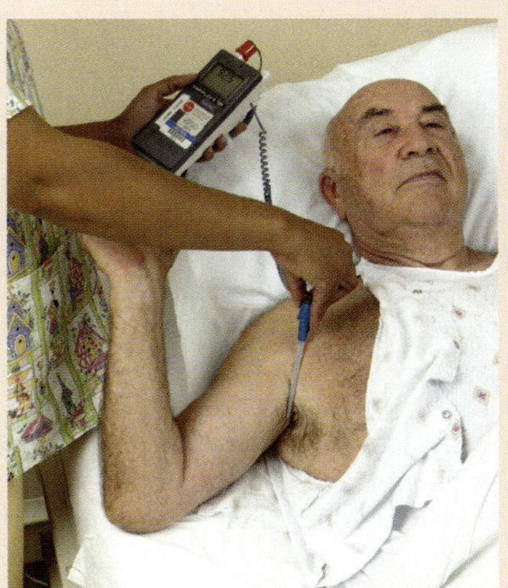

STEP 5d Place thermometer in axilla.

Continued

STEPS	RATIONALE

5. *Assess axillary temperature (electronic).*

a. Draw curtain around bed or close room door. Assist patient to supine or sitting position. Move clothing or gown away from shoulder and arm.

Maintains patient's privacy, minimizes embarrassment, and promotes comfort. Exposes axilla for correct thermometer probe placement.

b. Remove thermometer pack from charging unit. Attach oral thermometer probe stem (blue tip) to thermometer unit. Grasp top of thermometer probe stem, being careful not to apply pressure on ejection button.

Ejection button releases plastic cover from probe.

c. Slide disposable plastic probe cover over thermometer stem until cover locks in place.

Probe cover prevents transmission of microorganisms between patients.

d. Raise patient's arm away from torso. Inspect for skin lesions and excessive perspiration. Insert thermometer probe into center of axilla (see illustration), lower arm over probe, and place arm across patient's chest.

Maintains proper position of probe against blood vessels in axilla.

SAFE PATIENT CARE Do not use the axilla if skin lesions are present because local temperature may be altered, and the area may be painful to touch.

---

e. Once positioned, hold thermometer probe in place until audible signal indicates completion and patient's temperature appears on digital display. Remove thermometer probe from axilla.

Thermometer probe needs to stay in place until signal sounds to ensure accurate reading.

f. Push ejection button on thermometer stem to discard plastic probe cover into appropriate receptacle.

Reduces transmission of microorganisms.

g. Return thermometer stem to storage position/charger of recording unit.

Returning thermometer stem to storage position automatically causes digital reading to disappear. Storage position protects stem.

6. *Assess tympanic temperature.*

a. Assist patient in assuming comfortable position with head turned toward side, away from you. If patient has been lying on one side, use upper ear. Obtain temperature from patient's right ear if you are right-handed. Obtain temperature from patient's left ear if you are left-handed.

Ensures comfort and helps expose auditory canal for accurate temperature measurement. Heat trapped in ear facing down causes false-high temperature readings. Using the appropriate hand reduces the angle of approach. The less acute the angle, the better the probe seal.

b. Note if there is obvious earwax in patient's ear canal.

Earwax on the lens cover of the speculum blocks a clear optical pathway and lowers tympanic temperature. Switch to other ear, or select an alternative measurement site.

c. Remove thermometer handheld unit from charging base.

Base provides battery power. Removal of handheld unit from base prepares it to measure temperature.

d. Slide disposable speculum cover over otoscope-like tip until it locks into place. Be careful not to touch lens cover. Be careful not to apply pressure to ejection button.

Soft plastic probe cover prevents transmission of microorganisms between patients. Lens cover must be free of dust, fingerprints, and earwax to ensure clear optical path. Ejection button releases speculum cover from thermometer tip.

e. Insert speculum into ear canal, following manufacturer's instructions for tympanic probe positioning (see illustration).

Correct positioning of speculum probe tip with respect to ear canal allows maximum exposure of tympanic membrane.

(1) For children younger than 3 years old, point covered probe toward midpoint between eyebrow and sideburns. For children older than 3 years, pull pinna up and back (Hockenberry and Wilson, 2014).

The ear tug straightens the external auditory canal, allowing maximum exposure of the tympanic membrane to position speculum correctly in a young child.

STEPS	RATIONALE
(2) Fit speculum tip snugly into canal and do not move, pointing speculum tip toward nose.	Gentle pressure seals ear canal from ambient air temperature, which can alter readings 2.8°C (5°F). Operator error leads to false-low temperatures.
f. Once positioned, press scan button on handheld unit. Leave speculum in place until audible signal indicates completion and patient's temperature appears on digital display.	Pressing scan button causes detection of infrared energy. Speculum probe tip needs to stay in place until device has detected infrared energy, as noted by audible signal.
g. Carefully remove speculum from auditory canal.	Prevents rubbing of sensitive outer ear lining.
h. Push ejection button on handheld unit to discard speculum cover into appropriate receptacle.	Reduces transmission of microorganisms. automatically causes digital reading to disappear.
i. If temperature is abnormal or a second reading is necessary, replace speculum cover and wait 2 minutes before repeating the measurement in the same ear, or repeat measurement in other ear. Consider trying an alternative temperature site or instrument.	Time allows ear canal to regain usual temperature.
j. Return handheld unit to thermometer charger base.	Protects sensor tip from damage.

7. *Assess temporal artery temperature.*

a. Ensure that forehead is dry; wipe with towel if needed.	Moist skin interferes with thermometer sensor.
b. Place sensor flush on patient's forehead above eyebrow (see illustration).	Contact avoids measurement of ambient temperature.
c. Press red scan button with your thumb. Slowly slide thermometer straight across forehead while keeping sensor flush on skin.	Scanning for the highest temperature continues until you release the scan button.
d. Keeping the scan button pressed, lift sensor from forehead and touch sensor to skin on the neck, just behind the earlobe. Peak temperature occurs when clicking sound during scanning stops. Release scan button.	Sensor confirms highest temperature behind earlobe.
e. Clean sensor with alcohol swab.	Prevents transmission of microorganisms.
f. Return thermometer to charger or thermometer base.	Maintains battery charge of thermometer unit.

8. See Completion Protocol (inside front cover).

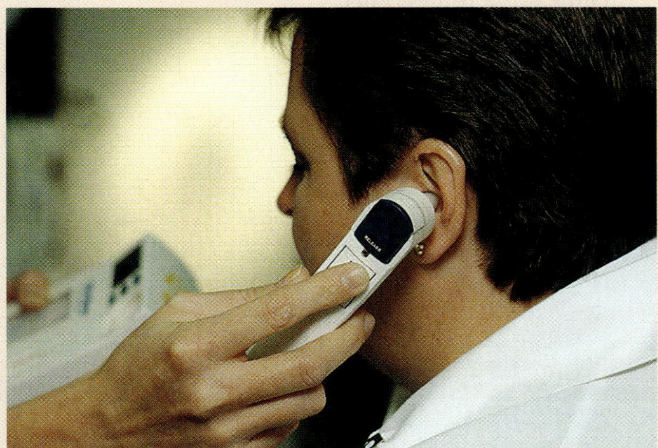

STEP 6e Tympanic membrane thermometer with probe cover placed in patient's ear.

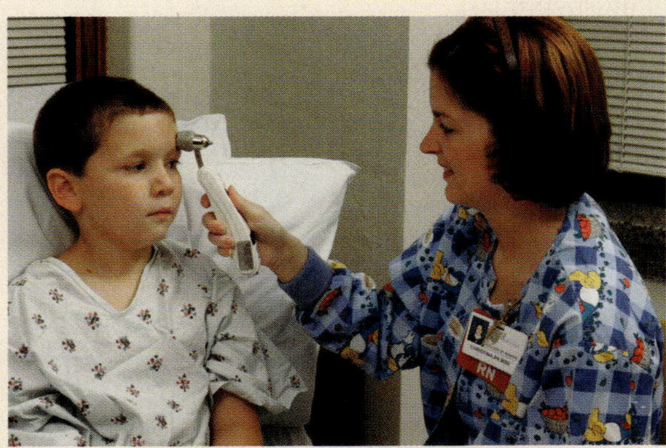

STEP 7b Scanning the forehead.

EVALUATION

1. Compare temperature measurement with patient's baseline and acceptable range.
2. If patient has a fever, take temperature approximately 30 minutes after administering antipyretics and every 4 hours until temperature stabilizes.
3. Use *Teach Back:* State to the patient, "I want to be sure I explained clearly the factors that can influence body temperature and ways to prevent your temperature from going too high or too low. Can you tell me what you could do to reduce your temperature on a hot day?" Evaluates what the patient is able to explain or demonstrate. Revise your instruction now or develop plan for revised patient teaching to be implemented at an appropriate time if patient is not able to teach back appropriately.

Unexpected Outcomes and Related Interventions

1. Patient has a temperature 1°C (1.8°F) or more above usual range.
   a. Assess possible sites for localized infection and related data suggesting systemic infection, including pain or tenderness; purulent drainage; local area of redness or unusual warmth; loss of appetite; headache; hot, dry skin; flushed face; thirst; general malaise; or chills.
   b. Reduce external covering on patient's body to promote heat loss. Conserve using a small room fan for cooling. Do not induce shivering.
   c. If fever persists or reaches an unacceptable level as defined by health care provider, administer antipyretics and antibiotics as ordered and institute cooling measures.
2. Patient has a temperature 1°C (1.8°F) or more below usual range.
   a. Remove any wet clothing or linen, replace with dry garments, and cover patient with warm blankets.
   b. Close room doors to eliminate drafts.
   c. Encourage warm liquids.
   d. Monitor apical pulse rate and rhythm (see Skill 6.2) because hypothermia causes bradycardia and dysrhythmias.

Recording and Reporting

- Record temperature and route in nurses' notes, vital sign flow sheet, or electronic medical record.
- Document your evaluation of patient learning.
- Record temperature after administration of specific therapies in narrative form in nurses' notes.
- Record in nurses' notes any signs or symptoms of temperature alterations.
- Report abnormal findings to nurse in charge or health care provider immediately.

Sample Documentation

1400 Temporal temperature 39.0°C (102.2°F). Patient reports fatigue. Skin flushed, dry. Acetaminophen 650 mg PO per order. Patient instructed to increase fluids.
1430 Temporal temperature 38.0°C (100.4°F). Patient napping. Skin pink, dry.

Special Considerations
Pediatric

- Axillary temperature cannot be relied on to detect fevers in infants and young children.
- For children who cry or become restless, take temperature last, after the other vital signs.

Geriatric

- Older adults without teeth or poor muscle control may be unable to close the mouth tightly to obtain accurate oral temperature readings.
- The temperature of older adults is at the lower end of the acceptable temperature range. Temperatures considered within normal range may reflect a fever in an older adult.
- A decrease in sweat gland reactivity in an older adult results in a higher threshold for sweating at high temperatures, which can lead to hyperthermia.
- Older adults are at high risk for hypothermia because of diminished sensation to cold, abnormal vasoconstrictor responses, and impaired shivering.

Home Care

- A temperature taken in the home may differ from the temperature assessed in a health care facility because the temperature routes differ.

SKILL 6.2   ASSESSING APICAL PULSE

- **Nursing Skills Online: Vital Signs, Lesson 3**

Assessing the apical pulse is the most accurate noninvasive method of determining a person's heart rate and rhythm.

Accurate assessment of the apical pulse requires correct use of a stethoscope (see Box 6-3).

ASSESSMENT

1. Identify medications or treatments that may influence pulse. *Rationale: Antiarrhythmics, antihypertensives, vasodilators, and vasoconstrictors affect pulse rate and rhythm.*
2. Identify factors affecting the patient that influence the pulse. *Rationale: Exercise and anxiety increase heart rate. An elevated temperature increases pulse rate and causes vasodilation, which can affect pulse strength. Certain conditions place patients at risk for pulse alterations, including a history of heart disease, cardiac arrhythmia, onset of sudden chest pain or acute pain from any site, invasive cardiovascular diagnostic tests, surgery, sudden infusion of a large volume of intravenous (IV) fluid, internal or external hemorrhage, or dehydration.*
3. Identify factors likely to interfere with accuracy of pulse rate. *Rationale: Caffeine and nicotine increase pulse rate. Smoking should be avoided within 30 minutes of measurement (Kaplan et al., 2014).*
4. Assess for signs and symptoms of altered cardiac function, such as dyspnea, fatigue, chest pain, orthopnea, syncope, palpitations (person's unpleasant awareness of heartbeat), edema of dependent body parts, cyanosis, or pallor of skin (see Chapter 7). *Rationale: Physical signs and symptoms indicate alteration in cardiac function, which affects pulse rate and rhythm.*
5. Assess pertinent laboratory values, including serum potassium and complete blood count. *Rationale: Low values for hemoglobin are associated with decreased oxygen transport, which can increase pulse rate. Low potassium or high potassium can cause arrhythmias.*
6. Determine if patient has a latex allergy. *Rationale: Allows you to protect the patient by verifying the stethoscope is latex-free.*
7. Determine previous baseline pulse rate from patient's record. *Rationale: Allows you to assess for change in condition and effect of cardiac medications.*

PLANNING

Expected Outcomes focus on identifying abnormalities and restoring homeostasis.
1. Patient's pulse rate is regular and within an acceptable range for age.
2. A baseline is established for patients with chronic diseases that alter pulse rate (e.g., atrial fibrillation or hypertension).

Delegation and Collaboration

The skill of apical pulse measurement can be delegated to nursing assistive personnel (NAP) if the patient is stable and not at high risk for acute or serious cardiac problems. The nurse instructs the NAP to:
- Obtain the appropriate frequency of measurement and consider factors related to the patient possibly having an abnormally slow or irregular pulse.
- Report any significant changes or abnormalities to the nurse.

Equipment
- Wristwatch with second hand or digital display
- Stethoscope
- Alcohol swab
- Pen and vital sign flow sheet or record or patient's electronic medical record

IMPLEMENTATION *for* ASSESSING APICAL PULSE

STEPS	RATIONALE
1. **See Standard Protocol (inside front cover).**	
2. Assist patient to supine or sitting position. Move bed linen and gown to uncover sternum and left side of chest.	Exposes portion of chest wall for selection of auscultatory site. Stethoscope must touch the skin for best sounds.
3. Locate anatomical landmarks to identify the apical impulse, also called the *point of maximal impulse.* The heart is located behind and to the left of the sternum with base at top and apex at bottom. Find the angle of Louis just below the suprasternal notch between the sternal body and manubrium; it feels like a bony prominence. Slip fingers down each side of the angle to find the second intercostal space. Carefully move fingers down the left side of the sternum to the fifth intercostal space and laterally to the left midclavicular line. A light tap felt within an area 1 to 2.5 cm ($\frac{1}{2}$ to 1 inch) of the apical impulse is reflected from the apex of the heart (see Fig. 6-1).	Use of anatomical landmarks allows correct placement of stethoscope over the apex of the heart. This position enhances the ability to hear heart sounds clearly. If unable to palpate the apical impulse, reposition patient on left side. In the presence of serious heart disease, locate the apical impulse to the left of the midclavicular line or at the sixth intercostal space.

Continued

STEPS	RATIONALE

4. Place diaphragm of stethoscope in palm of hand for 5 to 10 seconds.

Warming metal or plastic diaphragm prevents patient from being startled and promotes comfort.

5. Place diaphragm of stethoscope over the apical impulse at the fifth intercostal space, at the left midclavicular line, and auscultate for normal S_1 and S_2 heart sounds (heard as "lub dub") (see illustration). Allow stethoscope tubing to extend straight without kinks.

Normal S_1 and S_2 heart sounds are high-pitched and best heard with the diaphragm. Extended tubing does not distort sound transmission.

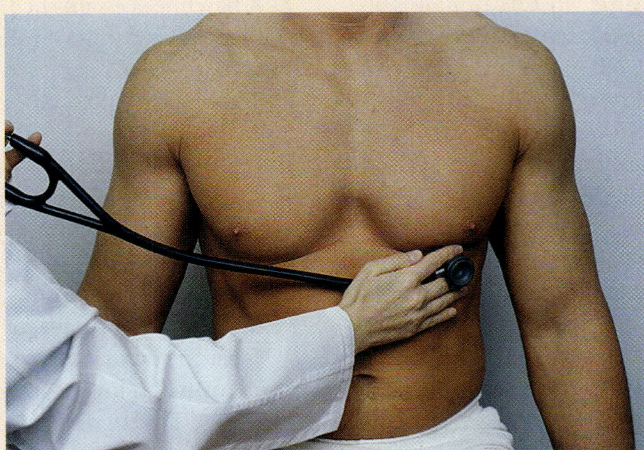

STEP 5 Stethoscope over the apical impulse at fifth intercostal space at left midclavicular line.

6. When you hear S_1 and S_2 with regularity, use second hand of watch and begin to count rate: when sweep hand hits number on dial, start counting with zero and then one, two, and so on.

Apical rate is accurate only after you are able to hear sounds clearly. Timing begins with zero. Count of one is first sound auscultated after timing begins.

7. If apical rate is regular, count for 30 seconds and multiply by 2. If heart rate is irregular or patient is receiving cardiovascular medication, count for 1 minute (60 seconds).

Monitor a regular apical rate for 30 seconds. You can assess irregular rate more accurately when measured over a longer interval, usually 60 seconds.

8. Note if heart rate is irregular, and describe pattern of irregularity (e.g., S_1 and S_2 occurring early or later after previous sequence of sounds—every third or every fourth beat is skipped).

Irregular heart rate indicates dysrhythmia. Regular occurrence of dysrhythmia within 1 minute indicates inefficient contraction of heart and alteration in cardiac function.

9. **See Completion Protocol (inside front cover).**

10. Clean earpieces and diaphragm of stethoscope with alcohol swab routinely after each use. Option: Simultaneously use hand foam to clean hands and stethoscope heads.

Stethoscopes are frequently contaminated with microorganisms. Regular disinfection controls hospital-acquired infections. Use of hand foam has been shown to reduce bacterial counts on stethoscopes (Uneke et al, 2014).

EVALUATION

1. Compare apical pulse rate with patient's baseline and acceptable range.

2. Correlate apical pulse rate with data obtained from radial pulse, blood pressure, and related signs and symptoms (chest pain, palpitations, dizziness).

Unexpected Outcomes and Related Interventions

1. Adult patient has an apical pulse greater than 100 beats/min (tachycardia).

   a. Identify related data, including pain, fear, anxiety, recent exercise, hypotension, blood loss, fever, or inadequate oxygenation.

b. Observe for signs and symptoms associated with abnormal cardiac function, including fatigue, chest pain, orthopnea, and cyanosis.

2. Adult patient has an apical pulse less than 60 beats/min (bradycardia).

   a. Assess for factors that alter heart rate such as digoxin (Lanoxin), beta blockers, and antiarrhythmics.

   b. Observe for signs and symptoms associated with abnormal cardiac function, including fatigue, chest pain, orthopnea, cyanosis.

3. Patient has an irregular rhythm.

   a. Observe for signs and symptoms associated with abnormal cardiac function, including fatigue, chest pain, orthopnea, and cyanosis.

   b. Report an irregular rhythm to the health care provider because patient may require an electrocardiogram or 24-hour heart monitor to detect heart abnormalities.

Recording and Reporting

- Record apical pulse rate in nurses' notes, vital signs flow sheet, or electronic medical record.
- Record apical pulse rate after administration of specific therapies, and document in narrative section of nurses' notes.

- Record any signs and symptoms of alteration in cardiac function in nurses' notes.
- Report abnormal findings to nurse in charge or health care provider immediately.

Sample Documentation

1200   Apical rate 64, regularly irregular. Health care provider aware.

Special Considerations
Pediatric

- Children often have a sinus arrhythmia, which is an irregular heartbeat that speeds up with inspiration and slows down with expiration. Breath holding in a child affects pulse rate.
- Apical or brachial pulse is the best site for assessing heart rate and rhythm in an infant or young child.

Geriatric

- An elevated pulse rate of an older adult takes longer to return to normal resting rate.
- Older adults have a reduced heart rate with exercise because of a decreased responsiveness to catecholamines.

SKILL 6.3   ASSESSING RADIAL PULSE

• **Nursing Skills Online: Vital Signs, Lesson 3**

The radial pulse in an adult is the easiest to access and provides a quick, accurate assessment of peripheral circulation and heart function.

ASSESSMENT

1. Identify medications or treatments that may influence pulse. *Rationale: Antiarrhythmics, antihypertensives, vasodilators, and vasoconstrictors affect pulse rate.*

2. Identify factors affecting the patient that influence pulse. *Rationale: Exercise and anxiety increase heart rate. An elevated temperature increases pulse rate and causes vasodilation, which can affect pulse strength.*

3. Identify factors likely to interfere with accuracy of pulse rate. *Rationale: Caffeine and nicotine increase pulse rate. Blood pressure should not be assessed if the patient has smoked within the previous 30 minutes (Kaplan et al., 2014).*

4. Assess for signs and symptoms of altered cardiac function, such as dyspnea, fatigue, chest pain, orthopnea, syncope, or palpitations. *Rationale: Physical signs and symptoms indicate alteration in cardiac function, which affects pulse rate and rhythm.*

5. Determine previous baseline pulse rate from patient's record. *Rationale: Allows you to assess for change in condition and effect of cardiac medications.*

PLANNING

Expected Outcomes focus on identifying abnormalities and restoring homeostasis.

1. Patient's pulse rate is regular and within an acceptable range for age.

2. A baseline is established for patients with chronic diseases that alter pulse rate, such as atrial fibrillation or hypertension.

Delegation and Collaboration

The skill of pulse measurement can be delegated to nursing assistive personnel (NAP) if the patient is stable and not at high risk for acute or serious cardiac or vascular problems. The nurse instructs the NAP to:

- Obtain the pulse using the appropriate site and frequency of measurement and considering factors related to the patient possibly having an abnormally slow or irregular pulse.
- Report any significant changes or abnormalities to the nurse.

Equipment

- Wristwatch with second hand or digital display
- Pen and vital sign flow sheet or record or patient's electronic medical record

IMPLEMENTATION *for* ASSESSING RADIAL PULSE

STEPS	RATIONALE
1. **See Standard Protocol (inside front cover).**	
2. Explain to patient that you will assess pulse or heart rate. Encourage patient to relax and not speak. If patient has been active, wait 5 to 10 minutes before assessing pulse.	Activity and anxiety elevate heart rate. Obtaining pulse rates at rest allows for objective comparison of values.
3. If patient is supine, place patient's forearm straight alongside or across lower chest or upper abdomen with wrist extended straight. If sitting, bend patient's elbow 90 degrees and support lower arm on chair or on your arm.	Relaxed position of lower arm and extension of wrist permit full exposure of artery to palpation.
4. Locate pulse by placing tips of first two or middle three fingers of your hand over groove along radial or thumb side of patient's inner wrist (see illustration). Slightly extend or flex the wrist with palm down until you note the strongest pulse.	Fingertips are the most sensitive parts of your hand to palpate arterial pulsation. Your thumb has a pulsation that interferes with accuracy.

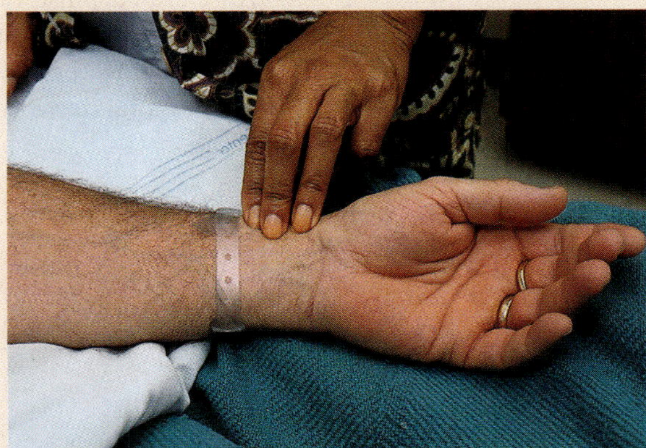

STEP 4 Hand placement for pulse assessment. (From Sorrentino SA, Remmert L: *Mosby's textbook for nursing assistants*, ed 8, St Louis, 2012, Mosby.)

STEPS	RATIONALE
5. Lightly compress the pulse against radius, losing the pulse initially, and then relax pressure so pulse becomes easily palpable.	Pulse is more accurate with moderate pressure. Too much pressure occludes pulse and impairs blood flow.
6. Determine strength of pulse. Note whether thrust of vessel against fingertips is bounding (4+); full or increased (+3); expected (+2); diminished or barely palpable (+1); or absent, nonpalpable (0).	Strength reflects volume of blood ejected against arterial wall with each heart contraction. Accurate description of strength improves communication among nurses and other health care providers.
7. After you feel pulse regularly, look at watch's second hand and begin to count rate: when sweep hand hits number on dial, start counting with zero and then one, two, and so on.	Timing begins with zero. Count of one is first beat palpated after timing begins.
8. If pulse is regular, count rate for 30 seconds and multiply total by 2.	A 30-second count is accurate for rapid, slow, or regular pulse rates.
9. If pulse is irregular, count rate for 60 seconds. Assess frequency and pattern of irregularity.	Inefficient contraction of heart fails to transmit pulse wave, resulting in irregular pulse. Longer time period promotes accurate count.
10. When pulse is irregular, compare radial pulses bilaterally.	A marked inequality indicates compromised arterial flow to one extremity, and you need to take action.
11. **See Completion Protocol (inside front cover).**	

EVALUATION

1. Compare pulse rate with patient's baseline and acceptable range.
2. Compare radial pulse strength and equality and note discrepancy. Differences between radial arteries indicate a compromised peripheral vascular system.
3. Correlate pulse rate with data obtained from apical pulse, blood pressure, temperature, and related signs and symptoms (e.g., chest pain, palpitations, dizziness).
4. Use **Teach Back:** State to the patient, "I want to be sure I demonstrated and explained clearly how to measure your own pulse rate. Can you show me by counting your pulse rate?" Evaluates what the patient is able to explain or demonstrate. Revise your instruction now or develop plan for revised patient teaching to be implemented at an appropriate time if patient is not able to teach back appropriately.

Unexpected Outcomes and Related Interventions

1. Patient has a weak, thready, or difficult-to-palpate radial pulse.
   a. Assess both radial pulses and compare findings. Assess for swelling in surrounding tissues or anything that may impede blood flow (e.g., dressing or cast).
   b. Observe for symptoms associated with altered peripheral tissue perfusion, including pallor or cyanosis of tissue distal to pulse and cold extremities.
2. Patient has an irregular radial pulse or pulse less than 60 beats/min (bradycardia) or greater than 100 beats/min (tachycardia).
   a. Auscultate the apical pulse.

Recording and Reporting

- Record pulse rate and rhythm with assessment site in nurses' notes, vital signs flow sheet, or electronic medical record.
- Document your evaluation of patient learning.
- Record pulse rate after administration of specific therapies, and document in narrative in nurses' notes.
- Record any signs and symptoms of alteration in cardiac function in nurses' notes.
- Report abnormal findings to nurse in charge or health care provider immediately.

Sample Documentation

1400 Right radial pulse +2; left radial pulse +1, left hand cool to touch, capillary refill >4 sec. Charge nurse notified.

Special Considerations

Pediatric

- Radial artery is difficult to assess in an infant. Apical or brachial pulse is the best site for assessing pediatric heart rate and rhythm until 2 years of age.

Geriatric

- An elevated pulse rate in an older adult takes longer to return to normal resting rate.
- Older adults have a reduced heart rate with exercise because of a decreased responsiveness to catecholamine.
- Peripheral vascular disease is more common among older adults, making radial pulse assessment difficult.

Home Care

- Patients taking certain prescribed cardiac or antiarrhythmic medications or their family caregivers should learn to assess radial pulse to detect side effects of medications.

PROCEDURAL GUIDELINE 6.1
Assessing Apical-Radial Pulse Deficit

The difference between pulses assessed from two different sites, or a pulse deficit, provides information about heart and blood vessel function. When a pulse deficit is assessed between the apical and radial pulses, the volume of blood ejected from the heart may be inadequate to meet the circulatory needs of the tissues, and intervention may be required. To assess for a pulse deficit, the nurse and a second health care provider assess a peripheral pulse rate and the apical pulse rate simultaneously and compare the measurements.

Delegation and Collaboration

The skill of assessing an apical-radial pulse deficit cannot be delegated to nursing assistive personnel (NAP) while the nurse assesses the apical pulse. Collaboration between the nurse and a second health provider is required.

Equipment

- Stethoscope
- Watch with second hand or digital display
- Pen and vital sign flow sheet or electronic medical record (EMR)
- Alcohol swab

Procedural Steps

1. Determine need to assess for pulse deficit. Irregular heart rate and signs and symptoms such as dyspnea, fatigue, chest pain, and palpitations may indicate abnormal cardiac function.
2. Perform hand hygiene.
3. Collect and bring appropriate supplies to the patient's bedside and draw curtain around bed and/or close door.

Continued

PROCEDURAL GUIDELINE 6.1
Assessing Apical-Radial Pulse Deficit—cont'd

4. Explain to the patient that two people will be assessing heart function at the same time.
5. Assist patient to supine or sitting position. Move aside bed linen and gown to expose sternum and left side of chest.
6. Locate apical and radial pulse sites. Nurse auscultates apical pulse (see Skill 6-2) while second health care provider palpates radial pulse (see Skill 6-3).
7. Nurse begins pulse count by calling out loud when to begin counting pulses.
8. Each nurse completes a 60-second pulse count simultaneously. The count ends when the nurse states, "Stop."

Sixty seconds is required when a discrepancy between pulse sites is expected or when the rhythm is irregular.

9. If the pulse count differs by more than 2, a pulse deficit exists. The pulse deficit reflects the number of ineffective cardiac contractions in 1 minute.
10. If a pulse deficit is noted, assess for other signs and symptoms of decreased cardiac output (see Chapter 7).
11. Discuss findings with patient as needed.
12. Perform hand hygiene.
13. Record apical pulse, radial pulse, and pulse deficit in nurses' notes. Inform the nurse in charge or health care provider of the presence of a pulse deficit.

SKILL 6.4   ASSESSING RESPIRATIONS

• **Nursing Skills Online: Vital Signs, Lesson 4**

Assessment of respirations includes determining respiratory rate, depth, and rhythm.

ASSESSMENT

1. Identify medications or treatments that may influence respiratory rate. *Rationale: Oxygen, bronchodilators, sedatives, or opioids can affect respiratory rate.*
2. Identify factors affecting the patient that influence respiratory rate, depth, and rhythm. *Rationale: Fever, pain, anxiety, diseases of the chest wall or muscles, constrictive chest or abdominal dressings, presence of abdominal incisions, pulmonary disease (emphysema, bronchitis, asthma), traumatic injury to the chest wall, presence of a chest tube, respiratory infection (pneumonia, acute bronchitis), pulmonary edema and emboli, head injury with damage to brainstem, and anemia all can affect respiratory assessment.*
3. Assess for signs and symptoms of altered respiratory function. *Rationale: Physical signs and symptoms indicate alterations in respiratory function that affect respiratory rate, depth, and rhythm.*
   • Restlessness, irritability, confusion, reduced level of consciousness
   • Pain during inspiration
   • Labored or difficult breathing
   • Orthopnea
   • Use of accessory muscles
   • Adventitious breath sounds (see Chapter 7)
   • Inability to breathe spontaneously
   • Thick, frothy, blood-tinged, or large amounts of sputum produced on coughing
   • Bluish or cyanotic appearance of nail beds, lips, mucous membranes, and skin

4. Identify that patient is in a comfortable position. *Rationale: Sitting erect promotes full ventilatory movement. A position of discomfort causes patient to breathe more rapidly.*
5. Determine previous baseline respiratory rate from patient's record. *Rationale: A baseline value allows you to assess for change in condition and effect of respiratory medications.*

PLANNING

Expected Outcomes focus on identifying abnormalities and restoring homeostasis.
1. Patient's respiratory rate is regular and within acceptable range for age.
2. A baseline is established for patients with chronic diseases such as obstructive lung disease that alter respiratory rate.

Delegation and Collaboration
The skill of counting respirations can be delegated to nursing assistive personnel (NAP). The nurse instructs the NAP to:
• Obtain the appropriate frequency of measurement as determined by the patient's history and factors related to it, such as labored breathing or complaints of breathing difficulty.
• Report any significant changes or abnormalities to the nurse.

Equipment
• Wristwatch with second hand or digital display
• Pen and vital sign flow sheet or record or patient's electronic medical record

IMPLEMENTATION *for* ASSESSING RESPIRATIONS

STEPS	RATIONALE
1. **See Standard Protocol (inside front cover).**	
2. Be sure that patient's chest is visible. If necessary, move bed linen or gown.	Ensures a clear view of chest wall and abdominal movements.
3. Place patient's arm in relaxed position across the abdomen or lower chest, or place your hand directly over patient's upper abdomen.	A similar position used during pulse assessment allows you to assess respiratory rate subtly. Patient's arm or your hand rises and falls during respiratory cycle.
4. Observe complete respiratory cycle (one inspiration and one expiration).	Viewing of the entire respiratory cycle is necessary for an accurate rate measurement.
5. After observing a cycle, look at watch's second hand and begin to count rate: when sweep hand hits number on dial, begin time frame, counting one with first full respiratory cycle.	Timing begins with count of one. Respirations occur more slowly than pulse; timing does not begin with zero.
6. If rhythm is regular, count number of respirations in 30 seconds and multiply by 2. If rhythm is irregular, less than 12, or greater than 20, count for 1 full minute.	Respiratory rate is equivalent to number of respirations per minute. Suspected irregularities require assessment for at least 1 minute (see Table 6-3).
7. Note depth of respirations, subjectively assessed by observing degree of chest wall movement while counting rate. You also objectively assess depth by palpating chest wall excursion or auscultating the posterior thorax (see Chapter 7) after you have counted the rate. Describe depth as shallow, normal, or deep.	Character of ventilatory movement reveals specific disease state that restricts volume of air from moving into and out of lungs.
8. Note rhythm of ventilatory cycle. Normal breathing is regular and uninterrupted. Do not confuse sighing with abnormal rhythm.	Character of ventilations reveals specific types of alterations. Periodically people unconsciously take single deep breaths or sighs to expand small airways prone to collapse.
9. Observe for any increased effort to inhale and exhale. Ask patient to describe subjective experience of breathing compared with usual breathing pattern.	Patients with chronic lung disease may experience difficulty breathing all the time and can best describe their own discomfort from shortness of breath.
10. **See Completion Protocol (inside front cover).**	

EVALUATION

1. Compare findings with previous baseline and acceptable range for patient's age.
2. Correlate respiratory rate with data obtained from auscultation, laboratory data, and related respiratory signs and symptoms.

Unexpected Outcomes and Related Interventions

1. Respiratory rate is less than 12 (bradypnea) or greater than 20 (tachypnea). Breathing pattern is irregular. Depth of respirations is increased or decreased; patient complains of dyspnea.
   a. Observe for related factors, including obstructed airway, noisy respirations, cyanosis, restlessness, irritability, confusion, productive cough, use of accessory muscles, and abnormal breath sounds (see Chapter 7).
   b. Assist patient to a supported sitting position (semi-Fowler's or high Fowler's) unless contraindicated.
   c. Provide oxygen as ordered (see Chapter 14).
   d. Assess for environmental factors that influence patient's respiratory rate, such as secondhand smoke, poor ventilation, or gas fumes.

Recording and Reporting

- Record respiratory rate and character in nurses' notes, vital sign flow sheet, or electronic medical record. Record type and amount of oxygen therapy if used by patient during assessment.
- Record abnormal depth and rhythm in narrative form in nurses' notes.
- Record respiratory rate after administration of specific therapies in narrative form in nurses' notes.
- Report abnormal findings to nurse in charge or health care provider immediately.

Sample Documentation

0750   Patient c/o dyspnea. RR 32, shallow and labored. SpO_2 92% with 2 L of oxygen via nasal cannula. Bilateral wheezing auscultated. BP 144/56 R arm, R radial pulse 112, strong. Respiratory therapy notified for prn nebulizer treatment. Charge nurse notified.

Special Considerations
Pediatric
- Assess respiratory rate before other vital signs and before child becomes anxious or fears other procedures.

Geriatric
- A change in lung function with aging results in respiratory rates that are generally higher in older adults, with a normal range of 16 to 25 breaths/min.

- Acceptable average respiratory rate for newborns is 30 to 60 breaths/min, for toddlers (2 years) is 24 to 40 breaths/min, and for children is 18 to 30 breaths/min (Marx et al., 2013).

SKILL 6.5   ASSESSING BLOOD PRESSURE

- **Nursing Skills Online: Vital Signs, Lesson 5**

Accurate blood pressure measurement is critical for making decisions about fluid volume replacement and need for medications and for assessing rapidly changing clinical conditions. This skill describes blood pressure assessment in upper and lower extremities using a sphygmomanometer and stethoscope.

ASSESSMENT

1. Consider normal daily fluctuations in blood pressure. *Rationale: Blood pressure varies throughout the day, with lower blood pressure during sleep and highest blood pressure in the afternoon.*
2. Identify patient's medications or treatments that may influence blood pressure. *Rationale: Opioids, sedatives, general anesthetics, antihypertensives, vasodilators, vasoconstrictors, blood, and IV fluids affect blood pressure.*
3. Identify factors affecting the patient that influence blood pressure. *Rationale: Exercise, pain, stress, anxiety, and hormone stimulation can increase blood pressure.*
4. Identify factors likely to interfere with accuracy of blood pressure measurements. *Rationale: Coffee, smoking, talking, movements, and patient position all affect blood pressure. Blood pressure should not be measured if patient has smoked or exercised within the previous 30 minutes (Kaplan et al., 2014).*
5. Assess for signs and symptoms of blood pressure alterations. *Rationale: Physical signs and symptoms sometimes indicate alterations in blood pressure. High blood pressure (hypertension) is often asymptomatic until pressure is very high. Assess for headache (usually occipital), flushing of face, nosebleed, and fatigue in older adults. Low blood pressure (hypotension) is associated with dizziness; confusion; restlessness; pale, dusky, or cyanotic skin and mucous membranes; and cool, mottled skin over extremities.*
6. Determine appropriate extremity and blood pressure cuff for patient. *Rationale: Inappropriate site selection results in poor amplification of sounds, causing inaccurate readings (see Table 6-4). Application of pressure from the inflated cuff temporarily impairs blood flow and further compromises circulation in an extremity that already has impaired blood flow. Avoid applying cuff to an extremity affected by the following situations: IV fluids are infusing; an arteriovenous shunt or fistula is present; breast or axillary surgery has been performed on that side; extremity has been traumatized or*
diseased or requires a cast or bulky bandage. Use the lower extremities when the brachial arteries are inaccessible.
7. Determine if patient has a latex allergy. *Rationale: If patient has a latex allergy, verify that blood pressure cuff is latex-free.*
8. Determine previous baseline blood pressure from patient's record.
9. If the patient monitors blood pressure in the home, assess patient's knowledge of blood pressure management and ability to obtain a measurement. If a family caregiver measures blood pressure in the home, assess the caregiver's competency as well.

PLANNING

Expected Outcomes focus on identifying abnormalities and restoring homeostasis.
1. Patient's blood pressure is within an acceptable range for age, gender, and ethnicity.
2. A baseline is established for patients with hypertension and chronic diseases that alter blood pressure.
3. Patient identifies factors that increase blood pressure.
4. Patient states strategies to reduce personal risk for hypertension.

Delegation and Collaboration
The skill of blood pressure measurement may be delegated to nursing assistive personnel (NAP) unless the patient is considered unstable (i.e., hypotensive). The nurse instructs the NAP to:
- Obtain the appropriate frequency of measurement and limb for measurement and to consider factors related to the patient's history, such as risk for orthostatic hypotension.
- Apply the appropriate size blood pressure cuff and equipment (electronic or manual) to be used.
- Report any significant changes or abnormalities to the nurse.

Equipment
- Calibrated aneroid sphygmomanometer
- Cloth or disposable vinyl pressure cuff of appropriate size for patient's extremity
- Stethoscope
- Alcohol swab
- Pen and vital sign flow sheet or record or patient's electronic medical record

IMPLEMENTATION *for* ASSESSING BLOOD PRESSURE

STEPS	RATIONALE

1. **See Standard Protocol (inside front cover).**

2. Explain to patient that you will assess blood pressure (BP). Have patient rest at least 5 minutes before measuring lying or sitting blood pressure and 1 minute before measuring standing blood pressure. Ask patient not to speak while measuring blood pressure.

   Reduces anxiety that falsely elevates readings. BP readings taken at different times can be compared more objectively when assessed with patient at rest. Exercise causes false elevations in BP. Talking to a patient when assessing the BP increases readings 8 to 15 mm Hg (Kaplan et al., 2014).

3. Be sure that patient has not ingested caffeine or smoked for 30 minutes before BP assessment.

   Caffeine and nicotine cause false elevations in BP. Smoking and caffeine intake can alter blood pressure (Kaplan et al., 2014).

4. Select appropriate cuff size:

   a. For arm circumference of 22 to 26 cm, cuff should be "small adult" size: 12 cm × 22 cm

   b. For arm circumference of 27 to 34 cm, cuff should be "adult" size: 16 cm × 30 cm

   c. For arm circumference of 35 to 44 cm, cuff should be "large adult" size: 16 cm × 36 cm

   d. For arm circumference of 45 to 52 cm, cuff should be "adult thigh" size: 16 cm × 42 cm (Kaplan et al., 2014).

   Improper cuff size results in inaccurate readings (see Table 6-4).

5. Clean stethoscope earpieces and diaphragm with alcohol swab. Option: Simultaneously use hand foam to clean hands and stethoscope heads.

   Reduces transmission of microorganisms. Use of hand foam has been shown to reduce bacterial counts on stethoscopes (Uneke et al., 2014).

6. Have patient assume sitting or lying position. Be sure that environment is warm, quiet, and relaxing.

   Sitting is preferred to lying if patient is mobile. Diastolic BP measured while supine is approximately 2 to 3 mm Hg lower than when measured sitting. A patient's perceptions that the physical or interpersonal environment is stressful affect BP measurement. Talking and background noise result in inaccurate readings.

7. Position patient's forearm, supported at heart level if needed, with palm turned up (see illustration); for thigh, position with knee slightly flexed. If sitting, instruct patient to keep feet flat on floor without legs crossed. If supine, support the patient's arm (e.g., on the mattress or with a pillow so that the cuff is at the level of the right atrium).

   If arm is extended and not supported, patient will perform isometric exercise that increases diastolic pressure. Placement of arm above the level of the heart causes false-low reading 2 mm Hg for each inch above heart level. Leg crossing falsely increases systolic BP. Even in the supine position a diastolic pressure increases BP up to 3 to 4 mm Hg for each 5-cm change in heart level.

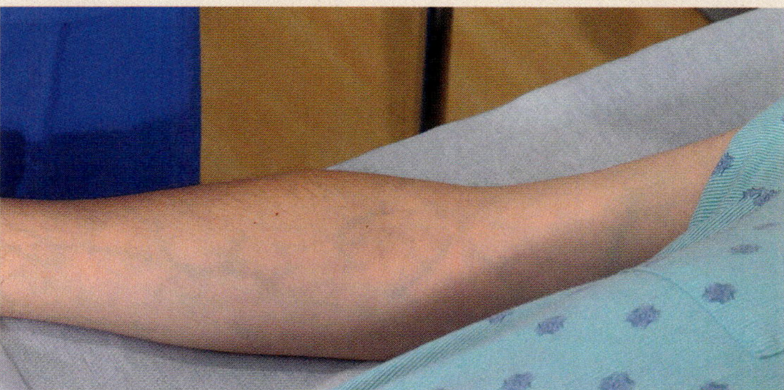

STEP 7 Patient's forearm supported in bed.

8. Expose extremity (arm or leg) fully by removing constricting clothing. The BP cuff may be applied over a sleeved arm, but a bare arm is preferred (Pinar et al., 2010; Kaplan et al., 2014).

   Ensures proper cuff application. Tight, constricted clothing causes congestion of blood and can falsely elevate BP readings. Sleeves have no effect on BP results.

Continued

STEPS	RATIONALE

9. Palpate brachial artery (arm) or popliteal artery (leg). With cuff fully deflated, apply bladder of cuff above artery by centering arrows marked on cuff over artery. If there are no center arrows on cuff, estimate the center of the bladder and place this center over artery. Position cuff 2.5 cm (1 inch) above site of pulsation (antecubital or popliteal space). With cuff fully deflated, wrap cuff evenly and snugly around extremity (see illustrations).

Inflating bladder directly over artery ensures that proper pressure is applied during inflation. A loose-fitting cuff causes false-high readings.

10. Position manometer gauge vertically at eye level. You should be no farther than 1 m (approximately 1 yard) away from the manometer gauge.

Looking up or down at the scale results in inaccurate readings.

11. Measure blood pressure.

   a. Two-step method:

     (1) Relocate brachial or popliteal pulse. Palpate the artery distal to the cuff with fingertips of nondominant hand while inflating cuff rapidly to a pressure 30 mm Hg above point at which pulse disappears. Slowly deflate cuff, and note point when pulse reappears. Deflate cuff fully and wait 30 seconds.

Estimating systolic pressure prevents false-low readings, which result in the presence of an auscultatory gap. Palpation determines maximal inflation point for accurate reading. If unable to palpate artery because of weakened pulse, use an ultrasonic stethoscope (see Chapter 7). Completely deflating cuff prevents venous congestion and false-high readings.

     (2) Place stethoscope earpieces in ears and be sure that sounds are clear, not muffled.

Ensures that each earpiece follows angle of ear canal to facilitate hearing.

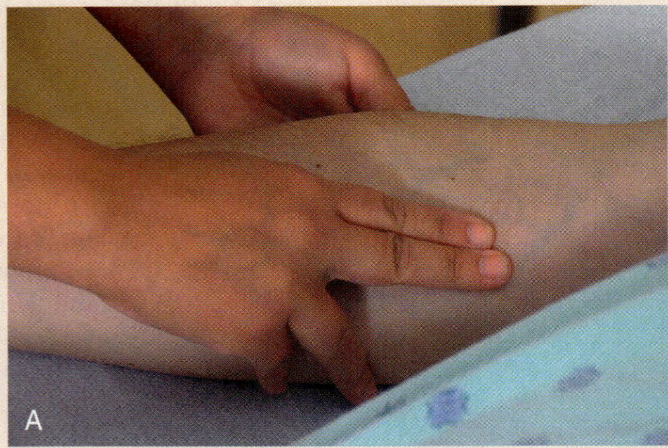
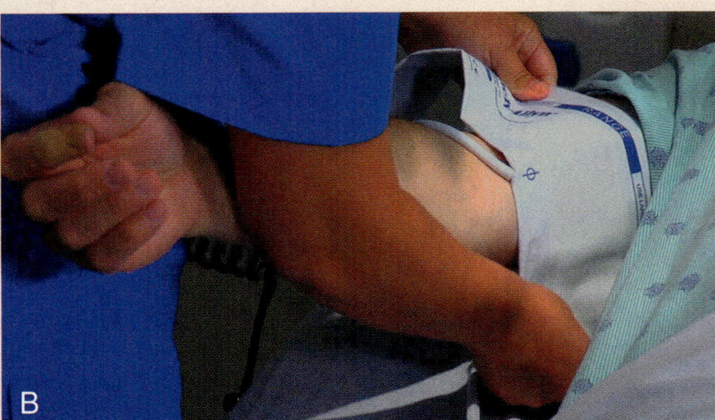

STEP 9 A, Palpating the brachial artery. **B,** Aligning blood pressure cuff arrow with brachial artery.

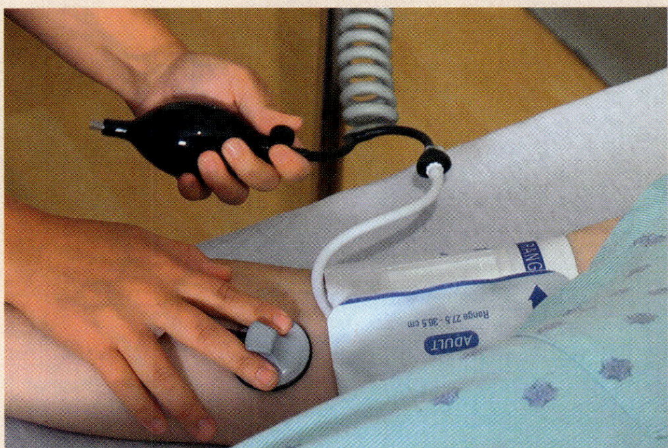

STEP 11a(3) Stethoscope over brachial artery to measure blood pressure.

STEPS	RATIONALE

(3) Relocate brachial or popliteal artery and place bell or diaphragm of stethoscope over it. Do not allow chest piece to touch cuff or clothing (see illustration).

Proper stethoscope placement ensures the best sound reception. The bell provides better sound reproduction, whereas the diaphragm is easier to secure with fingers and covers a larger area. An improperly positioned stethoscope causes muffled sounds that often result in false-low systolic and false-high diastolic readings.

(4) Close valve of pressure bulb clockwise until tight.

Tightening valve prevents air leak during inflation.

(5) Quickly inflate cuff to 30 mm Hg above patient's estimated systolic pressure.

Rapid inflation ensures accurate measurement of systolic pressure.

(6) Slowly release pressure bulb valve and allow manometer needle gauge to fall at rate of 2 to 3 mm Hg/sec.

A too-rapid or too-slow decline in pressure release causes inaccurate readings.

(7) Note point on manometer when the first clear sound is heard. The sound slowly increases in intensity.

First Korotkoff sound reflects systolic blood pressure.

(8) Continue to deflate cuff gradually, noting point at which sound disappears in adults. Note pressure to nearest 2 mm Hg. Listen for 20 to 30 mm Hg after the last sound, and then allow remaining air to escape quickly.

Beginning of the fifth Korotkoff sound is an indication of diastolic pressure in adults (Kaplan et al., 2014). Fourth Korotkoff sound involves distinct muffling of sounds and is an indication of diastolic pressure in children (Kaplan et al., 2014).

b. One-step method:

(1) Place stethoscope earpieces in ears and be sure that sounds are clear, not muffled.

Earpiece should follow the angle of ear canal to facilitate hearing.

(2) Relocate brachial or popliteal artery and place diaphragm of stethoscope over it. Do not allow chest piece to touch cuff or clothing.

Proper stethoscope placement ensures optimal sound reception.

(3) Close valve of pressure bulb clockwise until tight.

Tightening valve prevents air leak during inflation.

(4) Quickly inflate cuff to 30 mm Hg above patient's usual systolic pressure.

Inflation above systolic level ensures accurate measurement of systolic pressure.

(5) Slowly release pressure bulb valve and allow manometer needle to fall at rate of 2 to 3 mm Hg/sec. Note point on manometer when you hear the first clear sound. The sound slowly increases in intensity.

A too-rapid or too-slow decline in pressure release causes inaccurate readings. The first sound reflects the systolic pressure.

(6) Continue to deflate cuff gradually, noting point at which sound disappears in adults. Note pressure to nearest 2 mm Hg. Listen for 20 to 30 mm Hg after the last sound, and then allow remaining air to escape quickly.

The beginning of the last sound is an indication of diastolic pressure in adults. In children, the diastolic pressure is the beginning of the distinct muffling of sounds (Hockenberry and Wilson, 2014).

12. The American Heart Association recommends the average of two sets of BP measurements 2 minutes apart. Use the second set of BP measurements as the patient's baseline.

Two sets of BP measurements help to prevent false-positive measurements based on a patient's sympathetic response (alert reaction). Averaging minimizes the effect of anxiety, which often causes a first reading to be higher than subsequent readings (Kaplan et al., 2014).

13. Remove cuff from patient's extremity unless you need to repeat measurement. If this is the first assessment of patient, repeat procedure on the other extremity.

Comparison of BP in both extremities detects circulatory problems. (A normal difference of 5 to 10 mm Hg exists between extremities.)

14. **See Completion Protocol (inside front cover).** Clean earpieces, bell, and diaphragm of stethoscope with alcohol swab or use hand foam while cleansing hands.

Reduces transmission of microorganisms when nurses share stethoscopes.

EVALUATION

1. Compare reading with previous baseline and acceptable value of blood pressure for patient's age.
2. Compare blood pressure in both arms and both legs. If using upper extremities, use the arm with higher pressure for subsequent assessments unless contraindicated.
3. Correlate blood pressure with data obtained from pulse assessment and related cardiovascular signs and symptoms (e.g., dizziness, chest pain, excess fatigue).
4. Use *Teach Back:* State to the patient, "I want to be sure I explained clearly the factors that can increase your blood pressure and ways you can reduce your personal risk. Can you tell me how you can reduce your risk of high blood pressure?" Evaluates what the patient is able to explain or demonstrate. Revise your instruction now or develop plan for revised patient teaching to be implemented at an appropriate time if patient is not able to teach back correctly.

Unexpected Outcomes and Related Interventions

1. Blood pressure reading cannot be obtained.
   a. Verify technique by checking for correct selection and placement of cuff and correct elevation of extremity.
   b. Repeat the blood pressure measurement on the opposite extremity.
   c. Determine that no immediate crisis is present by assessing pulse and respiratory rate.
   d. Assess for signs and symptoms of altered cardiac function (e.g., chest pain, shortness of breath). If present, notify nurse in charge or health care provider immediately.
   e. Use alternative sites or procedures to obtain blood pressure: auscultate blood pressure in lower extremity, use an ultrasonic stethoscope, or use palpation method to obtain systolic blood pressure.
   f. Repeat any electronic blood pressure measurement with a sphygmomanometer. Electronic blood pressure measurements are less accurate in low blood flow conditions.
2. Blood pressure measurement is above acceptable range.
   a. Repeat blood pressure measurement in other extremity and compare findings.
   b. Verify correct selection of cuff size and placement of cuff.
   c. Ask nurse colleague to repeat measurement in 1 to 2 minutes.
   d. Observe for related symptoms, although symptoms sometimes are not apparent until blood pressure is extremely elevated.
3. Blood pressure value is insufficient for adequate perfusion and oxygenation of tissues.
   a. Compare blood pressure value with patient's baseline. A systolic reading of 90 mm Hg is an acceptable value for some patients.
   b. Position the patient in supine position to enhance circulation and restrict activity that may decrease blood pressure further.

   c. Assess for signs and symptoms associated with hypotension, including tachycardia; weak, thready pulse; weakness; dizziness; confusion; cool, pale, dusky or cyanotic skin.
   d. Assess for factors that would contribute to a low blood pressure, including hemorrhage, dilation of blood vessels resulting from hypothermia, anesthesia, or medication side effects.

Recording and Reporting

- Record blood pressure and the extremity assessed on vital sign flow sheet, nurses' notes, or electronic medical record.
- Document your evaluation of patient learning.
- Record any signs and symptoms of blood pressure alterations in narrative form in nurses' notes.
- Record measurement of blood pressure after administration of specific therapies in narrative form in nurses' notes.
- Report the following immediately to nurse in charge or health care provider: abnormal findings such as elevated or low blood pressure or if there is a difference of more than 20 mm Hg systolic or diastolic when comparing blood pressure measurements on upper extremities.

Sample Documentation

0400   BP 104/56 R arm, supine, decreased from baseline of 124/72. R radial pulse 112, weak, thready. RR 24, regular. SpO_2 95%. Temporal T 36.8°C (98.2°F). Patient c/o dizziness, nausea. Skin pale. Health care provider notified.

Special Considerations
Pediatric
- Blood pressure is not a routine part of assessment in children younger than 3 years.

Geriatric
- Older adults who have lost upper arm mass, especially a frail elderly adult, require special attention to selection of a smaller blood pressure cuff.
- Skin of older adults is more fragile and susceptible to cuff pressure when blood pressure measurements are frequent. More frequent assessment of the skin under the cuff or rotation of blood pressure sites is recommended.
- Instruct older adults to change position slowly and wait after each change to avoid postural hypotension and prevent injuries.

Home Care
- There is increasing evidence that home readings predict cardiovascular events and are particularly useful for monitoring the effects of treatment.
- Assess family's financial ability to afford a sphygmomanometer for regular measurement of blood pressure at home.
- Consider an electronic blood pressure cuff with large digital display for home if patient or family caregiver has hearing or vision difficulties.

PROCEDURAL GUIDELINE 6.2
Assessing Blood Pressure Electronically

• **Nursing Skills Online: Vital Signs, Lesson 5**

Electronic blood pressure (BP) machines are found in health care facilities and public places such as shopping malls. These machines rely on sound waves or vibrations that are interpreted electronically and converted into a blood pressure value. Verify an assessment of an abnormal blood pressure by an electronic machine with a sphygmomanometer and stethoscope. Automatic readings have been shown to record higher systolic readings (Suokhrie et al., 2013).

Delegation and Collaboration

The skill of blood pressure measurement using an electronic blood pressure machine can be delegated to nursing assistive personnel (NAP) unless the patient is considered unstable (i.e., hypotensive). The nurse instructs the NAP to:

- Obtain the appropriate frequency of measurement and extremity for measurement.
- Apply the appropriate size of blood pressure cuff for designated extremity and appropriate cuff for the machine.
- Report any significant changes or abnormalities to the nurse.

Equipment

- Electronic blood pressure machine
- Blood pressure cuff of appropriate size as recommended by manufacturer
- Source of electricity

Procedural Steps

1. **See Standard Protocol (inside front cover).**
2. Determine the appropriateness of using electronic BP measurement. Patients with irregular heart rate, seizures, tremors, and shivering are not candidates for this device.
3. Determine best site for cuff placement.
4. Assist patient to a comfortable position either lying or sitting with arm at heart level. Plug in the machine and place near patient, ensuring that the connector hose between the cuff and machine reaches easily.
5. Locate on/off switch and turn on machine to enable it to self-test computer systems.
6. Select an appropriate cuff size for patient's extremity and appropriate cuff for the machine (Table 6-5). An electronic BP cuff and machine are matched by manufacturer and are not interchangeable.
7. Expose the extremity for measurement by removing constricting clothing to ensure proper cuff application.
8. Prepare BP cuff by manually squeezing all the air out of the cuff and attaching the cuff to the connector hose.
9. Wrap flattened cuff snugly around extremity, verifying that only one finger fits between the cuff and patient's skin. Ensure that the "artery" arrow marked on the outside of the cuff is correctly placed (see illustration *B* for Skill 6.5, Step 9).
10. Verify that the connector hose between the cuff and the machine is not kinked. Kinking prevents proper inflation and deflation of the cuff.
11. Following the manufacturer's directions, set the frequency control to automatic or manual, and then press start button. The first BP measurement pumps the cuff to a peak pressure of about 180 mm Hg. After this pressure is reached, the machine begins a deflation sequence that determines the BP. The first reading determines the peak pressure inflation for additional measurements.
12. When deflation is complete, the digital display provides the most recent values and flashes time in minutes that has elapsed since the measurement occurred (see illustration).

TABLE 6-5	PROPER CUFF SIZE FOR ELECTRONIC MONITOR	
CUFF TYPE	**LIMB CIRCUMFERENCE (cm)**	
Small adult	17-25	
Adult	23-33	
Large adult	31-40	
Thigh	38-50	

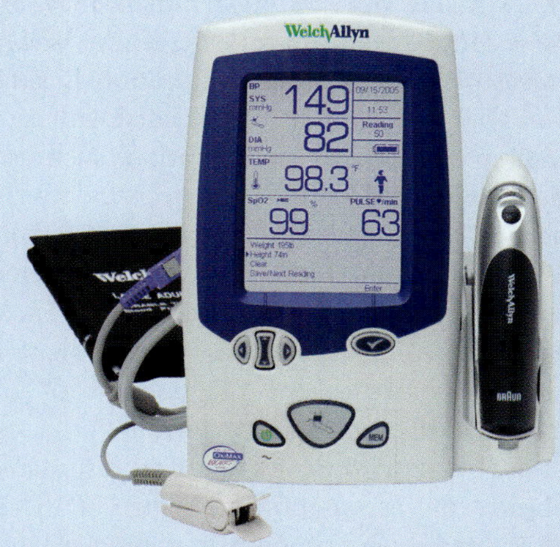

STEP 12 Monitor displays reading. Verify electronic alarm settings. (Image courtesy Welch Allyn.)

SAFE PATIENT CARE If unable to obtain BP with electronic device, verify machine connections (e.g., plugged into working electrical outlet, hose-cuff connections tight, machine on, correct cuff). Repeat electronic BP measurement; if unable to obtain, use auscultatory technique (see Skill 6.5).

Continued

PROCEDURAL GUIDELINE 6.2
Assessing Blood Pressure Electronically—cont'd

13. Set frequency of BP measurements and upper and lower alarm limits for systolic, diastolic, and mean BP readings. Intervals between BP measurements are set from 1 to 90 minutes. Determine frequency and alarm limits based on patient's acceptable range of BP, nursing judgment, facility standards, or health care provider order.

14. Obtain additional readings at any time by pressing the start button. (Sometimes you will need additional readings to assess unstable patients.) Pressing the cancel button immediately deflates the cuff.

15. If frequent BP measurements are required, leave the cuff in place. Remove the cuff every 2 hours to assess underlying skin integrity, and alternate BP sites if possible. Patients with abnormal bleeding tendencies are at risk for microvascular rupture from repeated inflations. When you are finished using the electronic BP machine, clean the cuff according to facility policy to reduce transmission of microorganisms.

16. Compare electronic BP readings with auscultatory BP measurements to verify accuracy of electronic BP measurement.

17. **See Completion Protocol (inside front cover).**

18. Record BP and site used to assess on vital sign flow sheet, nurses' notes, or electronic medical record. Record any signs of BP alterations in nurses' notes.

19. Report abnormal findings to nurse in charge or health care provider.

PROCEDURAL GUIDELINE 6.3
Measuring Oxygen Saturation (Pulse Oximetry)

• **Nursing Skills Online: Vital Signs, Lesson 6**

Pulse oximetry is the noninvasive measurement of arterial blood oxygen saturation, the percent to which hemoglobin is bound with oxygen. The assessment of oxygen saturation using pulse oximetry (SpO_2) is often included when obtaining vital signs. A pulse oximeter is a probe with a light-emitting diode (LED) connected by a cable to an oximeter. Normally, SpO_2 is greater than 95%. SpO_2 less than 90% is considered a clinical emergency (WHO, 2011).

The measurement of oxygen saturation is simple and painless and has few of the risks associated with more invasive measurements of oxygen saturation, such as arterial blood gas sampling. Conditions that decrease arterial blood flow, such as peripheral vascular disease, hypothermia, vasoconstrictors, hypotension, or peripheral edema, affect accurate measurement of oxygen saturation. Factors that affect light transmission, such as outside light sources, patient motion, or red-based nail polish, also affect the accurate measurement of oxygen saturation.

In adults, you can apply reusable and disposable oximeter probes to the earlobe, finger, bridge of the nose, or forehead. Oxygen saturation measurement using a forehead probe is quicker than finger probes (Yont, Korhan, and Khorshid, 2011) and more accurate in conditions that decrease arterial blood flow (Nesseler et al., 2012). Pulse oximetry is indicated in patients who have an unstable oxygen status or are at risk for impaired gas exchange.

Delegation and Collaboration

The skill of oxygen saturation measurement can be delegated to an NAP. The nurse instructs the NAP to:

- Consider the specific factors related to the patient that can falsely lower oxygen saturation.
- Obtain the appropriate frequency of oxygen saturation measurement.
- Apply the appropriate site and probe for measurement.
- Report any SpO_2 reading less than 95% to the nurse immediately.
- Refrain from using pulse oximetry as an assessment of heart rate because the oximeter will not detect an irregular pulse.

Equipment

- Oximeter
- Oximeter probe appropriate for patient and recommended by oximeter manufacturer
- Acetone or nail polish remover if needed
- Pen or pencil and vital sign flow sheet or record form

Procedural Steps

1. Determine the need to measure patient's oxygen saturation. Assess for risk factors for decreased oxygen saturation (e.g., acute or chronic respiratory problems, chest wall injury, monitoring during unconscious sedation, recovery from sedation or anesthesia).

2. Assess for signs and symptoms of alterations in oxygen saturation (e.g., altered respiratory rate, depth, or rhythm; adventitious breath sounds [see Chapter 7]; restlessness; difficulty breathing; cyanotic nail beds, lips, or mucous membranes).

3. Assess for factors that influence measurement of SpO_2: oxygen therapy, respiratory therapy treatments such as

PROCEDURAL GUIDELINE 6.3
Measuring Oxygen Saturation (Pulse Oximetry)—cont'd

postural drainage and percussion, hemoglobin level, hypotension, temperature, and medications such as bronchodilators.

4. Review patient's medical record for health care provider's order, or consult facility's procedure manual for oxygen saturation measurement standard of care.
5. Determine previous baseline SpO$_2$ (if available) from patient's record.
6. Determine most appropriate patient-specific site (e.g., finger, earlobe, bridge of nose, forehead) for sensor probe placement by measuring capillary refill. If capillary refill is greater than 2 seconds, select alternative site.
   a. Site must have adequate local circulation and be free of moisture.
   b. A finger free of polish or acrylic nail is preferred (Cicek et al., 2011).
   c. If patient has tremors or is likely to move, use earlobe or forehead.
   d. If patient is obese, clip-on probe may not fit properly; obtain a disposable (tape-on) probe.
7. **See Standard Protocol (inside front cover).**
8. Position patient comfortably. Instruct patient to breathe normally. If the finger is the monitoring site, support lower arm.
9. If using the finger, remove fingernail polish from digit with acetone or polish remover.
10. Attach the sensor to monitoring site. Instruct patient that the clip-on probe will feel like a clothespin on the finger but will not hurt.
11. When the sensor is in place, turn on oximeter by activating power. Observe pulse waveform/intensity display and audible beep. Correlate oximeter pulse rate with patient's radial pulse.
12. Leave the sensor in place until oximeter readout reaches a constant value and pulse display reaches full strength during each cardiac cycle. Inform patient that the oximeter alarm will sound if the sensor falls off or if patient moves the sensor. Read SpO$_2$ on digital display (see illustration).

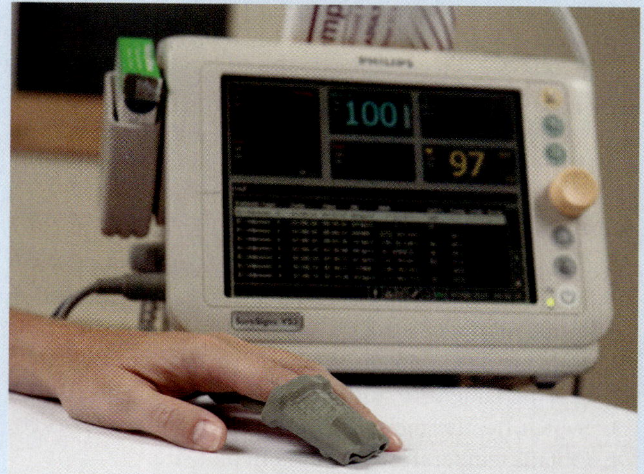

STEP 12 Obtain oximetry reading.

13. If you plan to monitor oxygen saturation continuously, verify that SpO$_2$ alarm limits are preset by the manufacturer at a low of 85% and a high of 100%. Determine limits for SpO$_2$ and pulse rate as indicated by patient's condition. Verify that alarms are on. Assess skin integrity under sensor probe every 2 hours; relocate sensor at least every 4 hours and more frequently if skin integrity is altered or tissue perfusion compromised.
14. If you plan on intermittent monitoring or spot-checking SpO$_2$, remove the probe and turn oximeter power off. Store the sensor in appropriate location.
15. **See Completion Protocol (inside front cover).**
16. Compare SpO$_2$ with patient's previous baseline and acceptable SpO$_2$. Note use of oxygen therapy, which can affect oxygen saturation.
17. Continue to monitor patient assessing for signs and symptoms of respiratory compromise if below baseline. If SpO$_2$ is below normal limits, apply oxygen, assess response, and notify the health care provider.

CRITICAL THINKING EXERCISES

Case Study

A 56-year-old woman has a history of cerebrovascular accident (stroke). She is able to use a walker to ambulate, even though her right arm is weaker than the left. She has drooping on the right side of her mouth but is able to eat and swallow safely. She is brought to the urgent care clinic by her daughter because of weakness, cough, dyspnea with activity, and general malaise. She appears alert and oriented and is cooperative.

1. When the nurse attempts to place an oral thermometer in the patient's mouth, she is unable to keep it positioned in the right sublingual pocket. What should the nurse do?
   1. Hold the thermometer in place with her gloved hand.
   2. Ask the patient to hold the thermometer herself.
   3. Switch the thermometer to the left sublingual pocket.
   4. Obtain temperature from a different site.
2. When the nurse assesses the patient's blood pressure, she obtains 140/76 mm Hg on the left arm and 128/72 mm Hg on the right arm. What action is appropriate at this time? Select all that apply.
   1. Notify the patient's primary health care provider immediately.
   2. Repeat the measurements on both arms after the other vital signs are obtained.
   3. Ask a nurse colleague to obtain the blood pressure.
   4. Ask the patient why she has not taken her blood pressure medications.
   5. Review the patient's medical record for her baseline vital signs.
   6. Conduct a complete assessment of the patient's vascular system.
   7. Obtain blood pressures on the lower extremities.
   8. Obtain a larger blood pressure cuff.
3. The nurse delegates the measurement of the radial pulse, respirations, and oxygen saturation. What instructions should the nurse provide to the NAP?
   1. Use the finger probe on the patient's right index finger.
   2. Notify the nurse of any SpO_2 value greater than 95%.
   3. Obtain the radial pulse rate from the pulse oximeter machine.
   4. Count respirations for a full 60 seconds.

Review Questions

1. What effect does acute postoperative pain have on a patient's initial set of vital signs?
   1. Decrease in heart rate
   2. Increase in blood pressure
   3. Decrease in respiratory rate
   4. Increase in temperature
2. Two hours after surgery, the NAP reports that a patient's vital signs are: BP R arm 112/72, L arm 124/96; HR 98, RR 22, temporal artery temp 36.4°C. Which of the following actions is appropriate by the nurse?
   1. Verify the blood pressure with sphygmomanometer and stethoscope.
   2. Direct the NAP to obtain the temperature using an alternative site.
   3. Conduct a focused respiratory assessment and obtain an apical heart rate.
   4. Report the right arm–to–left arm blood pressure difference to the health care provider.
3. A patient is admitted with pneumonia. Her vital signs are: BP 112/64 mm Hg, HR 102, RR 26, tympanic temperature 37.9°C (100.2°F). Which vital sign requires immediate attention?
   1. Heart rate
   2. Pulse pressure
   3. Respiratory rate
   4. Temperature
4. A patient arrives at the outpatient clinic complaining of a headache. His face is flushed, and blood pressure is 170/88 mm Hg in the right arm and 188/92 mm Hg in the left arm. He reports that he ran out of blood pressure medication last week and has been unable to afford to refill the prescription. What is the nurse's priority nursing action?
   1. Allow the patient to relax for 15 minutes and reevaluate the blood pressure measurements.
   2. Contact the social worker for financial assistance.
   3. Notify the health care provider.
   4. Retake the blood pressure in the left arm with a different-size cuff.
5. A high school student arrives at the school nurse's office complaining of headache, aches, pains, and general fatigue. The nurse observes the student's face is flushed and decides to obtain a set of vital signs. Which of the following vital signs is most likely to be abnormal?
   1. Blood pressure
   2. Temperature
   3. Radial pulse
   4. Oxygen saturation
   5. Respiratory rate
6. During report, the nurse obtains information on a 98-year-old patient who has terminal lung cancer and is admitted for palliative care. The nurse describes her breathing as labored, with periods of apnea alternating with deep breaths. The NAP reports the patient's respiratory rate as 12/min. After the nurse confirms these findings, how does the nurse describe this pattern?
   1. Kussmaul's respirations
   2. Cheyne-Stokes respirations
   3. Agonal respirations
   4. Hypoventilation

7. When taking frequent vital signs on a postoperative patient, the NAP uses an electronic blood pressure machine and obtains a blood pressure of 188/70 mm Hg. She appropriately notifies the nurse of the value, and the nurse checks the patient. The patient is awake and alert and offers no complaints. The nurse uses a stethoscope and obtains a blood pressure of 112/80 mm Hg. How does the nurse explain the difference in values?
   1. The blood pressure cuff used by the NAP was too small.
   2. The blood pressure cuff used by the NAP was too loose.
   3. The blood pressure cuff used by the NAP was too large.
   4. The blood pressure cuff used by the NAP was applied over the gown.
8. The nurse is caring for a patient after a motorcycle accident. He broke his left arm and right leg, both of which are in casts. An IV line is infusing in his right hand; the patient complains that his left hand is cool. Which of the following findings reported by the NAP would indicate the need for further assessment?
   1. Tympanic temperature of 36.2°C (97.2°F)
   2. Apical pulse rate of 92 beats/min
   3. Blood pressure in right arm of 118/84 mm Hg
   4. Left radial pulse 1+ strength
9. During a routine office visit, the NAP reports that a patient's blood pressure is 128/84 mm Hg. During previous visits, the patient's blood pressure was 110/70 to 114/74 mm Hg. What could account for the increase in blood pressure? Select all that apply.
   1. The patient was talking during the measurement.
   2. The patient was playing with the pulse oximeter with his other hand.
   3. The examination room was too warm.
   4. The blood pressure cuff was too small.
   5. The patient had just come from a workout at the gym.
   6. The NAP did not support the measurement arm.
   7. The patient had his legs crossed during measurement.
10. The nurse is taking the temporal artery temperature of a child. Place the following steps in appropriate order to obtain the temperature.
    1. Place sensor flush on forehead above the eyebrow.
    2. Touch sensor to skin just behind the earlobe.
    3. Press red scan button.
    4. Wipe forehead dry with towel.

REFERENCES

Cicek HS, et al: Effect of nail polish and henna on oxygen saturation determined by pulse oximetry in healthy young adult females, *Emerg Med J* 28(9):783, 2011.

Frese EM, Fick A, Sadowsky HS: Blood pressure measurement guidelines for physical therapists, *Cardiopulm Phys Ther J* 22(2):5, 2011.

Hockenberry MJ, Wilson D: *Wong's nursing care of infants and children*, ed 10, St Louis, 2014, Mosby.

James P, et al: 2014 Evidence based guideline for the management of high blood pressure in adults, *JAMA* 311(5):507, 2014.

Kaplan N, et al: Overview of hypertension in adults, *UpToDate* 2014. http://www.uptodate.com/contents/overview-of-hypertension-in-adults.

Marx J, et al: *Rosen's emergency medicine: concepts and clinical practice*, ed 8, Philadelphia, 2013, Saunders.

Nesseler N, et al: Pulse oximetry and high-dose vasopressors: a comparison between forehead reflectance and finger transmission sensors, *Intensive Care Med* 38(10):1718, 2012.

Pinar R, Ataalkin S, Watson R: The effect of clothes on sphygmomanometric blood pressure measurement in hypertensive patients, *J Clin Nurs* 19(13–14):1861, 2010.

Suokhrie L, et al: Differences in automated and manual blood pressure measurement in hospitalized psychiatric patients, *J Psychosoc Nurs Ment Health Serv* 51(3):32, 2013.

Uneke C, et al: Stethoscope disinfection campaign in Nigerian teaching hospital: results of a before-and-after study, *J Infect Develop Countries* 8(1):86, 2014.

World Health Organization (WHO): *WHO pulse oximetry training manual*, 2011, http://www.who.int/patientsafety/safesurgery/pulse_oximetry/who_ps_pulse_oxymetry_training_manual_en.pdf. Accessed August 15, 2013.

Yont GH, Korhan EA, Khorshid L: Comparison of oxygen saturation values and measurement times by pulse oximetry in various parts of the body, *Appl Nurs Res* 24(4):e39, 2011.

Health Assessment

Physical assessment findings are an important part of any assessment because of the behavioral cues and physical findings that lead nurses to make appropriate clinical decisions. Nurses perform systematic assessments on a regular basis in nearly every health care setting. In acute care settings, a brief 10- to 15-minute assessment at the beginning of each shift identifies any changes in a patient's status for comparison with the previous assessment. This assessment reveals information that adds to a patient's database (Box 7-1). In long-term care settings, nurses complete similar assessments weekly, monthly, or more frequently when a patient's health status changes. Continuity in health care improves when you make ongoing, objective, and comprehensive assessments.

PATIENT-CENTERED CARE

Nurses perform a more comprehensive assessment when a patient is admitted to a health care facility. This assessment involves a detailed review of a patient's condition and includes a nursing history and a behavioral and physical examination. The health history involves an interview with a patient to gather subjective data about the current state of health and any presenting conditions. It is important for the interview to be patient-centered for the nurse to learn about any problems through the patient's eyes. Patients are very helpful in describing their symptoms to allow nurses to focus their assessment appropriately.

A physical assessment includes a head-to-toe review of each body system that provides objective information about the patient. Use of examination techniques allows you to validate any subjective information the patient shared during the interview. For example, if a patient complains of shortness of breath, checking lung sounds and observing lung excursion help identify the nature of the problem. The patient's condition and response affect the extent of the examination. After gathering data, you make clinical decisions. Is there a change? If so, what should be your action? You will group significant findings into patterns of data (clusters) that reveal actual or potential nursing diagnoses or collaborative problems. Each abnormal finding directs you to gather additional data. Initial assessment and examination provides a baseline for the patient's functional status and serves as a comparison for future assessment findings. The information is useful in selecting the best nursing measures to manage a patient's health problems.

Respect patients' diversity and beliefs when conducting all aspects of a health assessment. It is important to remember that cultural, ethnic, and religious practice influence a patient's behavior. Consider the patient's health beliefs, use of alternative therapies, nutritional habits, relationships with

---

BOX 7-1   CHECKLIST FOR ROUTINE SHIFT ASSESSMENT

1. **Mental and neurological status**
   a. Level of consciousness (LOC)/responsiveness
   b. Alertness/orientation
   c. Pupils equal, round, and reactive to light and accommodation (PERRLA)
   d. Mood
   e. Behavior
   f. Facial expression
   g. Speech
2. **Vital signs**
   a. Blood pressure
   b. Pulse
   c. Respiration
   d. Temperature
   e. Pain and comfort level
   f. Pulse oximetry (if ordered for patient)
3. **Motor sensory function**
   a. Range of motion of major extremities
   b. Movement
   c. Strength
   d. Presence of numbness or tingling
4. **Integument (skin/mucous membranes)**
   a. Color
   b. Temperature
   c. Turgor
   d. Moisture
   e. Edema
   f. Integrity
5. **Cardiopulmonary system**
   a. Apical rate and rhythm
   b. Lung sounds
   c. Breathing pattern
   d. Peripheral pulses
   e. Capillary refill
6. **Gastrointestinal system**
   a. Bowel sounds
   b. Abdominal palpation
   c. Degree of abdominal distention
   d. Review for bowel elimination problems (e.g., diarrhea, constipation, flatulence)
7. **Genitourinary system**
   a. Presence of discharge, odor, or pain
   b. Review for urinary elimination problems (e.g., pain, difficulty with stream)
8. **Wounds**
   a. Appearance and character of any drainage
   b. Presence of swelling, redness, infection, or drainage
   c. Bandage/dressing, integrity of sutures
9. **Invasive tubes (e.g., intravenous [IV] lines, nasogastric [NG] tubes, wound drains, catheters)**
   a. Device and location
   b. IV line: Correct fluid/medication infusing
   c. Patency and position
   d. Presence of redness, swelling, or tenderness at IV site
   e. Drainage rate (wound drain) or infusion rate of IV or NG feeding
   f. Date of last tubing change
10. **Functioning of supportive devices**
    a. Oxygen
    b. Bed alarms
    c. Traction

---

family, and comfort with your physical closeness during all parts of the assessment. Be sensitive and avoid stereotyping based on culture, race, ethnicity, sexual preference, or age. Cultural behaviors are relevant to the health assessment, and you need to be aware of them before conducting an assessment on a patient. Consider how culture, ethnicity, heritage, and beliefs have an impact on patient needs and how you assess your patients. Each patient is an individual and may respond differently (Giger and Davidhizar, 2013). There is a difference between cultural and physical characteristics. Your recognition of cultural diversity helps you to respect a patient's uniqueness and provider a higher quality of individualized care. Improved patient outcomes can result from recognition and respect for cultural diversity (Giger and Davidhizar, 2013).

Nurses are often the first to detect changes in patients' conditions. For this reason, the ability to think critically and interpret patient behaviors and physiological changes is essential. The skills of physical assessment are powerful tools for detecting both subtle and obvious changes in a patient's health. The physical assessment is an ideal time to offer patient teaching and encourage promotion of health practices such as breast (Box 7-2) and genital (Box 7-3) self-examination. The American Cancer Society (ACS, 2013b, 2014a) recommends guidelines for early detection.

ASSESSMENT TECHNIQUES

Inspection, palpation, percussion, auscultation, and olfaction are the five basic assessment techniques. Each skill allows you to collect a broad range of physical data about patients. Nurses need experience to recognize normal variations among patients and ranges of normal for an individual. Cultural diversity is one factor that influences both normal variations and potential alterations that you may find during an assessment. It is very important to take the time needed to assess each body part carefully. Hurrying can cause you to overlook significant signs and form incorrect conclusions about a patient's condition.

Inspection is the visual examination of body parts or areas. An experienced nurse learns to make multiple observations almost simultaneously while becoming very perceptive of any abnormalities. It is important to recognize normal physical characteristics of patients of all ages before trying to distinguish abnormal findings.

Inspection requires adequate lighting and full exposure of body parts. Inspect each area for size, shape, color, symmetry, position, and the presence of abnormalities. If possible, inspect each area compared with the same area on the opposite side of the body. When necessary, use additional light such as a penlight to inspect body cavities such as the mouth

BOX 7-2 BREAST SELF-EXAMINATION

Women who are 20 years old and older should be told about the benefits and limitations of breast self-examination (BSE) (ACS, 2014a). Emphasize the importance of prompt reporting of any new breast symptoms to a health care provder. Women who choose to do BSE should receive instruction and have their technique reviewed. BSE should be done once a month so that the woman becomes familiar with the usual appearance and feel of her breast. Familiarity makes it easier to notice any changes in the breast from one month to another. Early discovery of a change from "normal" is the main idea behind BSE.

For women who menstruate, the best time to do BSE is the fourth through the seventh day of the menstrual cycle or right after the menstrual cycle ends, when the breasts are least likely to be tender or swollen. Women who no longer menstruate should pick a day such as the first day of the month to remind them to do BSE. Men should also examine their breast, areolas, nipples, and axillae for any swelling, nodules, or ulcerations.

When a woman has breast implants, it might be helpful for the surgeon to identify the edges of the implant. Women who are pregnant or breastfeeding should also do a breast examination (ACS, 2014a).

Procedure

1. Examine your right breast. Lie down on your back and place your right arm behind your head (see illustration A). The examination is completed lying down, not standing up (ACS, 2014a), because when you lie down the breast tissue spreads evenly over the chest wall and is as thin as possible, making it much easier to feel all the breast tissue.
2. Use finger pads of the three middle fingers on your left hand to feel for lumps in the right breast (see illustration B). Use overlapping dime-sized circular motions of the finger pads to feel the breast tissue. Use three different levels of pressure to feel all the breast tissue. Light pressure is needed to feel the tissue closest to the skin; medium pressure, to feel a little deeper; and firm pressure, to feel the tissue closest to

the chest and ribs. It is normal to feel a firm ridge in the lower curve of each breast, but you should tell your health care provider if you feel anything else out of the ordinary. If you are not sure how hard to press, discuss this with your health care provider. Use each pressure level to feel the breast tissue before moving on to the next spot.

3. Move around the breast in an up-and-down pattern starting at an imaginary line drawn straight down your side from the underarm and moving across the breast to the middle of the chest bone (sternum or breastbone). Be sure to check the entire breast area going down until you feel only ribs and up to the neck or collar bone (clavicle) (see illustration C). Evidence shows that the up-and-down pattern is the most effective pattern for covering the entire breast.
4. Repeat self-examination in the left breast, putting your left arm behind your head and examining the left breast as noted in Steps 1-3.
5. While standing in from of a mirror with your hands pressing firmly down on your hips, look at your breasts, observing for any changes in size, shape, contour, dimpling, or redness or scaliness of the nipple or breast tissue. Pressing down on your hips contracts the chest wall muscles and enhances any breast changes.
6. Examine each underarm while sitting or standing and with your arm only slightly raised so you can easily feel in this area any lumps or changes. Raising your arm straight tightens the tissue in this area making it harder to examine.
7. If implants are present, help the patient determine the edges of each implant and how to evaluate each breast.
8. Instruct patient to call the health care provider if she finds a lump or other abnormality.
9. **Use *Teach Back:*** State to the patient, "I want to be sure I explained to you how to do a breast self-examination. Can you show me how to examine both of your breasts?" Document your evaluation of patient learning. Revise your instruction now or develop plan for revised patient teaching to be implemented at an appropriate time if patient is not able to teach back correctly.

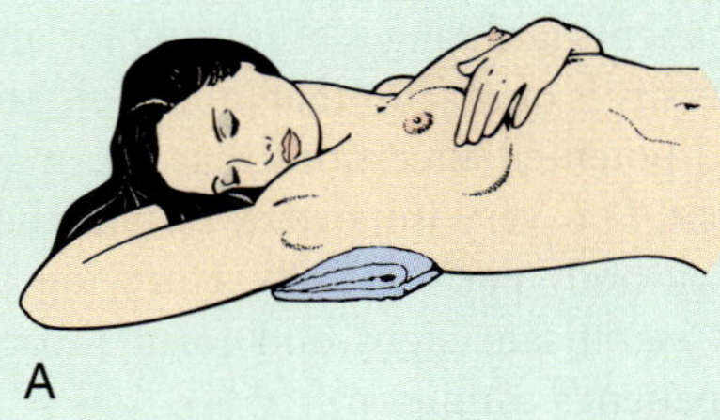

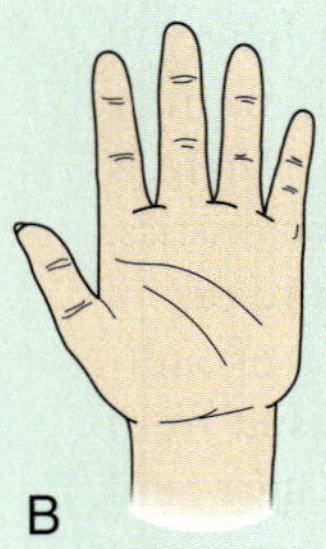

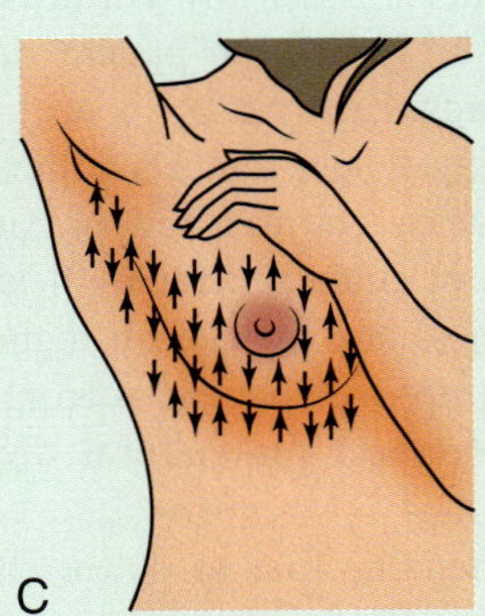

American Cancer Society (ACS): *Learn about Cancer, American Society recommendations for early breast cancer detection,* 2014a, http://www.cancer.org/Cancer/BreastCancer/DetailedGuide/breast-cancer-detection. Accessed May 27, 2014.

and throat. *Do not hurry. Pay attention to detail.* Verify and clarify all abnormalities with subjective patient data. In other words, ask the patient for further information about each abnormality or change, such as whether the change is recent.

Palpation uses the sense of touch. Through palpation, the hands make delicate and sensitive measurements of specific physical signs. Palpation detects resistance, resilience, roughness, texture, temperature, and mobility. You will often use palpation with or after visual inspection. You will also

BOX 7-3   GENITAL SELF-EXAMINATION

All men 15 years old and older should perform this examination monthly. Perform it after a warm bath or shower when the scrotal sac is relaxed. Call your health care provider if you find a lump or any other abnormality.

Penile Examination

1. Stand naked in front of a mirror and hold the penis in your hand and examine the head. Pull back the foreskin if uncircumcised.
2. Inspect and palpate the entire head of the penis in a clockwise motion, looking carefully for any bumps, sores, or blisters.
3. Look for any bumpy warts.
4. Look at the opening at the end of the penis for discharge (see illustration).
5. Look along the entire shaft of the penis for the same signs.
6. Separate pubic hair at the base of the penis and carefully examine the skin underneath.

Testicular Self-Examination

1. While looking in the mirror, look for swelling or lumps in the skin of the scrotum.
2. Use both hands, placing the index and middle fingers under the testicles and the thumb on top (see illustration).
3. Gently roll the testicle, feeling for lumps, thickening, or a change in consistency (hardening).
4. Find the epididymis (a cordlike structure on the top and back of the testicle; it is not a lump (ACS, 2013b).
5. Feel for small, pea-size lumps on the front and side of the testicle. The lumps are usually painless and are abnormal.
6. It is normal for one testicle to be slightly larger than the other and for one to hang lower (ACS, 2013b).
7. Instruct patient to call the health care provider if he finds a lump or other abnormality.
8. **Use *Teach Back:*** State to the patient, "I want to be sure I explained to you how to do a genital and testicular self-examination. Can you show me how to examine your penis and testicles?" Document your evaluation of patient learning. Revise your instruction now or develop plan for revised patient teaching to be implemented at an appropriate time if patient is not able to teach back correctly.

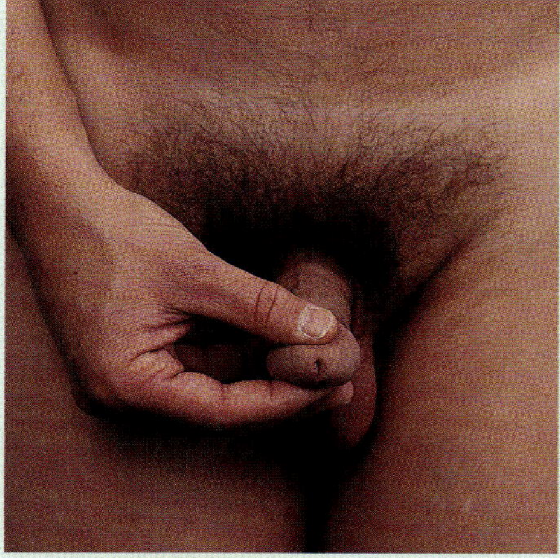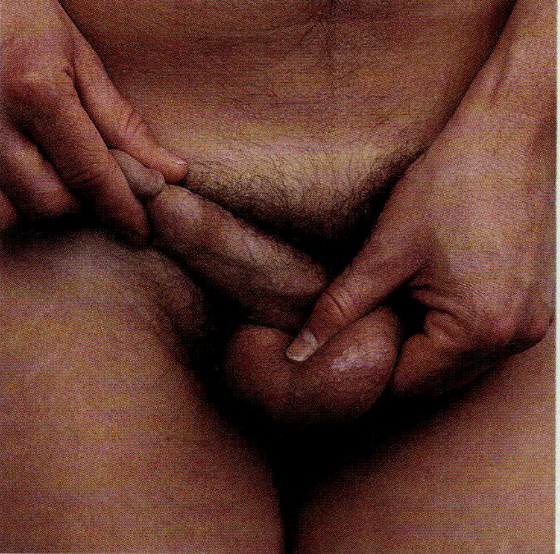

From American Cancer Society: *Testicular self-exam*, 2013b, http://www.cancer.org/cancer/testicularcancer/moreinformation/doihavetesticularcancer/do-i-have-testicular-cancer-self-exam. Accessed May 27, 2014; Seidel HM et al: *Seidel's guide to physical examination*, ed 8, St Louis, 2015, Mosby.

use different parts of the hand to detect specific characteristics. For example, the dorsum (back) of the hand is sensitive to temperature variations. The pads of the fingertips detect subtle changes in texture, shape, size, consistency, and pulsation of body parts. The palm of the hand is especially sensitive to vibration. You measure position, consistency, and turgor by lightly grasping the body part with the fingertips.

Assist the patient to relax and assume a comfortable position because muscle tension during palpation impairs the ability to palpate correctly. Asking a patient to take slow, deep breaths enhances muscle relaxation. Palpate tender areas last because they could cause a patient to become tense and hinder the assessment. Ask the patient to point out areas that are more sensitive, and note any nonverbal signs of discomfort. Patients appreciate clean, warm hands; short fingernails; and a gentle approach. Palpation is either light or deep and is controlled by the amount of pressure applied with the fingers or hand. Light palpation precedes deep palpation. Consider the patient's condition, the area being palpated, and the reason for using palpation. For example, when a patient is admitted to the emergency department after an automobile accident, consider the factors surrounding the injury, and inspect the chest wall carefully before performing any palpation around the area of the ribs.

For light palpation, apply pressure slowly, gently, and deliberately, depressing about 1 cm ($\frac{1}{2}$ inch). Check tender areas further, using light, intermittent pressure. After light palpation, you may use deeper palpation to examine the condition of organs (Fig. 7-1). Depress the area being examined approximately 2 cm (0.8 inch). Caution is the rule. Bimanual palpation involves one hand placed over the other while applying pressure. The upper hand exerts downward pressure as the other hand feels the subtle characteristics of underlying organs and masses. Seek the assistance of a qualified instructor before attempting deep palpation.

Percussion involves tapping the body with the fingertips to evaluate the size, borders, and consistency of body organs and to discover fluid in body cavities. The technique requires practice and skill and is typically used by advanced practice nurses.

Auscultation is listening with a stethoscope to sounds produced by the body. To auscultate correctly, listen in a quiet environment for both the presence of sound and its characteristics. To be successful in auscultation, you must first recognize normal sounds from each body structure, including the passage of blood through an artery, heart sounds, and movement of air through the lungs. These sounds vary according to the location in which they can most easily be heard. Likewise, you become familiar with areas that normally do not emit sounds. It is important for you to listen to many normal sounds to recognize abnormal sounds when they arise.

To auscultate, you need good hearing acuity, a good stethoscope, and knowledge of how to use the stethoscope properly (see Chapter 6). It is essential to place the stethoscope directly on a patient's skin because clothing obscures and changes sound. There are four characteristics of sound heard through auscultation:

Frequency: Number of sound wave cycles generated per second by a vibrating object. The higher the frequency, the higher the pitch of a sound, and vice versa.

Loudness: Amplitude of a sound wave. Auscultated sounds are either loud or soft.

Quality: Sounds of similar frequency and loudness from different sources. Terms such as *blowing* or *gurgling* describe quality of sound.

Duration: Length of time that sound vibrations last. Duration of sound is short, medium, or long. Layers of soft tissue dampen the duration of sounds from deep internal organs.

Olfaction uses the sense of smell to detect abnormalities that go unrecognized by any other means. Some alterations in body function and certain bacteria create characteristic odors (Table 7-1).

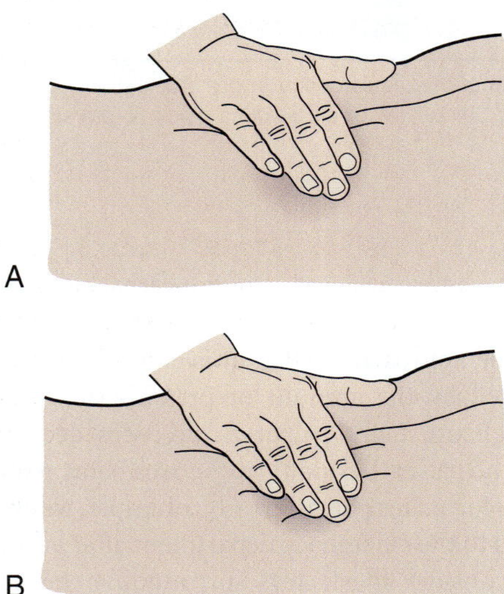

FIG 7-1 A, During light palpation, gentle pressure against underlying skin and tissues can be used to detect areas of irregularity and tenderness. **B,** During deep palpation, depressing tissue can assess the condition of underlying organs.

TABLE 7-1	ASSESSMENT OF CHARACTERISTIC ODORS	
ODOR	**SITE OR SOURCE**	**POTENTIAL CAUSES**
Alcohol	Oral cavity	Ingestion of alcohol
Ammonia	Urine	Urinary tract infection, renal failure
Body odor	Skin, particularly in areas where body parts rub together (e.g., underarms, beneath breasts)	Poor hygiene, excess perspiration (hyperhidrosis), foul-smelling perspiration (bromhidrosis)
	Wound site	Wound abscess; infection
	Vomitus	Abdominal irritation, contaminated food
Feces	Rectal area	Fecal incontinence; fistula
	Vomitus/oral cavity (fecal odor)	Bowel obstruction
Fetid, sweet odor	Tracheostomy or mucus secretions	Infection of bronchial tree (*Pseudomonas* bacteria)
Foul-smelling stools in infant	Stool	Malabsorption syndrome
Halitosis	Oral cavity	Poor dental and oral hygiene; gum disease; sinus infection
Musty odor	Casted body part	Infection inside cast
Stale urine	Skin	Uremic acidosis
Sweet, fruity ketones	Oral cavity	Diabetic acidosis
Sweet, heavy, thick odor	Draining wound	*Pseudomonas* (bacterial) infection

SAFETY

The process of assessment begins the moment that you see a patient and continues with each encounter. Always know a patient's health history and the reason for seeking care. Be alert for any changes or problems that may have developed since the last assessment. Changes in a patient's assessment findings affect priority assessments and care. Be organized, and follow a head-to-toe approach. Always identify a patient using at least two identifiers other than room number. For example, use the patient's name and date of birth, comparing them with the identification band or medical record (TJC, 2014). Always follow standard precautions for infection control. During an assessment, you may have contact or risk of contact with body fluids. Always wear clean gloves in these situations. In addition, consider the possibility of a latex allergy and wear latex-free gloves. When you complete your assessment, promptly record your findings in the patient's health care record.

PREPARATION FOR ASSESSMENT

Preparation of the environment, equipment, and patient facilitates a smooth assessment. Provide patients privacy to promote their comfort and the efficiency of the examination. In a health care facility, close the door and pull privacy curtains. In the home, examine the patient in the bedroom. A comfortable environment includes a warm, comfortable temperature; a loose-fitting gown or pajamas for the patient; adequate direct lighting; control of outside noises; and precautions to prevent interruptions by visitors or health care personnel. If possible, place the bed or examination table at waist level so that you can access the patient easily. During an assessment, you must protect patients from falls and injury; it is essential to return the bed to a safe height after an assessment (TJC, 2014).

Preparing a Patient

Prepare a patient both physically and psychologically for an accurate assessment. A tense, anxious patient may have difficulty understanding, following directions, or cooperating with your instructions. To prepare a patient:

1. Make the patient comfortable by allowing the opportunity to empty the bowel or bladder (a good time to collect needed specimens).
2. Provide privacy.
3. Minimize the patient's anxiety and fear by conveying an open, receptive, and professional approach. Using simple terms, thoroughly explain what will be done, what the patient should expect to feel, and how the patient can cooperate. Even if the patient appears unresponsive, it is still important to explain your actions.
4. Provide access to body parts while draping areas that are not being examined.
5. Reduce distractions. Turn down the volume or turn off the television or radio.
6. Eliminate drafts, control room temperature, and provide warm blankets.
7. Help the patient assume positions during the assessment so that body parts are accessible and the patient stays comfortable. A patient's ability to assume positions depends on physical strength and limitations. Some positions are uncomfortable or embarrassing; keep a patient in such a position no longer than is necessary.
8. Pace the assessment according to the patient's physical and emotional tolerance.
9. Use a relaxed tone of voice and facial expressions to put the patient at ease.
10. Encourage the patient to ask questions and report discomfort felt during the examination.
11. Have a third person of the patient's gender in the room during assessment of genitalia; this prevents the patient from accusing you of behaving in an unethical manner.
12. At the conclusion of the assessment, ask the patient if there are any concerns or questions.

Physical Assessment of Various Age-Groups
Children and Adolescents

1. Routine assessment of children focuses on health promotion and illness prevention, particularly for care of well children with competent parenting and no serious health problems (Hockenberry and Wilson, 2013). Focus on growth and development, sensory screening, dental examination, and behavioral assessment.
2. Children who are chronically ill, disabled, in foster care, or adopted after birth in a foreign country may require additional assessments because of their unique health risks.
3. When obtaining histories of infants and children, gather all or part of information from parents or guardians.
4. Parents may think the examiner is testing or judging them. Offer support during the examination, and do not pass judgment.
5. Call children by their preferred name, and address parents by their surnames (e.g., "Mr. and Mrs. Brown") rather than by first names.
6. Open-ended questions often allow parents to share more information and describe more of the child's problems.
7. Older children and adolescents respond best when treated as adults and individuals and often can provide details about their health history and severity of symptoms.
8. The adolescent has a right to confidentiality. After talking with parents about historical information, arrange to be alone with the adolescent to speak privately and perform the examination.

Older Adults

1. Do not assume that aging is always accompanied by illness or disability. Most older adults are able to adapt to change and maintain functional independence (Touhy and Jett, 2014).

2. A thorough assessment of an older adult provides critical information that can be used to maximize independence.
3. Provide adequate space for an examination, particularly if the patient uses a mobility aid.
4. Plan the history and examination, taking into account the older adult's energy level, physical limitations, pace, and adaptability. You may need more than one session to complete the assessment (Touhy and Jett, 2014).
5. Measure performance under the most favorable of conditions. Take advantage of natural opportunities for assessment (e.g., during bathing, grooming, and mealtime) (Touhy and Jett, 2014).
6. Be sure that an examination of an older adult includes review of mental status.

EVIDENCE-BASED PRACTICE

Dresser S: The role of nursing surveillance in keeping patients safe, *J Nurs Admin* 42(7/8):361, 2012.

Henneman EA et al: Surveillance: a strategy for improving patient safety in acute and critical care units, *Crit Care Nurse* 32(2):e9, 2012.

Shever LL: The impact of nursing surveillance on failure to rescue, *Res Theory Nurs Pract* 25(2):107, 2011.

Nurses play a vital role in keeping patients safe by continuously assessing their patients' entire situation. Taking physical assessment information and combining it with additional behavioral and cognitive actions, where nurses monitor, evaluate, and formulate a response on changes in a patient's condition, is surveillance. The purpose of surveillance is to detect changes in trends or patterns of data to initiate investigative or treatment measures. A key element for safe patient care is a high level of vigilance at all times (Dresser, 2012).

- Consider what you know about a patient. What risks and clinical conditions might result in an unexpected clinical change? Observe for that type of change.
- Conduct nursing surveillance greater than 12 times per day to reduce the rate of failure to rescue and avoid preventable complications (Shever, 2011).
- Identify the best time for systematic collection of information used to prevent or identify potential problems leading to nursing action that keeps patients safe (Henneman et al., 2012). Examples: immediate postoperative period for recovering patients, first hour of a blood transfusion.

SKILL GUIDELINES

1. Prioritize the assessment based on a patient's presenting signs and symptoms or health care needs. For example, when a patient develops sudden shortness of breath, first assess the lungs and thorax. If a patient is acutely ill, you may choose to assess only the involved body systems. Use judgment to ensure that an examination is relevant and inclusive.
2. Organize the examination. Compare both sides of the body for symmetry. If the patient becomes fatigued, offer rest periods. Perform painful or intrusive procedures near the end of the examination.
3. Use a head-to-toe approach following the sequence of inspection, palpation, and auscultation (except for abdominal assessment). This sequence facilitates an effective assessment.
4. Encourage the patient's active participation. Patients usually know about their physical condition. Often a patient can let you know when certain findings are normal or when there have been changes.
5. Always identify a patient using at least two patient identifiers other than the room number. For example, use the patient's name and date of birth, comparing with either the armband or the medical record (TJC, 2014). In long-term care settings, arm bands are not used; however, pictures are available for identification. Caution: Patients with difficulty hearing or altered level of consciousness (LOC) may answer to a name other than their own.
6. Record quick notes to facilitate accurate documentation. Inform the patient that you will be recording the data.
7. Use assessment skills during each patient contact, including activities such as bathing, administration of medications, other therapies, or while conversing with a patient.
8. Integrate health promotion and education into physical assessment activities. There are "teachable moments" when you can share findings and educate patients about health promotion.
9. Respect the patient's race, gender, age, and cultural beliefs. These important variables often influence assessment findings and examination approaches.
10. Record a summary of the assessment using appropriate medical terminology and in the sequence that findings are gathered. Be thorough and descriptive, especially for abnormal findings.

SKILL 7.1   GENERAL SURVEY

The general survey begins a review of the patient's primary health problems, and it includes assessment of a patient's vital signs, height and weight, general behavior, and appearance. It provides information about characteristics of an illness and the patient's hygiene, skin condition, body image, emotional state, recent weight changes, and developmental status. The survey reveals important information about a patient's behavior that can influence how you communicate instructions to the patient and continue the assessment.

ASSESSMENT

1. Note if patient has had any acute distress: difficulty breathing, pain, or anxiety. If such signs are present, defer the

general survey until later and focus immediately on body system affected. *Rationale: Acute distress establishes priorities for what part of the examination to conduct first.*

2. Review medical record graphic sheets for previous vital signs and consider factors or conditions that may alter values (see Chapter 6). *Rationale: Provides baseline data about patient's vital signs.*

3. Determine patient's primary language. If you identify a need for an interpreter, determine the availability of a professional interpreter. It is best to have an interpreter of the same gender who is older and more mature. Have the interpreter translate verbatim if possible. *Rationale: Facilitates patient understanding and promotes accuracy of information provided by patient.*

4. After reviewing history, confirm primary reason patient is seeking health care. *Rationale: Assessment is centered on the patient and the patient's health care expectations and needs.*

5. Identify patient's normal height, weight, and body mass index (BMI). If a sudden gain or loss in weight has occurred, determine the amount of weight change and period of time in which it occurred. Assess if patient has recently been dieting or is following an exercise program. Use growth charts for children younger than 18 years of age. *Rationale: A BMI of 18.5 to 24.9 is normal weight, a BMI of 25 to 29.9 for men and women is overweight, and a BMI of 30 and higher is obese (Seidel et al., 2015). Fluid retention is one factor that must be ruled out because a person's weight can fluctuate daily as a result of fluid loss or retention (1 L of water weighs 1 kg [2.2 pounds]).*

6. Review patient's past fluid intake and output (I&O) records. *Rationale: Fluid and electrolyte balance affects health and function in all body systems.*

7. Identify patient's general perceptions about personal health status. *Rationale: May help direct you to examine problem areas*

8. Ask if patient is allergic or sensitive to latex. Assess for evidence of latex allergy (e.g., contact dermatitis or systemic reactions [see Chapter 5]). Ask if patient has risk factors such as food allergies (papaya, avocado, banana, peach, kiwi, or tomato). *Rationale: Gloves are worn during certain aspects of the assessment. Repeated exposure may result in more serious reactions, including asthma, itching, and anaphylaxis (Seidel et al., 2015).*

PLANNING

Expected Outcomes focus on gathering accurate assessment data.

1. Patient demonstrates alert, cooperative behaviors without evidence of physical or emotional distress during assessment.
2. Patient provides appropriate subjective data related to physical condition.

Delegation and Collaboration

The general survey cannot be delegated to nursing assistive personnel (NAP). The nurse instructs the NAP to:
- Measure patient's height and weight.
- Obtain vital signs (not the initial set, but subsequent measurements if patient is stable).
- Monitor oral intake and urinary output.
- Report patient's subjective signs and symptoms to the nurse.

Equipment
- Stethoscope
- Sphygmomanometer and cuff
- Thermometer
- Digital watch or wristwatch with second hand
- Tape measure
- Clean gloves (use nonlatex if necessary)
- Tongue blade
- Appropriate electronic record or documentation form

IMPLEMENTATION *for* GENERAL SURVEY

STEPS	RATIONALE
1. **See Standard Protocol (inside front cover).**	
2. Throughout the assessment, note patient's verbal and nonverbal behaviors. Determine patient's LOC and orientation by observing and talking to patient. Use time to discuss any questions patient has about health status.	Behaviors may reflect specific physical abnormalities. Dementia and LOC influence patient's ability to cooperate.

> **SAFE PATIENT CARE** Timing of recent medications, especially pain medication and sedatives, may cause patient to be groggy or less responsive.

STEPS	RATIONALE
3. Obtain temperature, pulse, respirations, and blood pressure unless routinely taken within past 3 hours; or repeat if a serious potential change is noted (e.g., change in LOC or difficulty breathing [see Chapter 6]). Inform patient of vital signs.	Vital signs provide important information regarding physiological changes in relation to oxygenation and circulation.

Continued

STEPS	RATIONALE

4. Obtain patient's height and weight:

  a. Height: If patient is able to stand, use a stadiometer (attached to a standing scale). Have patient look straight ahead with his or her line of vision parallel to the floor. Once the patient is in position, lower the measuring rod until it firmly touches the crown of the head.

  Read the measurement on the scale at eye level. If patient cannot stand, measure length while the patient is lying supine. Have the patient lie on his or her back with arms at side and stretch as much as possible. Place a mark on the bottom sheet at the patient's heel and at the top of the patient's head. Use a tape measure to measure between these two marks on the taut bottom sheet.

  b. Weight: Weigh patient at the same time each day, with the same clothing and same scale. Be sure scale is calibrated. Have patient void before weighing if possible. Avoid weighing any equipment attached to patient (e.g., drainage bags, telemetry units). Hold the equipment while weighing patient. Some hospital beds contain a scale for weighing.

Rationale: Accurate height and weight are especially important when there is a need to calculate drug dosages or other treatments that depend on patient's body mass index.

> **SAFE PATIENT CARE** Measuring a patient's length while he or she is lying supine is the most accurate height estimate for patients who cannot stand (e.g., wheelchair users). Height estimates based on knee height and self-report may provide reasonable alternatives (Froehlich-Grobe, 2011).

5. Observe the following aspects of appearance: gender, race, and age. Note patient's physical features.

Rationale: Gender influences type of examination performed and manner in which assessments are made. Different physical characteristics and predisposition to illnesses are related to gender and race.

6. If uncertain whether patient understands a question, rephrase or ask a similar question.

Rationale: Inappropriate response from a patient may be caused by language barriers, deterioration of mental status, preoccupation with illness, or decreased hearing acuity.

7. If patient's responses are inappropriate, ask short, to-the-point questions regarding information patient should know (e.g., "Tell me your name," "Tell me where you live," "What day is this?" or "What season of the year is this?").

Rationale: Measures patient's orientation to person, place, time, and situation. You may note this in the documentation as "Oriented × 3." If disoriented in any way, include subjective or objective data, or both, rather than just documenting "disoriented."

8. If patient is unable to respond to questions of orientation, offer simple commands (e.g., "Squeeze my fingers" or "Move your toes").

Rationale: LOC exists along a continuum that includes full responsiveness, inability to initiate meaningful behaviors consciously, and unresponsiveness to stimuli.

9. Assess affect and mood. Note if verbal expressions match nonverbal behavior and if appropriate to situation.

Rationale: Reflects patient's mental and emotional status, consciousness, and feelings.

10. Watch patient interact with spouse or partner, older adult child, or caregiver. Be alert for indications of fear, hesitancy to report health status, or willingness to let caregiver control interview. Does partner or caregiver have a history of violence, alcoholism, or drug abuse? Is the person unemployed, ill, or frustrated with caring for patient? Note if patient has any obvious physical injuries.

Rationale: Suspect abuse in patients who have experienced obvious physical injury or neglect, show signs of malnutrition, or have ecchymosis (bruises) on the extremities or trunk. Health care providers are often the first to identify evidence of abuse because patients may be unable to tell family or friends. Partners or caregivers may have a history of abusive or addictive behaviors.

> **SAFE PATIENT CARE** If abuse is suspected, ask direct questions about abuse in private, where patient is more likely to reveal information. These questions may need to be delayed until partner or caregiver is not present. Asking about abuse in the presence of an abuser puts the patient at risk for further abuse.

11. Observe for signs of abuse:

    a. Child: Blood on underclothing, pain in genital area, pain on urination, vaginal or penile discharge, or difficulty sitting or walking. Physical injury inconsistent with parent's or caregiver's account of how injury occurred.

    Indicates child sexual abuse (Hockenberry and Wilson, 2013; Seidel et al., 2015). Suggests child physical abuse.

    b. Female patient: Injury or trauma inconsistent with reported cause or obvious injuries to face, neck, breasts, abdomen, and genitalia, such as black eyes, broken nose, lip lacerations, broken teeth, burns.

    May indicate intimate partner violence (IPV) or domestic abuse (Seidel et al., 2015). These signs also apply to a male patient being abused by a female partner.

    c. Older adult: Injury or trauma inconsistent with reported cause, injuries in unusual locations (e.g., neck or genitalia), pattern injuries (i.e., left when an object with which a person is struck leaves an imprint), parallel injuries (e.g., bilateral bruises on the upper arms suggesting that the person was held and shaken), burns (e.g., shaped like a cigarette, iron, rope), fractures, poor hygiene, and poor nutrition.

    Indicates elder abuse or neglect (Touhy and Jett, 2014). Prolonged interval between injury and time patient sought medical treatment also indicates older adult abuse or neglect.

> **SAFE PATIENT CARE** A pattern of findings indicating abuse usually mandates a report to a social service center (refer to state guidelines). Obtain an immediate consultation with health care provider, social worker, and other support staff to facilitate placement in a safer environment.

12. Assess posture, noting alignment of the shoulders and hips when patient stands and sits. Observe patient from the side in a standing position and note if patient has a slumped, erect, or bent posture. Then observe anteriorly and posteriorly. Also look sideways at cervical, thoracic, and lumbar curves (see illustrations).

    Reveals musculoskeletal problem, mood, fatigue, presence of pain, or difficulty breathing in certain positions. Normal standing posture is an upright stance with parallel alignment of hips and shoulders, even contour of shoulders, level scapulae, and iliac crests. Head is erect. Abnormal curves of posture include lordosis (swayback, increased lumbar curvature), kyphosis (hunchback, exaggerated posterior curvature of thoracic spine), and scoliosis (lateral spinal curvature).

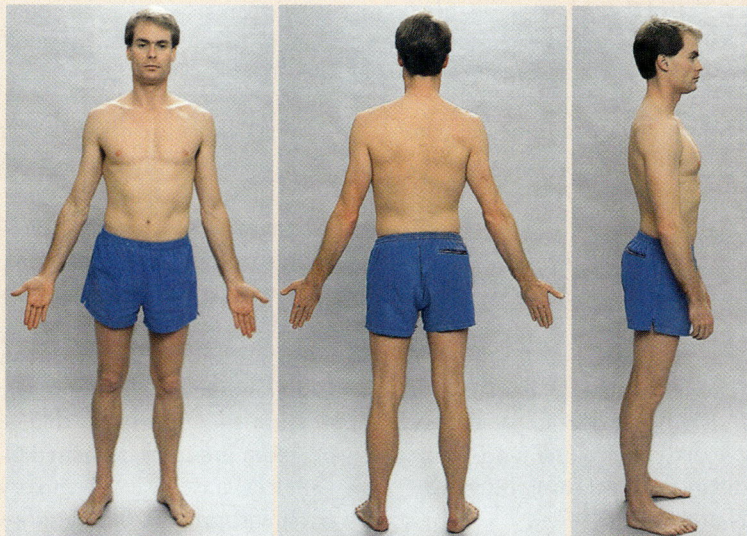

STEP 12 Inspection of overall body posture: anterior view *(left)*; posterior view *(middle)*; right lateral view *(right)*. (From Seidel HM et al: *Mosby's guide to physical examination,* ed 7, St Louis, 2011, Mosby.)

Continued

STEPS	RATIONALE

a. Assess body movements. Are they purposeful? Are there tremors of the extremities? Are any body parts immobile? Are movements coordinated or uncoordinated?

May indicate neurological or muscular problem or emotional stress (see Skill 7.7).

13. Assess speech. Is it understandable and moderately paced? Is there an association with the person's thoughts?

Alterations reflect neurological impairment, injury or impairment of mouth, improperly fitting dentures, or differences in dialect and language.

14. Observe hygiene and grooming for presence or absence of makeup, type of clothes (hospital or personal), and cleanliness. Hair, teeth, and nails are good places to assess for hygiene status.

Grooming may reflect activity level before examination, resources available to purchase grooming supplies, patient's mood, and self-care practices. May also reflect culture, lifestyle, and personal preferences.

a. Observe the color, distribution, quantity, thickness, texture, and lubrication of hair.

Changes in hair may reflect hormone changes, changes from aging, poor nutrition, or use of certain hair care products.

b. Inspect the condition of nails (hands and feet).

Changes indicate inadequate nutrition or grooming practices, nervous habits, or systemic diseases.

c. Assess the presence or absence of body odor.

Body odor may result from physical exercise, deficient hygiene, or physical or mental abnormalities.

15. Inspect exposed skin and ask if patient has noted any changes in the skin. Pay close attention to areas between the toes or under the breasts. Inspect for the following:

The incidence of melanoma in the United States has been increasing for at least 30 years (ACS, 2013c). It is an aggressive form of skin cancer. The cancer can spread to other parts of the body quickly. Early detection and prompt treatment are critical (Box 7-4).

a. Pruritus, oozing, bleeding

Itching could result from dry skin, oozing could indicate infection, and bleeding may indicate a blood disorder.

b. Change in the appearance of a mole (nevus), bump, or nodule; change in sensation, itchiness, tenderness, or pain

This is a key indicator of a lesion that may be cancerous.

c. Petechiae (pinpoint-size, red or purple spots on the skin caused by small hemorrhages in skin layers)

Petechiae may indicate a serious blood clotting disorder, drug reaction, or liver disease.

16. Inspect skin surfaces.

Changes in color can indicate pathological alterations (Table 7-2).

a. Compare color of symmetrical body parts, including areas unexposed to sun. Look for any patches or areas of skin color variation.

> **SAFE PATIENT CARE** Be alert for basal cell carcinomas, such as an open sore that does not heal, a shiny nodule, a pink or reddish growth, or a scarlike area. These often occur in sun-exposed areas, which frequently result in sun-damaged skin.

b. Carefully inspect color of face, oral mucosa, lips, conjunctivae, sclera, palms of hands, and nail beds.

Abnormalities are easier to identify in areas of body where melanin production is lowest.

17. Palpate skin surfaces

a. Use ungloved fingertips to palpate skin to feel texture and moisture of intact skin.

Changes in texture may be the first indication of skin rashes in dark-skinned patients. Hydration, body temperature, and environment affect the skin. Older adults are prone to xerosis, manifesting as dry, scaly skin (Touhy and Jett, 2014).

b. Using dorsum (back) of hand, palpate for temperature of skin surfaces. Compare symmetrical body parts and upper and lower body parts. Note distinct temperature differences and localized areas of warmth.

Skin on dorsum of hand is thin, which allows detection of subtle temperature changes. Cool skin temperature often indicates decreased blood flow. A stage I pressure ulcer causes warmth and erythema (redness) of an area. Environmental temperature and anxiety may also affect skin temperature.

STEPS	RATIONALE

c. Assess skin turgor by grasping fold of skin on the sternum, forearm, or abdomen with the fingertips. Release skin fold and note ease and speed with which skin returns to place (see illustration).

With reduced turgor, skin remains suspended or "tented" for a few seconds, then slowly returns to place, indicating decreased elasticity and possible dehydration. With altered turgor, provide measures for prevention of pressure ulcers (see Chapter 25).

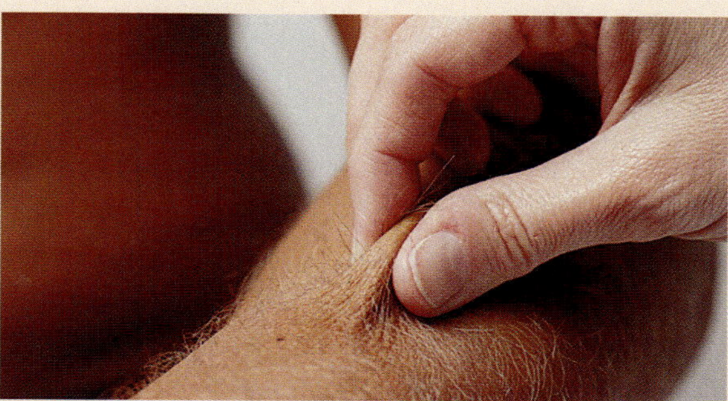

STEP 17c Assessment of skin turgor.

d. Apply clean gloves. Inspect character of any secretions; note color, odor, amount, and consistency (e.g., thin and watery or thick and oily). Remove gloves and perform hand hygiene.

Description of secretions helps to indicate whether infection is present or a wound is healing.

18. Assess condition of skin for pressure areas, paying particular attention to regions at risk for pressure (e.g., sacrum, greater trochanter, heels, occipital area, clavicles). If you see areas of redness, place fingertip over area, apply gentle pressure, and then release. Look at skin color.

Normal reactive hyperemia (redness) is a visible effect of localized vasodilation, the normal response of the body to lack of blood flow to underlying tissue. Affected area of skin normally blanches with fingertip pressure. If area does not blanch, suspect tissue injury.

> **SAFE PATIENT CARE** With evidence of normal reactive hyperemia, reposition the patient, and develop a turning schedule if patient is dependent (see Chapter 25).

19. When you detect a lesion, use adequate lighting to inspect color, location, texture, size, shape, and type (Box 7-5). Also note grouping (e.g., clustered or linear) and distribution (e.g., localized or generalized).

Observation of the lesion allows for accurate description and identification.

a. Apply clean gloves if lesion is moist or draining. Gently palpate any lesion to determine mobility, contour (flat, raised, or depressed), and consistency (soft or hard).

Gentle palpation prevents rupture of underlying cysts. Gloves reduce transmission of microorganisms.

b. Note if patient reports tenderness with or without palpation.

Tenderness may indicate inflammation or pressure on body part.

c. Measure size of lesion (length, width, and depth) with centimeter ruler. Length is measured in direction of head to toe. Remove gloves and perform hand hygiene.

Provides for baseline to assess changes in lesion over time.

20. See Completion Protocol (inside front cover).

BOX 7-4   ABCDE RULE OF MALIGNANT MELANOMA

This simple mnemonic helps you remember the characteristics that should alert you to the possibility of malignant melanoma (see illustration) (American Cancer Society, 2013c).

- **A**symmetry of lesion
- **B**orders: irregular
- **C**olor blue/black or variegated, pigmentation not uniform, variations or multiple colors (tan, black) with areas of pink, white, gray, blue, or red
- **D**iameter >6 mm
- **E**volving: Change in size, shape, color, itching, or bleeding

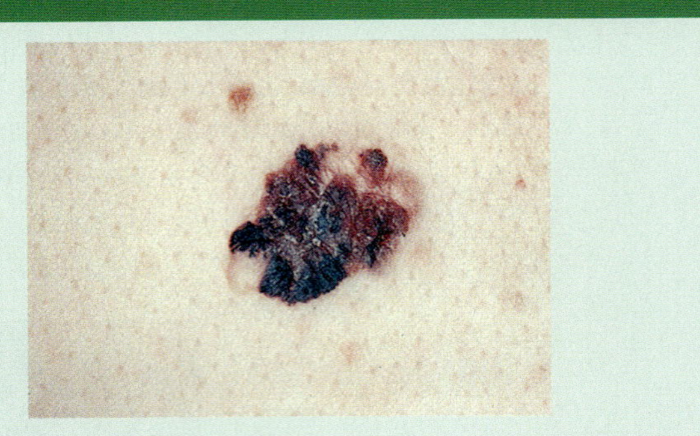

Source: American Cancer Society (ACS): *Can melanoma be prevented,* Atlanta, 2013c, The Society. Available at http://www.cancer.org/cancer/skincancer-melanoma/detailedguide/melanoma-skin-cancer-prevention. Accessed May 27, 2014.
Illustration from Ignatavicius DD, Workman ML: *Medical-surgical nursing: patient-centered collaborative care,* ed 6, St Louis, 2010, Mosby.

TABLE 7-2   SKIN COLOR VARIATIONS

COLOR	CONDITION	CAUSE	ASSESSMENT LOCATION
Bluish (cyanosis)	Related to hypoxia (late sign of decreased oxygen)	Heart or lung disease, cold environment	Nail beds, lips, base of tongue, skin (severe cases)
Pallor (decrease in color)	Reduced amount of oxyhemoglobin Reduced visibility of oxyhemoglobin resulting from decreased blood flow	Anemia Shock	Face, conjunctivae, nail beds, palms of hands Skin, nail beds, conjunctivae, lips
Red (erythema)	Increased visibility of oxyhemoglobin caused by dilation or increased blood flow	Fever, direct trauma, blushing, alcohol intake	Face, area of trauma, and areas at risk of pressure such as sacrum, shoulders, elbows, heels
Yellow-orange (jaundice)	Increased deposit of bilirubin in tissues	Liver disease, destruction of red blood cells	Sclerae, mucous membranes, skin
Loss of pigmentation	Vitiligo	Congenital autoimmune condition causing lack of pigment	Patchy areas on skin over face, hands, arms
Tan-brown	Increased amount of melanin	Suntan, pregnancy	Areas exposed to sun—face, arms; areolas, nipples

EVALUATION

1. Observe throughout the assessment for evidence of physical or emotional distress, which may alter assessment data.
2. Compare assessment findings with previous observations to identify changes.
3. Ask patient if there is information about physical condition that has not been discussed.
4. Use **Teach Back:** State to the patient, "We reviewed what to look for when you observe your skin each day. Can you tell me what changes in your skin should be reported to your doctor?" Evaluates what the patient is able to explain or demonstrate. Revise your instruction now or develop plan for revised patient teaching to be implemented at an appropriate time if patient is not able to teach back correctly.

Unexpected Outcomes and Related Interventions

1. Patient demonstrates acute distress (e.g., shortness of breath, acute pain, or severe anxiety).
   a. Respond immediately to identified issue, including assessment and intervention for complaint (e.g., vital signs, reposition patient with head of bed elevated, apply oxygen, or give medication as appropriate).
   b. Notify health care provider.

BOX 7-5   TYPES OF SKIN LESIONS

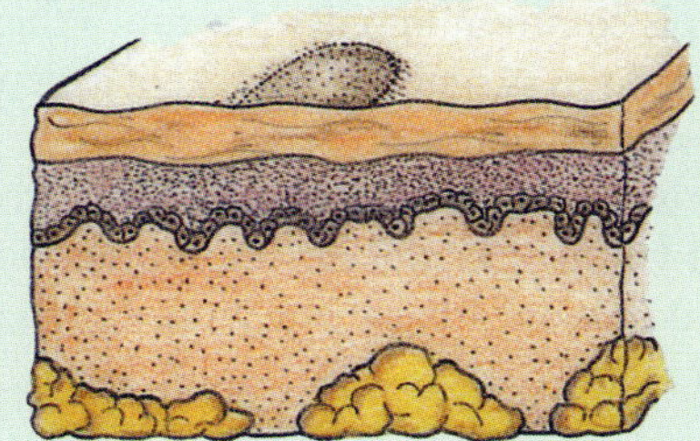

Macule: Flat, nonpalpable change in skin color; <1 cm (0.4 inch) (e.g., freckle, petechia)

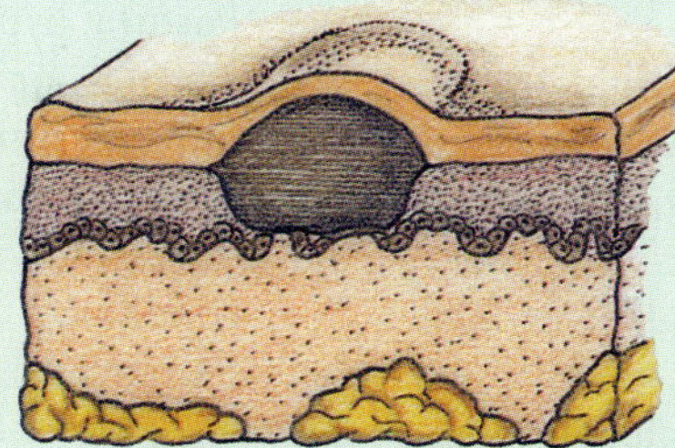

Papule: Palpable, circumscribed, solid elevation in skin; <0.5 cm (0.2 inch) (e.g., elevated nevus)

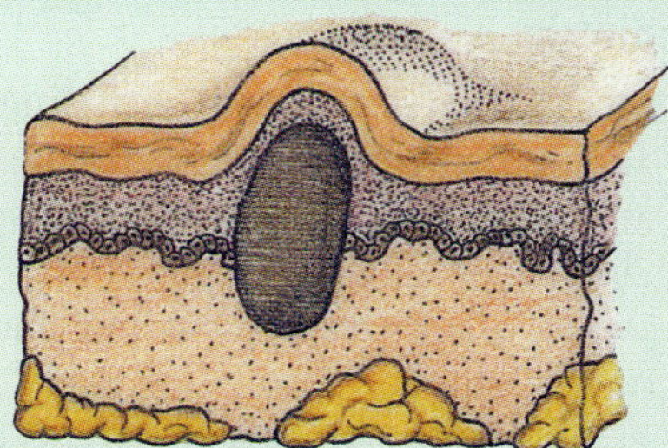

Nodule: Elevated solid mass; deeper and firmer than papule, 0.5 to 2 cm (0.2 to 0.8 inch) (e.g., wart)

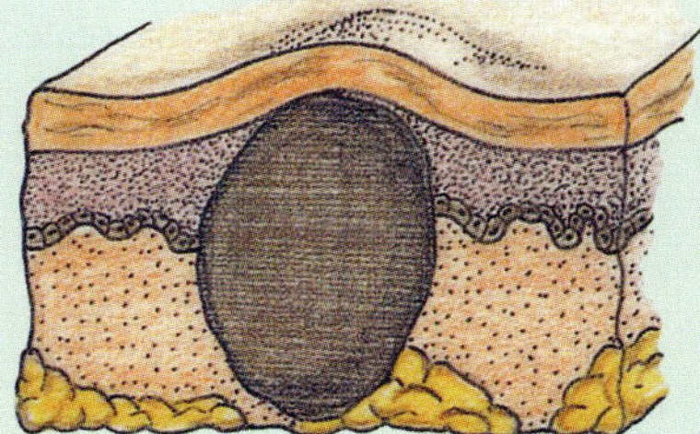

Tumor: Solid mass that may extend deep through subcutaneous tissue; >1 to 2 cm (0.4 to 0.8 inch) (e.g., epithelioma)

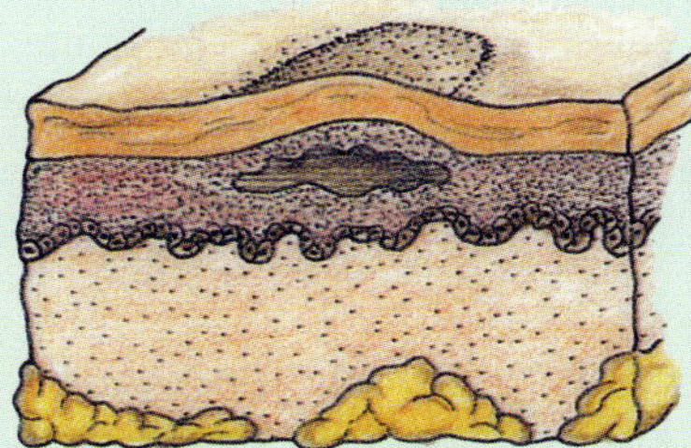

Wheal: Irregularly shaped, elevated area or superficial localized edema; varies in size (e.g., hive, mosquito bite)

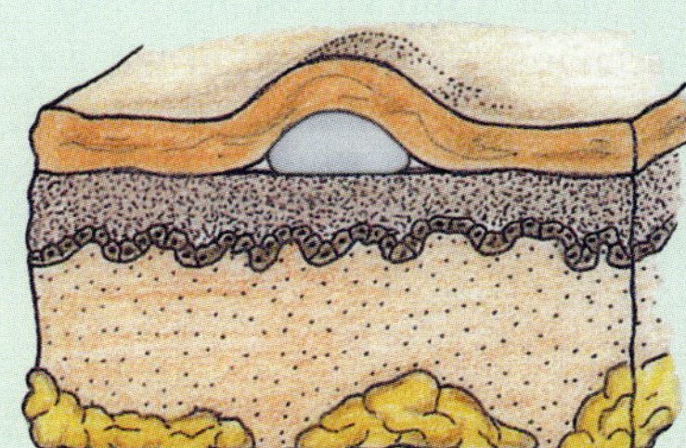

Vesicle: Circumscribed elevation of skin filled with serous fluid; <0.5 cm (0.2 inch) (e.g., herpes simplex, chickenpox)

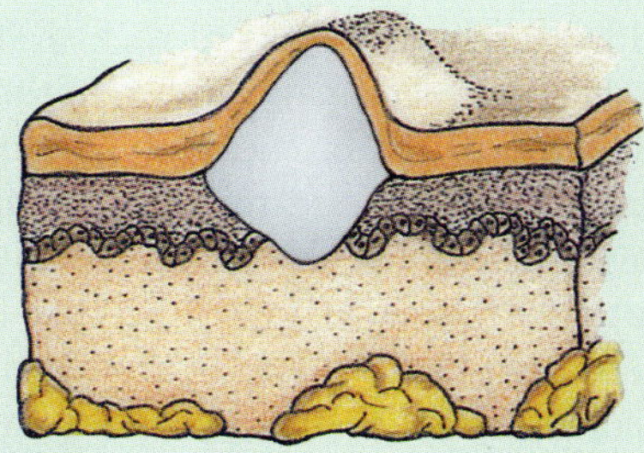

Pustule: Circumscribed elevation of skin similar to vesicle but filled with pus; varies in size (e.g., acne, staphylococcal infection)

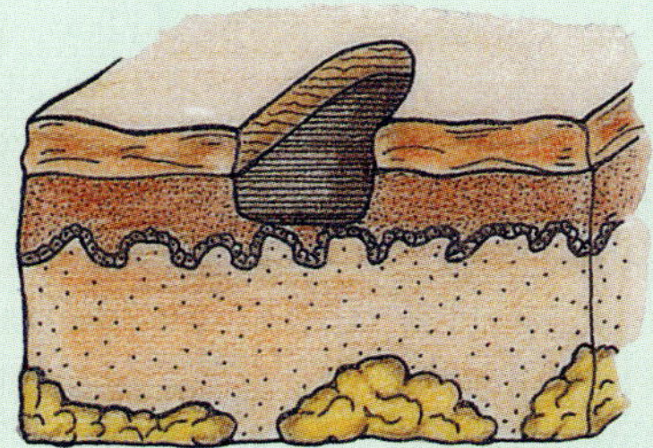

Ulcer: Deep loss of skin surface that may extend to dermis and frequently bleeds and scars; varies in size (e.g., venous stasis ulcer)

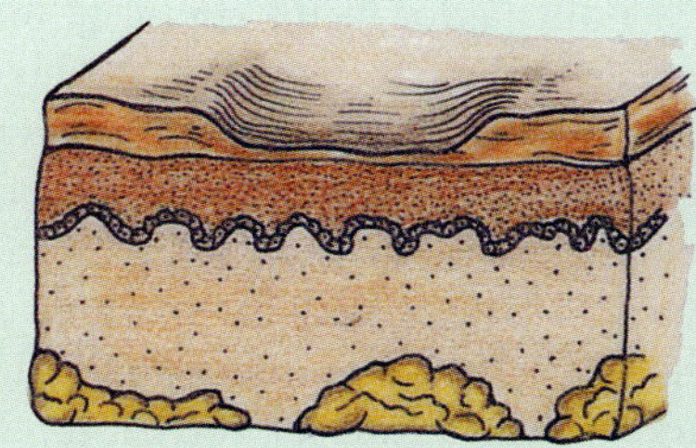

Atrophy: Thinning of skin with loss of normal skin furrow with skin appearing shiny and translucent; varies in size (e.g., arterial insufficiency)

2. Patient has abnormal skin condition (e.g., dry texture, reduced turgor, lesions, or erythema).
   a. Identify contributing factors and prevent continued irritation or damage as appropriate.
3. Patient is unwilling or unable to provide adequate information relating to identified concerns.
   a. Seek information from family members if present, and review patient's record for baseline data.

Recording and Reporting

- Record patient's vital signs on vital sign flow sheet.
- Record description of alterations in patient's general appearance.
- Describe patient's behavior using objective terminology. Include patient's self-report of any signs and symptoms.
- Document your evaluation of patient learning.
- Report abnormalities and acute symptoms to nurse in charge or health care provider.

Sample Documentation

0830 Patient reports a "painful bottom." A 2-cm (0.8-inch) flat, round, erythematous area is noted on sacrum. Skin is intact. Repositioned to left side and will be repositioned every 2 hours.

Special Considerations

Pediatric

- Measure physical growth, including height, weight, length, and head circumference, which are key elements in evaluation of a child's health status (Hockenberry and Wilson, 2013).
- Weigh infants nude. Children may be weighed in light underclothes or gown.
- A child's interactions with parents provide valuable information regarding the child's behavior.

Geriatric

- An older adult's presenting signs and symptoms can be deceiving. An older adult has a diminished physiological reserve that may mask the usual, or "classic," signs and symptoms of a disease. In older adults, signs and symptoms may be blunted or atypical (Touhy and Jett, 2014).
- Postural hypotension is common in older patients. When dizziness or lightheadedness is reported, check vital signs in lying, sitting, and standing positions.
- Inspection of the feet is critical in the presence of impaired circulation, impaired vision, and diabetes. Common foot conditions include ulceration, fungal infection, calluses, bunions, and plantar warts.

Home Care

- The focus may be on patient's ability to perform basic self-care tasks. Be sure that the assessment builds on all health concerns identified in other settings.
- The home health nurse takes a small portable scale to monitor weight changes.

PROCEDURAL GUIDELINE 7.1
Monitoring Intake and Output

Measuring and recording intake and output (I&O) during a 24-hour period helps complete the assessment database for fluid and electrolyte balance (Table 7-3). You are responsible for recording all intake (liquids taken orally, by enteral feeding, and parenterally) and all output (urine, diarrhea, vomitus, gastric suction, and drainage from surgical tubes). Placing a patient on I&O requires cooperation and assistance from the patient and family. I&O are monitored for patients with a fever or edema, receiving intravenous (IV) or diuretic therapy, or on restricted fluids. I&O monitoring is important when a patient has electrolyte losses associated with vomiting, diarrhea, gastrointestinal (GI) drainage, or extensive wounds such as burns. You total and evaluate I&O at the end of each shift or at specified times, such as every 24 hours.

Delegation and Collaboration

The skills of assessing I&O totals at the end of each shift; comparing 24-hour totals over several days; and monitoring and recording IV therapy, wound or chest tube drainage, and tube feeding cannot be delegated to nursing assistive personnel (NAP). The nurse emphasizes maintaining standard precautions relating to body fluids, accurately measuring and recording I&O, and using the metric system with standard containers. The nurse instructs the NAP to:

- Measure and record oral intake, urinary output, liquid diarrheal stool, vomitus, and wound drainage device output.
- Report changes in patient's condition such as alterations in intake or changes in color, amount, or odor of output.

TABLE 7-3	ADULT AVERAGE DAILY FLUID GAINS AND LOSSES		
FLUID INTAKE	**VOLUME (ML)**	**FLUID OUTPUT**	**VOLUME (ML)**
Oral fluids	1100-1400	Urine	1200-1500
Solid foods	800-1000	Skin	500-600
Oxidative metabolism	300	Insensible-lungs	400
Total gains	2200-2700	Gastrointestinal	100-200
		Total losses	2200-2700

From Hall, JE: Guyton and Hall textbook of medical physiology, ed. 12, Philadelphia, 2011, Saunders.

PROCEDURAL GUIDELINE 7.1
Monitoring Intake and Output—cont'd

Equipment

- Sign to alert personnel of I&O measurement
- Daily I&O record form or computer graphic
- Graduated measuring container
- Bedpan, urinal, bedside commode, or urine "hat" (a receptacle that fits under the toilet seat)
- Clean gloves
- Mask, eye protection, and gown (optional)

Procedural Steps

1. **See Standard Protocol (Inside front cover).**
2. Identify patients with conditions that increase fluid loss (e.g., fever, diarrhea, vomiting, surgical wound drainage, chest tube drainage, gastric suction, major burns, or severe trauma).
3. Identify patients with impaired swallowing or mobility and unconscious patients.
4. Identify patients on medications that influence fluid balance (e.g., diuretics and steroids).
5. Assess signs and symptoms of dehydration and fluid excess (e.g., bradycardia versus tachycardia, hypotension versus hypertension, and reduced skin turgor versus edema).
6. Weigh patients daily using the same scale, at the same time of day, and with comparable clothing.
7. Monitor laboratory results:
   a. Urine specific gravity (normal 1.010 to 1.030)
   b. Hematocrit (normal range is 38% to 47% for women and 40% to 54% for men).
8. Assess knowledge of patient and family of the purpose and process of I&O measurement.
9. Explain to patient and family the reasons that I&O are important.
10. Measure and record all intake of fluids:
    a. Liquids with meals, gelatin, custards, ice cream, popsicles, sherbets, ice chips (recorded as 50% of measured volume [e.g., 100 mL of ice chips equals 50 mL of water]). Convert household measures to the metric system: 1 ounce equals 30 mL; 12 ounces (soda can) equals 360 mL.
    b. Count liquid medications such as antacids as fluid intake, as are fluids taken with medications.
    c. Calculate fluid intake from tube feedings (see Chapter 12).
    d. Calculate fluid intake from parenteral fluids, blood components, and total parenteral nutrition (see Chapter 27).

11. Instruct patient and family to call you or NAP to empty contents of urinal, urine hat, or commode each time patient uses it. Patient and family also need to monitor incontinence, vomiting, and excessive perspiration and report it to the nurse.
12. Inform patient and family that Foley catheter drainage bag and wound, gastric, or chest tube drainage are closely monitored, measured, and recorded and who is responsible for this. Each patient must have a graduated container clearly marked with name and bed location and used only for the identified patient.
13. Apply clean gloves. Measure drainage at the end of the shift or as indicated, using appropriate containers and noting color and characteristics. If splashing is anticipated, wear mask, eye protection, and gown.
    a. Measure urine drainage using a "hat" into which the patient voids or a graduated container.
    b. Observe color and characteristics of urine in Foley tubing and drainage bag. Sometimes a measuring device is part of the drainage bag. Otherwise measure using a graduated container (see illustration).

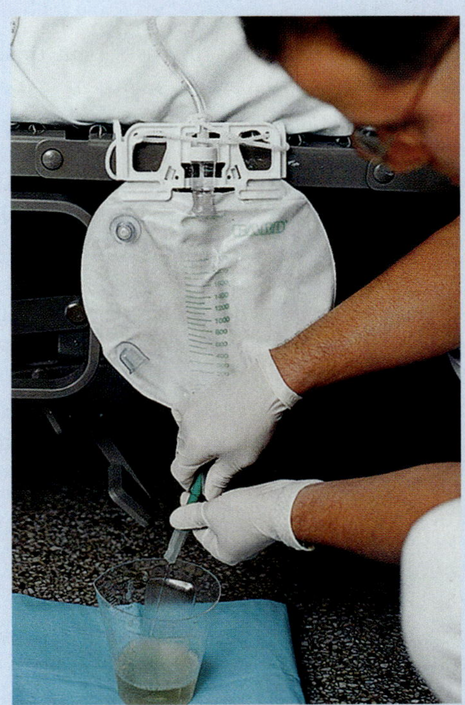

STEP 13b Device for measuring hourly urine output.

SAFE PATIENT CARE Record intake as soon as you measure it to maintain accuracy.

Continued

PROCEDURAL GUIDELINE 7.1
Monitoring Intake and Output—cont'd

   c. Measure chest tube drainage by marking and recording the time on the collection chamber at specified intervals. Empty chest tube drainage or change equipment *only* when container is nearly full. A closed system is necessary to maintain lung expansion.

   d. Measure Jackson-Pratt/Hemovac drainage using a measuring device (see illustration) (see Chapter 24).

   e. Measure gastric drainage or larger drainage pouches by opening clamp and pouring into graduated container with 240-mL capacity.

14. See Completion Protocol (inside front cover).

15. Note I&O balance or imbalance, and report to health care provider any urine output less than 30 mL/hr or significant changes in daily weight.

16. Document on I&O forms or computer record.

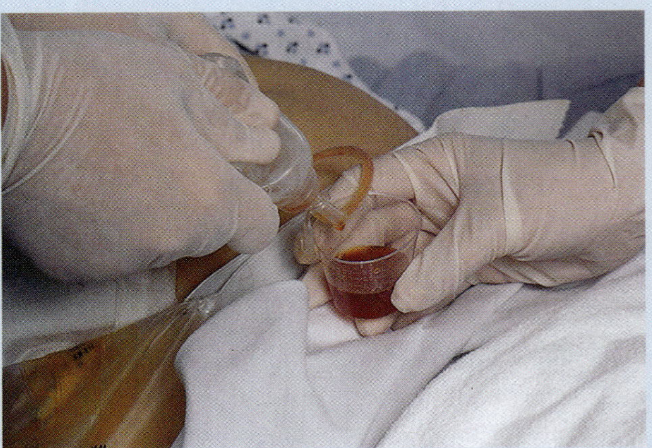

STEP 13d Measuring wound drainage from a Jackson-Pratt drain.

SKILL 7.2   ASSESSING THE HEAD AND NECK

Examination of the head and neck includes assessment of the head, eyes, ears, nose, mouth, and sinuses. Assessment of the head and neck uses inspection, palpation, and auscultation, with inspection and palpation often used simultaneously.

ASSESSMENT

1. Assess for history of headache, dizziness, pain, or stiffness. *Rationale: Headaches and dizziness may be a sign of stress, a symptom of another underlying problem such as high blood pressure, or a result of injury.*

2. Determine if patient has a history of eye disease, diabetes mellitus, or hypertension. *Rationale: Common conditions predispose patients to visual alterations requiring health care provider referral.*

3. Ask if patient has experienced blurred vision, flashing lights, or reduced visual field. *Rationale: These common symptoms indicate visual problems.*

4. Ask if patient has experienced ear pain, itching, discharge, vertigo, tinnitus (ringing in the ears), or change in hearing. *Rationale: These signs and symptoms indicate infection or hearing loss.*

5. Review patient's occupational history. *Rationale: Patient's occupation can create a risk of injury, potential for eye fatigue, or prolonged noise exposure.*

6. Ask if patient has a history of allergies, nasal discharge, epistaxis (nosebleeds), or postnasal drip. *Rationale: History is useful in determining source of nasal and sinus drainage.*

7. Determine if patient smokes or chews tobacco. *Rationale: Tobacco users have greater risk for mouth and throat cancer (ACS, 2013a).*

8. Ask if patient has regular or annual dental examinations. *Rationale: Annual examinations often detect abnormalities early.*

PLANNING

Expected Outcomes focus on identifying alterations in the head and neck.

1. Physical findings are within normal limits (oral mucosa are moist and pink, without lesions; patient able to see clearly without eye irritation and able to hear spoken word; lymph nodes are not palpable).

2. Patient recognizes warning signs and symptoms of eye, ear, sinus, and mouth disease.

3. Patient takes appropriate safety precautions for preventing occupational injury of the head and neck.

Delegation and Collaboration

The skill of assessing the head and neck cannot be delegated to nursing assistive personnel (NAP). The nurse directs the NAP to:

- Observe for nasal discharge and nasal bleeding.
- Report any findings found during routine care (e.g., oral care, bathing) to the nurse for further assessment.

EQUIPMENT

- Stethoscope
- Clean gloves (use nonlatex if necessary)
- Tongue blade
- Penlight

IMPLEMENTATION *for* ASSESSING THE HEAD AND NECK

STEPS	RATIONALE

1. **See Standard Protocol (inside front cover).**
2. Position patient sitting upright if possible.

   Provides for a more thorough examination of head and neck structures.

3. Inspect the head.
   a. Note head position and facial features.
   b. Note patient's facial features for symmetry.

   Head tilting to one side may indicate hearing or visual loss. Neurological disorders such as paralysis may affect symmetry of the face.

4. Assess the eyes (include discussion of signs and symptoms of eye disease)
   a. Inspect position of eyes, color and condition of sclera and conjunctivae, and movement.

   Asymmetrical positioning may reflect trauma or tumor growth. Changes in color may be due to local infection or symptomatic of another abnormality (e.g., pale conjunctiva is associated with anemia; yellow sclera is due to jaundice).

   b. Assess patient's near vision (ability to read newspaper or magazines) and far vision (ability to follow movement or read clock, watch television, or read signs at a distance).

   If patient has visual acuity or visual field loss, make adjustments to support self-care measures (e.g., feeding, bathing and hygiene, dressing) and teaching.

   c. Inspect pupils for size, shape, and equality (see illustration).

   Normal pupils are round, clear, and equal in size and shape.

   d. Test pupillary reflexes. To test reaction to light, dim room light. As patient looks straight ahead, move penlight from side of patient's face and direct light on pupil. Observe pupillary response of both eyes (consensual response), noting briskness and equality of reflex (see illustrations).

   Darkened room normally ensures brisk response of pupils to light. Pupil that is illuminated constricts. Pupil in other eye should constrict equally (consensual light reflex).

   (1) Test for accommodation by asking the patient to focus on a distant object, which dilates the pupil. Then have the patient shift to a near object about 7 to 8 cm (3 inches) from the nose, and observe for pupil constriction and convergence of the eyes. Note: Can also ask patient to follow an object (e.g., finger, pen) with eyes from a far to a near point.

   Absence of constriction or convergence or an asymmetric response requires further ophthalmologic assessment (Seidel et al., 2015).

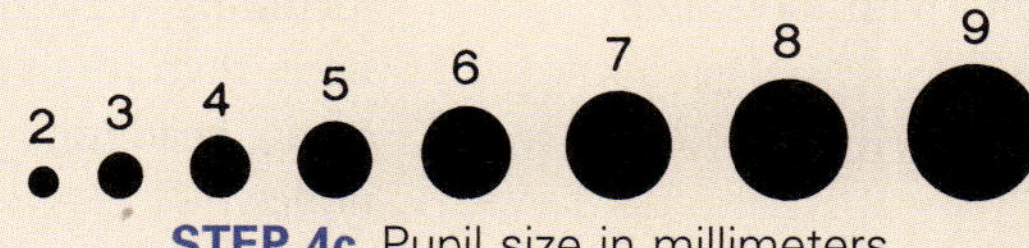

STEP 4c Pupil size in millimeters.

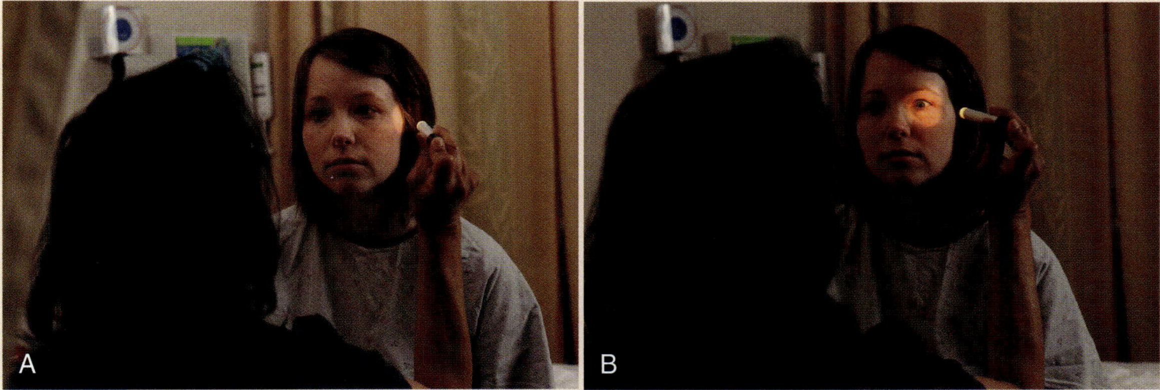

STEP 4d A, Hold penlight to side of patient's face. **B,** Illuminate pupil to cause pupil to constrict.

Continued

STEPS	RATIONALE

5. Assess hearing. Note patient's response to questions and presence and use of a hearing aid. If hearing loss is suspected, ask patient to repeat random numbers that you speak. Use one- or two-syllable words. Repeat, gradually increasing voice intensity until patient correctly repeats the words (use time to discuss hearing aid care [see Chapter 11]).

Patients normally hear numbers clearly when whispered, responding correctly at least 50% of the time. For a patient with obvious hearing impairment, speak clearly and concisely; stand so patient can see face; and speak toward patient's good ear, using a low pitch and without yelling (Seidel et al., 2015).

> **SAFE PATIENT CARE** If a hearing deficit is present, have a registered nurse inspect patient's ears because impaired hearing may be caused by impacted cerumen, external otitis, or swelling in ear canal owing to allergic reaction to material in hearing aid.

6. Inspect the nose externally for shape, skin color, alignment, drainage, and presence of deformity or inflammation. Note color of mucosa and any lesions, discharge, swelling, or presence of bleeding. If drainage appears infectious, consult health care provider about obtaining a specimen.

Character of discharge and inflammation indicates allergy or infection. Perforation and erosion of the septum and puffiness or increased vascularity of the mucosa may indicate habitual drug use.

7. In patients with a nasogastric (NG), nasointestinal, or nasotracheal tube, inspect the nares for excoriation, inflammation, or discharge. Using a penlight, look up into each nares. Stabilize tube as needed.

Swallowing or coughing reflex causes movement of tubes against nares, and pressure against tissues and mucosa can result in tissue erosion causing a medical device–related pressure ulcer (Norman, 2013).

8. Inspect the sinuses by palpation over frontal and maxillary areas (see illustration). Use pads of fingertips to palpate just above eyebrows (frontal sinus) and just below eyes (maxillary sinus).

Infection, allergy, or drug use sometimes causes tenderness.

9. Assess the mouth (include discussion of signs and symptoms of oral cancer).

   a. Use a tongue blade to depress the tongue, and inspect the oral cavity with a penlight. Inspect the oral mucosa, tongue, teeth, and gums for hydration, discoloration, and obvious lesions.

   Precancerous lesions can go unnoticed and progress rapidly.

   b. Determine if patient wears dentures or retainers and if they are comfortable. You may remove dentures to visualize and palpate gums.

   Ill-fitting dentures and retainers chronically irritate mucosa and gums and may pose a risk for mouth cancer.

10. Inspect and palpate the neck. Ask patient if there is a history of neck pain or difficulty with movement of the neck.

   This determines whether all neck structures are present, including neck muscles, lymph nodes of the head and neck, thyroid gland, and trachea. May indicate muscle strain, head injury, local nerve injury, or swollen lymph nodes.

   a. Neck muscles: Inspect neck for bilateral symmetry of muscles. Ask patient to flex and hyperextend neck and turn head side to side.

   Detects muscle weakness, strain, and range of motion (ROM).

   b. Lymph nodes:

   (1) With patient's chin raised and head tilted slightly, inspect area where lymph nodes are distributed and compare both sides (see illustration).

   Lymph nodes may be enlarged from infection or from various diseases such as cancer.

   (2) To examine lymph nodes, have patient relax with neck flexed slightly forward. To palpate, face or stand to the side of patient and use pads of middle three fingers of hand. Palpate gently in a rotary motion for superficial lymph nodes (see illustration).

   This position relaxes tissues and muscles.

   (3) Note if lymph nodes are large, fixed, inflamed, or tender.

   Large, fixed, inflamed, or tender lymph nodes indicate local infection, systemic disease, or neoplasm.

11. See Completion Protocol (inside front cover).

<table>
<tr><td>STEPS</td><td style="text-align:center">RATIONALE</td></tr>
</table>

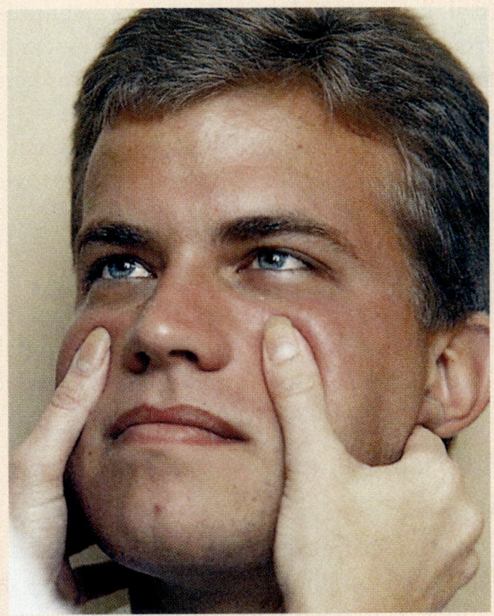

STEP 8 Palpation of maxillary sinuses.

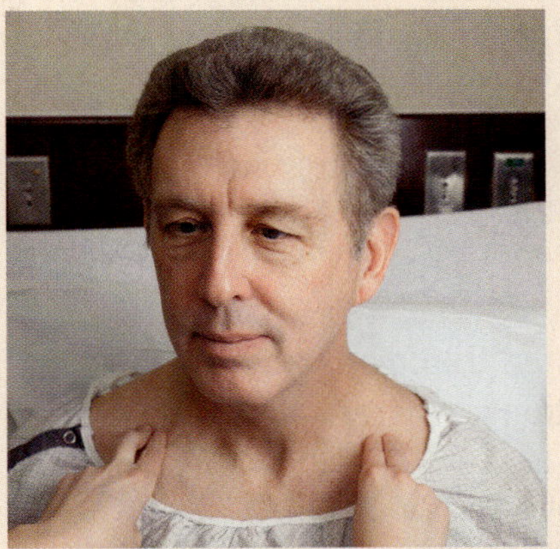

STEP 10b(2) Palpation of cervical lymph nodes.

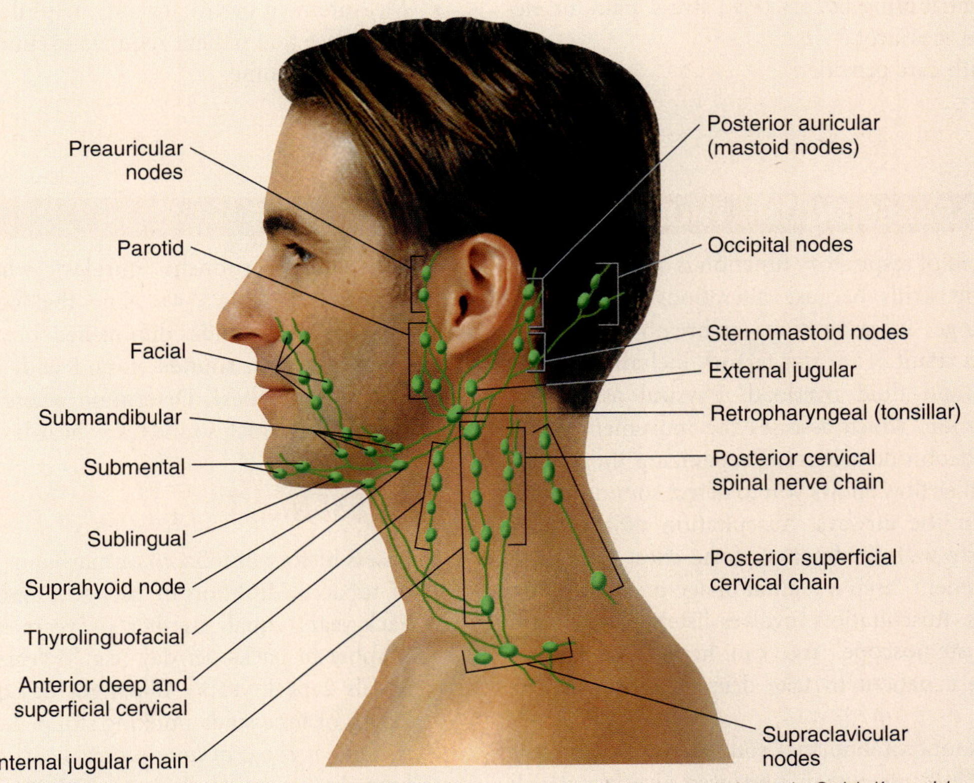

STEP 10b(1) Palpable lymph nodes of head and neck. (From Seidel HM et al: *Seidel's guide to physical examination,* ed 8, St Louis, 2015, Mosby.)

EVALUATION

1. Compare assessment with previous observations to identify changes.
2. Ask patient to describe common symptoms of eye, ear, sinus, or mouth disease.
3. Ask patient to list occupational safety precautions.
4. Use ***Teach Back:*** State to the patient, "We talked about signs of eye problems. Can you tell me some of the signs to notice that might mean you have a vision problem?" Evaluates what the patient is able to explain or demonstrate. Revise your instruction now or develop plan for revised patient teaching to be implemented at an appropriate time if patient is not able to teach back correctly.

Unexpected Outcomes and Related Interventions

1. Patient has yellow nasal discharge, sneezing, and complaint of sinus pain.
   a. Reposition into semi-Fowler's or other comfortable position to relieve sinus pain.
   b. Monitor temperature for fever.
   c. Notify health care provider if these are new findings.
2. Patient complains of severe headache and dizziness when standing.
   a. Immediately obtain vital signs, especially blood pressure (lying, sitting, and standing).
   b. Return patient to bed to minimize dizziness and relieve headache.
   c. Identify contributing factors (e.g., stress, pain, or elevated blood pressure).
   d. Notify health care provider.

Recording and Reporting

- Record all findings, including any abnormal findings such as hearing or visual loss, pain and its location, and current infection in nurses' notes or flow sheet. Record content of any patient education.
- Report increased headache, dizziness, or visual changes immediately to charge nurse or health care provider.
- Document your evaluation of patient learning.

Sample Documentation

1200   Copious, green, thick nasal discharge noted from both nares. No odor noted. Patient complains of frontal "headache." Blood pressure 110/70. Head of bed raised to 60 degrees. Health care provider notified.

Special Considerations
Pediatric

- Infants may resist eye examination by closing eyes. Holding the infant in an upright position over caregiver's shoulders may cause eyes to open (Hockenberry and Wilson, 2013).
- Headaches in children are usually caused by loss of sleep, poor nutrition, eye fatigue, and allergies (Hockenberry and Wilson, 2013).

Geriatric

- Older adults commonly have loss of peripheral vision caused by changes in the lens.
- Instruct patients older than age 65 to have regular hearing checks.
- Measurement of visual acuity helps determine the level of assistance that patient requires to function independently within the home.

SKILL 7.3   ASSESSING THE THORAX AND LUNGS

Routine assessment of respiratory function is one of the most critical assessment skills because alterations can be life-threatening. Changes in respirations or breath sounds can occur quickly as a result of various factors, including immobility, infection, and fluid overload. Physical assessment includes auscultation, which assesses the movement of air through the tracheobronchial tree. Recognizing the sounds created by normal airflow allows you to detect sounds caused by obstruction of the airways. Auscultation of the lungs requires familiarity with landmarks of the chest (Fig. 7-2). During the assessment, keep a mental image of the location of the lung lobes. Auscultation involves listening to breath sounds using a stethoscope. You can hear these sounds best by coaching a patient to take deep breaths with the mouth open.

Adventitious sounds (abnormal sounds) result from air passing through fluid, mucus, or narrowed airways; alveoli suddenly reinflating; or an inflammation between the pleural linings. The four types of adventitious sounds include crackles (rales), rhonchi (gurgles), wheezes, and pleural friction rubs (Table 7-4). Note the location and characteristics of the sounds, diminished breath sounds, or the absence of breath sounds (found with collapsed or surgically removed lobes). Determine where in the respiratory cycle the abnormal sounds are heard.

ASSESSMENT

1. Assess history of tobacco or marijuana use, including type of tobacco, duration of use, and amount in pack-years. Pack-years equal number of years smoking times the number of packs per day (e.g., 4 years × ½ pack per day equals 2 pack-years). If patient has quit, determine the length of time since smoking stopped. *Rationale: Smoking is a major cause of lung cancer, heart disease, and chronic lung disease (emphysema and chronic bronchitis) and is responsible for 15% of all lung cancers in the United States (ACS, 2013c).*

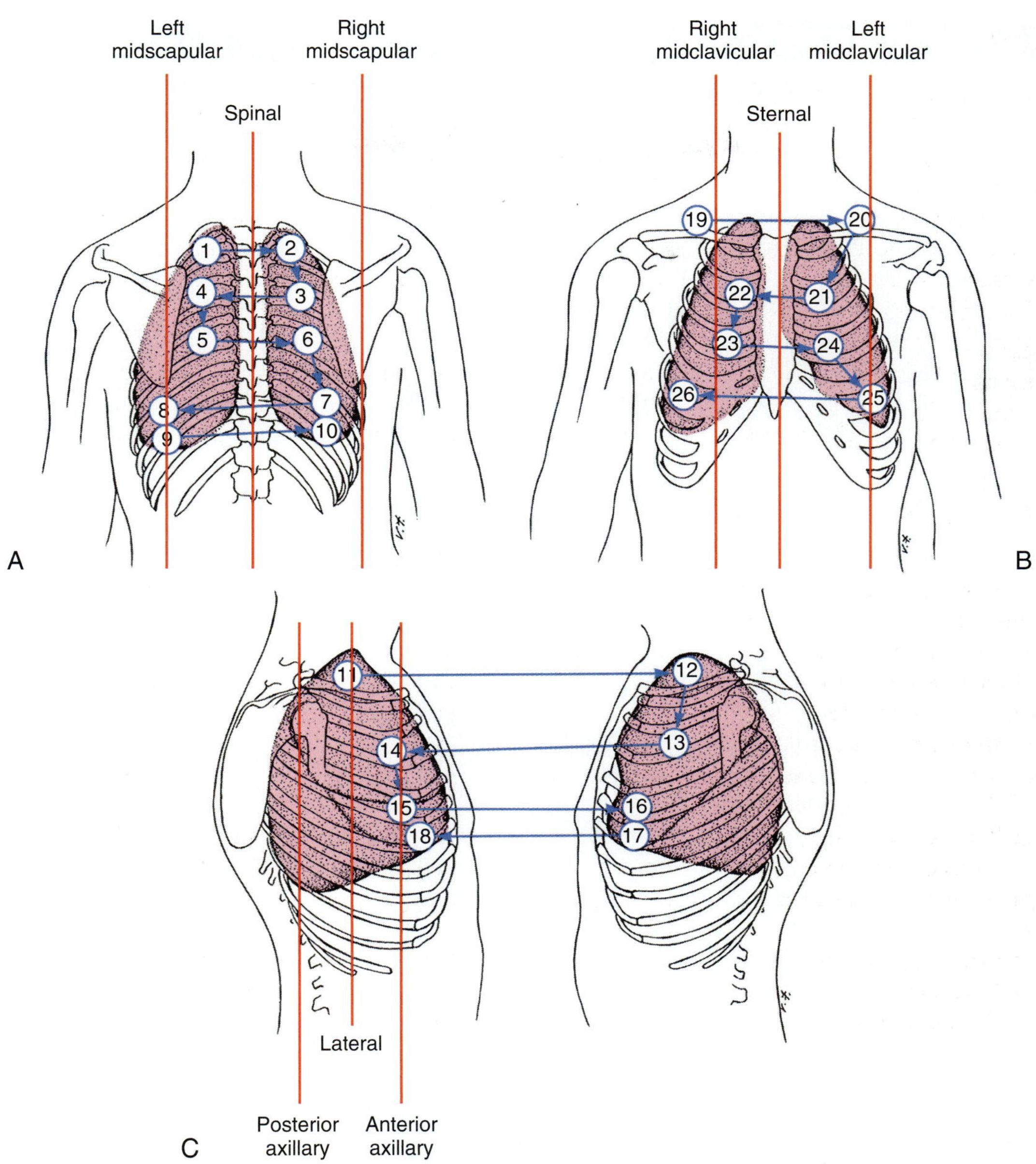

FIG 7-2 Anatomical landmarks and order of progression for examination of the thorax. **A,** Posterior thorax. **B,** Anterior thorax. **C,** Lateral thorax.

2. Ask if patient experiences any of the following: *persistent cough* (productive or nonproductive), sputum production, *blood-streaked sputum, chest pain,* shortness of breath, orthopnea, dyspnea during exertion, activity intolerance, or *recurrent attacks of pneumonia or bronchitis. Rationale: Symptoms of respiratory alterations help to localize objective physical findings. Warning signs of lung cancer are in italic type.*

3. Assess for history of allergies to pollens, dust, or other airborne irritants and to any foods, drugs, or chemical substances. *Rationale: Allergic response is associated with wheezing on auscultation, dyspnea, cyanosis, and diaphoresis.*

4. Determine if patient works in environment containing pollutants (e.g., asbestos, coal dust, or chemical irritants).

Does patient have exposure to secondhand cigarette smoke? *Rationale: Patients with chronic respiratory disease, particularly asthma, have symptoms aggravated by change in temperature and humidity, irritating fumes or smoke, emotional stress, and physical exertion.*

5. Review history for known or suspected human immuno-deficiency virus (HIV) infection, substance abuse, low income, residence or employment in nursing home or shelter, homelessness, recent imprisonment, or exposure to family member with tuberculosis (TB). *Rationale: These are known risk factors for exposure to or development of TB.*

6. Ask if patient has history of persistent cough, hemoptysis (bloody sputum), unexplained weight loss, fatigue, night sweats, or fever. *Rationale: These are signs and symptoms of both TB and HIV infection.*

TABLE 7-4 ADVENTITIOUS SOUNDS

SOUND	SITE AUSCULTATED	CAUSE	CHARACTER
Crackles (formerly called rales)	Most common in dependent lobes: right and left lung bases	Random, sudden reinflation of groups of alveoli; also related to increase in fluid in small airways	Fine, short, interrupted crackling sounds heard during end of inspiration, expiration, or both; may or may not change with coughing; sound like crushing cellophane; medium crackles are lower, more moist sounds heard during middle of inspiration, not cleared with coughing; coarse crackles are loud, bubbly sounds heard during inspiration, not cleared with coughing
Rhonchi (sonorous wheeze)	Heard primarily over trachea and bronchi; if loud enough, can be heard over most lung fields	Fluid or mucus in larger airways, causing turbulence; muscular spasm	Loud, low-pitched, continuous sounds heard more during expiration; sometimes cleared by coughing; sound like blowing air through fluid with a straw
Wheezes (sibilant wheeze)	Heard over all lung fields but more distinct over posterior lung fields	High-velocity airflow through severely narrowed or obstructed bronchus	High-pitched, musical sounds like a squeak heard continuously during inspiration or expiration; usually louder on expiration; do not clear with coughing
Pleural friction rub	Heard over anterior lateral lung field (if patient is sitting upright)	Inflamed pleura, parietal pleura rubbing against visceral pleura	Has grating quality heard best during inspiration; does not clear with coughing; heard loudest over lower lateral anterior surface

Data from Seidel HM et al: *Seidel's guide to physical examination*, ed 8, St Louis, 2015 Mosby.

7. Review family history for cancer, TB, allergies, or chronic obstructive pulmonary disease (COPD). *Rationale: Family history places patient at risk for lung disease.*

| PLANNING

Expected Outcomes focus on identifying alterations in respiratory function.

1. Physical findings are within normal limits (respirations passive, diaphragmatic or costal, and regular [12 to 20/min in adult] with symmetrical expansion; breath sounds clear to auscultation and equal in all lung fields).
2. Patient is able to describe own risks and factors that predispose to lung disease.

Delegation and Collaboration

The skill of assessing the lungs and thorax cannot be delegated to nursing assistive personnel (NAP). The nurse directs the NAP to:
- Measure patient's respirations after the nurse determines stability.
- Report any respiratory distress, difficulty breathing, and changes in rate or depth of respiration.

Equipment
- Stethoscope
- Clean gloves
- Drapes

IMPLEMENTATION *for* ASSESSING THE THORAX AND LUNGS

STEPS	RATIONALE

1. **See Standard Protocol (inside front cover).**
2. Position and prepare patient for examination.

   a. Position patient sitting upright. For bedridden patient, elevate head of bed 45 to 90 degrees. If patient is unable to tolerate sitting, use the supine position or side-lying position.

   Promotes full lung expansion during examination. Patients with chronic respiratory disease may need to sit up throughout the examination because of shortness of breath. May require assistance of another caregiver to help position unresponsive patients.

   b. Remove gown or drape first from posterior chest, keeping front of chest and legs covered. As examination progresses, remove gown from area being examined.

   Avoids unnecessary exposure and provides full visibility of thorax. Allows direct placement of diaphragm or bell of stethoscope on patient's skin, which enhances clarity of sounds.

   c. Explain all steps of procedure, encouraging patient to relax and breathe normally through the mouth.

   Anxiety alters respiratory function. Breathing through the mouth decreases extraneous sounds from air passing through the nose.

3. *Posterior thorax (if patient has risks for lung disease, discuss signs and symptoms of alterations).*

   a. If possible, stand behind patient. Inspect thorax for shape and deformities, position of the spine, slope of the ribs, retraction of intercostal spaces (ICS) during inspiration and bulging of ICS during expiration, and symmetrical expansion during inspiration.

   Allows for identification of impairment in chest expansion and any symptoms of respiratory distress. In the adults, the anteroposterior diameter is less than the lateral diameter (Seidel et al., 2015). Chronic lung disease causes the ribs to become more horizontal and increases the anteroposterior diameter, causing a "barrel chest."

> **SAFE PATIENT CARE** When a patient holds the chest wall during breathing, this indicates localized chest pain. Assess the nature of pain, including onset, severity, precipitating factors, quality, region, and radiation.

   b. Determine the rate and rhythm of breathing (see Chapter 6). Have patient relax.

   This is a good time to count respirations, with patient relaxed and unaware of inspection. Awareness could alter respirations.

   c. Systematically palpate posterior chest wall, costal spaces, and ICS, noting any masses, pulsations, unusual movement, or areas of localized tenderness (see Fig. 7-2, *B*, for numbered areas to palpate systematically). If you detect a suspicious mass or swollen area, palpate for size, shape, and typical qualities of lesion. Do not palpate painful areas deeply.

   Palpation assesses further characteristics and confirms or supplements findings from assessment. Localized swelling or tenderness may indicate trauma to ribs or underlying cartilage. A fractured rib fragment could be displaced.

   d. Standing behind patient, place thumbs along the spinal processes at the tenth rib, with the palms lightly contacting the posterolateral surfaces (see illustration *A*). Keep thumbs about 5 cm (2 inches) apart, with the thumbs pointing toward the spine and the fingers pointing laterally. Press hands toward patient's spine to form small skin fold between thumbs. After exhalation, patient takes deep breath. Note movement of thumbs (see illustration *B*) and symmetry of chest wall movement. Normally, symmetrical separation of the thumbs occurs during chest excursion—3 to 5 cm ($1\frac{1}{2}$ to 2 inches).

   Palpation of chest excursion assesses depth of patient's breathing. This technique is a good measure to evaluate patient's ability to perform deep-breathing exercises (see Chapter 28). Limited movement on one side may indicate that patient is voluntarily splinting during ventilation because of pain. Avoid allowing the hands to slide over the skin, which gives a false measure of excursion.

Continued

STEPS	RATIONALE

e. Auscultate breath sounds. Have patient take slow deep breaths with the mouth slightly open. For an adult, place diaphragm of stethoscope firmly on chest wall over ICS (see illustration). Listen to entire inspiration and expiration at each stethoscope position, anterior, posterior, and lateral (see Fig. 7-2, *C*). Systematically compare breath sounds over right and left sides. If sounds are faint, ask patient to breathe a little deeper temporarily.

Assesses movement of air through tracheobronchial tree (Table 7-5). Recognition of normal airflow sounds allows detection of sounds caused by mucus or airway obstruction. Characterize sound by length of inspiratory and expiratory phases.

f. If you auscultate adventitious sounds, have patient cough. Listen again with stethoscope to determine if sound has cleared with coughing. See Table 7-5 for a description of normal breath sounds.

Coughing may clear adventitious sound. Rhonchi often are eliminated or altered by coughing. Crackles and wheezes are not.

4. *Lateral thorax.*

a. Instruct patient to raise arms, and inspect chest wall for same characteristics as reviewed for posterior chest.

Improves access to lateral thoracic structures.

b. Extend palpation and auscultation of posterior thorax to lateral sides of chest except for excursion measurement (see Fig. 7-2, *C*).

Locates abnormalities in lateral lung fields.

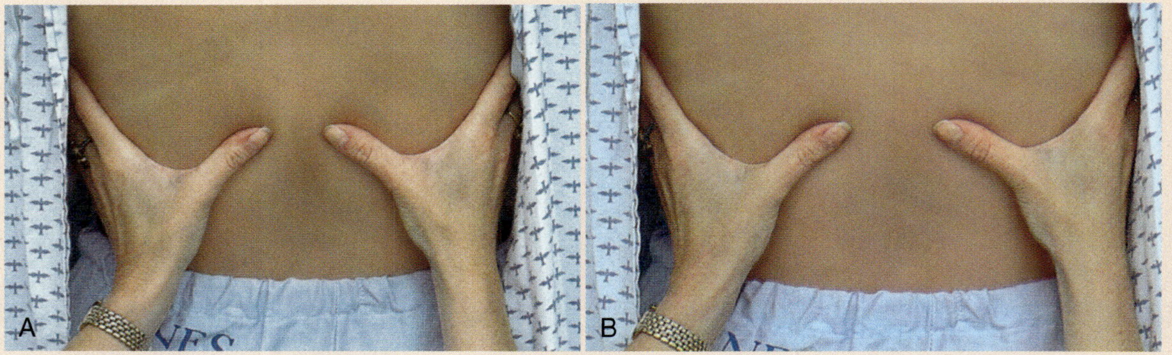

STEP 3d A, Position of hands for palpation of posterior thorax excursion. **B,** As patient inhales, movement of chest excursion separates nurse's thumbs.

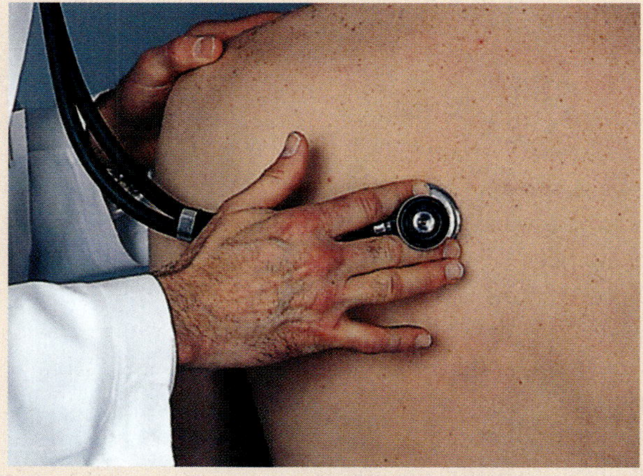

STEP 3e Use of diaphragm of stethoscope to auscultate breath sounds. (From Seidel HM et al: *Mosby's guide to physical examination,* ed 7, St Louis, 2011, Mosby.)

STEPS	RATIONALE

5. *Anterior thorax.*

a. Inspect accessory muscles of breathing: sternocleidomastoid, trapezius, and abdominal muscles, noting effort to breathe.

Extent to which accessory muscles are used reveals degree of effort to breathe. These muscles generally are not used for breathing.

b. Inspect width or spread of angle made by costal margins and tip of sternum. Angle is usually larger than 90 degrees between margins.

Indicates congenital, acquired, or traumatic alterations that may influence patient's chest expansion.

c. Observe patient's breathing pattern, observing symmetry and degree of chest wall and abdominal movement. Respiratory rate and rhythm are more often assessed on anterior chest wall.

Assesses patient's effort to breathe: symmetrical, passive movement indicates no respiratory distress.

d. Palpate anterior thoracic muscles and ribs for lumps, masses, tenderness, or unusual movement following pattern across and down.

Localized swelling or tenderness may indicate trauma to underlying ribs or cartilage.

e. Palpate anterior chest excursion. Place hands over each lateral rib cage, with thumbs approximately 5 cm (2 inches) apart and angled along each costal margin. As patient inhales deeply, thumbs should symmetrically separate approximately 3 to 5 cm ($1\frac{1}{2}$ to 2 inches), with each side expanding equally.

Assesses depth of patient's breathing and ability to perform deep-breathing exercises. Certain abnormalities are evident if expansion is not symmetrical.

f. With patient sitting, auscultate anterior thorax. Begin above clavicles and move across and then down as during palpation.

A systematic pattern of assessment comparing sides helps identify abnormal sounds.

6. See Completion Protocol (inside front cover).

TABLE 7-5 NORMAL BREATH SOUNDS

TYPE	DESCRIPTION	LOCATION	ORIGIN
Bronchial	Loud and high-pitched sounds with hollow quality; expiration lasts longer than inspiration (3:2 ratio)	Best heard over trachea	Created by air moving through trachea close to chest wall
Bronchovesicular	Medium-pitched and blowing sounds of medium intensity; inspiratory phase is equal to expiratory phase	Best heard posteriorly between scapulae and anteriorly over bronchioles lateral to sternum at first and second intercostal spaces	Created by air moving through large airways
Vesicular	Soft, breezy, low-pitched sounds; inspiratory phase is 3 times longer than expiratory phase	Best heard over periphery of lung (except over scapula)	Created by air moving through smaller airways

EVALUATION

1. Compare respiratory findings with assessment characteristics for thorax and lungs to identify changes.
2. Have patient identify factors leading to lung disease.
3. Use *Teach Back:* State to the patient, "Because you have been a smoker, we talked about the signs and symptoms of lung disease. Can you tell me the signs of lung disease?" Evaluates what the patient is able to explain or demonstrate. Revise your instruction now or develop plan for revised patient teaching to be implemented at an appropriate time if patient is not able to teach back correctly.

Unexpected Outcomes and Related Interventions

1. Patient has copious mucus production; audible inspiratory wheezing; or congested cough with thick, tenacious mucus, indicating an infection.
   a. Assist patient to cough by splinting chest; teach to inhale slowly through nose, exhale, and cough; encourage expectoration of sputum.
   b. Auscultate breath sounds before and after cough to evaluate cough effectiveness.
   c. Encourage increased oral fluid intake (if permitted).

   d. If unable to clear airway by coughing, suctioning is indicated (see Chapter 14).
   e. Monitor vital signs.
   f. Notify health care provider.
2. Patient demonstrates weakness, fatigue, dyspnea, altered vital signs, or dizziness with exertion.
   a. Provide bed rest and limited activity to conserve oxygen.
   b. Plan interventions to alternate with periods of rest.
   c. Monitor for restlessness, anxiety, confusion, and respiratory status.

Recording and Reporting

- Record patient's respiratory rate and character; condition of thorax; character of any mucous; breath sounds, including type, location, and presence on inspiration, expiration, or both; and changes noted after coughing in nurses' notes or on flow sheet. Record content of any patient education.
- Document your evaluation of patient learning.
- Report any abnormalities immediately to nurse in charge or health care provider.

Sample Documentation

0730   Inspiratory wheezing noted over anterior upper right lobe; lung sounds clear and equal bilaterally in all other lung fields. Respirations 26 and regular. Patient complaining of shortness of breath. Head of bed elevated to 90 degrees. Health care provider notified.

Special Considerations
Pediatric

- Infants and young children have thin chest walls, causing louder breath sounds and allowing breath sounds from one lung to be heard over entire chest (Hockenberry and Wilson, 2013).
- Children younger than 7 years old normally exhibit noticeable abdominal or diaphragmatic movement. Older children and adults exhibit more costal or thoracic movement. Use stethoscope bell to auscultate breath sounds in children.
- Observe for use of accessory muscles, which is a sign of respiratory distress and may involve intercostal, suprasternal, supraclavicular, or sternal muscles. Head bobbing and nasal flaring are signs of significant respiratory distress in infants (Hockenberry and Wilson, 2013).

Geriatric

- Older adults have a costal angle (anteriorly) of slightly less than 90 degrees. The anteroposterior diameter may be increased from kyphosis.
- Chest expansion is reduced in older adults because of calcification of rib cartilage and partial contraction of inspiratory muscles.
- Adults older than 65 years of age should receive influenza and pneumococcal vaccines (Touhy and Jett, 2014).

SKILL 7.4   CARDIOVASCULAR ASSESSMENT

A patient who presents with signs or symptoms of cardiac problems such as chest pain may have a life-threatening condition that requires immediate attention. In this situation you must act quickly and decide on the parts of the examination that are absolutely necessary. When a patient's condition is stable, a more thorough assessment can reveal baseline heart function and any risks for heart disease. The heart, neck vessels, and peripheral circulation are assessed together because the systems work together.

Your assessment can determine the integrity of the circulatory system. Inadequate tissue perfusion results in an inadequate delivery of oxygen and nutrients to cells, a condition called *ischemia*. This condition is caused by constriction of the vessels or occlusion (blockage) from clot formation. The effects of ischemia depend on the duration of the problem and the metabolic needs of the tissues. Ischemia results in pain. If lack of oxygen to tissues is unrelieved, tissue necrosis (death) occurs. An embolus is a blood clot that breaks loose and travels through the circulation.

The nurse assesses the heart after examining the lungs because the patient is already in a suitable position with the chest exposed. Assessment then proceeds to the neck vessels and ends with the peripheral circulation. Use the skills of inspection, palpation, and auscultation during the examination.

ASSESSMENT

1. Assess patient for history of smoking, alcohol intake, caffeine intake (coffee, tea, soft drinks, energy drinks, and chocolate), use of "recreational" drugs, exercise habits, and dietary patterns and intake. *Rationale: These substances can contribute to risk factors for cardiovascular disease. In addition, caffeine and alcohol may cause tachycardia.*
2. Determine if patient is taking medications for cardiovascular function (e.g., antiarrhythmics, antihypertensives, antianginals) and if patient knows their purpose, dosage, and side effects. *Rationale: Allows you to assess patient's compliance with and understanding of drug therapies. Medications for cardiovascular function cannot be taken intermittently.*
3. Ask if patient has experienced dyspnea, chest pain or discomfort, palpitations, excess fatigue, cough, leg pain or cramps, edema of the feet, cyanosis, fainting, or orthopnea. Ask if symptoms occur at rest or during exercise. *Rationale: These are the cardinal symptoms of heart disease. Cardiovascular function may be adequate during rest but not during exercise.*
4. If patient reports chest pain, determine onset (sudden or gradual), precipitating factors, quality, region, severity, and if pain radiates. Anginal pain is usually a deep pressure

or ache that is substernal and diffuse, radiating to one or both arms, neck, or jaw. *Rationale: Symptoms may reveal acute coronary syndrome or coronary artery disease.*

5. Assess family history for heart disease, diabetes mellitus, high cholesterol or lipid levels, hypertension, stroke, or rheumatic heart disease. *Rationale: Family history of these conditions increases risk for heart and vascular disease.*

6. Ask patient about a history of heart trouble (e.g., heart failure, congenital heart disease, coronary artery disease, dysrhythmias, murmurs), heart surgery, or vascular disease (e.g., hypertension, phlebitis, varicose veins). *Rationale: Knowledge reveals patient's level of understanding of condition. A preexisting condition influences which examination techniques to use and the expected findings.*

7. If patient experiences leg pain or cramping in lower extremities, ask if it is relieved or aggravated by walking or standing for long periods or if it occurs during sleep. *Rationale: Relationship of symptoms to exercise can help determine if problem is vascular or musculoskeletal. Musculoskeletal pain usually is not relieved when exercise ends.*

▌PLANNING

Expected Outcomes focus on identifying alterations in cardiovascular function.

1. Heart is in normal sinus rhythm with rate from 60 to 100 beats/min (adolescent through adult), without extra sounds or murmurs.
2. Point of maximal impulse (PMI) is palpable at fifth ICS at left midclavicular line in children older than age 7 and in adults (Fig. 7-3). PMI is at the fourth ICS at the left midclavicular line in children younger than age 7 (Hockenberry and Wilson, 2013).
3. Patient describes changes in own behavior that may improve cardiovascular function.
4. Patient describes schedule, dosage, purpose, and benefits of medications being taken for cardiovascular function.
5. Blood pressure is within normal limits for patient (see Chapter 6).
6. Carotid pulse is localized, strong, elastic, and equal bilaterally. No change occurs during inspiration or expiration and without carotid bruit. This indicates a patent vessel.

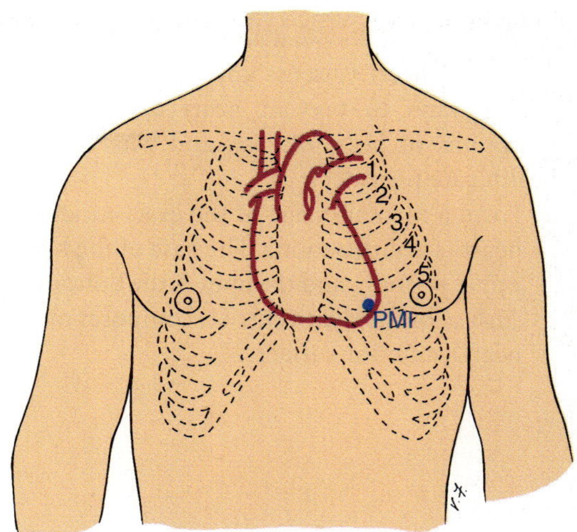

FIG 7-3 Location of point of maximal impulse (PMI) in an adult.

7. Peripheral pulses are equal and strong (2+), extremities are warm and pink with capillary refill less than 2 seconds. There is no dependent edema. Peripheral hair growth is symmetrical and evenly distributed, and the skin is free of lesions.

Delegation and Collaboration

Comprehensive cardiovascular assessment cannot be delegated to nursing assistive personnel (NAP). The nurse directs the NAP to:

- Count apical and peripheral pulses if patient is stable.
- Recognize skin temperature and color changes of affected extremities along with changes in peripheral pulses and report any changes to the nurse.

Equipment

- Stethoscope
- Doppler stethoscope (optional)
- Conducting gel (if a Doppler stethoscope is used)

▌IMPLEMENTATION *for* CARDIOVASCULAR ASSESSMENT

STEPS	RATIONALE
1. **See Standard Protocol (inside front cover).**	
2. Assist patient to be as relaxed and comfortable as possible.	An anxious or uncomfortable patient can have mild tachycardia, which alters findings.
3. Have patient assume semi-Fowler's or supine position.	Provides adequate visibility and access to left thorax and mediastinum.
4. Explain procedure. Avoid facial gestures reflecting concern.	Patient with previously normal cardiac history may become anxious if you show concern.
5. Be sure that room is quiet.	Subtle, low-pitched heart sounds are difficult to hear.

Continued

STEPS	RATIONALE

6. Assess the heart (discuss any medications patient is taking, ways to prevent heart disease, signs and symptoms of heart disease, and what to report to health care provider).

   a. Form a mental image of the exact location of the heart (see illustration). The base of the heart is the upper portion, and the apex is the bottom tip. The surface of the right ventricle composes most of the heart's anterior surface.

      Visualization improves ability to assess findings accurately and determine possible source of abnormalities.

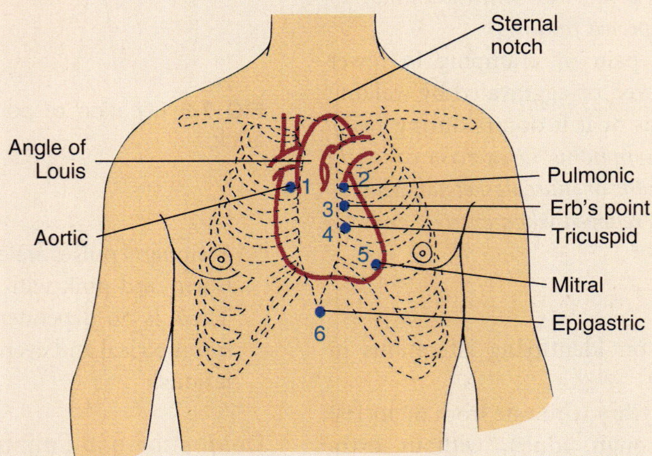

STEP 6a Anatomical sites for assessment of cardiac function.

   b. Locate the angle of Louis, felt as a ridge in the sternum approximately 5 cm (2 inches) below the suprasternal notch (between the sternal body and manubrium). Slip fingers down each side of angle to feel adjacent ribs. The ICS are just below each rib.

      Provides examiner with landmarks for locating and assessing heart sounds.

   c. Find the following anatomical landmarks (see illustration for Step 6a):

      Familiarity with landmarks allows clear description and may improve assessment.

     (1) The aortic area is at the second ICS, right of the sternum, close to the sternal border *(1)*.

      Listening to heart sounds from too far away from the sternal border decreases the ability to hear the sounds clearly.

     (2) The pulmonic area is at the second ICS, left of the sternum, close to the sternal border *(2)*.

     (3) The second pulmonic area is found by moving down the left side of sternum to the third ICS, close to the sternal border *(3)*; also referred to as Erb's point.

     (4) The tricuspid area *(4)* is located at the fourth left ICS along the sternum, close to the sternal border.

     (5) The mitral area is found by moving fingers laterally to patient's left to locate the fifth ICS at the left midclavicular line *(5)*.

     (6) The epigastric area *(6)* is at the inferior tip of the sternum.

STEPS	RATIONALE

d. Stand to patient's right to inspect and palpate the precordium with patient supine. Note any visible pulsations and more exaggerated lifts. Closely inspect at the area of the apex.

Reveals size and symmetry of the heart. The apical impulse may be visible at the midclavicular line in the fifth ICS. The apical impulse (PMI) may become visible only when the patient sits up, bringing the heart closer to the anterior wall. Obesity can easily obscure it. There should be no pulsations or vibrations.

e. Locate the PMI by palpating with fingertips along the fifth ICS in the midclavicular line. Note a light, brief pulsation in an area 1 to 2 cm ($\frac{1}{2}$ to 0.8 inch) in diameter at the apex. The PMI is less visible when there is more tissue covering the chest wall.

In the presence of serious heart disease, the PMI is located to the left of the midclavicular line related to the enlarged left ventricle. In chronic lung disease, the PMI may be to the right of the midclavicular line as a result of an enlarged right ventricle.

> **SAFE PATIENT CARE** A stronger-than-expected impulse may be a heave or lift, which may indicate increased cardiac output or left ventricular hypertrophy.

f. If palpating PMI is difficult, turn patient onto left side.

This maneuver moves the heart closer to the chest wall.

g. Inspect the epigastric area, and palpate the abdominal aorta. Note a localized strong beat.

Rules out reduced blood flow or diffuse pulse, which may indicate numerous abnormalities.

h. Auscultate heart sounds. Begin by having patient sit up and lean slightly forward (*A*); have patient lie supine (*B*); end the examination with patient in a left lateral recumbent position (*C*) (see illustrations *A*, *B*, and *C*). In a female patient it may be necessary to lift the left breast to hear heart sounds more effectively.

Different positions help to clarify type of sounds heard. Sitting position is best to hear high-pitched murmurs (if present). Supine is common position to hear all sounds. Left lateral recumbent is best position to hear low-pitched sounds. Listening through breast tissue diminishes sound and impairs assessment.

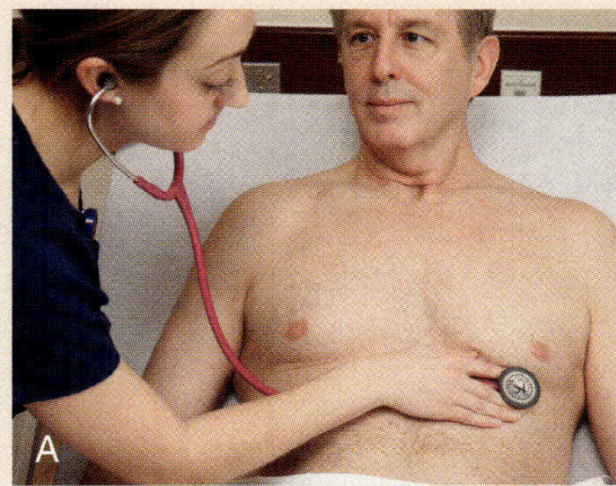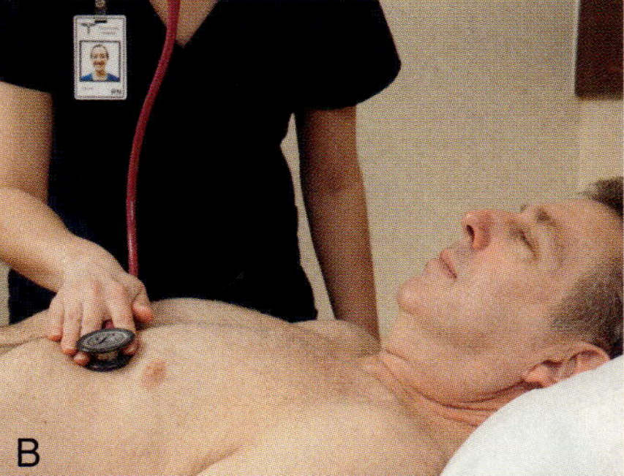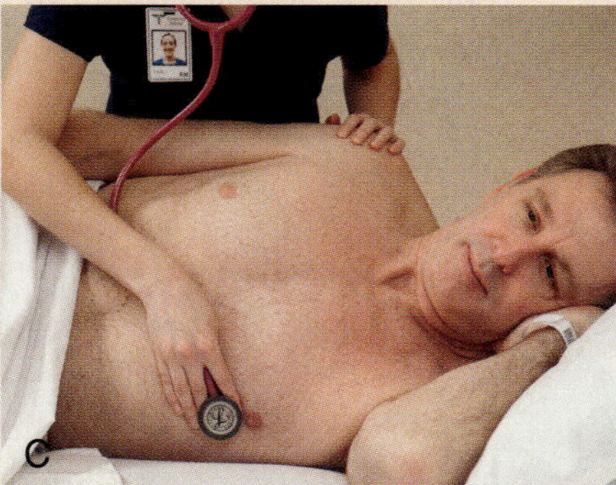

STEP 6h Patient positions for heart auscultation. **A,** Sitting. **B,** Supine. **C,** Left lateral.

(1) While auscultating sounds, ask patient not to speak but to breathe comfortably. Begin with the diaphragm of the stethoscope; then alternate with the bell. Use very light pressure for the bell. Inch the stethoscope along; avoid jumping from one area to another. Do not try to hear all heart sounds at once.

Auscultation requires the examiner to isolate each heart sound at all auscultation sites, especially in patients with soft heart sounds.

(2) Begin at the apex or PMI; move systematically to the aortic area, pulmonic area, Erb's point, tricuspid area, and mitral area (see illustration for Step 6h). (Note: Some examiners use reverse sequence.) S_1 is best heard at the apex and is simultaneous with the carotid pulse. Note: A helpful mnemonic for remembering heart sound locations: *A Pig Eats Too Much* (*A*ortic, *P*ulmonic, *E*rb's point, *T*ricuspid, *M*itral).

At normal slow rates, S_1 is high-pitched and dull in quality and sounds like "lub." This sound precedes the systolic phase of heart contraction.

Continued

STEPS	RATIONALE

(3) Listen for S_2 at each site. This sound is best heard at the aortic area. Heart sounds vary by pitch, loudness, and duration, depending on the auscultatory site.

Normal sounds S_1 and S_2 are high-pitched and best heard with a diaphragm. S_2 precedes the diastolic phase and sounds like "dub." For abnormal sounds, note physical location on chest wall and where in the cardiac cycle the sound is heard.

(4) After both sounds are heard clearly as "lub-dub," count each combination of S_1 and S_2 as one heartbeat. Count the number of beats for 1 minute.

Determines apical pulse rate.

(5) Assess heart rhythm by noting the time between S_1 and S_2 (systole) and the time between S_2 and the next S_1 (diastole). Listen to the full cycle at each auscultation area. Note regular intervals between each sequence of beats. There should be a distinct pause between S_1 and S_2.

Failure of heart to beat at regular intervals is a dysrhythmia, which interferes with the ability of the heart to pump effectively.

(6) When the heart rate is irregular, compare apical and radial pulses for a pulse deficit. Auscultate the apical pulse and then immediately palpate the radial pulse. A colleague can assess the radial pulse while you assess the apical pulse.

Determines if a pulse deficit (radial pulse is slower than apical) exists. Deficit indicates that ineffective contractions of the heart fail to send pulse waves to the periphery.

7. Assess neck vessels.

a. To assess carotid arteries, have patient remain in sitting position.

Allows easier mobility of neck to expose artery for inspection and palpation.

b. Inspect neck on both sides for obvious arterial pulsations. Ask patient to turn head slightly away from artery being examined. Sometimes pulse wave can be seen.

Carotids are the only sites to assess quality of pulse wave. Experience is required to evaluate wave in relation to events of cardiac cycle.

c. Palpate each carotid artery separately with index and middle fingers around medial edge of sternocleidomastoid muscle. Ask patient to raise chin slightly, keeping head straight (see illustration). Note rate and rhythm, strength, and elasticity of artery. Also note if the pulse changes as patient inspires and expires.

If both arteries were occluded simultaneously, patient could lose consciousness from reduced circulation to brain. Turning head improves access to artery. Change during respiratory cycle may indicate a sinus arrhythmia.

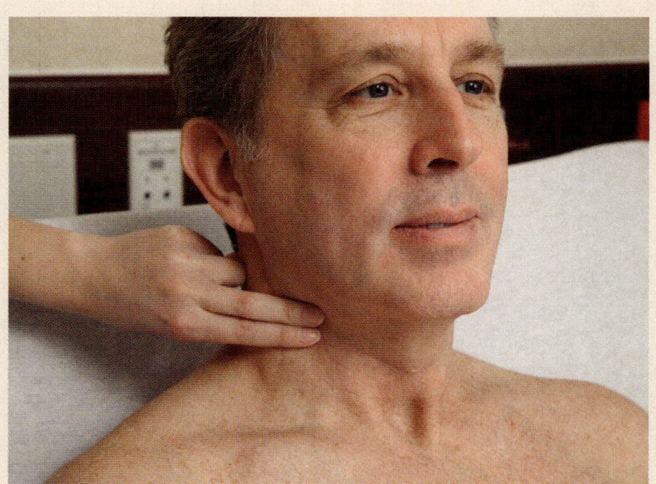

STEP 7c Palpation of internal carotid artery.

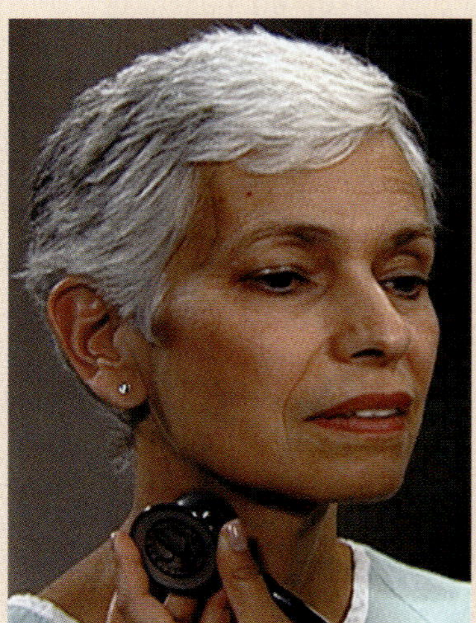

STEP 7d Auscultation for carotid artery bruit.

> **SAFE PATIENT CARE** Do not vigorously palpate or massage the artery. Stimulation of carotid sinus may cause a reflex drop in heart rate and blood pressure. Never palpate both arteries at same time.

d. Place bell of stethoscope over each carotid artery, auscultating for blowing sound (bruit) (see illustration). Ask patient to hold breath for a few heartbeats so respiratory sounds do not interfere with auscultation.

Narrowing of the lumen of the carotid artery by arteriosclerotic plaques causes disturbance in blood flow. Blood passing through narrowed section creates turbulence and emits blowing or swishing sound. Normally you do not hear a bruit.

8. Assess peripheral vascular area (discuss signs and symptoms of circulatory problems).

a. Inspect lower extremities for changes in color and condition of the skin (Table 7-6). Note skin and nail texture, hair distribution, venous patterns, edema, and scars or ulcers. Compare skin color in lying and standing positions.

Changes may reflect impaired peripheral circulation.

b. Palpate edematous areas, noting mobility, consistency, and tenderness.

Assists in determining extent of edema.

c. Assess for pitting edema by pressing area firmly for 5 seconds and then releasing. Depth of indentation determines severity (see illustration).

Unilateral edema of affected leg is the most common physical finding of deep vein thrombosis (DVT), although symptoms are similar to other conditions, making diagnosis difficult (Carter, 2010).

  2 mm: 1+ edema
  4 mm: 2+ edema
  6 mm: 3+ edema
  8 mm: 4+ edema

Measuring circumference establishes a baseline for future comparison.

Use tape measure to measure circumference of extremity.

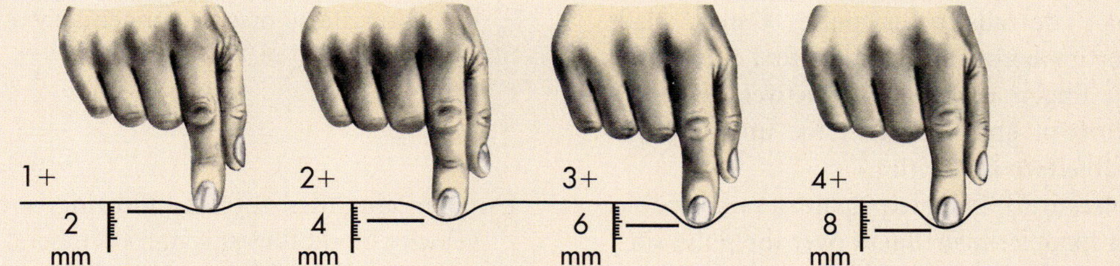

STEP 8c Assessing for pitting edema. (From Seidel HM et al: *Seidel's guide to physical examination,* ed 7, St Louis, 2015, Mosby.)

d. Check capillary refill by grasping patient's fingernail or toenail and noting color of nail bed. Next, apply gentle, firm pressure to the nail bed. Release quickly, watching for color change. Circulation is restored and pink color normally returns in less than 2 seconds.

Capillary refill is measured in seconds; less than 2 seconds is brisk, whereas greater than 4 seconds is sluggish. Cold environmental temperature with vasoconstriction and vascular disease can delay refill. Local pressure from a cast or bandage may also deter refill.

e. Ask if patient experiences pain or tenderness and then gently palpate for heat, firmness, or localized swelling of the calf muscle, which are signs of phlebitis or deep vein thrombosis (DVT).

Early recognition of DVT symptoms and complications (pulmonary embolism—new dyspnea, chest pain, and acute oxygen desaturation) can lead to better patient outcomes (Zrelak et al., 2012).

> **SAFE PATIENT CARE** Homans' sign (pain in calf on dorsiflexion of foot) is no longer a reliable indicator for the presence or absence of DVT and should not be considered a reliable test (Carter, 2010; Seidel et al., 2015). Trauma to vein or muscle, reduced mobility, and increased blood clotting are reliable risk factors. If the calf is swollen, red, or tender, notify patient's health care provider for further assessment and evaluation. If there is strong suspicion of DVT, testing for Homans' sign is contraindicated because if a clot is present, it may become dislodged from its original site. This could result in a pulmonary embolism.

Continued

f. Palpate peripheral arteries.

(1) Starting at the most distal part of each extremity, palpate each peripheral artery for equality, comparing side to side; elasticity of vessel wall (depress and release artery, noting ease with which it springs back to shape); and strength of pulse (force of blood against arterial wall) using the following rating scale (Seidel et al., 2015):

0 Absent, no pulse palpable

1+ Diminished, pulse barely palpable, weak and thready, and easy to obliterate

2+ Normal pulse, easy to palpate

3+ Full, easy to palpate, increased

4+ Strong, bounding against fingertips, and cannot be obliterated

Comparison of both arteries allows you to determine any localized obstruction or disturbance in blood flow. Pulses should be symmetrical side to side. If asymmetry is noted, look for other factors related to impaired circulation.

(2) Palpate radial pulse by lightly placing tips of first and second fingers in groove formed along radial side of forearm, lateral to flexor tendon of wrist (see illustration).

Pulse is relatively superficial and should not require deep palpation.

(3) Palpate ulnar pulse by placing fingertips along ulnar side of forearm (see illustration).

Palpated when arterial insufficiency to hand is expected or when nurse assesses for radial occlusion, which might affect circulation to hand.

(4) Palpate brachial pulse by locating groove between biceps and triceps muscles above elbow at antecubital fossa (see illustration). Place tips of first two fingers in muscle groove.

Artery runs along medial side of extended arm, requiring moderate palpation. If difficult to palpate, hyperextend arm to bring pulse site closer to the surface.

(5) Have patient lie supine with feet relaxed and palpate dorsalis pedis pulse. Gently place fingertips between great and first toe; slowly move fingers along groove between extensor tendons of great and first toe until pulse is palpable (see illustration).

Artery lies superficially and does not require deep palpation. Pulse may be congenitally absent.

(6) If pulses are difficult to palpate or not palpable, use a Doppler instrument over the pulse site.

(a) Apply conducting gel to patient's skin over the pulse site or onto transducer tip of probe.

(b) Turn Doppler on. Gently apply ultrasound probe to the skin, changing Doppler angle until pulsation is audible. Adjust volume as needed. Wipe off gel from patient and Doppler.

Doppler amplifies sounds, allowing you to hear low-velocity blood flow through peripheral arteries.

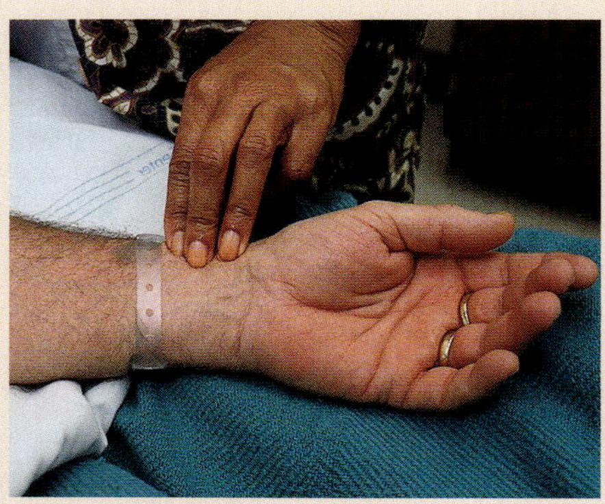

STEP 8f(2) Palpation of radial pulse.

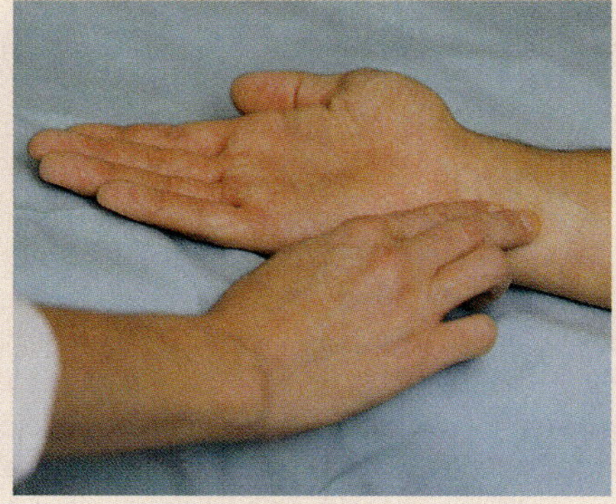

STEP 8f(3) Palpation of ulnar pulse.

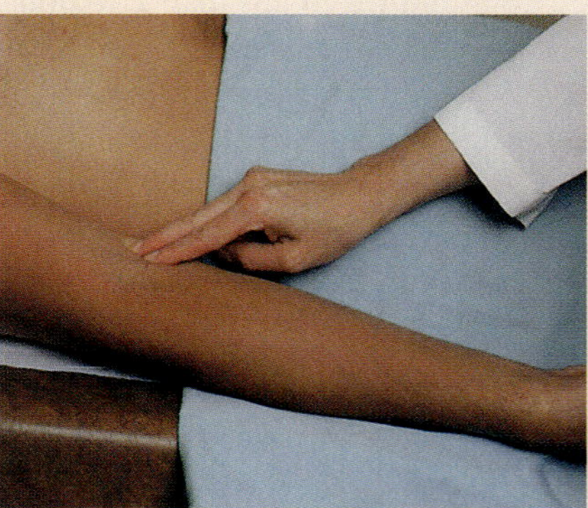

STEP 8f(4) Palpation of brachial pulse.

<table>
<tr><td>**STEPS**</td><td>**RATIONALE**</td></tr>
</table>

(7) Palpate posterior tibial pulse by having patient relax and slightly extend feet. Place fingertips behind and below medial malleolus (ankle bone) (see illustration).

Artery is easily palpable with foot relaxed.

(8) Palpate popliteal pulse by having patient slightly flex knee with foot resting on table or bed. Instruct patient to keep leg muscles relaxed. Palpate deeply into popliteal fossa with fingers of both hands placed just lateral to midline. Patient may also lie prone to achieve exposure of artery (see illustration).

Flexion of knee and muscle relaxation improve accessibility of artery. Popliteal pulse is one of the more difficult pulses to palpate.

(9) Apply clean gloves. With patient supine, palpate femoral pulse by placing first two fingers over inguinal area below inguinal ligament, midway between pubic symphysis and anterior superior iliac spine (see illustration).

Supine position prevents flexion in groin area, which interferes with artery access.

9. **See Completion Protocol (inside front cover).**

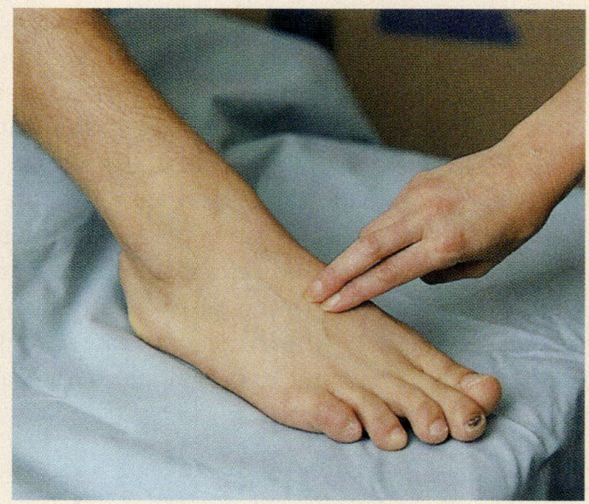

STEP 8f(5) Palpation of pedal pulse.

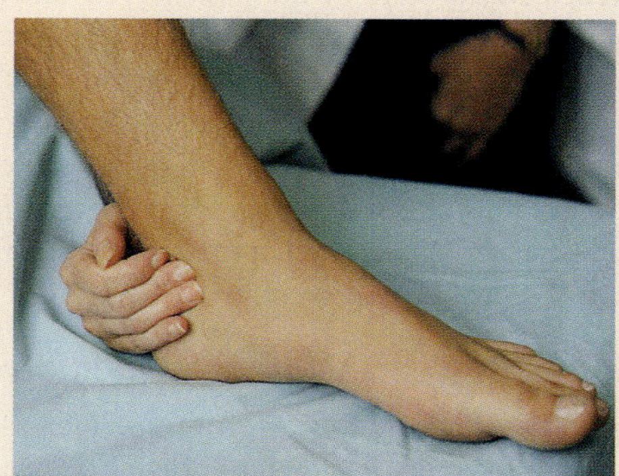

STEP 8f(7) Palpation of posterior tibial pulse.

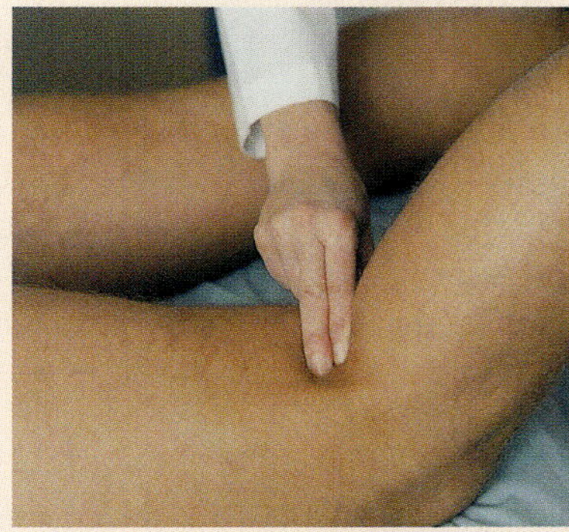

STEP 8f(8) Palpation of popliteal pulse with patient prone.

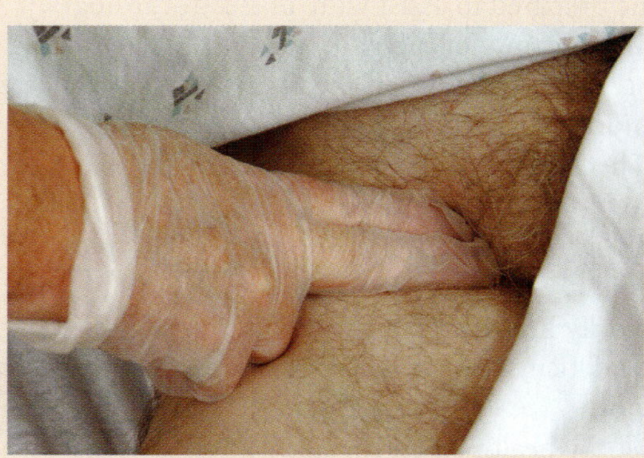

STEP 8f(9) Palpation of femoral pulse.

TABLE 7-6   SIGNS OF VENOUS AND ARTERIAL INSUFFICIENCY

ASSESSMENT CRITERION	VENOUS	ARTERIAL
Pain	Aching, increases in evening and with dependent position	Burning, throbbing, cramping, increases with exercise
Paresthesia	None	Numbness, tingling, decreased sensation
Temperature	Normal to touch	Cool to touch
Color	Normal or cyanotic	Pale; worsened by elevation of extremity; dusky red when extremity lowered
Capillary refill	Not applicable	>2 seconds
Pulse	Present	Decreased or absent
Skin changes	Brown pigmentation around ankles	Thin, shiny skin; decreased hair growth; thickened nails
Ulcerations	Shallow ulcers around ankles (chronic venous stasis); edema apparent	Deep, well defined at site of trauma or tips of toes

▌EVALUATION

1. Compare findings with normal assessment characteristics of heart and vascular system.
2. If heart sounds are not audible or pulses are not palpable, ask another nurse to confirm assessment.
3. Use *Teach Back:* State to the patient, "I want to be sure you understand the ways to improve your heart health. Can you tell me about the type of diet you should eat and what you learned about exercise?" Evaluates what the patient is able to explain or demonstrate. Revise your instruction now or develop plan for revised patient teaching to be implemented at an appropriate time if patient is not able to teach back correctly.

Unexpected Outcomes and Related Interventions

1. Abnormal findings that differ from previous assessments require you to notify health care provider. These include:
   - PMI is found left of the midclavicular line, suggesting cardiomegaly.
   - Extra heart sounds or a murmur is auscultated.
   a. Notify health care provider.
   b. Be prepared to assist with an electrocardiogram (ECG) and obtain vital signs.
2. Heart rate is irregular or the rate is less than 60 beats/min or more than 100 beats/min.
   a. Check blood pressure. If low, dysrhythmia is contributing to inadequate cardiac output.
   b. Observe for sensations or reports of dizziness or feeling "faint."
   c. Notify health care provider and prepare to order ECG.
3. Pulse deficit is noted. There is risk for inadequate cardiac output.
   a. Notify health care provider.
   b. Be prepared to assist with an ECG and obtain vital signs.
4. Previously palpable pedal pulses are diminished or absent.
   a. Notify health care provider.
   b. Elevate extremity.

Recording and Reporting

- Record quality (clear or muffled), intensity (weak or pounding), rate, and rhythm (regular, regularly irregular, or irregularly irregular) of heart sounds and peripheral pulses on nurses' notes or flow sheet. Document activity level and subjective data related to fatigue, shortness of breath, and chest pain. Document preferred position for rest, medications or treatments used, and patient's response. Record content of any patient education.
- Document your evaluation of patient learning.
- Report immediately to health care provider any irregularities in heart function and indications of impaired arterial blood flow. Report to health care provider any changes in peripheral circulation, which may indicate circulatory compromise; this can result in permanent nerve damage or tissue death if untreated.

Sample Documentation

0730   Apical pulse rate 104 and irregular. Pulse deficit 6/min. BP 110/70. Denies chest pain or other discomfort. Patient states, "I feel weak, but the pain I had last evening has not come back." Notified health care provider of pulse deficit.

Special Considerations
Pediatric

- Capillary refill in infants is usually less than 1 second.
- It is common for children to have third heart sounds (S3). Sinus arrhythmia occurs normally in many infants (Hockenberry and Wilson, 2013).
- Children have louder, higher pitched heart sounds because of thin chest walls.

Geriatric

- PMI may be difficult to find in an older adult because anteroposterior diameter of the chest deepens.
- Accidental massage of the carotid sinus during palpation of the carotid artery can be a particular problem for older adults, causing a sudden decrease in heart rate from vagal nerve stimulation.

Abdominal assessment is complex because of the multiple organs located within and near the abdominal cavity. This area of the body is associated with many health complaints, and many people are embarrassed by bowel or bladder dysfunction, reproductive problems, or urinary elimination problems. Abdominal pain is one of the most common symptoms patients report when seeking medical care. It can be caused by alterations in organs such as the stomach, pancreas, gallbladder, or intestines, or it may be the result of spinal or muscular injury. An accurate assessment requires matching a patient's history with a careful assessment of the location of physical symptoms (Table 7-7).

To perform an effective abdominal assessment, you need to know the location and function of the underlying structures involved, including the lower pelvis, kidneys, rectum, genitalia, liver, gallbladder, stomach, spleen, pancreas, intestines, and reproductive organs (Fig. 7-4). An abdominal assessment is routine after abdominal surgery and for any patient who has undergone invasive diagnostic tests of the GI tract (see Chapter 9). The order of an abdominal assessment differs from that of other assessments. You begin with inspection and follow with auscultation. It is important to auscultate before palpation because assessment maneuvers may alter the frequency and character of bowel sounds.

TABLE 7-7	COMMON CAUSES OF ABDOMINAL PAIN	
CONDITION	**PHYSICAL ALTERATION**	**PHYSICAL SIGNS AND SYMPTOMS**
Appendicitis	Obstruction of appendix associated with inflammation, perforation, and peritonitis; patient often lies on back or side with knees flexed to decrease pain	Sharp pain directly over irritated peritoneum 2-12 hours after onset. Often pain localizes in right lower quadrant between anterior iliac crest and umbilicus. Associated with rebound tenderness. Accompanied by anorexia, nausea, and vomiting.
Cholecystitis	Obstruction of the cystic duct causing inflammation or distention of gallbladder	*Murphy's sign:* Apply gentle pressure below right subcostal arch and below liver margin. Sharp pain and increased respiratory rate occur when patient takes a deep breath (Seidel et al., 2015).
Celiac disease	Damage to small intestinal mucosa from ingestion of barley, oats, rye, and wheat	Foul-smelling diarrhea, abdominal distention, and symptoms of malnutrition may be present.
Constipation	Disruption in normal bowel pattern that may occur with opioid use or inadequate fiber and fluid intake	Generalized discomfort accompanied by distention and palpation of a hard mass in left lower quadrant. Nausea and vomiting may begin after several days.
Crohn's disease	Chronic inflammatory lesion of the ileum	Steady colicky pain in right lower quadrant, with cramping, tenderness, flatulence, nausea, fever, and diarrhea. Often associated with bloody stools, weight loss, weakness, and fatigue.
Gastroenteritis	Inflammation of stomach and intestinal tract	Generalized abdominal discomfort accompanied by anorexia, nausea, vomiting, diarrhea, and abdominal cramping.
Pancreatitis	Inflammation of pancreas associated with alcoholism and gallbladder disease	Steady severe epigastric pain close to the umbilicus radiates to the back. Associated with abdominal rigidity and vomiting. Pain is unrelieved by vomiting and worsens by lying supine.
Paralytic ileus	Obstruction of small bowel that occurs after abdominal surgery or use of anticholinergic medications	Generalized severe abdominal distention, nausea, and vomiting. Decreased or absent bowel sounds.
Peptic ulcers (gastric and duodenal)	Damage of GI mucosa at any area of GI tract; may be caused by bacterial infection (*Helicobacter pylori*) or nonsteroidal antiinflammatory drugs; thought to be unrelated to stress; aggravated by smoking and excessive alcohol use	*Gastric ulcer:* Dull epigastric pain, localized midline. Early satiety; not usually relieved by food or antacids. *Duodenal ulcer:* Pain is episodic, lasting 30 minutes to 2 hours. Pain is located in midline epigastric region; described as aching, burning, or gnawing. Typically occurs 1-3 hours after meals and at night (12 midnight to 3 AM). Often relieved by food or antacid.

GI, Gastrointestinal.

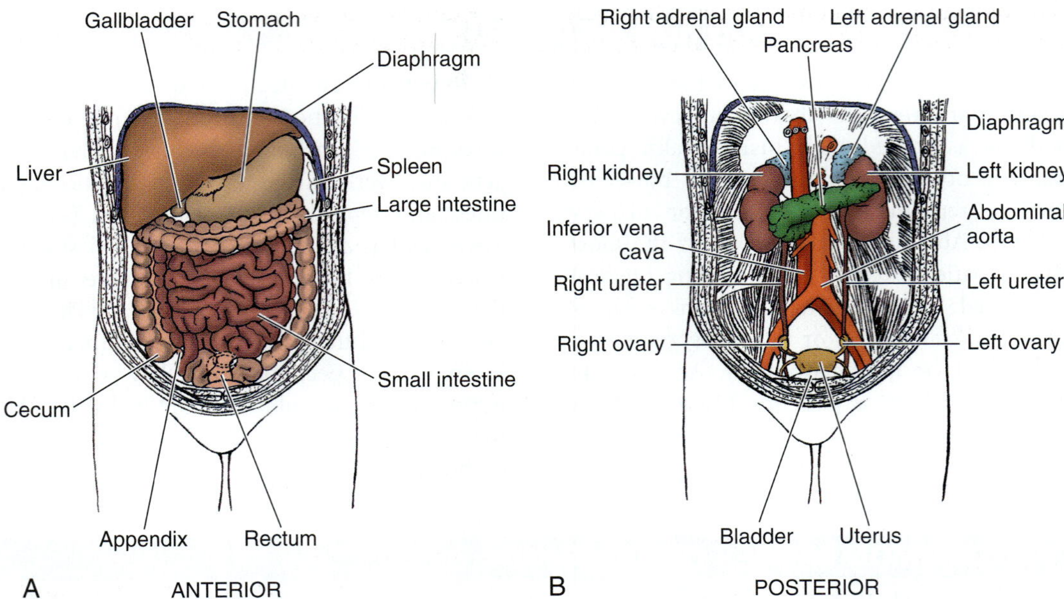

FIG 7-4 Location of organs in the abdomen. **A,** Anterior. **B,** Posterior. (Modified from *Mosby's expert 10 minute physical examinations,* ed 2, St Louis, 2005, Mosby.)

ASSESSMENT

1. If patient has abdominal or low back pain, assess the character of pain in detail (location, onset, frequency, precipitating factors, aggravating factors, type of pain, severity, course). *Rationale: Knowing the pattern of characteristics of pain helps determine its source.*

2. Carefully observe patient's movement and position, such as lying still with knees drawn up, moving restlessly to find a comfortable position, lying on one side, or sitting with knees drawn up to chest. *Rationale: Positions assumed by patient may reveal nature and source of pain (e.g., peritonitis, renal stone, pancreatitis). Patients with appendicitis often flex the trunk and draw knees up to the abdomen to reduce pain (Lewis et al., 2014).*

3. Assess patient's normal bowel habits: frequency and character of stools; recent changes in character of stools; measures used to promote elimination such as laxatives, enemas, and dietary intake; and eating and drinking habits. *Rationale: Compare data with information from physical assessment to identify cause and nature of elimination problems.*

4. Determine if patient has had abdominal surgery, trauma, or diagnostic tests of the GI tract. *Rationale: Surgery or trauma to abdomen may result in altered position of underlying organs. Diagnostic tests may change character of stool.*

5. Assess if patient has had recent weight changes or intolerance to diet (nausea, vomiting, or cramping, especially in past 24 hours). *Rationale: Changes may indicate alterations in upper GI tract (e.g., stomach, gallbladder) or lower colon.*

6. Assess for difficulty in swallowing, belching, flatulence, bloody emesis (hematemesis), black or tarry stools (melena), heartburn, diarrhea, or constipation. *Rationale: These indicate GI alterations.*

7. Determine if patient takes antiinflammatory medications (e.g., aspirin, steroids, nonsteroidal antiinflammatory drugs) or antibiotics. *Rationale: These medications may cause GI upset or bleeding.*

8. Review patient's history for health care occupation, hemodialysis, IV drug use, household or sexual contact with hepatitis B virus (HBV) carrier, sexually active heterosexual person (more than one sex partner in previous 6 months), sexually active homosexual or bisexual man, or international traveler in area of high HBV prevalence. *Rationale: These are risk factors for HBV exposure. Abdominal findings for hepatitis include jaundice, hepatomegaly, anorexia, abdominal discomfort, tea-colored urine, and clay-colored stool (Seidel et al., 2015).*

PLANNING

Expected Outcomes focus on identifying alterations in the abdomen.

1. Abdomen is soft and symmetrical with smooth and even contour. No mass, distention, or tenderness is palpable. No forceful visible pulsations are noted.

2. Bowel sounds are active and audible in all four quadrants.

3. Patient denies discomfort or worsening of existing discomfort after examination.

Delegation and Collaboration

The skill of abdominal assessment cannot be delegated to nursing assistive personnel (NAP). The nurse directs the NAP to:

- Report the development of abdominal pain and changes in the patient's bowel habits or dietary intake to the nurse.

Equipment
- Stethoscope
- Tape measure
- Examination light
- Water-based marking pen
- Drapes

IMPLEMENTATION *for* ASSESSING THE ABDOMEN

STEPS	RATIONALE
1. See Standard Protocol (inside front cover).	
2. Prepare patient.	
a. Ask if patient needs to empty bladder or defecate.	Palpation of full bladder can cause discomfort and feeling of urgency and make it difficult for patient to relax.
b. Keep upper chest and legs draped.	Exposes only areas to be examined and maintains patient comfort.
c. Be sure that room is warm.	Provides for patient comfort. Reduces risk of patient tensing muscles.
d. Have patient lie supine or in a dorsal recumbent position with arms down at sides and knees slightly bent. A small pillow may be placed under patient's knees.	Placing the arms under the head or keeping the knees fully extended can cause the abdominal muscles to tighten. Tightening of muscles prevents adequate palpation.
e. Move sheet or drape to expose area from just above the xiphoid process down to the symphysis pubis.	Exposes areas that you will examine during abdominal assessment.
f. Maintain conversation during assessment except during auscultation. Explain steps calmly and slowly.	When patient is relaxed, it improves accuracy of findings.
g. Ask patient to point to tender areas.	Assess painful areas last. Manipulation of body part can increase patient's pain and anxiety and make remainder of assessment difficult to complete.
3. Identify landmarks that divide abdominal region into quadrants. Boundary begins at tip of xiphoid process to symphysis pubis with line crossing and intersecting the umbilicus, dividing abdomen into four equal sections (see illustration).	Location of findings by common reference point helps successive examiners to confirm findings and locate abnormalities.

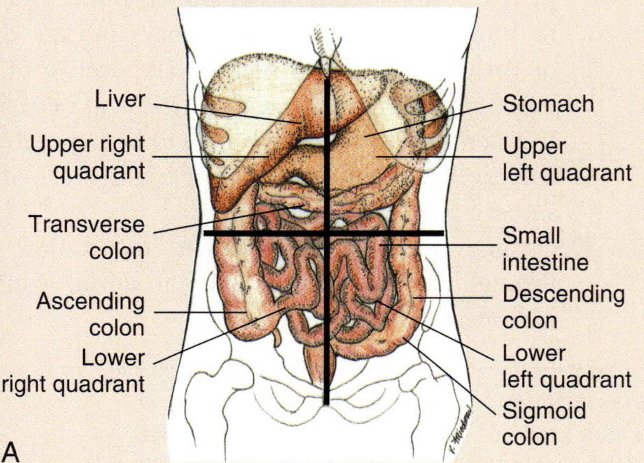

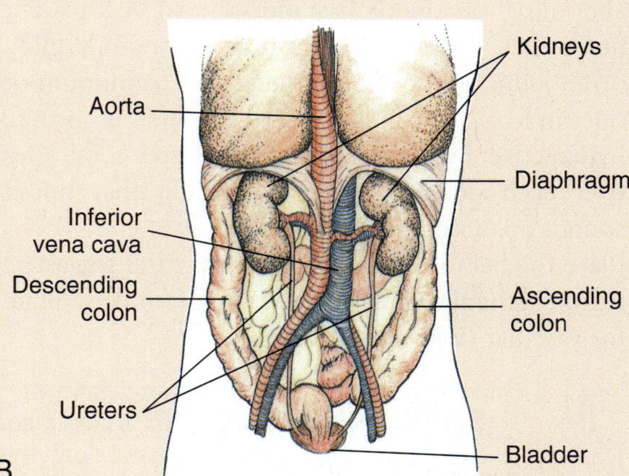

STEP 3 A, Anterior view of abdomen divided by quadrants. **B,** Posterior view of abdominal sections.

Continued

STEPS	RATIONALE

4. Inspect skin of surface of abdomen for color, scars, venous patterns, rashes, lesions, silvery white striae (stretch marks), and artificial openings (stomas). Observe lesions for characteristics described in Skill 7.1. (During exam, discuss factors to maintain normal bowel function and signs and symptoms of more common disorders.)

Scars reveal evidence that patient has past trauma or surgery. Striae indicate stretching of tissue from growth, obesity, pregnancy, ascites, or edema. Venous patterns may reflect liver disease (portal hypertension). Artificial openings indicate bowel or urinary diversion.

5. If you note bruising, ask if patient self-administers injections (e.g., heparin, insulin).

Frequent injections can cause bruising and hardening of underlying tissues.

> **SAFE PATIENT CARE** Bruising may also indicate physical abuse, accidental injury, or bleeding disorders. When bruising is noted, additional information may be needed from the patient.

6. Inspect contour, symmetry, and surface motion of abdomen. Note any masses, bulging, or distention. (Flat abdomen forms a horizontal plane from xiphoid process to symphysis pubis. Round abdomen protrudes in convex sphere from horizontal plane. Concave abdomen sinks into muscular wall. All are normal.)

Changes in symmetry or contour may reveal underlying masses, fluid collection, or gaseous distention. An everted (pouch extends outward) umbilicus indicates distention. A hernia can also cause the umbilicus to protrude upward.

7. If abdomen appears distended, note if distention is generalized. Look at flanks on each side.

Distention may be caused by the nine F's (*fat, flatus, feces, fluids, fibroid, full bladder, false pregnancy, fatal tumor,* and *fetus*) (Seidel et al., 2015). If gas causes distention, flanks do not bulge. If fluid causes distention, flanks bulge. A tumor may cause unilateral bulging or distention. Pregnancy causes symmetrical bulge in lower abdomen.

8. If you suspect distention, measure size of abdominal girth by placing tape measure around abdomen at level of umbilicus. Use marking pen to indicate where tape measure was applied.

Consecutive measurements show any increase or decrease in abdominal distention. Make all subsequent measurements at same level of umbilicus to provide objective means to evaluate changes. Use a water-based pen to make a mark on abdomen for subsequent measurements.

9. If patient has an NG or nasointestinal tube connected to suction, turn off momentarily.

Sound of suction obscures bowel sounds.

10. To auscultate bowel sounds, place the diaphragm of the stethoscope lightly over each of the four abdominal quadrants (see illustration). Ask patient not to talk. Listen until you hear repeated gurgling or bubbling sounds in each quadrant (minimum of once in 5 to 20 seconds). Describe sounds as normal, hyperactive, hypoactive, or absent. Listen 5 minutes over each quadrant before deciding that bowel sounds are absent.

Normal bowel sounds occur irregularly every 5 to 15 seconds. Absence of sounds indicates cessation of gastric motility. Hyperactive bowel sounds not related to hunger or a recent meal may indicate diarrhea or early intestinal obstruction. Hypoactive or absent bowel sounds may indicate paralytic ileus or peritonitis. It is common for bowel sounds to be hypoactive after surgery for 24 hours or more, especially after abdominal surgery.

11. Place the bell of the stethoscope over the epigastric region of the abdomen and each quadrant. Auscultate for vascular (whooshing) sounds.

Determines presence of turbulent blood flow (bruit) through thoracic or abdominal aorta, which can indicate an aneurysm.

> **SAFE PATIENT CARE** If aortic bruit is auscultated, suggesting the presence of an aneurysm, stop assessment and notify health care provider immediately. **Do not palpate or percuss this area.** Percussion or palpation over abdominal bruit can cause rupture of an already weakened vessel wall in the presence of an abdominal aneurysm.

STEPS	RATIONALE

12. Lightly palpate over each abdominal quadrant, laying the palm of the hand with fingers extended and approximated lightly on the abdomen. Keep the palm and forearm horizontal. The pads of the fingertips depress the skin no more than 1 cm (0.5 inch) in a gentle dipping motion (see illustration). Palpate painful areas last.

Detects areas of muscle spasm, localized tenderness, degree of tenderness, and presence and character of underlying masses or fluid. Palpation of sensitive area causes guarding (voluntary tightening of underlying abdominal muscles).

  a. Note muscular resistance, distention, tenderness, and superficial masses or organs while observing patient's face for signs of discomfort.

Patient's verbal and nonverbal cues may indicate discomfort from tenderness. Firm abdomen may indicate active obstruction with fluid or gas building up.

  b. Note if abdomen is firm or soft to touch.

Soft abdomen is normal or reveals that obstruction is resolving.

13. Just below umbilicus and above symphysis pubis, palpate for a smooth, rounded mass. While applying light pressure, ask if patient has sensation of need to void.

Detects presence of dome of distended bladder.

> **SAFE PATIENT CARE** Routinely check for distended bladder if patient has been unable to void, has been incontinent, if an indwelling Foley catheter is not draining well, or if patient recently had a Foley catheter removed.

14. If masses are palpated, note size, location, shape, consistency, tenderness, mobility, and texture.

Descriptive characteristics help to reveal type of mass.

15. When tenderness is present, test for rebound tenderness by pressing slowly and deeply into the involved area and then letting go quickly. Note if pain is aggravated.

Results are positive if pain increases. May indicate peritoneal irritation such as appendicitis (Seidel et al., 2015).

16. **See Completion Protocol (inside front cover).**

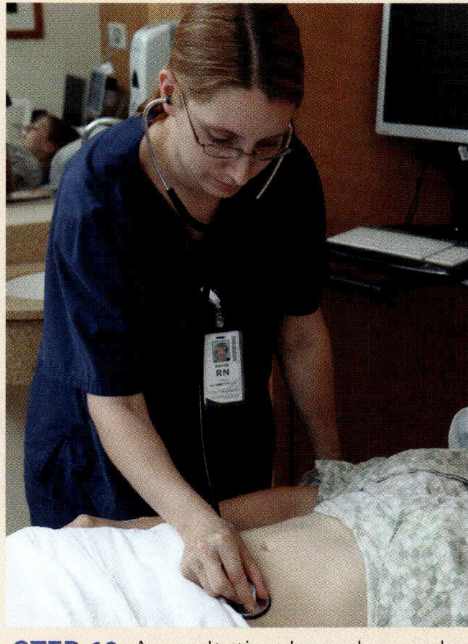

STEP 10 Auscultating bowel sounds.

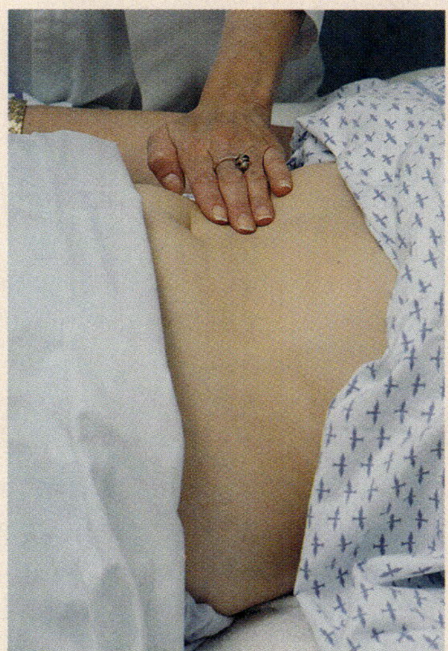

STEP 12 Light palpation of the abdomen.

EVALUATION

1. Observe throughout the assessment for evidence of discomfort.
2. Compare assessment findings with previous assessment to identify changes.
3. Use *Teach Back:* State to the patient, "We discussed ways to maintain good bowel function. Can you tell me the types of food and fluids to eat and drink?" Evaluates what the patient is able to explain or demonstrate. Revise your instruction now or develop plan for revised patient teaching to be implemented at an appropriate time if patient is not able to teach back correctly

Unexpected Outcomes and Related Interventions

1. Abdomen is asymmetrical, with palpable mass and hypoactive bowel sounds.
   a. Report to health care provider
2. Abdomen protrudes symmetrically, with skin taut; patient complains of tightness, or bowel sounds are absent. GI motility has ceased. Patient is vomiting.
   a. Place or keep patient on "nothing by mouth" (NPO) status and encourage ambulation.
   b. Notify health care provider; findings may indicate an obstruction.
   c. Gastric decompression with insertion of NG tube may become necessary.
3. Hyperactive bowel sounds are evident with GI motility, indicating possible anxiety, diarrhea, overuse of laxatives, inflammation of the bowel, or reaction of the intestines to certain foods.
   a. Patient may need to be NPO.
   b. Contact health care provider if patient may need antidiarrheal medications.
4. Rebound abdominal tenderness is found.
   a. Avoid palpating area.
   b. Notify health care provider if this is a new finding.
   c. Keep patient on NPO status until health care provider can evaluate.
5. Bladder is palpable over symphysis pubis. Bladder is distended.
   a. Facilitate voiding by placing patient in sitting position or encouraging patient to bear down; run water within hearing distance or have patient place hand in basin of warm water. Assist male patient to stand to void.
   b. Use a bladder scan to determine extent of bladder fullness.

Recording and Reporting

- Document quality of bowel sounds, presence of distention, abdominal circumference, and presence of tenderness on nurses' notes or flow sheet. Record patient's ability to void and defecate, including description of output. Record content of any patient education.
- Document your evaluation of patient learning.
- Report serious abnormalities such as absent bowel sounds or presence of mass or acute pain to nurse in charge and health care provider.

Sample Documentation

0800 Abdomen is distended, no masses palpated. No passage of flatus since surgery, and bowel sounds are hypoactive over all four quadrants. Encouraged to sip on warm fluids and ambulate frequently. Denies nausea, vomiting, or pain at this time.

Special Considerations
Pediatric

- Most common palpable mass in child is feces, usually felt in right lower quadrant (Hockenberry and Wilson, 2013).
- Have child stand erect and then lie supine during inspection of abdomen. Normal abdomen of infants and young children is cylindrical in erect position and flat in supine position. School-age children may have a rounded abdomen until 13 years of age when standing.
- Infants and children until 7 years of age are abdominal breathers.

Geriatric

- Older adults often lack abdominal tone; underlying organs are more easily palpable.
- A weakened intestinal musculature and decreased peristalsis affect the large intestine.
- Constipation, nausea, flatulence, and heartburn are common.
- Older adults may have increased fat deposits over the abdomen.

SKILL 7.6 ASSESSING THE GENITALIA AND RECTUM

You can perform an external genitalia examination during routine hygiene measures or when preparing to insert or care for a urinary catheter. An examination of female and male external genitalia is part of preventive health screenings. You examine adolescents and young adults because of the growing incidence of sexually transmitted infections (STIs). The average age of menarche among females has declined, and the average age that both males and females become sexually active is 19 (CDC, 2014). You can easily combine rectal and anal assessments with this examination because the patient assumes a lithotomy or dorsal recumbent position.

ASSESSMENT

1. Assessment of female patients:
   a. Determine if patient has signs and symptoms of vaginal discharge, painful or swollen perianal tissues, or genital

lesions. *Rationale: These signs and symptoms indicate the presence of an STI or other pathological condition.*

b. Determine if patient has symptoms or history of genitourinary problems, including burning on urination (dysuria), frequency, urgency, nocturia, hematuria, or incontinence. *Rationale: Urinary problems are associated with gynecological disorders, including STIs.*

c. Ask if the patient has had signs of bleeding outside of normal menstrual cycle or after menopause or has had unusual vaginal discharge. *Rationale: These are warning signs of cervical or endometrial cancer or a vaginal infection.*

d. Determine if patient has received human papillomavirus (HPV) vaccine. *Rationale: The CDC (2014) recommends routine HPV (Gardasil or Cervarix) for preteen girls and boys 11 to 12 years old. In addition, girls and women age 13 through 26 and males age 13 through 21 should get HPV vaccine if they have not received any or all doses when they were younger. All men should confer with their health care provider before receiving the vaccine (CDC, 2014).*

e. Determine if patient has history of HPV (condyloma acuminatum, herpes simplex, or cervical dysplasia); multiple sexual partners; smokes cigarettes; or has had multiple pregnancies. *Rationale: These are risk factors for cervical cancer (ACS, 2013d, 2014d; CDC, 2014).*

f. Determine if patient is older than 63 years of age; is obese; has a history of ovarian dysfunction, breast or endometrial cancer, or endometriosis; has a family history of reproductive cancer; has a history of infertility, nulliparity, or use of estrogen (alone) hormone replacement therapy. *Rationale: These are risk factors for ovarian cancer (ACS, 2014c).*

g. Determine if patient is postmenopausal, obese, or infertile; had early menarche or late menopause; has a history of hypertension, diabetes mellitus, gallbladder disease, or polycystic ovary disease; has a family history of estrogen-related exposure (estrogen replacement therapy, Tamoxifen use). *Rationale: These are risk factors for endometrial cancer (ACS, 2014c)*

h. Determine patient's knowledge of risk factors and signs of cervical and other gynecological cancers. *Rationale: Provides basis for patient education.*

2. Assessment of male patients:

a. Review normal elimination pattern, including frequency of voiding; history of nocturia; character and volume of urine; daily fluid intake; symptoms of burning, urgency, and frequency; difficulty starting stream; and hematuria. *Rationale: Urinary problems are directly associated with genitourinary problems because of anatomical structures of the male reproductive and urinary systems.*

b. Ask if patient has noted any penile pain or swelling, genital lesions, or urethral discharge. *Rationale: These are signs and symptoms of STIs.*

c. Determine if patient has noted any heaviness, painless enlargement, or irregular lumps of testis. *Rationale: These signs and symptoms are early warning signs of testicular cancer.*

d. Determine if patient reports any enlargement in inguinal area, and assess if it is intermittent or constant, associated with straining or lifting, and painful. Assess whether coughing, lifting, or straining at stool causes pain. *Rationale: Signs and symptoms indicate potential inguinal hernia.*

e. Ask if patient has experienced weak or interrupted urine flow, inability to urinate, difficulty in starting or stopping urine flow, polyuria, nocturia, dysuria, or hematuria. Determine if patient has continuing pain in lower back, pelvis, or upper thighs. *Rationale: These are warning signs of prostate cancer (ACS, 2013b). Symptoms also may indicate infection or prostate enlargement.*

f. Assess patient's knowledge of risk factors and signs of prostate and testicular cancer. *Rationale: Provides basis for patient education.*

3. Assessment of all patients:

a. Determine whether patient has experienced bleeding from rectum, black or tarry stools (melena), rectal pain, or change in bowel habits (constipation or diarrhea). *Rationale: These are warning signs of colorectal cancer (ACS, 2014b).*

b. Determine whether patient is over 50 years of age or has a personal or family history of colorectal cancer, polyps, or chronic inflammatory bowel disease. *Rationale: These are risk factors for colorectal cancer (ACS, 2014b).*

c. Determine if patient is obese, physically inactive, smokes cigarettes, or consumes alcohol. *Rationale: These are risk factors for colorectal cancer (ACS, 2014b).*

d. Assess medication history for use of laxatives or cathartics. *Rationale: Repeated use causes diarrhea and eventual loss of intestinal muscle tone.*

e. Assess for use of codeine or iron preparations. *Rationale: Codeine causes constipation. Iron turns stool black and tarry.*

f. Assess patient's knowledge of risks and signs of colorectal cancer. *Rationale: Provides basis for patient education.*

PLANNING

Expected Outcomes focus on accurate genitalia and rectal assessment data.

1. Patient demonstrates alert, cooperative behaviors without evidence of physical or emotional distress during assessment.

2. Patient is able to list warning signs of colorectal cancer; cervical, endometrial, and ovarian cancer (female patient); or testicular and prostate cancer (male patient).

Delegation and Collaboration

The skill of assessing the genitalia and rectum cannot be delegated to nursing assistive personnel (NAP). The nurse directs the NAP to:

- Report changes in patient's urinary or bowel pattern and presence of drainage in perineal area.

Equipment

- Stethoscope
- Examination light
- Clean gloves
- Linen or drapes

IMPLEMENTATION *for* ASSESSING THE GENITALIA AND RECTUM

STEPS	RATIONALE
1. See Standard Protocol (inside front cover).	
2. Prepare patient for assessment:	
a. Ask if patient needs to empty bladder or defecate.	Palpation of full bladder causes discomfort and feeling of urgency and makes it difficult for patient to relax.
b. Keep upper chest and legs draped and keep room warm.	Maintains patient's comfort.
c. Position patient: Female should lie in a dorsal recumbent position with arms down at sides and knees slightly bent. Place a small pillow under patient's knees. Male should lie supine with chest, abdomen, and lower legs draped *or* have patient stand during examination.	Placing the arms under the head or keeping knees fully extended causes tightening of abdominal muscles.
3. Apply clean gloves.	
4. *Female genitalia examination.* (Use time to discuss woman's risks for STIs and signs and symptoms of cervical, ovarian, and endometrial cancer).	
a. Reposition sheet to expose only perineal area	
b. Inspect surface characteristics of perineum and then retract labia majora; observe for inflammation, edema, lesions, or lacerations. Note if there is any vaginal discharge. Presence of discharge may indicate need for a culture.	Skin of perineum is smooth, clean, and slightly darker than other skin. Mucous membranes are dark pink and moist. Labia majora are symmetrical; may be dry or moist. Normally there is no vaginal discharge.
5. *Male genitalia examination.* (Use time to discuss man's risks for STIs and signs and symptoms of testicular cancer).	
a. Reposition sheet to expose only perineal area and observe genitalia for rashes, excoriations, or lesions.	Normally the skin is clear and without lesions.
b. Inspect and gently palpate penile surfaces.	
(1) Inspect the corona, prepuce (foreskin), glans, urethral meatus, and shaft. Retract the foreskin in uncircumcised males. Observe for discharge, lesions, edema, and inflammation. Return foreskin to normal position.	Glans should be smooth and pink along all surfaces. Urethral meatus is slitlike and positioned at the tip of the glans. The foreskin should retract easily. The area between the foreskin and glans is a common site for venereal lesions.
c. Inspect and palpate testicular surfaces.	
(1) Inspect size, color, shape, and symmetry; also gently palpate for lesions and edema.	The left testicle normally is lower than the right. Scrotal skin is usually loose, surface is coarse, and skin color is more deeply pigmented than body skin.
d. Palpate the testes.	
(1) Note size, shape, and consistency of tissue.	Testes are normally ovoid and approximately 2 cm × 4 cm (0.8 inches × 1.6 inches) in size, feel smooth and rubbery, and are free from nodules. Most common symptom of testicular cancer is an irregular, nontender, fixed mass.
(2) Ask if patient experiences tenderness with palpation.	Testes are normally sensitive but not tender.

STEPS	RATIONALE

6. Apply clean gloves. Assess rectum. (Use time to discuss signs and symptoms of colorectal cancer.)

a. Female patient remains in dorsal recumbent position or assumes a side-lying (Sims') position.

This position allows for optimal visualization of the rectum.

b. Male patient stands and bends forward with hips flexed and upper body resting across examination table; examine nonambulatory patient in Sims' position.

c. View the perianal and sacrococcygeal areas by gently retracting the buttocks using your nondominant hand.

Perianal skin is smooth, more pigmented, and coarser than skin covering the buttocks.

d. Inspect anal tissue for skin characteristics, lesions, external hemorrhoids (dilated veins that appear as reddened skin protrusions), ulcers, inflammation, rashes, and excoriation.

Anal tissues are moist and hairless; the voluntary sphincter holds the anus closed.

7. See Completion Protocol (inside front cover).

EVALUATION

1. Observe for evidence of physical or emotional distress, which may alter assessment data.
2. Compare assessment findings with previous assessment characteristics to identify changes.
3. Use *Teach Back:* State to the patient, "We discussed the signs and symptoms of genital cancer. This is important because of your risks. Tell me some of the signs to look for." Evaluates what the patient is able to explain or demonstrate. Revise your instruction now or develop plan for revised patient teaching to be implemented at an appropriate time if patient is not able to teach back correctly.

Unexpected Outcomes and Related Interventions

1. Patient is unable to list warning signs of colorectal cancer; cervical, endometrial, and ovarian cancer (female patient); or testicular and prostate cancer (male patient).
   a. Provide additional education.

Recording and Reporting

- Record results of assessment in nurses' notes or flow sheet. Record instruction and patient response. Record any abnormalities such as presence of a mass, drainage, or pain to nurse in charge and health care provider.
- Document your evaluation of patient learning.

Sample Documentation

0830   Patient reports "pain in groin when straining to move bowels." No swelling or inflammation noted in inguinal area on palpation. Patient able to lift groceries and granddaughter and cough with no pain. Health care provider notified.

Special Considerations

Pediatric

- Examination of the genitalia may cause anxiety in children. The best approach is to treat this examination the same as all other parts of the health assessment.
- In male infants, when examining the testes, avoid stimulating the cremasteric reflex, which causes the testes to pull higher into pelvic cavity.

Geriatric

- A weakened intestinal musculature and decreased peristalsis affect the large intestine.
- Adequate hydration (2000 to 3000 mL daily unless contraindicated) is the key to preventing constipation (Touhy and Jett, 2014).

Home Care

- General patient education should focus on the warning signs of colorectal cancer.
- Teach warning signs of STIs, the importance of self-examination for cancer, and the benefit of HPV vaccination in children and young women.

SKILL 7.7   MUSCULOSKELETAL AND NEUROLOGICAL ASSESSMENT

During the general survey (see Skill 7.1), you inspect a patient's gait, posture, and body position. A more thorough assessment of major bone, joint, and muscle groups and sensory, motor, and cranial nerve (CN) function is indicated in the presence of abnormalities. Use the skills of inspection and palpation during the musculoskeletal and neurological assessment. The assessment can be performed as you examine other body systems. For example, while assessing head and neck structures, assess neck ROM and examine selected CNs. Integrate assessment into routine activities of care (e.g., while bathing or positioning the patient). Always assess a patient who reports pain, loss of sensation, or impairment of muscle function. Prolonged illness or immobility may result in muscle weakness and atrophy. Neurological assessment is often conducted simultaneously because muscles may be weakened as a result of nerve involvement.

ASSESSMENT

1. Review patient history for use of alcohol or caffeine; cigarette smoking; constant dieting; calcium intake less than 500 mg daily; thin and light body frame; nulliparity (never been pregnant) in females; menopause before age 45; postmenopausal status; family history of osteoporosis; white, Asian, American Indian, or northern European ancestry; sedentary lifestyle; long-term use of certain medications (e.g., corticosteroids, heparin, phenytoin [Dilantin]); and lack of exposure to sunlight. *Rationale: These factors increase the risk for osteoporosis.*

2. Determine if patient has been screened for osteoporosis. *Rationale: Women 64 years old and older or with one or more risk factors need routine screening for osteoporosis (Touhy and Jett, 2014).*

3. Ask patient to describe history of alteration in bone, muscle, or joint function (e.g., recent fall, trauma, lifting heavy objects, bone or joint disease with sudden or gradual onset) and location of alteration. *Rationale: Assists in assessing nature of musculoskeletal problem. One in two women and one in four men 50 years old and older have an osteoporotic-related fracture (Touhy and Jett, 2014).*

4. Assess nature and extent of patient's musculoskeletal pain: location, duration, severity, predisposing and aggravating factors, relieving factors, and type of pain. If pain or cramping is reported in the lower extremities, ask if walking relieves or aggravates pain. Assess the distance walked and characteristics of pain before, during, and after activity. *Rationale: Pain frequently accompanies alterations in bone, joints, or muscle. Pain has implications for comfort and ability to perform activities of daily living. Pain caused by certain vascular conditions tends to increase with activity.*

5. Assess for height and weight (see Skill 7-1). Note if there is a decrease in height in a woman older than 50 by subtracting current height from recall of maximum adult height. *Rationale: BMI less than 22 is a risk factor, and a loss of height of more than 3 cm (1.2 inches) is one of the first clinical signs of osteoporosis (Touhy and Jett, 2014).*

6. Determine if patient uses analgesics, antipsychotics, antidepressants, nervous system stimulants, or recreational drugs. *Rationale: These medications alter LOC or cause behavioral changes.*

7. Determine if patient has recent history of seizures or convulsions: clarify sequence of events (aura, loss of muscle tone, falling, motor activity, loss of consciousness); character of any symptoms; and relationship to time of day, fatigue, or emotional stress. *Rationale: Seizure activity often originates from central nervous system (CNS) alteration. Characteristics of seizure help determine its origin.*

8. Screen patient for headache, tremors, dizziness, numbness, or tingling of body part; visual changes; weakness; pain; or changes in speech. *Rationale: These symptoms commonly result from CNS dysfunction. Identifying patterns may assist in diagnosis.*

9. Discuss with spouse, family member, or friends any recent changes in patient's behavior (e.g., increased irritability, mood swings, memory loss, change in energy level). *Rationale: Behavioral changes may result from intracranial pathology.*

10. Determine if patient notices any change in vision (cranial nerve I), hearing (cranial nerve VIII), smell (cranial nerve I), taste (cranial nerve VII), or touch. *Rationale: Major sensory nerves originate in the brainstem. Changes in sensory perception may help locate the nature of a problem.*

11. If patient displays sudden acute confusion (delirium), review history for drug toxicity (e.g., anticholinergics, digoxin, antihistamines, opioid analgesics); infections, fever, metabolic disturbances (low glucose); heart failure; and severe anemia. *Rationale: Delirium is a common mental disorder in older adults. It often results from a variety of causes (Touhy and Jett, 2014).*

12. Review history for frequent head injury, frequency of injury in contact sports, meningitis, and psychiatric illnesses. *Rationale: Neurological and behavioral symptoms may result from head injuries sustained in accidents or contact sports or may be the result of severe neurological infections; psychiatric illnesses may also be the cause of behavioral changes.*

PLANNING

Expected Outcomes focus on identifying deficits in musculoskeletal and neurological function.

1. Patient demonstrates strong grasp and steady gait with arms swinging freely at side.

2. There is bilateral symmetry of extremities in length, circumference, alignment, position, and skin folds.

3. Full active ROM is present in all joints with good muscle tone and absence of contractures, spasticity, or muscular weakness.

4. Patient is alert and oriented to person, place, and time. Behavior and appearance are appropriate for condition or situation.

5. Patient demonstrates normal pupil reaction to light and accommodation (see Skill 7.2); external ocular muscles intact; facial sensation intact; symmetrical facial expressions; soft palate and uvula midline and rise on phonation; gag reflex intact; speech clear without hoarseness; no difficulty swallowing.

6. Patient distinguishes between sharp and dull sensations and light touch on symmetrical areas of extremities.

7. Gait is coordinated and steady. Romberg test is negative.

Delegation and Collaboration

The skill of assessing musculoskeletal and neurological function cannot be delegated to nursing assistive personnel (NAP). The nurse directs the NAP to:

- Report patient problems with gait, ROM, and muscle strength.
- Take precautions during ROM exercises to avoid forcing a joint beyond patient's current ROM.
- Be informed of patients at risk for falls (unsteady gait, foot dragging, weakness of lower extremities).
- Assist patients with muscular weakness with transfer and ambulation.

Equipment

- Cotton balls or cotton-tipped applicators
- Penlight
- Opposite tip of cotton swab or tongue blade broken in half
- Tongue blade
- Watch with second hand or digital display

IMPLEMENTATION *for* MUSCULOSKELETAL AND NEUROLOGICAL ASSESSMENT

STEPS	RATIONALE
1. See Standard Protocol (inside front cover).	
2. Prepare patient:	
a. Integrate musculoskeletal and neurological assessment during other portions of physical assessment or during care. (Discuss any risks patient may have for falls or other injuries from changes in mobility/sensation).	You can conduct an assessment as the patient moves in bed, rises from chair, walks, or goes through movements required during complete physical exam. Integration with care conserves patient's energy and allows observation of patient performing activities more naturally.
b. Plan time for short rest periods during assessment.	Movement of body parts and various maneuvers may fatigue patient. Always plan rest periods with older adults and very ill patients.
3. Assess musculoskeletal system.	
a. Observe ability to use arms and hands for grasping objects (e.g., utensils, pen).	Assesses fine motor coordination and muscle strength.
b. To assess hand grasp strength, cross your hands and have patient grasp index and middle fingers of both of your hands and squeeze them simultaneously as hard as possible.	It is common for patient's dominant hand to be slightly stronger than nondominant hand. By crossing your hands, patient's right hand grasps your right hand and vice versa. This helps you recall which is patient's right or left hand.
c. Assess muscle strength by having patient assume a stable position. Then have patient demonstrate strength of each major muscle group (e.g., flexion and extension of arm, flexion and extension of lower leg [while sitting]). Have patient first flex the muscle against resistance when you apply opposing force against flexion. Have patient maintain resistance until told to stop. Compare symmetrical muscle groups. Note weakness, and compare right with left.	Compares strength of symmetrical muscle groups. Rate muscle strength on scale of 0 to 5. Grade as follows: **0** No voluntary contraction **1** Trace of movement **2** Full ROM, passive **3** Full ROM against gravity but not against resistance **4** Full ROM against gravity, some against resistance but weak **5** Full ROM against gravity and full resistance
d. Observe body alignment for sitting, supine, prone, or standing positions. Muscles and joints should be exposed and free to move to allow for accurate measurement.	Each joint or muscle group may require a different position for measurement.
e. Inspect gait as patient walks. Have patient use assistive device (cane, walker) if appropriate. Observe for foot dragging, shuffling or limping, balance, presence of obvious deformity in lower extremities, and position of trunk in relation to legs.	Gait is more natural if patient is unaware of your observation. Observations may indicate a neuromusculoskeletal disorder.

Continued

STEPS	RATIONALE

f. Perform the get-up-and-go test: Have adult wear regular footwear, sit back in comfortable chair, and use normal assist device (if needed). Have a watch with second hand. On the word "GO" have the patient: Stand from a sitting position without using chair arms for support; stand still momentarily; walk 10 feet (3 meters) in a line; turn around, return to chair; and sit back in chair without using arms for support. Observe gait and ability to sit or stand.

The get-up-and-go test is an assessment that should be conducted as part of a routine evaluation of older adults. The test helps to detect people at risk for falling. Normally a person completes the task in less than 10 seconds; over 20 seconds is abnormal.

g. Observe the extremities for overall size, gross deformity, bony enlargement, alignment, and symmetry.

General review helps to pinpoint areas requiring in-depth assessment.

h. Gently palpate bones, joints, and surrounding tissue in involved areas. Note any heat, tenderness, redness, edema, or resistance to pressure.

Reveals changes resulting from trauma, chronic disease, or acute or chronic inflammation (e.g., arthritis). Do not try to move joint when fracture is suspected or when joint apparently is "frozen" by lack of movement over a long period.

i. Ask patient to put major joint through its full ROM (Table 7-8). Observe equality of motion in same body parts:

Assessment of patient's normal ROM provides baseline for assessing later changes after surgery or inactivity. Patients with deformities, reduced mobility, joint fixation, or weakness often require passive ROM assessment.

(1) *Active motion* (patient needs no support or assistance and is able to move joint independently): Instruct patient in moving each joint through its normal range. Sometimes it is necessary to demonstrate movements and ask patient to mimic your movements.

Identifies muscle strength and detects limited ROM.

(2) *Passive motion* (joint has full ROM, but patient does not have the strength to move it independently): Have patient relax and move the same joints passively until the end of the range is felt. Support extremity at joint. Do not force the joint if there is pain or muscle spasm.

Determines ability to perform joint motion in the presence of muscle weakness. Forcing joint causes pain and injury.

j. Assess muscle tone in major muscle groups. Normal tone causes mild, even resistance to movement through entire ROM.

If muscle has increased tone (hypertonicity), any sudden movement of joint is met with considerable resistance. Hypotonic muscle moves without resistance. Muscle feels flabby.

4. Neurological assessment:

a. Assess LOC and orientation: ask patient to identify name, location, day of week, and year; note behavior and appearance. This can be performed during general survey.

A fully conscious patient responds to questions spontaneously. As consciousness declines, patient may show irritability, short attention span, or unwillingness to cooperate. As consciousness continues to deteriorate, patient becomes disoriented to name, time, and place. Behavior and appearance reveal information about patient's mental status.

b. Assess cranial nerves (CNs). **Note:** See Assessment, Step 10.

(1) For CN III (oculomotor), IV (trochlear), and VI (abducens), assess extraocular movement. Ask patient to follow movement of your finger through the six cardinal positions of gaze; measure pupillary reaction to light and accommodation (CN III) (see Skill 7.2).

These CNs are most likely affected by increased intracranial pressure, which causes changes in response or size of pupil; pupils may change shape (more oval) or react sluggishly. Intracranial pressure impairs movement of external ocular muscles. Accommodation is ability of the eye to adjust vision from near to far.

STEPS	RATIONALE
(2) For CN V (trigeminal), apply light sensation with a cotton ball to symmetrical areas of face.	Sensations should be symmetrical; unilateral decrease or loss of sensation may be caused by CN V lesion.
(3) For CN VII (facial), note facial symmetry. Have patient frown, smile, puff out cheeks, and raise eyebrows.	Expressions should be symmetrical; Bell's palsy causes drooping of upper and lower face; cerebrovascular accident causes asymmetry.
(4) For CN IX (glossopharyngeal) and CN X (vagus), have patient speak and swallow. Ask patient to say "ah" while using tongue blade and penlight. Check for midline uvula and symmetrical rise of uvula and soft palate. Use tongue blade and place on posterior tongue to elicit gag reflex.	Damage to CN IX causes impaired swallowing, loss of gag reflex, hoarseness, and nasal voice. When palate fails to rise and uvula pulls toward normal side, this indicates a unilateral paralysis.
c. Assess extremities for sensation. Perform all sensory testing with patient's eyes closed so patient is unable to see when or where a stimulus strikes the skin.	
(1) *Pain:* Ask patient to indicate when sharp or dull sensation is felt as you alternately apply sharp and blunt ends of tongue blade to skin surface. Apply in symmetrical areas of extremities.	Patient should be able to distinguish sharp or dull sensations. Impaired sensations may indicate disorders of the spinal cord or peripheral nerve roots.
(2) *Light touch:* Apply light wisp of cotton to different points along surface of skin in symmetrical areas of extremities.	Patient should be able to distinguish when touched.
d. Assess motor and cerebellar function:	
(1) *Gait:* Have patient walk across room, turn, and come back. If an assistive device is present, this is a good time to instruct patient on proper use of the device.	Neurological and musculoskeletal disorders may impair gait and balance.
(2) *Romberg's test:* Have patient stand with feet together, arm at sides, both eyes open and closed (for 20 to 30 seconds). Protect patient's safety by standing at side; observe for swaying.	Romberg's test should be negative; slight swaying is considered normal.
5. **See Completion Protocol (inside front cover).**	

EVALUATION

1. Compare gait, muscle condition, strength and tone, and ROM with previous physical assessment.
2. Compare neurological status with previous physical assessment.
3. Use **Teach Back:** State to the patient, "We discussed your risks for falls related to your heart medications. Tell me some of the risks and how your risk for falls increases." Evaluates what the patient is able to explain or demonstrate. Revise your instruction now or develop plan for revised patient teaching to be implemented at an appropriate time if patient is not able to teach back correctly.

Unexpected Outcomes and Related Interventions

1. Joints are prominent, swollen, and tender with nodules or overgrowth of bone in distal joints, indicating signs of arthritis.
   a. Instruct patient in proper ROM.
   b. Determine patient's knowledge regarding antiinflammatory medications and nonpharmacological measures.
2. ROM is reduced in one or more major joints: shoulder, elbow, wrist, fingers, knee, hip.
   a. Assess further for pain during movement or if joint is unstable, stiff, swollen or with obvious deformity.
   b. Notify health care provider.
   c. Reduce mobility in extremity until cause of abnormal joint motion is determined.
3. Patient demonstrates weakness in one or more major muscle groups or has difficulty with gait or ability to walk and get-up-and-go test greater than 20 seconds, indicating a fall risk.
   a. Provide for patient safety when ambulating.
   b. Place patient on fall precautions.
4. Patient has changes in mental status and pupillary response or other neurological deficits.

TABLE 7-8	**ASSESSING RANGE OF MOTION***	
BODY PART	**ASSESSMENT PROCEDURE**	**ROM**
Upper Extremities		
Neck	Bend head forward and then backward. Bend neck side to side. Turn head to look over each shoulder.	Flexion; hyperextension; lateral flexion; rotation
Shoulders	Raise both arms to vertical position level at the sides of the head.	Flexion
	Bring arm across upper chest to touch opposite shoulder.	Adduction
	Place both hands behind the neck, with elbows out to the sides.	External rotation and abduction
	Place both hands behind the small of the back.	Internal rotation
	Have patient make small circles with hands with arms extended at shoulder level.	Circumduction
Elbows	Bend and straighten elbows.	Flexion and extension
	Place hands at waist with elbows flexed.	Internal rotation
Wrists	Flex and extend wrist (bend and straighten).	Flexion and extension
	Bend wrist to radial then ulnar side.	Radial and ulnar deviation
	Turn palm upward and then downward.	Supination and pronation
Hands	Make a fist with both hands; open hand.	Flexion and extension
	Extend and spread fingers and thumb outward; bring back together.	Adduction and abduction
Lower Extremities		
Hips (with patient supine)	With knees extended, raise one leg upward.	Flexion: expect 90 degrees
	Cross leg over other leg.	Abduction: expect 45 degrees
	Swing legs laterally.	Abduction: expect 30 degrees
	With knee flexed, hold ankle and rotate leg inward and outward.	Internal and external rotation: expect 40-45 degrees
Knees (with patient sitting)	Raise foot, keeping knee in place.	Extension: expect full extension and up to 15 degrees hyperextension
Ankles	With foot held off the floor, point toes downward, and then bring toes back toward knee.	Plantar flexion: expect 45 degrees; Dorsiflexion: expect 20 degrees
Toes	Turn sole of foot inward and then outward.	Inversion and eversion: expect to reach 5 degrees
	Bend toes down and back.	Flexion and hyperextension: expect to reach 40 degrees

*This may be done actively by the patient (active ROM) or passively by the nurse (passive ROM).
ROM, Range of motion.

a. Notify health care provider immediately.
b. Place on fall precautions.
c. Assess vital signs and patient's LOC closely.

Recording and Reporting

- Record posture, gait, muscle strength, ROM, LOC, orientation, pupillary response, CN status, and sensation in nurses' notes or appropriate assessment flow sheet.
- Document your evaluation of patient learning.
- Report to nurse in charge or health care provider any acute pain or sudden muscle weakness, change in LOC, or change in size or pupillary reaction, which require immediate treatment.

Sample Documentation

1530 Patient ambulated 10 feet from bed to chair, gait steady. Denies any complaints of weakness, dizziness, or pain.

Special Considerations
Pediatric

- Examine infants carefully for musculoskeletal anomalies resulting from genetic or fetal insults. An examination includes review of posture, generalized movement, symmetry, and skin creases of the extremities, muscle strength, and hip alignment.

- Normally the back of a newborn is rounded or C-shaped from the thoracic and pelvic curves.
- Scoliosis, lateral curvature of the spine, is an important childhood problem, especially in girls, apparent at puberty. (For closer examination, have child stand erect, wearing only underclothes. Observe from behind, looking for asymmetry of shoulders and hips. Then observe from the back as the child bends forward.) Uneven dress hems or pant leg hems or uneven fit of clothing at the waist may be noted.

Geriatric

- Instruct older adults about fall risks and precautions to take.
- Older adults tend to assume a stooped, forward-bent posture, with hips and knees flexed and arms bent at the elbows and the level of the arms raised (Touhy and Jett, 2014).
- Instruct older adults and patients with osteoporosis in proper body mechanics, ROM exercises, and moderate weight-bearing exercises (e.g., swimming, walking) to minimize trauma.
- Functional assessment is a measurement of the older person's ability to perform basic self-care tasks (Touhy and Jett, 2014). When the patient is unable to perform self-care easily, determine the need for assistive devices (e.g., zippers on clothing instead of buttons, elevation of toilet seat or chairs to minimize bending of knees and hips).

Home Care

- Make modifications in the home for any patient at risk for falls (see Chapter 31).

CRITICAL THINKING EXERCISES

Case Study

A new postoperative patient has an IV infusion, an abdominal dressing, a Foley catheter to gravity, and a Jackson-Pratt surgical drain in place.

1. What body systems would the nurse assess for this patient? Describe key elements for this patient.
2. The nurse assesses unilateral lower extremity swelling around the calf. What additional body system should be assessed and why?
3. The nurse auscultates the patient's abdomen. After listening for 60 seconds at a site below and to the left of the umbilicus, the nurse is unable to hear bowel sounds. What is the best assessment of this situation?

Review Questions

1. In conducting a general survey of a patient, the nurse knows that the survey should include which of the following? Select all that apply.
   1. Appearance
   2. Obtaining peripheral pulses
   3. Measuring chest excursion
   4. Conducting a detailed history
   5. Behavior
   6. Pupillary response
   7. Posture
2. In teaching a patient about skin lesions, the nurse knows that teaching has been successful when the patient identifies which lesion as abnormal?
   1. A symmetrical lesion
   2. A lesion with regular edges and borders
   3. One that is blue-black or varied in color
   4. One that is less than 7 mm in diameter
3. On respiratory assessment, the nurse notes high-pitched, musical sounds on auscultation. The nurse interprets these sounds as:
   1. Normal; vesicular
   2. Rhonchi
   3. Crackles
   4. Wheezes
4. The nurse determines that the patient has an audible S_2 on auscultation during cardiovascular assessment. After documenting this finding, the nurse should:
   1. Reposition the patient for comfort.
   2. Report the finding to the health care provider.
   3. Initiate fluid restriction.
   4. Do nothing because this is a normal finding.
5. Fill in the Blank: The assessment skill of ___________ in the abdominal assessment is done following inspection.
6. The patient has an IV line infusing in the left arm. The skin looks reddened at the site. Which of the following techniques is most appropriate for the nurse to use to check if there is warmth at the site?
   1. Place palm of hand over site
   2. Grasp skin at site with fingers
   3. Apply dorsum of hand over site
   4. Place pads of fingertips above site
7. Which of the following does the nurse document as an abnormal finding during a muscular-neurological assessment? Select all that apply.
   1. Strength in right arm during flexion is Grade 1.
   2. Uses hands to sit down in chair during get-up-and-go test
   3. Negative Romberg's test
   4. Uvula rises symmetrically

8. Calculate the patient's intake in milliliters based on the following fluids: 3 ounces of apple juice, ¼ carton of milk (250 mL per carton), 6 ounces of soda, and 8-ounce cup of ice.

9. When is the best time for a menstruating woman to complete a breast self-examination and why?

10. Select all the characteristics that can be heard through auscultation.
    1. Adaptability
    2. Quality
    3. Loudness
    4. Vibration
    5. Duration
    6. Frequency

REFERENCES

American Cancer Society (ACS): *Cancer prevention and early detection facts and figures 2013*, Atlanta, 2013a, The Society. Available at: http://www.cancer.org/research/cancerfactsfigures/cancerpreventionearlydetectionfactsfigures/index. Accessed May 27, 2014.

American Cancer Society (ACS): *Testicular self-exam*, 2013b, http://www.cancer.org/cancer/testicularcancer/moreinformation/doihavetesticularcancer/do-i-have-testicular-cancer-self-exam. Accessed May 27, 2014.

American Cancer Society (ACS): *Can melanoma be prevented*, Atlanta, 2013c, The Society. Available at: http://www.cancer.org/cancer/skincancer-melanoma/detailedguide/melanoma-skin-cancer-prevention. Accessed May 27 2014.

American Cancer Society (ACS): *Recommendations for human papilloma virus (HPV) vaccine use to prevent cervical cancer and pre-cancers*, Atlanta, 2013d, The Society. Available at: http://www.cancer.org/cancer/cancercauses/othercarcinogens/infectiousagents/hpv/acs-recommendations-for-hpv-vaccine-use. Accessed May 27, 2014.

American Cancer Society (ACS): *Learn about Cancer, American Society recommendations for early breast cancer detection*, 2014a, http://www.cancer.org/Cancer/BreastCancer/DetailedGuide/breast-cancer-detection. Accessed May 27, 2014.

American Cancer Society (ACS): *What are the risk factors for colorectal cancer? Can melanoma be prevented*, Atlanta, 2014b, The Society. Available at: http://www.cancer.org/cancer/colonandrectumcancer/detailedguide/colorectal-cancer-risk-factors. Accessed May 27, 2014.

American Cancer Society (ACS): *What are the risk factors for ovarian cancer?* Atlanta, 2014c, The Society. Available at: http://www.cancer.org/cancer/ovariancancer/detailedguide/ovarian-cancer-risk-factors. Accessed May 27, 2014.

American Cancer Society (ACS): *What are the risk factors for endometrial ovarian cancer?* Atlanta, 2014d, The Society. Available at: http://www.cancer.org/cancer/endometrialcancer/detailedguide/endometrial-uterine-cancer-risk-factors. Accessed May 27, 2014.

Carter K: Identifying and managing deep vein thrombosis, *Prim Health Care* 20(1):30, 2010.

Centers for Disease Control and Prevention: *HPV vaccination*, Atlanta, 2014, Centers for Disease Control and Prevention. Available at: http://www.cdc.gov/vaccines/vpd-vac/hpv/default.htm. Accessed May 27, 2014.

Froehlich-Grobe K, et al: Measuring without a Standiometer: Empirical investigation of Four Height Estimates among Wheelchair Users, *Am J Phys Med Rehabil* 90(8):658–666, 2011.

Giger J, Davidhizar R: *Transcultural nursing: assessment and intervention*, ed 6, St Louis, 2013, Mosby.

Henneman EA, et al: Surveillance: a strategy for improving patient safety in acute and critical care units, *Crit Care Nurse* 32(2):e9, 2012.

Hockenberry MJ, Wilson D: *Wong's essentials of pediatric nursing*, ed 9, St Louis, 2013, Mosby.

Lewis S, et al: *Medical-surgical nursing*, ed 9, St Louis, 2014, Mosby.

Norman J: MDR pressure ulcer: who thought plastic tubing could be harmful, *Healthy Skin* 24, 2013.

Seidel HM, et al: *Seidel's guide to physical examination*, ed 8, St Louis, 2015, Mosby.

Shever LL: The impact of nursing surveillance on failure to rescue, *Res Theory Nurs Pract* 25(2):107, 2011.

The Joint Commission (TJC): *National Patient Safety Goals*, Oakbrook Terrace, IL, 2014, The Commission. Available at: http://www.jointcommission.org/standards_information/npsgs.aspx. Accessed May 24, 2014.

Touhy T, Jett K: *Ebersole & Hess' gerontological nursing & healthy aging*, ed 4, St Louis, 2014, Mosby.

Zrelak PA, et al: Using the Agency for Healthcare Research and Quality patient safety indicators for targeting nursing quality improvement, *J Nurs Care Qual* 27(2):99, 2012.

Specimen Collection

Laboratory test results aid in the diagnosis of health care problems, provide information about the stage and activity of diseases, and measure patient responses to therapy. Proficiency and judgment in obtaining specimens minimize patient discomfort, ensure patient safety, and ensure accuracy and quality of diagnostic procedures. Nurses are accountable for correctly collecting specimens, monitoring patient outcomes, and ensuring that these tests are collected in a timely manner.

When questions arise about laboratory tests, consult the facility's procedure manual or call the laboratory. You can find normal values for laboratory tests in reference books. However, be aware that each laboratory may also establish its own values for each test. It is important to know the significance of abnormal findings so that you can report and discuss with the patient's health care provider.

PATIENT-CENTERED CARE

Patients often experience embarrassment or discomfort when giving a sample of body excretions or secretions. It is important to handle excretions discreetly and to provide a patient with as much privacy as possible. Psychosocial characteristics of patients, including age, gender, ethnicity, and values and beliefs, must be taken into consideration when collecting specimens (Pagana and Pagana, 2013).

Given clear instructions, patients are able to obtain their own specimens of urine, stool, and sputum without unnecessary exposure. Choose words that are clearly understood; many patients, especially children, do not understand the terms *void, urine,* or *stool.*

Cultural considerations are important when collecting specimens. Health beliefs, previous experiences, and a patient's literacy level are examples of factors that can affect a patient's willingness to participate in various diagnostic procedures. Ethnicity may also be a factor; for example, a patient of Southeast Asian descent may consider the blood as a vital life force that should not be wasted. Whenever possible, use same-gender caregivers when collecting vaginal, rectal, or urinary specimens from patients whose cultural values demand modesty and distinct separation of gender roles. Provide privacy both when giving instructions and when collecting the specimen.

SAFETY

When collecting any specimen, know the purpose of the test, how much of the specimen is needed, the appropriate collection technique, and how the specimen is to be transported to the laboratory (Pagana and Pagana, 2013). A completed laboratory requisition is needed for each specimen to instruct laboratory personnel on the test to be performed and to facilitate accurate reporting of the results. Each requisition includes patient identification (e.g., name and birthday or name and account number, according to facility policy), the date and time the specimen is obtained, the name of the test, and the source of the specimen or culture for each container (TJC, 2014).

The 2014 *National Patient Safety Goals* by The Joint Commission (2014) requires the use of at least two identifiers when providing care, treatment, and services. The intent is to identify the individual reliably as the patient for whom the service or treatment is intended and match the service or treatment to that patient (TJC, 2014). After you collect the specimen and in the presence of the patient, you must label the container itself (not the lid) with the same two identifiers (e.g., name and birthday or name and account number, according to facility policy), specimen source, collection date and time, series number (if more than one specimen), and anatomical site if appropriate (e.g., wound culture from knee versus abdominal incision).

Everyone who handles body fluids is at risk for exposure to body fluids. The use of hand hygiene and clean gloves is necessary when collecting a specimen. Use a plastic bag marked "biohazard" to enclose the specimen for delivery to the laboratory (Fig. 8-1). Deliver specimens to the laboratory promptly. Specimens left at room temperature are at risk for additional bacterial growth, altering the results of the test, and so need timely delivery to the laboratory.

EVIDENCE-BASED PRACTICE

Heyer NJ, et al: Effectiveness of practices to reduce blood sample hemolysis in EDs: a laboratory medicine best practices systematic review and meta-analysis, *Clin Biochem* 45(13–14):1012, 2012.

Stauss M, et al: Hemolysis of coagulation specimens: a comparative study of intravenous draw methods, *J Emerg Nurs* 38(1):15, 2012.

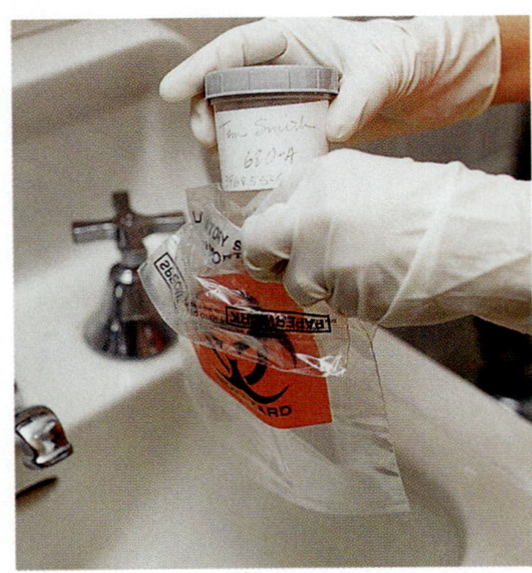

FIG 8-1 Enclose all specimens in a biohazard plastic bag.

Use of straight needle venipuncture instead of an intravenous (IV) device is effective in reducing hemolysis rates of blood samples collected in emergency departments and is recommended as an evidence-based best practice (Heyer et al., 2012; Stauss et al., 2012). When IV starts must be used, observed rates of hemolysis may be substantially reduced by placing the IV at the antecubital site (Heyer et al., 2012; Stauss et al., 2012). Additional best practices, including tourniquet use and care of the specimen after venipuncture, assist in reducing hemolysis rates:

- Venipuncture is recommended over the use of obtaining a blood sample from an IV site to prevent hemolysis.
- Hemolysis may result from vigorous shaking of a blood sample and may invalidate test results.
- Collect a blood specimen from the arm without an IV device if possible.
- Do not fasten the tourniquet for longer than 1 minute. Prolonged tourniquet application can cause stasis, localized acidemia, and hemoconcentration.
- Because the blood cells continue to live in the collection tubes, they will metabolize some of the components in the blood, which can result in alterations in the concentration of some blood components before analysis in the laboratory. Blood specimens should be promptly delivered to the laboratory for processing within 1 hour, depending on the test.

SKILL 8.1   URINE SPECIMEN COLLECTION—MIDSTREAM (CLEAN-VOIDED) URINE, STERILE URINARY CATHETER

• Nursing Skills Online: Specimen Collection, Lessons 1 and 2

A urinalysis provides information about kidney or metabolic function, nutrition, and systemic diseases. Urine collection uses a variety of methods, depending on the purpose of the urinalysis and the presence or absence of a urinary catheter. Regardless of the method of collection, guidelines for assessment, planning, and evaluation are similar. Routine urinalysis includes measurement of nine or more elements, including urine pH, protein and glucose levels, ketones, blood, specific gravity, white blood cell (WBC) count, and presence of bacteria and casts (Pagana and Pagana, 2013).

TYPES OF URINE TESTS AND SPECIMENS

A *random urine specimen for routine urinalysis* in the hospital is usually collected using a specimen "hat" (Fig. 8-2), which you place under a toilet seat to collect voided urine. In an outpatient setting such as a clinic, a patient is instructed to void directly into a specimen container. You place approximately 120 mL of urine in a specimen container, properly label it, and send to the laboratory.

A *culture and sensitivity (C&S) of urine* is performed to identify bacteria causing a urinary tract infection (UTI) (culture) and to determine the most effective antibiotic for treatment (sensitivity). Use sterile technique to ensure that any microorganisms present originate in the urine and not from the patient's skin, the hands, or the environment. You collect specimens for C&S either as a clean-voided midstream specimen or under sterile conditions from a urinary catheter.

A *timed urine specimen for quantitative analysis* requires urine to be collected over 2 to 72 hours. The 24-hour timed collection (see Procedural Guideline 8.1) is most common and allows for measurement and quantitative analysis of elements such as amino acids, creatinine, hormones, glucose, and adrenocorticosteroid excreted.

Chemical properties of urine are tested by immersing a specially prepared strip of paper (Chemstrip) into a clean urine specimen. The test detects the presence of glucose, ketones, protein, or blood *not* normally present in the urine (see Procedural Guideline 8.2). When the screening test for the presence of substances in the urine is positive, additional laboratory tests are used to determine the patient's diagnosis or to measure the effectiveness of treatment.

ASSESSMENT

1. Identify patient using two identifiers (e.g., name and birth date or name and account number) according to facility policy. Compare identifiers with information on the patient's MAR or medical record. *Rationale: Ensures correct patient. Complies with The Joint Commission standards and improves patient safety (TJC, 2014).*
2. Assess patient's understanding of need for the specimen. *Rationale: This determines the need for health teaching. Patient's understanding of purpose promotes cooperation.*

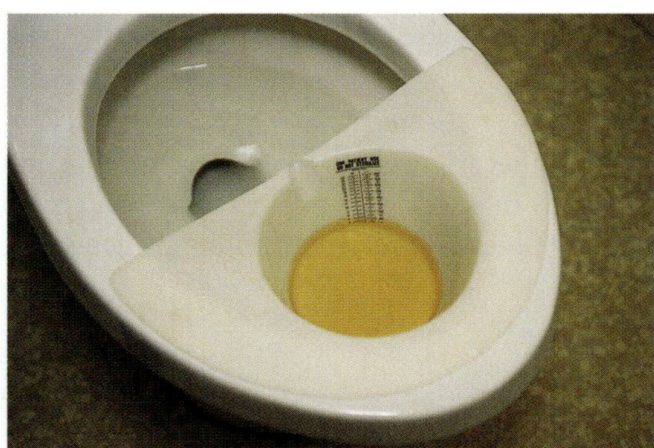

FIG 8-2 Specimen "hat."

3. Assess patient's ability to assist with urine specimen collection: able to position self and hold container. *Rationale: This determines the degree of assistance patient requires.*
4. Determine if you need to administer or add fluids, dietary requirements, or medications in conjunction with the test. *Rationale: Certain substances affect excretion and levels of urinary constituents. Specific amounts of fluid may be required for concentration or dilution tests. Drugs such as cortisone preparations, diuretics, and anesthetics increase glucose levels. Anticoagulants increase risk of blood in the urine.*
5. Assess for signs and symptoms of UTI (frequency, urgency, dysuria, hematuria, flank pain, cloudy urine with sediment, foul odor, fever). *Rationale: These are indicators of UTI.*
6. Assess patient's current urinary elimination pattern. *Rationale: Indicates possibility of UTI. Knowledge of frequency of urination facilitates effective planning of specimen collection.*

PLANNING

Expected Outcomes focus on collecting an appropriate uncontaminated specimen with patient knowledgeable of the purpose of the specimen examination.
1. Patient explains procedure for specimen collection.
2. Patient explains purpose of specimen analysis.
3. A specimen free of contaminants is collected.

Delegation and Collaboration
The skill of collecting urine specimens can be delegated to nursing assistive personnel (NAP). The nurse instructs the NAP to:
- Obtain the specimens at a specified time when appropriate.
- Report to the nurse if the urine is not clear (e.g., contains blood, cloudiness, or excess sediment).
- Report to the nurse if a patient is unable to initiate a stream or has pain or burning on urination.

Equipment
- Completed identification labels with appropriate patient identifiers
- Completed laboratory requisition, including appropriate patient identification, date, time, name of test, and source of culture
- Small plastic biohazard bag for delivery of specimen to laboratory (or container as specified by facility)

Clean-Voided Urine Specimen
- Commercial kit for clean-voided urine (Fig. 8-3) containing:
  - Sterile cotton balls or antiseptic towelettes
  - Antiseptic solution (usually chlorhexidine or povidone-iodine solution)
  - Sterile water or normal saline
  - Sterile specimen container
  - Urine cup

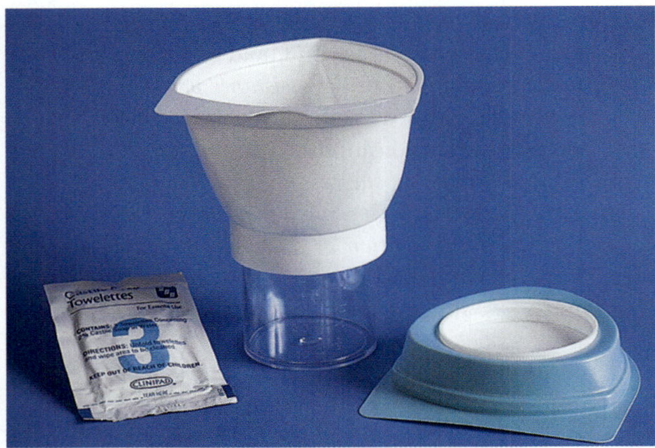

FIG 8-3 Clean-voided urine kit.

- Clean gloves if assisting patient
- Sterile gloves
- Soap, water, washcloth, and towel
- Bedpan for nonambulatory patient or specimen hat for ambulatory patient.

Sterile Urine Specimen from Urinary Catheter

- 20-mL Luer-Lok safety syringe for routine urinalysis or a 3-mL safety Luer-Lok syringe for culture
- Clean gloves
- Clamp or rubber band
- Alcohol, chlorhexidine, or other disinfectant swab
- Specimen container (nonsterile for routine urinalysis; sterile for culture)

IMPLEMENTATION *for* URINE SPECIMEN COLLECTION—MIDSTREAM (CLEAN-VOIDED) URINE, STERILE URINARY CATHETER

STEPS	RATIONALE
1. See Standard Protocol (inside front cover).	
2. Provide privacy for patient; close curtains around bed or close room door. Explain to patient or family caregiver reason specimen is necessary, how patient can assist (when applicable), and how to obtain a specimen that is free of tissue and stool.	Promotes cooperation and patient participation. In some cases, patient can collect clean-voided specimen independently. Minimizes contamination of specimen and need for repeat collection.
3. *Collect clean-voided urine specimen.*	
a. Give patient or family caregiver towel, cleaning towelette or washcloth, and soap to cleanse perineum or assist with cleansing perineum. If assisting bedridden patient, apply clean gloves before helping onto bedpan to facilitate access to the perineum. Remove and dispose of gloves.	Patients usually prefer to wash their own perineal area when possible. Cleansing prevents contamination of specimen after urine passes the urethra.
b. Using surgical asepsis, open outer package of commercial specimen kit.	Maintains sterility of specimen container.
c. Apply sterile gloves.	Prevents contact of microorganisms on your hands.
d. Pour antiseptic solution over cotton balls (unless kit contains prepared antiseptic towelette).	Cotton ball or gauze pad is used to cleanse perineum.
e. Open specimen container, maintaining sterility of inside of specimen container, and place cap with sterile inside surface up. Do not touch inside of cap or container.	Prevents accidental contamination of specimen.
f. Assist patient to cleanse perineum antiseptically, and collect specimen or allow patient to do so independently. The amount of assistance needed varies with each patient. Inform patient that the antiseptic solution will feel cold.	Maintains patient's dignity and comfort.
(1) Male patient:	
(a) Hold penis with one hand; using circular motion and antiseptic towelette, cleanse meatus, moving from center to outside (see illustration). Have uncircumcised male patient retract foreskin for effective cleansing of urinary meatus and keep retracted during voiding. Return foreskin when done.	Reduces number of microorganisms at urethral meatus and moves from areas of least to most contamination. Return of foreskin prevents stricture of penis.

(b) If facility procedure indicates, rinse area with sterile water and dry with cotton balls or gauze pad.

Prevents contamination of specimen with antiseptic solution.

(c) Have patient initiate urine stream into toilet or bedpan; then have either you or the patient pass urine specimen container into stream and collect 90 to 120 mL of urine (see illustration).

Initial urine flushes microorganisms that normally accumulate at urinary meatus and prevents collection in specimen.

(2) Female patient:

(a) Either nurse or patient spreads labia minora with fingers of nondominant hand.

Provides access to urinary meatus.

(b) With dominant hand, cleanse urethral area with antiseptic swab, cotton ball, or gauze. Move from front (above urethral orifice) to back (toward anus). Use a fresh swab each time; cleanse *three times;* begin with labial fold farthest from you, then labial fold closest, and then down center (see illustration).

Prevents contamination of urinary meatus with fecal material. Move from cleanest to most soiled.

(c) If facility procedure indicates, rinse area with sterile water and dry with cotton ball.

Prevents contamination of specimen with antiseptic solution.

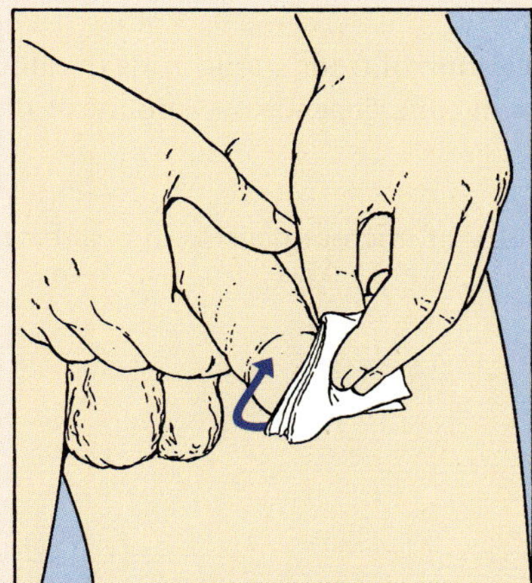

STEP 3f(1)(a) Cleanse penis with a circular motion. (Modified from Grimes D: *Infectious diseases, Mosby's clinical nursing series,* St Louis, 1991, Mosby.)

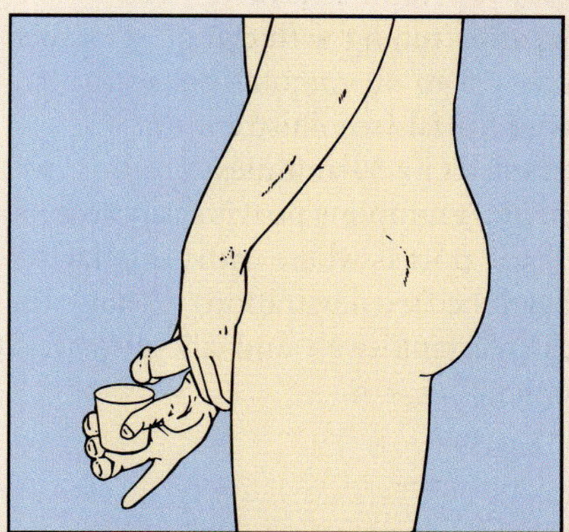

STEP 3f(1)(c) Position of male patient for collecting midstream urine specimen.

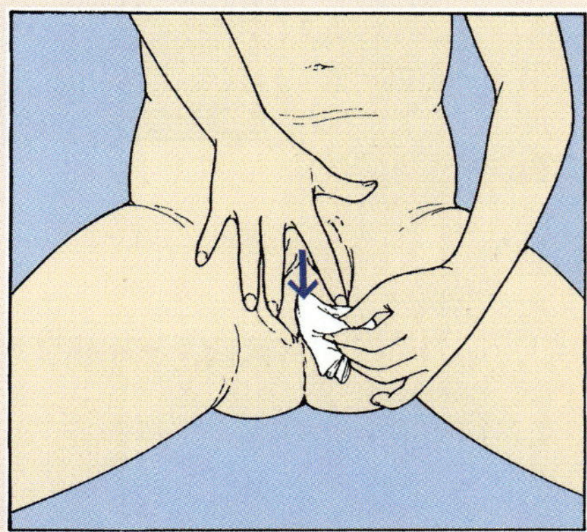

STEP 3f(2)(b) Cleanse from front to back, holding labia apart. (Modified from Grimes D: *Infectious diseases, Mosby's clinical nursing series,* St Louis, 1991, Mosby.)

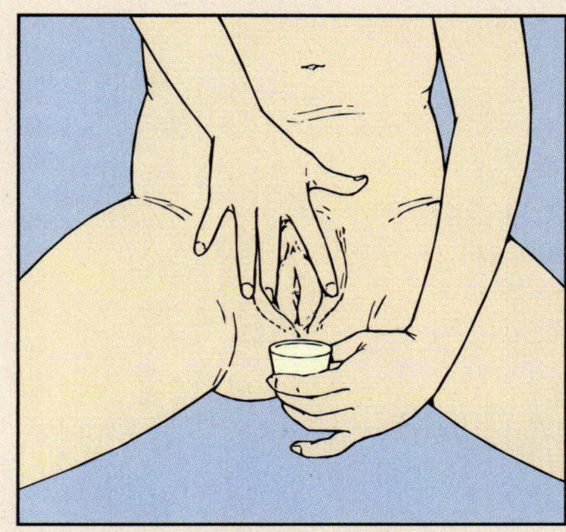

STEP 3f(2)(d) Collection of midstream urine specimen (female patient).

Continued

STEPS	RATIONALE

(d) While continuing to hold labia apart, have patient initiate urine stream into the toilet or bedpan; after stream is achieved, have you or the patient pass the specimen container into stream and collect 90 to 120 mL of urine (Pagana and Pagana, 2013) (see illustration).

Initial urine flushes out microorganisms that normally accumulate at the urinary meatus and provides uncontaminated urine from the bladder itself.

g. Remove specimen container before flow of urine stops and before releasing penis or labia. Patient finishes voiding into bedpan or toilet. Offer to help with perineal hygiene as appropriate.

Prevents contamination of specimen with skin flora.

h. Replace cap securely on specimen container, touching outside only.

Retains sterility of inside of container and prevents spillage of urine.

i. Cleanse urine from exterior surface of container. Remove and dispose of gloves.

Prevents transfer of microorganisms to others.

4. *Collect urine from an indwelling urinary catheter.*

a. Explain that you will use a syringe without a needle to remove the urine through the catheter port and patient will not experience discomfort.

Minimizes anxiety when nurse manipulates catheter and aspirates urine with syringe from the catheter port.

b. Explain that you need to clamp the catheter for approximately 15 to 30 minutes before obtaining a urine specimen and that urine cannot be obtained from drainage bag.

A time span of 15 to 30 minutes allows urine to accumulate in catheter (Pagana and Pagana, 2013). Urine in drainage bag is not considered sterile.

c. Apply clean gloves. Clamp drainage tubing with clamp or rubber band for at least 15 to 30 minutes below the site chosen for withdrawal (see illustration).

Permits collection of fresh, sterile urine in catheter tubing. Amount of time depends on amount of urine patient produces.

d. After 15 to 30 minutes, position patient so that catheter sampling port is easily accessible. Location of the port is where catheter attaches to drainage bag tube (see illustration). Cleanse the port with a disinfectant swab and allow to dry (see facility policy).

Prevents entry of microorganisms into catheter.

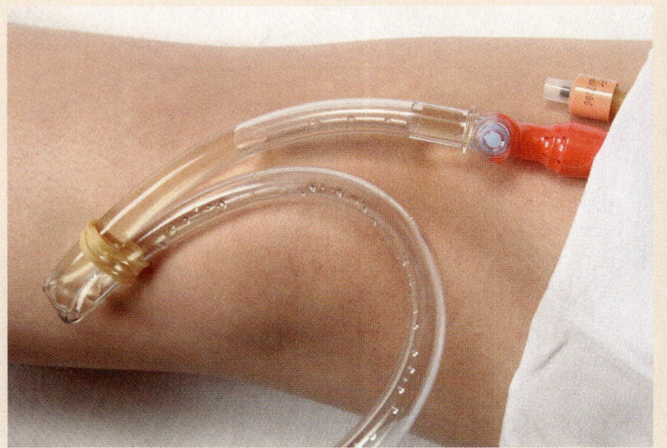

STEP 4c Rubber band used to clamp catheter drainage tube.

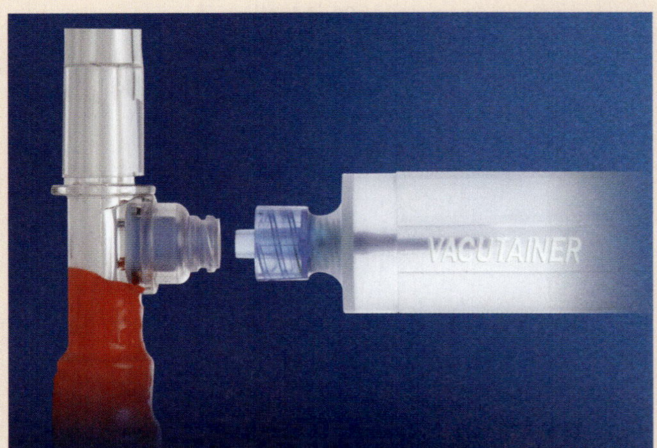

STEP 4d Port with syringe attached. (Courtesy and © Becton, Dickinson and Company.)

STEPS	RATIONALE

e. Attach a needleless Luer-Lok syringe to the built-in catheter sampling port (see illustration).

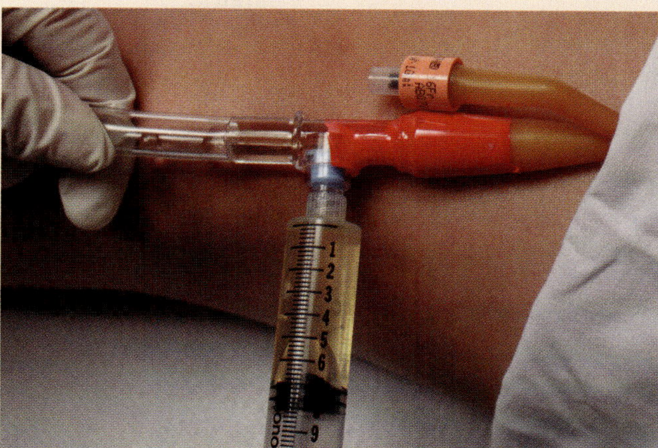

STEP 4e Access urinary catheter port with Luer-Lok syringe or syringe with blunt plastic valve.

f. Withdraw 3 mL for a culture or 20 mL for routine urinalysis.

Allows collection of urine without contamination. Obtains proper volume for testing.

g. Transfer urine from syringe into clean urine container for routine urinalysis or into a sterile urine container for culture.

Prevents contamination of urine during transfer procedure.

h. Place lid tightly on container.

Prevents contamination of specimen by air and loss by spillage.

i. Unclamp catheter and allow urine to flow into drainage bag. Ensure that urine flows freely.

Allows urine to drain by gravity and prevents stasis of urine in bladder.

5. Securely attach label to container (not the lid). In patient's presence, complete label with two identifiers, specimen source, and collection date and time. If patient is female, indicate if patient is menstruating.

Ensures that specimen is identified correctly for proper diagnosis (TJC, 2014).

6. Send specimen and completed requisition to laboratory within 20 minutes. Refrigerate if delay cannot be avoided.

Delay of analysis may alter test results significantly (Pagana and Pagana, 2013).

7. See Standard Completion Protocol (inside front cover).

EVALUATION

1. Ask patient to describe midstream (clean-voided) urine specimen collection procedure.
2. Inspect clean-voided specimen for contamination with toilet tissue or stool.
3. Observe urinary drainage system in catheterized patient to ensure that it is intact and patent.
4. Use *Teach Back:* State to the patient, "I want to be sure I explained the way to obtain a clean-voided specimen. Can you repeat the steps back to me?" Evaluates what the patient is able to explain or demonstrate. Revise your instruction now or develop plan for revised patient teaching to be implemented at an appropriate time if patient is not able to teach back correctly.

Unexpected Outcomes and Related Interventions

1. Patient is unable to void or urine does not collect in drainage tube.
   a. Offer fluids (if permitted) to enhance urine production.
2. Patient's urine specimen is contaminated with stool or toilet tissue or both.
   a. Reinforce importance of obtaining specimen free of contaminants.
   b. Collect a new specimen and assist patient with specimen collection; place specimen hat as close to front of commode as possible for midstream (clean-voided) specimens.

3. Lumen that leads to balloon holding catheter in bladder is punctured.
   a. Notify health care provider and prepare for insertion of new catheter.
   b. Obtain new specimen.
4. Patient unable to teach back.
   a. Allow patient to ask questions.
   b. Revise your instructions and clarify misconceptions or directions.

Recording and Reporting

- Record method used to obtain specimen, date and time collected, type of test ordered, laboratory receiving specimen, characteristics of specimen, and patient's tolerance to procedure of specimen collection.
- Report any abnormal findings to health care provider.
- Document your evaluation of patient learning.

Sample Documentation

1125   Patient able to teach back the correct procedure to obtain a clean-voided specimen.
1135   Clean-voided specimen of 130 mL dark amber urine obtained and sent to lab. Reports frequent urge to void, burning sensation with voiding, and voiding small amounts. Health care provider notified.

Special Considerations
Pediatric

- It is impossible to obtain a midstream urine collection on a child who has not been toilet-trained; consequently, obtain urine for culture by straight catheterization. Consider age-appropriate fears, especially with preschool and school-age children (Hockenberry and Wilson, 2013).

Geriatric

- Older adults may need assistance in positioning to obtain specimen. In confused patients, NAP may be necessary to assist the patient in collecting a specimen (Touhy and Jett, 2014).

Home Care

- Instruct a patient collecting a sample at home to keep the specimen on ice until it reaches the laboratory to minimize bacterial growth before applying it to a culture medium in a laboratory setting.

PROCEDURAL GUIDELINE 8.1
Collecting a Timed Urine Specimen

Some tests of renal function and urine composition require urine to be collected over 2 to 72 hours. The 24-hour timed collection is used most often and measures elements such as amino acids, creatine, hormones, glucose, and adrenocorticosteroids. To ensure the accuracy of a 24-hour timed urine specimen, the patient and staff must work together to collect all voided urine in a 24-hour period. Obtain an appropriate container with or without preservative from the laboratory. The type of analysis for the 24-hour timed specimen determines the need for any preservative. You may place the specimen container in the patient's bathroom or the "soiled" utility room. Post a sign to remind the patient and staff that a test is in progress. Label the specimen container with all appropriate identification information and the number of containers sequentially if more than one container is needed. Also note if toxic material is used as a preservative. Documentation and collection of all urine are necessary for an accurate test result.

Delegation and Collaboration

The skill of collecting a timed urine specimen can be delegated to nursing assistive personnel (NAP). Instruct the NAP by:

- Explaining the time to begin specimen collection, how to store collected urine, where to place signs that a timed urine collection is in progress, and to save all urine.
- Reviewing what to observe for and to report blood, mucus, or foul odors present in the specimen or if there is a break in the collection procedure.

Equipment

- Large collection bottle with cap that usually contains a chemical preservative
- Bedpan, urinal, specimen hat, bedside commode, or pediatric potty-chair
- Graduated measuring cup for intake and output (I&O) measurement
- Large basin to hold collection bottle (surrounded by ice if immediate refrigeration is required)
- Instructional signs that remind patient and staff of timed urine collection
- Clean gloves
- Completed identification labels and laboratory requisition (with appropriate patient identifiers and specimen information)
- Plastic biohazard bag or container (see facility policy).

Procedural Steps

1. **See Standard Protocol (inside front cover).**
2. Identify patient using two identifiers (e.g., name and birth date or name and account number) according

PROCEDURAL GUIDELINE 8.1
Collecting a Timed Urine Specimen—cont'd

to facility policy. Compare identifiers with information on the patient's MAR or medical record (TJC, 2014).

3. Explain the reason for specimen collection, how patient can assist, and that urine must be free of feces and toilet tissue.

4. Place signs indicating timed urine specimen collection on patient's door and toileting area. If patient leaves unit for another test or procedure, be sure that personnel in that area collect and save all urine.

5. If possible, have patient drink two to four glasses of water about 30 minutes before timed collection to facilitate ability to void at the appropriate time for the test to begin.

6. Apply clean gloves. Discard the first voided specimen as test begins. Print time that test began on laboratory requisition. For accurate results, the patient must begin the test with an empty bladder. Restart timed period if urine is accidentally lost, discarded, or contaminated.

7. Measure volume of each voiding if I&O is being recorded. Place all voided urine in labeled specimen bottle with appropriate additive.

8. Unless instructed otherwise, keep specimen bottle in specimen refrigerator or in container of ice in bathroom to prevent decomposition of urine.

9. Encourage patient to drink 2 glasses of water 1 hour before timed urine collection ends. Encourage patient to empty bladder during the last 15 minutes of the urine collection period.

10. Apply clean gloves. At end of collection period, collect final specimen, label specimen (two identifiers, specimen source, collection date and time, number of bottle) in patient's presence, and attach appropriate requisition (patient identification, date, time, name of test, and specimen source) and send to laboratory.

11. Remove signs and inform patient that specimen collection period is completed.

12. **See Completion Protocol (inside front cover).**

PROCEDURAL GUIDELINE 8.2
Urine Screening for Glucose, Ketones, Protein, Blood, and PH

Tests for chemical properties of urine are part of the routine urinalysis completed in the laboratory, as point-of-care at the bedside, or in the home. The use of a Multistix reagent test strip may simultaneously assess for up to nine chemical properties, including specific gravity, pH, protein, glucose, ketones, blood bilirubin, urobilinogen, leukocytes, and nitrates. The test is easy to perform and causes no pain. This type of screening is used when more detailed laboratory testing is not readily available (e.g., in a health care provider's office or clinic and in the outpatient, long-term care, or home setting). It may also be done for pregnant women on admission to the hospital in labor. The use of urine testing for managing blood glucose is no longer recommended but continues to be useful in detecting the presence of ketones in patients with diabetes (ADA, 2013a).

Delegation and Collaboration

The skill of urine screening for chemical properties can be delegated to nursing assistive personnel (NAP). Instruct the NAP by:

- Explaining when to obtain the specimen (e.g., before meals, following a "double-voided" specimen).
- Reviewing the need to report to the nurse the results of the test or any blood, mucus, or odor in the specimen.

Equipment

- Specimen hat, bedpan, urinal, bedside commode, or pediatric potty-chair
- Container for urine from urinary catheter (if needed)
- Watch with second hand or digital counter
- Clean gloves
- Reagent test strip (check expiration date on container)
- Test strip color chart

Procedural Steps

1. **See Standard Protocol (inside front cover).**

2. Identify patient using two identifiers (e.g., name and birth date or name and account number) according to facility policy. Compare identifiers with information on the patient's MAR or medical record (TJC, 2014).

3. Determine if a "double-voided" specimen is needed for glucose testing. If required, ask patient to void, discard urine, and then drink a glass of water.

4. Apply clean gloves. Assist or ask patient to collect a fresh random urine sample (see Skill 8.1). If patient is catheterized, remove a 5-mL urine specimen from the catheter port.

5. Immerse end of reagent test strip into urine container. Remove the strip immediately and tap it gently against the side of the container to remove excess urine.

Continued

PROCEDURAL GUIDELINE 8.2
Urine Screening for Glucose, Ketones, Protein, Blood, and PH—cont'd

6. Hold strip in horizontal position to prevent mixing of chemical reagents (see illustration).
7. Precisely time the number of seconds specified on container, and then compare color of strip with color chart on container.
8. When appropriate, discuss test results with patient. Record test results immediately on appropriate testing flow sheet. Report findings to health care provider.
9. **See Completion Protocol (inside front cover).**

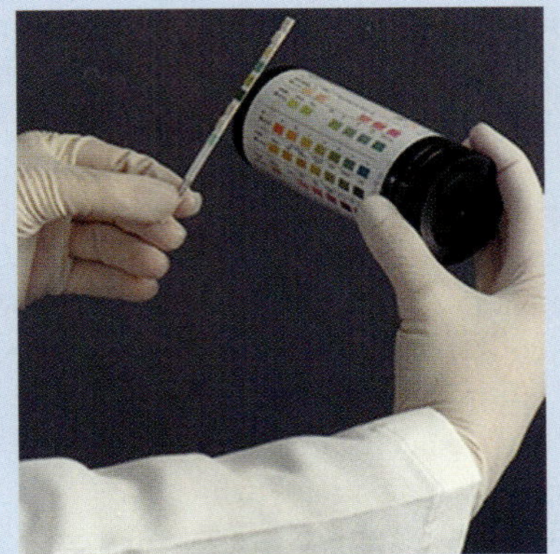

STEP 6 Testing urine using reagent strip.

SKILL 8.2   TESTING FOR GASTROINTESTINAL ALTERATIONS—GASTROCCULT TEST, STOOL SPECIMEN, AND HEMOCCULT TEST

• **Nursing Skills Online: Specimen Collection, Lessons 3 and 4**

The collection of gastric secretions involves obtaining a specimen from an existing nasogastric (NG) or nasointestinal (NI) tube. When a patient has emesis, you test the material for the presence of blood. Analysis of stool or gastric secretions from the gastrointestinal (GI) tract provides useful information about pathological conditions including the presence of tumors, infection, and malabsorption problems.

Patients can often assist in providing stool specimens. The term *occult blood* refers to blood that is not visible but is present in microscopic amounts. Tests done to detect the presence of occult blood in stool (guaiac test) or emesis and gastric secretions (Gastroccult test) reveal bleeding in the esophagus, stomach, small intestine, or large intestine. The tests verify the presence of blood when the nurse notices red or black coloration of stool or gastric contents or a "coffee grounds" appearance of gastric contents in emesis or with NG suction.

Hemoccult testing is useful for screening for the presence of occult (invisible) blood in the stool for conditions such as colon cancer, bleeding GI ulcers, and localized gastric or intestinal irritation. Instruct the patient to avoid red meats for 3 days before testing (Pagana and Pagana, 2013; Van Leeuwen et al., 2011). The animal hemoglobin of ingested animal meat may instigate the guaiac peroxidation process and cause false-positive results. When blood is present, further testing is indicated to determine the source of the bleeding. A single positive test does not confirm bleeding or indicate colorectal cancer. To confirm positive results, repeat the test.

ASSESSMENT

1. Identify patient using two identifiers (e.g., name and birth date or name and account number) according to facility policy. Compare identifiers with information on the patient's MAR or medical record. *Rationale: Ensures correct patient. Complies with The Joint Commission standards and improves patient safety (TJC, 2014).*
2. Assess patient's medical history for GI disorders (e.g., history of bleeding, hemorrhoids, colitis, malabsorption disorders).
3. Determine patient's understanding of need for test and the ability to cooperate with procedure and collect specimen.
4. Assess female patient's menstrual cycle. *Rationale: A woman who is menstruating may have a stool specimen contaminated with blood.*
5. Review medications for drugs that can contribute to GI bleeding. *Rationale: Anticoagulants, steroids, nonsteroidal antiinflammatory drugs (NSAIDs), ascorbic acid (vitamin C), antiinflammatory agents, and alcohol commonly cause bleeding tendency or irritation of GI mucosa (Pagana and Pagana, 2013).*
6. Check health care provider's orders for dietary restrictions before testing. *Rationale: Diets rich in red meats and peroxidase-rich vegetables (turnips, horseradish, artichokes, mushrooms, radishes, broccoli, bean sprouts, cauliflower, oranges, bananas, cantaloupes, and grapes) may affect results (Pagana and Pagana, 2013).*

PLANNING

Expected Outcomes focus on the collection of an appropriate specimen, with patient knowledgeable of the purpose of the specimen test.

1. Patient discusses the purpose of test.
2. Patient maintains a high-residue diet that is free of red meat for specified period.
3. Patient's specimen is appropriate for testing analysis.

Delegation and Collaboration

Assessment of the patient's condition cannot be delegated. The skills of obtaining and testing gastric secretions from an NG or NI tube may not be delegated. The skill of obtaining stool specimens may be delegated to nursing assistive personnel (NAP). Instruct the NAP by:

- Explaining when to obtain stool specimen.
- Reviewing with personnel to report immediately if blood is detected, *not to discard stool from a positive test,* and to report immediately if blood is observed in patient emesis or NG tube drainage.

Equipment

- Clean gloves
- Soap, water, washcloth, and towel

Gastroccult Test

- Facial tissues
- Emesis basin
- Wooden applicator or 3-mL syringe
- 60-mL bulb or catheter tip syringe
- Cardboard Gastroccult slide and developing solution (Fig. 8-4)

Stool Specimens

- Plastic container with lid
- Two tongue blades
- Paper towel
- Bedpan, specimen hat, or bedside commode
- "Save stool" signs (24-hour timed specimen)
- Sterile test tube and swab (for culture)
- Identification labels and completed laboratory requisition, including appropriate patient identification, date, time, name of test, and source of culture
- Small plastic bag for delivery of specimen to laboratory (or container as specified by facility)

Hemoccult (Guaiac Test)

- Paper towel
- Wooden applicator
- Cardboard Hemoccult slide and Hemoccult developing solution (Fig. 8-5)

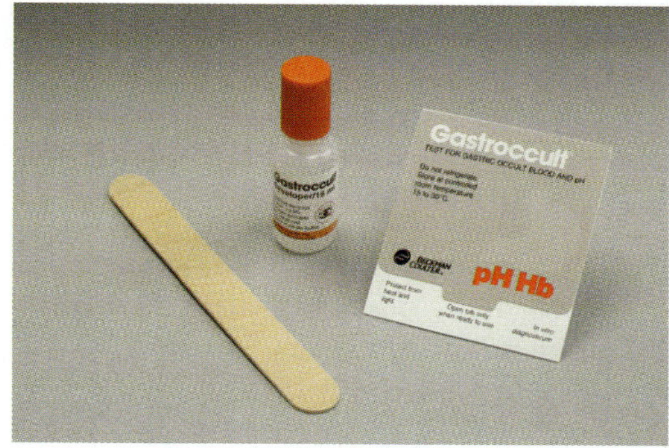

FIG 8-4 Cardboard Gastroccult slide and developing solution.

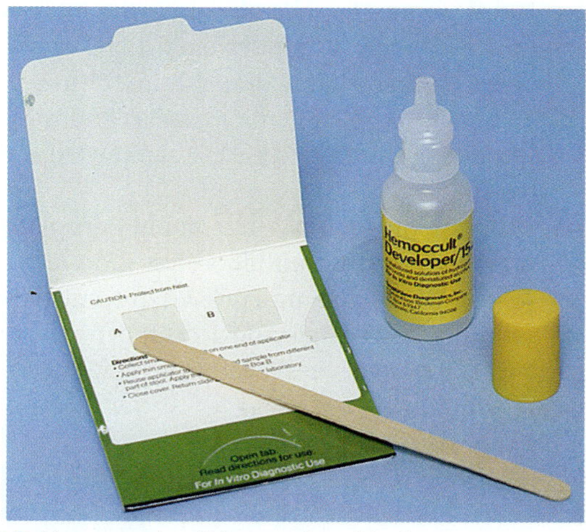

FIG 8-5 Hemoccult slide testing kit for measuring occult blood.

IMPLEMENTATION *for* TESTING FOR GASTROINTESTINAL ALTERATIONS—GASTROCCULT TEST, STOOL SPECIMEN, AND HEMOCCULT TEST

STEPS	RATIONALE
1. **See Standard Protocol (inside front cover).**	
2. Arrange for dietary or medication restrictions as indicated.	Increases accuracy of test results.
3. Discuss reason specimen is necessary, how patient can assist in collecting an uncontaminated specimen (for stool specimen), and how you will obtain the gastric specimen.	Promotes patient cooperation.

Continued

STEPS	RATIONALE

4. *Point-of-Care Gastroccult test.*

> **SAFE PATIENT CARE** Gastroccult and Hemoccult slides and developers are *not* interchangeable.

a. To obtain specimen of gastric contents from NG or NI tube, position patient in high-Fowler's position in bed or chair.

Minimizes chance of aspiration of gastric contents. Position relieves pressure on abdominal organs. If patient is nauseated, flat position in bed or one in which patient cannot sit straight may cause abdominal discomfort.

b. Apply clean gloves. Verify enteral tube placement (see Chapter 12).

Ensures aspiration of gastric or intestinal contents.

c. Collect GI contents via NG or NI tube by disconnecting tube from suction or gravity drainage. Draw 30 mL of air (for NG tube) or 10 mL of air (for NI tube) into the bulb or slip-tipped syringe, attach syringe to NG or NI tube, inject air, and aspirate 5 to 10 mL of fluid.

Only small amount of specimen is needed for pH and occult blood testing.

d. To obtain sample of emesis, use a 3-mL syringe or wooden applicator to gather sample from emesis basin.

e. Using applicator or syringe, apply 1 drop of gastric sample to Gastroccult blood test slide.

Sample must cover test paper for test reaction to occur.

f. Apply 2 drops of commercial Gastroccult developer solution over sample and 1 drop between positive and negative performance monitors (see illustration).

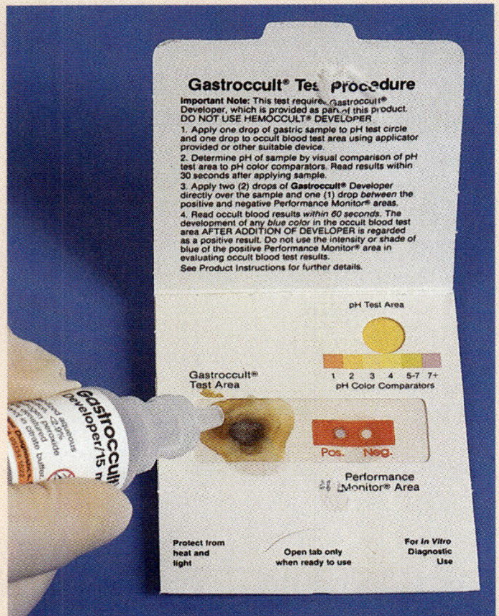

STEP 4f Apply developing solution to Gastroccult test area.

g. Verify that performance monitor turns blue after 30 seconds.

Indicates proper function of the testing paper.

h. After 60 seconds, compare color of gastric sample with that of performance monitors.

If sample turns blue, test is positive for occult blood. If sample turns green, test is negative for occult blood.

i. Explain test results to patient if appropriate or contact health care provider if positive.

j. If needed, reconnect enteral tube to drainage system, suction, or clamp as ordered.

Ensures proper function of enteral tube.

STEPS	RATIONALE

5. Collect stool specimen.

a. 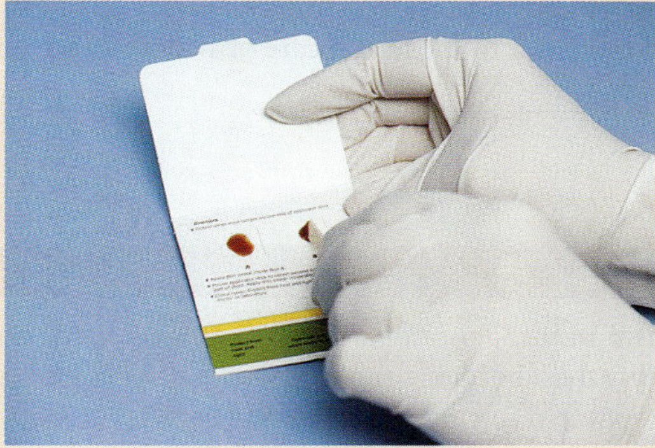 Apply clean gloves. Assist patient as needed into bathroom or to commode or bedpan. Instruct patient to void into toilet or urinal before collecting specimen in container. Provide a clean, dry bedpan or specimen hat in which to defecate.

Feces must not be mixed with urine, water, or toilet tissue. Urine inhibits fecal bacterial growth. Toilet tissue contains bismuth, which interferes with test results.

b. If needed, assist patient in washing after toileting and leave in a comfortable position.

c. Transport specimen container with stool to bathroom or utility room and gather specimen.

   (1) Culture:

      Remove swab from sterile test tube, gather bean-size piece of stool, and return swab to tube. If stool is liquid, soak swab in it and return to tube.

Use of sterile swab prevents introduction of bacteria.

   (2) Timed stool specimen:

      Place stool from each collection in waxed cardboard container for specific time ordered and keep in specimen refrigerator.

Tests for dietary products and digestive enzymes such as fat content or bile require analysis of all feces over select time period.

     (a) For timed test, place signs that read "Save all stool" (with appropriate date or time) over patient's bed, on bathroom door, and above toilet.

Helps prevent any accidental disposal of stool.

     (b) After obtaining the specimen for the laboratory, immediately place lid tightly on container.

Prevents spread of microorganisms by air or contact with other articles.

   (3) All other tests to laboratory:

      Obtain specimen by using tongue blades and transfer portion of stool to container (2.5 cm [1 inch] of formed stool or 15 mL of liquid stool).

   (4) Point-of-Care Hemoccult test (guaic):

     (a) 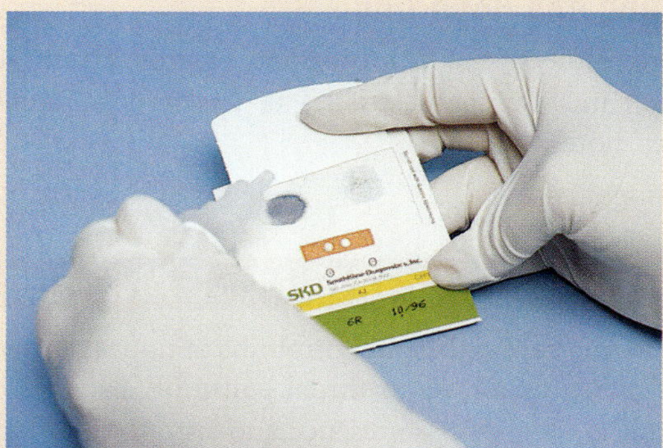 Apply clean gloves. Use tip of wooden applicator to obtain small portion of feces.

     (b) Open flap of Hemoccult slide. Apply thin smear of stool on paper in first box.

Guaiac paper inside box is sensitive to fecal blood content.

     (c) Obtain a second fecal specimen from different portion of stool and apply thinly to second box of slide (see illustration).

Occult blood from upper GI tract is not always dispersed equally throughout stool. Findings of occult blood are more conclusive when entire specimen is found to contain blood.

STEP 5c(4)(c) Apply stool to both spots on Hemoccult slide.

STEP 5c(4)(d) Apply developing solution to Hemoccult slide.

Continued

STEPS	RATIONALE
(d) Close slide cover and turn slide over to reverse side. Open cardboard flap, and apply 2 drops of Hemoccult developing solution on each box of guaiac paper (see illustration).	Developing solution penetrates underlying fecal specimen. Blood is indicated by change in color of guaiac paper.
(e) Read results of test after 30 to 60 seconds. Note color changes.	Bluish discoloration indicates occult blood (guaiac positive). No change in color of guaiac paper indicates negative results.
6. For timed specimen, stool culture, and other laboratory tests, label specimen (two identifiers, specimen source, collection date and time, number of bottle) in patient's presence, attach appropriate requisition (patient identification, date, time, name of test, and specimen source), and send to laboratory.	
7. See Standard Completion Protocol (inside front cover).	

EVALUATION

1. Observe quantity, character, and color of stool, emesis, or GI secretions.
2. Compare test findings with normal expected results.
3. Use **Teach Back:** State to the patient, "You will need to check your stool two more times for blood when you go home. I want to be sure I explained the procedure correctly. Can you repeat the steps back to me?" Evaluates what the patient is able to explain or demonstrate. Revise your instruction now or develop plan for revised patient teaching to be implemented at an appropriate time if patient is not able to teach back correctly.

Unexpected Outcomes and Related Interventions

1. Occult blood test results are positive.
   a. Continue to monitor patient and notify health care provider.
2. Patient unable to teach back.
   a. Allow patient to ask questions.
   b. Revise your instructions and clarify misconceptions or directions.

Recording and Reporting

- Record results of test in appropriate records (check facility policy); include characteristics of specimen contents in nurses' notes.
- Report positive results to health care provider.
- Document your evaluation of patient learning.

Sample Documentation

1600 Large, liquid, dark brown stool tested positive for occult blood. Health care provider notified. Patient informed that test is to be repeated × 2.

1630 Patient able to teach back procedure for testing stool for occult blood.

Special Considerations
Pediatric

- Children of school age and older are concrete thinkers, are often curious, and ask many questions about tests. Answer honestly and at child's level of understanding. Allow child to watch, if desired, while test is performed (Hockenberry and Wilson, 2013).

Home Care

- Patients are instructed to collect Hemoccult specimens at home. To collect stool specimen, a piece of plastic wrap can be draped over the toilet. If possible the specimen should not be contaminated with urine. Patient or family caregiver prepares slide with feces, closes cardboard slide, and returns it to the health care provider's office or clinic.

SKILL 8.3   COLLECTING NOSE AND THROAT SPECIMENS

When patients have signs and symptoms of upper respiratory or sinus infection, a nose or throat culture is a simple diagnostic tool to identify the presence and type of microorganisms. You should obtain cultures before antibiotic therapy is started because the antibiotic may interrupt the growth of the organism in the laboratory. If a patient is receiving antibiotics, notify the laboratory and explain what specific antibiotics the patient is receiving (Pagana and Pagana, 2013).

Collection of a specimen from the nose and throat can cause a patient discomfort and gagging because of sensitive mucosal membranes. It is important to collect a throat culture before mealtime or at least 1 hour after eating or drinking to lessen the chance of inducing vomiting and risk for aspiration.

ASSESSMENT

1. Identify patient using two identifiers (e.g., name and birth date or name and account number) according to facility policy. Compare identifiers with information on the patient's MAR or medical record. *Rationale: Ensures correct patient. Complies with The Joint Commission standards and improves patient safety (TJC, 2014).*
2. Assess patient's understanding of purpose of procedure and ability to cooperate. You may need assistance to obtain throat cultures from confused, combative, or unconscious patients. *Rationale: Provides basis to determine need for health teaching, need for assistance, and prevention of injury.*
3. Assess condition of and drainage from nasal mucosa and sinuses. *Rationale: Reveals physical signs that may indicate infection or allergic irritation.*
4. Determine if patient has experienced postnasal drip, sinus headache or tenderness, nasal congestion, or sore throat. *Rationale: Further clarifies nature of problem.*
5. Assess condition of posterior pharynx (see Chapter 7).
6. Assess for systemic indications of infection, including fever, chills, and malaise.

PLANNING

Expected Outcomes focus on obtaining an uncontaminated specimen in the appropriate amount for diagnosis and appropriate treatment.

1. Patient verbalizes understanding of purpose of specimen and how specimen is to be obtained.
2. Culture specimen is obtained without contamination from adjacent skin or tissues.
3. Patient does not experience bleeding of nasal mucosa.

Delegation and Collaboration

The skill of obtaining specimens from the nose and throat cannot be delegated to nursing assistive personnel (NAP). The nurse instructs the NAP to:

- Report any complaints of shortness of breath, difficulty breathing, and other signs of respiratory distress.

Equipment

- Two sterile swabs in sterile culture tubes (flexible wire swab with cotton tip may be used for nose cultures)
- Nasal speculum (optional)
- Tongue blades
- Penlight
- Emesis basin or clean container (optional)
- Facial tissues
- Gauze
- Clean gloves
- Identification labels and completed laboratory requisition, including appropriate patient identification, date, time, name of test, and source of culture
- Small plastic biohazard bag for delivery of specimen to laboratory (or container as specified by facility)

IMPLEMENTATION *for* COLLECTING NOSE AND THROAT SPECIMENS

STEPS	RATIONALE
1. **See Standard Protocol (inside front cover).**	
2. Ask patient to sit erect in bed or on a chair facing you. Acutely ill patient may lie supported at 45-degree angle in semi-Fowler's position. Explain that patient may have tickling sensation or gag during swabbing of throat. Nasal swab may create urge to sneeze. State that procedure takes only a few seconds.	Provides easy access to oral structures.
3. Have swab in tube ready for use. You may want to loosen top so that swab can be removed easily.	Most commercial tubes have a top that fits securely over end of swab, which allows you to touch outer top without contaminating swab stick.
4. *Collect throat culture.*	
a. Apply clean gloves. Schedule procedure when patient's stomach is empty. With patient in sitting position, have patient tilt head backward. For patients in bed, place pillow behind shoulders.	Obtaining specimen on empty stomach reduces risk of vomiting and aspiration.
b. Ask patient to open mouth and say "ah."	Permits exposure of pharynx, relaxes throat muscles, and minimizes gag reflex.

Continued

STEPS	RATIONALE

    c. Depress tongue with tongue blade if unable to expose pharynx and note inflamed areas of pharynx or tonsils. Depress anterior third of tongue only, and illuminate with penlight as needed.

Area to be swabbed should be clearly visualized.

    d. Insert swab without touching lips, teeth, tongue, or cheeks (see illustration).

Ensures collection of infected drainage.

    e. Gently but quickly swab tonsillar area side to side, making contact with inflamed or purulent sites.

Collects microorganisms from the throat tissues without contamination from mouth or tongue.

    f. Carefully withdraw swab without touching oral structures.

5. *Collect nasal culture.*

    a. Apply clean gloves. Ask patient to blow nose and then check nostrils for patency with penlight. Select nostril with greatest patency.

Clears nasal passage of mucus that contains resident bacteria.

    b. With patient in sitting position, have patient tilt head backward. Patients in bed should have pillow behind shoulders.

    c. Gently insert nasal speculum in one nostril *(optional).*

Improves ability to view nasal mucosa and reach back of naris.

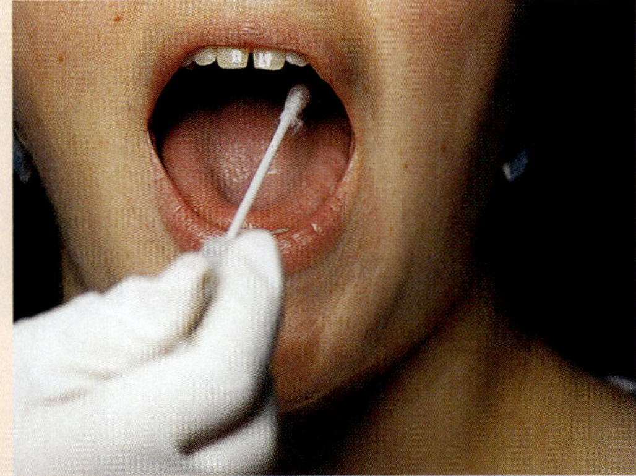

STEP 4d Collection of specimen from posterior pharynx. (From Pagana KD, Pagana TJ: *Mosby's manual of diagnostic and laboratory tests*, ed 4, St Louis, 2010, Mosby.)

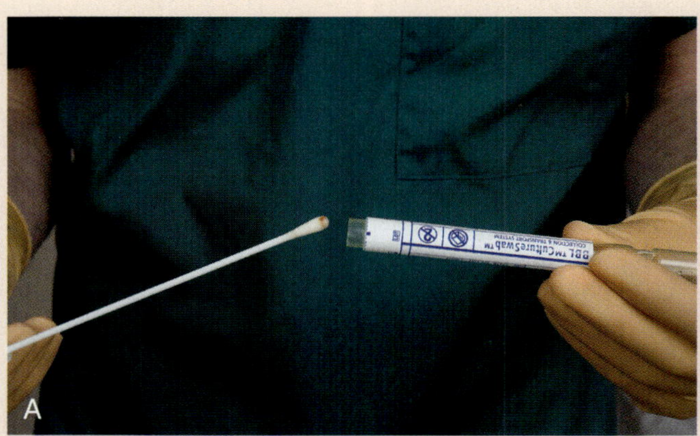
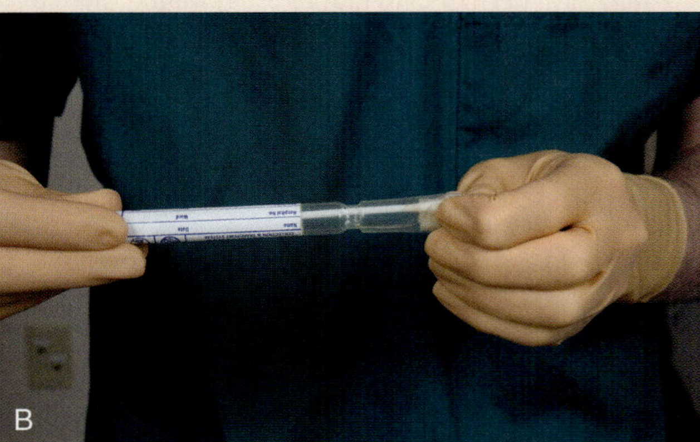

STEP 6 Activating culture tube. **A,** Place swab into tube. **B,** Crush end of tube to release liquid.

STEPS	RATIONALE
d. Carefully pass swab into nostril until it reaches the portion of mucosa that is inflamed or contains exudate. Rotate swab quickly. Note: If you need to obtain a nasopharyngeal culture, use a special swab on a flexible wire that can be flexed downward to reach nasopharynx.	Swab should remain sterile until it reaches area to be cultured. Rotating swab covers all surfaces where exudate is present.
e. Remove swab without touching sides of speculum or nasal canal.	Prevents contamination by resident bacteria.
f. Carefully remove nasal speculum (if used) and place in basin. Offer patient facial tissue.	
6. Insert swab into culture tube. Using gauze to protect your fingers, crush ampule at bottom of tube to release culture medium (see illustration).	Placing tip within culture medium maintains life of bacteria for testing.
7. Push tip of swab into liquid medium.	Preserves specimen for testing.
8. Place top on tube securely.	
9. In presence of patient, complete identification label (two identifiers, specimen source, collection date and time) and attach to tube. Attach properly completed laboratory requisition to tube. Enclose specimen in plastic biohazard bag (according to facility policy) and send immediately to laboratory.	Incorrect identification of specimen could result in diagnostic or therapeutic errors. Specimen not sent to laboratory immediately or refrigerated allows growth of organisms and inaccurate results.
10. See Standard Completion Protocol (inside front cover).	Reduces transmission of microorganisms.

EVALUATION

1. Monitor technique of culture collection process for potential contamination.
2. Inspect specimen for traces of blood, and reinspect mucosa if bleeding is apparent.
3. Check laboratory report for test results.
4. Use *Teach Back:* State to the patient, "I want to be sure I explained the purpose and why I need to perform a throat culture. Let's review it one more time and then you explain it to me in your own words." Evaluates what the patient is able to explain or demonstrate. Revise your instruction now or develop plan for revised patient teaching to be implemented at an appropriate time if patient is not able to teach back correctly.

Unexpected Outcomes and Related Interventions

1. Cultures reveal heavy bacterial growth.
   a. Notify health care provider of results.
   b. Administer antibiotics as ordered.
2. Culture was contaminated by bacteria from adjacent skin or tissues.
   a. Notify health care provider and repeat collection of cultures.
3. Patient experiences minor nasal bleeding.
   a. Apply mild pressure and ice pack over bridge of nose.
   b. Notify health care provider of patient's condition.

4. Patient unable to state teach back.
   a. Allow patient to ask questions.
   b. Revise your instructions and clarify misconceptions or directions.

Recording and Reporting

- Record type of specimen obtained, source, and time and date sent to laboratory; describe appearance of site and presence or absence of signs of local or systemic infection; note any unusual patient response to procedure.
- Report unusual test results to health care provider.
- Document your evaluation of patient learning.

Sample Documentation

0930   Report of sore throat, oral temp 101° F. Pharynx "red hot" with green-colored exudate noted on inspection.
0955   Explained purpose of a throat culture and what to expect during the procedure. Patient able to teach back procedure for throat culture. Stated that her throat was very sore but agreed to have specimen collected.
1000   Obtained throat culture per order. Tolerated without gagging or discomfort. Specimen sent to lab.

Special Considerations
Pediatric

- Immobilization of child's head and arms is important when obtaining nose or throat culture and should be done

in a firm, gentle, kind manner. Ask another nurse or ask and instruct a parent to assist if necessary.
- Showing tongue blade and penlight to child and demonstrating how to say "ah" helps to decrease anxiety.

- Do not attempt throat cultures if you suspect acute epiglottitis because trauma from swab might cause increase in edema and resulting occlusion of airway (Hockenberry and Wilson, 2013).

SKILL 8.4   COLLECTING A SPUTUM SPECIMEN

Sputum is mucus secretions produced by the cells of the lungs, bronchi, and trachea. You collect a specimen either by having a patient cough and expectorate into a sterile specimen container or by suctioning into a sterile sputum trap. In a normal health state, sputum production is minimal; a disease state can increase the amount and character of sputum. Sputum specimens are collected for three purposes:
1. Cytology to identify cancer cells
2. Culture and sensitivity (C&S) to identify specific pathogens and determine the antibiotics to which they are most sensitive
3. Acid-fast bacillus to support the diagnosis of pulmonary tuberculosis

Nasotracheal suctioning is required to collect a sputum specimen when a patient cannot expectorate sputum. Suctioning can provoke violent coughing, which can induce vomiting and constriction of pharyngeal, laryngeal, and bronchial muscles. Suctioning can also cause direct stimulation of vagal nerve fibers, resulting in cardiac arrhythmias and increased intracranial pressure.

ASSESSMENT

1. Identify patient using two identifiers (e.g., name and birth date or name and account number) according to facility policy. Compare identifiers with information on the patient's MAR or medical record. *Rationale: Ensures correct patient. Complies with The Joint Commission standards and improves patient safety (TJC, 2014).*
2. Check health care provider's orders for number and type of specimens needed and time and method of collection.
3. Assess patient's understanding of procedure and its purpose.
4. Assess patient's ability to cough and expectorate sputum. *Rationale: Suction is unnecessary when a patient can expectorate mucus.*
5. Determine when patient last ate a meal. *Rationale: It is best to obtain the specimen 1 to 2 hours after or 1 hour before a meal to minimize gagging, which can cause vomiting and aspiration.*
6. Assess patient's respiratory status, including respiratory rate, depth, and pattern; lung sounds; and lung color. *Rationale: Changes in respiration may indicate the presence of secretions in tracheobronchial tree and potential need for supplementary oxygenation.*
7. Assess patient's anxiety level. *Rationale: This procedure may be contraindicated in patients who cannot cooperate or remain still during the procedure (Pagana and Pagana, 2013).*

PLANNING

Expected Outcomes focus on collecting an uncontaminated specimen while maintaining a patent airway, adequate oxygenation, and patient comfort.
1. Patient's respirations are same rate and character before and after procedure.
2. Patient verbalizes understanding of the purpose and process of specimen collection.
3. Patient maintains comfort level and experiences minimal anxiety.
4. Sputum is not contaminated by saliva or oropharyngeal flora.

Delegation and Collaboration

Collection of a sputum specimen by suction may not be delegated. Collection of expectorated sputum specimens can be delegated to nursing assistive personnel (NAP). Instruct the NAP to:
- Notify nurse if patient expectorates bloody sputum.
- Notify nurse if patient has difficulty breathing

Equipment
- Completed identification labels with appropriate patient identifiers
- Completed laboratory requisition, including appropriate patient identification, date, time, name of test, and source of specimen
- Small plastic biohazard bag for delivery of specimen to laboratory (or container as specified by facility)

Sputum Collected by Expectoration
- Clean gloves
- Sterile specimen container with cover
- Oxygen therapy equipment if indicated
- Protective eyewear (if required)
- Facial tissue

Sputum Collected by Suction
- Suction device (wall or portable)
- Sterile suction catheter (size 13, 16, or 18 Fr [not large enough to cause trauma to nasal mucosa]) or suction catheter with sleeve
- Sterile gloves (a single glove if suction catheter has a sleeve)
- Sterile water 100-mL container
- In-line specimen container (sputum trap)
- Oxygen therapy equipment if indicated
- Protective eyewear (if required)
- Facial tissue

IMPLEMENTATION *for* COLLECTING A SPUTUM SPECIMEN

STEPS	RATIONALE

1. **See Standard Protocol (inside front cover).**
2. Position patient in high-Fowler's or semi-Fowler's position.

Promotes full lung expansion and facilitates ability to cough.

3. Explain steps of procedure and purpose. Instruct patient not to use mouthwash or toothpaste before procedure. During procedure have patient breathe normally to reduce hyperventilation.

Toothpaste and mouthwash may decrease the viability of microorganisms and alter culture results.

4. *Collect sputum specimen by expectoration.*

   a. Apply clean gloves. Provide sputum cup and instruct patient not to touch inside of container.

Decreases contamination, which can alter results.

   b. Instruct patient to take three to four deep slow breaths with full exhalation. Then take full inhalation followed immediately by a forceful cough, expectorating sputum directly into specimen container (see illustration). Repeat until 5 to 10 mL of sputum has been collected.

Sputum must come from tracheobronchial tree, and expectorant must not simply be saliva in mouth.

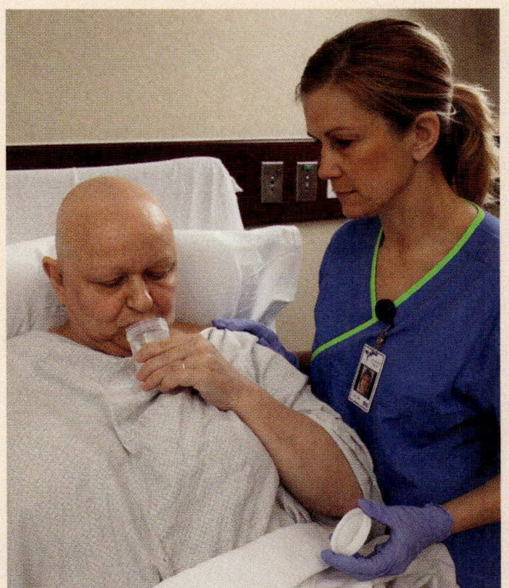

STEP 4b Expectorating sputum.

   c. Secure lid on specimen container.
5. If any sputum is present on outside of container, wipe it off with disinfectant.

Prevents spread of infection to persons handling specimen.

6. Offer patient tissues.
7. In presence of patient, complete label (two identifiers, specimen source, collection date and time) and attach to container. Attach completed laboratory requisition to container. Enclose specimen in a plastic biohazard bag and send immediately to laboratory.

Incorrect patient identification could lead to diagnostic or therapeutic error. Bacteria multiply quickly. Specimen should be analyzed promptly for accurate results.

Continued

STEPS	RATIONALE

8. Offer patient mouth care.

9. *Collect sputum specimen by suctioning.*

   a. If necessary, apply protective eyewear. Apply clean glove to nondominant hand. Prepare suction machine or device and make sure that it is functioning properly.

Adequate amount of suction is necessary to aspirate sputum.

   b. Connect suction tube to adapter on sputum trap. Open sterile water.

   c. Apply sterile glove to dominant hand or use clean glove if suction catheter has sterile plastic sleeve.

Allows handling of suction catheter without introducing microorganisms into sterile tracheobronchial tree.

   d. Connect sterile suction catheter to rubber tubing on sputum trap.

Aspirated sputum goes directly to trap instead of to suction tubing.

   e. Lubricate suction catheter tip with sterile water **(with suction off)**. Gently insert tip of suction catheter through nasopharynx, endotracheal tube, or tracheostomy without applying suction (see Chapter 14) (see illustration).

Minimizes trauma to airway as catheter is inserted. Lubrication allows for easier insertion.

   f. Gently and quickly advance catheter into trachea. Warn patient to expect to cough.

Placement of a catheter into larynx and trachea triggers cough reflex.

   g. As patient coughs, apply suction for 5 to 10 seconds, collecting 2 to 10 mL of sputum.

Suctioning longer than 10 seconds can cause hypoxia and mucosal damage (see Chapter 14).

   h. Release suction, remove catheter, and turn off suction. Detach and dispose of catheter into appropriate receptacle.

Releasing suction avoids unnecessary trauma to mucosa as catheter is withdrawn.

   i. Connect rubber tubing on sputum trap to plastic adapter (see illustration).

10. **See Standard Completion Protocol (inside front cover).**

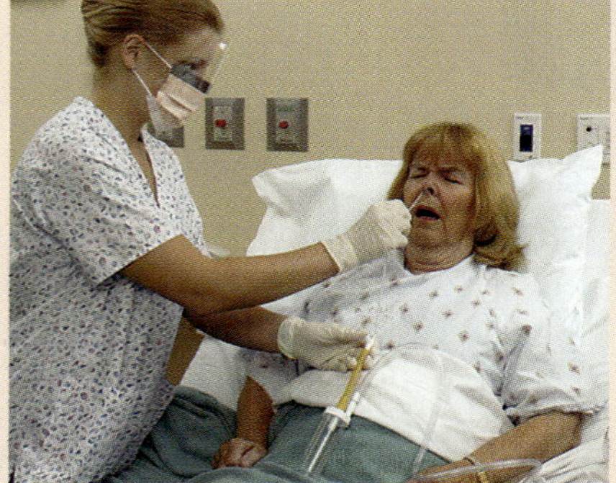

STEP 9e Insert catheter through nasopharynx.

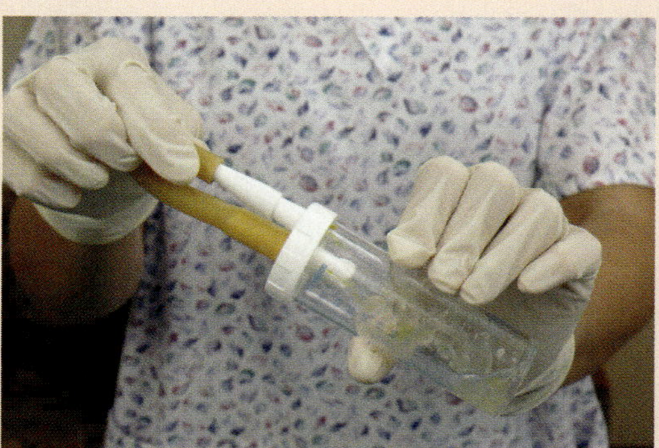

STEP 9i Closing sputum trap.

EVALUATION

1. Observe respiratory and oxygenation status throughout procedure, especially during suctioning.

2. Note behaviors suggesting anxiety or discomfort.

3. Observe character of sputum, color, consistency, odor, volume, viscosity, or presence of blood.

4. Refer to laboratory reports for test results.

5. Use *Teach Back:* State to the patient, "I want to be sure I explained the process of collecting a sputum specimen by coughing correctly. Let's review it one more time and then you can demonstrate for me." Evaluates what the patient is able to explain or demonstrate. Revise your instruction now or develop plan for revised patient teaching to be implemented at an appropriate time if patient is not able to teach back correctly.

Unexpected Outcomes and Related Interventions

1. Patient becomes hypoxic with increased respiratory rate and shortness of breath.
   a. Discontinue suctioning immediately.
   b. Administer oxygen (if ordered).
   c. Monitor vital signs and oxygen saturation.
   d. Notify health care provider if distress is unrelieved.
2. Inadequate amount of sputum is collected, or specimen contains saliva.
   a. Repeat collection procedure after patient has rested.
   b. Encourage patient to deep breathe and cough.
3. Patient remains anxious or complains of discomfort from suction catheter.
   a. Discontinue procedure until patient is stable.
   b. Provide oxygen as needed (if ordered).
   c. Notify health care provider of patient's condition.
   d. Continue to monitor patient's vital signs. Consider measuring oxygen saturation.
4. Patient unable to teach back.
   a. Allow patient to ask questions.
   b. Revise your instructions and clarify misconceptions or directions. Demonstrate difference between clearing throat and coughing.

Recording and Reporting

- Record method used to obtain specimen, date and time collected, type of test ordered, and transport to the laboratory. Describe characteristics of sputum specimen and patient's tolerance of procedure.
- Report any unusual findings such as bloody sputum or patient response such as increased dyspnea.
- Document your evaluation of patient learning.

Sample Documentation

0730 Patient unable to expectorate enough sputum for culture.

0740 Repeated explanation of procedure. Patient able to teach back procedure for expectorating sputum. Encouraged patient to deep breathe and cough.

0745 Patient expectorated 15 mL thick green sputum for culture; immediately transported to lab for C&S. Reports slight shortness of breath. Respirations 26 and unlabored.

Special Considerations
Home Care

- If patient is to obtain a sputum specimen at home, instruct patient or family caregiver regarding proper technique and importance of having sputum (not saliva) specimen sent to laboratory in timely manner.
- Discuss ways to avoid contaminating specimen (e.g., handwashing, using appropriate equipment).

• **Nursing Skills Online:** Specimen Collection, Lesson 5

When caring for a patient with a wound, you will regularly assess the condition of the wound and observe for the development of infection. Localized inflammation, tenderness, warmth at the wound site, and purulent drainage are signs and symptoms of wound infection. Infection is best treated with antibiotics after the causative organism or organisms are confirmed from a wound culture. Considerations when obtaining a wound culture are the following (Pagana and Pagana, 2013):

- Cultures of specimens from the skin edge yield much less accurate results than cultures of the suppurative material in the wound.
- If a patient is to undergo wound irrigation, obtain the culture before the wound is irrigated.
- If any antibiotic ointment or solution has been previously applied, remove it with sterile water or saline, wait several hours, and then obtain the culture.

Use separate techniques to collect specimens for measuring aerobic versus anaerobic microorganism growth. Aerobic organisms grow in superficial wounds exposed to the air. Anaerobic organisms grow deep within body cavities, where oxygen is not normally present.

ASSESSMENT

1. Identify patient using two identifiers (e.g., name and birth date or name and account number) according to facility policy. Compare identifiers with information on the patient's MAR or medical record. *Rationale: Ensures correct patient. Complies with The Joint Commission standards and improves patient safety (TJC, 2014).*
2. Assess patient's understanding of need for wound culture and ability to cooperate with procedure.
3. Assess patient for fever, chills, malaise, and elevated WBC count. *Rationale: Signs and symptoms indicate systemic infection.*
4. Assess severity of pain at wound site (scale of 0 to 10). *Rationale: If patient requires analgesic before dressing change or a wound culture, ideally medication is given 30 minutes before dressing change to reach peak effect.*

PLANNING

Expected Outcomes focus on obtaining an uncontaminated specimen while maintaining patient comfort.

1. Culture swab is free of contaminants.
2. Patient denies discomfort during procedure.
3. Patient can discuss purpose and procedure for specimen collection.

Delegation and Collaboration

The skill of obtaining wound drainage for culture cannot be delegated to nursing assistive personnel (NAP). The nurse instructs the NAP to:

- Report foul odor, increase in drainage, and increase in temperature or patient complaint of discomfort.

Equipment

- Culture tube with swab and transport medium for aerobic culture
- Anaerobic culture tube with swab (tubes contain carbon dioxide or nitrogen gas)
- 5- to 10-mL safety syringe and 19-gauge needle
- Clean and sterile gloves
- Protective eyewear
- Antiseptic swab
- Sterile dressing materials (determined by type of dressing)
- Paper or plastic disposable bag
- Completed identification labels with appropriate patient identifiers
- Completed laboratory requisition, including appropriate patient identification, date, time, name of test, and source of culture
- Small plastic biohazard bag for delivery of specimen to laboratory (or container as specified by facility)

IMPLEMENTATION *for* COLLECTING WOUND DRAINAGE SPECIMENS

STEPS	RATIONALE
1. **See Standard Protocol (inside front cover).**	
2. Apply clean gloves. If indicated, apply protective eyewear. Remove old dressing. Assess drainage. Fold soiled sides of dressing together and dispose in appropriate receptacle.	Provides baseline for condition of wound.
3. Cleanse area around wound edges with antiseptic swab. Wipe from edges outward. Remove old exudate.	Removes skin flora, preventing possible contamination of specimen.
4. Discard swab; remove and dispose of soiled gloves in trash bag. Perform hand hygiene.	
5. Open packages containing sterile culture tube and dressing supplies. *Apply sterile gloves.*	Provides sterile field from which nurse can handle supplies.
6. Obtain cultures.	
a. Aerobic culture	
(1) Take swab from culture tube, insert tip into wound in area of drainage, and rotate swab gently. Remove swab from wound and return to culture tube (wrap outside of ampule with gauze to prevent injury to your fingers). Crush ampule of medium and push swab into fluid (see illustration for Skill 8-3, Step 6).	Swab should be coated with fresh secretions from within wound. Medium keeps bacteria alive until analysis is complete.
b. Anaerobic culture	
(1) Take swab from special anaerobic culture tube, swab deeply into draining body cavity, and rotate gently. Remove swab from wound and return to culture tube.	Specimen is taken from deep cavity where oxygen is not present. Carbon dioxide or nitrogen gas keeps organisms alive until analysis is complete. Air injected into tube would cause organisms to die.
Or	
(2) Insert tip of syringe (without needle) into wound and aspirate 5 to 10 mL of exudate. Attach 19-gauge needle, expel all air, and inject drainage into special culture tube.	Sterile large-bore needle (19-gauge) allows exudate to transfer from sterile syringe into anaerobic culture tube without contamination or exposure to air.
7. In presence of patient, complete label (two identifiers, specimen source, collection date and time) and attach to tube. Attach completed laboratory requisition to tube. Note: Indicate on specimen requisition if patient is receiving antibiotics. Send specimens to laboratory immediately, no more than 30 minutes after collection (Pagana and Pagana, 2013).	Ensures correct results for correct patient. Bacteria grow rapidly. Prepare cultures quickly for accurate results.

STEPS	RATIONALE
8. Clean wound per health care provider's orders. Apply new sterile dressing (see Chapter 24). Secure dressing with tape or ties.	Protects wound from further contamination and aids in absorbing drainage and débriding wound.
9. See Standard Completion Protocol (inside front cover).	

EVALUATION

1. Observe character of wound drainage and edges of wound for redness and bleeding.
2. Ask patient to describe any discomfort during procedure.
3. Obtain laboratory report for results of cultures.
4. Use **Teach Back:** State to the patient, "I want to be sure I explained the purpose and process of collecting a small amount of drainage from your abdominal wound for a culture test. Let's review it one more time and then describe the purpose and process in your own words." Evaluates what the patient is able to explain or demonstrate. Revise your instruction now or develop plan for revised patient teaching to be implemented at an appropriate time if patient is not able to teach back correctly.

Unexpected Outcomes and Related Interventions

1. Wound cultures reveal heavy bacterial growth.
   a. Monitor patient for fever, chills, and increased WBC count.
   b. Inform health care provider of findings.
2. Laboratory report indicates wound culture is contaminated with superficial skin cells.
   a. Monitor patient for fever and pain.
   b. Inform health care provider.
   c. Repeat collection of specimen as ordered.
3. Patient unable to teach back.
   a. Allow patient to ask questions.
   b. Revise your instructions and clarify misconceptions or directions.

Recording and Reporting

- Record type of specimen obtained, source, and time and date specimen sent to laboratory; describe appearance of wound and characteristics of drainage; describe patient's tolerance to procedure and response to analgesia.
- Report any evidence of infection to health care provider.
- Document your evaluation of patient learning.

Sample Documentation

1320 Patient reports pain from surgical site. Dressing change reveals 4-cm right lower quadrant (RLQ) abdominal wound, separated at top with yellow purulent drainage. Lower half of incision remains well approximated.

1345 Order received to culture abdominal wound. Patient reports that he is very anxious and confused about what this "culture" means. Explained procedure and purpose of the need for the culture. Patient able to teach back procedure for wound culture and agrees to procedure.

1400 Aerobic culture obtained from site of drainage, sent to laboratory as ordered.

Special Considerations
Pediatric

- In some facilities, if you anticipate that the procedure will be painful for the child, perform procedure in area other than child's room, keeping child's room a safe place (Hockenberry and Wilson, 2013).

Home Care

- Risks for wound infections are different in the home setting than in the hospital setting because a patient is less susceptible to infections from microorganisms in the home environment. Careful handwashing and clean technique are usually adequate for performing dressing changes by patients and family caregivers in the home.

SKILL 8.6   BLOOD GLUCOSE MONITORING

A blood glucose meter is an effective and efficient method for assessing glucose control in a patient with diabetes mellitus. In the health care setting, the monitor used may be different from the type the patient uses at home. The patient needs to know about the general principles for accurate glucose monitoring and reporting results. It is often helpful to request that a family caregiver bring the meter from home to assess the patient's skill. Blood glucose monitoring (BGM) checks glucose levels in a sample of capillary blood, usually obtained by using the fingertip method. The results are used to direct lifestyle changes such as diet, medication, and physical activity. Regular BGM is an essential component of any diabetes self-management program (ADA, 2013b).

Blood glucose meters available today are portable, lightweight, and battery powered. They provide fast results, usually in 1 minute or less and some in 5 seconds (Diabetes

Forecast, 2013). Most meters now allow for the use of alternate site or forearm capillary blood testing. Many believe that this is less painful than fingerstick testing. Alternate-site testing is most accurate and correlates best to fingerstick testing when blood glucose levels are not changing rapidly, such as during the period when fasting blood glucose levels are being checked.

Improved technology introduced two methods for glucose measurement now available on the market. A minimally invasive glucose meter uses a very small, fine plastic sensor inserted through the abdomen and provides continuous readings of blood glucose levels. A biosensor is taped on the external abdomen. Using a handheld wireless meter, a patient activates the biosensor to transmit the blood glucose level at any time without puncturing the skin. Another model, considered a noninvasive glucose meter, does not prick the skin with a needle but uses precise laser technology or light beam to puncture the skin, resulting in less damage to tissue. For the patient with diabetes mellitus who requires assessment of trends and patterns, these systems are ideal.

This skill describes the technique used to measure blood glucose with a specific style of glucose meter. Specific steps in using meters vary, depending on the make and model of the equipment used. Always follow manufacturer instructions and facility policy and procedure when performing BGM.

ASSESSMENT

1. Identify patient using two identifiers (e.g., name and birth date or name and account number) according to facility policy. Compare identifiers with information on the patient's MAR or medical record. *Rationale: Ensures correct patient. Complies with The Joint Commission standards and improves patient safety (TJC, 2014).*
2. Assess patient's understanding of the procedure and the purpose and importance of BGM. *Rationale: Provides baseline on which to provide necessary teaching. Adult patients learn best when the teaching and learning relate to what the patient already knows.*
3. Review all medications that the patient is receiving. *Rationale: Drugs such as corticosteroids, diuretics, and anesthetics increase blood glucose levels. Anticoagulants increase risk for local ecchymosis or excessive bleeding from puncture site.*
4. Determine if specific conditions need to be met before or after glucose level is checked (e.g., fasting or postprandial status; medication administration, including insulin). *Rationale: Dietary intake, especially of carbohydrates, alters*

blood glucose levels. Doses of short-acting or rapid-acting insulin before a meal are based on current blood glucose levels.

5. Assess area of skin to be used at puncture site. Inspect fingers or forearms for edema, inflammation, or open cuts or sores. Avoid areas of bruising or open lesions and the hand on the side of a mastectomy. *Rationale: The puncture site should not be edematous, inflamed, or recently punctured because these factors cause increased interstitial fluid and blood to mix, which increases the risk for infection (Pagana and Pagana, 2013). The sides of the fingertips have fewer nerve endings and good vascularity.*
6. Review the health care provider's order for timing and frequency of blood glucose measurement. *Rationale: Test schedule is based on patient's physiological status, risk for glucose imbalance, and any established facility protocols.*

PLANNING

Expected Outcomes focus on minimizing tissue damage at the puncture site, achieving accurate results, and maintaining blood glucose levels within the patient's goal range.

1. Puncture site shows no evidence of excessive or prolonged bleeding or tissue damage.
2. Blood glucose measurements are accurate.
3. Patient can verbalize procedure for self-monitoring of blood glucose and provide feedback on possible causes of results that are out of the target range.

Delegation and Collaboration

When the patient's condition is stable, the skill of obtaining and testing a sample of blood for blood glucose level can be delegated to nursing assistive personnel (NAP). Instruct the NAP by:

- Explaining what sites to use for the puncture and when to obtain glucose levels.
- Reviewing expected values and reminding to report all unexpected glucose levels to the nurse.

Equipment

- Antiseptic swab
- Lancet device, either self-activating or button activated
- Sterile single-use lancet specific to lancet device
- Blood glucose meter (e.g., OneTouch, FreeStyle Freedom)
- Blood glucose test strips appropriate for meter brand used
- Clean gloves

IMPLEMENTATION *for* BLOOD GLUCOSE MONITORING

STEPS	RATIONALE
1. **See Standard Protocol (inside front cover).**	
2. Instruct patient to wash hands and forearm (if applicable) thoroughly with soap and warm water. Rinse and dry.	Reduces presence of microorganisms and any food residue. Food residue can contaminate blood drop and cause false reading. Warmth promotes vasodilatation at puncture site. Establishes practice for patient when test is performed at home.

STEPS	RATIONALE

3. Position patient comfortably in chair or in semi-Fowler's position in bed.

Ensures easy accessibility to puncture site.

4. Remove reagent strip from vial and tightly recap.

Protects strips from accidental discoloration caused by exposure to air or light.

5. Check the code on the test strip vial. Use test strips recommended for the glucose meter. Some newer meters do not require entering the code or have a disk or drum with 10 or more test strips.

Code on test strip must match code entered into the glucose meter to generate accurate results.

6. Insert the test strip into the meter. Do not bend the strip. The meter turns on automatically.

A bent strip does not measure blood sample accurately.

7. Apply clean gloves. Prepare lancet device. Two types of lancet devices are used to perform skin punctures: single-use and multiple-use.

   a. Single-use lancet (see illustration).

Decreases cross-contamination between patients.

   b. Multiple-use lancet device is prepared with a new lancet (see illustration). *NOTE: Some meters recommend that this step be completed before preparing the test strip.* Remove cap from lancet device. Insert new lancet. Some lancet devices have a disk or cylinder that rotates to a new lancet.

Never reuse a lancet because of risk of infection.

   (1) Twist off protective cover on the tip of the lancet. Replace cap of the lancet device.

   (2) Cock the lancet device, adjusting for proper puncture depth.

Each patient varies as to depth of insertion needed for lancet to produce blood drop.

8. Obtain blood sample.

   a. Wipe finger or forearm lightly with antiseptic swab. Choose a vascular area for puncture site. In stable adults, select lateral side of finger; be sure to avoid central tip of finger, which has a denser nerve supply (Pagana and Pagana, 2013).

Removes resident microorganisms. Too much alcohol can cause blood to hemolyze. Side of finger is less sensitive to pain and has a dense nerve supply. Do not use alternate site when patients are hypoglycemic, prone to hypoglycemia (during peak activity of an injected basal insulin or 2 hours after injecting rapid-acting insulin), after exercise, during illness, or when blood glucose levels are rapidly increasing or decreasing.

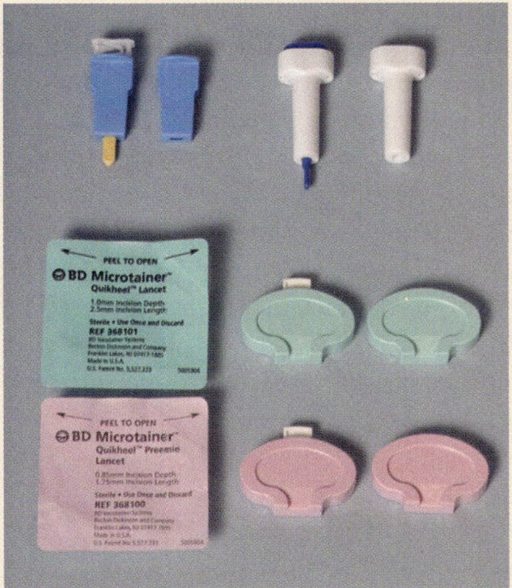

STEP 7a Single-use lancet devices. (Courtesy Zack Bent. From Garrels M, Oatis CS: *Laboratory testing for ambulatory settings: a guide for health care professionals,* Philadelphia, 2006, Saunders.)

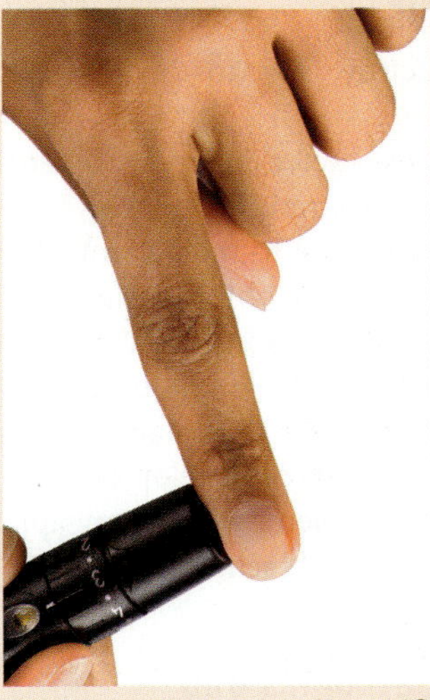

STEP 7b Multiple-use lancet device. (Courtesy Accu-Chek Multiclix.)

Continued

STEPS	RATIONALE

b. Hold area to be punctured in a dependent position. Do not milk or massage the finger site.

Increases blood flow to area before puncture. Milking may hemolyze the specimen and introduce excess tissue fluid (Pagana and Pagana, 2013).

c. Hold the tip of the lancet device against the area of skin chosen for a test site (see illustration). Press the release button on the device. Some devices allow you to see the blood sample forming. Remove the device.

Placement ensures that lancet enters skin properly.

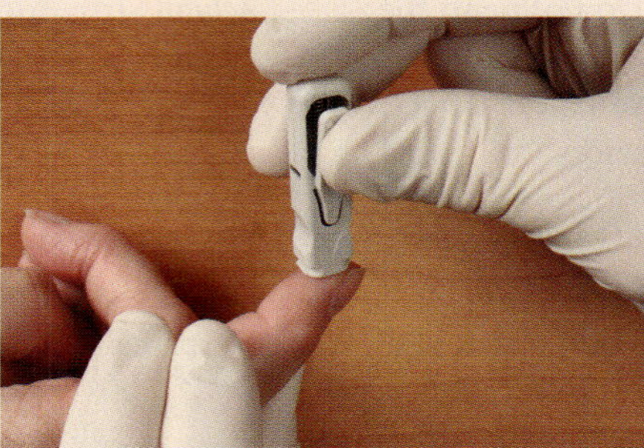

STEP 8c Prick side of finger with lancet.

9. Obtain test results.

   a. Be sure that meter is still on. Bring the test strip in the meter to the drop of blood. The blood will be wicked onto the test strip. Follow specific meter directions to be sure that you obtain a full sample. Do not scrape or apply blood to wrong side of test strip.

Blood enters strip, and glucose device shows message on screen to signal that enough blood is obtained. Scraping or use of wrong side of test strip prevents proper glucose measurement.

   b. The blood glucose test result appears on the screen. Some devices beep when completed. Share result with patient.

Supports patient's self-management of blood glucose.

10. Turn meter off. Some meters automatically turn off.

Meter is battery powered.

11. See Standard Completion Protocol (inside front cover).

EVALUATION

1. Observe puncture site for evidence of bleeding or bruising.

2. Compare glucose meter reading with target blood glucose levels and prior test results.

3. Use *Teach Back:* State to the patient, "I want to be sure I explained the way to obtain your blood glucose. Let's review it one more time and then you show me how to do the technique on your blood glucose monitor." Evaluates what the patient is able to explain or demonstrate. Revise your instruction now or develop plan for revised patient teaching to be implemented at an appropriate time if patient is not able to teach back correctly.

Unexpected Outcomes and Related Interventions

1. Puncture site continues to bleed or is bruised.
   a. Apply pressure to site.
   b. Notify health care provider.

2. Glucose meter malfunctions.

   a. Repeat test, following directions.
   b. Follow manufacturer's directions for malfunctions.

3. Blood glucose level above or below target range.
   a. Continue to monitor patient.
   b. Follow facility protocol for laboratory confirmation testing of very high or very low results. Laboratory testing generally is considered more accurate.
   c. Check medical record to see if there is a medication order for deviations in glucose level; if not, notify health care provider.
   d. Administer insulin or carbohydrate source as ordered (depending on glucose level).
   e. Notify health care provider of patient's response.

4. Patient unable to teach back.
   a. Allow patient to ask questions.
   b. Revise your instructions and clarify misconceptions or directions.

Recording and Reporting

• Record glucose results on appropriate flow sheet and describe response, including presence or absence of pain or excessive oozing of blood at puncture site.

- Report blood glucose levels out of target range and take appropriate action for hypoglycemia or hyperglycemia.
- Document your evaluation of patient learning.

Sample Documentation

0730   Patient able to teach back and demonstrate use of new glucose monitor for home use.
0800   Patient correctly obtained blood glucose level of 110; able to teach back about normal and abnormal blood glucose levels. Denies questions at this time.

Special Considerations
Geriatric

- Older adults who have difficulty seeing the readings on the meter display screen may use a device with a larger display screen and lighted background or an audio blood glucose meter that gives verbal instructions to guide the patient through the procedure and give an audio result.
- Older adults with musculoskeletal alterations may not have the fine-motor coordination necessary to manipulate the device and place blood samples on test strips or insert strips in meter. Some models can be loaded with multiple strips.

Home Care

- Patients should usually assess blood glucose levels before meals, before taking medication, and at bedtime to monitor effectiveness of treatment plan.
- One or more family caregivers should be able to monitor blood glucose levels in the event that the patient is unable to do so independently.

<table><tr><td>SKILL 8.7   COLLECTING BLOOD AND CULTURE SPECIMENS BY VENIPUNCTURE (SYRINGE AND VACUTAINER METHOD)</td></tr></table>

Blood tests are one of the most commonly used diagnostic measures that yield valuable information about a patient's nutritional, hematological, metabolic, immune, and bio-chemical status. These tests allow health care providers to screen patients for early signs of physical illness, monitor changes in acute or chronic diseases, and evaluate responses to therapies.

Because larger veins are sources of blood for both laboratory tests and routes for IV fluid or blood administration, maintaining their integrity is essential. It is important to use the most distal sites first and retain one or more appropriate sites for IV access. Do not draw blood from a site proximal to an IV insertion site.

After obtaining a specimen, place it directly into the appropriate blood tube. A color-coding system for the tops of the collection tubes indicates the types of specimens that can be collected within each tube (see facility procedure). Special blood tubes may contain an additive. For example, a tube with an anticoagulant is used for a test that requires blood not to be clotted or hemolyzed.

Venipuncture is the most common method of obtaining blood specimens. This method involves insertion of a hollow-bore needle into the lumen of a large vein to obtain a specimen using either a needle and syringe or a Vacutainer device that allows the drawing of multiple samples.

Blood cultures aid in the detection of bacteria in the blood. It is important that at least two culture specimens be drawn from two different sites. Because fever and chills may accompany bacteremia, blood cultures may be drawn when symptoms are present (Pagana and Pagana, 2013). If only one culture produces bacteria, the assumption is that the bacteria were skin contaminants rather than the infecting agent.

Bacteremia exists when both cultures grow the infectious agent.

ASSESSMENT

1. Identify patient using two identifiers (e.g., name and birth date or name and account number) according to facility policy. Compare identifiers with information on the patient's MAR or medical record. *Rationale: Ensures correct patient. Complies with The Joint Commission standards and improves patient safety (TJC, 2014).*
2. Determine patient's understanding of purpose of test and ability to cooperate with procedure. *Rationale: Procedure can appear threatening to patient and is uncomfortable.*
3. Determine if special conditions need to be met for specimen collection (e.g., patient allowed nothing by mouth [NPO], a specific time for collection in relation to time medication is given, need to ice specimen). *Rationale: Some patients have special conditions for accurate measurement of blood elements (e.g., fasting blood sugar, drug peak and trough, ammonia levels).*
4. Assess patient for possible risk factors for venipuncture, which include anticoagulant therapy, low platelet count, or bleeding disorder. Review medication history. *Rationale: Abnormal clotting caused by low platelet count, hemophilia, or medications increases risk for bleeding and hematoma formation.*
5. Assess patient for contraindicated sites for venipuncture: presence of IV infusion, hematoma at potential site, arm on side of mastectomy or axillary surgery, or hemodialysis shunt. *Rationale: Drawing specimens from such sites can result in false test results or may injure patient.*

6. Identify latex allergies, tape sensitivity, or povidone-iodine (Betadine) allergy. *Rationale: Determines the need for avoiding exposure to these items.*
7. Before drawing blood cultures, assess for systemic evidence of bacteremia, including fever and chills. *Rationale: Three blood samples should be drawn at least 1 hour apart beginning at the earliest sign of sepsis (Pagana and Pagana, 2013).*
8. Review health care provider's order for type of blood tests. *Rationale: Order is required. Type of test determines blood tubes to use and amount of specimen.*

PLANNING

Expected Outcomes focus on the collection of an uncontaminated, appropriate blood specimen.
1. Patient explains purpose of blood collections before collection is attempted.
2. Venipuncture site shows no evidence of continued bleeding or hematoma.
3. Patient denies anxiety or discomfort.
4. An adequate sample is collected for testing (see facility report or appropriate laboratory manual).

Delegation and Collaboration

The skill of collecting blood specimens by venipuncture can be delegated to trained nursing assistive personnel (NAP). In some settings, phlebotomists are available. Instruct the NAP by:
- Explaining patient's condition (e.g., presence of IV therapy, edema that affects extremity or vein for venipuncture selection).
- Instructing personnel to report patient's discomfort or signs of excessive bleeding to the nurse.

Equipment
All Procedures
- Chlorhexidine or antiseptic swab (check facility policy for use of 70% alcohol or other antiseptic solution)
- Clean gloves
- Small pillow or folded towel
- Sterile gauze pads (2 × 2 inch)
- Tourniquet
- Adhesive bandage or adhesive tape
- Appropriate blood tubes
- Completed identification labels with appropriate patient identifiers
- Completed laboratory requisition, including appropriate patient identification, date, time, name of test, and source of specimen
- Small plastic biohazard bag for delivery of specimen to laboratory (or container as specified by facility)
- Sharps container

Venipuncture with Syringe
- Sterile safety needles (20- to 21-gauge for adults; 23- to 25-gauge for children)
- Sterile 10- to 20-mL Luer-Lok safety syringe
- Needle-free blood transfer device

Venipuncture with Vacutainer
- Vacutainer and safety access device with Luer-Lok adapter
- Sterile double-ended needles (20- to 21-gauge for adults; 23- to 25-gauge for children)

Blood Cultures
- Two 20-mL sterile syringes
- Sterile safety needles (20- to 21-gauge for adults; 23- to 25-gauge for children)
- Anaerobic and aerobic culture bottles (check facility policy)

IMPLEMENTATION *for* COLLECTING BLOOD AND CULTURE SPECIMENS BY VENIPUNCTURE (SYRINGE AND VACUTAINER METHOD)

STEPS	RATIONALE
1. **See Standard Protocol (inside front cover).**	
2. Assist patient with lying supine or sitting in semi-Fowler's position or in a chair with arm supported and elbow extended. Place small pillow or towel under upper arm. (Option: Lower arm briefly to fill hand and lower arm with blood.)	Helps to stabilize extremity. Supported position in bed reduces chance of injury to patient if fainting occurs.
3. Apply tourniquet so that it can be removed by pulling an end with a single motion.	Tourniquet blocks venous return to heart from extremity, causing veins to dilate for easier visibility.
a. Position the tourniquet 5 to 10 cm (3 to 4 inches) above venipuncture site selected.	
b. Cross the tourniquet over patient's arm (see illustration). May place tourniquet over gown sleeve to protect skin.	Older adult's skin is very fragile.

STEPS	RATIONALE

c. Hold tourniquet between your fingers close to the arm. Tuck a loop between the patient's arm and the tourniquet so you can grasp the free end easily (see illustration).

Pull free end to release tourniquet after the venipuncture.

> **SAFE PATIENT CARE** Palpate distal pulse (e.g., radial) below tourniquet. If pulse is not palpable, the tourniquet is too tight and impeding arterial blood flow. If this happens, remove and wait 60 seconds before reapplying tourniquet more loosely or using other extremity. Keeping the tourniquet in place no longer than 1 minute minimizes effects of hemoconcentration and hemolysis (Pagana and Pagana, 2013). Prolonged time may alter test results and cause pain and venous stasis (e.g., falsely elevated serum potassium level) (Metheny, 2012).

4. Inspect extremity for best venipuncture site, looking for straight, prominent vein without swelling or hematoma. Of the three veins located in the antecubital area, the median cubital vein is preferred (see illustration).

This vein is large, well anchored (does not easily move), closer to the surface of the skin, and less painful to puncture. Straight and intact veins are easiest to puncture. The veins of the lower arm and hand are preferred for administering IV fluids.

5. Palpate selected vein with finger. Note if vein is firm and rebounds when palpated or if it feels rigid and cordlike and rolls when palpated. Avoid vigorously slapping vein because this can cause vasospasm.

A healthy vein is elastic and rebounds on palpation. Thrombosed vein is rigid, rolls easily, and is difficult to puncture.

6. Apply clean gloves. Obtain blood specimen.

a. Syringe method

(1) Have syringe with appropriate needle securely attached.

(2) Cleanse venipuncture site with antiseptic swabs, the first swab moving back and forth on horizontal plane, then another swab on a vertical plane, and the last swab in a circular motion from site outward for about 5 cm (2 inches). Allow to dry.

Antimicrobial agent cleanses skin surface of resident bacteria so that organisms do not enter puncture site. Allowing antiseptic to dry completes its antimicrobial task and reduces "sting" of venipuncture. Alcohol left on skin can cause hemolysis of sample.

(a) If drawing sample for blood alcohol level or blood cultures, use antiseptic swab only rather than alcohol swab.

Ensures accurate test results.

(3) Remove needle cover and inform patient of "stick" lasting only a few seconds.

Prepares patient and prevents sudden movement from the needle.

> **SAFE PATIENT CARE** Observe needle for defects such as burrs, which can cause increased discomfort and damage to patient's veins (McCall and Tankersley, 2012).

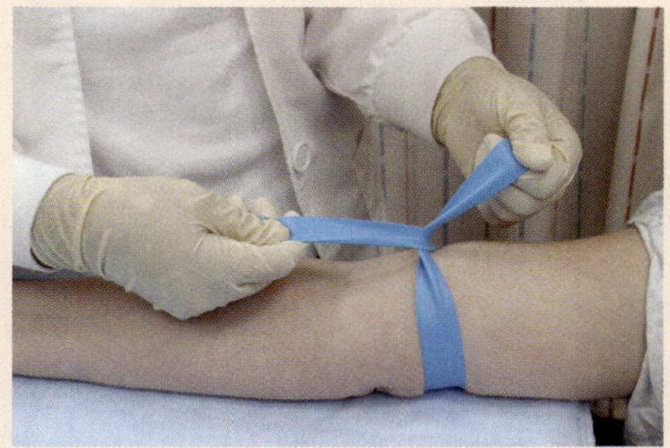

STEP 3b Cross tourniquet over the arm.

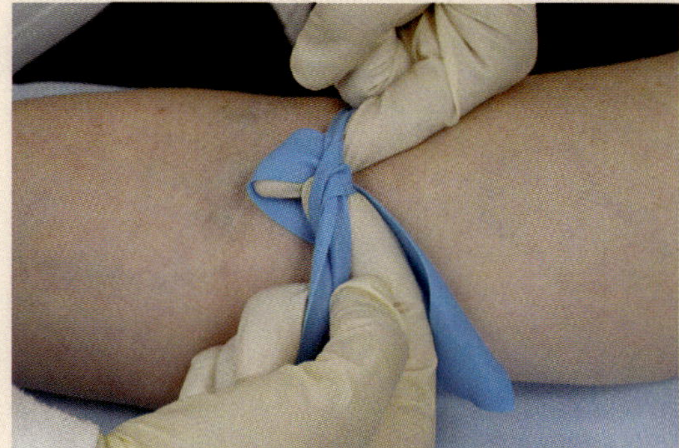

STEP 3c Tuck a loop between patient's arm and tourniquet.

Continued

<table>
<tr><td>STEPS</td><td>RATIONALE</td></tr>
</table>

(4) Place thumb or forefinger of nondominant hand 2.5 cm (1 inch) below site, and gently pull skin taut. Stretch skin steadily until vein is stabilized.

Stabilizes vein and minimizes rolling during needle insertion.

(5) Hold syringe and needle at a 15- to 30-degree angle from patient's arm with bevel up.

Angle and bevel-up position facilitate entry of the needle into the vein.

(6) Slowly insert needle into vein, stopping when a "pop" is felt as needle enters vein (see illustration).

Prevents puncture through the opposite side of the vein.

(7) Hold syringe securely and pull back gently on plunger.

Creates a vacuum for withdrawal of blood specimen.

(8) Observe for blood return and withdraw until you obtain the desired amount of blood.

Verifies placement in the vein.

(9) Release tourniquet before removing needle.

Reduces bleeding at site.

(10) Apply 2 × 2–inch gauze pad over puncture site without pressure (see illustration). Quickly but carefully withdraw needle, and apply pressure after removal of needle. If patient is on anticoagulants, hold site for several minutes.

Minimizes discomfort and trauma to vein. Prevents bruising and oozing of blood at venipuncture site.

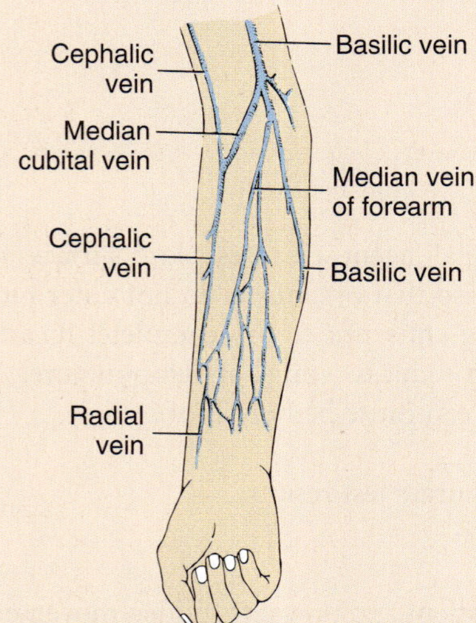

STEP 4 Location of antecubital veins.

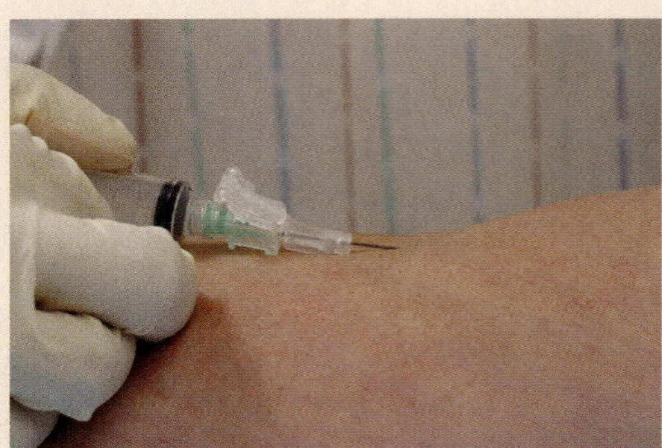

STEP 6a(6) Inserting needle into vein.

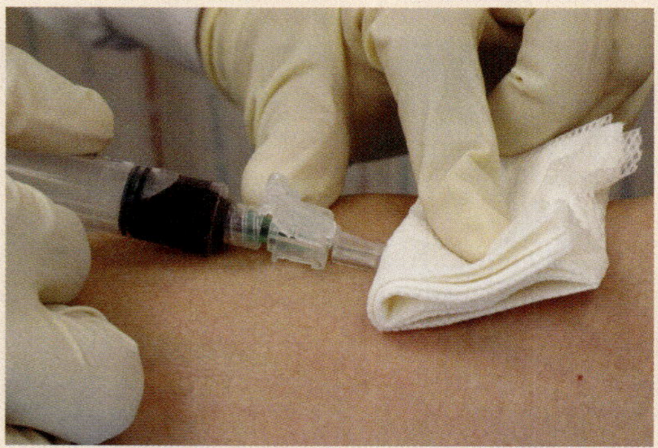

STEP 6a(10) Apply gauze over puncture site.

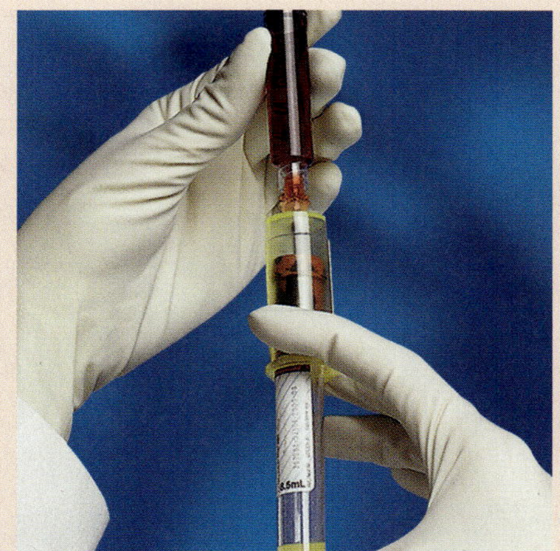

STEP 6a(12) Attach blood-filled syringe to needle-free blood transfer device. (Courtesy and © Becton, Dickinson and Company.)

STEPS	RATIONALE

(11) Activate needle safety cover and immediately discard needle in proper receptacle.

Phlebotomy equipment must include needle safety devices. Reduces risk of needlestick injury (OSHA, 2012).

(12) Attach blood-filled syringe to needle-free blood transfer device. Attach tube and allow vacuum to fill tube to specified level. Remove and fill other tubes as appropriate (see illustration). Gently rotate each tube back and forth 8 to 10 times.

Prevents needlestick injury. Tubes with additives should be inverted as soon as possible. Prevents clotting as additives are mixed with blood.

b. Vacutainer system method

(1) Attach double-ended needle to Vacutainer tube (see illustration).

Long end of needle is used to puncture vein, and short end fits into blood specimen tube.

(2) Have proper blood specimen tube resting inside Vacutainer device, but do not puncture rubber stopper.

Tubes are color coded to indicate intended use based on size of tube and presence or absence of a chemical additive. Puncture of stopper results in loss of vacuum.

(3) Cleanse venipuncture site with antiseptic swabs, the first swab moving back and forth on horizontal plane, then another swab on a vertical plane, and the last swab in a circular motion from site outward for about 5 cm (2 inches). Allow to dry.

Antimicrobial agent cleanses skin surface of resident bacteria so that organisms do not enter puncture site. Allowing alcohol to dry reduces "sting" of venipuncture. If using an alcohol swab, the risk of hemolysis increases from the alcohol left on the skin.

(4) Remove needle cover and inform patient that he or she will feel "stick" lasting only a few seconds.

Explanation of what to expect reduces anxiety.

(5) Place thumb or forefinger of nondominant hand 2.5 cm (1 inch) *below* site and pull skin taut. Stretch skin down until vein is stabilized.

Position of finger below site prevents accidental needlestick. Stretching helps to stabilize vein and prevents rolling during needle insertion.

(6) Hold Vacutainer needle at 15- to 30-degree angle from arm with bevel of needle up.

Reduces chance of penetrating both sides of vein during insertion and is less traumatic to the vein.

(7) Slowly insert needle into vein (see illustration).

Prevents puncture on opposite side.

(8) Grasp Vacutainer securely and advance specimen tube into needle of holder (do not advance needle in vein).

Pushing needle through stopper breaks vacuum and causes flow of blood into tube. Advancing needle into vein may puncture vein.

(9) Note flow of blood into tube, which should be fairly rapid (see illustration).

Failure of blood to appear indicates that vacuum in tube is lost or needle is not in vein.

(10) After filling specimen tube, grasp Vacutainer firmly and remove tube. Insert additional specimen tubes as needed. Gently rotate each tube back and forth 8 to 10 times.

Prevents needle from advancing or dislodging. Tubes with additives should be inverted as soon as possible. Prevents clotting as additives are mixed with blood.

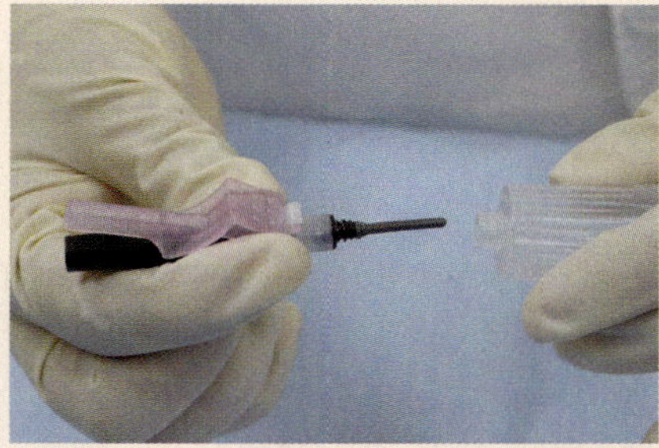

STEP 6b(1) Attach double-ended needle.

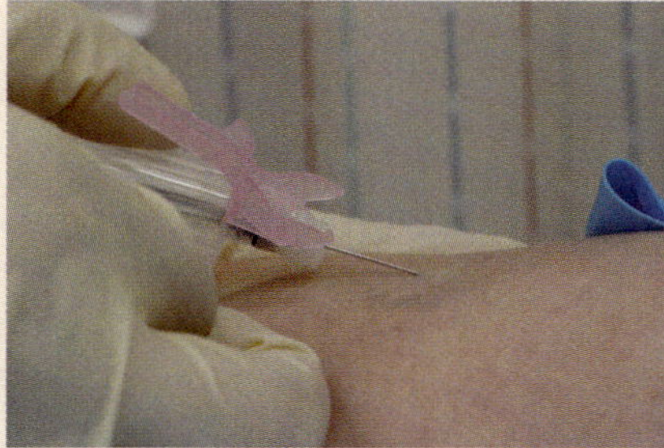

STEP 6b(7) Insert Vacutainer needle into vein.

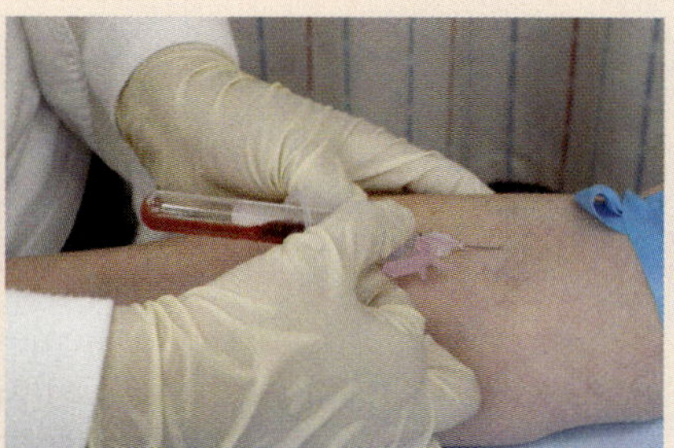

STEP 6b(9) Note rapid flow of blood into tube.

Continued

STEPS	RATIONALE
(11) Release tourniquet before removing needle. Immediately apply pressure over venipuncture site for 2 to 3 minutes or until bleeding stops. Apply gauze dressing securely.	Reduces bleeding at site when needle is withdrawn.
c. Blood culture	
(1) Cleanse venipuncture site with antiseptic swab (check facility policy). Allow to dry.	Antimicrobial agent cleanses skin surface so that organisms do not enter puncture site or contaminate culture. Drying ensures complete antimicrobial action.
(2) Clean bottle tops of culture bottles for 15 seconds with either alcohol or antiseptic swab. Check facility policy regarding cleaning solution.	Ensures that specimen is sterile.
(3) Collect 10 to 15 mL of venous blood using syringe method from first venipuncture site and repeat procedure in other arm.	Specimens must be obtained from two sites to confirm culture growth.
(4) With each specimen, activate needle safety cover, discard needle on syringe, and replace with new sterile needle before injecting blood sample into culture bottles.	Maintains sterile technique and prevents contamination of specimen.
(5) If both aerobic and anaerobic cultures are needed, fill the anaerobic container first (Pagana and Pagana, 2013).	Anaerobic organisms may take longer to grow.
(6) Gently mix blood in each culture bottle.	Mixes medium and blood.
(7) Release tourniquet, apply gauze over puncture site, and withdraw needle.	
7. Observe for any sign of blood on outside of tube; decontaminate with 70% alcohol.	
8. Double needles have built-in safety cover; activate and then discard in proper receptacle for disposal.	One-handed technique and activation of safe needle devices helps to avoid needlestick injuries and exposure to potentially fatal bloodborne pathogens (OSHA, 2012).
9. In presence of patient, label the specimen with patient identifiers, date, and time. Label each tube noting the arm from which specimen was drawn. Attach the proper completed requisition to specimen container.	Ensures diagnostic information reported on correct patient.
10. Place all specimens in plastic biohazard bag and send to laboratory. Send cultures immediately to laboratory (Pagana and Pagana, 2013).	Minimizes spread of microorganisms.
11. See Standard Completion Protocol (inside front cover).	

▍EVALUATION

1. Reinspect venipuncture site for hemostasis.
2. Determine if patient is anxious or fearful.
3. Check laboratory report for test results.
4. Use **Teach Back:** State to the patient, "I want to be sure I explained the purpose of drawing your blood for a complete blood count and why we need these results. Let's review it one more time and then you explain it to me in your own words." Evaluates what the patient is able to explain or demonstrate. Revise your instruction now or develop plan for revised patient teaching to be implemented at an appropriate time if patient is not able to teach back correctly.

Unexpected Outcomes and Related Interventions

1. Hematoma forms at venipuncture site.
   a. Apply pressure using 2 × 2–inch gauze dressing.
   b. Continue to monitor patient for pain and discomfort.

2. Bleeding at site continues.
   a. Apply pressure and have patient help to maintain pressure on site; continue to monitor.
3. Laboratory tests reveal significantly abnormal blood results (see laboratory report or laboratory manual for normal limits).
   a. Report to health care provider.
4. Patient unable to teach back.
   a. Allow patient to ask questions.
   b. Revise your instructions and clarify misconceptions or directions.

Recording and Reporting

- Record method used to obtain blood specimen, date and time collected, type of test ordered, site (for blood cultures), and laboratory receiving specimen; describe venipuncture site after specimen collection and patient's response to procedure.
- Report abnormal results to health care provider.
- Document your evaluation of patient learning.

Sample Documentation

1000 Patient refused to have blood drawn for CBC. Explained purpose and need for the information obtained from results.
1015 Patient able to teach back reason for obtaining CBC and agreed to have blood drawn.

1025 CBC specimen drawn from left median cubital vein. Specimen sent to laboratory.

Special Considerations
Pediatric

- Explain procedure to child using developmentally appropriate language.
- Apply EMLA cream over planned puncture site 60 minutes before procedure; other local anesthetic cream may be ordered to reduce pain in infants and young children (Hockenberry and Wilson, 2013).
- When performing venipuncture on children, explore a variety of sources for vein access (e.g., scalp, antecubital fossa, saphenous veins, hand veins) to ensure access.
- Vacutainers are not recommended for children younger than 2 years of age because of possible vein collapse (Hockenberry and Wilson, 2013).

Geriatric

- Older adults have fragile skin and veins that are easily traumatized during venipuncture. Sometimes application of warm compresses may help in obtaining samples.
- A small-bore needle or catheter also may be beneficial.

CRITICAL THINKING EXERCISES

Case Study

An 82-year-old woman was admitted to the medical-surgical unit 3 days ago for uncontrolled diabetes mellitus. She lives with her eldest daughter. Her fasting blood sugar has been decreasing with new medications and moving toward desired level of 110. At 7:00 A.M., the NAP reports that the patient seems confused and is complaining of frequency and burning with urination. Vital signs are BP 98/80, pulse 86, respiratory rate 20, temperature 38.4°C (101.2°F), and fasting blood sugar 165. You recheck the vital signs and fasting blood sugar. You check her indwelling catheter bag and note that her urine is cloudy, pink-tinged, and foul-smelling. When you ask the patient if she knows what this building is called, she is unable to state that she is in a hospital. She is also unable to state her date of birth.

1. The nurse calls the health care provider and receives an order for a urine culture and sensitivity (C&S). The nurse takes the urine sample from the needleless port of the catheter. Place the following steps for obtaining a sterile urine specimen in the correct order:
   1. Withdraw 3 to 5 mL of urine, and instill into a sterile urine container using sterile technique.
   2. Perform hand hygiene and apply gloves.
   3. Attach completed requisition and send immediately to the laboratory.
   4. Wipe needleless port with antiseptic wipe and attach 3-mL Luer-Lok syringe.
   5. Attach label to sterile urine container and double bag.
      1. 4, 2, 1, 3, 5
      2. 2, 4, 3, 1, 5
      3. 4, 2, 3, 5, 1
      4. 2, 4, 1, 5, 3
2. Which of the following indicates that the patient's daughter understands the importance of having a C&S test done on her mother's urine?
   1. "The C&S test is necessary if her diabetes is under control."
   2. "She always gets the same medication for her urine infections, so she doesn't need a test."
   3. "The C&S test is important so the doctor can order the correct medication if there is bacteria in the urine."
   4. "The C&S test is necessary only when she has a catheter."

Review Questions

1. A patient with a new diagnosis of diabetes performs her blood glucose test before meals and at bedtime. She tells the nurse that her fingers are getting sore, and she has trouble getting a droplet of blood large enough for testing. Which of the following interventions would be most appropriate for the nurse?
   1. Instruct her to use the forearm for a blood droplet.
   2. Apply pressure to the puncture site for at least 1 minute before a puncture.
   3. Cleanse site with warm water and allow to dry.
   4. Place the lancet firmly against the site to ensure an appropriate depth of puncture.

2. Which is the preferred vein for venipuncture to obtain a blood specimen?
   1. The antecubital vein, which is less painful
   2. The basilic vein, which is straight
   3. The cephalic vein, which is in the hand and well anchored
   4. The median cubital vein, which is larger and closer to the surface

3. A patient is scheduled to obtain a stool sample for occult blood several days from now. Which food should be avoided before the stool sample is obtained because it can alter the results of the test?
   1. Red meat
   2. Cheese
   3. Yogurt
   4. Pasta

4. The laboratory results for a wound specimen indicated contamination with superficial skin cells. Which of the following actions would the nurse take?
   1. Begin antibiotic therapy.
   2. Monitor patient.
   3. Repeat wound specimen collection.
   4. Cleanse wound with sterile water.

5. A female patient started on a 24-hour urine collection at 0800. At 1200, the nurse notes that the hat for collection of urine is on the floor in the bathroom and empty. Questioning indicates that the patient has been voiding in the toilet and flushing. Which is the nurse's most appropriate initial intervention?
   1. Assess patient's understanding of a 24-hour urine collection.
   2. Continue to collect urine for the remainder of the 24 hours.
   3. Stop the procedure and restart urine collections.
   4. Have patient drink at least one glass of water every hour.

6. The nurse is preparing to obtain a throat culture. All of the following are contraindications to obtaining a throat culture except which one?
   1. Suspected epiglottitis
   2. Elevated body temperature
   3. Extreme combativeness, anxiety, and restlessness
   4. Immediately after lunch

7. The nurse is preparing to obtain a throat culture. Which steps would facilitate collecting an accurate specimen? Select all that apply.
   1. Place patient in a sitting position or with head elevated at a 45-degree angle.
   2. Have patient lean the head forward.
   3. Have patient swallow a small amount of water to rinse away food from the culture site before swabbing the area.
   4. Swab the tonsillar area.
   5. Swab the uvula.
   6. Have patient blow the nose.

8. This is the third admission for a male patient in 4 months for hyperglycemia. He has insulin-dependent diabetes and has been instructed to perform fingersticks before each meal and at bedtime. Which statement indicates that the patient understands and does not need further teaching? Select all that apply.
   1. "My sight is poor, so I need to have my son Jeff help me read the meter."
   2. "My friend said I should do like he does and poke my finger only in the morning to save money."
   3. "I need to be sure that I take my blood sugar before I eat and before bed."
   4. "I take the same amount of insulin every morning but still need to do the fingerstick."

9. The nurse plans to collect a blood specimen. After placing the tourniquet above the elbow, she palpates absence of the radial pulse. Which nursing intervention should be completed first?
   1. Remove the tourniquet impeding venous blood flow, wait 60 minutes, and then reapply.
   2. Continue performing the phlebotomy; the blood specimen is from the venous system.
   3. Remove the tourniquet to allow arterial blood flow to return, wait 60 seconds, and then reapply the tourniquet.
   4. Palpate for the brachial pulse above the tourniquet.

10. A urine specimen for culture and sensitivity is being collected from a male patient. Which steps would be used to obtain an accurate specimen? Select all that apply.
    1. Two patient identifiers are checked.
    2. Help patient to perform perineal care before the sterile part of the procedure.
    3. Wipe the head of the penis back and forth three times with each swab.
    4. Collect 10 to 20 mL for the sample.
    5. Have the patient initially void into a bedpan or clean container.
    6. Have patient hold the penis above the sterile specimen cup without touching the container.

REFERENCES

American Diabetes Association (ADA): *Living with diabetes,* 2013a, http://www.diabetes.org/living-with-diabetes/complications/ketoacidosis-dka. Accessed July 22, 2013.

American Diabetes Association (ADA): *Checking your blood glucose,* 2013b, http://www.diabetes.org/living-with-diabetes/treatment-and-care/blood-glucose-control/checking-your-blood-glucose.html. Accessed July 28, 2013.

Diabetes Forecast: *Blood glucose meters 2013,* Alexandria, VA, 2013, American Diabetes Association. Available at: http://www.diabetesforecast.org/2013/jan/blood-glucose-meters-2013.html.

Hockenberry MJ, Wilson D: *Wong's essentials of pediatric nursing,* ed 9, St Louis, 2013, Mosby.

McCall R, Tankersley C: *Phlebotomy essentials,* ed 5, Philadelphia, 2012, Lippincott Williams & Wilkins.

Metheny N: *Fluid and electrolyte balance nursing considerations,* ed 5, Sudbury, MA, 2012, Jones & Bartlett.

Occupational Safety and Health Administration (OSHA): *Bloodborne pathogens and needlestick injuries, 77 FR 19934,* 2012, http://www.osha.gov/pls/oshaweb/owadisp.show_document?p_table=STANDARDS&p_id=10051. Accessed July 29, 2013.

Pagana KD, Pagana TJ: *Mosby's diagnostic and laboratory tests reference,* ed 11, St Louis, 2013, Mosby.

Stuart B, Stuart J, Cherry C: *Pocket guide to culturally sensitive health care,* Philadelphia, 2011, FA Davis.

The Joint Commission (TJC): *National Patient Safety Goals,* Oakbrook Terrace, IL, 2014, The Commission. Available at: http://www.jointcommission.org/standards_information/npsgs.aspx.

Touhy T, Jett K: *Ebersole and Hess's gerontological nursing and healthy aging,* ed 4, St Louis, 2014, Mosby.

Van Leeuwen A, et al: *Davis's comprehensive handbook of laboratory and diagnostic tests with nursing implications,* ed 4, Philadelphia, 2011, FA Davis.

Diagnostic Procedures

Diagnostic procedures are necessary to determine the cause or nature of patients' health problems and often to determine the need for surgery. Follow-up diagnostic procedures document the progression of a medical condition or determine the effectiveness of a treatment plan. The procedures are typically performed at a patient's bedside or in specially equipped procedure rooms within a hospital or in an outpatient setting. For many diagnostic procedures, patients undergo a series of activities before the procedure either in the hospital or while still at home. Informed consent is legally required and is performed by the health care provider. As the nurse, ask a patient if there are questions. If so, refer the patient to the health care provider. During diagnostic procedures, you are responsible for assessing patients' knowledge of their procedure, preparing them, providing a safe environment, and performing preprocedure and postprocedure assessment. In addition, nurses provide postprocedure care and instruction on any postprocedure restrictions or activities patients must follow.

PATIENT-CENTERED CARE

Diagnostic procedures are often confusing, frightening, and embarrassing. Anticipate that patients will have concerns. Learn about their expectations or fears, and give them the opportunity to ask questions. Previous experiences, beliefs about health care (e.g., value of screening or disease prevention), and existing knowledge significantly affect how patients respond to these procedures. Educating patients about the purpose of preprocedure activities helps to ensure the procedures will be completed correctly. For example, if a patient does not limit fluid intake before a procedure that requires him or her to "have nothing by mouth" (NPO), the procedure could be canceled. A delay of a test occurs if preprocedure activities are omitted or not performed correctly.

Learn why a patient is having a diagnostic test and the types of outcomes that are expected. Anxiety commonly develops when a patient does not understand the preparation before a procedure, the procedure itself, or the potential outcome of a test. For example, a colonoscopy is a routine examination to screen for early-stage colon cancer in adults older than age 50. When a patient has had signs and symptoms such as a change in bowel habits or rectal bleeding, the potential of receiving a diagnosis of colon cancer may cause fear and anxiety.

Family members will have similar concerns as your patients. Include family members when appropriate in any discussion or instruction, unless patients request they not be involved. A family caregiver may be the one to provide postprocedure care or monitoring in the home.

SAFETY

Certain diagnostic procedures require patients to receive moderate intravenous (IV) sedation. Moderate sedation/analgesia produces a minimally depressed level of consciousness. It is induced by the administration of medications. With moderate sedation/analgesia, a patient retains a continuous and independent ability to maintain protective reflexes (cough and swallow) and a patent airway and is aroused by physical or verbal stimulation. Procedural sedation is classified as "minimal," "moderate," or "deep" sedation/analgesia.

Minimal IV sedation is given to reduce patients' anxiety. Patients are able to respond normally to verbal commands during procedures (e.g., dental procedure); however, cognitive function and coordination may be impaired. Ventilation and cardiovascular function are unaffected with minimal sedation.

Moderate IV sedation, commonly used in procedures such as endoscopy and cardiac catheterization, depresses a patient's consciousness; however, patients are able to respond purposefully to a health care provider's verbal commands. It often raises a patient's pain threshold and provides amnesia about the actual procedural events. It is not necessary to provide an artificial airway (e.g., endotracheal tube). A patient should be able to breathe spontaneously, and cardiovascular function is also usually maintained (ASA, 2013). Deep sedation is one risk associated with moderate sedation during a procedure when a patient's level of consciousness (LOC) decreases past the point where a patent airway cannot be maintained. Because of this risk, the use of IV moderate sedation is closely controlled, and it normally can be administered only by physicians and registered nurses specially trained or credentialed (AORN, 2011).

In procedures that require sedation, health care facilities maintain standards for preassessment, preparation, and procedural monitoring. Before a patient receives sedation, the American Society of Anesthesiologists (ASA, 2013) and American Society for Gastrointestinal Endoscopy (2011) recommend these standards for preprocedure assessment: A presedation assessment must be completed within 30 days of the procedure and documented in the patient's medical record. The assessment should include the following (Practice Advisory for Preanesthesia Evaluation, 2012):

- Physical status assessment
- Past and present drug history including drug allergies
- Previous adverse experience with sedation and analgesia and with regional and general anesthesia
- Results of relevant diagnostic studies
- History of tobacco, alcohol, and substance use/abuse
- Verification of patient NPO status
- Plan and choice of sedation
- Transport arrangements on discharge

When a patient requires moderate sedation for a procedure, maintaining a patent airway during and after the procedure is a primary safety concern. During and after a procedure, patients need continuous monitoring of vital

TABLE 9-1	MODIFIED RAMSAY SEDATION SCALE		
Minimal sedation (anxiolysis)	1	Anxious and agitated or restless or both
	2	Cooperative, oriented, and tranquil
Moderate sedation/ analgesia (conscious sedation)	3	Responds to commands spoken in a normal voice
Deep sedation/analgesia	4	Brisk response to a light forehead tap or loud auditory stimulus
	5	Sluggish response to a light forehead tap or loud auditory stimulus
	6	No response to a light forehead tap or loud auditory stimulus

Data from Ramsay MA et al: Controlled sedation with alphaxalone-alphadolone, *Br Med J* 2(920):656, 1974; American Society of Anesthesiologists: *Continuum of depth of sedation definition of general anesthesia and levels of sedation/analgesia*, Oct 27, 2004.

signs, airway patency, heart rhythm, lung sounds, level of consciousness (LOC), and responsiveness (Table 9-1). Most facilities monitor oxygen saturation (SaO_2), but measurement of end-tidal CO_2 ($ETCO_2$) is becoming more common. $ETCO_2$ is helpful in detecting hypoventilation during procedural sedation. As a patient recovers from sedation, it is imperative that accurate assessments document a patient's level of recovery before he or she can be safely discharged. When using IV sedation, know the facility policy for recommended and maximum doses of medications and monitoring and documentation requirements.

The most common types of medications used to achieve moderate sedation include benzodiazepines and opiates. Benzodiazepines reduce anxiety and promote muscle relaxation. Midazolam (Versed), in particular, also produces an amnesic effect. Opiates such as morphine sulfate or fentanyl (Sublimaze, Duragesic) help control pain while achieving sedation. Propofol (Diprivan), a safe, rapid-acting hypnotic, is also commonly used and may offer a faster recovery time than the combination of benzodiazepine and opiates (Muller and Wehrmann, 2011).

Patient risks during IV sedation include hypoventilation, airway compromise, aspiration, hemodynamic instability, and altered LOC that can include an overly depressed LOC or agitation and combativeness. Emergency equipment appropriate for the patient's age and size (see Chapter 29) and staff with skill in airway management, oxygen delivery, and use of resuscitation equipment are essential. Reversal agents must be readily available: naloxone (Narcan) to reverse the effects of opioids and flumazenil (Romazicon) to reverse the effects of benzodiazepines (Lilly et al., 2012).

When an outpatient procedure requires sedation, a patient must come to the diagnostic center with a designated driver.

Instruct patients not to drive, consume alcohol, or take over-the-counter medications (e.g., aspirin-containing drugs) without a health care provider's approval for 24 hours after the procedure. If you are admitting a patient to a diagnostic center, verify that there is a designated driver or that the patient has arranged for transportation before the procedure begins.

Another safety concern associated with invasive procedures involves injection of radiopaque dye. Some patients are allergic to dye contrast material used in some diagnostic procedures to enhance visualization of the internal structures and organs. The health care provider is responsible for providing an explanation of what is involved with a diagnostic test, probable outcomes, and the risks involved (including possibility of allergic reaction). During your nursing assessment, determine if a patient is allergic to iodine or dye contrast, latex, any foods, antiseptic, tape, or anesthetic solutions. Ensure that any allergies or conditions are noted on the patient's chart and identified according to facility policy. Last, be sure that the health care provider performing the diagnostic test is aware of the allergy before starting an IV or administering any sedation. In some situations, when dye is necessary to obtain accurate results and the patient has an allergy to the dye or iodine, the patient is premedicated with an antihistamine such as diphenhydramine (Benadryl) to reduce the chance of an allergic reaction.

In addition to dye-related allergies, patients with a history of cardiac or renal failure may experience acute kidney injury (AKI), contrast-induced nephropathy (CIN), or acute renal failure (ARF). The best prevention for AKI, CIN, or ARF in patients with a history of cardiac or renal failure is hydration before and after the procedure and the discontinuation of nephrotoxic medications (Maioli et al., 2011). Be sure the health care provider performing the diagnostic test with contrast media is aware of the past medical history for cardiac or renal failure, ensuring time for adequate preprocedure hydration or consultation with specialists as required.

EVIDENCE-BASED PRACTICE

Frank R, Wolfson A, Grayzel J: Procedural sedation in adults, 2014, *UpToDate*, http://www.uptodate.com/contents/procedural-sedation-in-adults

Aspiration of stomach contents during anesthesia is rare but is usually of great concern to health care providers. The importance of fasting to prevent aspiration during procedural sedation remains unclear. The guidelines list the same fasting recommendations for patients undergoing elective procedures as for patients undergoing general anesthesia. To prevent aspiration for patients undergoing procedural sedation in emergency situations the following guidelines are recommended (Frank et al., 2014):

- It is reasonable to wait if the patient's stomach is full if possible, especially if there may be anticipated airway issues.
- Avoid deep sedation.
- Do not administer pre-procedural mobility agents or antacids.
- It may be preferable to use general anesthesia.

SKILL 9.1   CONTRAST MEDIA STUDIES: ARTERIOGRAM (ANGIOGRAM), CARDIAC CATHETERIZATION, INTRAVENOUS PYELOGRAM

Contrast media studies involve visualization of blood vessel structures of the body by intravascular injection of a radiopaque medium. An arteriogram (angiogram) permits visualization of the vasculature and arterial system of an area of the body or an organ. Arteriography is most frequently performed by an interventional radiologist or cardiologist to diagnose venous or arterial occlusions, stenosis, emboli, thromboses, aneurysms, tumors, congenital malformations, or trauma anywhere in the body.

Cardiac catheterization is a specialized form of angiography. The interventionist inserts a catheter introducer into a femoral artery or vein and threads the tip of a long thin catheter into the right or left side of the heart (Fig. 9-1). The brachial artery or vein can also be used. A contrast medium is injected through the catheter allowing for assessment of the structures and functions of the heart, including blood flow. The test studies pressures and blood flow in the heart chambers and large arteries, oxygen levels, cardiac volumes, valve function, and patency of coronary arteries. Cardiac catheterization also allows for collection of blood samples and biopsy of heart muscle. Cardiac catheterizations are performed in specially equipped laboratories.

Cardiac catheterizations are usually contraindicated in patients who refuse needed surgery, are allergic to iodine contrast media, are uncooperative or cannot lie still during the entire procedure, or are susceptible to dye-induced renal failure. When a cardiac catheterization is essential for patients with allergies to iodine contrast media, a nonionic medium is used, or the patient is pretreated with medications to reduce the allergic reactions. Precautions to help prevent dye-induced renal failure are controversial and include ensuring a patient is well hydrated using bicarbonate solution or sodium chloride with or without prophylactic acetylcysteine (Mucomyst) before, during, and after the procedure and using nonionic (instead of ionic) contrast media (Lewis et al., 2014).

Intravenous pyelography (IVP) is an examination of the flow of radiopaque contrast medium that shows how the kidneys remove the dye and how it collects in the urine. IVP helps to identify obstruction, hematuria, stones, bladder injury, or renal artery occlusion. Dye is injected via a catheter

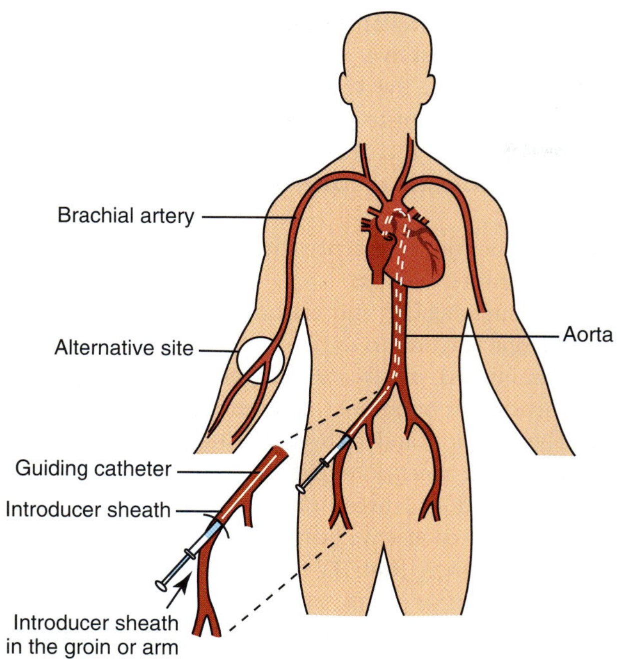

FIG 9-1 A catheter introducer placed into a femoral artery or vein allows for threading the tip of a long thin catheter into the right or left side of the heart during cardiac catheterization.

through a peripheral artery, and serial radiographs are taken over the subsequent 30 minutes.

ASSESSMENT

1. Identify patient using two identifiers (e.g., name and birthday or name and account number) according to facility policy. Compare identifiers with information on the patient's MAR or medical record. *Rationale: Ensures correct patient. Complies with The Joint Commission standards and improves patient safety (TJC, 2014).*

2. Verify the type of procedure that the physician will perform and procedure site with patient and medical record. *Rationale: Verifies correct patient receives correct procedure.*

3. Verify that informed consent was obtained before administering a sedative. Ask patient if there are questions. *Rationale: Federal regulations, many state laws, and accreditation agencies require informed consent for procedures.*

4. Determine if patient is taking anticoagulants, antiplatelets, aspirin, acetaminophen, or nonsteroidal medications. *Rationale: Medications and disease conditions may affect liver or kidney function, leading to increased risk of bleeding. The drugs need to be stopped before the procedure. Acetaminophen is found in many over-the-counter medications.*

5. Assess patient's liver and kidney function, bleeding and coagulation status (e.g., liver profile, BUN, creatinine, urine specific gravity, complete blood count [CBC], platelet count, prothrombin time [PT], international normalized ratio [INR]). *Rationale: Abnormal clotting factors contraindicate the procedure because of increased risk for bleeding. Abnormal liver or kidney values may indicate liver or kidney failure.*

6. Assess patient for allergies to iodine dye, latex, or any food and whether patient has had a previous reaction to a contrast agent (Schabelman and Witting, 2010). If allergies are present, notify the cardiologist or radiologist. *Rationale: Allergy to shellfish in particular does not increase the risk of reaction to IV contrast medium any more than other allergies. Risk of anaphylactic reaction to contrast medium ranges from 0.2% to 17% depending on contrast medium used and prior history of any allergy (Schabelman and Witting, 2010). An alternative hypoallergenic contrast medium may sometimes be used.*

7. Review medical record for contraindications.

    a. All contrast media: Pregnancy unless the benefits to the tests outweigh the risks to the infant. *Rationale: Contrast media crosses the blood-placental barrier.*

    b. Angiography: Anticoagulant therapy, bleeding disorders, thrombocytopenia, dehydration, uncontrolled hypertension, renal insufficiency or failure, congestive heart or cardiac failure, type 1 or type 2 diabetes. *Rationale: Anticoagulants and bleeding disorders interfere with blood clotting abilities and may cause blood loss. Dehydration and renal insufficiency are contraindications to the use of ionic radiographic contrast media because the patient has an impaired ability to excrete the contrast media via the kidneys (Chernecky and Berger, 2013). Hydration provided before and after the procedure to break down and excrete dye may worsen congestive heart failure and diabetes.*

    c. Cardiac catheterization: Severe cardiomyopathy, severe dysrhythmias, uncontrolled congestive heart failure, renal failure. *Rationale: Introduction of a catheter into the myocardium irritates myocardial tissue and increases the risk for dysrhythmias and heart failure (Pagana and Pagana, 2013).*

    d. IVP: Dehydration, known renal insufficiency. *Rationale: Impair the ability to excrete the contrast media via the kidneys (Chernecky and Berger, 2013).*

    e. Assess if patient took metformin hydrochloride within the past 48 hours. If so, notify health care provider immediately. *Rationale: Metformin taken within 48 hours before receiving iodinated contrast media can lead to renal failure and lactic acidosis. Metformin is contained in the drugs metformin hydrochloride (Glumetza), and glyburide and metformin (Glucovance)* (Lilly et al., 2012).

8. Obtain vital signs and peripheral pulses. For arterial procedures, mark the patient's peripheral pulses before the procedure. Auscultate heart and lungs, and obtain weight. *Rationale: Provides baseline data for postprocedural assessments.*

9. Assess patient's hydration status, including condition of mucous membranes and recent 24-hour intake. *Rationale: Severe dehydration can lead to renal failure (Pagana and Pagana, 2013).*

10. Assess patient's level of understanding of procedure, including any concerns. *Rationale: Determines extent of preprocedure understanding or level of additional instruction or support needed.*
11. Determine that preprocedure preparation is complete (check facility policy).
    a. For cardiac catheterization: Determine whether the site of catheter insertion needs to be clipped to remove hair and prepared with antiseptic just before the procedure. Allow antiseptic to dry. *Rationale: Reduces risk of site-related infection.*
    b. For IVP: Verify that patient has taken the orally administered bowel evacuation medication 24 hours before the test or completed an evacuation enema 8 hours before the test. *Rationale: An evacuated lower intestine and bowel improve visualization.*
11. Determine and document time of last ingested fluid, medication, or food. *Rationale: Patient needs to be NPO for 6 to 8 hours before the procedure because of risk of nausea and associated aspiration from sedation and effects of iodine. Excessive hydration dilutes contrast medium, making structures more difficult to visualize.*
12. Remove metal objects and all of patient's jewelry or body piercings. *Rationale: Eliminates objects that interfere with radiography visualization of blood vessels.*
13. Review physician's orders for preprocedure medications, hydration, antihistamines, and IV sedation. *Rationale: Increased hydration is often required for renal insufficiency, antihistamines for possible allergic reaction, or sedation for anxious or confused patients.*
    a. Atropine decreases salivary secretions and increases heart rate when bradycardia is present.
    b. Diphenhydramine blocks histamine and decreases allergic response. Often used prophylactically.
    c. Preprocedure sedative decreases anxiety and promotes relaxation.
    d. Have drugs available for treatment of anaphylactic reactions, such as IV Solu-Medrol, diphenhydramine, and epinephrine. For reversal of opioids or benzodiazepines, have naloxone (opioid) and flumazenil (benzodiazepine) available (check facility policy). *Rationale: These medications are needed immediately in the case of an allergic reaction to dye or oversedation.*

PLANNING

Expected Outcomes focus on prevention of respiratory side effects from sedation and cardiovascular complications from catheter placement, puncture site complications, and reactions to contrast dye.

1. Patient assumes the correct position and remains still throughout the entire procedure.
2. Patient has pain less than 4 (on a scale of 0 to 10) that is limited to soreness at catheter insertion site and possible backache.
3. Patient does not experience complications during or after the procedure, such as:
    a. Flushing, itching, and urticaria, which signify possible allergic reaction to dye.
    b. Diminished or absent peripheral pulses, signifying thrombosis or embolism at puncture site.
    c. Hypotension and tachycardia, signifying hemorrhage or allergic reaction to dye.
    d. Decreased or absent urine output related to renal failure or congestive heart failure.
4. Patient recovers from IV sedation without respiratory complications or change in LOC.
5. Patient tolerates increased fluid intake after procedure and voids sufficiently to excrete radiographic dye.

Delegation and Collaboration

The skill of assisting with angiography and IVP may be delegated to nursing assistive personnel (NAP) if the patient is stable and if no IV sedation is used. Assessment cannot be delegated. The nurse instructs the NAP about:
- When to obtain and report vital signs, urinary output, and weight.
- What signs and symptoms to observe for and report to the nurse.
- Accompanying the patient to the procedure room and assisting specially trained and licensed interventional radiology personnel with the specific angiography procedure.

Equipment
- Personal protective equipment: Mask, goggles, sterile gown, and sterile gloves
- Sterile packs containing catheters and equipment for performing procedures
- Equipment for IV access
- Medications for IV sedation
- Emergency equipment: Oxygen, emergency cart, defibrillator, cardiac monitor, intubation/airway maintenance equipment, medication to treat anaphylaxis, and sedative reversal agents
- Sphygmomanometer, pulse oximetry, $ETCO_2$ monitor

IMPLEMENTATION *for* CONTRAST MEDIA STUDIES: ARTERIOGRAM (ANGIOGRAM), CARDIAC CATHETERIZATION, INTRAVENOUS PYELOGRAM

STEPS	RATIONALE
1. **See Standard Protocol (inside front cover).**	
2. Have patient empty bowels and bladder before procedure.	Ensures that patient will not need to void during procedure.

STEPS	RATIONALE

3. Prepare cardiac monitor, pulse oximetry, and $ETCO_2$ monitor.

Provides easy access to equipment for monitoring patient status during and after procedure.

4. Apply clean gloves. Provide IV access using large-bore cannula (see Chapter 27). Remove gloves. Perform hand hygiene.

Provides access for delivery of IV fluids or drugs. Reduces transmission of microorganisms.

5. Assist patient in assuming a comfortable supine position on fluoroscopy table. Some patients undergoing IVP may be in a supine or in a slight Trendelenburg's position. Immobilize the extremity that will be injected. Pad any bony prominences.

For arterial procedures, the patient may need to maintain the position for 1 to 3 hours. Padding of bony prominences reduces the risk for impaired skin integrity.

6. Take "Time Out" to verify the patient's name, type of procedure to be performed, and procedure site with the patient.

"Time Out" verification before the start of an invasive procedure includes the physician and all involved personnel. Safety precaution prevents wrong patient, wrong site, and wrong procedure errors (TJC, 2014).

7. Inform patient that it is common during the injection of the dye to experience some chest pain and a severe hot flash, but it usually lasts only a few seconds.

Dye causes a sensation of warmth, flushing, or a metallic taste shortly after injection.

8. Certified nurse, Certified Registered Nurse Anesthetist (CRNA), or physician will administer IV moderate sedation as ordered.

9. Support health care providers in performing all media studies.

   a. Physician or nurse cleanses site for catheter insertion (femoral, carotid, or brachial) with antiseptic.

Reduces transmission of infection.

   b. Members of the team apply mask and goggles, sterile gown, head cover, and sterile gloves. Drape patient with sterile drapes, leaving puncture site exposed.

Maintains surgical asepsis.

   c. Physician anesthetizes the skin over the arterial puncture site.

Provides local anesthesia to incision or puncture site.

> **SAFE PATIENT CARE** The physician may end the procedure early in the event of severe unrelieved chest pain, neurological symptoms of a cerebrovascular accident, cardiac arrhythmias, or hemodynamic changes (Pagana and Pagana, 2013).

10. For arterial procedures the physician does the following:

   a. Punctures artery; inserts introducer sheath into artery, inserts guidewire through introducer, and inserts flexible catheter over guidewire and advances it into heart. Different catheters may be inserted and removed during procedure.

Permits access to artery and prevents coiling of catheter in the artery. Permits radiographic visualization of structures, aneurysms, occlusions, or anomalies. Sheath provides support at the puncture site and reduces arterial trauma during multiple catheter exchanges.

   b. Advances catheter to desired artery or cardiac chamber and injects contrast dye or collects volume and pressure measurements. If procedure is interventional, catheter used to open arterial occlusions.

11. For all procedures, nurse administering IV sedation monitors level of sedation, LOC, airway, and vital signs. Note: Some facilities require the presence of an anesthetist (physician or CRNA) to administer sedation during procedures of this type.

IV sedation should not cause loss of consciousness or ability of the patient to maintain airway and spontaneous respirations.

Continued

STEPS	RATIONALE
12. During dye injection, specialized machinery takes real-time video images of the dye as it travels through the visualized area (fluoroscopy).	Provides radiographic records of dye through the artery or cardiac chamber and documents any abnormalities.
13. If iodinated dye is administered, observe patient for signs of anaphylaxis, including respiratory distress, palpitations, itching, and diaphoresis.	Allergic reactions can be life-threatening.
14. During cardiac catheterization, the nurse assists with measuring cardiac volumes and pressures.	Provides data related to cardiac output, central venous pressure, ventricular pressures, and pulmonary artery pressure.
15. Completion of procedure:	
a. The physician withdraws catheter and applies pressure to puncture site until hemostasis occurs (5 to 15 minutes or longer). A VCD commonly may be used. Use of devices is weighed against risk of complications.	Pressure on puncture site promotes clotting and prevents bleeding and hematoma formation. A hematoma can compromise arterial blood blow. Types of VCDs each have a unique method for providing closure of an arterial site. A passive closure device provides compression using clamps, tamping devices, and sealants. Active closure devices provide immediate closure with sutures, clips, or collagen plugs.
16. In certain procedures (e.g., percutaneous transluminal cardiac angiography) during a cardiac catheterization, a femoral sheath is often left in place and removed in 2 to 3 hours by the nurse caring for the patient.	Sheaths left in place after intervention provide emergency access to the vasculature in the event that the coronary artery occludes and allow time for anticoagulants to wear off.

> **SAFE PATIENT CARE** Timing of the removal of the femoral sheath depends on location of the access site, size of the sheath, use of anticoagulants, and facility protocols. Manual pressure applied to the groin can stimulate the baroreceptors and cause a vasovagal reaction in which the patient becomes bradycardic and hypotensive. Vasovagal reactions are usually brief and self-limiting. When applying pressure to the groin after sheath removal, be alert for a vasovagal reaction and be prepared to treat it by lowering the head of the bed to the flat position and giving a bolus of IV fluids. Have emergency resuscitation equipment available during sheath removal.

STEPS	RATIONALE
17. Remove and discard personal protective equipment. Perform hand hygiene.	Reduces transmission of microorganisms.
18. Postprocedure precautions:	
a. Keep affected extremity immobilized for 2 to 6 hours after removal of catheter (see facility policy). Use urinal or orthopedic bedpan as needed while on bed rest. Log roll patient onto bedpan. Provide ongoing comfort measures.	Studies show that prolonged bed rest after angiographic procedures may not be necessary to ensure hemostasis at an arterial puncture site. In patients undergoing coronary interventional or diagnostic procedures, 2 hours of bed rest has been shown to be safe and significantly effective in reducing back pain (Hoglund et al, 2011).
b. During bed rest, explain the reason patient must lie flat (possibly overnight if the catheters are left in the groin). Consider prn pain or antianxiety medications.	Helps prevent disruption of hemostasis at the puncture site. Reduces discomfort or anxiety related to prolonged immobility or bed rest.
c. Encourage patient to drink 1 to 2 L of fluid after procedure or administer oral and IV fluids as ordered.	Facilitates elimination of contrast material and prevents renal damage (Pagana and Pagana, 2013).
19. See Completion Protocol (inside front cover).	

EVALUATION

1. Evaluate patient's body position and comfort (using a pain rating scale) during procedure.
2. Monitor vital signs, pulse oximetry, $ETCO_2$, and urinary output, and evaluate for cardiac complications every 15 minutes for 1 hour, every 30 minutes for 2 hours, or until vital signs are stable (see facility policy).
3. Monitor for complications:
   a. Assess arterial access site for bleeding and hematoma. Assess for back, lower abdominal, or catheter site discomfort or pain; anxiety; tachycardia; and loss of distal pulses and observe under the patient for blood (retroperitoneal or site hemorrhage).
   b. If ordered, monitor postprocedure laboratory values (CBC, electrolytes, creatinine, activated partial thromboplastin time, PT).
   c. Perform neurovascular checks: Palpate peripheral pulses in affected extremity, assess skin temperature, and note color of skin. Compare with unaffected extremity. Use Doppler ultrasonic stethoscope if pulses are not palpable.
   d. Auscultate heart and lungs, and compare findings with preprocedure findings.
   e. Monitor electrocardiogram (ECG) recording as appropriate.
   f. Monitor patient for allergic reactions: Assess patient for flushing, itching, and urticaria, and assess patient's respiratory status for sudden, severe shortness of breath. Delayed allergic reaction may occur several hours after procedure.
   g. Monitor for complications of sedation (e.g., excessive sleepiness, inability to arouse patient, confusion, combativeness).
   h. Measure vital signs; compare with baseline and subsequent values.
   i. Measure pulse oximetry and $ETCO_2$, and compare with baseline.
   j. Use Modified Ramsay Sedation Scale (see Table 9-1).
4. Use **Teach Back:** State to the patient, "It is important for you to lie flat now that the procedure is over. I want to be sure you understand. Can you tell me what may happen if you are not able to lie still?" Evaluates what the patient is able to explain or demonstrate. Revise your instruction now or develop plan for revised patient teaching to be implemented at an appropriate time if patient is not able to teach back correctly.

Unexpected Outcomes and Related Interventions

1. Patient experiences vasovagal response (occurs at time of femoral puncture or after procedure when femoral pressure applied). Symptoms include feeling faint, dizzy, lightheaded, and possible loss of consciousness for a few seconds. Bradycardic pulse is caused by stimulation of the vagus nerve via baroreceptors.
   a. Support airway, breathing, and circulation.
   b. Lower table or head of bed to the Trendelenburg's position.
   c. Administer IV fluid bolus if ordered.
2. Patient's pedal pulses are nonpalpable bilaterally 2 hours after an angiogram.
   a. Assess pulses (with a Doppler scope), extremity skin temperature, color, and capillary refill time.
   b. Notify physician immediately.
3. Patient develops hematoma or hemorrhage at catheter insertion site.
   a. Maintain direct pressure over insertion site.
   b. Contact physician immediately. Follow specific postprocedure orders related to findings.
   c. Monitor catheter site per facility policy or as ordered.
4. Oversedation occurs (e.g., decreased $SaO_2/ETCO_2$, shallow respirations, decreased blood pressure, tachycardia).
   a. Support patient's airway and breathing.
   b. Immediately notify patient's physician (call Rapid Response Team if available).
   c. Be prepared to administer emergency medications or reversal agents (e.g., naloxone [Narcan] for reversal of opioids or flumazenil [Romazicon] for reversal of benzodiazepines).
5. Retroperitoneal bleeding occurs (when femoral access site is used). A hallmark sign is low back pain radiating to both sides of the body.
   a. Immediately notify patient's physician (call Rapid Response Team if available).
   b. Prepare patient for emergency surgery.
   c. Monitor vital signs every 5 minutes and monitor distal pulses.

Recording and Reporting

- Record in medical record patient's condition: Vital signs, pulse oximetry, $ETCO_2$, peripheral pulses for equality and symmetry, blood pressure, temperature and color of catheterized extremity, condition of access/puncture site including any drainage and presence of any VCD, status of IV.

- Document your evaluation of patient learning.
- Report to physician or charge nurse immediately: Changes in vital signs, pulse oximetry, ETCO$_2$, arrhythmias, excessive bleeding or increasing hematoma at access/puncture site, decreased or absent peripheral pulses, urine output less than 30 mL per hour (0.5 mL/kg/hr) for adults and 1 mL/kg/hr for children, and decreased level of patient responsiveness.

Sample Documentation

0800-0900   Returned from angiogram via stretcher awake and alert. Vital signs obtained every 15 minutes, remain stable with BP 132/84, HR 88 and regular. Dorsalis pedis and posterior tibial pulses are palpable and equal bilaterally. No bleeding, swelling, or discoloration noted at catheter insertion site in left groin. Left leg extended with soft restraint in place. Complains of mild discomfort at left groin equal to 2 on a 0 to 10 pain scale but denies need for analgesics.
0900-1000   Vital signs obtained every 30 minutes remained stable. Dorsalis pedis and posterior tibial pulses are palpable and equal bilaterally. No bleeding, swelling, or discoloration noted at catheter insertion site in left groin. Left leg extended without soft restraint. Rates pain at 0 on a 0 to 10 pain scale.

Special Considerations
Pediatric

- Infants and children are susceptible to the diuretic effects of radiocontrast dyes because of their small body size. Pediatric patients with congenital cardiac anomalies develop compensatory erythrocytosis and experience complications from dehydration very quickly. Emphasize the importance of fluid intake with the child and parent (Hockenberry and Wilson, 2013).

Geriatric

- Slight alterations in vital signs or behavior (confusion) in older adults are signs of impending problems; close monitoring is critical.
- Physical exposure and room temperature contribute to hypothermia in frail adults. Use heated blankets or forced air heat to maintain core temperature at comfortable, safe levels.
- Renal insufficiency contributes to prolonged sedation.
- An older adult with preexisting dehydration or renal insufficiency in combination with NPO status is at risk for dye-induced renal failure. Carefully monitor intake and output.

Home Care

- Instruct patient to contact the physician (or affiliated emergency department) if any of the following occur after cardiac catheterization:
  - Chest pain or shortness of breath.
  - Blood in the urine.
  - Bleeding from the catheterization puncture site: Apply gentle pressure with clean gauze or cloth.
  - Formation of a knot or lump under the skin that increases in size.
  - Worsening of a bruise or its movement down the extremity rather than disappearing.
  - Increased pain at puncture site or in the extremity used for the catheterization.
  - Extremity with arterial puncture that is pale and cool to touch.
  - Appearance of redness, swelling, or warmth of the affected extremity.
  - Although bathing or showering is allowed the day after the catheterization, the leg used as the access site is often stiff, which increases risk of slipping in the bath or shower.

SKILL 9.2   CARE OF PATIENTS UNDERGOING ASPIRATIONS: BONE MARROW, LUMBAR PUNCTURE, PARACENTESIS, THORACENTESIS

Aspirations are sterile invasive procedures involving removal of body fluids or tissue for diagnostic purposes. The nurse assists the health care provider during an aspiration procedure (Table 9-2).

Bone marrow aspiration is the removal of a small amount of the liquid organic material in the medullary canals of selected bones. The bones used for aspiration in adults include the sternum and the posterior superior iliac crests. In children, the anterior or posterior iliac crests are used, and in infants, the proximal tibia is used (Hockenberry and Wilson, 2013; Pagana and Pagana, 2013). A biopsy is the removal of a core of marrow cells for laboratory analysis. Both aspiration and biopsy diagnose and differentiate leukemia, certain cancerous tumors, anemia,

and thrombocytopenia. Laboratory analysis of the marrow reveals the number, size, shape, and development of red blood cells and megakaryocytes (platelet precursors). Bone marrow cultures help differentiate infectious diseases such as tuberculosis or histoplasmosis. This procedure takes approximately 20 minutes.

A lumbar puncture (LP), called a *spinal puncture* or *tap,* involves the introduction of a needle into the subarachnoid space of the spinal column. The purpose of the test is to measure pressure in the subarachnoid space and obtain cerebrospinal fluid (CSF) for visualization and laboratory testing. LP is also used to inject anesthetic, diagnostic, or therapeutic agents. Laboratory testing of CSF helps diagnose spinal cord tumors, central nervous system (CNS) infections,

TABLE 9-2 SUMMARY OF ASPIRATION PROCEDURES

ASPIRATION PROCEDURE	PREPARATION/ ASSESSMENT SPECIFIC TO TEST	POSITION OR SITE PRONE OR SUPINE POSITION	SPECIAL CONSIDERATIONS
Bone marrow aspiration	Assess complete blood count and clotting studies for abnormalities. For sternal biopsy, place adult patient in supine position. For iliac crest biopsy, place in prone or lateral recumbent position.	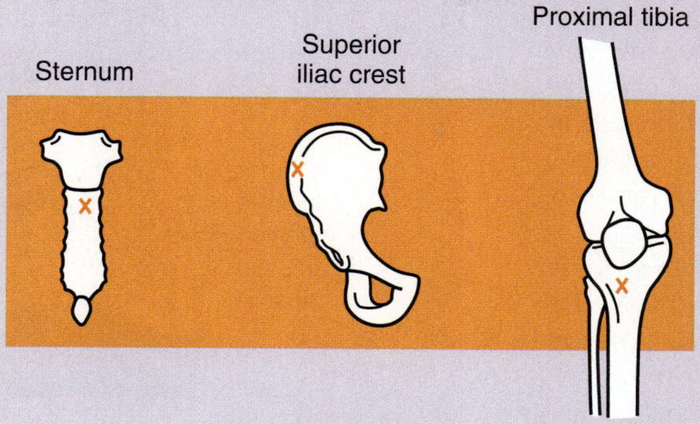	Patients with arthritis or orthopnea may have difficulty assuming the positions. Apply pressure to aspiration site after the procedure.
Lumbar puncture	Assess neurological status, including movement, sensation, and muscle strength of legs to provide a baseline for comparison. Assess bladder for distention and determine last voiding. Allow patient to void before procedure.	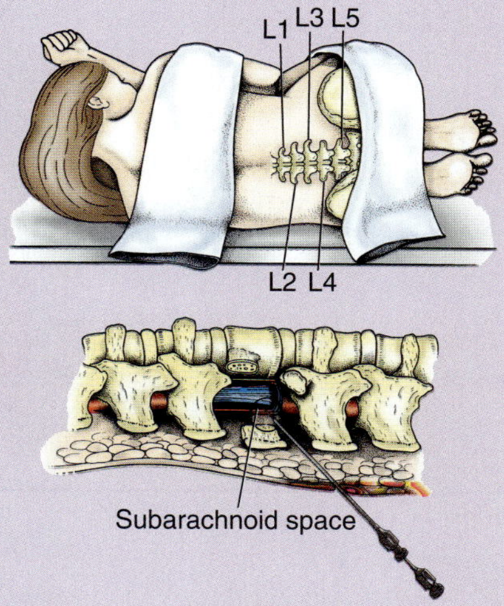	*Risk of spinal headache:* Some physicians still order patients to remain flat and log roll after procedure. Administer NSAIDs or opioids for mild headache and try nonpharmacological relief measures. *Risk of infection:* Observe for excessive drainage at the site.
Paracentesis	Assess bladder for distention and determine last voiding. Weigh patient, assess abdomen, and measure abdominal girth at largest point. Mark location.	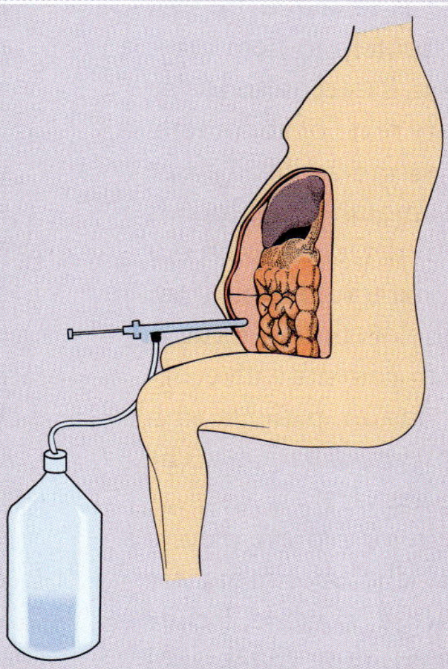	After removing fluid, pressure on diaphragm is released, and breathing becomes much easier. *Risk of trauma:* Have patient empty urinary bladder before procedure.

For the bone marrow aspiration diagram:

For the lumbar puncture diagram:

(From Ignatavicius DD, Workman ML: *Medical-surgical nursing: patient-centered collaborative care,* ed 7, Philadelphia, 2012, Saunders.)

(From Ignatavicius DD, Workman ML: *Medical-surgical nursing: patient-centered collaborative care,* ed 7, Philadelphia, 2012, Saunders.)

Continued

	TABLE 9-2 **SUMMARY OF ASPIRATION PROCEDURES—cont'd**		
ASPIRATION PROCEDURE	**PREPARATION/ ASSESSMENT SPECIFIC TO TEST**	**POSITION OR SITE PRONE OR SUPINE POSITION**	**SPECIAL CONSIDERATIONS**
Thoracentesis	Assess respiratory rate and depth, symmetry of chest on inspiration and expiration, cough, and sputum. Assist patient with remaining still during the procedure to prevent trauma to the visceral pleura. Patient needs to hold breath and avoid coughing during the procedure.	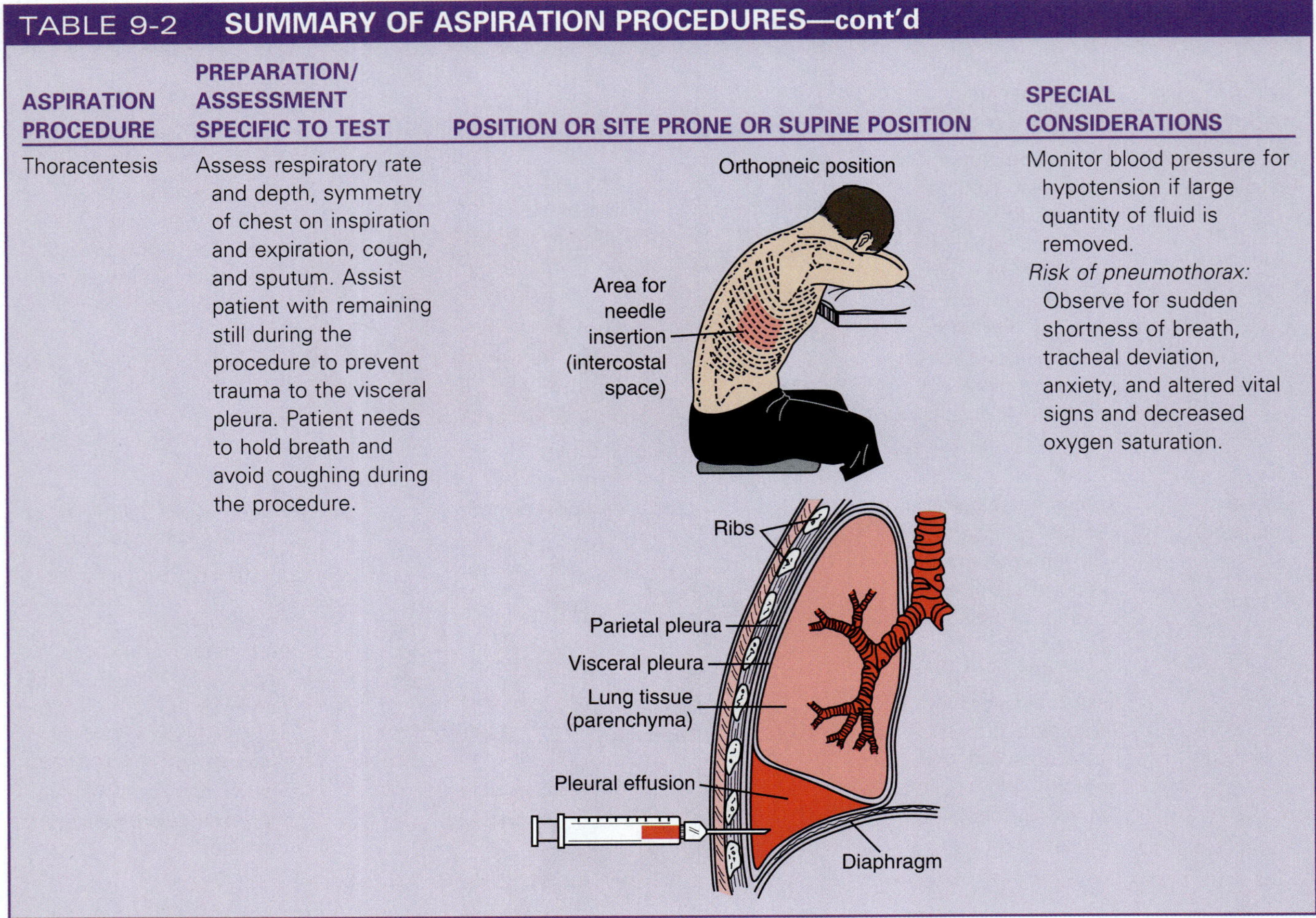	Monitor blood pressure for hypotension if large quantity of fluid is removed. *Risk of pneumothorax:* Observe for sudden shortness of breath, tracheal deviation, anxiety, and altered vital signs and decreased oxygen saturation.

NSAIDs, Nonsteroidal antiinflammatory drugs.

hemorrhage, and degenerative brain disease. The procedure takes approximately 30 minutes.

Abdominal paracentesis involves aspiration of peritoneal fluid from the abdomen. The aspirate is analyzed for cell cytology, bacteria, blood, glucose, and protein to help diagnose the causes of an abdominal effusion. Paracentesis is also a palliative measure to provide temporary relief of abdominal and respiratory discomfort caused by severe ascites. Lavage paracentesis, a process in which a large amount of solution is instilled and then withdrawn, is done to detect the presence of bleeding, as in cases of blunt abdominal trauma, or tumor cells when cancer is suspected. Although not contraindicated, paracentesis is performed with caution in patients with coagulopathies, patients with portal hypertension, patients with abdominal collateral circulation, and pregnant patients. The procedure takes approximately 30 minutes.

Thoracentesis is performed to analyze or remove pleural fluid or instill medications intrapleurally. Specimens are examined for cell cytology, blood, glucose, amylase, lactate dehydrogenase (LD), and cellular composition. Cytological specimens are examined for malignancy and cultured for pathogens. Therapeutic thoracentesis relieves pain, dyspnea, and signs of pleural pressure. The procedure takes approximately 30 minutes.

ASSESSMENT

1. Identify patient using two identifiers (e.g., name and birthday or name and account number) according to facility policy. Compare identifiers with information on the patient's MAR or medical record. *Rationale: Ensures correct patient. Complies with The Joint Commission standards and improves patient safety (TJC, 2014).*

2. Verify the type of procedure that the physician will perform and procedure site with the patient and medical record. *Rationale: Verifies correct patient receives correct procedure.*

3. Verify that informed consent was obtained. Ask patient if there are questions. *Rationale: Federal regulations, many state laws, and accreditation agencies require informed consent for procedures.*

4. Review medical record for contraindications.
   a. Bone marrow biopsy: Patient cannot maintain position or lie still during procedure.
   b. LP: Increased intracranial pressure and spinal deformities.
   c. Paracentesis: Clotting disorders, intestinal obstructions, and pregnancy.

d. Thoracentesis: Patient cannot maintain position during procedure.

5. Determine patient's ability to assume position required for procedure and ability to remain still (see Table 9-2). *Rationale: Movement during the procedure can cause complications such as bleeding and injury to nerves or tissue.*

6. Before procedure: Obtain vital signs, SaO_2/$ETCO_2$, and weight. For paracentesis, obtain an abdominal girth measurement. (Use ink pen to mark location of position of abdominal girth measurement.) For LP, obtain baseline assessment of lower extremity movement, sensation, and muscle strength. *Rationale: Provides baseline for comparison with patient's postprocedure status. Patients have decreased abdominal girth and lose weight after paracentesis.*

7. Instruct patient to empty bladder. *Rationale: Reduces risk for bladder trauma during paracentesis. Promotes patient comfort.*

8. Assess patient's coagulation status: Use of anticoagulants, platelet count, and PT. *Rationale: Invasive procedures are contraindicated in patients with coagulation disorders because of risk of bleeding (Pagana and Pagana, 2013).*

9. Determine whether patient is allergic to antiseptic, latex, or anesthetic solutions. *Rationale: Decreases chance of allergic reactions.*

10. Assess patient's level of understanding of procedure, including any concerns. *Rationale: Determines extent of instructions and level of support required.*

11. Obtain baseline pain level. *Rationale: Determines need for preprocedure analgesia. Pain control helps patients maintain proper position and tolerate aspiration procedure.*

▌PLANNING

Expected Outcomes focus on proper positioning, patient's ability to follow directions, comfort, and absence of complications.

1. Patient assumes the correct position and remains still throughout the entire procedure.

2. There is no bleeding at needle insertion site.

3. The amount of aspirate is sufficient to perform laboratory testing.

4. Patient's level of pain is 4 or less on a pain scale of 0 to 10.

5. Patient's respiratory rate, heart rate, and blood pressure are within normal limits during and after aspiration procedure.

Delegation and Collaboration

The skill of assisting with aspirations may be delegated to nursing assistive personnel (NAP) if the patient is stable (check facility policy). Assessment of the patient's condition cannot be delegated. The nurse instructs the NAP about:

- How to position properly the patient during the procedure.
- Obtaining baseline and postprocedure vital signs and reporting them to the nurse.
- Which signs and symptoms experienced by the patient to report immediately to the nurse.

Equipment

- Personal protective equipment: Masks, goggles, gowns, sterile gloves, head cover for health care personnel
- Test tubes, sterile specimen containers, laboratory requisitions, and labels
- Analgesia if ordered, given 30 minutes before procedure
- Antiseptic solution
- Gauze pads (4 × 4 inch), tape, band aid
- Sphygmomanometer, pulse oximeter/$ETCO_2$ monitor
- Aspiration tray: Most facilities provide trays specific to the aspiration procedure; standard equipment includes antiseptic solution (e.g., chlorhexidine), gauze sponges (4 × 4 inch), sterile towels, local anesthetic solution (e.g., lidocaine 1%), two 3-mL sterile syringes with 16- to 27-gauge needles

Additional equipment may be required (refer to facility policy or health care provider preference).

IMPLEMENTATION *for* CARE OF PATIENTS UNDERGOING ASPIRATIONS: BONE MARROW, LUMBAR PUNCTURE, PARACENTESIS, THORACENTESIS

STEPS	RATIONALE
1. **See Standard Protocol (inside front cover).**	
2. Premedicate patient 30 minutes before procedure as ordered.	Reduces pain and anxiety associated with procedure.
3. Explain steps of skin preparation, anesthetic injection, needle insertion, and position required. Note: For bone marrow biopsy, explain to patient that pain may occur when the bone marrow is aspirated.	Explanation reduces anxiety.
4. Set up sterile tray or open supplies to make accessible for health care provider.	Reduces risk of contamination of sterile field, and promotes prompt completion of procedure.

Continued

5. Take "Time Out" to verify the patient's name, type of procedure to be performed, and procedure site with patient.

"Time Out" verification before start of an invasive procedure includes the health care provider and all involved personnel. Safety precaution prevents wrong patient, wrong site, and wrong procedure errors (TJC, 2014).

6. Assist patient in maintaining correct position (see Table 9-2). Reassure patient while explaining procedure.

Decreases chance of complications during procedure. Explanations increase patient comfort and relaxation.

> **SAFE PATIENT CARE** Emphasize importance of staying immobile during procedure to prevent trauma. Encourage patient to try not to sneeze, cough, or breathe too deeply because these actions may cause needle displacement.

7. Health care providers apply appropriate personal protective equipment. Physician cleanses insertion site with antiseptic solution and drapes site with sterile drape.

Removes surface bacteria from skin. Creates sterile field.

8. Explain to patient that pain can occur when local anesthetic is injected into the tissues. Pressure may also occur when the tissue of fluid is aspirated.

Aspiration is painful but lasts for only a few minutes. Preprocedure analgesia decreases discomfort. If the patient is having a bone marrow aspirate, a deep pressure feeling is frequently experienced as the bone marrow is withdrawn (Pagana and Pagana, 2013).

9. Health care provider injects local anesthetic and waits for area over site to become numb.

Minimizes pain during needle insertion. Discomfort and pressure may still occur when deep tissues are disrupted.

10. Physician inserts needle or trocar into spinal space or body cavity involved (see Table 9-2). To aspirate tissue or body fluids for specimen analysis, a syringe is attached to the trocar or needle, and aspirate is placed into a specimen container.

Successful placement depends on positioning, accurate insertion site, and patient remaining still.

   a. For a thoracentesis or paracentesis, a vacuum container with tubing is attached to the needle or trocar to collect large volumes of fluid. A needless system connected to a collection bag or catheter may also be used.

11. Assess patient's condition during procedure, including respiratory status, vital signs if indicated, and complaints of pain.

Changes indicate complications.

> **SAFE PATIENT CARE** For patients who have a paracentesis or thoracentesis, increased abdominal or thoracic pain is significant. Severe abdominal pain after a paracentesis indicates a possible bowel perforation. Abdominal pain after a thoracentesis may result from diaphragmatic, liver, or spleen perforation. Inspiratory chest pain may result from perforation of the lung.

12. Note characteristics of aspirate.
   a. **Bone marrow aspirate:** Marrow is red or yellow.

Normal marrow.

   b. **Lumbar puncture:** Record opening pressure; observe fluid for color, cloudiness, or blood.

Normal CSF is clear and colorless. Cloudy color is the result of protein, which indicates an infection.

   c. **Paracentesis:** Fluid is yellow, cloudy, bile-stained green, or blood tinged. Gastric lavage fluid may appear bright red.

Blood-tinged fluid results from a traumatic tap.

   d. **Thoracentesis:** Pleural fluid is clear yellow, puslike, or cloudy.

Transudates and exudates are typically yellow, straw color. Blood-stained fluid indicates a malignancy, pulmonary infarction, or severe inflammation. Puslike fluid indicates an infection (empyema); milky fluid indicates a leak from the thoracic duct resulting in lymphatic drainage in the pleural cavity.

13. Properly label specimen in presence of patient (see Chapter 8). Transport tubes with filled-out test requisitions to the laboratory immediately.

You are responsible for labeling tubes with required patient identification, collection date and time, and tests desired. Test tubes are numbered in sequence of collection (e.g., 1 through 4).

STEPS	RATIONALE
14. Physician removes needle or trocar and applies pressure over insertion site until drainage ceases. Assist with placement of closure device or direct pressure and gauze dressing. Continue to apply pressure for a specific time period as ordered.	Assists with homeostasis and secures insertion site.
15. Assist patient to comfortable position per procedure protocol. Resume activity per health care provider order.	
16. **See Completion Protocol (inside front cover).**	

▌EVALUATION

1. Monitor vital signs; pulse oximetry, $ETCO_2$; symmetry of chest wall movements (thoracentesis and paracentesis); and lower extremity movement, sensation, and muscle strength according to facility policy or as ordered.
2. Inspect dressing over puncture site for bleeding, swelling, tenderness, and erythema. Inspect area under patient for bleeding. Avoid disrupting a healing clot at the site if a pressure dressing is present.
3. Ask patient to describe level of pain using a scale of 0 to 10.
4. Following paracentesis, obtain patient weight and measure abdominal girth.
5. Use *Teach Back:* State to the patient, "I want to be sure you understand the instructions I gave. Tell me what activities you are not able to do now that your (procedure) is done." Evaluates what the patient is able to explain or demonstrate. Revise your instruction now or develop plan for revised patient teaching to be implemented at an appropriate time if patient is not able to teach back correctly.

Unexpected Outcomes and Related Interventions

1. Oversedation occurs (e.g., decreased SaO_2, shallow respirations, tachycardia).
   a. Support patient's airway and breathing (administer oxygen as needed).
   b. Immediately notify patient's physician (call Rapid Response Team if available).
   c. Be prepared to administer emergency medications or reversal agents (e.g., naloxone [Narcan] for reversal of opioids or flumazenil [Romazicon] for reversal of benzodiazepines).
2. Postprocedural headache after LP (frontal or occipital, "burning" that radiates into the neck and shoulders, blurred vision, and tinnitus).
   a. Medicate for pain as ordered.
   b. Notify physician, who may choose to inject a blood patch into the epidural space.
   c. IV caffeine sodium benzoate has been used with limited success in relieving mild PPH.
3. Hematoma develops internally at LP site (lower extremity tingling, decreased peripheral pulse).
   a. Notify physician.
   b. Continue frequent evaluation.
4. Patient after LP develops excessive loss of CSF (large amount of CSF drainage from site and reduced LOC, dilated pupils, and increased blood pressure).
   a. Maintain airway and monitor vital signs.
   b. Notify health care provider immediately (call Rapid Response Team if available).
   c. Prepare for transfer to intensive care setting.
5. Patient after paracentesis develops leakage of fluid at the aspiration site as evidenced by continuously saturated dressings.
   a. Reinforce dressing. Place collection bag over the site if needed.
   b. Notify health care provider, who may place a small suture to stop the drainage.
6. Pneumothorax (sudden dyspnea and tachypnea and asymmetrical chest excursion).
   a. Administer oxygen as needed.
   b. Monitor vital signs and respiratory status frequently.
   c. Notify health care provider immediately (call Rapid Response Team if available).
   d. Anticipate chest x-ray film and possible chest tube insertion.

Recording and Reporting

- Record in medical record name of procedure; preprocedure preparation; location of puncture site; amount, consistency, and color of fluid drained or specimen obtained; duration of procedure; patient's tolerance of procedure (e.g., vital signs, SaO_2) and comfort level; laboratory tests ordered; specimen sent; type of dressing; postprocedure activities (e.g., chest x-ray film); and other procedure-specific assessments (e.g., extremity assessment, abdominal girth, LOC).
- Document your evaluation of patient learning.
- Immediately report to health care provider or charge nurse any unexpected drainage or significant changes in vital signs or SaO_2/$ETCO_2$ status. (For significant changes in vital signs or decrease in SaO_2, call Rapid Response Team if available.)

Sample Documentation

0930 Voided 300 mL. Abdominal girth measures 42 inches (106 cm) at umbilicus preprocedure. Preprocedure weight 72.7 kg (160 pounds). Assisted with sitting on side of bed. Physician completed abdominal paracentesis with 1100 mL cloudy liquid aspirated. Respirations 18 with moderate depth, pulse 98, and blood pressure 138/86. Rates pain at 6 on scale of 0 to 10. 22-inch gauze dressing applied to puncture site; remains dry and intact.

0940 Morphine sulfate 4 mg IV push given through IV in right forearm for abdominal pain.

1010 States pain has decreased to 2, which is tolerable. Abdominal girth measures 38 inches at umbilicus. Weight decreased to 71.8 kg (158 pounds).

Special Considerations

Pediatric

- Conscious or unconscious sedation is recommended for children because of the risk of injury caused by movement during procedures. Very young children may receive IV moderate sedation or general anesthetic.
- Prepare child of preschool age before the procedure; make a game out of having child recall the next procedural step, using a doll as a model. This can distract the child (Hockenberry and Wilson, 2013).
- Provide parental/family teaching, emotional support, and coaching before, during, and after procedure.

Geriatric

- Older adults with arthritis may have difficulty sustaining the position required for the procedure and need help during the procedure.
- During thoracentesis, be aware of ineffective breathing patterns in older adults because of age-related changes, such as reduced elastic lung recoil, declining chest expansion, reduced cough efficiency, and weaker thoracic and diaphragmatic muscles.
- Be aware of need to change positions slowly to minimize risks for postural hypotension.

Home Care

- Explain that some patients experience tenderness at the puncture site for several days, and the physician may order a mild analgesia.
- Instruct patient to get medical attention immediately if he or she suddenly experiences severe headache or has change in LOC.
- Inform patient after paracentesis to notify physician of fever or any swelling, pain, or drainage at puncture site. Instruct men to report scrotal pain, edema, or discoloration to the physician.
- Teach the patient after paracentesis symptoms of complications related to liver and spleen perforation that may not be present for several days after procedure and to notify the physician. Instruct patient to report any new abdominal pain to the physician.

SKILL 9.3 **CARE OF PATIENTS UNDERGOING BRONCHOSCOPY**

Bronchoscopy is the examination of the tracheobronchial tree through a lighted tube containing mirrors (Fig. 9-2). The tube most commonly used is a flexible fiberoptic bronchoscope that allows both visualization and simultaneous administration of oxygen. The fiberoptic bronchoscope has lumens for visualization and for obtaining sputum, foreign bodies, and biopsy specimens. Laser ablation of endotracheal lesions may be performed through the bronchoscope.

Bronchoscopy is an emergency or elective procedure performed for diagnostic and therapeutic reasons. The main purposes of this procedure are to aspirate excessive sputum or mucous plugs that airway suctioning cannot remove; to visualize the tracheobronchial tree for assessment of abnormalities of the mucosa, abscesses, aspiration pneumonia, strictures, and tumors; to obtain deep-tissue biopsy and sputum specimens; and to remove foreign bodies. Potential complications of bronchoscopy include fever, infection, hypoxemia, bronchospasm and laryngospasm, pneumothorax, aspiration, dysrhythmias and hypotension, hemorrhage (after biopsy), and cardiac arrest. The procedure is performed at the bedside or in a specially equipped endoscopy room. Usually a pulmonary specialist or surgeon performs this procedure in approximately 30 to 45 minutes.

ASSESSMENT

1. Identify patient using two identifiers (e.g., name and birthday or name and account number) according to facility policy. Compare identifiers with information on the patient's MAR or medical record. *Rationale: Ensures correct patient. Complies with The Joint Commission standards and improves patient safety (TJC, 2014).*
2. Verify the type of procedure that the physician will perform with the patient and medical record. *Rationale: Verifies correct patient receives correct procedure.*
3. Verify that informed consent was obtained. Ask patient if there are questions. *Rationale: Federal regulations, many state laws, and accreditation agencies require informed consent for procedures.*
4. Assess patient's history and cardiopulmonary status, including inability to tolerate interruption of high-flow oxygen. Report this to the health care provider. *Rationale: Determines need for oxygen administration during procedure.*
5. Obtain vital signs, pulse oximetry, and ETCO$_2$ level. *Rationale: Provides baseline data to compare with findings during and after procedure.*

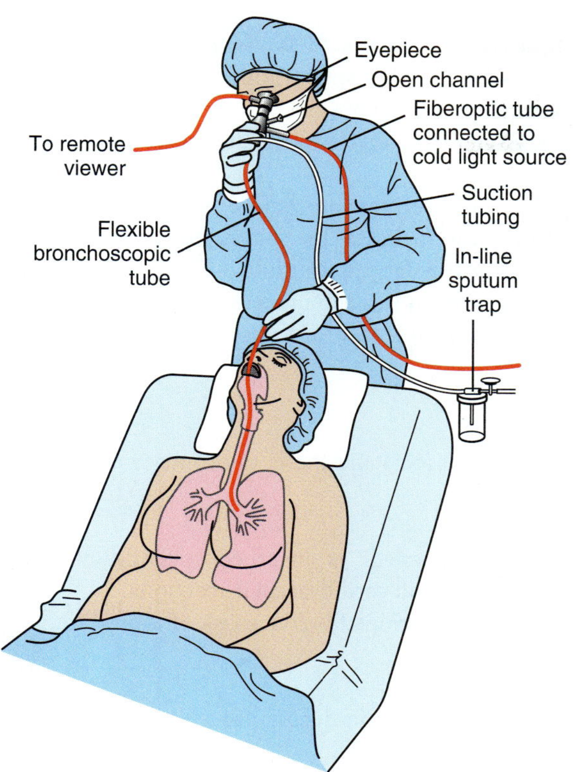

FIG 9-2 Flexible fiberoptic bronchoscopy.

6. Perform respiratory assessment, including lung sounds, chest wall symmetry, pain on inspiration, type of cough, and sputum quantity and color. *Rationale: Provides baseline of respiratory status for comparison during and after procedure.*

7. Review medical record for purpose of procedure: Sputum aspiration, tissue biopsy, sputum culture, removal of foreign object. *Rationale: Anticipates equipment and patient needs.*

8. Determine if patient is allergic to local anesthetic (usually lidocaine) for spraying throat. *Rationale: Allergy produces laryngospasm and laryngeal edema.*

9. Assess time patient last ingested fluids or food. Patients should be NPO 8 hours before bronchoscopy. *Rationale: NPO status decreases chance of aspiration of stomach contents.*

10. Assess patient's knowledge of procedure to determine level of teaching required. *Rationale: Determines level of understanding and level of support needed.*

PLANNING

Expected Outcomes focus on improving patient's knowledge of the procedure, reducing anxiety regarding the procedure and results, and detecting potential complications early.

1. Patient recovers from sedation without respiratory complications or change in LOC.
2. Patient's pain level is 4 or less on a pain scale of 0 to 10.
3. Patient explains what to expect during the procedure before it begins.
4. Patient's vital signs remain within baseline values.

Delegation and Collaboration

The skill of assisting with bronchoscopy cannot be delegated to nursing assistive personnel (NAP). Respiratory therapists typically assist in the procedure; however, they are not licensed to give IV medications or perform the assessments required during the procedure. Some facilities may use CRNAs or anesthesiologists to administer sedation and to monitor the patient during the procedure. The NAP may take baseline and postprocedure vital signs and assist with patient positioning as long as a nurse is present continuously during the procedure. The nurse instructs the NAP about:

- How to assist with patient positioning.

Equipment

- Bronchoscopy tray, if available from central supply, which may include: Flexible fiberoptic bronchoscope (Fig. 9-2), gauze sponges (4 × 4 inch), local anesthetic spray (lidocaine), sterile tracheal suction catheters
- Diazepam (Valium), midazolam (Versed), or other sedatives for IV sedation
- Oxygen, resuscitative equipment
- Sphygmomanometer, SaO_2/$ETCO_2$ monitor, cardiac monitor
- Sterile gloves
- Sterile water-soluble lubricating jelly (Note: Petroleum-based lubricants are not used because of the hazard of aspiration and subsequent pneumonia.)
- Personal protective equipment: Mask, gown, sterile gloves, and goggles for all health care providers
- Emesis basin
- Tongue depressor
- Tracheal suction equipment

IMPLEMENTATION *for* CARE OF PATIENTS UNDERGOING BRONCHOSCOPY

STEPS	RATIONALE
1. **See Standard Protocol (inside front cover).**	
2. Remove and safely store patient's dentures and eyeglasses (if applicable).	Bronchoscope may be inserted into oropharynx.
3. Assess current IV access or establish new IV access using large-bore cannula (see Chapter 27).	Provides access for IV fluids or medications if an emergency occurs.

Continued

STEPS	RATIONALE
4. Assist patient in maintaining position desired by physician, usually semi-Fowler's.	Provides maximal visualization of lower airways and adequate lung expansion.
5. Premedicate patient 30 minutes before procedure as ordered.	Reduces pain and anxiety associated with procedure.
6. Take "Time Out" to verify patient's name, type of procedure to be performed, and procedure site with the patient.	"Time Out" verification before start of an invasive procedure includes the physician and all involved personnel. Safety precaution prevents wrong patient, wrong site, and wrong procedure errors (TJC, 2014).
7. Team members perform hand hygiene and apply appropriate protective equipment.	Prevents transmission of infection.
8. Certified nurse, CRNA, or physician will administer IV moderate sedation when ordered.	
9. Physician sprays nasopharynx and oropharynx with topical anesthetic 0 to 15 minutes before the procedure.	Provides swift local anesthesia to oropharynx.
10. Instruct patient not to swallow local anesthetic; provide an emesis basin.	Swallowed anesthetic is absorbed systemically and can cause CNS and cardiovascular reactions.
11. Apply clean gloves. Position tip of suction catheter for easy access in patient's mouth as physician prepares to begin.	Drains oral secretions to reduce risk of aspiration.
12. Another physician or nurse attaches bronchoscope to machine light source.	Enhances visualization during procedure.
13. Physician introduces bronchoscope into mouth to pharynx and passes through glottis and into trachea and bronchi (see Fig. 9-2). The physician may use more anesthetic spray at glottis to prevent cough reflex or gagging. For intubated patients, the flexible bronchoscope is introduced through the endotracheal tube.	Bronchoscope must pass through upper airway structures to promote visualization of lower airways. Trachea and bronchi are observed for lesions and obstructions.
14. Physician suctions mucus, performs bronchial washing, and collects cytological specimens with a wire brush or curette. Biopsy specimens may also be obtained.	Cytological specimens are obtained to diagnose carcinoma.
15. Assist patient by giving explanations, verbal reassurance, and support.	Premedicated and drowsy patients need reminders not to change position and to cooperate.
16. Assess patient's vital signs, pulse oximetry, $ETCO_2$, cardiac monitor, and breathing capacity every 5 minutes during procedure. (This will be done by personnel delivering sedation.)	Establishes monitoring for oversedation (see Skill 9.1).
17. Observe degree of restlessness, respiratory rate, capillary refill, and color of nail beds.	Bronchoscope may cause feelings of suffocation; also, because airway is partially occluded, patient may become hypoxic during observations.
18. Note characteristics of suctioned material. Expect a small amount of blood mixed with the aspirate as a result of tissue trauma. Report anything unusual.	Alerts physician to any developing problem.
19. Physician will remove bronchoscope. Use your gloved hand to wipe patient's nose to remove lubricant.	Promotes hygiene and comfort.
20. Instruct patient not to try to swallow sputum until gag reflex returns and tracheobronchial anesthesia has worn off (usually 2 hours). Patient will be NPO until reflex returns. Provide emesis basis or hand-controlled Yankauer suction device for expectoration of sputum. If patient still sedated, place in side-lying position.	Helps prevent aspiration pneumonia, which is a risk until gag reflex returns.

STEPS	RATIONALE
21. Properly label specimen in presence of patient (see Chapter 8). Transport tubes with filled-out test requisitions to the laboratory immediately.	You are responsible for labeling tubes with required patient identification, collection date and time, and tests desired. Test tubes are numbered in sequence of collection (e.g., 1 through 4).
22. See Completion Protocol (inside front cover).	

EVALUATION

1. Closely monitor patient's vital signs, SaO_2/$ETCO_2$ and respiratory status, including auscultation of lung fields. Monitor for sudden dyspnea indicating laryngospasm or bronchospasm.
2. Evaluate level of sedation and LOC; use Modified Ramsay Sedation Scale (see Table 9-1).
3. Monitor for return of gag reflex, which usually returns within 2 hours. Use tongue depressor to touch pharynx to test for presence of reflex.
4. Observe character and amount of sputum. Physician may order serial sputum collection for 24 hours for cytological examination.
5. Assess patient's level of pain.
6. Use *Teach Back:* State to the patient, "It is important you know what to do now that the test is over. I want to be sure you understand what I explained. Tell me why you cannot have any fluid or food for the next 2 hours. What may happen if you do?" Evaluates what the patient is able to explain or demonstrate. Revise your instruction now or develop plan for revised patient teaching to be implemented at an appropriate time if patient is not able to teach back correctly.

Unexpected Outcomes and Related Interventions

1. Laryngospasm and bronchospasm (sudden, severe shortness of breath, stridor, and intercostal retractions).
   a. Call physician immediately (call Rapid Response Team if available).
   b. Prepare emergency resuscitation equipment, and administer oxygen as needed.
   c. Anticipate possible cricothyrotomy.
2. Presence of hypoxemia (decreased SaO_2/$ETCO_2$, gradual shortness of breath, and decreasing LOC).
   a. Maintain airway and oxygenation (administer oxygen as needed).
   b. Notify physician immediately (call Rapid Response Team if available).
   c. Monitor SaO_2.
3. Vasovagal response during bronchoscope insertion: Vasovagal response is caused by stimulation of the baroreceptors, causing bradycardia. Symptoms include feeling faint, dizzy, and light-headed and being diaphoretic with a slow, steady pulse. Patient may become unconscious for a few seconds.
   a. Lower head of table as ordered.
   b. Support airway.

c. Be prepared to administer emergency medications as ordered: Atropine (up to 0.03 mg/kg) to increase heart rate or epinephrine (0.1 mg/kg).
4. Hemorrhage.
   a. Call physician immediately (call Rapid Response Team if available).
   b. Emergency resuscitation equipment must be readily available.
   c. Follow specific postprocedure orders related to findings.
5. Oversedation occurs (e.g., decreased SaO_2, shallow respirations, tachycardia).
   a. Support patient's airway and breathing (administer oxygen as needed).
   b. Immediately notify patient's physician (call Rapid Response Team if available).
   c. Be prepared to administer emergency medications or reversal agent (e.g., naloxone [Narcan] for reversal of opioids or flumazenil [Romazicon] for reversal of benzodiazepines).

Recording and Reporting

- Record name of procedure (include biopsy if performed), duration of procedure, patient's tolerance of procedure and any complications, and collection and disposition of specimen. Document return of gag reflex.
- Document your evaluation of patient learning.
- Report excessive bleeding, hemoptysis, or respiratory difficulty after procedure or changes in vital signs beyond patient's normal limits to physician immediately. Report results of procedure to appropriate health care personnel.

Sample Documentation

0900 To bronchoscopy via stretcher.
1030 Returned from bronchoscopy. Alert and oriented. Vital signs stable. SaO_2 88% on room air. Resting in semi-Fowler's position. Denies dyspnea. Color pale. Respirations 28; rhonchi noted bilaterally at bases, clears some with cough. Occasional cough noted productive of small amount of bright red sputum. No gag reflex present.
1130 Vital signs stable and recorded every 15 minutes $\times$ 4. No change in assessment.
1230 Vital signs stable. Gag reflex present. No cough or sputum production since 1130. Taking sips of clear liquids without difficulty.

Special Considerations
Pediatric

- Bronchoscopy is performed in children to remove foreign bodies from larynx or trachea and is done under general anesthesia.
- Children are at higher risk of hypoxemia than adults because of their smaller bronchus and because the bronchoscope decreases the available breathing space (Pagana and Pagana, 2013).
- Provide parental/family teaching, emotional support, and coaching before, during, and after procedure.

Geriatric

- Postprocedure restlessness in the older adult patient often indicates hypoxemia or pain. Thoroughly assess oxygenation status before administration of an opioid analgesic.
- Physical exposure and room temperature contribute to hypothermia in frail older adults, who are unable to communicate that they are cold. Use heated blankets or forced air heat to maintain core temperature at comfortable, safe levels.

Home Care

- Instruct patient to notify the physician if the following symptoms develop: fever, chest pain, dyspnea, wheezing, or hemoptysis.
- Throat discomfort is normal after this procedure. Warm saline gargles or throat lozenges are helpful.

SKILL 9.4 CARE OF PATIENTS UNDERGOING GASTROINTESTINAL ENDOSCOPY

Endoscopy is any study that allows direct visualization of an internal organ or structure via a long, flexible fiberoptic scope with a light source attached (Fig. 9-3). An esophagoscopy, gastroscopy, gastroduodenojejunoscopy, or duodenoscopy visualizes the upper gastrointestinal (GI) tract; more frequently, these procedures are combined, which permits visualization of the esophagus, stomach, and duodenum (esophagogastroduodenoscopy [EGD]) in one examination. A proctoscopy, sigmoidoscopy, or colonoscopy visualizes the lower GI tract. Endoscopy enables visualization of the lining of the GI tract for polyps and bleeding, biopsy of suspicious tissue, polyp removal, and performance of procedures requiring direct visual guidance (e.g., fine-needle aspiration biopsies and dilation and stenting of strictures). For visualization of the hepatobiliary tree and pancreatic ducts, endoscopic retrograde cholangiopancreatography is performed during EGD. Typically, these patients receive IV moderate sedation.

The most common risks after upper GI colonoscopy include abnormal reaction (cardiovascular and pulmonary) to sedatives, bleeding from biopsy, and accidental puncture of the upper GI tract (NDDIC, 2012). Similar complications are common with lower GI procedures. Infection can occur but is rare unless intestinal perforation occurs. Both upper and lower GI endoscopic examinations are performed in a specially equipped endoscopic unit.

2. Verify the type of procedure that the physician will perform and the procedure site with the patient. *Rationale: Ensures correct patient receives correct procedure.*
3. Verify that informed consent was obtained. Ask patient if there are questions. *Rationale: Federal regulations, many state laws, and accreditation agencies require informed consent for procedures.*
4. Obtain baseline vital signs and SaO_2/$ETCO_2$ levels.
5. Determine if signs of GI bleeding are present by observing the character of emesis, stool, and nasogastric tube drainage for frank blood or black material that looks like coffee grounds. *Rationale: Procedure is contraindicated in patients with severe upper GI bleeding because the viewing lens is covered with blood clots, preventing visualization (Pagana and Pagana, 2013).*

ASSESSMENT

1. Identify patient using two identifiers (e.g., name and birthday or name and account number) according to facility policy. Compare identifiers with information on the patient's MAR or medical record. *Rationale: Ensures correct patient. Complies with The Joint Commission standards and improves patient safety (TJC, 2014).*

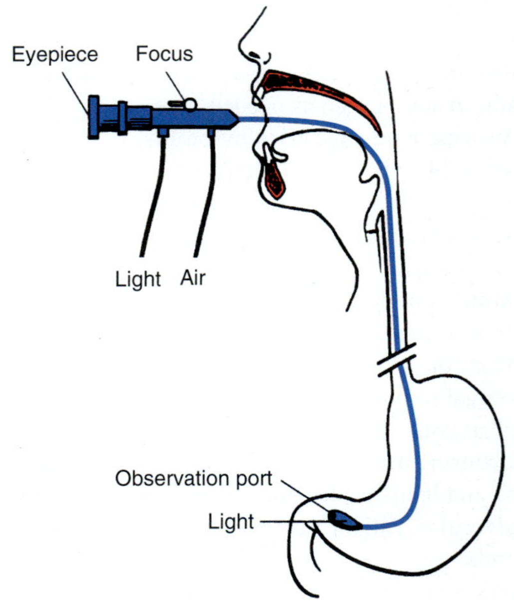

FIG 9-3 Flexible endoscope to visualize stomach.

> **SAFE PATIENT CARE** If patient is bleeding actively, the physician may order lavage of the stomach and aspiration to clear clots so that procedure can be performed.

6. Determine the purpose of procedure: Biopsy, examination, or coagulation of bleeding sites. *Rationale: Anticipates appropriate equipment needs.*

7. Assess patient's knowledge and explain the steps of the procedure. *Rationale: Determines level of teaching required.*

8. Verify that patient has followed the "2-6-8 rule" for preprocedure fasting—a minimum fasting period of 2 hours is required for clear liquids; 6 hours, for a light meal (toast and liquids but no fatty foods or butter); and 8 hours, for full meal (Lewis and Cohen, 2013). *Rationale: Reduces chances of vomiting and resultant aspiration during and immediately after procedure.*

9. For lower GI studies (proctoscopy, sigmoidoscopy, or colonoscopy), verify that the patient has followed a clear liquid diet for 2 days and has completed any ordered bowel cleansing regimen. *Rationale: An empty intestinal tract is necessary to allow insertion of the endoscope and good visualization of the interior walls.*

10. Assess patient's ability to understand and follow directions. *Rationale: Procedures require patient to follow directions closely and assume proper position.*

11. Identify designated driver after procedure. *Rationale: Patients are not allowed to drive for 24 hours after sedation anesthesia.*

PLANNING

Expected Outcomes focus on preventing complications, promoting patient's ability to follow instructions, and protecting patient's airway.

1. Patient does not aspirate and has no postprocedure bleeding.
2. Patient's level of pain is 4 or less on a pain scale of 0 to 10.
3. Patient is without respiratory complications or change in LOC.
4. Vital signs remain within baseline.

Delegation and Collaboration

The skill of assisting with endoscopy cannot be delegated to nursing assistive personnel (NAP). Some facilities may use CRNAs or anesthesiologists to administer sedation and to monitor the patient during the procedure. The NAP may take baseline and postprocedure vital signs and assist with patient positioning as long as a nurse is present continuously. The nurse instructs the NAP about:

- How to assist with patient positioning.

Equipment

- Personal protective equipment: Mask, gown, gloves, goggles for all health care personnel
- Endoscopy tray
- Fiberoptic endoscope and camera (see Fig. 9-3) and carbon dioxide source (for lower GI procedures)
- Solutions for biopsy specimens
- Local anesthetic spray
- Tracheal suction equipment (see Chapter 14)
- Vital signs monitoring equipment
- Water-soluble jelly
- Sterile gloves for physician
- Emesis basin
- IV fluid and equipment for IV start (optional)
- Diazepam (Valium), midazolam (Versed), or other sedative for IV sedation (optional)
- Oxygen, resuscitative equipment, and pulse oximetry and $ETCO_2$ monitors

IMPLEMENTATION *for* CARE OF PATIENTS UNDERGOING GASTROINTESTINAL ENDOSCOPY

STEPS	RATIONALE
1. **See Standard Protocol (inside front cover).**	
2. Administer any preprocedure medication.	Promotes relaxation and reduces anxiety.
3. Apply clean gloves. Remove patient's eyeglasses, dentures, or other dental appliances.	Prevents damage to glasses and dislodgment of dental structures during procedure.
4. Take "Time Out" to verify patient's name, type of procedure to be performed, and procedure site with the patient.	"Time Out" verification before start of an invasive procedure includes the physician and all involved personnel. Safety precaution prevents wrong patient, wrong site, and wrong procedure errors (TJC, 2014).
5. Assess current IV access or establish new IV access using large-bore cannula (see Chapter 27).	Provides access for IV fluids or medications if an emergency occurs.
6. All staff participating in procedure will perform hand hygiene and apply appropriate personal protective gear.	Reduces transmission of infection.
7. Assist patient through procedure:	Helps to minimize patient's anxiety.
a. Anticipate needs and promote comfort.	Patient unable to speak if endoscope is passed into throat.

Continued

STEPS	RATIONALE

    b. Tell patient what will happen during each phase.

Reassures patient.

8. Position patient.

    a. *Upper GI procedures:* Assist patient in maintaining left lateral Sims' position.

Sims' position allows easy passage of upper or lower endoscope. Provides for airway clearance if patient gags and vomits gastric contents.

    b. *Lower GI procedures:* Assist patient in maintaining left lateral decubitus position. Drape patient for privacy and comfort.

Left lateral decubitus position provides access to lower GI tract.

9. Certified nurse, CRNA, or physician will administer IV moderate sedation as ordered. Atropine is typically given for upper GI studies.

Ensures safe delivery of sedation. Atropine reduces quantity of secretions, reducing risk of aspiration.

10. Position tip of suction cannula for easy access in patient's mouth (upper GI studies).

Drains oral secretions to reduce risk for aspiration.

11. *Upper GI studies:* The physician administers local anesthetic spray to the oropharynx, then slowly passes the endoscope into mouth, esophagus, stomach, or duodenum and advances to desired depth while visualizing the organ lining.

Provides visualization of structures.

12. *Lower GI studies:* A lubricant-coated flexible fiberoptic endoscope is inserted through the anus and slowly advanced through the rectum and colon, visualizing the linings.

13. Physician insufflates air through endoscope into upper GI tract. Carbon dioxide is used for colonoscopies. Physician examines, photographs, or performs biopsy of structures. Physician slowly removes the endoscope.

Distends GI structures for better visualization. Carbon dioxide insufflation produces less postprocedure abdominal cramping than air insufflation (Shi et al., 2013).

14. Properly label specimen in presence of patient (see Chapter 8). Transport tubes with filled-out test requisitions to the laboratory immediately.

You are responsible for labeling tubes with required patient identification, collection date and time, and tests desired. Test tubes are numbered in sequence of collection (e.g., 1 through 4).

15. Assist patient to comfortable position. If sedated, place in a side-lying position.

Promotes rest and relaxation.

16. Suction airway if patient begins to vomit or accumulate saliva. Remove and discard gloves.

Prevents aspiration of gastric contents or oral secretions.

17. Prepare to discharge patient only after return of gag reflex. Explain that patient will feel "woozy" and may notice abdominal cramping. Patient should not drive for 24 hours.

Absence of gag reflex increases risk of aspiration. When the gag reflex is absent, the patient needs continuous monitoring.

18. See Completion Protocol (inside front cover).

▌EVALUATION

1. Monitor vital signs for signs of bleeding (tachycardia and hypotension) every 15 minutes for 2 hours (see facility protocol). Evaluate emesis or aspirate for frank or occult blood.
2. Evaluate level of sedation; use the Modified Ramsay Sedation Scale (see Table 9-1).
3. Ask patient to describe pain using a 0 to 10 pain scale.
5. Evaluate for return of gag reflex, usually within 2 hours. Assess breath sounds, labor of respirations, and SaO_2/$ETCO_2$. Patient NPO until return of gag reflex.
6. Use **Teach Back:** State to the patient, "I want to be sure you have no problems once you go home. Can you tell me what we discussed about the things you should not do after your procedure?" Evaluates what the patient is able to explain or demonstrate. Revise your instruction now or develop plan for revised patient teaching to be implemented at an appropriate time if patient is not able to teach back correctly.

Unexpected Outcomes and Related Interventions

1. Presence of hypoxemia (decreased SaO_2/$ETCO_2$, gradual shortness of breath, and decreasing LOC).
   a. Maintain airway and oxygenation (administer oxygen as needed).
   b. Notify physician immediately (call Rapid Response Team if available).

c. Monitor SaO_2/$ETCO_2$, and have sedative reversal agents available.

2. Hemorrhage (hypotension and tachycardia and decreasing LOC with or without visible signs of hemorrhage). Note: Hemorrhage may occur immediately or after several weeks.

   a. Take vital signs and notify physician immediately. Hemorrhage can be life-threatening (call Rapid Response Team if available).
   b. Prepare emergency resuscitation equipment (administer oxygen as needed).
   c. Observe and auscultate the abdomen.
   d. Follow specific postprocedure orders related to findings.

3. Perforation (sharp intense pain in chest, stomach, or abdomen; abdominal distention; and cool, pale skin).

   a. Notify physician immediately (call Rapid Response Team if available).
   b. Prepare for order of chest computed tomography scan.
   c. Maintain patent, functioning IV.

4. Vasovagal response caused by stimulation of the baroreceptors during endoscope insertion, as evidenced by feeling faint, dizzy, and light-headed; diaphoresis with a slow, steady pulse; or a few seconds of unconsciousness.

   a. Lower head of table.
   b. Support airway.

Reporting and Recording

- Record the procedure, duration, patient's tolerance, complications and interventions, and collection and disposition of specimen.
- Document your evaluation of patient learning.
- Report onset of difficulty to arouse, bleeding, abdominal pain, dyspnea, and vital sign changes to physician.

Sample Documentation

0800   Patient NPO since midnight. Transported to endoscopy department via wheelchair for EGD. Vital signs within normal limits. Consent signed. Reports that physician explained procedure and he has no questions at present.
1000   Returned from endoscopy. Reports no discomfort. Vital signs at baseline level. No apparent bleeding. Gag reflex present.

Special Considerations
Pediatric

- Children require deep sedation or general anesthesia for this procedure.
- Introduction of the endoscope in infants and small children who have a narrow and collapsible airway can result in respiratory distress.
- Provide parental/family teaching, emotional support, and coaching before, during, and after procedure.

Geriatric

- The risk of cardiopulmonary events associated with endoscopy is increased with advanced age and presence of comorbidities (other illnesses).
- Older adults are at risk for prolonged sedation because of age-related decreased glomerular filtration rate and decreased hepatic function. Monitor urine output closely.
- Physical exposure and room temperature contribute to hypothermia in frail older adults. Use heated blankets or forced air heat to maintain core temperature at comfortable, safe levels.
- Older adults are at risk for dehydration, electrolyte imbalance, and exhaustion from test preparation combined with NPO status. If the procedure is done on an ambulatory care basis, it is helpful to have someone stay with the patient.

Home Care

- Instruct ambulatory care patients to notify the physician if the following symptoms develop: swallowing difficulties; throat, chest, and abdominal pain that worsens; vomiting; bloody or very dark stool; fever; dyspnea and wheezing (NDDIC, 2012).
- Manage throat discomfort with throat lozenges. Avoid commercial alcohol-based mouthwashes, which further irritate throat discomfort.
- After colonoscopy, a warm tub bath minimizes rectal discomfort.

SKILL 9.5   **OBTAINING AN ELECTROCARDIOGRAM**

A 12-lead electrocardiogram (ECG or EKG) is a graphic representation of the electrical activities, or conduction system, of the heart. The normal sequence of electrical impulses, called normal sinus rhythm, is transmitted through the heart and displayed in an ECG wave (Fig. 9-4). The electrical activity of the heart's conduction system is recorded to determine baseline cardiac function, to evaluate response to cardiac medications, to monitory recovery after a myocardial infarction (MI), or to evaluate a patient who has chest discomfort. An ECG monitors the regularity and path of an electrical impulse through the conduction system; however, it does not reflect muscular work of the heart. Continuous ECG monitoring is common in emergent situations when there is a need for ongoing cardiac monitoring. In this case, a health care provider will run either a three- or five-lead ECG.

ASSESSMENT

1. Identify patient using two identifiers (e.g., name and birthday or name and account number) according to

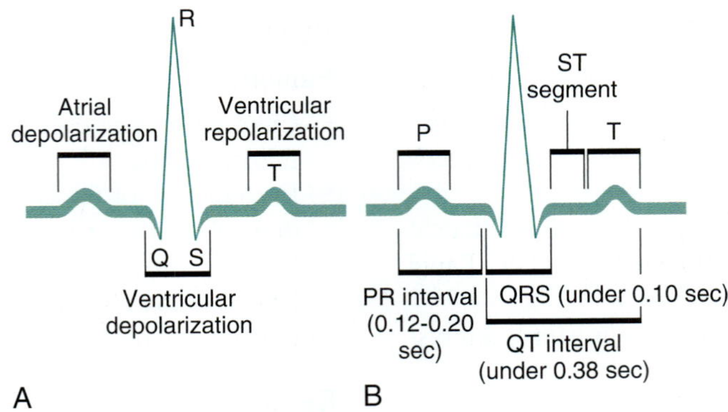

FIG 9-4 A and **B,** Normal ECG waveform. (From Pagana KD, Pagana TJ: *Mosby's manual of diagnostic and laboratory tests,* ed 5, St Louis, 2014, Mosby.)

facility policy. Compare identifiers with information on the patient's MAR or medical record. *Rationale: Ensures correct patient. Complies with The Joint Commission standards and improves patient safety (TJC, 2014).*

2. Assess patient's history and cardiopulmonary status, including response to previous procedures. *Rationale: Determines need for oxygen administration during procedure if the patient must lay flat or if the head of bed should be elevated during the procedure.*

3. Verify type of ECG ordered. Review medical record for purpose of procedure (e.g., baseline assessment or diagnostic). *Rationale: Anticipates timing for when to perform procedure. Onset of chest pain requires immediate testing.*

4. Assess patient's knowledge of procedure to determine level of teaching required.

5. Assess patient's ability to follow instructions and remain still in supine position. *Rationale: Provides clear, accurate recording without electrical artifacts.*

- Patient tolerates procedure without anxiety or discomfort.
- Clear recording of ECG waveform is obtained.

Delegation and Collaboration

The skill of assisting or performing the ECG may be delegated to NAP. The nurse instructs the NAP about:
- How to position the patient.
- To notify the nurse immediately if the patient experiences any chest pain or appears anxious.

Equipment
- Twelve-lead ECG machine
- ECG leads and electrodes appropriate for machine
- Alcohol wipes for skin preparation
- Electrode gel (optional depending on type of electrodes)
- Hair clippers (optional depending on hair at electrode sites)
- Sphygmomanometer
- Tape (optional)

PLANNING

Expected Outcomes focus on reducing patient's anxiety regarding the procedure and obtaining accurate test results.

IMPLEMENTATION *for* OBTAINING AN ELECTROCARDIOGRAM

STEPS	RATIONALE
1. **See Standard Protocol (inside front cover).**	
2. Assist the patient with the removal of clothing or reposition patient's clothing to expose only patient's chest and arms. Keep pelvis and thighs covered.	Minimizes patient embarrassment. Facilitates correct lead placement.
3. Explain to patient what the test involves, the sensation of electrode application, and the importance of lying still during the tracing.	Promotes patient cooperation.

STEPS	RATIONALE
4. Place patient in the supine position. Monitor for dyspnea or anxiety related to the procedure. Some patients may need to have the head of bed elevated to promote comfort or reduce anxiety. If patient is having chest pain, obtain vital signs.	Makes it easier for application of electrodes across chest and arms.
5. Clean and prepare the skin; wipe sites where electrodes will be placed with alcohol pads. Clip hair from the chest or extremities if the electrodes will not secure to the skin. Bony structures or prominence may prevent the electrode from adequately adhering to the skin requiring the use of tape to secure the electrode to the area.	Skin preparation removes oils that prevent adherence of electrodes.
6. Apply self-sticking electrodes. Use pressure on perimeter only and attach leads. (If self-sticking leads are unavailable, apply electrode paste and suction cup electrodes to skin.) **a.** Chest (precordial leads) (see illustration):	Positioning of leads promotes accurate display of ECG.

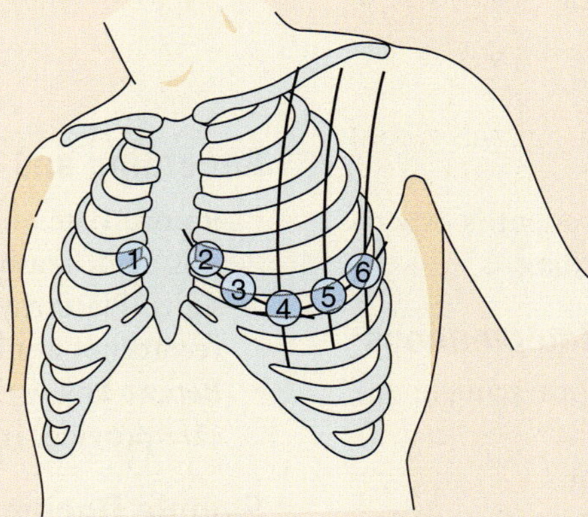

STEP 6a Anatomical placement of precordial leads. (From Pagana KD, Pagana TJ: *Mosby's manual of diagnostic and laboratory tests,* ed 5, St Louis, 2014, Mosby.)

V_1—fourth intercostal space (ICS) at right sternal border
V_2—fourth ICS at left sternal border
V_3—midway between V_2 and V_4
V_4—fifth ICS at midclavicular line
V_5—left anterior axillary line at level of V_4 horizontally
V_6—left midaxillary line at level of V_4 horizontally

b. Extremities—one lead on each extremity. Place on lower portion of each extremity, avoiding any bony prominences.
aV_r—right wrist
aV_l—left wrist
aV_f—left ankle
$aV_?$—right ankle

Continued

STEPS	RATIONALE

7. Turn on ECG machine, enter required demographic information into computer, and obtain tracing as ordered. Transmit or print ECG tracings for analysis.
  a. Simultaneous 12-lead recording:
    (1) Obtain simultaneous tracing of all 12 leads. Reposition leads as needed if artifacts or poor-quality tracing. If patient experiences chest pain, document on ECG printout.
  b. Continuous interpretation/monitoring:
    (1) Apply limb electrodes. Apply gel over location for a single chest lead where designated by facility policy or as ordered.
    (2) Maintain either two upper limb electrodes (three-lead), or four limb electrodes (five-lead).	

8. On completion of tracing, disconnect leads and wipe off any gel or adhesive. If serial tracings are expected, mark where leads were placed.	Promotes comfort and hygiene. Health care provider may desire subsequent tracings from same electrode site.
9. Deliver ECG tracing (if not computerized) to appropriate health care provider. Send electronic ECG to laboratory for analysis.	Provides for review of ECG by cardiologist.
10. **See Completion Protocol (inside front cover).**	

EVALUATION

1. Although procedure is painless, note if patient is experiencing any chest discomfort during recording.

Unexpected Outcomes and Related Interventions

1. ECG cannot be interpreted because of poor tracing in one or more leads and presence of artifacts.
   a. Inspect electrodes for secure placement.
   b. Reposition lead that moves secondary to patient movement and repeat tracing.
   c. Remind patient to lie still for accurate tracing.
2. Patient has chest pain or is very anxious.
   a. Continue to monitor ECG.
   b. Reassess factors contributing to anxiety or pain.
   c. Notify health care provider.

Recording and Reporting

- Record date and time ECG was obtained, where tracing was sent, reason for obtaining ECG, and baseline vital signs. Place rhythm strip in patient's chart (if electronic record not available).
- Report any arrhythmias or patient chest pain to health care provider immediately.

Sample Documentation

0900   Explained procedure to patient positioned in bed. 12-lead ECG performed and transmitted to cardiology laboratory. Skin cleansed, no irritation at electrode sites. Patient stated no complaints of pain or discomfort during or after ECG.

CRITICAL THINKING EXERCISES

Case Study

A 67-year-old African-American man is scheduled for a cardiac catheterization under moderate sedation. The prescription for the procedure faxed from the health care provider's office lists "new-onset chest pain" as the clinical indication for the procedure. The patient is currently taking medication to control blood pressure and cholesterol and is taking warfarin (Coumadin) for chronic atrial fibrillation. His personal health care provider instructed him to stop his warfarin 2 nights before the procedure. The patient followed the health care provider's recommendation and has not had warfarin for 2 days.

1. What laboratory data would the nurse review to prepare the patient for his procedure? Select all that apply.
   1. Complete blood count (CBC) and levels of prealbumin and blood gases
   2. CBC, PTT, and PT
   3. Lipid panel, blood glucose level, and electrolyte levels
   4. Blood urea nitrogen (BUN), creatinine, and urine specific gravity

2. When the nurse reviews the patient's chart, he sees that the consent form for the procedure is unsigned. When he inquires whether the health care provider explained the procedure and the risks and asks if the patient has any questions, the patient replies, "I was told that I needed this to find out why I have chest pain. But I don't know how risky it is." What should the nurse do?
   1. Ask the patient to sign the consent form and tell him to ask about the risks when the health care provider arrives.
   2. Hold the consent form until the health care provider arrives to speak with the patient.
   3. Hold the preprocedure laboratory tests until after the health care provider arrives to speak with the patient.
   4. Administer preprocedure diazepam (Valium) to help patient relax.

Review Questions

1. The nurse is assessing a patient after a cardiac catheterization. What assessments indicate possible bleeding? Select all that apply.
   1. Catheter site pain and loss of distal pulses
   2. Anxiety, backache, and heart rate increase from 90 to 105 beats/min
   3. Atrial fibrillation and drowsiness
   4. Pooling of blood under patient
   5. Fever and bradycardia
2. The nurse has four patients scheduled for interventional radiology procedures that require the use of radiopaque dye. For which patient is the procedure contraindicated?
   1. The patient with renal failure
   2. The patient with urinary tract infection
   3. The patient with possible kidney stones
   4. The patient with one kidney
3. The nurse's pediatric patient with leukemia is scheduled for a bone marrow aspiration. What nursing intervention is *not* appropriate?
   1. Apply topical anesthetic to the bone marrow aspiration site 10 minutes before the procedure is scheduled to begin.
   2. Verify that parental informed consent has been obtained.
   3. Use a doll to demonstrate the steps of the procedure for the child.
   4. Check emergency equipment for pediatric sizes.
4. Place the following steps of bronchoscopy preprocedure care in correct order.
   1. Perform the preprocedure "Time Out."
   2. Instruct patient not to swallow anesthetic
   3. Establish new IV access.
   4. Verify that informed consent has been obtained.
   5. Remove and store patient's dentures.

5. The nurse's patient is unresponsive and febrile, and acute meningitis is suspected. An emergent LP has been ordered. Appropriate delegation of care to NAP includes:
   1. Staying with registered nurse during the procedure to help maintain the patient's side-lying position
   2. Assisting the physician during the procedure and notifying you if the patient's vital signs deteriorate
   3. Monitoring patient's airway during the procedure and administering oxygen as needed
   4. Preparing the site and setting up the sterile tray
6. An abdominal paracentesis is performed on a patient, and 1500 mL of fluid is drained. Which of the following outcomes indicates a successful procedure?
   1. Increased abdominal girth, decreased respiratory effort, increased respiratory rate
   2. Increased abdominal girth, increased respiratory effort, decreased respiratory rate
   3. Decreased abdominal girth, decreased respiratory effort, decreased respiratory rate
   4. Decreased abdominal girth, increased respiratory effort, increased respiratory rate
7. The nurse is preparing the patient for a colonoscopy. Which of the following are necessary for preprocedure preparation? Select all that apply.
   1. Assist patient into a left side-lying position.
   2. Complete bowel preparation the morning of the procedure.
   3. NPO from midnight the day of the procedure.
   4. Come to the procedure with a designated driver.
8. Following an endoscopy, the patient is nauseated and vomits 200 mL of bright red blood. What are the nurse's correct actions? Select all that apply.
   1. Obtain the patient's vital signs.
   2. Notify the physician (call Rapid Response Team if available).
   3. Observe and auscultate the abdomen.
   4. Instruct the NAP to obtain next set of vital signs.
   5. Administer oxygen as needed.
   6. Observe the vomitus.
9. A nurse working in a procedure area receives a patient following a bronchoscopy. The patient is breathing shallow respirations at 8 per minute, HR is 100 beats/min and regular, BP is 110/68 mm Hg, and the patient does not arouse easily when the nurse speaks in a normal voice. It is likely this patient is experiencing:
   1. Hypotension
   2. Shock
   3. Oversedation
   4. Allergic reaction to lidocaine spray
10. A patient who exhibits signs and symptoms of oversedation after receiving fentanyl would likely receive which of the following reversal agents?
    1. Flumazenil
    2. Midazolam
    3. Naloxone
    4. Morphine

REFERENCES

American Society of Anesthesiologists (ASA): *Distinguishing monitored anesthesia (MAC) from moderate sedation/analgesia (Conscious Sedation)*, 2013, https://www.asahq.org/For-Members/Standards-Guidelines-and-Statements.aspx. Accessed June 13, 2014.

American Society for Gastrointestinal Endoscopy (ASGE): Complications of colonoscopy, *Gastrointest Endosc* 74(4):745, 2011.

Association of periOperative Registered Nurses (AORN): *Standards, recommended practices, and guidelines*, Denver, 2011, The Association.

Chernecky CC, Berger BJ: *Laboratory tests and diagnostic procedures*, ed 6, Philadelphia, 2013, Saunders.

Frank R, Wolfson A, Grayzel J: Procedural sedation in adults, *UpToDate*. http://www.uptodate.com/contents/procedural-sedation-in-adults.

Hockenberry MJ, Wilson D: *Wong's essentials of pediatric nursing*, ed 9, St Louis, 2013, Mosby.

Hoglund J, et al: The effect of early mobilization for patient undergoing coronary angiography: a pilot study with a focus on vascular complications and back pain, *Eur J Cardiovasc Nurs* 10(2):136, 2011.

Lewis S, et al: *Medical-surgical nursing*, ed 9, St Louis, 2014, Mosby.

Lewis JR, Cohen LB: Update on colonoscopy preparation, premedication and sedation, *Exp Rev Gastroenterol Hepatol* 7(1):77, 2013.

Lilly LL, et al: *Pharmacology and the nursing process*, ed 7, St Louis, 2012, Mosby.

Maioli M, et al: Effects of hydration in contrast-induced acute kidney injury after primary angioplasty: a randomized-controlled trial, *Circ Cardiovasc Interv* 4(5):456, 2011.

Muller M, Wehrmann T: How best to approach endoscopic sedation?, *Nat Rev Gastroenterol Hepatol* 8(9):481, 2011.

National Digestive Diseases Information Clearinghouse (NDDIC): Upper GI Endoscopy, 2012. http://digestive.niddk.nih.gov/ddiseases/pubs/upperendoscopy/#risks. Accessed March 22, 2014.

Pagana KD, Pagana TJ: *Mosby's diagnostic and laboratory tests*, ed 11, St Louis, 2013, Mosby.

Practice Advisory for Preanesthesia Evaluation: An Updated Report by the American Society of Anesthesiologist Taskforce on Preanesthesia Evaluation, *Anesthesiology* 116(3):3, 2012.

Schabelman E, Witting M: The relationship of radiocontrast, iodine, and seafood allergies: a medical myth exposed, *J Emerg Med* 39(5):701, 2010.

Shi H, et al: Carbon dioxide insufflation during endoscopic retrograde cholangiopancreatography: a review and meta-analysis, *Pancreas* 42(7):1093, 2013.

The Joint Commission (TJC): *National Patient Safety Goals*, Oakbrook Terrace, IL, 2014, The Commission. Available at: http://www.jointcommission.org/standards_information/npsgs.aspx.

CHAPTER

10

Bathing and Personal Hygiene

EVOLVE WEBSITE/EVOLVE RESOURCES LIST

http://evolve.elsevier.com/Perry/nursinginterventions
Audio Glossary • Checklists • Review Questions

Hygiene is important to the health and well-being of patients. Good hygiene supports physical and mental health. Personal hygiene provides an opportunity for a nurse and patient to discuss health-related concerns and allows the nurse to perform a physical assessment. Personal hygiene maintains skin integrity by promoting adequate circulation and hydration. The functions of intact skin include (1) defense against infection, (2) sensory perception, and (3) regulation of body temperature. Bathe the patient and change linens when any body part or linen becomes soiled. Problems such as incontinence, wound drainage, or diaphoresis may require frequent bathing. In addition to cleansing the skin, bathing a patient has benefits such as stimulating circulation, promoting range of motion (ROM), reducing body odors, and improving self-image.

PATIENT-CENTERED CARE

Hygiene requires close contact with a patient; ensure as much privacy as possible, and convey sensitivity and respect for personal beliefs and cultural customs. Take time to talk with patients to identify their personal and cultural preferences for the best methods to perform hygiene. When possible, ask friends or family members to bring in appropriate hygiene soaps, oils, and creams that are not available in the health care setting. Performing hygienic care gives you an opportunity to communicate with patients and assess their physical and psychological conditions. Bathing is a very personal experience, and taking into consideration each person's preferences promotes patient-centered care. If a patient is anxious, use a calm and gentle manner when talking to him or her. Use a reassuring tone of voice so that the patient feels safe and comfortable during bathing. Before performing any aspect of hygiene care, inform the patient of the procedure and acknowledge his or her preferences. Promote independence by encouraging the patient to participate in self-care activities.

SAFETY

Some patients lack the physical energy or functional status to perform self-care and are temporarily dependent on others to enhance the healing and recovery process. Although these patients may want to try to assist with their hygiene, do not leave them unattended because there is an increased risk for falls. If the patient cannot participate, the family or significant other may want to assist if appropriate. Assist the patient and family to understand that a full bath 3 times a week may be adequate for many older patients. Bathing older patients too frequently may contribute to dry skin and cause breaks in the skin. Normal skin is elastic, well hydrated, firm, and smooth. With age, the skin undergoes numerous changes internally and externally (Cowdell, 2011). The skin becomes thinner, dry, less vascular, more fragile, and prone to bruising and tears. The skin is also affected by decreased mobility, sensation changes, and poor nutrition (Cowdell, 2011). Bathing is an excellent opportunity to assess the skin for common skin problems or pressure points, which are potential risks for pressure ulcers (Table 10-1). Be aware of other factors, such as incontinence, friction, shear, immobility, loss of sensory perception, level of activity, and poor nutrition, that contribute to formation of pressure ulcers. It is imperative to identify risk factors and begin interventions immediately to reduce or eliminate the negative effects of each factor (see Chapter 25).

Before using showers or baths in health care settings, be sure that patients have the physical energy and functional status to use the tub or shower. Fully assess the patient's activity tolerance, and instruct the patient on how to use the emergency call device. In the home setting, assess the patient's bath or shower facilities for a safety bar, setting on hot water heaters, and the physical layout of the bathroom. Teach family caregivers for a dependent patient how to give a bath safely in the home.

EVIDENCE-BASED PRACTICE

American Association of Critical-Care Nurses (AACN): *American Association of Critical-Care Nurses Updates Patient Bathing Practices,* 2013, http://www.aacn.org/wd/publishing/content/pressroom/pressreleases/2013/april-bathing-practice-alert-press-release.pcms?menu=. Accessed December 13, 2013.

Climo MW et al: Effect of daily chlorhexidine bathing on hospital-acquired infection, *N Engl J Med* 368:533–542, 2013

Graling P, Vasaly F: Effectiveness of 2% CHG cloth bathing for reducing surgical site infections, *AORN J* 97(5):547, 2013.

Sievert D et al: Chlorhexidine gluconate bathing: does it decrease hospital-acquired infections? *Am J Crit Care* 20(2):166, 2011.

A study by Graling and Vasaly (2013) proved the use of chlorhexidine gluconate (CHG) cloths along with surgical preparation could reduce surgical site infections. Graling and Vasaly found a statistically significant overall reduction of surgical site infection in patients who received the 2% CHG cloth bath before surgery.

Climo et al. (2013) studied 7727 critical care patients comparing chlorhexidine bathing with non-antimicrobial cleansers. The overall rate of multidrug-resistant microorganism acquisition and the overall rate of hospital-acquired bloodstream infections were lower for patients bathed with chlorhexidene. No serious skin reactions were noted during the study. Sievert et al. (2011) examined current evidence on the effect of bathing with chlorhexidine and reducing colonization, surgical site infection, and

central line–associated bloodstream infections. Review of evidenced-based research showed that evidence does exist that bathing with chlorhexidine is an option to consider to reduce central line–associated bloodstream infection. There is a lack of research with use of CHG on pediatric and neonatal patients.

Based on the latest available evidence, the expected practice related to bathing adult patients includes:

- Provide a daily bath for bed-bound patients to improve hygiene and promote comfort. More frequent baths may be performed on patient request or in response to individual patient needs.

TABLE 10-1	**COMMON SKIN PROBLEMS AND RELATED INTERVENTIONS**
PROBLEM	**INTERVENTIONS**
Dry skin: Flaky, rough texture to skin, which may crack and become infected.	Bathe less frequently; rinse away all soap or use a waterless cleanser rather than soap and water; increase fluid intake; use moisturizing lotion.
Acne: Inflammatory papulopustular skin eruption, usually involving bacterial breakdown of sebum, typically on face, neck, shoulders, and back.	Wash hair daily. Wash skin twice daily with warm water and soap to remove oils and cosmetics (if used); cosmetics that can accumulate in pores should be used sparingly. If prescribed, topical antibiotics may minimize problems.
Rashes: Skin eruption from overexposure to sun or moisture or from allergic reaction; may be flat, raised, localized, or systemic; may be associated with pruritus (itching).	Wash and rinse thoroughly; apply antiseptic spray or lotion (as ordered) to prevent further itching and to aid in healing process; warm or cold soaks relieve inflammation.
Contact dermatitis: Inflammation of skin characterized by abrupt onset with erythema, pruritus, pain, and scaly, oozing lesions; usually results from contact with substance difficult to identify and eliminate.	Wash and rinse thoroughly. Identify and avoid contributing agents; provide linens rinsed and sterilized to minimize irritation.
Abrasion: Scraping or rubbing away of epidermis (e.g., a sheet burn) that results in localized bleeding and later weeping of serous fluid; easily infected.	Wash with mild soap and water; observe dressings for retained moisture, which can increase risk of infection.

- Determine bath time based on patient preference and clinical condition.
- It is important to use a basin dedicated to bathing only and not for the storage of supplies.
- Avoid use of unfiltered tap water. Alternatives include prepackaged bathing products, sterile or distilled water, or filtered water from faucets.
- Use no-rinse pH-balanced cleansers, which are superior to alkaline soaps that require cycles of wash and rinse.
- Apply emollients compatible with CHG after each non-prepackaged bathing product when available.

- Bathe patients at high risk for skin colonization and infection daily using a disposable cloth that is prepackaged with a 2% solution of CHG. Use of CHG is associated with significant reductions in colonization of specific bacteria and infections with multidrug-resistant organisms (AACN, 2013). Use of 2% CHG liquid in a basin of water is also acceptable.
- Do not use CHG if a patient has an allergy or sensitivity to CHG. Report any sensitivities as an adverse event.

SKILL 10.1 COMPLETE BATHING

The type of bath, the extent of the bath, and the methods for bathing depend on a patient's ability to participate, the condition of the patient's skin, and in some settings time of day (Box 10-1). Whether to use a basin for bathing or a bag bath often depends on availability of the bag bath.

BOX 10-1   TYPES OF BATHS

Complete Bed Bath
Bath administered to totally dependent patient in bed.

Partial Bed Bath
Bed bath that consists of bathing only body parts that would cause discomfort if left unbathed, such as the hands, face, axilla, and perineal area. Partial bath also includes washing back and providing back rub. Dependent patients in need of partial hygiene or self-sufficient bedridden patients who are unable to reach all body parts receive a partial bed bath.

Sponge Bath at the Sink
Involves bathing from a bath basin or sink with patient sitting in a chair. Patient is able to perform a portion of the bath independently. Assistance is needed from the nurse for hard-to-reach areas.

Tub Bath
Involves immersion in a tub of water that allows more thorough washing and rinsing than a bed bath. Some patients require the nurse's assistance. Some facilities have tubs equipped with lifting devices or panels that swing open to facilitate entry and positioning of dependent patients in the tub.

Shower
Patient sits or stands under a continuous stream of water. Shower provides more thorough washing than a bed bath but can be fatiguing.

Bag Bath (Travel Bath)
Bag bath contains several soft, nonwoven cotton cloths that are premoistened in a solution of no-rinse surfactant cleanser and emollient. The bag bath is an appealing alternative because of the ease of use, shorter bathing time, and patient comfort. Several commercial body cleansing systems are available that contain the same ingredients as the bag bath.

ASSESSMENT

1. Assess degree of assistance needed for bathing. Factors include vision, ability to sit without support, hand grasp, ROM of extremities, and cognitive ability. *Rationale: Determines patient's ability to perform bathing.*
2. Assess patient's fall risk, tolerance of activity, level of discomfort with movement, and presence of shortness of breath or chest pain with exertion. *Rationale: Determines type of cleansing bath appropriate for patient and degree of assistance needed for bathing.*
3. Assess patient's bathing preferences, including time of day, products used, usual frequency of bathing, and type of bath. *Rationale: Patient participates in plan of care. Promotes patient's comfort, dignity, and willingness to cooperate.*
4. Ask if patient has noticed any problems related to skin and genitalia. *Rationale: Provides information to direct physical assessment of skin and genitalia during the bath. Also aids in determining the type of cleansing agent to use.*
5. Assess patients at risk for skin breakdown; use a pressure ulcer assessment tool for patients at risk for pressure ulcers (see Chapter 25). *Rationale: Provides baseline for comparison over time in determining if bathing improves skin condition. Assessment also influences selection of skin care products. Pressure ulcer assessment tools also identify patient's risk for skin impairment.*
   a. Immobilization or decreased mobility (e.g., patients with paralysis, immobilized extremities, traction; weakened or disabled patients). *Rationale: These patients are more prone to pressure spots in dependent areas.*
   b. Reduced sensation (e.g., paresthesia, circulatory insufficiency, neuropathies).
   c. Excessive moisture on skin, particularly on skin surfaces that rub against each other (e.g., under breasts, in perineal area. *Rationale: Skin folds trap moisture and cause friction between surfaces, which can lead to breaks in the skin and result in infection.*
   d. Vascular insufficiencies. *Rationale: Result in poor circulation to skin.*
   e. External devices applied to or around skin (e.g., casts, braces, restraints, dressings, catheters, tubes). *Rationale: Improperly placed medical devices or devices that move*

after placement provide pressure or friction that can result in a wound.

f. Older-adult patients. *Rationale: Older adults have decreased appetite, which contributes to deficits in caloric intake, nutrients, vitamins, and fluids. Decrease in nutrition and hydration affect the condition of the skin with decreases in skin turgor, thickness, and elasticity.*

g. Shear or friction (sliding down in bed). *Rationale: Causes damage to underlying tissues.*

h. Incontinence (bowel or bladder). *Rationale: Accumulation of fluid causes skin maceration.*

7. Identify presence of devices (e.g., catheters, drains, dressings, restraints) and any prescribed limitations of activity or positioning required by patient's illness or treatment plan. *Rationale: Determines patient's safety needs to prevent injury and identifies medical devices that may contribute to breakdown.*

8. Assess patient for allergy or sensitivity to CHG. *Rationale: In cases in which a patient is allergic or sensitive to CHG, an alternative cleansing agent is needed.*

9. Assess room environment for temperature level. *Rationale: Promotes patient comfort.*

PLANNING

Expected Outcomes focus on promoting comfort, mobility, and self-care abilities.

1. Patient's skin is clean and free of excretions, drainage, and odor.

2. Patient's skin shows decreased redness, cracking, flaking, and scaling.

3. Patient maintains functional ROM of hands and shoulders.

4. Patient demonstrates ability to wash face, hands, and chest independently.

5. Patient expresses comfort and relaxation.

Delegation and Collaboration

Assessment of the patient's skin, pain level, and ROM cannot be delegated to nursing assistive personnel (NAP). The skill of bathing can be delegated. The nurse instructs the NAP about:

- Reporting early signs of impaired skin integrity, including redness or pallor.
- Reporting perineal drainage, discomfort, or tenderness.
- Proper ways to position male and female patients with musculoskeletal limitations and indwelling catheters.
- Reporting fatigue or pain during hygiene care.

Equipment

- Four to six washcloths
- Bath towels
- Bath blanket
- Soap and soap dish/liquid soap, CHG cloths or 2% solution, or disposable bag bath cloths
- Toilet tissue or hygiene wipes
- Warm water
- Toiletry items (e.g., deodorant, powder)
- Body lotion (Note: if using CHG soap, use a lotion that is hospital approved, such as Aloe Vesta)
- Clean hospital gown or patient's own pajamas or gown
- Laundry bag
- Clean gloves (when risk for contacting body fluids)
- Wash basin (use for bath water only)
- Disposable bed bath if available

IMPLEMENTATION *for* COMPLETE BATHING

STEPS	RATIONALE

1. **See Standard Protocol (inside front cover).**

> **SAFE PATIENT CARE** Refer to hospital policy regarding bathing with bath basin and soap and water or use of CHG. Research suggests that bath basins holding soap and water can easily become contaminated with infectious microorganisms. CHG soap can be used successfully in bath basins without increasing infection risk.

2. Apply clean gloves. Offer patient bedpan or urinal. Provide toilet tissue. Discard gloves.

Provides comfort and prevents interruption of bath.

a. Raise bed to comfortable working height. Lower side rail closest to you, and help patient assume comfortable supine position, maintaining body alignment. Bring patient toward side closest to you.

Prevents bed from moving. Helps you reach patient without stretching and reaching across bed, minimizing strain on back muscles.

b. Use time during bath to discuss patient's condition, health care needs, and concerns and to offer appropriate instruction as needed.

Use of time during bathing allows you to conduct thorough assessments and engage in instruction.

3. Apply clean gloves. Place bath blanket over patient, and remove top sheet without exposing patient. Have patient hold top of bath blanket while removing linen.

Blanket provides warmth and privacy.

STEPS	**RATIONALE**

4. Place soiled linen in laundry bag, taking care not to allow it to contact uniform.

Prevents transmission of microorganisms.

5. Remove patient's gown or pajamas. If an extremity is injured or has limited mobility, begin removal from unaffected side first. For patients with an intravenous (IV) line, use a gown with sleeves that have shoulder snaps if possible.

Reduces risk of increased pain or injury.

a. When the gown does not have shoulder snaps, remove it from the arm without the IV line first. Then slide it off the other shoulder and arm toward the wrist, keeping the IV line carefully secured (see illustration).

Reduces risk of accidental dislodgment of IV line.

b. Remove bag from IV pole (see illustration).

c. Slide IV bag and tubing through sleeve (see illustration).

d. Rehang bag, check flow rate, and regulate if necessary (see illustration).

Manipulation of tubing and container may disrupt flow rate.

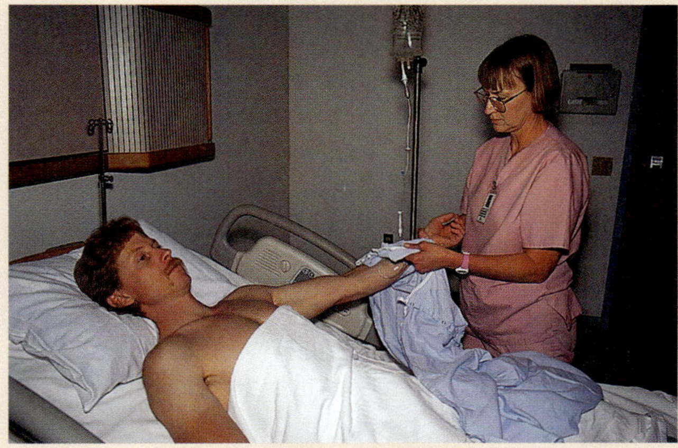

STEP 5a Remove patient's gown.

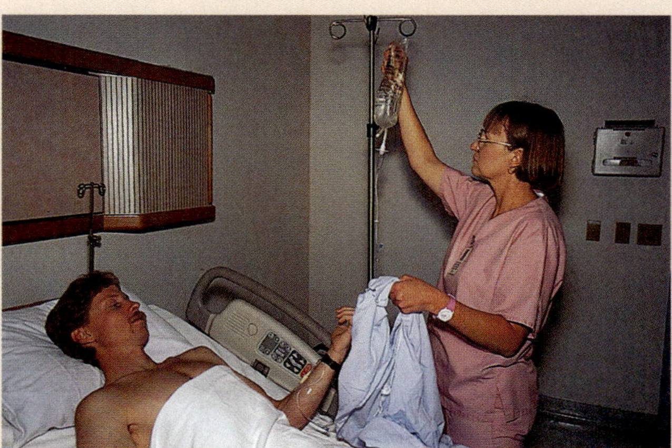

STEP 5b Remove IV bag from pole.

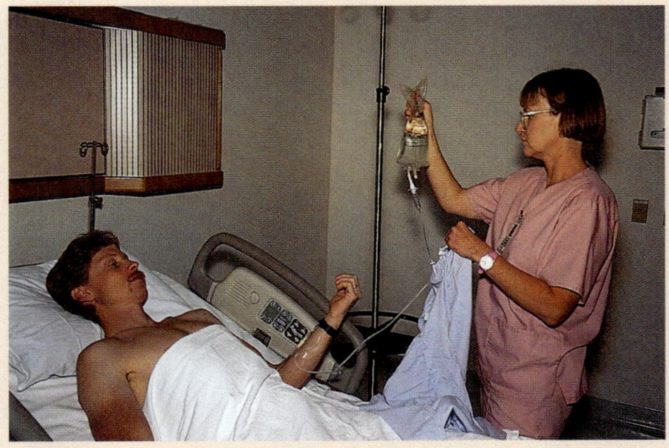

STEP 5c Slide IV tubing and bag through arm of patient's gown.

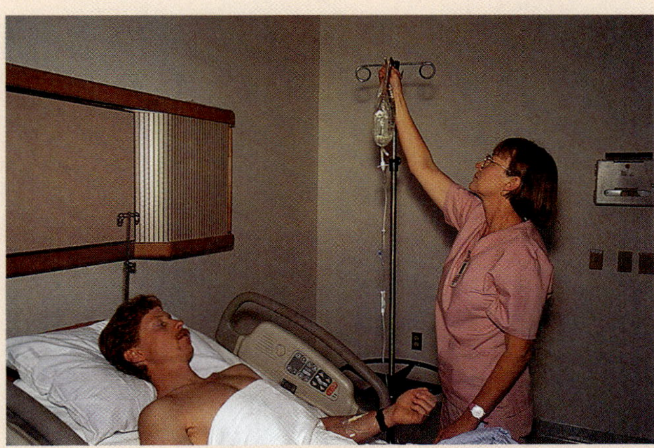

STEP 5d Rehang IV bag.

Continued

STEPS	RATIONALE

e. If IV pump is in use, with the assistance of a registered nurse, turn pump off, clamp tubing, remove tubing from pump, and proceed as in Steps a to d. Once gown is removed, insert tubing into pump, unclamp tubing, and turn pump on at correct rate. Observe flow rate and regulate if necessary.

Sterility, patency, and correct rate of infusion must be maintained.

> **SAFE PATIENT CARE** For debilitated patients at risk for falls, provide safety by using side rails as appropriate if at any time it is necessary to leave the patient unattended. Check temperature of bath water throughout the bath, and change as needed to maintain warmth.

6. Fill wash basin two thirds full with warm water. Adjust water temperature to be comfortably warm to your wrist, and allow patient to test temperature tolerance. Place wash basin and supplies within easy reach.

Warm water promotes comfort, relaxes muscles, and prevents chilling.

7. Lower side rail, remove pillow if tolerated, and raise head of bed 30 to 45 degrees if allowed. Place bath towel under patient's head. Place second bath towel over patient's chest. Remove pillow. Place one bath towel under patient's head and another over chest.

Removing pillow facilitates bathing ears and neck. Towels absorb moisture and prevent soiling of linen.

8. Wash face.

a. Inquire if patient is wearing contact lenses.

Prevents accidental injury to eyes.

b. Apply clean gloves. Form a mitt with washcloth (see illustration). Immerse in water and wring thoroughly.

Mitt retains heat better and prevents loose ends from dripping or annoying patient.

> **SAFE PATIENT CARE** Do not use CHG around face or any wound surfaces.

c. Wash patient's eyes with plain warm water using clean area of mitt for each eye and bathing from inner to outer canthus (see illustration). Soak any crusts on eyelid for 2 to 3 minutes with damp cloth before washing and rinsing eyes. Dry eyes thoroughly but gently.

Soap irritates eyes. Use of separate sections of mitt reduces infection transmission. Bathing eye from inner to outer canthus prevents secretions from entering nasolacrimal duct.

d. Wash, rinse, and dry forehead, cheeks, nose, neck, and ears without using soap. Ask men if they want to be shaved (see Procedural Guideline 10.4)

Soap can be used if patient prefers; however, soap tends to dry face, which is exposed to air more than other body part. If patient has a preferred facial wash, use it.

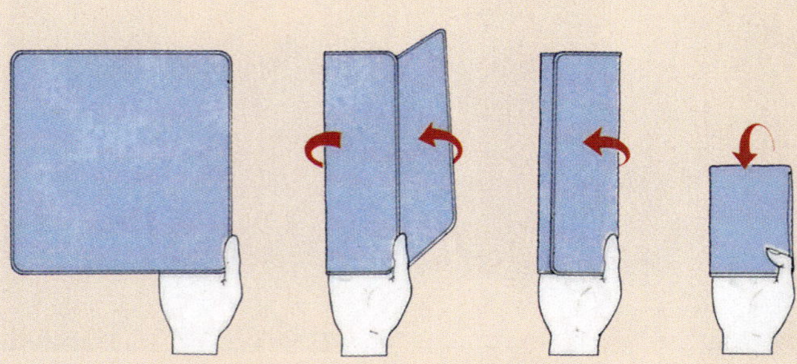

STEP 8b Steps for folding washcloth to form a mitt.

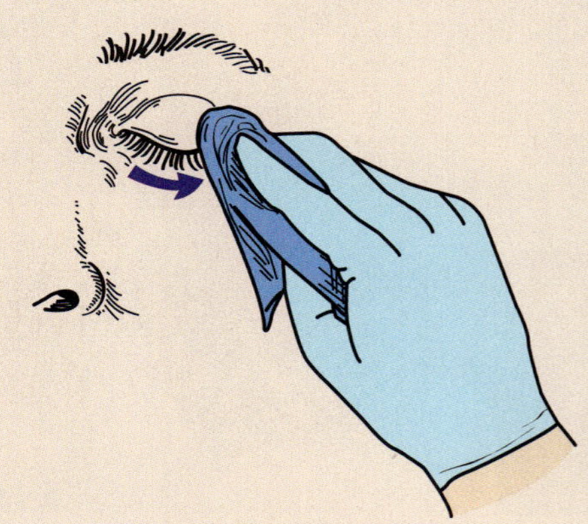

STEP 8c Wash eye from inner to outer canthus.

<table>
<tr><td>**STEPS**</td><td>**RATIONALE**</td></tr>
</table>

> **SAFE PATIENT CARE** Patients who are unconscious have lost the normal blink reflex of the eye, which increases their risk for corneal drying, corneal abrasions, scarring, and eye infections. Obtain a health care provider's order or follow facility policy to instill eyedrops or ointment to help keep a patient's eyes moist. Reassess eyes every 2 to 4 hours for dryness. In the absence of a blink reflex, keep the eyelids closed and covered with an eye patch or shield. Do not tape the eyelid closed because this can injure tissues.

9. Wash trunk and upper extremities.

   a. Expose patient's arm. Place bath towel lengthwise under arm. Bathe with soap or CHG and water using long, firm strokes from distal to proximal (fingers to axilla).

Promotes venous blood return to heart.

   b. Raise and support arm above head (if possible) to wash, rinse, and dry axilla thoroughly (see illustration).

Raising arm promotes ROM and facilitates thorough cleansing.

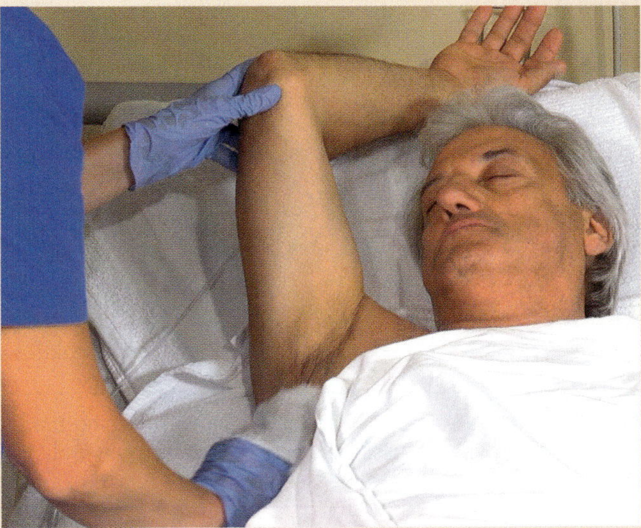

STEP 9b Positioning the arm to wash the axilla.

   c. Move to the opposite side of the bed and repeat Steps 9a and 9b. Apply deodorant or powder sparingly to underarms, following patient preference.

Deodorant and powder control body odor.

   d. Cover patient's chest with bath towel and fold bath blanket down to umbilicus. Bathe chest using long, firm strokes, lifting breast upward if necessary. Rinse and dry well.

Skin under breasts is vulnerable to excoriation and fungal infections if not kept clean and dry.

10. Wash hands and nails.

   a. Fold bath towel in half and lay it on bed beside patient. Place basin on towel. Immerse patient's hand in water. Allow hand to soak for 3 to 5 minutes before cleaning fingernails. Remove basin and dry hand well. Repeat for other hand.

Soaking softens cuticles and calluses of hand, loosens debris beneath nails, and enhances feeling of cleanliness. Thorough drying removes moisture from between fingers.

   b. Check temperature of bath water, and change water when cool or soapy.

Warm water maintains patient's comfort. Alkaline soap residue is irritating to skin and can decrease normal protectiveness of acid pH.

> **SAFE PATIENT CARE** When using CHG in water, do not discard water (unless in the original basin you filled ½ full with water and used ½ bottle of CHG). One bottle of CHG soap is sufficient for a complete bath.

Continued

STEPS	RATIONALE

11. Wash the abdomen.

  a. Place bath towel over chest and abdomen and fold bath blanket down to just above the pubic region. Bathe, rinse, and dry abdomen with special care to umbilicus and skin folds of abdomen and groin.

Keeping skin folds clean and dry helps prevent odor and skin irritation. Moisture and sediment that collect in skin folds predispose skin to maceration and fungal infections.

12. Wash legs.

  a. Expose patient's leg nearest to you, leaving perineum covered.

Provides privacy and promotes patient comfort.

  b. Place bath towel under leg, supporting leg at knee and with foot flat on bed.

Keeps linen dry.

  c. Place patient's foot in a basin to soak while washing and rinsing. If patient is unable to support leg, assistance is needed, or soaking is omitted.

> **SAFE PATIENT CARE**
> Do not soak the feet of patients with diabetes mellitus. Soaking of feet softens tissue and increases susceptibility to breaks and tears (Anastasi et al., 2013).

  d. Wash leg using short, light strokes. Dry leg thoroughly from ankle to knee and knee to thigh (see illustration). Assess for redness, swelling, tenderness, or pain. Wash between toes. Rinse and dry thoroughly.

Promotes circulation and venous return. Assessing for redness, entire leg swelling, tenderness, pitting edema, unilateral calf swelling, and pain in the lower extremities is important because these may be early signs of deep venous thromboembolism (VTE; i.e., blood clots) (Tabei et al., 2012). Secretions and moisture are often present between toes, predisposing patient to maceration, breakdown, and infection.

> **SAFE PATIENT CARE** Use short, light strokes when washing the legs of a patient at risk of VTE. Long, firm strokes can dislodge a clot, resulting in an embolism (Tabei et al., 2012).

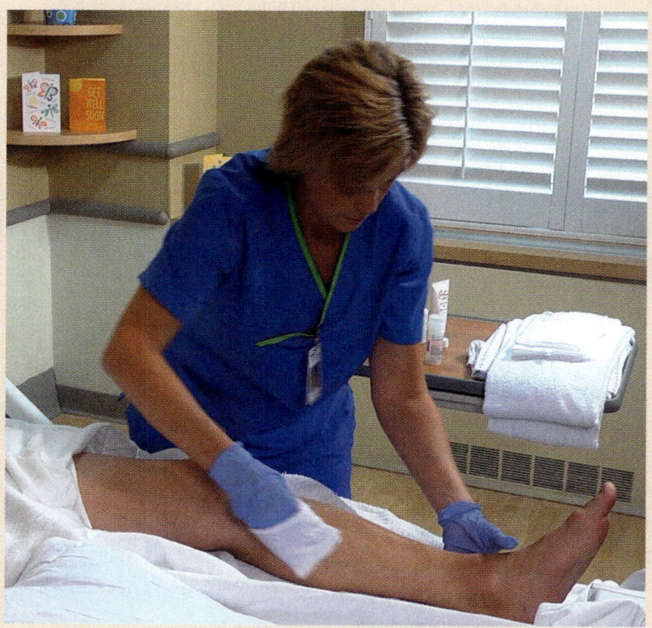

STEP 12d Washing the leg.

STEPS	RATIONALE

e. Raise side rail (if used), move to opposite side, lower side rail, and repeat with other leg and foot. If skin is dry, apply lotion.

Promotes good body mechanics for the nurse. Lotions are effective in moisturizing skin.

f. Cover with bath blanket and raise side rail (if used). Change bath water if appropriate.

Provides patient warmth and safety.

13. Wash back.

a. Raise bed to working height. Lower side rail and help patient assume prone or side-lying position. Place towel lengthwise along patient's side.

Exposes back and buttocks for bathing. Protects bed from moisture and soiling.

b. Keep patient draped by sliding bath blanket over shoulders and thighs during bathing. Wash, rinse, and dry back from neck to buttocks using long, firm strokes.

Maintains warmth and prevents unnecessary exposure.

c. Cleanse buttocks and anus, washing from front to back (see illustration). Cleanse, rinse, and dry areas thoroughly. Pay special attention to folds of buttocks and anus. If fecal material is present, enclose in a fold of underpad or toilet tissue and cleanse with disposable wipes. If needed place a clean pad under patient's buttocks.

Cleansing buttocks and anus prevents contamination of back. Skin folds near buttocks and anus may contain fecal excretions and microorganisms.

d. Remove gloves, perform hand hygiene.

Promotes patient relaxation.

e. Position patient supine; cover patient with bath blanket, raise side rail, lower bed, and provide call light before leaving bedside to change bath water.

Provides for patient safety. Clean water reduces microorganism transmission to perineal structures.

14. Apply clean gloves. Provide perineal care (see Procedural Guideline 10.1).

15. Cover patient with bath blanket when completed.

16. Dispose of water and store basin appropriately. Remove gloves and perform hand hygiene.

17. Apply body lotion to skin as needed and topical moisturizing agents to dry, flaky, or scaling areas. Replace gown.

Dry skin results in reduced pliability and cracking. Moisturizers help prevent skin breakdown.

18. Massage back.

a. Position patient prone if possible. Side-lying position is used frequently

b. Using lotion, begin at sacral area and massage in circular motion, stroking upward from buttocks to shoulders and upper arms and over scapulae with smooth, firm strokes (see illustration). Keep hands on skin and continue massage pattern for 3 to 4 minutes.

Massage stimulates circulation and relaxation.

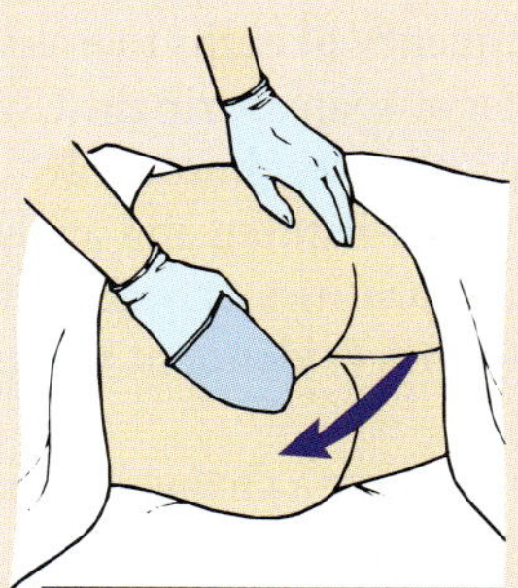

STEP 13c Cleanse buttocks from front to back.

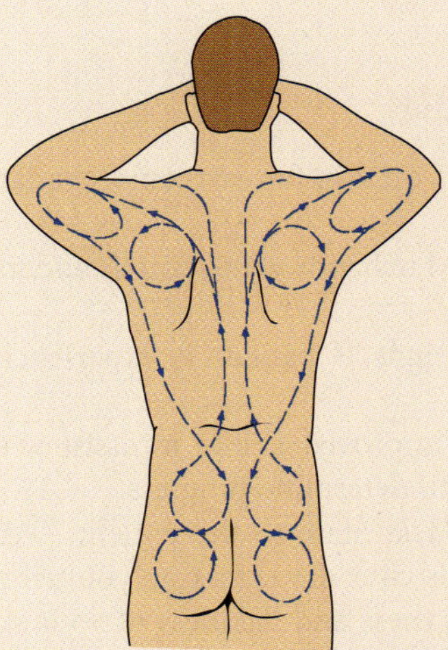

STEP 18b Massage in circular motion upward from buttocks.

Continued

STEPS	RATIONALE

c. Knead muscles of upper back and shoulders by grasping tissue between thumb and fingers. Ask the patient if your grasp is uncomfortable. Knead upward along each side of spine and around muscles of neck, avoiding bony prominences.

These muscles are thick and can be massaged vigorously.

> **SAFE PATIENT CARE** Do not massage reddened areas over bony prominences. Evidence suggests that firm massage over these areas may result in decreased blood flow and tissue damage (EPUAP and NPUAP, 2009).

d. End massage with long, stroking movements, and tell patient that you are ending massage.

Long strokes promote comfort and relaxation.

e. Observe and report any redness or skin breakdown, paying particular attention to bony prominences.

Assessment is a key intervention to identification of early signs of skin breakdown.

f. Remove excess lotion from back with bath towel.

Excess lotion could promote maceration of skin.

19. Option: CHG cleansing cloths or commercial bag bath/cleansing pack

a. A cleansing pack contains 5 to 10 premoistened towels for cleansing.

Provides soothing heat.

b. Use single towel for each general body part cleansed. Follow same order of cleansing as total or partial bed bath.

Reduces transmission of microorganisms.

c. Allow skin to air dry for 30 seconds. It is permissible to cover patient lightly with bath towel or blanket to prevent chilling.

Drying skin with towel removes emollient that is left behind after water/cleanser solution evaporates.

d. If there is excessive soiling (e.g., in perineal region), use an extra bag bath or conventional washcloths, soap, water, and towels.

To ensure removal of secretions.

20. Assist patient with grooming, oral hygiene, shaving, hair care, and application of makeup if desired (see Procedural Guidelines 10.2 through 10.4).

Promotes patient's body image.

21. Make patient's bed (see Procedural Guideline 10.6).

22. See Completion Protocol (inside front cover).

EVALUATION

1. Observe areas on skin for erythema, exudate, drainage, or breakdown.
2. Measure ROM in hands, arms, and shoulders, and compare with baseline.
3. Assess vital signs if patient is experiencing distress or restlessness.
4. Observe for improved ability to assist with self-bathing and hygiene to determine progress.
5. Use **Teach Back:** State to the patient, "We talked about what to do for your dry skin. Can you tell me the ways to reduce the dryness and flakiness of your skin?" Evaluates what the patient is able to explain or demonstrate. Revise your instruction now or develop plan for revised patient teaching to be implemented at an appropriate time if patient is not able to teach back correctly.

Unexpected Outcomes and Related Interventions

1. Patient's skin on lower extremities is dry, flaky, and itchy.
   a. Limit the frequency of baths to every other day or less.
   b. Use antibacterial soap sparingly. Use a mild soap that is nondrying and rinse thoroughly.
   c. Blot skin dry after bathing and apply lotion to skin.
   d. Administer antipruritics as ordered to control itching.
2. The patient's skin has evidence of rashes, redness, scaling, or cracking.
   a. Evaluate the need for a change in frequency of bathing and soap product used.
   b. Collaborate with the health care provider regarding application of ointments or creams to provide a protective barrier and help maintain moisture within the skin.

c. For obese patients with fungal growth between skin folds, consider antifungal powders to minimize moisture and treat irritations.

3. The rectum, perineum, or genital region is inflamed, swollen, or has foul-smelling discharge.
   a. Bathe area frequently enough to keep clean and dry.
   b. Apply protective barrier or antiinflammatory cream.
   c. Report to health care provider.

Recording and Reporting

- Routine documentation may include completion of flow sheet. Record observations made during the bath, which may include type of bath given, patient's ability to assist or cooperate, condition of patient's skin, patient's knowledge of hygiene practices, and any nursing interventions for improving skin integrity.
- Document your evaluation of patient learning.
- Record patient's response to bathing and any concerns voiced by patient regarding self-care needs.

Sample Documentation

0900   Cooperative with turning during bed bath. Stated he felt "very weak." Both legs dry and flaking. Complained of severe itching. Bath oil added to bath water. Emollient lotion applied after bath. States itching is less now.

Special Considerations

Pediatric

- Infants chill easily; keep body covered and work quickly.
- Use only mild soap for bathing infants and children.
- Families need to be involved in a child's care; children feel more secure in the presence of their family.

Geriatric

- Older adults may chill easily.
- Older adults with urinary incontinence need meticulous skin care to reduce skin irritation from urine and feces.
- Older adults have dry skin and do not need frequent bathing. Avoid use of harsh soaps that can increase skin pH, which can cause drying, itching, and breakdown (Cowdell, 2011).

Home Care

- Type of bath chosen depends on assessment of the home, availability of running water, and condition of bathing facilities.
- Adhesive strips on bottom of tub or shower, hand rails, chairs, or stools in tub or shower help protect patients from falls and injury. Patient also may use portable shower seat.

PROCEDURAL GUIDELINE 10.1
Perineal Care

Perineal care involves thorough cleansing of the patient's external genitalia and surrounding skin. A patient routinely receives perineal care during a complete bath (see Skill 10.1). However, patients who have fecal or urinary incontinence or an indwelling Foley catheter or are recovering from rectal or genital surgery or childbirth need more frequent perineal hygiene. Wear gloves during perineal care because of the risk of contacting infectious organisms present in fecal, urinary, or vaginal secretions. Perineal care may be embarrassing for you and the patient. Always act in a professional and sensitive manner, and provide privacy at all times.

Delegation and Collaboration

The skill of perineal care can be delegated to nursing assistive personnel (NAP). The nurse instructs the NAP about:

- Any physical restrictions that affect proper positioning of patient.
- The proper ways to position male and female patients with an indwelling Foley catheter during perineal care.
- Notifying the nurse of any perineal drainage, excoriation, or rash observed.

Equipment

- Washcloths, bath towels, and bath blankets
- Cleansing product for bath (CHG can be used for perineal and catheter care; however, some institutions do not use CHG because of the risk of irritation to mucous membranes. See facility policy.)
- Disposable wipes and wash basin
- Warm water
- Laundry bag
- Waterproof pad or bedpan
- Clean gloves

Procedural Steps

1. **See Standard Protocol (inside front cover).**
2. Provide perineal care:
   a. *For a female patient:*
      (1) If patient is able to maneuver and handle washcloth, allow cleansing perineum on own.
      (2) Assist patient in assuming dorsal recumbent position. Note restrictions or any limitation in patient's positioning. Be sure to position waterproof pad under buttocks.
      (3) Apply clean gloves. Drape patient with bath blanket placed in the shape of a diamond.
      (4) Fold both outer corners of the bath blanket up around patient's legs onto abdomen and under hip (see illustration). Then you can lift the lower tip of the bath blanket when you are ready to expose the perineum.

Continued

PROCEDURAL GUIDELINE 10.1
Perineal Care—cont'd

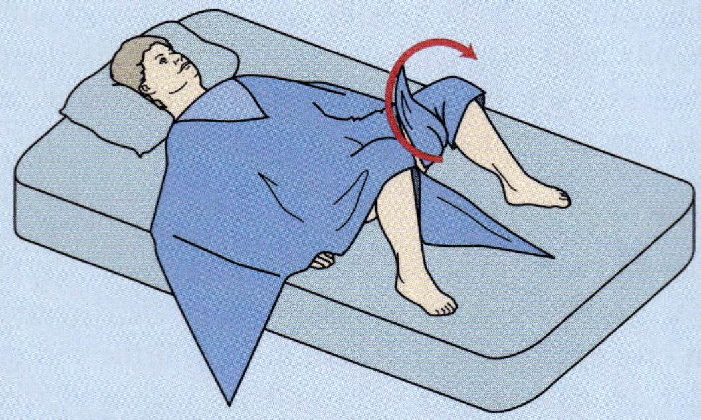

STEP 2a(4) Drape patient for perineal care.

(5) Wash and dry the patient's upper thighs.

(6) Wash labia majora. Use nondominant hand to retract labia gently from thigh; with dominant hand, wash carefully in skin folds. Wipe in direction from perineum to rectum (front to back). Repeat on opposite side using separate section of washcloth. Rinse and dry area thoroughly. Discard washcloth.

(7) Gently separate labia with nondominant hand to expose urethral meatus and vaginal orifice. With dominant hand, use a new washcloth to wash downward from pubic area toward rectum in one smooth stroke (see illustration). Use separate section of cloth for each stroke. Cleanse thoroughly over labia minora, clitoris, and vaginal orifice. Avoid placing tension on indwelling catheter if present and clean around it thoroughly (see Procedural Guideline 18.3 for care of catheter).

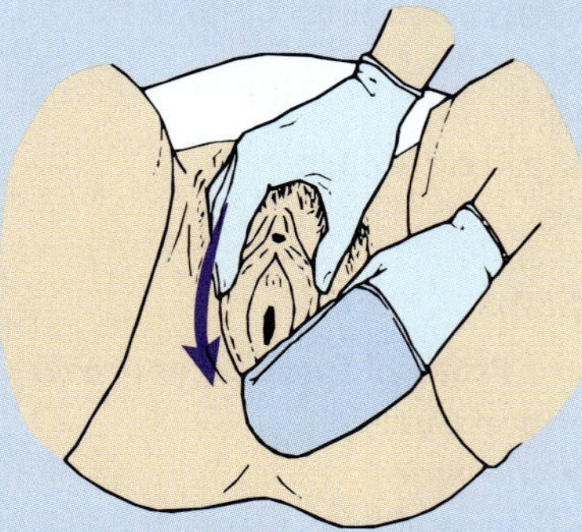

STEP 2a(7) Cleanse from perineum to rectum (front to back).

(8) Rinse area thoroughly. If patient uses a bedpan, an option is to have patient on the pan and to pour warm water over perineum.

(9) Ask patient to lower legs and assume comfortable position.

b. For a male patient:

(1) If patient is able to maneuver and handle washcloth, allow cleansing perineum on own.

(2) Assist patient to supine position. Note any mobility restrictions.

(3) Apply clean gloves. Place bath blanket over patient. Then fold lower half of bath blanket up to expose upper thighs. Wash and dry thighs.

(4) Cover thighs with bath towels. Raise bath blanket to expose genitalia. Gently raise penis and place bath towel underneath. Gently grasp shaft of penis. If patient is uncircumcised, retract foreskin. If patient has an erection, defer procedure until later.

(5) Wash tip of penis at urethral meatus first. Using circular motion, cleanse from meatus outward (see illustration). Repeat, using a separate section of the cloth until the penis is clean. Rinse and dry carefully. Discard the washcloth.

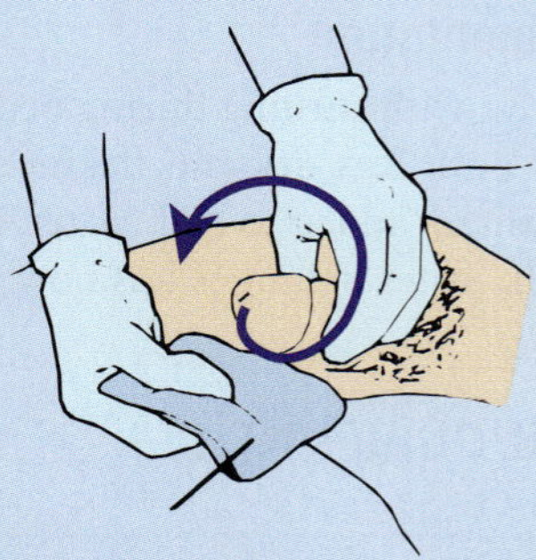

STEP 2b(5) Wash penis in a circular motion.

(6) Return foreskin to its natural position.

> **SAFE PATIENT CARE** If foreskin is not returned to its natural position, tightening of foreskin around shaft of penis can cause local edema; discomfort; and, if not corrected, permanent urethral damage.

(7) Take a new washcloth and gently cleanse the shaft of penis and the scrotum by having patient abduct legs. Pay special attention to underlying surface of penis. Lift scrotum carefully and wash underlying skin folds. Rinse and dry thoroughly.

(8) Avoid placing tension on indwelling catheter if present, and clean around it thoroughly (see Procedural Guideline 18.3 for care of catheter).

3. Remove all towels, and fold bath blanket back over patient's perineum and assist patient to comfortable position.

4. Observe perineal area for any irritation, redness, or drainage that persists after perineal hygiene.

5. **See Completion Protocol (inside front cover).**

PROCEDURAL GUIDELINE 10.2
Oral Care for a Debilitated Patient

Oral hygiene maintains the integrity of oral cavity mucosa and helps control plaque-associated oral diseases. Oral hygiene promotes comfort, prevents infection, and aids in nutrition. Adequate daily oral hygiene includes brushing, flossing, and rinsing. Many factors influence oral hygiene (Box 10-2). Encouraging dependent or chronically ill patients to attend to their own oral hygiene creates a general sense of comfort and improves appetite. Frequency of oral care depends on the condition of the oral cavity and the patient's comfort. Oral hygiene may be required every 1 to 2 hours. For unconscious patients, first assess the patient's gag reflex, and determine the type of suction apparatus needed to prevent aspiration. Unconscious patients are at risk for oral infections because of the absence of saliva movement and production, which leads to large numbers of gram-negative bacteria in the oral cavity.

Critically ill patients with endotracheal tubes and who are on mechanical ventilation are at risk for ventilator-associated pneumonia (VAP) if the saliva is aspirated (see Skill 14.5). Many patients have no gag reflex. Proper hygiene requires keeping the mucosa moist and removing secretions. A study that involved using a toothbrush to clean the teeth of critically ill patients with sodium monoflurophosphate 0.7% paste, rinsing the teeth with tap water, and applying a 0.12% chlorhexidine gluconate solution twice daily at 12-hour intervals has been shown to reduce the incidence of VAP (Sona et al., 2009). Mechanical cleansing and oral hygiene reduce plaque and oropharyngeal colonization, which is associated with VAP (Weigand, 2011). A comprehensive oral care program is recommended by the Centers for Disease Control and Prevention to reduce VAP (CDC, 2012).

Delegation and Collaboration

The skill of providing oral hygiene (including toothbrushing, flossing, and rinsing) can be delegated to nursing assistive personnel (NAP). However, the nurse is responsible for the assessment of a patient's gag reflex to determine if the patient is at risk for aspiration. The nurse instructs the NAP about:

- The patient's level of consciousness, presence or absence of gag reflex, proper positioning, and whether oral suction apparatus is needed for clearing oral secretions.
- Reporting any changes in oral mucosa to the nurse.
- Reporting excessive coughing or choking during or after oral care.

Equipment

- Clean gloves
- Goggles
- Soft-bristled toothbrush or Toothette sponges for patients when a toothbrush is contraindicated.
- Nonabrasive fluoride toothpaste or dentifrice
- Antiseptic or chlorhexidine (CHG) mouth rinse (check facility policy)
- Water-based mouth moisturizer
- Glass of water
- Emesis basin
- Tongue blade
- Face towel, paper towels
- Penlight
- Suction equipment (optional): Suction machine or Yankauer suction
- Water-soluble lubricant
- Oral airway (uncooperative patient or patient who shows bite reflex)

Procedural Steps

1. **See Standard Protocol (inside front cover).**
2. Apply clean gloves. Assess for presence or absence of gag reflex by placing tongue blade on back of tongue. Absence of reflex increases risk for aspiration of fluids in mouth.

BOX 10-2 FACTORS INFLUENCING ORAL HYGIENE

- Patient lacks upper extremity strength or dexterity to perform oral hygiene (e.g., is paralyzed, has limited ROM).
- Patient is unable or unwilling to attend to personal hygiene needs (e.g., is unconscious, depressed, confused).
- Patient has diabetes and is prone to dryness of mouth, gingivitis, periodontal disease, and loss of teeth.
- Patient is prone to dehydration, has a fever, or is NPO (unable to take food or fluids). Thick secretions develop on tongue and gums. Lips become cracked and reddened.
- Radiation therapy causes soreness, mild erythema, swollen mucosa, dysphagia, dryness, taste changes, and possible oral infection.
- Chronic inflammatory disease may be caused by bacterial, viral, or fungal infections or ineffective oral hygiene.
- Chemotherapy causes ulcerations and inflammation of mucosa and possible oral infection. Chemical injury may result from irritating substances such as alcohol, tobacco, or acidic foods or side effects of medications, including chemotherapy, antibiotics, steroids, and antidepressants. Mucositis (inflammation of the mucous membranes in the mouth) is a common complication in patients receiving radiation or chemotherapy.
- Trauma to oral cavity from oral tubes, suctioning, hot foods, broken teeth, or ill-fitting dentures causes swelling, ulcerations, inflammation, and possible bleeding.
- Mouth breathing and use of oxygen may result in dry mucous membranes.

Continued

PROCEDURAL GUIDELINE 10.2
Oral Care for a Debilitated Patient—cont'd

3. Inspect lips, teeth, gums, buccal mucosa, palate, and tongue using tongue depressor and penlight if necessary (see Chapter 7). Observe for color, texture, moisture, lesions or ulcers, and condition of teeth or dentures.

4. Position a responsive patient in a sitting position. Position an unconscious patient in side-lying position with bed flat and head turned toward mattress. Place towel under chin. Have emesis basin available.

5. Remove dentures or partial plates if present (see Procedural Guideline 10.3).

6. If patient is uncooperative or having difficulty keeping mouth open, insert an oral airway. Insert it upside down into the mouth, and turn it sideways as you insert it toward the back of the pharynx and then over the tongue to keep teeth apart. Insert when patient is relaxed. Do not use force (see illustration).

7. Clean mouth using brush moistened in water. Apply toothpaste or use antiinfective solution first to loosen crusts. Hold toothbrush bristles at 45-degree angle to gum line. Brush inner and outer surfaces of upper and lower teeth by brushing from gum to crown of tooth. Clean biting surface of teeth by holding top of bristles parallel with teeth and brushing back and forth. Brush sides of teeth moving bristles back and forth (see illustration). A Toothette may be used for patients who have no teeth or have sensitive gums. Use brush or Toothette to clean roof of mouth, gums, and inside cheeks. Gently brush tongue, but avoid stimulating gag reflex (if present). Moisten the brush or Toothette to rinse; repeat, rinsing several times. As a last step, moisten brush with antiseptic mouthwash or CHG solution to rinse (check facility policy).

> **SAFE PATIENT CARE** Suction should be on and ready for use if gag reflex is absent (see Chapter 14).

8. Suction oral secretions as they accumulate to reduce risk of aspiration.

9. Apply a thin layer of water-soluble jelly to lips (see illustration).

10. **See Completion Protocol (inside front cover).**

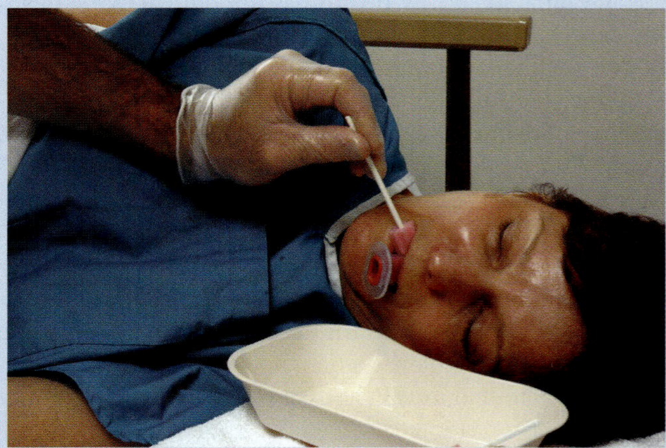

STEP 6 Placement of oral airway; nurse cleans lips with moistened Toothette.

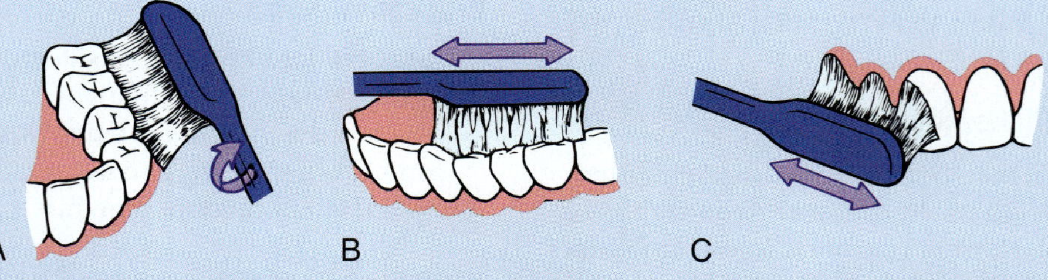

STEP 7 Directions of toothbrush. **A,** A 45-degree angle brushes gum line. **B,** Parallel position brushes biting surfaces. **C,** Lateral position brushes side of teeth.

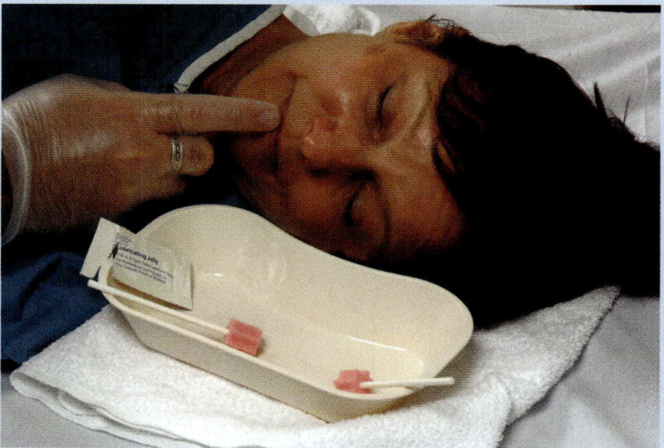

STEP 9 Apply water-soluble moisturizer to lips.

PROCEDURAL GUIDELINE 10.3
Care of Dentures

Clean dentures as regularly as natural teeth to prevent gingival infection and irritation. Loose dentures can cause discomfort and make it difficult for patients to chew food and speak clearly. Loose dentures may result from weight loss. Refer patients to their dentist as needed. Dentures can be easily lost or broken. Store them in an enclosed, labeled cup, and soak when not worn (e.g., at night, during surgery or a diagnostic procedure). Reinsert dentures as soon as possible. The change in appearance when they are not worn may be of major concern to a patient.

Delegation and Collaboration

The skill of denture care can be delegated to nursing assistive personnel (NAP). The nurse instructs the NAP to:
- Avoid use of hot or excessively cold water when caring for dentures.
- Inform the nurse if there are cracks in the dentures.
- Inform the nurse if the patient complains of any oral discomfort.

Equipment

- Clean gloves
- Soft-bristled toothbrush or denture toothbrush
- Denture cleaning agent or toothpaste, denture adhesive (optional)
- Glass of water
- Emesis basin or sink
- Washcloth
- 4 × 4–inch gauze
- Denture cup (if dentures are to be stored after cleaning)

Procedural Steps

1. **See Standard Protocol (inside front cover).**
2. Ask patient if dentures fit and if there is any gum or mucous membrane tenderness or irritation.
3. Ask patient about preferences for denture care and products used.
4. Encourage patient to provide denture care independently if able. If patient is unable, it is important for the nurse to provide care.
5. Provide denture care during routine mouth care.
6. Fill emesis basin with tepid water or, if using sink, place washcloth in bottom of sink and fill sink with 1 inch of water.
7. Apply clean gloves. Ask patient to remove dentures. Grasp upper plate at front with thumb and index finger wrapped in gauze, and pull downward. Gently lift lower denture from jaw and rotate one side downward to remove from patient's mouth. Hold dentures over emesis basin or sink lined with washcloth and containing 1 inch of water.
8. Apply cleaning agent to brush, and brush surfaces of dentures. Hold dentures close to water (see illustration). Hold brush horizontally and use back-and-forth motion to cleanse biting surfaces. Use short strokes from top of denture to biting surfaces to clean outer teeth surfaces. Hold brush vertically and use short strokes to clean inner tooth surfaces. Hold brush horizontally and use back-and-forth motion to clean undersurface of dentures.

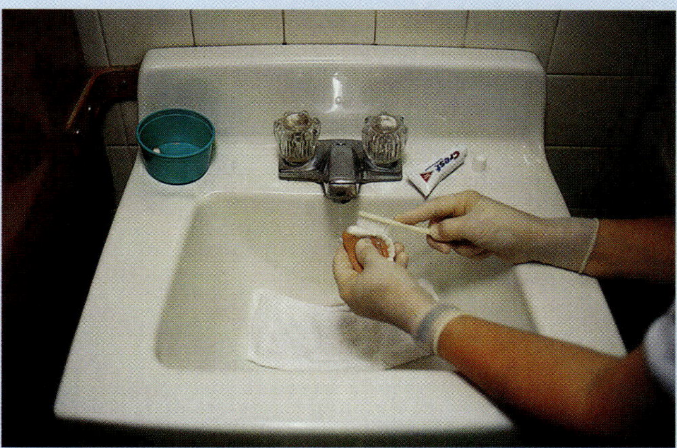

STEP 8 Cleansing dentures in sink.

9. Rinse thoroughly in tepid water.
10. Some patients use an adhesive to seal dentures in place. Apply a thin layer to undersurface of each denture before inserting.
11. If patient needs assistance with insertion of dentures, moisten upper denture and press firmly to seal it in place. Then insert moistened lower denture. Ask if dentures feel comfortable.
12. Some patients prefer to have their dentures stored to give the gums a rest and reduce risk of infection. Keeping dentures moist prevents warping and facilitates easier insertion. Store in tepid water in denture cup. Label the denture cup with patient's name, using either a permanent marker or the patient's identification label, and keep in a secure place.
13. **See Completion Protocol (inside front cover).**

PROCEDURAL GUIDELINE 10.4
Hair Care—Combing, Shampooing, and Shaving

Brushing, combing, and shampooing hair are basic measures for all patients unable to provide self-care. Having the hair groomed makes a person feel more comfortable. Many facilities have a beauty shop where patients can go for professional hair care. Fever, malnutrition, some medications, emotional stress, and depression affect the condition of hair. Diaphoresis leaves hair oily and unmanageable. Table 10-2 describes common hair and scalp conditions and nursing interventions.

Frequency of shampooing depends on the condition of the hair and the person's personal preferences. Dry hair requires less frequent shampooing than oily hair. Hospitalized patients who have excess perspiration or treatments that leave blood or solutions in the hair may need a shampoo. Positioning with the neck hyperextended over the edge of a sink is contraindicated for patients who have had neck injuries or back pain. Patients may be placed on a stretcher with their head extended over a sink. Bedridden patients use a plastic shampoo trough that drains into a bedside container. Dry shampoos or a shampoo cap are available, making it easy to offer a shampoo with less physical stress for the patient.

Dependent patients with beards or mustaches need assistance keeping the facial hair clean, especially after eating. Food particles easily collect in the hair. Shaving facial hair is a task most men prefer to do for themselves daily. Shaving of hair must take into consideration patient preference and cultural and spiritual needs.

Delegation and Collaboration

Assessment of the patient's condition may not be delegated to nursing assistive personnel (NAP). The skills of combing, shampooing, and shaving can be delegated to NAP. The nurse instructs the NAP about:
- How to position patients with mobility restrictions properly.
- Reporting patient's tolerance of the procedure and any concerns (e.g., neck pain).
- Any patient at risk for bleeding and the need to use an electric razor.

Equipment

Hair care
- Clean gloves
- Brush and comb
- Shampoo board
- Shampoo and conditioner (optional)

TABLE 10-2	COMMON HAIR AND SCALP CONDITIONS AND RELATED INTERVENTIONS
PROBLEM	**INTERVENTIONS**
Alopecia (hair loss): Chemotherapeutic agents kill cells that rapidly multiply, including both tumor and normal cells.	Some patients wear scarves. Some prefer hairpieces. Referral may be necessary for professional consultation for long-term interventions.
Dandruff: Scaling of scalp accompanied by itching; if severe, may involve eyebrows.	Shampoo regularly with medicated shampoo.
Pediculosis *Head lice:* Parasites attached to hair strands. Eggs look like oval particles. Bites or pustules may be found behind ears and at hairline. May spread to furniture and other people.	Check the entire scalp. Centers for Disease Control and Prevention recommends treatment for persons diagnosed with an active infection (CDC, 2013). Over-the-counter or prescription treatment may be needed. Machine wash and dry clothing and linens in hot water. Nit combs can be used in combination with medicated shampoo. Change bed linens according to facility policy and follow facility infection prevention guidelines. Lindane is no longer recommended by American Academy of Pediatrics.
Body lice: Parasites tend to cling to clothing. Patient itches. Hemorrhagic spots may appear on skin where lice are sucking blood. Lice may lay eggs on clothing and furniture.	Have patient bathe or shower thoroughly. Good hygiene and regular changes of clothes, bedding, and towels constitute the only treatment needed for body lice (CDC, 2013). Bag infested clothing or linen until laundered. Follow facility infection prevention policy.
Crab lice: Found in pubic hair. Are grayish white with red legs. May spread via sexual contact.	For pubic lice, shave hair off affected area, cleanse as for body lice, use medicated product for lice, and notify sexual partner of proper treatment.

PROCEDURAL GUIDELINE 10.4
Hair Care—Combing, Shampooing, and Shaving—cont'd

- Towels (two or more)
- Dry shampoo or shampoo cap as an alternative

Shaving
- Disposable or electric razor
- Shaving cream (patient preference)
- Basin of very warm water
- Mirror
- Bath towels

Procedural Steps

1. **See Standard Protocol (inside front cover).**
2. *Shampoo for bed-bound patient*
   a. Before washing patient's hair, determine that there are no contraindications to procedure, such as head and neck injuries, spinal cord injuries, and arthritis. Often a health care provider's order is required to wash a patient's hair (check facility policy). If exposure to moisture is contraindicated, use a dry shampoo.
   b. Apply clean gloves. Inspect condition of hair and scalp. Note distribution of hair, oiliness, and texture. Inspect scalp for abrasions, lacerations, lesions, inflammation, and infestation. If draining head wounds are suspected, apply clean gloves. If lice are present, wear disposable gown and follow facility procedure.
   c. Ask if there are any product preferences or personal items that the patient wants to use.
   d. Explain procedure to patient and family.
   e. Place a towel and waterproof pad under patient's shoulders, neck, and head.
   f. Wet shampoo
      (1) Position patient supine with head and shoulders at top edge of bed. Place plastic trough under head and wash basin at end of trough spout (see illustration). Be sure that spout extends beyond edge of mattress.

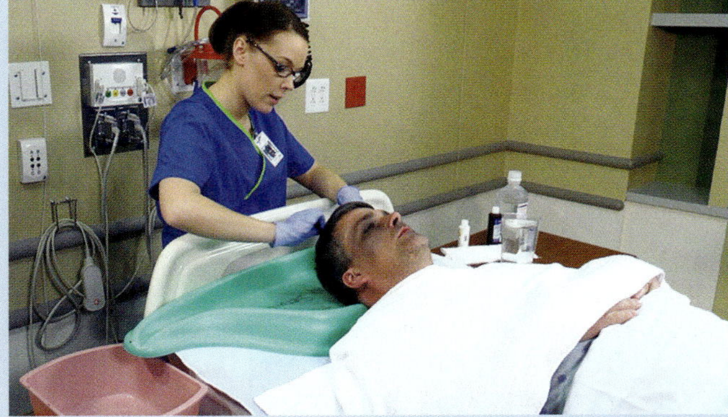

STEP 2f(1) Patient with waterproof pad under shoulders, neck, and head with shampoo board.

      (2) Obtain warm water, testing temperature with your wrist. Allow patient to feel water temperature for comfort.

      (3) Slowly pour warm water from water pitcher over hair until it is completely wet (see illustration). Protect patient's face with towel or washcloth over eyes as needed. If hair contains matted blood, apply hydrogen peroxide; then rinse hair with saline.

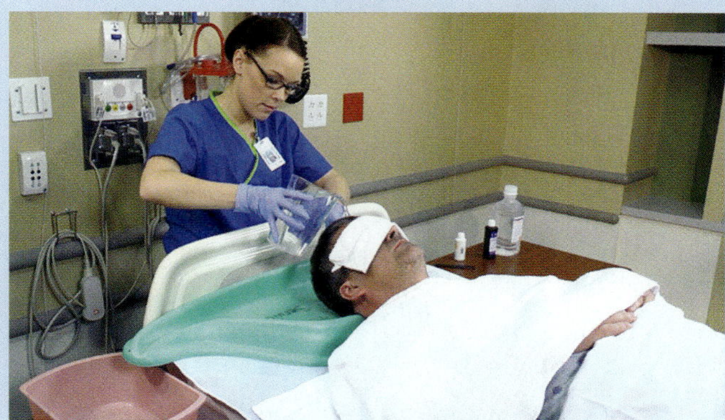

STEP 2f(3) Pour water over hair.

      (4) Apply small amount of shampoo and work up lather with both hands. Start at hairline and work toward back of neck. Lift head slightly with one hand to wash back of head. Shampoo sides of head. Massage scalp gently by applying pressure with fingertips.
      (5) Rinse thoroughly and repeat if necessary until hair is free of soap. Apply conditioner if requested and rinse thoroughly. Dry hair using a second towel if needed or hair dryer (if available).
   g. Shampoo cap
      (1) Some shampoo caps can be heated in a microwave before use. When warming shampoo cap in a microwave, follow package directions, and never heat for more than 15 seconds to prevent burning the patient. Microwave heating times will vary according to wattage.
      (2) After heating, place shampoo cap on head (longer hair requires bundling patient's hair on top of head before placement). Massage hair through cap until hair feels saturated (approximately 1 to 2 minutes for shorter hair, 2 to 3 minutes for longer hair).
      (3) Use longer massage time or use another shampoo cap if patient has excessive tangles or foreign matter in hair.
   h. Remove gloves and dispose in proper receptacle.
   i. Assist patient to a comfortable position and complete styling of hair. Braids may be helpful for patients with very long hair.
3. *Combing and brushing hair*
   a. Part the hair into two sections, and then separate it into two more sections (see illustration).
   b. Brush or comb from the scalp toward the hair ends.

Continued

PROCEDURAL GUIDELINE 10.4
Hair Care—Combing, Shampooing, and Shaving—cont'd

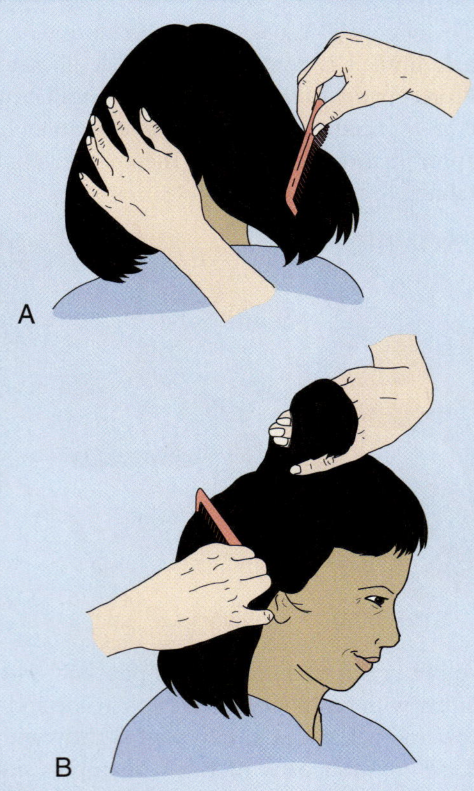

STEP 3a Parting hair. **A,** Part hair down the middle and divide into two main sections. **B,** Part the main section into two smaller sections.

   c. Moisten hair lightly with water, conditioner, or an alcohol-free detangle product before combing.

   d. Move fingers through hair to loosen any larger tangles.

   e. Using a wide-tooth comb, start on either side of the head and insert the comb with the teeth upward to the hair near the scalp. Comb through the hair in a circular motion by turning the wrist while lifting up and out. Continue until all hair is combed through, and then comb into place to shape and style.

4. *Shaving a patient*

   a. Before shaving patient with a disposable razor, assess for risk of bleeding. Review medical history and laboratory values, including platelet count, prothrombin time, and activated partial thromboplastin time. If risk of bleeding is present, use an electric razor.

   b. If patient prefers to shave himself, assess ability to manipulate razor.

   c. Assist patient to sitting position if possible, and place towel over chest and shoulders.

   d. Place a warm, moist washcloth over patient's face for several seconds.

   e. Apply clean gloves. Shave using appropriate tools available.

     (1) Apply shaving cream, using product patient prefers. With a disposable or safety razor at a 45-degree angle, shave in direction of hair growth using short strokes. Hold skin taut with nondominant hand (see illustration). Ask patient to tell you if it becomes uncomfortable. Dip razor blade in water; shaving cream accumulates on edge of blade.

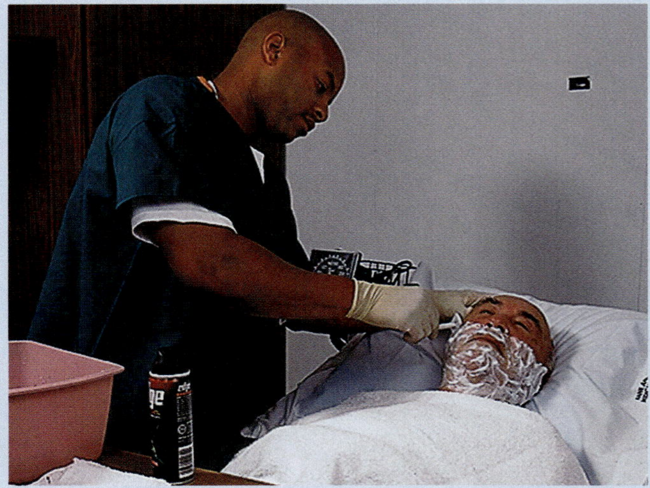

STEP 4e(1) Shaving a patient.

     (2) Apply conditioner for electric razor. Turn electric razor on and shave across side of face using a gentle downward stroke in direction of hair growth.

     (3) If necessary, gently comb mustache or beard. Allow patient to use mirror and direct areas to trim with scissors.

5. Rinse and dry face. Apply aftershave if desired.

6. **See Completion Protocol (inside front cover).**

PROCEDURAL GUIDELINE 10.5
Foot and Nail Care

Care of the nails is important to prevent the occurrence of pain and infection. Foot and nail care should be incorporated into the patient's daily hygiene. Changes also occur in the shape, color, and texture of nails, which may result from various nutritional, infectious, and circulatory disorders such as diabetes (Table 10-3). Patients with peripheral vascular disease such as diabetes may have inadequate arterial or venous circulation or both. These patients are at high risk for neuropathy, a degeneration of peripheral nerves with loss of sensation. These patients cannot sense pressure or

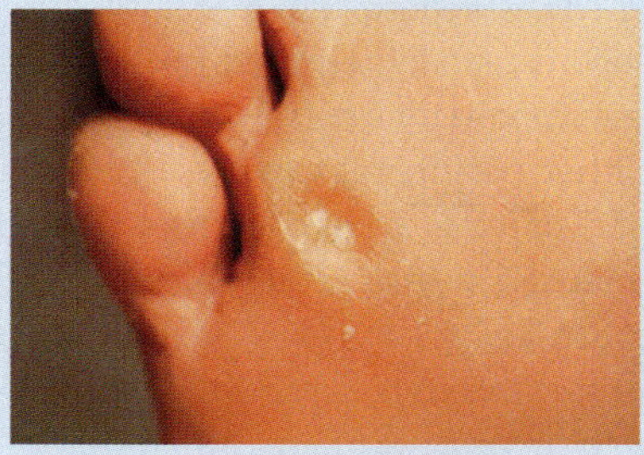

FIG 10-1 Corn. (From Weston WL, Lane AT: *Color textbook of pediatric dermatology*, ed 4, St Louis, 2007, Mosby.)

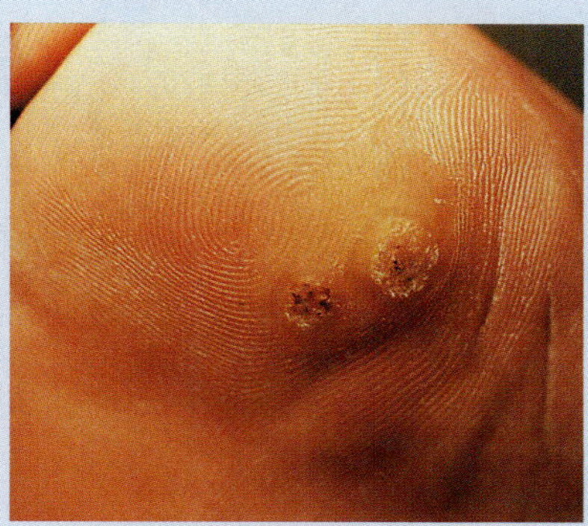

FIG 10-2 Plantar warts. (From Zitelli BJ, Davis HW: *Atlas of pediatric physical diagnosis*, ed 3, St Louis, 1997, Mosby.)

TABLE 10-3   COMMON FOOT AND NAIL PROBLEMS AND RELATED INTERVENTIONS

PROBLEM	PREVENTION	INTERVENTIONS
Callus: Thickened epidermis, usually flat, painless, and on underside of foot; caused by friction or pressure.	Wear proper footwear and always wear clean socks or stockings.	Soak callus in warm water to soften. Creams or lotions can help prevent reformation. Refer patient with diabetes or peripheral vascular disease to a podiatrist.
Corns: Caused by friction and pressure from shoes, mainly on toes, over bony prominence; usually cone-shaped, round, raised, and tender; may affect gait (Fig. 10-1).	Wear proper footwear; pain is aggravated by tight shoes. Always wear clean socks or stockings.	Surgical removal may be necessary. Use oval corn pads carefully because they increase pressure on toes and reduce circulation. Refer patient to podiatrist.
Plantar warts: Fungating lesions on sole of foot caused by papillomavirus (Fig. 10-2).	Warts are contagious. Avoid going barefoot, especially in public places.	Treatment ordered by a podiatrist may include applications of acid, burning, or freezing for removal.
Athlete's foot: Fungal infection of foot; scaling and cracking of skin occur between toes and on soles of feet; may have small blisters containing fluid. Apparently induced by tight footwear (Fig. 10-3).	Feet should be well ventilated. Avoid tight footwear. Dry feet well after bathing; apply powder. Wear clean socks.	Treat with medicated powder or cream. Refer to physician if condition does not improve with medicated products.
Ingrown nails: Toenail or fingernail grows inward into soft tissue around nail; may be painful (Fig. 10-4).	Cut with a nail clipper and file toenails straight across after bathing when they are soft. If nails are thick or vision is poor, have toenails trimmed by a podiatrist.	Treat with frequent warm soaks in antiseptic solution. Surgical removal of portion of nail that has grown into skin may be necessary. Refer patients with diabetes or peripheral vascular disease to podiatrist.
Fungus infection: Thick, discolored nails with yellow streaks.	Keep feet and nails clean and dry. Check feet and nails daily.	Refer to podiatrist.

Continued

PROCEDURAL GUIDELINE 10.5
Foot and Nail Care—cont'd

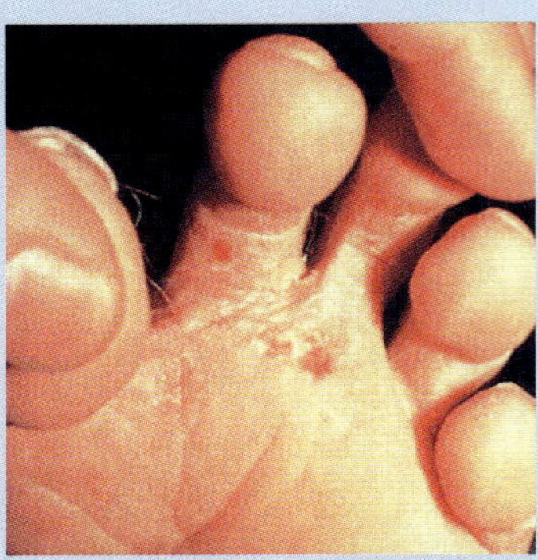

FIG 10-3 Athlete's foot (tinea pedis). (From Greenberger NJ, Hinthorn DR: *History taking and physical examination: essentials and clinical correlates,* St Louis, 1993, Mosby; courtesy Dr Loren Amundson, University of South Dakota, Sioux Falls, SD.)

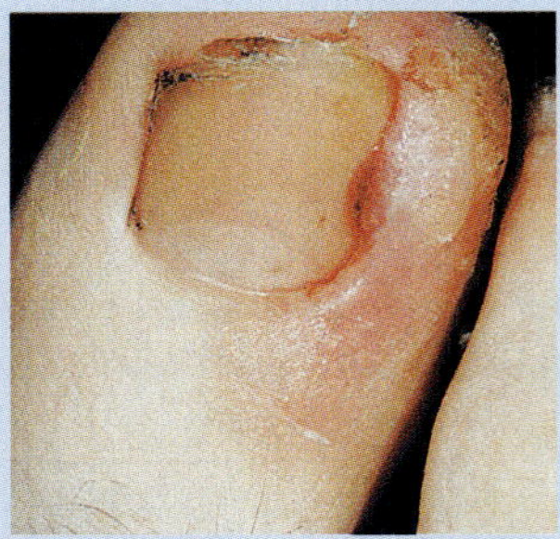

FIG 10-4 Ingrown toenail. (From Habif TP: *Clinical dermatology: a color guide to diagnosis and therapy,* ed 2, St Louis, 1990, Mosby.)

pain from foot lesions. Instruct these patients or their family caregivers on how to inspect the feet daily for cuts, blisters, temperature change, color, swelling, pain, dry cracking skin, sweaty skin, signs and symptoms of infection, corns, and calluses (Anastasi et al, 2013). Check facility policy for requirement of a health care provider order before cutting nails.

Delegation and Collaboration

The skill of foot and nail care may be delegated to nursing assistive personnel (NAP) *except* for patients with diabetes or patients with peripheral vascular disease or circulatory compromise. The nurse instructs the NAP about:
- Reporting any breaks in skin, redness, numbness, swelling, or pain.
- Not trimming patient's nails.

Equipment
- Clean gloves
- Basin (appropriate size for soaking)
- Washcloth
- Bath or face towel
- Nail clippers (check facility policy)
- Plastic applicator stick or soft brush, emery board, or nail file
- Soft nail or cuticle brush
- Lotion
- Disposable bath mat

Procedural Steps

1. **See Standard Protocol (inside front cover).**
2. Review medical record for a health care provider's order, which is usually required for cutting nails, especially when impaired circulation is suspected (e.g., diabetes mellitus, peripheral vascular disease, leg ulcers).
3. Identify if patient is at risk for foot or nail problems, such as reduced visual acuity, history of diabetes, or history of stroke.
4. Inspect all surfaces of toes, feet, and nails. Pay particular attention to areas of dryness, inflammation, or cracking. Also inspect areas between toes, heels, and soles of feet.
5. Palpate the dorsalis pedis pulse of both feet simultaneously, comparing the strength of pulses. Note color and warmth of toes and feet. Observe for capillary refill of nails. (Refill of less than 3 seconds indicates reduced circulation.)
6. Assess sensation in the feet by checking for light touch or discrimination between warm and cold.
7. Determine patient's ability to perform self-care.
8. Assess patient's foot and nail care practices for existing foot problems (e.g., home remedies such as cutting corns with razor blade or scissors, applying adhesive tape on foot, or using oval corn pads on toes). Use this time to instruct patients about foot care.
9. Assess type of footwear worn by patients, including type and cleanliness of socks worn, type and fit of shoes, and restrictive garters or knee-high hose.
10. Soak feet and fingers.
    a. Explain that soaking requires 10 to 20 minutes.
    b. Assist ambulatory patient to sit in chair with disposable bath mat under feet. If confined to bed, assist to a semi-Fowler's position with a waterproof pad and bath towel under feet.
    c. Fill wash basin and emesis basin with warm water. Test temperature of water with back of hand.
    d. Place wash basin on bath mat or towel, and help patient place one foot in basin. Place emesis basin on over-bed table in front of patient and have him or her immerse the fingers. Place call light within patient's reach. Offer diversional activity.

SAFE PATIENT CARE Patients who have diabetes mellitus or peripheral vascular disease should *not* soak their feet because of potential of increased dryness of skin and decrease in ability to assess temperature variations related to decreased sensations (ADA, 2014).

PROCEDURAL GUIDELINE 10.5
Foot and Nail Care—cont'd

11. Foot and nail care:
    a. Allow patient's feet and fingers to soak for 10 to 20 minutes. If necessary, rewarm water after 10 minutes.
    b. Apply clean gloves. Begin care on fingernails. Clean gently under nails with plastic applicator stick or soft brush while immersing fingers (see illustration).

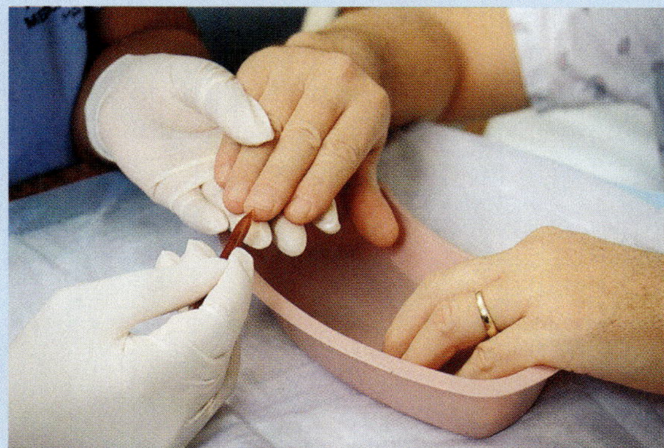

STEP 11b Clean under fingernails.

    c. Remove hands from basin and dry thoroughly.
    d. File fingernails straight across and even with tops of fingers. Or use nail clippers and clip fingernails straight across and even with tops of fingers (see illustration) and then smooth nail using file.

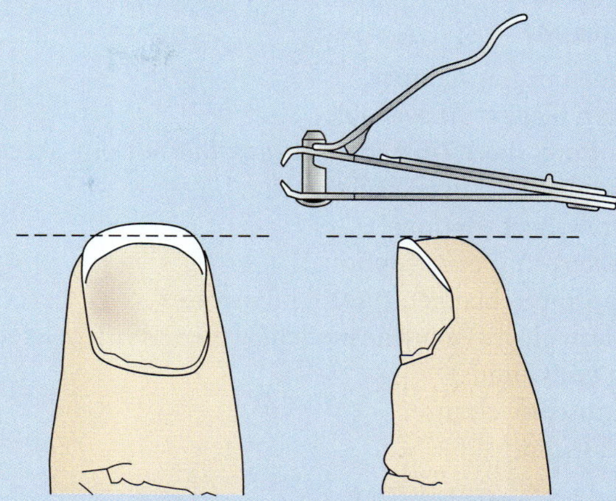

STEP 11d File or clip fingernails straight across.

    e. Use soft cuticle brush or nail brush to clean around cuticles.
    f. Move over-bed table away from patient.
    g. Remove feet from basin and scrub callused areas with washcloth or soft brush.
    h. Clean gently under nails with plastic stick applicator or soft brush.
    i. Clean and file toenails as in Steps 11d and 11e.
12. Apply thin layer of lotion to feet and hands. Lotion lubricates the skin and retains moisture.
13. **See Completion Protocol (inside front cover).**

PROCEDURAL GUIDELINE 10.6
Making an Occupied Bed

Because the bed is the piece of equipment most often used by a patient, it should be comfortable, safe, and adaptable to various positions. The typical hospital bed consists of a firm mattress on a metal frame that you can raise or lower horizontally. The frame of the bed is divided into three sections so that the operator can raise and lower the head and foot of the bed separately, in addition to inclining the entire bed with the head up or down. Each bed is set on four rollers or casters, which allows you to move the bed easily. See Table 10-4 for common bed positions.

Bed making may be done with the patient out of the bed (unoccupied) or in the bed (occupied). In some settings, bed linen is not changed every day; however, you always need to change any wet or soiled linen promptly.

Occupied bed making is limited to patients who cannot tolerate being out of bed. In addition, some patients have activity or positioning restrictions ordered by their health care provider; thus it is important to understand which position a patient can assume while the bed linens are changed. Plan the procedure carefully and perform it in a way that conserves time and the patient's energy. Patient condition and stability determines if it is appropriate to make the bed occupied. If a patient experiences severe pain with movement, an analgesic administered 30 to 60 minutes before the procedure is helpful in controlling pain and maintaining comfort. Even though the patient is unable to get out of bed, encourage self-help if possible, which helps maintain the patient's strength and mobility. For example, depending on restrictions, have the patient turn, assist in moving up in bed, or hold top sheets while linen is applied.

Delegation and Collaboration

The skill of bed making is delegated to nursing assistive personnel (NAP). The nurse instructs the NAP about:
- The patient's activity or position restrictions.
- What to do if the patient becomes fatigued or short of breath.
- Immediately reporting any unexpected concerns (e.g., excess wound drainage, dislodged IV tubing).

Continued

PROCEDURAL GUIDELINE 10.6
Making an Occupied Bed—cont'd

Equipment

- Linen bag or hamper
- Bath blanket (if available)
- Bottom sheet (in most settings the bottom sheet is a fitted sheet; check facility policy)
- Drawsheet (optional)
- Waterproof pads (optional)
- Top sheet, blanket, spread, pillowcases
- Clean gloves (if linen is soiled or there is risk of exposure to body fluids)
- Antiseptic cleanser
- Washcloth

Procedural Steps

1. **See Standard Protocol (inside front cover).**
2. Apply clean gloves. If patient has been incontinent or if drainage is present from dressings, gloves are necessary to reduce contact with infectious microorganisms.
3. Assess restrictions in mobility and positioning of patient. Explain procedure to patient, noting that you will need to ask the patient to turn over layers of linens.
4. Raise bed to comfortable working height. Loosen all top linens. Remove spread and blanket separately, leaving patient covered with top sheet. If soiled, place in linen bag. If to be reused, fold into square and place over back of chair.
5. Cover patient with bath blanket. Unfold bath blanket over top sheet. Ask patient to hold top edge of bath blanket. If patient is unable to help, tuck top of bath blanket under shoulders. Grasp top sheet under bath blanket at patient's shoulders and bring sheet down to foot of bed. Remove sheet and discard in linen bag.
6. Position patient on the far side of the bed, turned onto side and facing away from you. Encourage use of side rail to aid in turning. Adjust pillow under patient's head. Check that any tubing is not being stretched or pulled.
7. Loosen used bottom linens, moving from head to foot. Fanfold any cloth bed pad, bottom sheet, and drawsheet (if present) toward patient—first pad, then drawsheet, and then bottom sheet. Tuck edges of used linens just under buttocks, back, and shoulders (see illustration). Do not fanfold mattress pad (if it is to be reused). Remove any nonlinen items such as disposable pads and discard in appropriate receptacle.

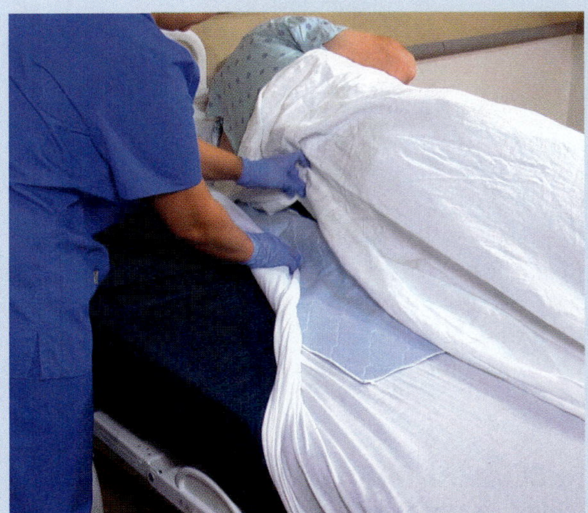

STEP 7 Old linen tucked alongside patient.

TABLE 10-4	COMMON BED POSITIONS	
POSITION	**DESCRIPTION**	**USES**
Fowler's	Head of bed raised to angle of 45 degrees or more; semi-sitting position; foot of bed may also be raised at knee	Used during meals, nasogastric tube insertion, and nasotracheal suction; promotes lung expansion
Semi-Fowler's	Head of bed raised approximately 30 degrees; incline is less than Fowler's position; foot of bed may also be raised at knee	Promotes lung expansion; used when patients receive gastric feedings to reduce regurgitation and risk for aspiration
Trendelenburg's	Entire bed tilted with head of bed down	Used for postural drainage; facilitates venous return in patients with poor peripheral venous perfusion
Reverse Trendelenburg's	Entire bedframe tilted with foot of bed down	Used infrequently; promotes gastric emptying; prevents esophageal reflux
Flat/supine	Entire bedframe horizontally parallel with floor	Used for patients with vertebral injuries and in cervical traction; used for patients who are hypotensive; generally preferred by patients for sleeping

PROCEDURAL GUIDELINE 10.6
Making an Occupied Bed—cont'd

8. Clean, disinfect, and dry mattress surface if it is soiled or has moisture (follow facility policy).

9. Apply clean linens to exposed half of bed; in separate layers.

   a. If applying a new mattress pad, place clean pad on bed by folding it lengthwise with center crease in middle of bed. Fanfold layer to center of bed alongside patient. (If reusing a pad, simply smooth out wrinkles.)

   b. Next apply bottom sheet. For a fitted sheet, pull corners of sheet smoothly over mattress ends and fanfold remainder toward center of bed. If bottom sheet is not fitted, place flat sheet lengthwise with center crease in middle of bed and fanfold to center of bed alongside patient (see illustration).

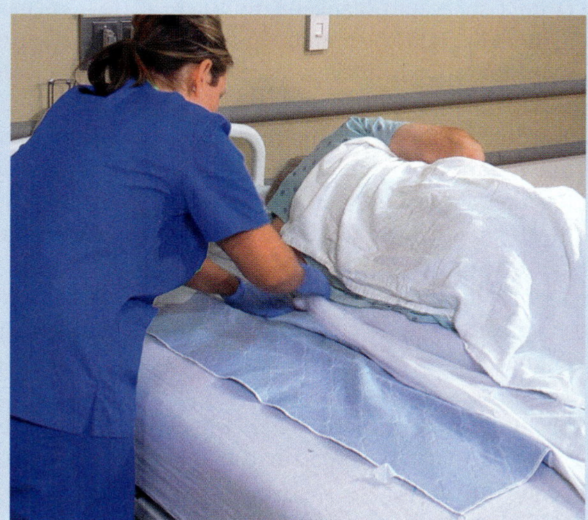

STEP 9b Clean linen applied to bed.

   c. Allow edge of flat unfitted sheet to hang about 25 cm (10 inches) over mattress edge. Lower hem of bottom flat sheet should lie seam down and even with bottom edge of mattress.

10. If flat sheet is used, miter bottom flat sheet at head of bed:

   a. Face head of bed diagonally. Place hand away from head of bed under top corner of mattress, near mattress edge, and lift.

   b. With other hand, tuck top edge of bottom sheet smoothly under mattress so that side edges of sheet above and below mattress meet when brought together.

   c. Face side of bed and pick up top edge of sheet at approximately 45 cm (18 inches) from top end of mattress (see illustration).

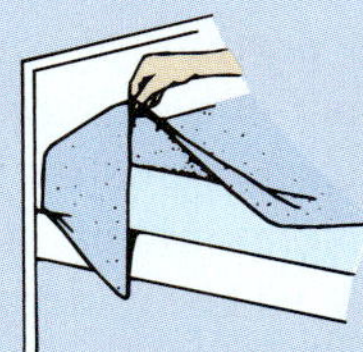

STEP 10c Top edge of sheet picked up.

   d. Lift sheet, and lay it on top of mattress to form a neat triangular fold, with lower base of triangle even with mattress side edge (see illustration).

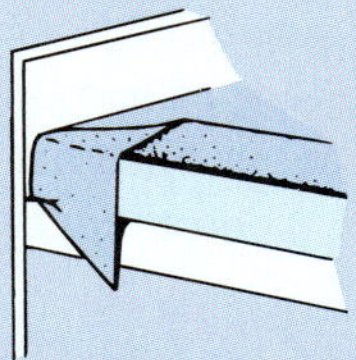

STEP 10d Sheet on top of mattress in a triangular fold.

   e. Tuck lower edge of sheet, which is hanging free below the mattress, under mattress. Tuck with palms down, without pulling triangular fold (see illustration).

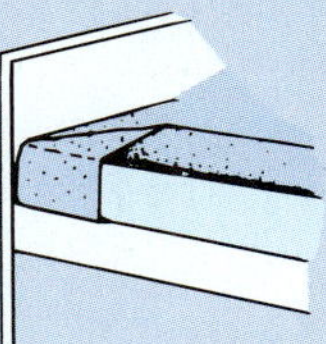

STEP 10e Lower edge of sheet tucked under mattress.

   f. Hold portion of sheet covering side of mattress in place with one hand. With the other hand, pick up top of triangular linen fold and bring it down over side of mattress (see illustrations). Tuck under mattress with palms down without pulling fold (see illustration).

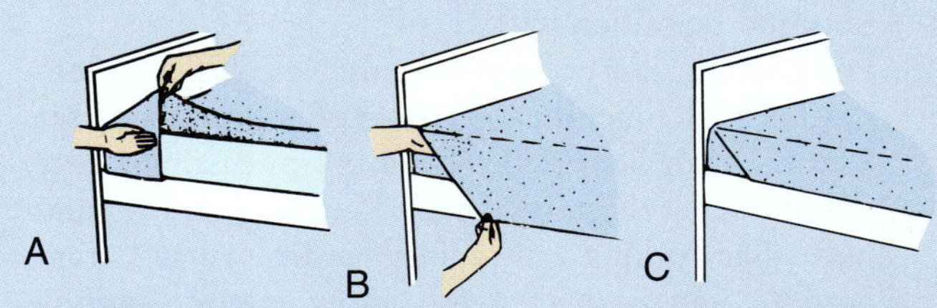

STEP 10f **A** and **B**, Triangular fold placed over side of mattress. **C,** Linen tucked under mattress.

Continued

PROCEDURAL GUIDELINE 10.6
Making an Occupied Bed—cont'd

11. Tuck remaining portion of sheet under mattress, moving toward foot of bed. Keep linen smooth.

12. If needed, open clean drawsheet so it unfolds in half. Lay center fold along middle of bed lengthwise and position sheet so it will be under patient's buttocks and torso. Fanfold top layer toward patient with edge along patient's back. Smooth over mattress and tuck excess edge under mattress. Add waterproof pad (absorbent side up) over drawsheet with seam side down. Fanfold toward patient. Keep clean and soiled linen separate.

13. Advise patient that he or she will be rolling over a thick layer of linens. Keeping patient covered, ask patient to roll toward you slowly, over the layers of linen. Do not let patient raise hips; simply roll. Raise side rail before moving to other side of bed.

14. Move to opposite side of bed and lower side rail. Assist patient in positioning on other side, over linen folds (see illustration). Loosen edges of soiled linen from under mattress.

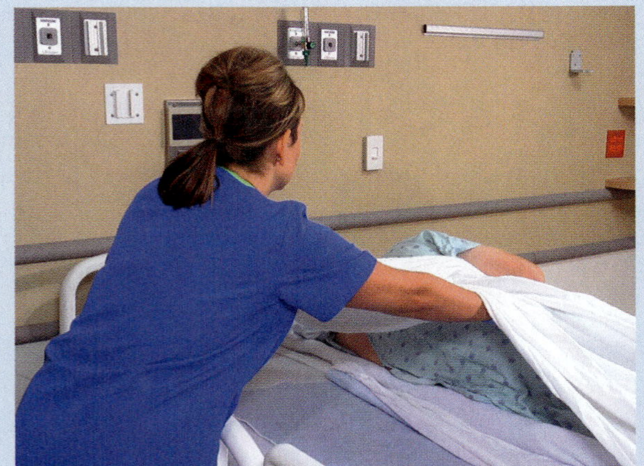

STEP 14 Nurse assists patient with rolling over linen folds.

15. Remove soiled linen by folding into a ball or square, with soiled side turned in. Hold linen away from your body and place in a linen bag.

16. Clean, disinfect, and dry other half of mattress as needed.

17. Pull clean, fanfolded linen out from beneath patient toward you and smooth it out over mattress from head to foot of bed. Assist patient to roll back to supine position, and reposition pillow.

18. Pull fitted sheet over mattress ends. Note: If flat bottom sheet is used, miter the top corner of bottom sheet (see Step 10), then, facing side of bed, grasp remaining edge of bottom flat sheet. Lean back. Keep back straight and pull while tucking excess linen under mattress from head to foot of bed. Avoid lifting mattress during tucking.

19. Smooth fanfolded drawsheet over bottom sheet. (Tucking is optional.) Smooth out waterproof pads.

20. Place top sheet over patient with center fold lengthwise down middle of bed and with seam side of hem facing up. Open sheet out from head to foot and unfold over patient. Be sure that top edge of sheet is even with top edge of mattress.

21. Ask patient to hold clean top sheet (if able). Remove bath blanket and discard in linen bag.

22. Place clean or reused bed blanket or spread on bed with crease running lengthwise along middle of bed. Unfold to cover patient. Make sure top edge is parallel with edge of top sheet and 15 to 20 cm (6 to 8 inches) from edge of top sheet.

23. Make a cuff by turning edge of top sheet down over top edge of blanket.

24. Make horizontal toe pleat; stand at foot of bed and fanfold sheet and blanket 5 to 10 cm (2 to 4 inches) across bed. Pull sheet and blanket up from bottom to make fold approximately 15 cm (6 inches) from bottom edge of mattress.

25. Tuck in remaining portion of sheet and blanket/spread under foot of mattress. Tuck top sheet and blanket together. Ensure that toe pleats are not pulled out.

26. Make modified mitered corner with top sheet and blanket/spread.
    a. Pick up side edge of top sheet and blanket and spread about 45 cm (18 inches) from foot of mattress. Lift linen to form a triangular fold, and lay it on bed.
    b. Tuck lower edge of sheet, which is hanging free below mattress, under mattress. Do not pull triangular fold.
    c. Pick up triangular fold, and bring it down over mattress while holding linen in place alongside of mattress. Do not tuck in lower edge of triangle (see illustration).

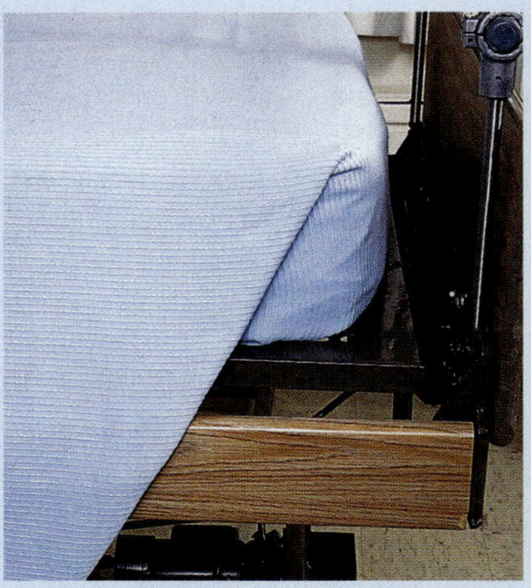

STEP 26c Modified mitered corner.

PROCEDURAL GUIDELINE 10.6
Making an Occupied Bed—cont'd

27. Change pillowcase. Have patient raise head. While supporting neck with one hand, remove pillow. Allow patient to lower head. Remove soiled case and place in linen bag. Grasp clean pillowcase at center of closed end. Gather case, turning it inside out over the hand holding it. With the same hand, pick up middle of one end of pillow. Pull pillowcase down over pillow with other hand. Do not hold pillow against your uniform. Be sure pillow corners fit evenly into corners of case.

28. During procedure, inspect skin for areas of irritation. Observe patient for signs of fatigue, dyspnea, pain, or discomfort.

29. **See Completion Protocol (inside front cover).**

PROCEDURAL GUIDELINE 10.7
Making an Unoccupied Bed

Bed making may be done with the patient out of the bed (unoccupied) or in the bed (occupied). An unoccupied bed is one left open with the top sheets fanfolded down. A post-operative surgical bed is prepared for patients returning from the operating room or procedural area. The bed is left with the top sheets fanfolded lengthwise and not tucked in to facilitate the patient's transfer from a stretcher. A closed bed, which is made with the top sheets pulled up to the head of the bed, is used after a patient is discharged and housekeeping cleans the unit.

Delegation and Collaboration

The skill of making an unoccupied bed can be delegated to nursing assistive personnel (NAP). The nurse instructs the NAP about:

- Use of special linen instructions if the patient is on an airflow or specialty mattress.

Equipment

- Linen bag or hamper
- Bottom sheet (in some settings the bottom sheet is a fitted sheet; check facility policy)
- Drawsheet (optional)
- Waterproof pads (optional)
- Top sheet, blanket, spread, pillowcases
- Clean gloves (if linen is soiled or there is risk of exposure to body fluids)
- Antiseptic cleanser
- Washcloth

Procedural Steps

1. **See Standard Protocol (inside front cover).**
2. Assist patient to bedside chair or recliner or encourage ambulation if appropriate.
3. Raise bed to comfortable working position with side rails lowered.
4. Apply clean gloves if linen is soiled with body fluids. Remove all soiled linen and place in laundry bag, taking care not to contact uniform. Avoid shaking or fanning linen. Cleanse mattress with antiseptic solution if soiled.
5. Apply all bottom linen on one side of bed before moving to opposite side. Make mitered corners at the top corner of the mattress when using a flat sheet (see Procedural Guideline 10.6). Place fitted sheet smoothly over mattress.
6. Optional: Apply waterproof pad or drawsheet, laying center fold along middle of bed lengthwise. Smooth pad or drawsheet over bottom sheet and tuck under mattress.
7. Move to the opposite side of the bed. Repeat Steps 5 and 6.
8. Smooth pad or drawsheet over mattress and tuck excess edge under mattress, keeping palms down.
9. Place top sheet over bed with vertical center fold lengthwise down middle of bed. Open sheet out from head to foot, being sure that top edge of sheet is even with top edge of mattress. Optional: Spread a blanket or spread evenly over bed in same fashion.
10. Standing on one side at foot of bed, lift mattress corner slightly with one hand and with other hand tuck top sheet and blanket or spread under mattress.
11. Make modified mitered corner with top sheet, blanket, and spread. After triangular fold is made, leave tip of triangle untucked (see Procedural Guideline 10.6, Step 26).
12. Go to other side of bed. Complete Step 11 to make a modified corner.
13. Make a horizontal toe pleat with all top layers of linen:
    a. Stand at foot of bed and fanfold in sheet 5 to 10 cm (2 to 4 inches) across bed.
    b. Pull sheet up from bottom to make fold approximately 15 cm (6 inches) from bottom edge of mattress.
14. Make a cuff at top of bed by turning edge of top sheet down over top edge of blanket and spread.

Continued

PROCEDURAL GUIDELINE 10.7
Making an Unoccupied Bed—cont'd

15. Apply clean pillowcase. Open bed by fanfolding top covers to foot of bed. Leave bed in low position.
16. *Surgical bed (variation):*
    a. Fold all top linen from foot of bed toward center of mattress, even with foot of mattress.
    b. Fold corners toward opposite side of bed, forming a triangle.
    c. Fanfold linen toward you on side of bed away from where patient will be transferred.
17. Leave all side rails down and place bed in high position to match height of stretcher.
18. **See Completion Protocol (inside front cover).**

■ CRITICAL THINKING EXERCISES

Case Study

An 80-year-old man with a history of heart failure and diabetes mellitus was admitted to the hospital because of increasing shortness of breath, especially on exertion. He has had diabetes mellitus for 30 years, and recently his blood glucose levels have been out of control. He recently had all of his teeth pulled and now wears dentures.

1. Place the steps for assisting a patient with denture care in the correct order.
   a. Rinse dentures thoroughly in tepid water.
   b. Perform hand hygiene and don clean gloves; remove upper denture plate by applying gentle downward pressure with 4 × 4–inch gauze.
   c. Hold dentures over an emesis basin or sink lined with a washcloth and containing 1 inch of water.
   d. Gently lift lower denture from jaw and rotate one side downward to remove from patient's mouth.
   e. Ask patient about preferences for denture care and products used.
   f. Apply cleaning agent to brush, and brush surfaces of dentures.
   g. Store dentures in a denture cup with patient's identification label.
   1. b, d, e, a, c, f, g
   2. e, b, d, c, f, a, g
   3. d, b, a, e, f, c, g
   4. g, e, b, d, c, a, f
2. The patient states that he is feeling uncomfortable and wants a bath. Which type of bath would be most appropriate at this time?
   1. Complete bath
   2. Partial bath
   3. Tub bath
   4. Shower

Review Questions

1. Which of the following actions are steps used when making an unoccupied bed? Select all that apply.
   1. Raise bed to working height.
   2. Wear gloves at all times.
   3. Apply all bottom linen on one side of bed before moving to opposite side.
   4. Remove soiled linen and place on the floor.
   5. Tuck top sheet and spread in at bottom of bed using a modified mitered corner.
   6. Keep top covers at head of bed when procedure is completed.
   7. Make horizontal toe pleat with all top layers of linen.
2. Which of the following is an appropriate guideline when providing perineal care for a patient?
   1. Leave the foreskin in an uncircumcised male patient retracted after cleansing.
   2. Cleanse from the most contaminated to the least contaminated area for a female patient.
   3. Wash the tip of the penis at the meatus outward in a circular motion.
   4. A patient with a Foley catheter needs minimal perineal care.
3. A patient who has a decreased level of consciousness needs mouth care. When performing mouth care, in what position should the patient be placed?
   1. Supine
   2. Semi-Fowler's
   3. High-Fowler's
   4. Side-lying
4. The nurse begins to prepare a patient for a partial bed bath. The nurse brings a bag bath packet into the room and prepares to bathe the patient. The patient asks, "Why aren't you using soap and water?" The nurse's best response would be:
   1. The bag bath is a bit quicker and causes less discomfort.
   2. The bag bath is easier for me to use.
   3. The bag bath is what our facility uses.
   4. The bag bath poses less risk of infection than using a basin of water.

5. What is the most important reason that the nurse washes the patient's extremities from distal to proximal?
   1. Enhance patient comfort
   2. Prevent skin irritation
   3. Promote venous return
   4. Reduce any noticeable swelling
6. Which steps should the nurse take to facilitate the shaving of a male patient's facial hair with a disposable razor? Select all that apply.
   1. Use the disposable razor at a 45-degree angle.
   2. Place a cool, moist washcloth over the patient's face.
   3. Shave in the direction of hair growth.
   4. Use long, downward strokes while shaving.
7. The nurse is providing a bed bath to a patient. Place the steps for bathing the patient in the correct order.
   1. Eyes, face, arms, chest, abdomen, legs, back
   2. Face, eyes, arms, legs, back, chest, abdomen
   3. Eyes, arms, face, chest, back, abdomen, legs
   4. Arms, chest, abdomen, legs, back, eyes, face

8. A patient with diabetes mellitus wants to have his nails trimmed. What is the nurse's first step on hearing this request?
   1. Clip the nails to fit the contour of his fingers.
   2. Use manicure scissors to cut the nails straight across.
   3. Use an emery board to shape the nails before being trimmed.
   4. Make sure that there is a health care provider's order to cut the nails.
9. A NAP asks you if it is okay to trim facial hair on one of your patients. What is the first thing you should do before allowing the NAP to trim his facial hair?
   1. Ask the patient his preference or cultural beliefs
   2. Ensure cleanliness of beard
   3. Tell the NAP that we do not trim patients' beards
   4. Encourage patient to shave himself
10. Which of the following are signs and symptoms of a VTE?
    1. Unilateral calf swelling
    2. Pitting edema
    3. Pain
    4. All of the above

REFERENCES

American Association of Critical-Care Nurses (AACN): *American Association of Critical-Care Nurses Updates Patient Bathing Practices*, 2013. http://www.aacn.org/wd/publishing/content/pressroom/pressreleases/2013/april-bathing-practice-alert-press-release.pcms?menu=. Accessed December 13, 2013.

American Diabetes Association (ADA): *Foot complications*, 2014. http://www.diabetes.org/living-with-diabetes/complications/foot-complications/. Accessed June 15, 2014.

Anastasi J, et al: HIV peripheral neuropathy and foot care management: a review of assessment and relevant guidelines, *AJN* 113(12):34, 2013.

Centers for Disease Control and Prevention (CDC): *Parasites/lice*, 2013. http://www.cdc.gov/parasites/lice/. Accessed September 8, 2014.

Centers for Disease Control and Prevention (CDC): *Healthcare associated infections: Ventilator associated pneumonia*, 2012. http://www.cdc.gov/HAI/vap/vap.html. Accessed September 8, 2014.

Climo MW, et al: Effect of daily chlorhexidine bathing on hospital-acquired infection, *N Engl J Med* 368:533–542, 2013.

Cowdell F: Older people, personal hygiene, and skin care, *Medsurg Nurs* 20(5):235, 2011.

European Pressure Ulcer Advisory Panel (EPUAP) and National Pressure Ulcer Advisory Panel (NPUAP): *Treatment of pressure ulcers: quick reference guide*, Washington, DC, 2009, NPUAP. http://www.epuap.org/guidelines/Final_Quick_Treatment.pdf. Accessed September 14, 2014.

Sona C, et al: The impact of a simple, low-cost oral care protocol on ventilator-associated pneumonia rates in a surgical intensive care unit, *J Intens Care Med* 24(1):54–62, 2009.

Tabei L, et al: Accuracy in diagnosing deep and pelvic vein thrombosis in primary care, *Dtsch Arztebl Int* 109(45):761, 2012.

Weigand D: *AACN procedure manual for critical care*, ed 6, St Louis, 2011, Saunders.

Care of the Eye and Ear

Meaningful sensory stimuli helps a person learn about the environment. Perceiving and understanding environmental stimuli are necessary for healthy functioning. In addition, how well a patient hears also affects health literacy. When there are alterations in vision and hearing, people often seek artificial sensory devices to replace or restore sensory function. Artificial sensory devices must fit and work properly if patients are to function optimally within their environment. Eyeglasses and contact lenses help to restore visual loss, and hearing aids improve sound reception. Breakage or loss of sensory devices is expensive and may result in serious impairment that places a patient at risk for injury, interferes with communication, socially isolates a patient, and affects patient independence and self-esteem.

PATIENT-CENTERED CARE

Any intervention or device to improve sensory perception must fit and work properly. It is important to know patients' preferences and have a discussion with them about how to use and care for their eyewear or hearing aid.

When a patient is acutely ill or has mobility limitations, provide more direct care and supervision, and communicate the patient's sensory loss to other health care professionals. For example, when patients have a hearing deficit, be sure they understand what you communicate. Always face the patient before beginning to speak, and make sure there is enough light for the patient to see your lips. Eliminate external noises; speak in a slow, clear, normal tone of voice. Ask patients what communication styles they prefer. Never talk over or exclude a patient from conversation or decisions. Optimal outcomes are hampered when patients are unable to hear or are excluded from instructions (Hardin, 2012).

Hospitals, rehabilitation centers, and skilled nursing facilities are poor listening environments. Hard flooring surfaces, medical equipment, televisions, and the constant need to speak with other health care professionals all produce noise. This increased background noise makes hearing even more difficult for hearing-impaired individuals.. When patients have auditory impairments, the increased background noise in an unfamiliar environment often makes them more anxious and decreases their ability to adjust to new surroundings.

Communication is vital to all persons from all cultures. Discuss what a loss in hearing or vision means to a patient. In some cultures, limited eye contact is the norm and demonstrates a nonverbal form of respect (Zerwekh and Garneau, 2015). Changes in the ability to move the eyes, as with a prosthesis, present a social difficulty because the patient is unable to lower the eyes.

Some cultures are more comfortable with the soft-spoken word and silence (Zerwekh and Garneau, 2015). Hearing impairments may force the patient's family and friends to speak louder. In addition, because of the comfort with silence, you can easily mistake a patient's silence as a measure of comfort and never correctly assess what the patient is able to hear or if the information was heard correctly. You may sometimes use touch to get the attention of a patient with decreased hearing; however, in some cultures, it is unacceptable for caregivers of the opposite sex to touch a patient. Remember to learn a patient's preferences before using touch to gain the attention of a patient with sensory impairment.

SAFETY

Health literacy is becoming increasingly more important in preparing patients and caregivers to be proactive in areas of health promotion and disease prevention as well as providing aspects of physical care in the home environment. Sensory impairments make it difficult for patients and caregivers to communicate health care needs, and these impairments affect health literacy. Health literacy, which is the capacity to obtain, process, and understand basic health information and services to make appropriate health decisions, is an important aspect of patient care, and it is important to identify resources to improve health literacy (CDC, 2014).

Whenever you care for patients with sensory alterations, safety is a priority. Anticipate how the sensory alteration places the patient at risk for injury. Orient the patient to any new environment or changes within an existing environment to minimize safety hazards. In addition, educate family and friends regarding the best way they can help the patient adapt to sensory loss.

When patients have visual impairments, they may have difficulty with tasks requiring visual detail (e.g., reading prescriptions or syringes). This difficulty increases the risk of improper administration of medications in the home setting. In addition, certain eye conditions, such as cataracts and macular degeneration, cause the patient difficulty when adjusting to changes in contrast and brightness. Individuals with diabetic retinopathy have changes related to distorted vision, changes in acuity, and loss of depth and contrast cues (Kergoat and Chriqui, 2011). These changes leave the patient at risk for accidents in the home or health care environments.

Hearing aids require regular cleaning to ensure function and prevent injury. Most patients have an established routine for cleaning their hearing aids. When a patient is unable to care for the hearing aid, you must understand the correct way to clean, handle, and store the device. Careful handling of prostheses is vital to avoid damage to these devices or injury to the patient's eyes or ears.

EVIDENCE-BASED PRACTICE

Gopinath B et al.: Dual sensory impairment in older adults increases the risk of mortality: a population based study, *PLoSOne* 8(3):e55054, 2013.

Roets-Merken LM, et al.: Screening for hearing, visual and dual sensory impairment in older adults using behavioural cues: a validation study. *Int J Nurs Stud* 51, 2014.

Vision and hearing impairments occurring together are significant and are referred to as dual sensory impairment (DSI). DSI has the potential to cause a decline in cognitive function or contribute to acute confusion or depression. DSI in rehabilitation or long-term care settings affects a patient's success in learning how to use assistive devices safely. DSI diminishes communication and well-being and can cause social isolation, depression, reduced independence, cognitive impairment, and mortality (Gopinath et al., 2013). Guidelines for management of patients with DSL include early identification of sensory loss and prompt interventions to improve vision or hearing loss or both are beneficial in reducing confusion, improving orientation, and increasing patient independence (Roets-Merken et al., 2014).

- Visual impairment:
  - Understand the type of visual impairment; for example, if a patient has a visual field loss, approach the patient on the opposite side.
  - Orient the patient to the room and location of furniture. In the bathroom, orient the patient to the location of the fixtures and the emergency call bell
- Hearing impairment:
  - Routinely assess the patient's ears to determine if sudden changes in hearing acuity are related to a buildup of cerumen.
  - Know the patient's usual method for dealing with sensory loss, what type of hearing aid care is needed, and what type of assistance is required to enhance communication.
  - Determine that sound outlet is not blocked by wax or moisture.

SKILL 11.1 EYE IRRIGATION

Eye irrigations are necessary following a chemical exposure to the eye. Such exposures can occur in the home but commonly occur in the workplace. Employers are required to comply with Occupational Safety and Health Administration standards for material safety data sheets (MSDS). All employees must have access to MSDS related to chemicals present in their work environment. With MSDS available, in the case of an exposure, the employee and health care providers know the specific chemical exposure and immediate treatment requirements.

Eye irrigations effectively flush out exudates, irritating solutions, or foreign bodies from the eye. Ocular chemical burns are commonly sustained after exposure to chemicals found in cleaning agents, fertilizers, bleaches, or plaster (Chau et al., 2012). When a chemical or irritating substance contaminates the eye, irrigate immediately with copious amounts of cool water for at least 15 minutes to minimize corneal damage (NLM, 2013a). The procedure typically is used in emergency situations when a foreign object or some other substance has entered the eye.

When a chemical injury to the eye occurs, the priority is flushing the eye with copious amounts of irrigation fluid. Immediate eye irrigation takes priority over a comprehensive ocular assessment (Chau et al., 2012). Although irrigating solutions are usually normal saline or lactated Ringer's solution, cool tap water is effective during the emergent phase until the person can seek medical help (Chau et al., 2012; NLM, 2013a). When the acute phase is over, an irrigation solution that buffers alkali or acid chemical is selected (Chau et al., 2012).

ASSESSMENT

1. Identify patient using two identifiers (e.g., name and birthday or name and account number, according to facility policy). Compare identifiers with information on the patient's MAR or medical record. *Rationale: Ensures correct patient. Complies with The Joint Commission standards and improves patient safety (TJC, 2014).*
2. Review health care provider's medication order, including solution to be instilled and the affected eye (left, right, or both) to receive irrigation. *Rationale: Ensures safe and correct administration of irrigant.*
3. Unless this is an emergent chemical exposure, assess reason for eye irrigation by obtaining a history of the injury from the patient. *Rationale: Knowing if the chemical exposure is alkali versus acid determines type and amount of irrigating solution and the frequency of irrigation (Chau et al., 2012).*

> **SAFE PATIENT CARE** Determine if patient is wearing contact lens. Do not remove contact lens unless there is a rapid swelling, there is a chemical injury, or you cannot get rapid medical attention. *Rationale: If the contacts did not flush out during the immediate rapid irrigation, have the patient try to remove them after the initial irrigation (NLM, 2013a).*

4. Determine patient's ability to open affected eye. *Rationale: Spasm of the eyelid or pain makes opening the eye difficult. Local anesthetics, such as proparacaine or tetracaine, cause topical numbness and are used before eye examination procedures.*
5. Conduct an eye examination (NLM, 2013a). Ask patient about itching, burning, pain, blurred vision, or photophobia. Assess eye for redness, excessive tearing, and discharge. Assess pupils are round and react to light and accommodation (PERRLA) and condition of eyelids and lacrimal glands for edema. Assess visual acuity before and after treatment. *Rationale: Provides baseline for condition of eye. You may need to obtain topical anesthetic drops to provide comfort and perform a detailed eye examination.*
6. Ask patient to rate pain level using a scale of 0 to 10. *Rationale: Provides baseline to evaluate response to irrigation later.*
7. Assess patient's ability to cooperate. *Rationale: Extra assistance may be necessary.*

PLANNING

Expected Outcomes focus on patient's physical and psychological comfort and improving vision.
1. Patient demonstrates minimal anxiety during and after irrigation.
2. Patient verbalizes reduced pain, burning, or itching and improved visual acuity after eye irrigation.
3. Patient maintains normal pupillary reaction and eye movements after irrigation.

Delegation and Collaboration

The skill of eye irrigation cannot be delegated to nursing assistive personnel (NAP). The nurse instructs the NAP to:
- Report any patient complaint of discomfort or excess tearing after the irrigation.

Equipment

- Prescribed irrigating solution: volume usually 30 to 180 mL at about 32° to 38°C (90° to 100°F). (For chemical flushing, use normal saline or lactated Ringer's solution in volume to provide continuous irrigation over 15 minutes.)
- Sterile basin or bag of intravenous (IV) solution
- Curved emesis basin
- Waterproof pad or towel
- 4 × 4–inch gauze pads
- Soft bulb syringe, eyedropper, or IV tubing
- Clean gloves
- Penlight
- Medication administration record (MAR)

IMPLEMENTATION *for* EYE IRRIGATION

STEPS	RATIONALE
1. **See Standard Protocol (inside front cover).**	
2. Check accuracy and completeness of each MAR with health care provider's written medication or procedure order. Check patient's name, irrigation solution name and concentration, route of administration, and time for administration. Compare MAR with label of eye irrigation solution.	The order sheet is the most reliable source and only legal record of drugs or procedure the patient is to receive. Ensures that patient receives correct medication.

3. Assist patient to side-lying position, turn patient's head so that the injured eye is down and to the side (NLM, 2013a). If both eyes are injured, have patient take a shower if possible or place patient supine for simultaneous irrigation of both eyes.

Irrigation solution flows from inner to outer canthus, preventing contamination of unaffected eye and nasolacrimal duct.

4. Apply clean gloves. If patient reports sensation of foreign body in the eye, remove contact lenses (if possible) before initial irrigation (Box 11-1).

Prompt removal of contact lenses is needed to irrigate small foreign bodies, such as dust and sand particles, safely and completely from the eye (NLM, 2013a).

> **SAFE PATIENT CARE** In an emergency, such as first aid for chemical burns, do not delay treatment by removing patient's contact lens before irrigation.

5. Explain to patient that the eye can be closed periodically and that no object will touch the eye.

Informing patients what to expect decreases anxiety and reassures them.

6. Place towel or waterproof pad under patient's face, and place curved emesis basin just below patient's cheek on side of affected eye.

Catches irrigation fluid.

7. With 4 × 4–inch gauze moistened in prescribed solution (or normal saline), gently clean eyelid margins and eyelashes from inner to outer canthus.

Minimizes transfer of debris from lids or lashes into eye during irrigation.

8. Explain next steps to patient and encourage relaxation.

   a. With gloved finger, gently retract upper and lower eyelids to expose conjunctival sacs.

Retraction minimizes blinking and allows irrigation of conjunctiva.

   b. To hold lids open, apply gentle pressure to lower bony orbit and bony prominence beneath eyebrow. *Do not apply pressure over eye.*

9. Hold irrigating syringe, dropper, or IV tubing approximately 2.5 cm (1 inch) from the inner canthus.

Direct contact with irrigation equipment may injure the eye.

10. Ask patient to look toward brow and tell patient when you are starting the irrigation. Gently irrigate with a steady stream toward lower conjunctival sac, moving from inner to outer canthus (see illustration).

Minimizes force of stream on patient's cornea. Flushes irrigant out and away from the other eye and nasolacrimal duct.

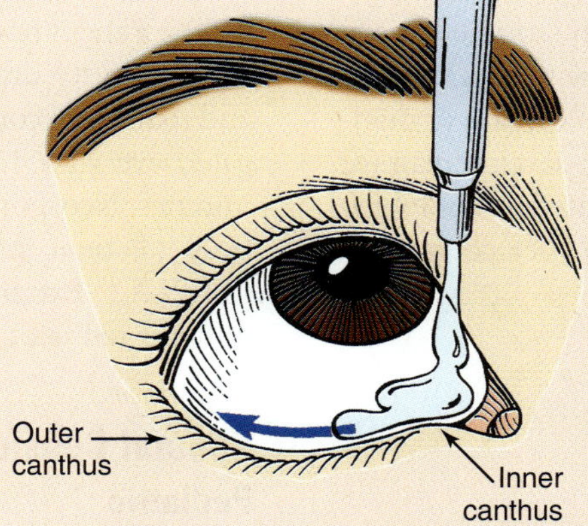

STEP 10 Irrigation of eye from inner to outer canthus.

11. Reinforce the importance of the procedure, and encourage patient to lie still by using calm, confident, soft voice.

Reduces anxiety.

12. Allow patient to blink periodically.

Lid closure moves secretions from upper conjunctival sac.

13. Continue irrigation with prescribed solution, volume, or time or until secretions are cleared. (Note: An irrigation of ≥15 minutes is needed to flush chemicals.)

Ensures complete removal of irritant. Assessment of pH of eye secretion may be necessary if eye was exposed to an acidic or basic solution during injury (NLM, 2013a).

14. Blot excess moisture from eyelids and face with gauze or towel.

15. **See Completion Protocol (inside front cover).**

Continued

BOX 11-1   REMOVAL OF CONTACT LENSES

Soft Lenses
- Wash hands. Apply powder-free gloves. Place a towel just below patient's face.
- *Option:* Add 2 to 3 drops of sterile saline solution to patient's eye.
- If possible, have patient look straight ahead. Retract lower eyelid and expose lower edge of lens.
- Using pad of index finger, slide lens off cornea down onto white of eye.
- Pull upper eyelid down gently with thumb of other hand and compress lens slightly between thumb and index finger.
- Gently pinch lens and lift out without allowing edges to stick together.
- If lens edges stick together, place lens in palm and soak thoroughly with sterile saline.
- Place lens in storage case.
- Follow procedure for cleansing, disinfecting, and disposing lens.

Rigid Lenses
- Wash hands. Apply powder-free gloves. Place a towel just below patient's face.
- Ensure lens is positioned directly over cornea. If it is not, have patient close eyelids. Place index and middle fingers of one hand on eyelid just beside the lens and gently but firmly massage lens back over cornea. If lens cannot be repositioned, referral to an ophthalmologist is needed.
- Place index finger on outer corner of patient's eye and draw skin gently back toward ear.
- Ask patient to blink. Do not release pressure on lid until blink is completed.
- If lens fails to pop out, gently retract eyelid beyond edges of lens. Press lower eyelid gently against lower edge of lens to dislodge it.
- Allow both eyelids to close slightly and grasp lens as it rises from the eye. Cup lens in hand.
- If patient is unable to assist, use a specially designed suction cup. Place cup on center of lens and, while applying suction, gently remove lens off patient's cornea.
- Place lens in storage case.
- Follow procedure for cleansing and disinfecting.

EVALUATION

1. Observe for verbal and nonverbal signs of anxiety during irrigation.
2. Assess patient's comfort level after eye irrigation.
3. Inspect eye for presence of discharge and assess PERRLA.
4. Ask patient about improved visual acuity or blurred vision.
5. Use **Teach Back:** State to the patient, "I want to be sure I explained how to irrigate your eye safely, so you can do this at home. Can you show me now how to irrigate your eye?" Evaluates what the patient is able to explain or demonstrate. Revise your instruction now or develop plan for revised patient teaching to be implemented at an appropriate time if patient is not able to teach back correctly.

Unexpected Outcomes and Related Interventions

1. Anxiety:
   a. Reinforce rationale for irrigation.
   b. Allow patient to close eye periodically during irrigation.
   c. Instruct patient to take slow, deep breaths.
2. Patient complains of pain and foreign body sensation in eye after irrigation. Excessive tearing and photophobia are noted.
   a. Advise patient to close the eye and avoid eye movement.
   b. Notify health care provider of specific assessment findings.

Recording and Reporting

- Record in nurses' notes condition of eye and patient's report of pain and visual symptoms. Record the type and amount of irrigation solution on patient's MAR. Document your evaluation of patient demonstration of an eye irrigation.
- Document your evaluation of patient learning.
- Report continued symptoms of pain or blurred vision.

Sample Documentation

0800   Patient notes blurred vision and tenderness in left eye. Yellow, crusty drainage noted on eyelids with slight edema and redness of conjunctiva. Patient correctly cleaned and irrigated eye with 120 mL warm, sterile, normal saline for 15 minutes. Neosporin ophthalmic ointment applied.

0900   Patient states that eye "feels better." Vision clearer. PERRLA. Extraocular movements intact. Conjunctiva remains red with slight edema, no drainage.

Special Considerations
Pediatric

- Children with foreign bodies or chemicals in the eye often panic. You may need to use a mummy restraint (see Chapter 4) so you can irrigate the eye safely and quickly, reducing the risk of injury (Hockenberry and Wilson, 2013).

Geriatric

- Because of changes in fine motor coordination or mobility, an older adult who needs eye irrigations in the home setting may need the assistance of a family member or friend. The significant other must be present for patient teaching (Touhy and Jett, 2014).

PROCEDURAL GUIDELINE 11.1
Eye Care for the Comatose Patient

A complication of sedation and coma is that some patients are unable to maintain effective eyelid closure (Werli-Alvarenga et al., 2013). These patients lose their natural protective mechanisms to protect the cornea. When the cornea is unprotected, there is an increased risk of corneal dehydration, abrasion, perforation, and infection. Normal protective mechanisms include blinking with lubrication of the eye (Douglas and Berry, 2011). Blinking provides a mechanical barrier to injury and prevents dehydration. Tears maintain a moist environment, lubricate the eyelids, wash away foreign material and cell debris, prevent organisms from adhering to the ocular surface, and transport oxygen to the outer eye surface.

Preventive nursing care is essential for patients in the intensive care unit (Kocaçal Güler et al., 2011). The nurse is responsible for providing eye care when patients are in a coma. Left unprotected, damage to the cornea can occur. Damage ranges from corneal scarring to premature cataract formation or vision changes. Depending on the patient's condition, moisture chambers, lubrication, and corneal surface protection are the best interventions to protect the corneas (Werli-Alvarenga et al., 2013).

Delegation and Collaboration

The skill of providing eye care for the comatose patient can be delegated to nursing assistive personnel (NAP). However, it is the nurse's responsibility to assess the condition of the patient's eyes and administer the sterile lubricant. The nurse instructs the NAP to:
- Adapt the skill for specific patients (e.g., using skin-sensitive tape to affix eye pads for patients with sensitive skin).
- Report immediately any eye drainage or irritation to the nurse for further assessment.

Equipment
- Clean gloves
- Water or normal saline solution
- Clean washcloth
- Cotton balls
- Eye pads or patches
- Paper tape
- Eyedropper bulb syringe
- Sterile lubricant or eye preparations as ordered

NOTE: A moisture chamber (e.g., polyethylene covers or polyacrylamide hydrogel dressings seal off the eye from the environment) is often used (Kocaçal Güler et al., 2011). Check facility policy.

Procedural Steps

1. **See Standard Protocol (inside front cover).**
2. Observe patient's eyes for drainage, irritation, redness, and lesions. Apply clean gloves if drainage is present.
3. Continually explain each step of the procedure. It is unknown how much a comatose patient can hear; it is important to orient continually and explain any procedure to a patient.
4. Assess for blink reflex.
5. Perform pupillary examination to determine if pupils are PERRLA (see Chapter 7).
6. Observe patient's eye movements, noting symmetry.
7. Explain procedure to patient and family members.
8. Position patient in supine position.
9. Use clean washcloth or cotton balls moistened with water or saline and gently wipe each eye from inner to outer canthus. Use a separate, clean cotton ball or corner of the washcloth for each eye.
10. Use an eyedropper to instill the prescribed lubricant (e.g., saline, methylcellulose, liquid tears) as ordered. Wipe away any excess lubricant, moving from inner to outer canthus.
11. If blink reflex is absent, gently close patient's eyes and apply eye patches, pads, or a moisture chamber. Secure patch, being careful not to tape patient's eyes.
12. **See Completion Protocol (inside front cover).**
13. Remove eye pad or patches every 4 hours or as ordered and observe condition of patient's eye for drainage, irritation, redness, and lesions. Remove moisture chamber as ordered, and assess the eye as noted previously.
14. Notify health care provider if signs of irritation or infection are present.

SKILL 11.2 EAR IRRIGATION

Common indications for irrigation of the external ear canal are presence of foreign bodies, local inflammation, and buildup of cerumen. The procedure is not without potential hazards. Usually irrigations are performed with liquid warmed to body temperature to avoid vertigo or nausea in patients. The greatest danger during ear irrigation is rupture of the tympanic membrane caused by forcing irrigant into the canal under pressure. Damage to the external auditory meatus may also occur by scratching the lining of the canal if the patient suddenly moves or if there is inadequate control of the irrigating syringe (NLM, 2013b). Improperly drying the ear may lead to acute otitis externa (infection of the outer ear).

Ear emergencies include the presence of foreign bodies, insect bites, or percussion injuries. In addition, the patient can have damage from inside the ear, which includes blood and drainage. Sometimes the cause of bloody drainage may be the result of a head or neck injury. If you suspect a head or neck injury, (1) do not move the patient, (2) cover the outside of the ear with a sterile dressing (if available), (3) get medical help immediately, and (4) do not irrigate the ear (NLM, 2013c). In addition, the ear should not be irrigated if vegetable matter or an insect is present in the canal; the tympanic membrane is ruptured; or the patient has otitis externa, myringotomy tubes, or a mastoid cavity (Hockenberry and Wilson, 2013).

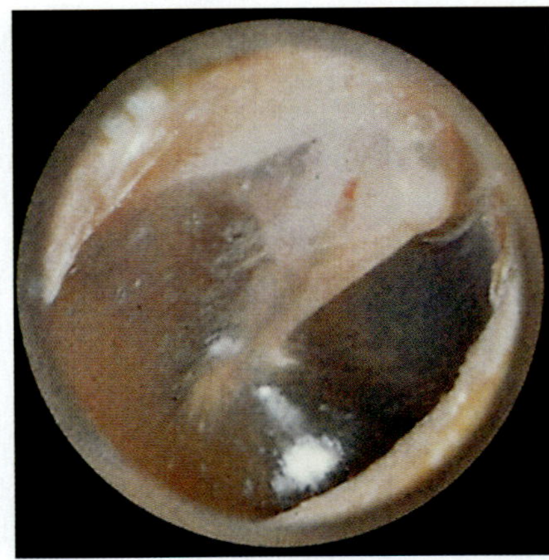

FIG 11-1 Normal tympanic membrane.

ASSESSMENT

1. Identify patient using two identifiers (e.g., name and birthday or name and account number, according to facility policy). Compare identifiers with information on the patient's MAR or medical record. *Rationale: Ensures correct patient. Complies with The Joint Commission standards and improves patient safety (TJC, 2014).*
2. Identify possible causes for ear occlusion (e.g., use of Q-Tips, child playing with small rocks, vegetables, beads).
3. Assess for history of ruptured tympanic membrane, placement of myringotomy tubes, or surgery of auditory canal. *Rationale: These factors contraindicate ear irrigation.*
4. Inspect pinna and external auditory meatus for redness, swelling, drainage, abrasions, and presence of cerumen or foreign objects. Wear clean gloves if drainage is present. *Rationale: Provides baseline information to monitor effects of irrigation.*
   a. Attempt to remove foreign object in ear by straightening ear canal. *Rationale: Straightening of canal may cause object to fall out and negate need for irrigation.*

> **SAFE PATIENT CARE** If vegetable matter (e.g., dried bean or pea) is occluding canal, do not perform irrigation because the object may absorb the solution and swell, causing further damage (NLM, 2013c).

5. Use an otoscope to inspect deeper portions of the auditory canal and tympanic membrane (Fig. 11-1). *Rationale: If the patient's tympanic membrane (eardrum) is not intact, irrigation is contraindicated.*
6. Assess patient's comfort level using a scale of 0 to 10. *Rationale: Provides baseline to evaluate changes in patient's condition. Presence of pain is symptomatic of ear infection or inflammation.*
7. Assess patient's hearing ability in the affected ear. *Rationale: Occlusion of canal by cerumen or foreign object can impair hearing.*
8. Assess patient's knowledge of proper ear care. *Rationale: May indicate need for instruction regarding hygiene.*

PLANNING

Expected Outcomes focus on patient comfort and improved auditory perception.

1. Patient denies increased pain, using a scale of 0 to 10, during instillation.
2. Patient's ear canal is clear of discharge, cerumen, or foreign material after irrigation.
3. Patient demonstrates improved hearing acuity in affected ear after irrigation.
4. Patient describes proper ear care techniques.

Delegation and Collaboration

The skill of irrigating the external ear cannot be delegated to nursing assistive personnel (NAP). The nurse instructs the NAP to:
- Report any ear drainage or patient's report of ear discomfort.
- Help patient ambulate or sit up because some light-headedness might occur, which increases a patient's risk for falling.

Equipment
- Clean gloves
- Otoscope
- Irrigation or bulb syringe
- Basin for irrigating solution (Use sterile basin if sterile irrigating solution is used.)
- Emesis basin for drainage or irrigating solution exiting the ear
- Towel
- Cotton balls or 4 × 4–inch gauze
- Prescribed irrigating solution warmed to body temperature
- Mineral oil or an over-the-counter earwax softener
- MAR or computer printout

STEPS	RATIONALE

1. **See Standard Protocol (inside front cover).**

2. If patient is found to have impacted cerumen, instill 1 to 2 drops of mineral oil or over-the-counter softener into ear twice a day for 2 to 3 days before irrigation.

   Loosens cerumen for easier removal.

3. Check accuracy and completeness of each MAR with health care provider's written medication or procedure order. Check patient's name, drug name and dosage, route of administration, and time for administration. Compare MAR with label of ear irrigation solution.

   The order sheet is the most reliable source and only legal record of drugs or procedure that the patient is to receive. Ensures that patient receives correct medication.

4. Apply clean gloves. Assist patient to a sitting or lying position with head tilted forward and toward the affected ear. Place towel or waterproof pad under patient's head and shoulder. If possible, have patient help hold basin under affected ear.

   Position minimizes leakage of fluids around neck and facial area. Solution flows from ear canal to basin.

5. Pour prescribed irrigating solution into basin. Check the temperature of the solution (37° C [98.6° F]) by pouring a small drop on your inner forearm. Note: If a sterile solution is prescribed, use a sterile basin.

   Warming ear irrigating solutions to body temperature helps to avoid vertigo or nausea.

SAFE PATIENT CARE To prevent trauma to the ear or tympanic membrane during irrigation, instruct patient not to make any sudden moves.

---

6. Apply clean gloves. Gently clean auricle and outer ear canal with moistened gauze or cotton balls. Do not force drainage or cerumen into ear canal.

   Prevents infected material from reentering ear canal.

7. Fill irrigating syringe with approximately 50 mL of solution, and expel air.

   Prevents sudden expulsion of fluid.

8. For adults and children over 3 years-of-age, gently pull pinna up and back. In children 3 years or younger, pinna should be pulled down and back (Hockenberry and Wilson, 2013). Adults can lie supine. Leave space around irrigating tip and the ear canal.

   Pulling pinna straightens external ear canal and prevents obstruction of canal with device, which can lead to increased pressure on tympanic membrane.

9. Slowly instill irrigating solution by holding tip of syringe 1 cm (½ inch) above opening to ear canal. Leave space between tip and canal; do not occlude canal with syringe. Direct the fluid toward the superior aspect of the ear canal. Allow fluid to drain out during instillation into the basis. Continue until canal is cleansed or solution is used (see illustration).

   Prevents occlusion of ear canal with syringe tip. Slow instillation prevents buildup of pressure in ear canal and ensures contact of solution with all canal surfaces.

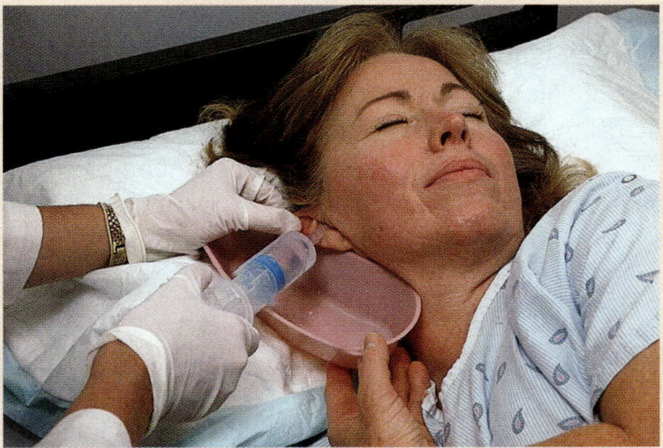

STEP 9 Irrigation of affected ear.

Continued

STEPS	RATIONALE
10. Maintain the flow of irrigation in a steady stream until you see pieces of cerumen flow from the canal.	Constant flow of fluid loosens cerumen.
11. Periodically ask if patient is experiencing pain, nausea, or vertigo.	Symptoms indicate irrigating solution is too hot, too cold, or instilled with too much pressure.
12. Drain excessive fluid from ear by having patient tilt head toward affected side.	Excess fluid may promote microorganism growth.
13. Dry outer ear canal gently with a cotton ball. Leave cotton ball in place for 5 to 10 minutes.	Drying prevents buildup of moisture that can lead to otitis externa.
14. **See Completion Protocol (inside front cover).**	

EVALUATION

1. Ask patient if discomfort is noted during instillation of solution.
2. Ask patient about any sensations of dizziness or feeling light-headed.
3. Reinspect condition of external meatus and ear canal.
4. Evaluate hearing acuity in affected ear after irrigation.
5. Use *Teach Back:* State to the patient, "I want to be sure I explained the purpose of irrigation and proper ear care. Can you explain to me and show me how to irrigate your ear?" Evaluates what the patient is able to explain or demonstrate. Revise your instruction now or develop plan for revised patient teaching to be implemented at an appropriate time if patient is not able to teach back correctly.

Unexpected Outcomes and Related Interventions

1. Patient complains of increased ear pain during irrigation.
   a. Discontinue irrigation and notify health care provider.
2. Foreign body remains in the ear canal.
   a. Repeat irrigation.
   b. Refer patient to an otolaryngologist.
3. Patient's ear canal remains occluded. Patient's hearing acuity has not improved in the affected ear.
   a. Repeat irrigation if prescribed.
   b. If condition persists, notify health care provider.

Recording and Reporting

- Record procedure, noting which ear and record appearance of external ear and patient's hearing acuity after procedure. Record the type and amount of solution, time of administration, and the ear receiving the irrigation on patient's MAR.
- Document your evaluation of patient learning.
- Report adverse effects and patient response to health care provider.

Sample Documentation

1000 Patient reports difficulty hearing in right ear. Cerumen plug noted in canal. Irrigated right ear with 50 mL warm normal saline. Return fluid clear with brown particles. No complaints of pain or discomfort. States that hearing "is fine." Responds appropriately to normal conversation tone. Right ear canal clear. Instructed on ear hygiene.

Special Considerations
Pediatric

- Be certain that child's head is immobilized to prevent puncturing eardrum. Ask parent to help calm child during procedure.

Geriatric

- Older adults often require ongoing ear care for cerumen removal. Use of an oil-based softening agent such as slightly warmed mineral oil twice daily for several days before irrigation is helpful (Touhy and Jett, 2014; NLM, 2013b).
- Older adults with higher risk of cerumen impaction include individuals with large amounts of ear canal hair, individuals with benign growths that narrow the ear canal, and individuals who habitually wear hearing aids (Touhy and Jett, 2014; NLM, 2013b).

Home Care

- Instruct patient to clean ears with a damp washcloth wrapped around a finger. Do not use a cotton-tipped applicator.
- If patient uses a ceruminolytic agent, instruct that these are softening products and that they will not remove the impaction.

SKILL 11.3 CARING FOR A HEARING AID

Hearing is vital for normal communication and orientation to sounds in the environment. Hearing loss affects 360 million people worldwide, and one third of people over 65 years of age have a disabling hearing loss (WHO,

2014). The National Institute on Deafness and Other Communication Disorders also notes that only one of five people who actually need a hearing aid wear one (NIDCD, 2010). People who choose not to wear a hearing aid often dislike the type of sound they hear, or they have trouble keeping the hearing aid functional. Sensorineural hearing loss or nerve deafness is more prevalent in the older-adult population.

Any hearing loss has social implications, with the person often avoiding social activities. There are also many safety considerations. People with hearing loss have difficulty hearing or locating the direction of car horns and emergency sirens. There is a potential for a decline in a patients' health literacy because there is difficulty understanding patient education, and, as a result, patients may not safely manage their symptoms or therapies (Wallhagen, 2010).

For people with hearing loss, a proper hearing aid improves the ability to hear and understand spoken words. Hearing aids do not restore hearing, but rather improve a person's ability to hear because the aid amplifies sound so it is heard at a more effective level (Harkin and Kelleher, 2011). All hearing aids have four basic components:

1. A microphone, which receives and converts sound into electrical signals
2. An amplifier, which increases the strength of the electrical signal
3. A receiver, which converts the strengthened signal back into sound
4. A power source (batteries)

In addition, programmable hearing aids are now available. They are in analog and digital formats. Digital technology uses a tiny processor to convert the sound before it is amplified (Mayo Clinic, 2011). This conversion allows the signal to be analyzed to remove background noise and adjust the volume automatically. Patients seeking these hearing aids need to be evaluated by a licensed audiologist to determine the type of aid and which frequencies are needed for the individual patient. These hearing aids are adjusted to accommodate the range of the patient's residual hearing. Programmable aids independently amplify high-frequency (soft-spoken consonants) from low-frequency (loudly spoken vowels) sounds; this process occurs rapidly and continuously (Harkin and Kelleher, 2011). Several styles of hearing aids are available to patients (Table 11-1).

ASSESSMENT

1. Determine whether patient can hear clearly with use of hearing aid by talking slowly and clearly in normal tone of voice. *Rationale: Inability to hear may indicate faulty function of hearing aid or that aid is no longer effective for patient's auditory loss.*
2. If patient wears a hearing aid, determine if he or she is able to manipulate the hearing aid and batteries. Watch patient insert aid independently. *Rationale: Determines level of assistance required.*
3. Assess if hearing aid is working by removing from patient's ear. Close battery case and turn volume slowly to high. Cup hand over hearing aid. If you hear a squealing sound (feedback), it is working. If no sound is heard, replace batteries and test again. *Rationale: May indicate malfunctioning of hearing aid.*
4. Assess patient for any unusual physical or auditory signs and symptoms (pain, itching, redness, discharge, odor, tinnitus, decreased hearing acuity) (see Chapter 7). *Rationale: May indicate injury, infection, or cerumen accumulation.*
5. Inspect ear mold for cracked or rough edges. *Rationale: Poorly fitting hearing aids cause irritation or discomfort to external ear canal.*
6. Inspect for accumulation of cerumen around hearing aid and plugging of opening in aid. *Rationale: Cerumen can block sound reception (NLM, 2013b).*
7. Assess patient's knowledge of and routines for cleaning and caring for hearing aid. *Rationale: Determines compliance with and knowledge of self-care.*

PLANNING

Expected Outcomes focus on facilitating communication and promoting comfort and appropriate self-care.
1. Patient hears conversation spoken in normal tone of voice and responds appropriately.
2. Patient responds appropriately to environmental sounds.
3. Patient demonstrates proper care of hearing aid.
4. Patient verbalizes that hearing aid fits comfortably.

Delegation and Collaboration

The skill of caring for a hearing aid can be delegated to nursing assistive personnel (NAP). The nurse instructs the NAP about:

- Using patient preferences when cleaning aid.
- Communication tips to use for individual patient while aid is being cleaned.
- Reporting signs and symptoms of hearing loss, pain, excessive itching, ear odor, or presence of ear drainage.

Equipment
- Soft towel and washcloth
- Warm soap and water
- Brush or wax loop
- Storage case
- Clean gloves (if drainage is present)
- Spare battery (optional) or stationary charger for specific device if available
- Facial tissue

TYPE	ADVANTAGES	DISADVANTAGES	CAUTIONS
In-the-ear (ITE) hearing aids fit completely in the outer ear and are used for mild-to-severe hearing loss (illustration *A*).	Design of the aid can improve sound transmission through telephone calls.	Damaged by earwax and ear drainage, and small size can cause adjustment problems and feedback.	They are not usually worn by children because the casings need to be replaced as the ear grows.

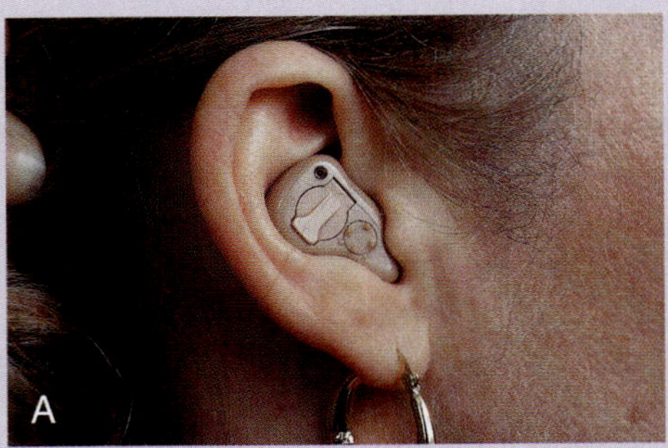

A, In-the-ear hearing aid.

Behind-the-ear (BTE) hearing aids are worn behind the ear and are connected to a plastic ear mold that fits inside the outer ear (illustration *B*).	Sound travels through the ear mold into the ear. People of all ages wear BTE aids for mild to profound hearing loss.	Poorly fitting BTE ear molds can cause feedback, a whistling sound caused by the fit of the hearing aid.	May not be appropriate for children or adults who are active in sports because of the potential for damage of the device.

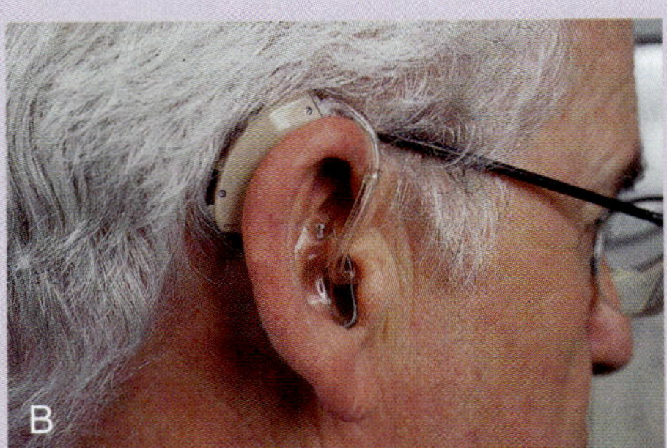

B, Behind-the-ear hearing aid.

Completely in canal (CIC) hearing aids are customized to fit the size and shape of the ear canal (illustration *C*).	Used for mild to moderately severe hearing loss and are largely concealed in the ear canal.	Because of their small size, CIC aids may be difficult for the user to adjust and remove and may not be able to hold additional devices, such as a telecoil.	Expensive and not recommended for children. CIC aids can also be damaged by earwax and ear drainage.

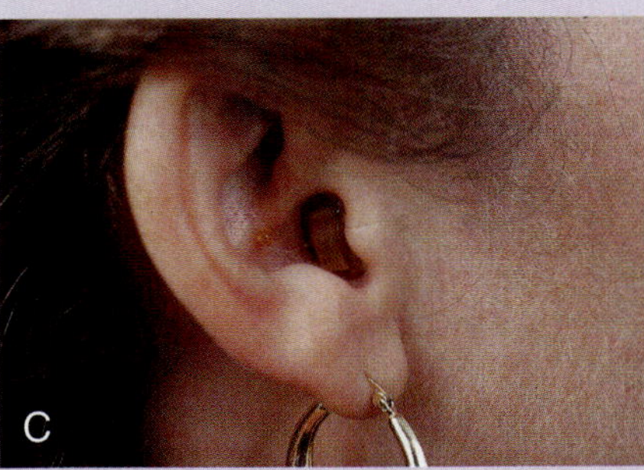

C, Completely-in-canal hearing aid.

Digital hearing aids (illustration *D*).	Analyzes sounds to remove background noise. Programs for low-frequency and high-frequency sounds.	Need to be programmed and adjusted by a licensed audiologist.	Digital aids can be damaged by earwax and ear drainage.

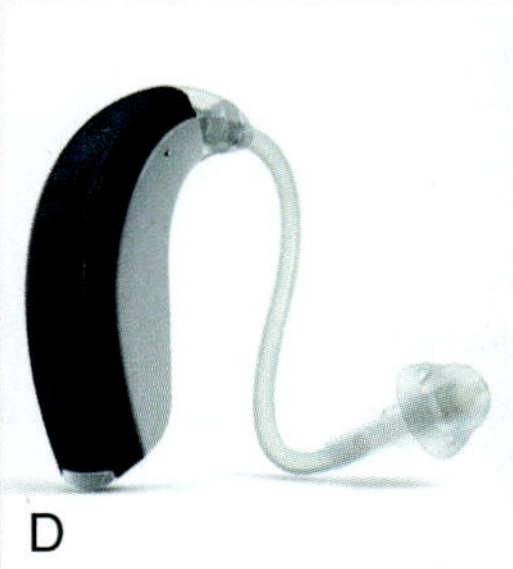

D, Digital hearing aid.

STEPS	RATIONALE

1. **See Standard Protocol (inside front cover).**
2. *Removing and cleaning hearing aid:*

   a. Apply clean gloves if drainage is present. — Reduces transmission of microorganisms.

   b. Have patient turn hearing aid volume off (or assist as needed). Usually you rotate the volume control toward the nose to increase volume and away from the nose to lower volume. Grasp aid securely and gently remove device following natural ear contour. Note: Some in-the-ear (ITE) and completely in canal (CIC) devices do not have a volume control but are turned off by opening the battery door. CIC devices have a clear plastic handle for removal. Grasp handle and gently pull straight out. — Prevents feedback (whistling) during removal, dropping hearing aid, or injury to ear.

   c. Hold hearing aid over towel and wipe exterior with tissue to remove cerumen. — Prevents breakage if dropped. Impaction of cerumen blocks normal sound transmission.

   d. Inspect all openings in aid for accumulated cerumen. Carefully remove cerumen with wax loop or brush (supplied with aid) to clean holes in hearing aid. — Cerumen may block sound from receiver. It may also block pressure equalization channel and create feeling of ear pressure.

   e. Inspect ear mold for rough edges.

   f. Open battery door, remove battery, place it in labeled storage container, and allow it to air dry. — Increases battery life and allows moisture to evaporate.

   g. Wash ear canal with washcloth moistened in soap and water. Rinse and dry. — Removes cerumen from ear canal. Removes soap residue and water that may harbor microbes or damage hearing aid.

   h. If you will be storing the hearing aid, place it in a dry storage case. Most come with a desiccant material for drying. Label case with patient's name and room number. If more than one aid, note right or left. — Protects hearing aid against damage, moisture, and breakage.

3. *Inserting hearing aid:*

   a. Perform hand hygiene and apply clean gloves if drainage is present. — Reduces transmission of microorganisms.

   b. Remove hearing aid from storage case and check battery (see Assessment). Make sure hearing aid volume off. — Turning volume off prevents feedback (whistling) during insertion.

   c. Identify hearing aid as either right (marked "R" or red color coded) or left (marked "L" or blue color coded). — Proper orientation prevents damage and injury.

   d. Allow patient to reinsert aid, if possible. Otherwise, hold hearing aid with thumb and index finger of dominant hand so that canal—long portion with hole(s)—is at the bottom. Insert pointed end of ear mold into ear canal. Follow natural ear contours to guide aid into place. — Proper orientation is important for hearing aid insertion. Ensures correct positioning of aid within ear canal.

   e. Adjust or have patient adjust volume gradually to comfortable level for talking to patient in regular voice 3 to 4 feet away. Rotate volume control toward nose to increase volume and away from nose to decrease volume.

SAFE PATIENT CARE Programmable hearing aids have the volume control located on the remote. Be sure patient knows the importance of ensuring that the volume is on the off position when the aid is not in use. For most patients, hearing aids work best at lower volume settings.

---

4. **See Completion Protocol (inside front cover).**

EVALUATION

1. Ask patient to rate comfort level after removal or insertion.
2. Use **Teach Back:** State to the patient, "I want to be sure I explained how to remove and insert your hearing aid. Can you show me how you would remove and then insert your hearing aid?" Evaluates what the patient is able to explain or demonstrate. Revise your instruction now or develop plan for revised patient teaching to be implemented at an appropriate time if patient is not able to teach back correctly.

Unexpected Outcomes and Related Interventions

1. Patient is unable to hear conversations or environmental sounds clearly. Patient's verbal responses are inappropriate.
   a. Remove hearing aid and check battery for power and correct placement.
   b. Inspect ear mold and ear canal for cerumen blockage.
   c. Change volume setting as needed.
   d. If problems persist, contact audiologist or hearing aid specialist.
2. Patient is unable to perform care of hearing aid.
   a. Demonstrate correct aid care and offer return demonstration.
   b. Include family caregiver who will be available to patient.
3. Patient complains of ear discomfort and may complain of whistling sound.
   a. Remove aid and reinsert.
   b. Assess external ear for signs of inflammation.
   c. If problems persist, contact audiologist or hearing aid specialist.

Recording and Reporting

- Record that hearing aid is removed and stored if patient is going for surgery or special procedure. Be sure to document where or with whom aid is stored. Record patient's preferred communication techniques.
- Document your evaluation of patient learning.
- Record and report any signs or symptoms of infection or injury or sudden decrease in hearing acuity to health care provider.
- Report to nursing staff and document on plan-of-care tips that promote communication with patient.

Sample Documentation

1000   Patient responds inappropriately to questions. Unable to hear normal conversation tone. States he hears "an echo." Volume turned down on the ITE aid in right ear. Daughter states that patient frequently turns the volume up so he can "hear better." Reviewed proper volume settings and improved listening techniques with patient and daughter.

Special Considerations
Pediatric

- As children grow older, they can become self-conscious of a hearing aid. Changes in hairstyle may help some children overcome self-consciousness (Hockenberry and Wilson, 2013).
- Store batteries away from children's reach. Batteries are toxic when swallowed.

Geriatric

- The small size of some hearing aids may make it difficult for older adults to handle and manipulate the devices. Patients should contact their hearing aid specialist for assistance. Family members may be able to assist with care of device.
- High-pitched signals associated with consonants *f, p, t, k, ch, sh,* and *st* are more difficult to hear clearly as people age (Touhy and Jett, 2014).
- Inappropriate responses to questions or situations, irritation when spoken to, asking to have a statement repeated, inattentiveness, or difficulty following instructions should alert you or family members that the patient may have some hearing loss that needs to be evaluated. People incorrectly may assume that the patient is confused (Touhy and Jett, 2014).
- Be alert for patient assessment findings that may indicate depression. Hearing loss and depression are common, and correction of hearing loss may resolve depression in some patients (Wallhagen, 2010).

Home Care

- Initial use of hearing aid should be restricted to quiet situations in the home. Patients need to adjust gradually to voices and household sounds (Touhy and Jett, 2014).
- Avoid exposure of hearing aid to extreme heat, cold, or moisture. Do not leave in case near stove, heater, or sunny window. Do not use with hair dryer on hot settings or with sunlamp. Do not wear when bathing, during excess sweating, or when shampooing at a hair stylist.
- Do not use hairspray or other hair care products while wearing hearing aids.
- Store batteries in a dry safe place away from pets and children. Always keep a set of unused batteries in the home.
- Be sure the person cleans the ears daily. Likewise, a hearing aid should be cleaned daily.

CRITICAL THINKING EXERCISES

Case Study

An older adult patient has worn bilateral in-the-ear hearing aids for the last 10 years. He knows how to care for his aids. He notes that when the aids are working well, he hears his family and co-workers clearly, has minimal distortion in large gatherings, and is able to distinguish emergency sirens and car horns when he is driving.

1. He now complains of diminished hearing in the left ear and senses drainage from the ear. The nurse decides to check the functioning of the hearing aid. Place the following steps in appropriate order for cleaning the hearing aid.
   a. Wash ear canal.
   b. Place hearing aid in storage case.
   c. Apply clean gloves.
   d. Grasp aid securely and remove from ear following natural ear contour.
   e. Use brush to clean holes in the aid.
   f. Have patient turn hearing aid volume off.
      1. f, d, c, a, b, e
      2. c, f, d, e, a, b
      3. c, f, d, a, e, b
      4. f, d, c, e, a, b

2. The patient's preschool-age grandchildren visit frequently and are curious about the hearing aids. What preschool safety concerns should the nurse teach? Select all that apply.
   1. Batteries are toxic if swallowed.
   2. Tell the children to face grandpa when speaking.
   3. Keep batteries and aids out of children's reach.
   4. Show the children how the aid fits in the ear.

Review Questions

1. The nurse should question an order for an ear irrigation if the patient has which of the following conditions?
   1. Foreign body such as a pea
   2. Migraine headaches
   3. Cerumen accumulation
   4. Hearing impairment

2. How should the nurse position a 26-month-old child's ear during irrigation?
   1. Without pulling on the pinna
   2. While pulling the pinna down and back
   3. While pulling the tragus down and back
   4. While pulling the auricle up and back

3. Which statement best explains nursing actions during an irrigation of the left ear?
   1. Lean the patient's head toward right side.
   2. Hold the irrigation syringe approximately 1 cm (½ inch) above opening to ear canal.
   3. Delegate the procedure to NAP.
   4. Place the patient in supine position with head elevated.

4. A patient is being discharged after care for severe conjunctivitis related to noncompliance with the prescribed lens care regimen. Which patient statement indicates a need for further teaching?
   1. "I should discard my open lens care solutions when I get home."
   2. "Cloudy solutions should be discarded even if they haven't expired."
   3. "Plain soap is the best thing for washing my hands before I touch my contacts."
   4. "I'm switching to disposable contacts so I won't have to worry about getting another infection."

5. A patient calls the nurse at the health care provider's office about increasing pain in her left ear. What should be the nurse's initial response?
   1. "Clean your ears daily with soap and water."
   2. "Try to get as much earwax out of your ear as possible."
   3. "Put a drop or two of mineral oil in your left ear."
   4. "Tell me more about the ear pain you're having."

6. A young man enters the emergency department with a chemical burn from household bleach. His wife ran tap water over his eyes before bringing him to the emergency department. Which represents the nurse's immediate actions in this situation?
   a. Assess the injured eye.
   b. Determine the patient's level of pain.
   c. Prepare to initiate eye irrigation.
   d. Teach eye safety.
   e. Wait for the health care provider because the patient irrigated the eye at home.
      1. a, b, c
      2. a, b, e
      3. a, c, d
      4. b, c, d
      5. b, d, e

7. Routine eye care for a comatose patient facilitates which of the following?
   1. Blinking
   2. Visual acuity
   3. Lubrication
   4. Scleral integrity

8. The NAP informs the nurse that while providing eye care to a comatose patient, she observed yellowish drainage. What is the nurse's immediate reaction?
   1. Instruct her to continue eye care.
   2. Explain that the environmental contact with eye secretions causes yellow drainage.
   3. Contact the health care provider.
   4. Completely assess the patient's eyes.

9. A patient with bilateral hearing aids is experiencing some discomfort in his right ear. What should the nurse initially do for this patient?
  1. Make sure the patient understands how to care for his hearing aids.
  2. Check the patient's ears for any signs of irritation.
  3. Teach the patient how to reposition his hearing aids if they are uncomfortable.
  4. Reduce the volume of the hearing aid in his left ear.

10. A patient who wears contact lenses for 20/150 vision in each eye is scheduled for hand surgery and will have her hand in a cast for 6 weeks. What is the priority nursing diagnosis for this patient?
  1. Anxiety
  2. Self-care deficit
  3. Imbalanced nutrition: less than body requirements
  4. Disturbed sensory perception

REFERENCES

Centers for Disease Control and Prevention (CDC): *Health literacy: accurate, accessible, and actionable health information for all*, Atlanta, GA, 2014, Centers for Disease Control and Prevention. www.cdc.gov/healthliteracy. Accessed January 30, 2014.

Chau JP, Lee DT, Lo SH: A systematic review of methods of eye irrigation for adults and children with ocular chemical burns, *Worldviews Evid Based Nurs* 9(3):129, 2012.

Douglas L, Berry S: Developing clinical guidelines in eye care for intensive care units, *Nurs Child Young People* 23(5):14, 2011.

Gopinath B, et al: Dual sensory impairment in older adults increases the risk of mortality: A population based study, *PLoS ONE* 8(3):e55054, 2013.

Hardin SR: Hearing loss in older critical care patients: participation in decision making, *Crit Care Nurse* 32(6):43, 2012.

Harkin H, Kelleher C: Caring for older adults with hearing loss, *Nurs Older People* 23(9):22, 2011.

Hockenberry MJ, Wilson D: *Wong's essentials of pediatric nursing*, ed 9, St Louis, 2013, Mosby.

Kergoat H, Chriqui E: Vision and eye care in the nursing home setting, *Canadian Nursing Home* 22(2):9, 2011.

Kocaçal Güler EK, et al: Effectiveness of polyethylene covers versus carbomer drops (Vicotears) to prevent dry eye syndrome in the critically ill, *J Clin Nurs* 20(13–14):1916, 2011.

Mayo Clinic: *Hearing aids: how to choose the right one*, 2011. www.mayoclinic.com/health/hearing-aids/HQ00812. Accessed February 1, 2014.

National Institute on Deafness and Other Communication Disorders (NIDCD): *Quick statistics*, 2010. http://www.nidcd.nih.gov/health/statistics/quick.htm. Accessed February 1, 2014.

National Library of Medicine (NLM): *Medline Plus: eye emergencies*, 2013a. http://www.nlm.nih.gov/medlineplus/ency/article/000054.htm. Accessed February 1, 2014.

National Library of Medicine (NLM): *Medline Plus: ear wax*, 2013b. http://www.nlm.nih.gov/medlineplus/ency/article/000979.htm. Accessed February 1, 2014.

National Library of Medicine (NLM): *Medline Plus: ear emergencies*, 2013c. http://www.nlm.nih.gov/medlineplus/ency/article/000052.htm. Accessed February 1, 2014.

Roets-Merken LM, et al: Screening for hearing, visual and dual sensory impairment in older adults using behavioural cues: a validation study, *Int J Nurs Stud* 51, 2014.

The Joint Commission (TJC): *National Patient Safety Goals*, Oakbrook Terrace, IL, 2014, The Commission. Available at: http://www.jointcommission.org/standards_information/npsgs.aspx.

Touhy TT, Jett T: *Ebersole and Hess's gerontological nursing and healthy aging*, ed 5, St Louis, 2014, Mosby.

Wallhagen MI: The stigma of hearing loss, *Gerontologist* 50(1):66, 2010.

Werli-Alvarenga A, et al: Nursing interventions for adult intensive care patients with risk for corneal injury: a systematic review, *Int J Nurs Knowl* 24(1):25, 2013.

World Health Organization (WHO): *Deafness and hearing loss*, 2014, WHO. http://www.who.int/mediacentre/factsheets/fs300/en/.

Zerwekh J, Garneau A: *Nursing today: transitions and trends*, ed 8, St Louis, 2015, Elsevier.

Promoting Nutrition

 **EVOLVE WEBSITE/EVOLVE RESOURCES LIST**

http://evolve.elsevier.com/Perry/nursinginterventions
Audio Glossary • Checklists • Review Questions

Nutrition is a basic component of health. It affects patients' recovery from short-term and chronic illness, surgery, and injury. Your role is to assess patients' risks for nutritional problems, assist patients with oral feeding when needed, and administer enteral nutritional therapies while protecting patients from the risk of aspiration. Routine identification of malnutrition with screening of patients in health care settings is a requirement of The Joint Commission (2014a). Nutritional screening involves identifying patient characteristics associated with nutritional problems and risk factors for malnutrition (Hammond and Litchford, 2012). You conduct an initial nutritional screening with every patient, including a history and physical examination (Table 12-1). Findings determine if there is a need for consultation with a registered dietitian (RD). Box 12-1 provides a list of risk factors for nutritional problems. No single objective measure alone is an effective predictor for nutritional risk. Work closely with RDs to discuss a patient's situation such as resources for buying food and availability of family assistance to devise an appropriate nutritional plan.

PATIENT-CENTERED CARE

Multiple factors affect a patient's nutritional needs. Using a patient-centered approach to care ensures a relevant and

appropriate nutritional plan for your patients. In addition to a thorough screening of a patient's physical status, ability to take in nutrients, and nutritional knowledge level (see Skill 12.1), your assessment should include a patient's eating patterns and food choices. Ethnicity, culture, income, and religious practices all influence what a person eats and the manner in which he or she plans meals and eats socially. Cultural awareness helps you to include patients' preferences in their diet (Box 12-2). Foods are often associated with caring and love, health promotion, maintenance, and restoration. Food preferences are a major factor in patient adherence to modification of safe oral intake. A patient must be part of the decision-making process when dietary modifications are required.

SAFETY

Difficulty swallowing, or dysphagia, involves losing control over the ability to chew, move food into a bolus at the back of the mouth, and swallow. Dysphagia is a symptom or complication of numerous conditions, including stroke, advanced dementia, cerebral palsy, multiple sclerosis, Parkinson's disease, and oral cancer. Physical impairment of muscles and nerves within the mouth and cognitive conditions that affect concentration and selective attention alter

TABLE 12-1	PHYSICAL SIGNS OF NUTRITIONAL STATUS	
BODY AREA	**NORMAL APPEARANCE**	**INDICATORS OF MALNUTRITION**
General appearance	Alert, responsive	Listless, apathetic, cachectic
Weight	Normal for height, age, body build	Overweight, obese, or underweight (special concern for underweight); weight trend, including weight loss over a period of time
Posture	Erect; arms and legs straight	Sagging shoulders, sunken chest, humped back
Muscles	Well-developed, firm, good tone; some fat under skin	Flaccid, poor tone; undeveloped, tender, "wasted" appearance; impaired ability to walk
Nervous conduction and mental status	Good attention span, not irritable or restless, normal reflexes, psychological stability	Inattentive, irritable, confused, burning and tingling of hands and feet (paresthesia), loss of position and vibratory sense, weakness and tenderness of muscles (may result in inability to walk), decrease or loss of ankle and knee reflexes
Gastrointestinal function	Good appetite and digestion, normal regular elimination, no palpable (perceptible to touch) organs or masses	Anorexia, indigestion, constipation or diarrhea, liver or spleen enlargement; distention, firmness, audible air with percussion
Cardiovascular function	Normal heart rate and rhythm, no murmurs, normal blood pressure for age	Rapid heart rate (>100 beats/min), enlarged heart, abnormal rhythm, elevated blood pressure
General vitality	Endurance, energetic, sleeps well, vigorous	Easily fatigued, no energy, falls asleep easily, looks tired, apathetic
Hair	Shiny, lustrous, firm, not easily plucked; healthy scalp	Stringy, dull, brittle, dry, thin and sparse, depigmented; easily plucked
Skin (general)	Smooth, slightly moist, good color	Rough, dry, scaly, pale, pigmented, irritated, bruises, petechiae
Face and neck	Skin color uniform; smooth, healthy appearance; not swollen	Greasy, discolored, scaly, swollen, skin dark over cheeks and under eyes, lumpiness or flakiness of skin around nose and mouth
Lips	Smooth, good color, moist, not chapped or swollen	Dry, scaly, swollen, redness and swelling (cheilosis); angular lesions at corners of the mouth or fissures or scars (stomatitis)
Gums	Good pink color, healthy, red, no swelling or bleeding	Spongy, bleed easily, marginal redness, inflamed, receding
Tongue	Good pink color or deep reddish in appearance, not swollen or smooth, surface papillae present, no lesions	Swelling, scarlet and raw, magenta color, beefy (glossitis), hyperemic and hypertrophic or atrophic papillae
Teeth	No pain, no sensitivity	Missing teeth, broken teeth
Eyes	Bright, clear, shiny; no sores at corner of eyelids, membranes moist and healthy pink color, no prominent blood vessels, no fatigue circles beneath	Eye membranes pale (pale conjunctivae), redness of membranes (conjunctival infection), dryness or infection, redness and fissuring of eyelid corners (angular palpebritis), Bitot's spots, dryness of eye membrane (conjunctival xerosis), dull appearance of cornea (corneal xerosis), soft cornea (keratomalacia)
Neck (glands)	No enlargement	Thyroid or lymph nodes enlarged
Nails	Firm, pink	Spoon-shaped (koilonychia), brittle, ridged
Legs and feet	No tenderness, weakness, or swelling; good color	Edema, tender calf, tingling, weakness, lesions
Skeleton	No malformation	Bowlegs, knock-knees, chest deformity at diaphragm, beaded ribs, prominent scapulae

Adapted from Mahan LK et al, editors: *Krause's food nutrition and the nutrient care process,* ed 13, Philadelphia, 2012, Saunders.

BOX 12-1	RISK FACTORS FOR POTENTIAL NUTRITIONAL PROBLEMS

- Clear-liquid or full-liquid diets for >3 days without nutrient supplementation or inappropriate or insufficient nutrient supplementation
- Intravenous feeding (dextrose or saline) or nothing by mouth (NPO) for >3 days without supplementation
- Low intake of prescribed diet or tube feeding
- Weight 20% above or 10% below desirable body weight (accounting for edema)
- Pregnancy weight gain deviating from normal patterns
- Diagnoses that increase nutritional needs or decrease nutrient intake or both: alcoholism, burns, cancer, dementia, diarrhea, hemorrhage, hyperthyroidism, infected or draining wounds, systemic infection, malabsorption, major trauma, postoperative status
- Chronic use of drugs, especially alcohol, which affects nutritional intake
- Alterations in chewing, swallowing, appetite, taste, and smell
- Body temperature consistently >37° C (98.6° F) for >2 days
- Hematocrit <43% in men, <37% in women; hemoglobin <14 g/dL in men, <12 g/dL in women
- Absolute decrease in lymphocyte count (<1500 cells/mm^3)
- Elevated (>250 mg/dL) or decreased (<130 mg/dL) total plasma cholesterol
- Serum albumin <3 g/dL in patients without renal or liver disease, generalized dermatitis, overhydration
- Older adult living in long-term care facility

Adapted from Grodner M et al: *Nutritional foundations and clinical applications of nutrition: a nursing approach,* ed 5, St Louis, 2013, Mosby.

BOX 12-2	CULTURAL CONSIDERATIONS TO ENHANCE PATIENT NUTRITION

Cultural sensitivity is the ability to interact effectively with people of different cultural, religious, and ethnic backgrounds. Food is essential to one's identity, and dietary descriptions must be as objective as possible to prevent criticism of the culture (Kitler et al., 2012). As a nurse, you should seek out the opportunity to assess patients' preferences for nutrition while they are under your care.

Assess religious and cultural influences on nutritional practices.

- Many Orthodox Jews adhere to kosher food preparation methods and are prohibited from eating pork, predatory fowl, shellfish (i.e., crab, shrimp), blood, and meat dishes mixed with milk or dairy products. No cooking is done on the Sabbath (sundown Friday through sundown Saturday).
- Buddhists and Hindus are generally vegetarians because of their respect for life and belief in transmigration of the soul.
- Vegetarians and vegans prefer meat substitutes.

Collect information on the types of foods that are generally eaten for different conditions.

- Some cultures believe in the hot-and-cold theory of health and illness. Foods are classified as cold or hot based on their characteristics, independent of the temperature at which they are served.
- There is no universal agreement across cultures about which foods are hot and which foods are cold.
- Some African-Americans believe that certain foods build blood, preventing anemia.

Understand food practices, and collaborate to develop healthy alternatives. Use cultural food guides developed for specific populations.

- Assess which ingredient or food content you need to reduce.
- Patients from cultures that use soy sauce as a primary ingredient may need to use a low-sodium version if they are on a low-sodium diet.

---

swallowing. A person with dysphagia is at risk for aspiration, the inhalation of food particles and saliva into the lower respiratory tract. When bacteria growing in oral secretions reach the lung, pneumonia develops. Dysphagia leads to disability, decreased functional status, increased length of stay and cost of care, increased likelihood of discharge to institutionalized care, and increased mortality (Tanner, 2010). As a nurse, assess if your patients are at risk for dysphagia. If dysphagia is present, nursing strategies that include safe feeding techniques and following aspiration precautions can be used (see Skill 12.2).

When educating patients and families, food safety and preparation are important topics. Food safety is a public health issue. Germs enter food from improper cleansing or preparation or poor handwashing practices. Persons most at risk for developing foodborne illnesses are older adults, infants and very young children, and individuals with lowered resistance to infection. The food safety tips in Box 12-3 help prevent foodborne infections such as *Escherichia coli, Listeria monocytogenes,* and *Salmonella.*

EVIDENCE-BASED PRACTICE

Choban P et al: A.S.P.E.N. clinical guidelines: nutrition support of hospitalized adult patients with obesity, *JPEN J Parenter Enteral Nutr* 37(6):714, 2013.

As nurses care for more patients with obesity, we must understand the implications for safe nutritional support. A group of health care professionals performed an extensive review of the literature to provide clinical guidelines for the management of nutrition in bariatric hospitalized patients. Strong recommendations were made for patients with bariatric considerations (Choban et al., 2013).

- Critically ill patients with obesity experience more complications than patients with optimal body mass index.
- Nutritional support assessment and development of a nutritional support plan are recommended within 48 hours of intensive care unit admission.

BOX 12-3 FOOD SAFETY TIPS

- Wash hands, food-preparation surfaces, and utensils with warm soapy water before touching food.
- Cook meat, poultry, fish, and eggs until well done (180° F).
- Wash all fresh fruits and vegetables thoroughly.
- Do not eat raw meats or drink unpasteurized milk or juices.
- Do not use food past the expiration date on a package.
- Keep foods properly refrigerated.
- Refrigerate foods at 40° F within 2 hours of cooking.
- Thaw frozen foods in the refrigerator.
- Discard food that you suspect is spoiled.
- Do not use wooden cutting boards. Instead use plastic laminate or solid surface cutting boards that can be disinfected.
- Wash dishcloths, towels, and sponges regularly or run in a dishwasher cycle, or use paper towels.
- Clean the inside of the refrigerator and microwave regularly with bleach or soap.

Modified from Nix S: *Williams' basic nutrition and diet therapy,* ed 14, St Louis, 2013, Mosby.

- All hospitalized patients, regardless of body mass index, should be screened for nutritional risk within 48 hours of admission, using nutritional assessment for patients who are considered at risk.
- In critically ill obese patients, energy requirements should be based on predictive equations, such as equations developed by Penn State University or Mifflin-St. Joer.
- Collaboration between staff from nursing, medicine, dietetics, and pharmacy is necessary to provide optimal caloric intake for obese patients in the hospital setting.

SKILL 12.1 FEEDING DEPENDENT PATIENTS

• Nursing Skills Online: Safety, Lesson 4

Patients with severe illness, debility, and fatigue may be unable to feed themselves adequately and require assistance with feeding. Some patients have trouble chewing or swallowing, poor vision, or difficulty holding eating utensils. As a nurse, you are responsible for preparing patients and offering the type of assistance needed to help them successfully eat an adequate amount of food at a comfortable pace. Patients should be involved in selecting food preferences that fit dietary guidelines, choosing where to eat (bed or chair), and selecting the time to eat. It can be difficult to provide meals at times other than when meal trays are delivered in health care facilities. If patients are not hungry at that time, ensuring sufficient food intake is difficult. Use dietary resources in the facility to provide nutritional snacks between meals. Use common sense when feeding adults, and provide a socially meaningful mealtime experience. It is important to encourage independence when possible with the use of adaptive devices or finger foods and with comfortable and safe positioning for swallowing.

Patients frequently receive therapeutic diets, which require a health care provider's order. A therapeutic diet treats many disease states, complementing and at times replacing drug therapy. Therapeutic diets are available in modified consistencies or texture. For example, patients initially may require a liquid diet for 1 to 2 days after surgery. A mechanical soft diet is used for patients without teeth. When there are no restrictions, the order may be diet as tolerated or regular diet. Table 12-2 summarizes therapeutic diets. For specific information about special diets, see the facility dietary manual or contact an RD.

ASSESSMENT

1. Conduct a diet history, review current medications, previous surgeries, food allergies, coexisting medical conditions compromising nutrition, and recent dietary intake. *Rationale: Provides a baseline to determine appropriate therapeutic diet, food options, and educational needs of patient.*
2. Assess if patient is without nausea. Ask patient about bowel patterns and passing flatus. Auscultate bowel sounds. *Rationale: Determines baseline assessment of gastrointestinal (GI) functioning.*
3. On initial assessment and routinely as ordered, measure patient's weight and assess pertinent laboratory values (e.g., albumin, prealbumin, and transferrin; complete blood count). *Rationale: Provides baseline of nutritional status.*
4. Assess food tolerance, cultural and religious preferences, and food likes and dislikes. *Rationale: Determines type of foods that can potentially improve oral intake and the desire to feed independently.*
5. Review diet orders by health care provider. *Rationale: Ensures that patient receives proper diet. Patients with chronic diseases may need alterations in nutrient content or flavoring.*
6. Place a tongue blade on the back of the patient's tongue to elicit the gag reflex. This may be done on initial assessment. *Rationale: Patients who do not gag are at risk for aspiration (see Skill 12.2).*
7. Place fingers on neck at level of larynx, ask patient to swallow saliva, and feel for laryngeal movement.

TABLE 12-2 THERAPEUTIC DIETS

DIET	DESCRIPTION
Clear-liquid	Foods that are clear and liquid at room or body temperature (e.g., chicken broth, tea, soda, gelatin, and apple or cranberry juice) and that leave little residue and are easily absorbed; commonly ordered for short-term use (24 to 48 hours) after surgery, before diagnostic tests, and after episodes of vomiting or diarrhea
Full-liquid	Includes foods on clear-liquid diet plus addition of smooth-textured dairy products (e.g., milk and ice cream), strained soups and custard, refined cooked cereals, vegetable juice, and pureed vegetables; commonly ordered before or after surgery for patients who are acutely ill from infection or for patients who cannot chew or tolerate solid foods; must verify that patients are lactose tolerant before providing dairy products
Pureed	Includes food on clear-liquid and full-liquid diets plus easily swallowed foods that do not require chewing (e.g., scrambled eggs; pureed meats, vegetables, and fruits; mashed potatoes); ordered for patients with head and neck abnormalities or who have had oral surgery; can be modified for low sodium, fat, or calorie count
Mechanical or dental-soft	Includes foods on all previous diets plus addition of lightly seasoned ground or finely diced meats, flaked fish, cottage cheese, cheese, rice, potatoes, pancakes, light breads, cooked vegetables, cooked or canned fruit, bananas, and peanut butter; avoids tough meats, nuts, bacon, and fruits with tough skins or membranes; ordered for patients who have chewing problems or mild GI problems; used as transition diet from liquids to regular
Soft/low-residue	Addition of low-fiber, easily digested foods such as pastas, casseroles, moist tender meats, and canned cooked fruits and vegetables; includes foods that are easy to chew and simply cooked; does not permit fatty, rich, and fried foods; is sometimes referred to as low-fiber diet
High-fiber	Addition of fresh uncooked fruits, steamed vegetables, bran, oatmeal, and dried fruits; includes sufficient amounts of indigestible carbohydrate to relieve constipation, increase GI motility, and increase stool weight
Regular or diet as tolerated	No restrictions; permits patients' preferences and allows for postoperative diet progression
Sample Therapeutic Diets Restricted fluids	Required in severe heart failure and kidney failure
Sodium-restricted	Allows low levels of sodium and may include a 4-g (no added salt), 2-g (moderate), 1-g (strict), or 500-mg (very strict) diet; may be ordered for patients with heart failure, renal failure, cirrhosis, or hypertension
Fat-modified	Low total and saturated fat and low cholesterol; cholesterol intake limited to <300 mg daily and fat intake to 30% to 35%; eliminates or reduces fatty foods for hypercholesterolemia, malabsorptive disorders, and diarrhea
Diabetic	Essential treatment for patients with diabetes mellitus; provides patients with a diet recommended by American Diabetes Association, which allows for patients to select set amount of food from basic food groups. Meal planning tools include carbohydrate counting, the plate method, and glycemic index. It is important that food intake is balanced with patient's exercise and medications for safe management of patient's blood glucose levels

Modified from Grodner M et al: *Nutritional foundations and clinical applications of nutrition: a nursing approach,* ed 5, St Louis, 2013, Mosby.

Rationale: Movement of larynx normally occurs during swallowing.

8. Assess physical motor skills (ability to grasp utensil, hold cup, and move utensil to mouth), level of consciousness or ability to attend to feeding, and visual acuity. *Rationale: Determines appropriate positioning for meals and level of assistance required.*

9. Assess patient's energy level (ability to sit up). *Rationale: Patients eat better when well rested.*

10. Assess need for toileting, handwashing, and oral care (including dentures) before feeding. *Rationale: Reduces interruptions and improves patient's appetite during the meal.*

PLANNING

Expected Outcomes focus on increased independence with eating, improved nutritional intake, and safe intake of food.

1. Patient's body weight remains stable or trends toward the desired level.

2. Patient's nutrition-related laboratory values are within expected limits for patient.

3. Patient demonstrates increased ability to self-feed or open items on tray as appropriate.

4. Patient coughs appropriately when eating with no new signs of respiratory compromise.

5. Patient completes meal.

6. Patient able to describe foods allowed within any prescribed diet.

Delegation and Collaboration

The skill of assisting a patient with oral nutrition may be delegated to nursing assistive personnel (NAP). The nurse instructs the NAP by:

- Explaining how to position patient to avoid any swallowing problems.
- Reviewing need to observe for coughing, gagging, or other signs of dysphagia and to report information back to the nurse.

Equipment

- Stethoscope and tongue blade for assessment
- Meal tray
- Over-bed table
- Adaptive utensils if appropriate (Fig. 12-1)
- Damp washcloth
- Towel
- Oral hygiene supplies

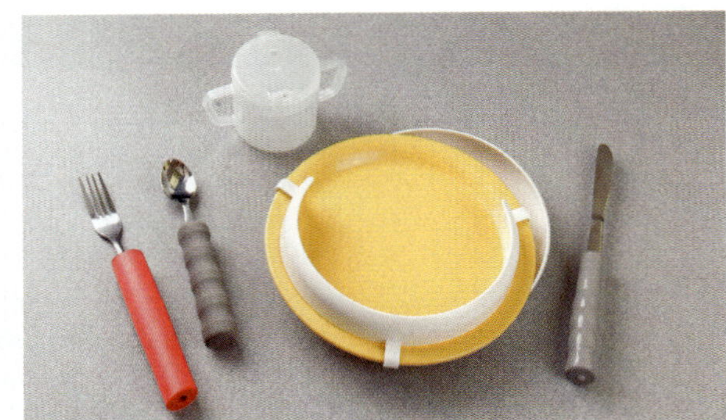

FIG 12-1 Adaptive equipment. *Clockwise from upper left:* Two-handled cup with lid, plate with plate guard, utensils with splints, and utensils with enlarged handles.

IMPLEMENTATION *for* FEEDING DEPENDENT PATIENTS

STEPS	RATIONALE
1. See Standard Protocol (inside front cover).	
2. Prepare patient for meal.	
a. Offer toileting and then handwashing before meal.	Increases level of comfort. Prevents transmission of infection.
b. Place patient in high-Fowler's position (bed or chair). If unable to sit, turn on side with head elevated.	Upright position helps patient keep food toward front of mouth before swallowing, reducing risk for aspiration.
c. Offer oral hygiene. If patient has dentures, remove and rinse thoroughly and reinsert.	Moist, clean oral mucosa and teeth improve taste and appetite.
d. Patients with stomatitis (inflammation of mucous membranes) benefit from rinsing with solutions such as saline, saline-sodium bicarbonate mouthwash, sodium bicarbonate solution, or topical anesthetics (NCI, 2014). Consult with health care provider to determine the most appropriate therapy for patient (Lalla et al., 2011).	The pain of stomatitis causes some patients to avoid eating.
e. Help patient put on eyeglasses or insert contact lenses if used.	Promotes ability to self-feed and makes meal more visually appealing.
3. Check the environment for distractions. Reduce the noise level if possible. *Option:* If patient enjoys music, play a soothing, low-volume selection.	Pleasant environment enhances mealtime experience.
4. Obtain special assistive devices as needed (see Fig. 12-1) and instruct on use. For example:	Devices facilitate self-feeding by improving ability to grasp, pick up foods with utensils, and drink liquids.
a. Two-handled cup with spout in lid makes it easier to drink and hold and lift a cup. Spills are avoided. Cup has wide base, which prevents tipping over.	
b. Plate with plate guard and nonskid bottom helps a person with limited flexibility of hands or poor motor coordination or who has use of only one hand.	
c. Knife, fork, and spoon with large handles or attached splints help a person with limited hand function or a weak grip.	

STEPS	RATIONALE
5. Assess tray for completeness and correct diet. Use this time (and during actual feeding) to instruct patient about diet, rationale for diet, and food options.	Prevents intake of incomplete or incorrect diet.
6. Assist patient with setting up meal tray if patient is unable to do so. Open packages, cut up food, apply seasonings or condiments, butter bread, and place napkin.	Reduces effort needed to self-feed.
7. Watch patient successfully swallow first bites of food and drink. If patient is able to eat independently, stop here. Return after 10 to 20 minutes or stay at side for communication and additional teaching time.	Aim is to make patient as self-sufficient as possible for self-feeding.

> **SAFE PATIENT CARE** If patient is at risk for aspiration, stay at his or her side during feeding.

STEPS	RATIONALE
8. Assist patient who cannot eat independently.	
a. Assume a comfortable position.	Being comfortable prevents you from rushing the patient through a meal.
b. If patient is visually impaired, identify food location on plate as if it were a clock (e.g., the chicken is at 12 o'clock) (see illustration).	Visually impaired patient may be able to feed self when given adequate information about food placement on tray.

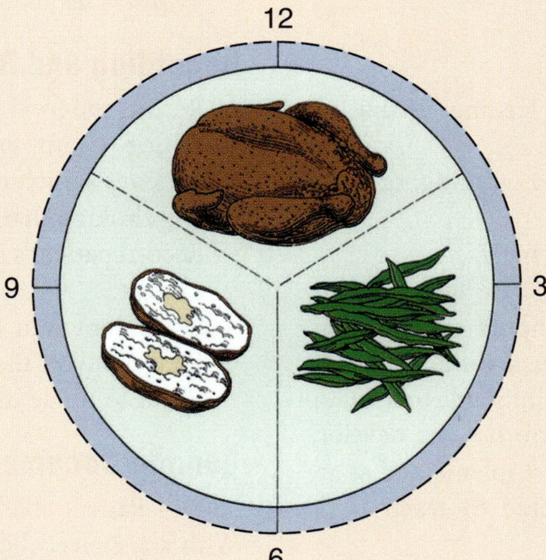

STEP 8b Orient patient to position of food on plate as if it were a clock face.

STEPS	RATIONALE
c. Ask patient in what order he or she would like to eat and cut food into bite-size pieces.	Gives patient more independence and control. Small bites reduce risk of aspiration.
d. Provide fluids as requested. Discourage patient from drinking all fluids at beginning of meal.	Promotes swallowing. Prevents patient from filling up on fluids.
e. Pace feeding to avoid patient fatigue. Interact with patient during mealtime. Verbally encourage self-feeding attempts.	Social interaction may improve appetite.
f. Use meal as an opportunity to educate patient on nutrition topics and discharge plan.	Offers extended time for teaching.
g. Use appropriate feeding techniques for patients with special needs.	

Continued

STEPS	RATIONALE
(1) *Older-adult patients:* Observe biting, chewing, swallowing. Ensure that patient has swallowed food between bites. Offer a variety of foods and frequent rest periods.	Decreased saliva production in older adults impairs swallowing. Aspiration results from decreased or absent gag reflex.
(2) *Neurologically impaired patients:* Feed small amounts at a time. Observe ability to chew, manipulate tongue to form bolus of food, and swallow. Ask patient to open mouth and check for pocketed food. Give small amount of thin liquids between bites.	Patients with limited tongue strength and control are unable to move bolus for swallowing. Checking for pocketed food reduces risk of aspiration.
(3) *Patients with cancer:* Check for food aversions before and during meal.	Strong, abnormal sense of taste and smell are side effects of chemotherapy.
9. Assist patient with washing hands and mouth care after meal is completed.	
10. Help patient to resting position. If in bed, leave head elevated at least 45 degrees for 30 minutes after meal.	Reduces risk of aspiration from regurgitation.
11. Monitor intake and output (I&O) (see Procedural Guideline 7.1), and complete intake measurement (e.g., observed intake, calorie count).	Health care provider's orders may require identifying the specific number of calories consumed. The RD usually completes this; however, the nurse is vital in recording percentages of menu items consumed.
12. See Completion Protocol (inside front cover).	

EVALUATION

1. Monitor body weight daily or weekly.
2. Monitor laboratory values as ordered.
3. Observe patient's technique for self-feeding: intake of certain items, part or all of meal.
4. Observe patient for choking, coughing, gagging, or food left in the mouth during eating.
5. Observe amount of food on tray after meal.
6. Use **Teach Back:** State to the patient, "We talked about your diet and the type of foods you should eat. Can you give me some examples of what you should eat for a dinner meal?" Evaluates what the patient is able to explain or demonstrate. Revise your instruction now or develop plan for revised patient teaching to be implemented at an appropriate time if patient is not able to teach back correctly.

Unexpected Outcomes and Related Interventions

1. Patient is unable to eat entire meal or refuses to eat.
   a. Determine if patient has other food preferences, cultural influences, or religious restrictions.
   b. Determine if patient's ability and desire to eat are better at other times of the day.
   c. Determine if patient is in pain, nauseated, or has constipation.
   d. If repeated problem, consult with health care provider.
2. Patient chokes on food.
   a. Position patient on side with head forward and suction food and secretions from mouth and airway.
   b. If choking occurs repeatedly, stop feeding and notify health care provider.

   c. Make appropriate referrals (e.g., RD or speech therapist) (see Skill 12.2).

Recording and Reporting

- Record the food and fluids actually consumed (including calorie count and I&O), extent of patient self-feeds, patient's ability to swallow and tolerance of diet (including any choking that occurs).
- Record patient's ability to describe types of food he or she can eat.
- Document your evaluation of patient learning.
- Report any swallowing difficulties, food dislikes, or refusal to eat to nurse in charge and the RD.

Sample Documentation

0800: Patient able to feed self 5 bites with encouragement. With assistance, able to consume 60% of meal. Stated, "That is all I can do." No difficulty swallowing and no coughing noted during feeding. Discussed food preferences to include in next meal.

Special Considerations
Pediatric

- Human milk is the most desirable complete diet for infants during first 12 months. Infants who are breastfed or bottle-fed with formula do not require additional fluids (e.g., water or juice) during the first 6 months. Excessive water intake causes water intoxication, failure to thrive, and hyponatremia. Infants usually do not consume solid foods until 6 months. A common sequence for introducing solid food is one new food every 5 to 7 days (AAP, 2012).

Geriatric

- A priority of nutritional care in older adults is to ensure consumption of enough food to prevent unintended weight loss and malnutrition. Therapeutic diets, such as the diabetic diet or the low-sodium diet, can restrict flavors and reduce intake. Collaborate with health care providers and RDs to provide optimal nutrition to older adults (Touhy and Jett, 2014).
- Changes in taste and smell, oral mucus and saliva production, and dentition with aging may affect the patient's food choices, appetite, and ability to chew or swallow.
- Thirst sensation may diminish in older adults, leading to inadequate fluid intake or dehydration.

Home Care

- Homebound older adults may benefit from Meals on Wheels, which can provide three meals per day, depending on the community services (Meals on Wheels Association of America, 2013).
- Educate family caregivers on skills for assisting patients with feeding.
- Patients who are unable to feed themselves independently may eat better if other family caregivers participate at mealtimes to avoid social isolation.

SKILL 12.2   ASPIRATION PRECAUTIONS

• Nursing Skills Online: Safety Module, Lesson 4

Aspiration in adults usually occurs as a result of dysphagia (difficulty swallowing). The condition is associated with muscular, nerve, and obstructive causes (Box 12-4). Dysphagia is a decreased ability to pass fluids or solids voluntarily from the mouth to the stomach. Swallowing is complex, requiring the coordination of cranial nerves and the muscles of the tongue, pharynx, larynx, and jaw. Know patients at risk. For example, assess patients with neuromuscular diseases involving the brain, brainstem, cranial nerves, or muscles of swallowing before feeding. The National Stroke Association (2013) has identified characteristics of dysphagia that are most predictive of aspiration risk (Box 12-5).

Dysphagia often causes a decrease in food intake, which leads to malnutrition. In most cases, malnutrition is caused by difficulty in consuming an adequate volume of solids or liquids. Dietary intake may be affected for long periods as a result of dysphagia. The malnutrition that occurs is secondary to insufficient protein, calorie, and micronutrient intake (Touhy and Jett, 2014).

In some patients, aspiration from dysphagia occurs silently—a patient aspirates without any outward signs of swallowing difficulty. Conditions associated with silent aspiration include local weakness of the pharyngeal muscles, reduced laryngopharyngeal sensation, and impaired ability to cough reflexively. Research studies are evaluating strategies to identify silent aspiration (Miles et al., 2013). Silent aspiration is most often identified following a chest x-ray film.

There are three techniques for identifying dysphagia: bedside screening tests, videofluoroscopy, and fiberoptic endoscopy. An initial bedside swallow assessment is a brief examination that a nurse can administer with basic clinical swallowing training. A water test with pulse oximetry evaluating coughing, choking, and voice alteration is the best method to screen patients with neurologic disorders for dysphagia. Dysphagia screening by nurses is an important initial step in the care of patients with acute neurological impairment, but to achieve the best outcomes, screening should be followed up with a more formal evaluation and safe management of food and fluid intake (Hines et al., 2011). If

---

BOX 12-4   CAUSES OF DYSPHAGIA

Myogenic (Muscle)
- Aging
- Muscular dystrophy
- Myasthenia gravis
- Polymyositis

Neurogenic (Nerve)
- Amyotrophic lateral sclerosis (Lou Gehrig's disease)
- Cerebral palsy
- Diabetic neuropathy
- Guillain-Barré syndrome
- Multiple sclerosis
- Parkinson's disease
- Stroke

Obstructive
- Anterior mediastinal masses
- Candidiasis
- Cervical spondylosis
- Benign peptic stricture
- Head and neck cancer
- Inflammatory masses
- Lower esophageal ring
- Trauma/surgical resection

Other
- Connective tissue disorders
- Gastrointestinal or esophageal resection
- Rheumatological disorders
- Vagotomy

BOX 12-5   CHARACTERISTICS PREDICTIVE OF ASPIRATION

Oropharyngeal dysphagia (difficulty moving food or liquid from mouth to upper esophagus):
- Weak voice
- Drooling
- Difficulty initiating swallow
- Choking, coughing, or gagging with food
- Poor tongue control
- Loss of gag reflex
- Nasal regurgitation

Esophageal dysphagia (difficulty moving food from esophagus to stomach):
- Pain with swallowing
- Feeling of food stuck in throat
- Burping
- Chest pressure/heartburn

you suspect dysphagia, a trained swallowing technician (e.g., speech pathologist) conducts a more thorough assessment. Videofluoroscopy is an x-ray procedure in which the patient swallows food or liquid with barium, and films are taken of the mouth, esophagus, and stomach. Fiberoptic endoscopy is a procedure in which a small tube with a camera is inserted into the nose down through the esophagus into the stomach.

A priority for patients with dysphagia is safe management of oral nutrition and adequate hydration (Hines et al., 2011). Common diet modifications include changes in food or liquid consistencies and elimination of oral intake and initiation of tube feedings. Have a dietitian determine the viscosity of foods that the patient tolerates best through the use of trials of different consistencies of food and fluids. The American Dietetic Association published the National Dysphagia Diet Task Force's diet to provide uniformity of diets offered to patients with dysphagia (NDDTF, 2002). There are four levels of diet: dysphagia pureed, dysphagia mechanically altered, dysphagia advanced, and regular. The four levels of liquid are thin liquids (low viscosity), nectar-like liquids (medium viscosity), honey-like liquids (honey-like viscosity), and spoon-thick liquids (viscosity of pudding) (Academy of Nutrition and Dietetics, 2012; NDDTF, 2002). After placing a patient on a thickened-liquids diet, carefully monitor and assist as needed at each meal or snack to prevent the patient from choking or aspirating. Encouragement may be needed to help the patient adjust to thickened liquids. The consistency and taste may be altered from the patient's normal eating before experiencing dysphagia. In 2011, the U.S. Food and Drug Administration issued a warning for the use of certain thickeners in infants born before 37 weeks of gestational age because it can cause necrotizing enterocolitis. There are many forms of thickeners. Collaborate with the health care provider and RD to determine which type of thickener is safe for your patient population.

ASSESSMENT

1. Perform a nutritional screening (see Skill 12.1). *Rationale: Patients with aspiration from dysphagia may alter their eating patterns or choose foods that do not provide adequate nutrition (Touhy and Jett, 2014).*
2. Identify patient's risk for aspiration (see Box 12-4). Use a dysphagia screening tool if available. *Rationale: Allows you to identify if patient requires precautionary measures during feeding to prevent aspiration.*
3. Measure patient's oxygen saturation. *Rationale: Provides baseline to assess for aspiration during meal.*
4. Observe patient during mealtime for signs of dysphagia and allow patient to try to feed self. Note at end of meal

if patient tires, has wet voice, or coughs after trying to swallow. *Rationale: Detects abnormal eating patterns, increasing risk of aspiration.*
5. Ask patient about any difficulties with chewing or swallowing various textures of food.
6. Assess patient's swallowing reflex before initial feeding by placing fingers on patient's throat at level of the larynx and asking patient to swallow saliva. Feel for movement of larynx. *Rationale: Movement of the larynx normally can be palpated.*
7. Take tongue blade and while asking patient to say "ah," notice movement of tongue. Then gently elicit gag reflex. *Rationale: Tongue movement may reveal weakness on one side of mouth, impairing swallowing. This should be done on initial assessment of the patient or if there is a concern for a change in swallowing ability.*
8. Place identification on patient's chart or in the electronic health record indicating that dysphagia/aspiration risk is present. *Rationale: Identification reduces risk of patient receiving oral nutrition without supervision.*

PLANNING

Expected Outcomes focus on adequate food and fluid intake to prevent malnutrition and dehydration while avoiding aspiration.
1. Patient exhibits no symptoms of aspiration or new respiratory distress.
2. Patient maintains stable weight.
3. Patient understands reason he or she is at risk for aspirating.

Delegation and Collaboration

The assessment of patients' risk for aspiration and determination of positioning cannot be delegated to nursing assistive personnel (NAP). However, the NAP may feed patients after receiving instruction in aspiration precautions. The nurse instructs the NAP to:
- Report immediately to the nurse in charge any onset of coughing, gagging, a wet voice, or pocketing of food.

Equipment

- Upright chair or bed in high-Fowler's position
- Thickener agent (rice, cereal, yogurt, gelatin, commercial thickener)
- Tongue blade
- Oral hygiene supplies, including antimicrobial mouthwash
- Penlight
- Pulse oximeter
- Suction equipment

IMPLEMENTATION for ASPIRATION PRECAUTIONS

STEPS	RATIONALE
1. **See Standard Protocol (inside front cover).**	
2. Provide thorough oral or denture hygiene (see Chapter 10), including brushing of tongue before meal.	Tongue coating is associated with buildup of bacterial cells in the saliva and aspiration pneumonia (Tada and Miura, 2011).

STEPS	RATIONALE
3. Apply pulse oximeter to patient's finger.	Oxygen desaturation and hypoxia occur with aspiration.
4. Position patient upright in a chair or in bed at a 90-degree angle or to highest position allowed by patient's medical condition.	Position aims to prevent gastric reflux and reduces occurrence of aspiration (Grodner et al., 2013; Metheny and Frantz, 2013). Side-lying position is an option if patient cannot have head elevated.
5. Using penlight and tongue blade, gently inspect mouth for pockets of food.	Pocketing food indicates that the patient has difficulty moving food from the mouth into the pharynx (Remig and Weeden, 2012).
6. Have patient assume a chin-tuck position. Begin by having patient try sips of water. Monitor for swallowing and respiratory difficulties continuously. If patient tolerates water, offer a larger volume of water and then different consistencies of foods and liquids.	Chin-tuck or chin-down position helps reduce aspiration (Terre and Mearin, 2012). Giving liquids and foods of different textures assesses patient's ability to swallow safely. Gradual increase in types and textures, coupled with monitoring, ensures that patient is able to eat safely.
7. Add thickener to liquids, if ordered, creating the consistency of mashed potatoes.	Thin liquids are easily aspirated (Remig and Weeden, 2012). Progress to the consistency of thickness that the patient can tolerate.
8. Place ½ to 1 teaspoon of food on unaffected side of mouth, allowing utensils to touch the mouth or tongue.	Provides tactile cue to begin eating. Placing the food on the affected (or weakened side) can put the patient at risk for aspiration.
9. Provide verbal coaching and redirection while feeding patient. Use this time to explain why patient is at risk for aspirating.	Keeps patient focused on swallowing and minimizes distractions (Metheny, 2012). Prepares patient for understanding importance of precautions.
10. Observe for coughing, choking, gagging, and drooling food; suction airway as necessary.	Indicators of dysphagia and aspiration risk (National Stroke Association, 2013).
11. Do not rush a patient during feeding. Allow time for adequate chewing and swallowing. Alternate solids and liquids. Inspect contents of patient's mouth after swallowing for food pocketing.	Enhances swallowing. Checking for pocketed food can prevent aspiration. Limit environmental distractions and conversations to reduce the risk of aspiration (Chang and Roberts, 2011).
12. If needed, demonstrate chewing for patients with dementia.	
13. Have patient remain sitting upright for at least 30 to 60 minutes after the meal.	Reduces risk of gastroesophageal reflux, which causes aspiration (Metheny, 2012).
14. Provide mouth care after meals. Consider using an antimicrobial mouthwash.	Dislodges any food or fluids that may have accumulated inside patient's cheeks. Swallow training with oral care can reduce the risk of pneumonia (Tada and Miura, 2011).
15. Advance diet to thicker foods that require more chewing and finally to thin liquids as tolerated.	RD or speech pathologist can direct safest advancement of diet.
16. **See Completion Protocol (inside front cover).**	

EVALUATION

1. Observe patient's ability to swallow foods of various textures and thicknesses.
2. Observe for signs of aspiration, including choking, coughing, and wet voice.
3. Monitor I&O, calorie count, weight, and food eaten from tray.
4. Monitor pulse oximetry readings.
5. Use **Teach Back:** State to the patient, "During the meal we discussed the reason why it is easy for you to choke on food. To review and to be sure you understand, tell me why you choke on food easily and what can be done to minimize this." Evaluates what the patient is able to explain or demonstrate. Revise your instruction now or develop plan for revised patient teaching to be implemented at an appropriate time if patient is not able to teach back correctly.

Unexpected Outcomes and Related Interventions

1. Patient coughs, gags, develops a wet voice, or complains of food "stuck in throat"; has pocketed food in mouth.
   a. Stop feeding patient.
   b. Be sure that patient is in high-Fowler's position, or if unable to assume high-Fowler's position, place patient in side-lying position.
   c. Suction airway until clear.
   d. Notify health care provider.

2. Patient avoids certain textures of food.
  a. Change consistency of food in diet.
3. Patient loses weight.
  a. Consult with RD on increasing frequency of meals or providing nutritional supplements.

Recording and Reporting

- Record patient's tolerance of liquids and food textures, amount of assistance required, response to instruction, position during meal, absence or presence of any symptoms of dysphagia, fluid intake, and amount of food eaten.
- Document your evaluation of patient learning.
- Report any coughing, gagging, choking, or swallowing difficulties to nurse in charge or health care provider.

Sample Documentation

1200 Fed half of pureed diet and 4 oz juice with 1 teaspoon of thickener added. Patient needs much encouragement. Tires easily during feeding. Benefits from coaching to swallow. No coughing or aspiration noted.

Special Considerations
Pediatric

- Infants and children have swallowing problems because of anatomical, neuromuscular, GI, and other physiological impairments. Once confirmed with diagnostic testing, it is critical to prevent aspiration in pediatric patients at risk. Positioning, modifications in utensils or bottles, adding thickening agents, and exercises to improve swallow function are some interventions nurses may perform to prevent aspiration (Tutor and Gosa, 2012).

Geriatric

- Aspiration is a common cause of pneumonia in older adults. No one intervention has been identified to reduce an older adult's risk.

SKILL 12.3 INSERTION AND REMOVAL OF A SMALL-BORE FEEDING TUBE

• Nursing Skills Online: Enteral Nutrition Module, Lessons 1 and 2

Enteral nutrition, commonly called tube feeding, refers to the delivery of nutritional formulas through a tube that has been placed into the gastrointestinal (GI) tract. Gastric tubes, such as nasogastric (NG) tubes, gastrostomy tubes, or G-buttons, supply enteral feedings directly into the stomach. Small bowel tubes, such as nasojejunal (NJ) or gastrojejunal (G-J) tubes, place food directly into the jejunum of the small intestine. Tubes placed into the small bowel are thought to reduce the incidence of pulmonary aspiration of stomach contents because the tube goes beyond the natural sphincters controlling reflux. However, research shows that even NJ tubes can migrate back into the stomach.

The selection of tube and placement method depends on the anticipated duration of feeding and other patient-related factors such as gastric emptying. For short-term feeding, nasal or oral feeding tubes are appropriate. When the duration of tube feeding extends beyond 4 weeks or in situations in which access to the GI tract through the nose or mouth is contraindicated, direct enteral access through the abdominal wall is the best choice.

NG and NJ tubes are composed of either silicone or polyurethane. They are more flexible and reportedly more comfortable for patients. These tubes are more difficult to insert than large-bore NG tubes used for decompression (see Chapter 19). Some tubes are weighted, and research shows that weighted tubes are superior to nonweighted tubes. Temporary tubes are generally coated with a hydrophilic substance that is activated when exposed to water, making it slippery and easier to insert. A nurse activates the substance immediately before insertion by simply flushing the tube inside and out with water. Wire stylets are included with some, but not all, tubes. Stylets are thought to improve insertion success but have also been associated with increased risk for nasopulmonary intubation. You can pass a feeding tube without the use of a stylet.

Besides inserting a tube, nursing responsibilities include verifying and maintaining proper positioning of a tube, keeping it patent, administering nutrient feedings, and preventing complications. Placement of a temporary feeding tube requires a health care provider's order. Nasal and oral insertion of feeding tubes is commonly performed at a patient's bedside. Confirmation of the correct position of a newly inserted tube is mandatory before any feeding or medication administration. Nurses use a variety of bedside tests to determine tube placement. However, the gold standard for confirming correct placement of a blindly inserted enteral tube is a chest x-ray film that visualizes the entire course of the tube. Assessing the color and pH of gastric aspirate for ongoing monitoring of tube location has been shown to be effective and less costly (AACN, 2012; Proehl et al., 2011). A nurse, registered dietitian (RD), and health care provider collaborate to select an enteral feeding formula based on a patient's protein and caloric requirements and digestive ability.

Adverse events related to enteral nutrition administration include enteral tube misconnections (e.g., connecting an enteral tube to an intravenous [IV] site), access device misplacements (e.g., intubation of the lung instead of GI tract), bronchopulmonary aspiration, and GI intolerance to formulas. The practice of inserting enteral tubes and administering tube feedings requires great care and attention to practice guidelines.

ASSESSMENT

1. Verify health care provider's order for type of tube and enteric feeding schedule. Order should indicate delivery site and device, patient's name and identifying information (see facility policy), formula type, and administration method and rate (see Skill 12.5). *Rationale: Health care provider's order is needed to intubate patients with feeding tube.*

2. Identify patient using two identifiers (e.g., name and birthday or name and account number) according to facility policy. *Rationale: Ensures correct patient. Complies with The Joint Commission standards and improves patient safety (TJC, 2014b).*

3. Assess patient's height, weight, hydration status and I&O, electrolyte balance, and caloric needs. *Rationale: Provides baseline information to measure nutritional improvement after enteral feedings are initiated.*

4. Have patient close each nostril alternately and breathe. Examine each naris for patency and skin breakdown. *Rationale: Determines if nasal passage is obstructed or irritated or if septal defect or facial fractures are present.*

5. Review patient's medical history (e.g., for basilar skull fractures, nasal problems, nosebleeds, facial trauma, nasal-facial surgery, deviated septum, anticoagulant therapy, bleeding tendency). If a tube is inserted in the presence of these conditions, it should be done under fluoroscopy by a gastroenterologist. *Rationale: History of these problems may require nurse to consult with health care provider to select alternative route (e.g., gastrostomy) for nutritional support.*

6. Assess patient's mental status (ability to cooperate with procedure, sedation level), presence of cough and gag reflex, ability to swallow, and presence of artificial airway. *Rationale: These are risk factors for inadvertent tube placement into the tracheobronchial tree (Krenitsky, 2011).*

SAFE PATIENT CARE Recognize situations in which blind placement of a feeding tube poses an unacceptable risk for placement. Devices for detecting accidental insertion of a tube into the airway, such as carbon dioxide sensors or electromagnetic tracking devices, enhance patient safety. Electromagnetically guided nasointestinal (NI) tubes enhance placement with real-time tip tracking verifying tube placement (Taylor et al., 2010). Only clinicians trained in the use of visualization or imaging techniques should perform blind placement of tubes (AACN, 2010; Krenitsky, 2011).

---

7. Assess abdomen (Chapter 7). *Rationale: Absence of bowel sounds or the presence of abdominal pain, tenderness, or distention may indicate GI problem, contraindicating feedings.*

8. Check medical record orders to determine if health care provider wants a prokinetic agent (e.g., metoclopramide) administered before placement of tube. *Rationale: Prokinetic agents given before tube placement may help advance the tube into the intestine.*

9. Assess patient's knowledge of procedure. *Rationale: Determine level of instruction needed.*

PLANNING

Expected Outcomes focus on proper placement of small-bore feeding tube into GI tract.

1. Tube is successfully placed in stomach or intestine.
2. Patient has no respiratory distress (e.g., increased respiratory rate, coughing, poor color) or signs of discomfort or nasal trauma during tube insertion.

Delegation and Collaboration

The skill of small-bore feeding tube insertion cannot be delegated to nursing assistive personnel (NAP). However, the NAP may assist with patient positioning and comfort measures during tube insertion.

Equipment

Insertion
- Small-bore NG or nasoenteric feeding tube with or without stylet (select the smallest diameter possible to enhance patient comfort) (Fig. 12-2)
- 60-mL slip tip, catheter-tip, or Luer-Lok syringe
- Stethoscope and pulse oximeter
- Hypoallergenic tape, semipermeable (transparent) dressing, or tube fixation device
- Tincture of benzoin or other skin barrier protectant
- pH indicator strip (scale 1.0 to 11.0)
- Cup of water and straw (for patients able to swallow)
- Emesis basin
- Towel or disposable pad
- Facial tissues
- Clean gloves
- Suction equipment in case of aspiration
- Penlight to check placement in nasopharynx
- Tongue blade
- Capnograph (optional)

Removal
- Towel
- Facial tissue
- Oral hygiene supplies
- 30-mL Luer-Lok catheter tip syringe

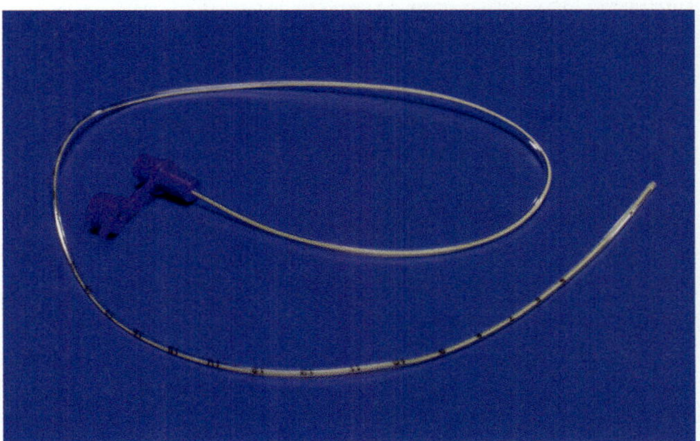

FIG 12-2 Small-bore feeding tube. (Used with permission from Covidien.)

IMPLEMENTATION *for* INSERTION AND REMOVAL OF A SMALL-BORE FEEDING TUBE

STEPS	RATIONALE

1. **See Standard Protocol (inside front cover).**

Tube Insertion

2. Position patient upright in high-Fowler's position unless contraindicated. If patient is comatose, place in semi-Fowler's position with head propped forward using a pillow. If necessary, have the NAP help with positioning of confused or comatose patients. If patient must lie supine, place in reverse Trendelenburg's position.

   Reduces risk for pulmonary aspiration in event patient should vomit. Head propped assists with closure of airway and passage of the tube into the esophagus.

3. Verify capnography or pulse oximetry to confirm oxygenation status.

   Permits objective assessment of respiratory status during tube insertion.

   a. If the patient experiences an increase in end-tidal carbon dioxide or decrease in pulse oximetry measurements, the tube should be removed and reinserted if applicable. If end-tidal carbon dioxide decreases, the patient may be hyperventilating. Stop and encourage slow breathing or remove and reinsert tube if applicable.

4. Determine length of tube to be inserted, and mark location with tape or indelible ink.

   Length approximates distance from nose to stomach.

   a. Measure distance from tip of nose to earlobe to xiphoid process of sternum (see illustration).

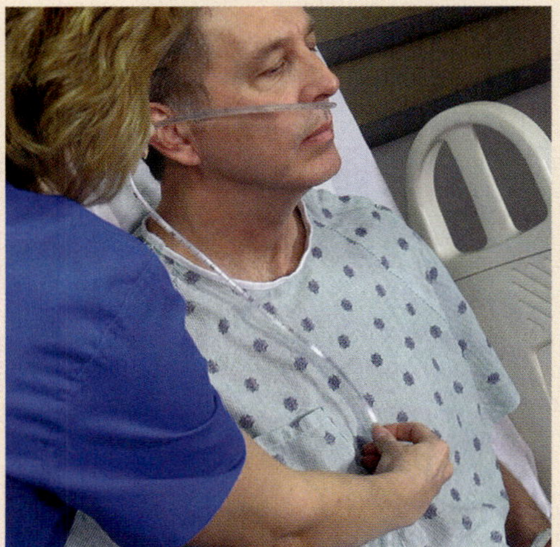

STEP 4a Determine length of tube to be inserted.

   b. Measure distance from tip of nose to earlobe to mid-umbilicus for pediatric patients.

   c. Add an additional 20 to 30 cm (8 to 12 inches) for NI tubes

5. Prepare NG or NI tube for intubation.

   a. If tube has a guidewire or stylet, inject 10 mL of water from the Luer-Lok or catheter-tip syringe into the tube.

   Ensures the tube is patent. Aids in guidewire or stylet removal. Activates lubrication of tube for easier passage and ensures that tube is patent.

   b. If using stylet, ensure that it is securely positioned against tube tip and that both Luer-Lok connections are snugly fit.

   Promotes smooth passage of tube into GI tract. Improperly positioned stylet can induce serious trauma.

STEPS	RATIONALE

6. Cut hypoallergenic tape 10 cm (4 inches) long or prepare membrane dressing or other tube fixation device.

Anchors tube after insertion.

7.  Apply clean gloves.

Prevents transmission of microorganisms.

8. *Option:* Dip tube with surface lubricant into glass of room-temperature water or apply water-soluble lubricant (see manufacturer's directions).

Activates lubricant or applies lubricant to facilitate passage of tube into naris and GI tract.

9. Hand alert patient a cup of water with straw (if able to swallow).

Patient is asked to swallow water to facilitate tube passage.

10. Explain the next steps and gently insert tube through nostril to back of throat (posterior nasopharynx). This may cause patient to gag. Aim back and down toward ear.

Natural contours facilitate passage of tube into GI tract.

11. Have patient flex head toward chest after tube has passed through nasopharynx. Then encourage patient to swallow by giving small sips of water. Advance tube as patient swallows. Rotate tube 180 degrees while inserting.

Closes off glottis and reduces risk for tube entering trachea. Swallowing facilitates passage of tube past oropharynx.

12. Emphasize need to mouth breathe and swallow during the procedure. You do not want to advance the tube during inspiration or coughing because it is more likely to enter the respiratory tract. Monitor pulse oximetry readings.

Helps facilitate passage of tube and alleviates patient's fears during the procedure.

13. Advance tube each time patient swallows until desired length has been passed as long as it advances without resistance (see illustration).

Resistance may indicate kinking of the tube or anatomic irregularity.

SAFE PATIENT CARE Do not force the tube or push against resistance. If patient starts to cough or has a drop in oxygen saturation or increased CO_2, withdraw the tube into the posterior nasopharynx until normal breathing resumes.

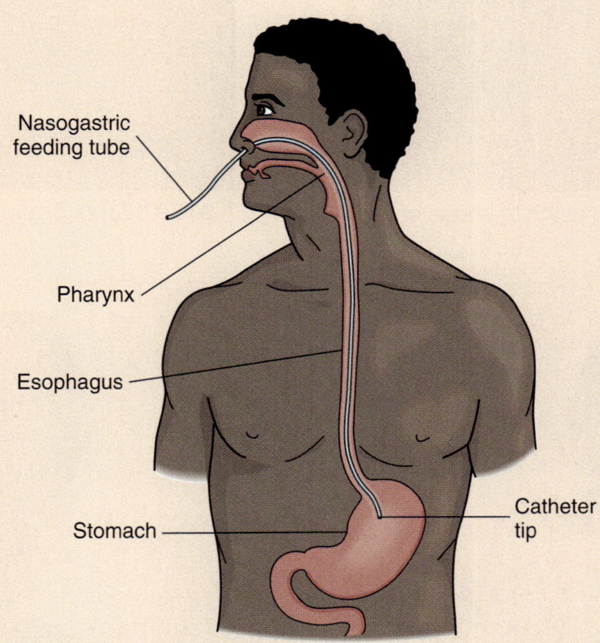

STEP 13 Nasogastric feeding tube inserted through nose and esophagus into stomach.

Continued

STEPS	RATIONALE

14. Check to be sure tube is not positioned in back of throat with penlight and tongue blade.

Tube may be coiled, kinked, or entering trachea.

15. Temporarily anchor tube to the nose with a small piece of tape.

Movement of the tube stimulates gagging. Allows for assessment of position before anchoring tube more securely.

16. Keep tube secure. Attach syringe to end of feeding tube and obtain gastric aspirate: assess amount, color and quality of return (see Skill 12.4). Measure pH of return.

Proper tube position is essential before initiating feeding. Properly obtained pH of 1.0 to 4.0 is a good indication of gastric placement (Proehl et al., 2011).

17. After you obtain gastric aspirates, anchor the tube to nose, avoiding pressure on naris. Mark exit site with indelible ink. Use one of the following options for anchoring:

A properly secured tube allows the patient more mobility and prevents trauma to nasal mucosa.

  a. Apply tube fixation device with shaped adhesive patch.

Secures tube and reduces friction on naris.

    (1) Apply wide end of patch to bridge of nose (see illustration).

    (2) Slip connector around feeding tube as it exits nose (see illustration).

Decreases risk for patient's inadvertent extubation.

  b. Apply hypoallergenic tape to nose.

Prevents pulling of tube. Frequent change may be required if tape becomes soiled.

    (1) *Optional:* Apply tincture of benzoin or other skin adhesive on tip of patient's nose and allow it to become "tacky."

Helps tape adhere better. Protects skin.

    (2) Remove and dispose of gloves and split one end of tape lengthwise 5 cm (2 inches).

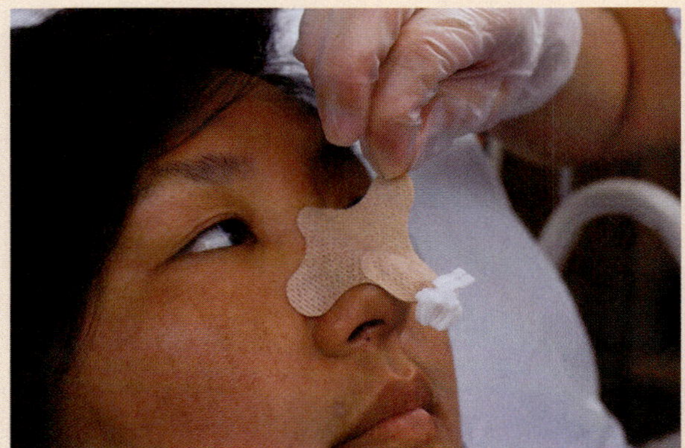

STEP 17a(1) Applying tube fixation patch to bridge of nose.

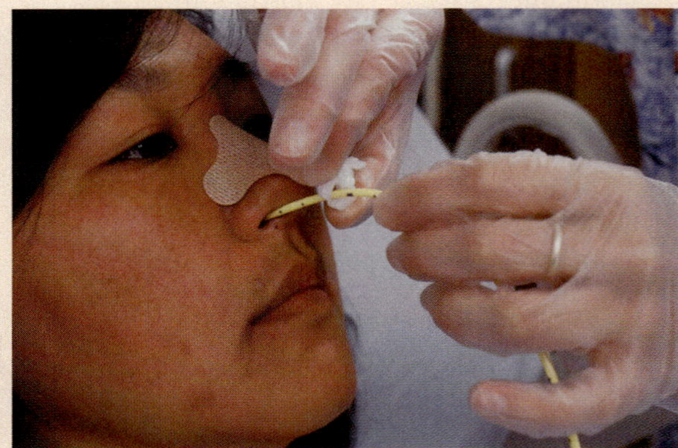

STEP 17a(2) Slip connector around feeding tube.

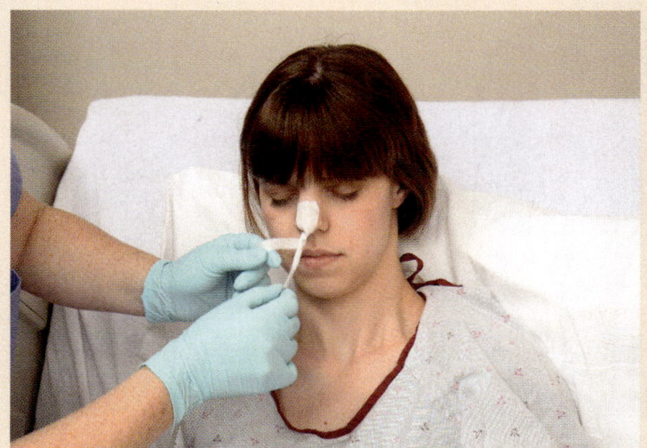

STEP 17b(3) Wrapping tape to anchor nasoenteral tube.

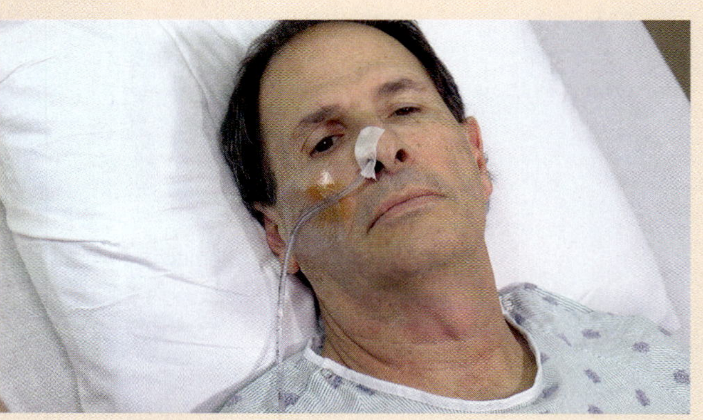

STEP 17b(4) Tube attached to cheek using transparent dressing.

STEPS	RATIONALE

(3) Place the intact end of tape over bridge of patient's nose. Wrap each of the 5-cm (2-inch) strips in opposite directions around tube as it exits nose (see illustration), taking care that it is not secured against side of naris too tightly.

Secures tube firmly. Securing tape against naris can increase chance of pressure ulcer.

(4) *Optional:* Use transparent membrane to secure tube to cheek. Be sure skin is clean and not oily. Apply dressing to cheek, and then apply second dressing, overlapping the first to ensure tube is secure (see illustration).

Securing tube to cheek relieves downward pulling of tube in naris, which increases risk of pressure ulcer.

18. Fasten tube to patient's gown using a clip (see illustration) or piece of tape. Do not use safety pins to secure tube to patient's gown.

Reduces traction on tube and its securement (McGinnis, 2011).

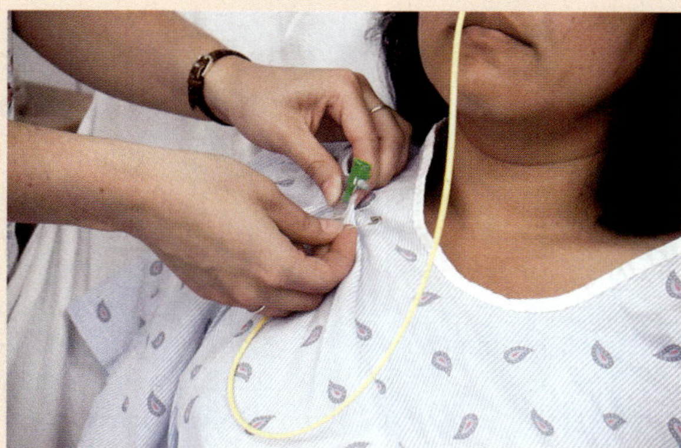

STEP 18 Fasten feeding tube to patient's gown.

19. Keep head of the bed elevated at least 30 degrees (preferably 45 degrees) unless contraindicated (Metheny and Frantz, 2013). For intestinal tube placement, place patient on right side when possible until radiographic confirmation of correct placement.

Promotes patient comfort. Placing patient on right side promotes passage of tube into the small intestine.

> **SAFE PATIENT CARE** Leave guidewire or stylet in place until x-ray verifies tube placement. Never try to reinsert a partially or fully removed guidewire or stylet; this could perforate the tube and injure the patient.

20. Obtain x-ray film of chest and abdomen. Once obtained, confirm results with health care provider.

X-ray film confirmation is most accurate method to determine tube placement (Tho et al., 2011).

21. After proper tube placement is verified, measure the amount of tube that is external and mark the exit of the tube at the naris with indelible marker as a guide for displacement.

This mark can alert nurses to possible displacement of the tube, which will require confirmation of placement before further use.

22. Apply clean gloves. Administer oral hygiene (see Chapter 10). Cleanse tubing at nostril with washcloth dampened in mild soap and water.

Promotes patient comfort and integrity of oral mucous membranes.

Tube Removal

23. Verify health care provider's order for tube removal.

24. Gather equipment and explain procedure to patient.

Informs patient and enhances cooperation.

25. Perform hand hygiene and apply clean gloves.

Reduces transmission of microorganisms.

26. Position patient upright in high-Fowler's position unless contraindicated.

Reduces risk of aspiration in the event the patient vomits.

Continued

STEPS	RATIONALE
27. Place disposable pad or towel on patient's chest. If present, disconnect tube from feeding administration set.	Prevents mucus and secretions from soiling patient's gown.
28. Remove tube fixation device or tape from patient's nose. Unclip tube from patient's gown.	Allows tube to be easily removed.
29. Instruct patient to take deep breath and hold it.	Prevents inadvertent aspiration of gastric contents during tube removal.
30. Kink end of tubing securely by folding it over on itself. Then completely withdraw tube by pulling it out steadily and smoothly. Dispose of tubing in proper receptacle.	Prevents residual leakage of fluid from tube. Minimizes patient discomfort. Reduces transmission of microorganisms.
31. Offer tissues to patient to blow nose. Clean nares and provide mouth care.	Provides patient comfort.
32. **See Completion Protocol (inside front cover).**	

EVALUATION

1. Observe patient's response to NG or NI intubation. Have patient speak. Check vital signs. *Option:* Use capnography in critical care settings to determine if tip of tube is in trachea or lung.
2. Remove guidewire or stylet (if used) after x-ray film verification of correct placement.
3. Routinely check condition of naris for signs of irritation or pressure.
4. Check location of external exit site marking on the tube and color and pH of fluid withdrawn from the tube.
5. After tube removal, ask patient about level of comfort.

Unexpected Outcomes and Related Interventions

1. Tube tip is placed into the respiratory tract. This may not be discovered until the x-ray film report. A small-bore tube can enter the airway without causing obvious respiratory symptoms, particularly in a semiconscious or an unconscious patient.
   a. Remove the tube and report the incident to the health care provider.
   b. Obtain order for reinsertion.
2. Stomach contents were aspirated into respiratory tract (immediate response) in alert patient, evidenced by regurgitation with coughing, dyspnea, cyanosis, or decreases in oxygen saturation during the procedure.
   a. Position patient on side to protect the airway.
   b. Suction patient nasotracheally or orotracheally to remove aspirated substance (see Chapter 14).
   c. Report event immediately to health care provider.
3. Stomach contents were aspirated into respiratory tract (delayed response or small-volume aspiration), evidenced by auscultation of crackles or wheezes, dyspnea, or fever.
   a. Report change in patient condition to the health care provider; if there has not been a recent chest x-ray film, suggest ordering one.
   b. Prepare for possible initiation of antibiotics.

Recording and Reporting

- Tube insertion: Record and report type and size of tube placed, location of distal tip of tube, patient's tolerance of procedure, and confirmation of tube position by x-ray film examination.
- Report any type of unexpected outcome and the interventions performed to health care provider.
- Tube removal: Record patient's level of comfort and condition of naris.

Sample Documentation

0800   Small-bore nasogastric feeding tube inserted into left naris, exit site marked at 52 cm. Patient tolerated insertion well. pH of 3.0 for gastric aspirate. Tube secured with fixation device. Abdominal x-ray obtained, position confirmed by health care provider.

Special Considerations
Pediatric

- Colorimetric carbon dioxide detector can detect inadvertent tube placement of tubes in the lung at the bedside (Gilbert and Burns, 2012). X-ray confirmation is the most accurate method to determine placement (Metheny and Meert, 2013).
- Observe for vagal stimulation during tube insertion in infants by assessing for decreased heart rate.

Geriatric

- Ensure adequate lubrication of tube to decrease discomfort for older adults because of the potential for decreased oral or nasopharyngeal secretions.

Home Care

- Assess ability of patient or family caregiver to maintain tube for a feeding program.
- Assess the environmental safety and sanitation of patient's home environment.
- Teach the family caregiver correct method for resecuring feeding tube and checking tube placement.

SKILL 12.4   VERIFYING PLACEMENT AND IRRIGATING A FEEDING TUBE

• Nursing Skills Online: Enteral Nutrition Module, Lesson 3

Once a feeding tube is inserted (see Skill 12.1), it is essential to routinely check its location and keep the tube patent. It is possible for the tip of a feeding tube to move or migrate into a different location (e.g., from the stomach to the intestine or esophagus, from the intestine into the stomach) without any external evidence that the tube has moved. The risk for aspiration of regurgitated gastric contents into the respiratory tract increases when the tip of the tube accidentally dislocates upward into the esophagus.

After initial x-ray film verification that a tube is positioned correctly (either in the stomach or in the small intestine), you are responsible for ensuring that the tube has remained in the intended position before administering formula or medications. You must verify tube position every 4 to 6 hours and as needed (see facility policy). Because it is not practical to take x-ray films that often, other methods of determining placement have been used. The pH testing of gastric aspirate is easy and reliable to distinguish between gastric and intestinal tube placement, but medications can alter the pH levels (Simons and Abdallah, 2012). Characteristics of fluid from feeding tubes may contribute to your assessment of the aspirate but cannot be used solely to determine placement. Visualization of the external tube length can indicate if the tube has shifted but does not indicate the placement of the tube tip (Simons and Abdallah, 2012). Air auscultation is no longer a standard of practice for checking tube placement because of its unreliability (Bankhead et al., 2009). To ensure a high confirmation rate for a correctly placed NG tube, the pH of gastric aspirate should be less than or equal to 4. When pH levels are greater than 5, further confirmation of placement should be conducted with an x-ray (Gilbertson et al., 2011).

A feeding tube must remain patent to ensure adequate nutrition. You routinely irrigate a feeding tube while it is in place and after the administration of medications and feedings. Plain water is the preferred flush solution. However, the American Society for Parenteral and Enteral Nutrition recommends use of sterile water for flushing before and after medication administration and in immunocompromised and critically ill patients (Bankhead et al., 2009). All types of feeding tubes require routine irrigation, including gastrostomy and jejunostomy tubes (see Skill 12.5). Question the patency of a tube when you cannot instill air or fluid through the tube.

ASSESSMENT

1. Review facility policy and procedures for frequency and method of checking tube placement and frequency of irrigation. *Rationale: Maintains quality of care.*
2. Review patient's medical record for history of prior tube displacement. *Rationale: Patients with prior tube displacement are at increased risk for repeated tube displacement.*

3. Identify patient using two identifiers (e.g., name and birthday or name and account number) according to facility policy. *Rationale: Ensures correct patient. Complies with The Joint Commission standards and improves patient safety (TJC, 2014b).*
4. Observe for signs and symptoms of respiratory distress including coughing, choking, or cyanosis. *Rationale: Signs and symptoms indicate accidental migration of feeding tube into the airway. However, absence of signs and symptoms does not ensure that respiratory migration has not occurred, especially in a patient with altered level of consciousness or altered gag and cough reflexes.*
5. Identify conditions that increase the risk for spontaneous tube migration or dislocation, including retching and vomiting, nasotracheal suctioning, or severe bouts of coughing. *Rationale: Feeding tubes migrate by increases in intraabdominal pressure or coughing.*
6. Observe the external portion of the tube for movement of the ink mark away from the mouth or naris (see Skill 12.3). *Rationale: Increased external length of a tube indicates that the distal tip is no longer in the correct position.*
7. Review patient's medication record for continuous feeding or a gastric acid inhibitor or proton pump inhibitor. *Rationale: Feeding or medications can increase pH values (Simons and Abdallah, 2012).*
8. For irrigation, inspect previous volume color and character of aspirates. *Rationale: Thick secretions and a reduced volume of secretions indicate need to irrigate tube. Excess volume of secretions (>200 mL) may indicate delayed gastric emptying.*
9. For irrigation, monitor volume of tube-feeding formula administered during a shift and compare with ordered amount. *Rationale: Indicates whether sufficient volume of feeding is infusing.*

PLANNING

Expected Outcomes focus on correct placement and maintaining patency of feeding tubes.
1. Color, pH, and appearance of gastric aspirate are consistent with initial placement.

Delegation and Collaboration

The verification of tube placement and irrigation may not be delegated to nursing assistive personnel (NAP). The nurse instructs the NAP to:
* Inform the nurse immediately if patient's respirations change or if shortness of breath, coughing, or choking develops.
* Inform the nurse immediately if the patient vomits or the NAP notices vomitus in patient's mouth during oral hygiene.

- Inform the nurse immediately if a change in the external length of the feeding tube occurs, which could indicate displacement.
- Report when a continuous tube feeding stops infusing.

Equipment
- 60-mL catheter-tip syringe
- Clean gloves
- pH indicator strip (scale of 1.0 to 11.0)
- Small medication cup
- Tap water or sterile water (for immunocompromised and critically ill patients)
- Towel

IMPLEMENTATION *for* VERIFYING PLACEMENT AND IRRIGATING A FEEDING TUBE

STEPS	RATIONALE
1. See Standard Protocol (inside front cover).	
2. *Verify tube placement.*	
a. Verify tube placement at the following times:	
(1) For intermittently tube-fed patients, test placement immediately before each feeding (usually a period of at least 4 hours will have elapsed since previous feeding).	Each administration of feeding can lead to aspiration if the tube is displaced. More frequent checking has been associated with increased clogging of small-bore tubes.
(2) Follow facility policy regarding pH testing for patients receiving continuous tube feeding. AACN (2010) recommends that continuous feedings be stopped for several hours to obtain reliable pH readings. It may be helpful to measure when feedings are interrupted for procedures.	Determines if tube migration has occurred. Placement confirmed at same time of routine tube irrigation. Enteral formula buffers pH of gastric secretions.
(3) Wait to verify placement at least 1 hour after medication administration by tube or mouth.	Premature aspiration of contents removes unabsorbed medication, reducing dose delivered to patient. Medication interferes with pH testing and appearance of aspirate (Simons and Abdullah, 2012).
b. Apply clean gloves. If an existing tube feeding is infusing, turn off the feeding temporarily. Close clamp or kink feeding tube while disconnecting it from feeding-bag tubing or while removing plug at end of tube.	Prevents leakage of gastric contents.
c. Draw up 30 mL of air into syringe. Attach syringe tip to end of feeding tube. Release kink, and flush tube with 30 mL of air before attempting to aspirate fluid. If there is resistance, reposition the patient from side to side. In some cases, more than one bolus of air is necessary.	It is more difficult to aspirate fluid from the small intestine than from the stomach or from a smaller bore feeding tube. A bolus of air aids in aspirating fluid more easily by forcing ports of tube away from mucosal folds of stomach or intestine (AACN, 2010).
d. Draw back on syringe slowly and obtain 5 to 10 mL of gastric aspirate (see illustration). Observe appearance of aspirate. Aspirates from continuous tube feeding often have the appearance of curdled enteral formula. Aspirates from intermittent tube feeding are not typically bile-stained (unless intestinal fluid has refluxed into the stomach).	Drawing back quickly or using a smaller syringe may cause the tube to collapse. Appearance of aspirate helps to assess the position of the tube.
e. Gently mix aspirate in syringe. Expel a few drops into a clean medicine cup. Measure pH by dipping a pH strip into the fluid or applying a few drops of the fluid to the strip. Compare the color of the strip with the color on the chart (see illustration) provided by the manufacturer.	Mixing ensures equal distribution of contents for testing.
(1) Gastric fluid from patient who has fasted for at least 4 hours usually has pH range of 5.0 or less.	Range of 5.0 or less is a reliable indicator of stomach placement, even when a gastric acid inhibitor is being used (Bankhead et al., 2009).

STEPS	RATIONALE

(2) Fluid from NI tube in fasting patient usually has pH greater than or equal to 6.0.

Intestinal contents are more alkaline than stomach contents (AACN, 2010; Gilbertson et al., 2011).

(3) Patient with continuous tube feeding may have pH of 5.0 or higher.

Formulas contain solutions that are alkaline.

(4) The pH of pleural fluid from the tracheobronchial tree is generally greater than 6.0.

pH values of pleural contents are more alkaline and typically are greater than 6 (AACN, 2010; Gilbertson et al., 2011).

f. If it is impossible after repeated attempts to aspirate fluid from a tube that was confirmed by x-ray film to be in desired position and if (1) there are no risk factors for tube dislocation, (2) tube has remained in original taped position, and (3) patient is not in respiratory distress, assume tube is correctly placed. Continue with irrigation (Bankhead et al., 2009; Stepter, 2012).

It is reasonable to assume that tube is correctly placed. When abdominal x-ray films are obtained for clinical reasons, you can take advantage of reports to monitor tube location.

3. Tube Irrigation

a. Apply clean gloves. Elevate patient's head of bed 45 to 90 degrees. Kink tube while it is disconnected from feeding-bag tubing or while plug is removed (see illustration).

Upright position helps to minimize reflux. Prevents leakage of gastric secretions.

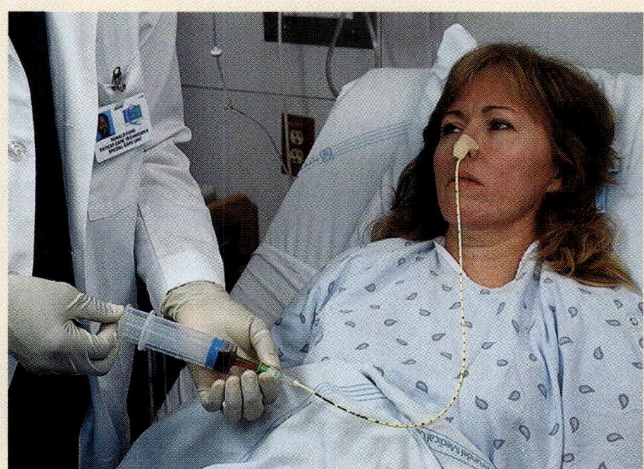

STEP 2d Obtain gastric aspirate.

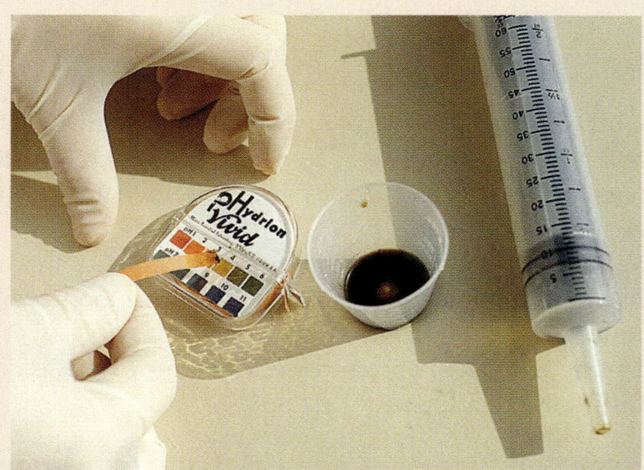

STEP 2e Compare color on test strip with color on pH chart.

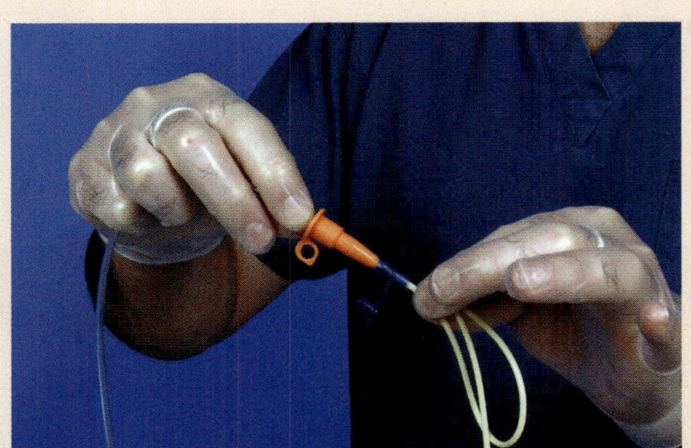

STEP 3a Kink tubing while unplugging feeding tube.

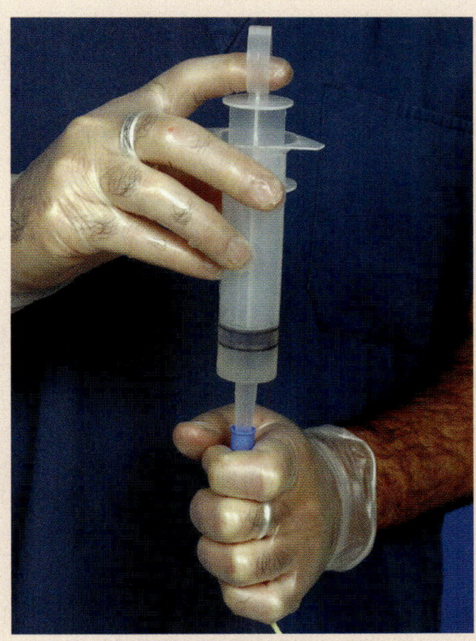

STEP 3c Irrigate feeding tube.

Continued

STEPS	RATIONALE
b. Draw up 30 mL of water into the syringe. Use sterile water before and after medication administration or in immunocompromised and critically ill patients (Bankhead et al., 2009). Do not use irrigation fluids from multidose bottles that are used on other patients. Patient should have personal bottle of solution. Change irrigation bottle every 24 hours.	This amount of solution flushes length of tube. Using sterile water prevents contamination of fluids. Not using fluids from multidose bottles ensures sterile solution.
c. Insert tip of syringe into end of feeding tube. Release kink and slowly instill irrigating solution (see illustration).	Infusion of fluid clears tubing.
d. If unable to instill fluid, reposition patient on left side and try again.	Tip of tube may be against stomach wall. Changing patient's position may move tip away from stomach wall.
e. When water has been instilled, remove syringe. Reinstitute tube feeding or administer medication as ordered. Irrigate before, between, and after the final medication (before feedings are reinstituted).	Tubing is clear and patent. Certain formulas may predispose to tube clogging. Irrigation prevents mixing medications in the tube, which may cause clogging, and flushes medications through the tube so that medications do not mix with formula.

  4. See Completion Protocol (inside front cover).

EVALUATION

1. Observe patient for respiratory distress including persistent gagging, paroxysms of coughing, and respiratory patterns (e.g., rate and depth) inconsistent with baseline measures.
2. Verify that color, pH, and appearance of aspirate are consistent with initial tube placement according to x-ray film results.
3. During irrigation, observe ease with which tube feeding instills through tubing.

Unexpected Outcomes and Related Interventions

1. Red or brown coloring ("coffee grounds" appearance) of fluid aspirated from a feeding tube indicates new blood or old blood, respectively, in the GI tract.
   a. If the color is not related to medications recently administered, notify the health care provider.
2. Patient develops severe respiratory distress.
   a. Stop any enteral feeding and notify health care provider.
   b. Prepare to obtain chest x-ray film as ordered.
3. Tube cannot be irrigated and remains obstructed.
   a. Reattempt irrigation but do not force fluid; if unsuccessful, notify health care provider.
   b. Tube may need to be removed, and a new tube may need to be placed.

Recording and Reporting

- Record the pH and appearance of aspirate. Report findings if displacement is suspected.
- Record time of irrigation, amount and type of fluid instilled, and patient's tolerance.
- Report if tubing is clogged.

Sample Documentation

1400   Dobhoff feeding tube placement confirmed, aspirate pH 3.0, dark green bile–colored fluid. Tube irrigated easily with 30 mL of sterile water; continuous feeding reconnected and infusing at 60 mL/hr.

Special Considerations
Pediatric

- Decrease the amount of air insufflated before gastric aspiration according to size of patient (e.g., an infant may need only 1 mL of air; a small child may need 5 mL).

Home Care

- Instruct patient or family caregiver not to proceed with feedings or medication administration via the tube if there is any doubt as to proper placement of tube.

SKILL 12.5   ADMINISTERING ENTERAL NUTRITION: NASOGASTRIC, GASTROSTOMY, OR JEJUNOSTOMY TUBE

• Nursing Skills Online: Enteral Nutrition Module, Lesson 4

Enteral nutrition, or tube feeding, is a method for providing nutrients to patients who are unable to meet their own nutritional needs orally. When making the decision regarding enteral access, the health care provider considers a patient's rate of gastric emptying, GI anatomy, risk for gastric reflux and aspiration, anticipated duration of feeding, and disease state. Nasal tubes used for short periods of time are associated with sinusitis, otitis, vocal cord paralysis, pressure ulcers of the nose and sinuses, and potential displacement. Feeding tubes that end in the stomach are used for gravity bolus or continuous infusion feedings. The small intestine does not have the storage capability of the stomach, and therefore a tube feeding administered into the small intestine is delivered more slowly and continuously with an infusion pump.

Patients with long-term needs or who have no easy access to the GI tract through the nose or mouth require more invasive access to the GI tract in the form of gastrostomy and jejunostomy tubes. A gastrostomy tube is surgically placed in the stomach; it is sutured in place and exits through an incision typically in the upper left quadrant of the abdomen. A more current practice is a percutaneous endoscopic gastrostomy tube, which is inserted during endoscopic viewing of the stomach. A tube is placed in the stomach and exits through the incision, where an external bumper holds it in place (Fig. 12-3). When patients develop a gastric ileus (decreased or absent peristalsis of the stomach but not intestine), have documented gastroparesis (delayed gastric emptying), or gastric resection, enteral nutrition is given via a percutaneous endoscopic jejunostomy tube. Jejunostomy tubes are inserted most often by endoscopy through the abdomen and fed into the jejunum of the large intestine. Always know whether the patient has a gastric or jejunal tube or both. General indications for enteral feeding include the following:

1. Patients who cannot eat because of surgery, injury, or disease process
2. Nutritional deficit resulting from reduced food ingestion, even when patients are physically able to eat
3. Patients with impaired swallowing or gag reflex

Aspiration into the lung can occur as a result of reflux of gastric content, including tube feeding formula. Aspiration of material foreign to the lung irritates the bronchial mucosa and provides a growth medium for pneumonia or other infections. Common conditions that increase the risk of aspiration include severity of illness and interventions that compromise the gag reflex. Specific risk factors for aspiration include sedation, mechanical ventilation, nasotracheal suctioning, neurologic compromise, lying flat, and sepsis (Makic et al., 2011). Reduce the risk of aspiration by keeping a patient's head of bed elevated unless medically contraindicated and by checking routinely for gastric residual volume (GRV). The amount of GRV in a patient's stomach is not predictive of aspiration. Aspiration has been shown to occur with 5 to 500 mL of GRV (McClave et al., 2009).

ASSESSMENT

1. Review and verify health care provider's order for formula, concentration, route, method of delivery (continuous versus intermittent), and frequency or rate of infusion. *Rationale: Ensures that correct formula will be administered in the appropriate volume.*
2. Identify patient using two identifiers (e.g., name and birthday or name and account number) according to facility policy. *Rationale: Ensures correct patient. Complies with The Joint Commission standards and improves patient safety (TJC, 2014b).*
3. Assess patient's need for tube feedings, such as decreased level of consciousness, a nutritional deficit, head or neck surgery, facial trauma, or impaired swallowing; consult with nutrition support team or health care provider. *Rationale: Identify candidates for enteral nutrition before they become nutritionally depleted.*
4. Assess patient for food allergies or intolerances. *Rationale: Prevents patient from developing localized or systemic allergic responses to feeding.*
5. Perform physical assessment of abdomen (Chapter 7). *Rationale: Absent bowel sounds are not a contraindication to feeding, but you need to report a change from baseline in abdominal examination, particularly if tenderness or distention develop, to determine if feeding can proceed safely (Bankhead et al., 2009)*
6. Obtain baseline weight, and review serum electrolytes and capillary blood glucose measurement. Assess patient for fluid volume excess or deficit, electrolyte abnormalities, and metabolic abnormalities (e.g., hyperglycemia). *Rationale: Provides baseline to measure patient's response to enteral nutrition.*
7. For feeding tubes placed through the abdominal wall, assess insertion site for breakdown, irritation, drainage, discomfort, or presence of an external disk that it is not excessively snug. Monitor that length of external tube remains the same as when originally placed. *Rationale: Infection, pressure from gastrostomy tube, or drainage can cause skin breakdown. A disk that is too snug may cause skin breakdown. Internal tube migration may block pylorus and cause patient distress.*

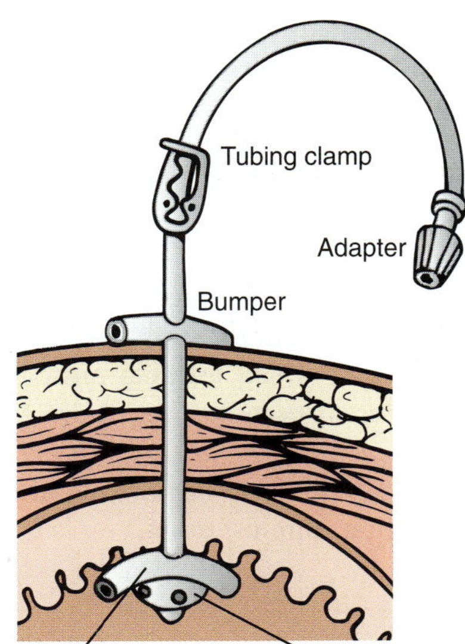

FIG 12-3 Placement of gastrostomy tube into stomach.

PLANNING

Expected Outcomes focus on safe administration of tube-feeding formula, patient tolerance of formula, and avoidance of administration complications.

1. Patient experiences slow increase in nutritional status and weight over time.
2. Patient has no sign of respiratory distress.
3. Patient has no fluid or electrolyte imbalance.
4. Patient has no GI distress.

Delegation and Collaboration

The skill of administration of NG, NI, gastrostomy, and jejunostomy tube feeding can be delegated to trained nursing assistive personnel (NAP) (check facility policy). However, the nurse must first verify tube placement and patency and that the feeding product and fluid (water) to be administered are correct. The nurse must monitor the patient for effectiveness and tolerance of the feeding being delivered. The nurse instructs the NAP to:

- Elevate the head of the bed to a minimum of 30 degrees (45 degrees is preferred) or sit patient up in bed or in chair.
- Infuse the feeding as ordered.
- Report any difficulty infusing the feeding or patient report of abdominal pain or cramping.
- Report any gagging, paroxysms of coughing, or choking.

Equipment

- Disposable feeding bag, tubing, and formula or ready-to-hang system with formula
- 60-mL or larger Luer-Lok or catheter-tip syringe
- Stethoscope
- Enteral infusion pump (required for continuous or intestinal feeding); use pump designed for tube feedings.
- Prescribed enteral feeding
- pH indicator strip (scale 1.0 to 11.0)
- Cup of tap water or sterile water (immunocompromised and critically ill patients)
- Clean gloves
- Equipment to obtain blood glucose level by fingerstick, if ordered
- Labels for marking tube connections

IMPLEMENTATION *for* ADMINISTERING ENTERAL NUTRITION: NASOGASTRIC, GASTROSTOMY, OR JEJUNOSTOMY TUBE

STEPS	RATIONALE
1. **See Standard Protocol (inside front cover).**	
2. 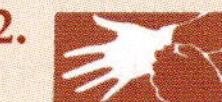 Apply clean gloves. Obtain formula to administer:	
a. Verify correct formula, check expiration date on formula and integrity of container.	Ensures you administer correct formula and checks integrity of formula. Tube feeding administered within designated shelf life from an intact container reduces risk of GI infection. Prevents leakage of tube feeding.
b. Be sure that tube feeding is at room temperature.	Cold formula causes gastric cramping and discomfort because the liquid is not warmed by mouth and esophagus.
3. Prepare formula for administration:	
a. Use aseptic technique when manipulating feeding system or touching can tops, container openings, spike, and spike port.	Bag, connections, and tubing must be free of contamination to prevent bacterial growth (Bankhead et al., 2009).
b. Shake formula container well (prepackaged or can). Clean top of canned formula with alcohol swab before opening (Bankhead et al., 2009).	Ensures integrity of formula; prevents transmission of microorganisms.
c. For closed systems, connect administration tubing to prepared feeding container. If using an open system, connect administration tubing to feeding bag and then pour formula from brick pack or can into bag (see illustration).	Formulas are available in closed system containers that contain a 24- to 48-hour supply of formula or in an open system, in which formula must be transferred from brick packs or cans to a bag before administration.
d. Label bag with feeding formula, patient name, date, time, and your initials. Open clamp on tubing and fill tubing with formula to remove air (prime tubing). Clamp off tubing with roller clamp. Hang bag or container on feeding pump pole.	Filling the tubing with formula prevents air from entering GI tract during administration.

STEPS	RATIONALE

4. Place patient in high-Fowler's position, or elevate head of bed at least 30 degrees (preferably 45 degrees) (unless contraindicated).

Elevated head helps to prevent aspiration (AACN, 2012; Metheny and Frantz, 2013).

5. Verify tube placement (see Skill 12.4).

   a. Nasoenteric tube: Attach syringe and aspirate 5 mL of gastric contents. Observe appearance of aspirate and note pH.

Verifies if tip of tube is in stomach or intestine. Feedings instilled in a misplaced tube can cause serious injury or death.

   b. Gastrostomy tube: Attach syringe and aspirate 5 mL of gastric contents. Observe appearance of aspirate and note pH.

Gastric fluid for a patient who has fasted for at least 4 hours usually has a pH of 1.0 to 4.0 (especially when patient is not receiving gastric acid inhibitor). Continuous administration of tube feeding elevates pH (Simons and Abdullah, 2012).

   c. Jejunostomy tube: Aspirate 5 mL of intestinal secretions; observe appearance. If significant amounts are returned or resemble gastric secretions, check pH.

Presence of intestinal fluid indicates that the end of the tube is in the small intestine. If the fluid tests acidic on the pH test or looks like gastric fluid, the tube may be displaced into the stomach.

6. Check gastric residual volume (GRV):

   a. Draw up 10 to 30 mL of air into syringe and connect tip to feeding tube. Inject the air slowly. Pull back slowly and aspirate the total amount of gastric contents you can aspirate (see illustration).

GRV may not be easy to obtain from a small-bore feeding tube. A 60-mL syringe prevents gastric tube collapse (Makic et al., 2011).

> **SAFE PATIENT CARE** Numerous factors affect measurement accuracy of GRV, including size of gastric tube, position of the tube port in the gastric antrum, patient's position, and whether tube location is near the gastroesophageal junction. Best evidence suggests that a single high GRV should be monitored for the following hour, but enteral feeding should not be stopped or withheld for an isolated high GRV (see facility policy) (Makic et al., 2011).

   b. Return aspirated contents to stomach unless volume exceeds 250 mL (check facility policy) (Metheny, 2010).

Prevents loss of nutrients and electrolytes in discarded fluid. Some questions exist on the safety of returning high volumes of fluid into the stomach (Metheny et al., 2010).

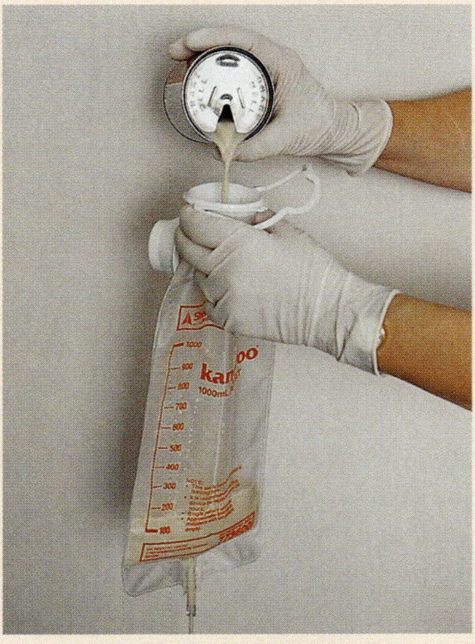

STEP 3c Pour formula into feeding container.

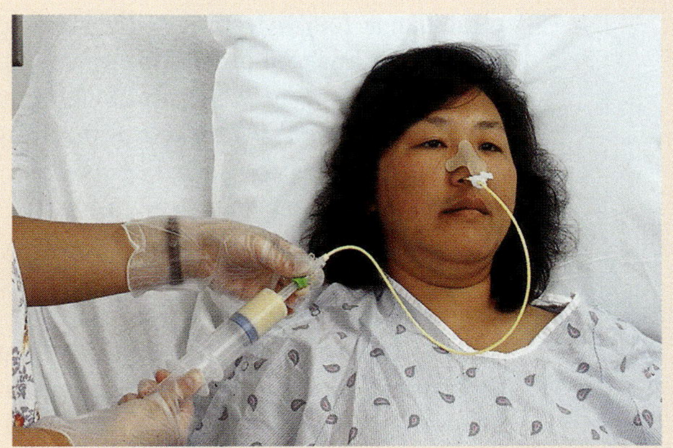

STEP 6a Check for gastric residual volume.

Continued

STEPS	RATIONALE

c. Do not administer feedings when a single GRV measurement is greater than 500 mL or when two measurements taken 1 hour apart each exceed 250 mL (Bankhead et al., 2009) (check facility policy).

Some controversy exists regarding the ability of elevated GVRs to identify risk for pulmonary aspiration. However, frequent interruptions of feeding based on GVR levels is a recognized reason for failure to meet nutritional goals (Bankhead et al., 2009; DeLegge, 2011).

> **SAFE PATIENT CARE** Intestinal residual is usually very small, so if a residual volume is greater than 10 mL, displacement of the tube into the stomach may have occurred. Notify the health care provider.

7. Flush feeding tube:

Ensures that tube is patent and reduces risk of occlusion (Bankhead et al., 2009). Irrigation is routinely performed before, between, and after final medication; before each intermittent feeding; and before initial continuous feeding.

a. After measuring GRV, kink feeding tube to prevent leakage of fluid. Draw up 30 mL of water into syringe. Do not use irrigation fluids from bottles that are used for other patients.

Amount of water will flush length of tube. Water is most effective in preventing tube clogging (Bankhead et al., 2009; Dandeles and Lodolce, 2011).

b. Insert tip of syringe into feeding tube. Release kink and slowly instill irrigation solution.

Irrigation fluid clears tubing.

c. If unable to instill water, reposition patient on left side and try again.

Tip of tube may be against stomach wall.

d. When water has been instilled, remove syringe. Cap tube.

Tubing is clear.

8. Before attaching feeding administration set to feeding tube, trace tube to its point of origin. Label administration set "Tube Feeding Only."

Avoids misconnections between feeding set and IV systems or other medical tubing or devices (Bankhead et al., 2009; Simmons et al., 2011).

9. Initiate tube feeding (use time to instruct patient about feedings).

a. Intermittent gravity feeding:

(1) Pinch proximal end of feeding tube and remove cap. Connect distal end of administration set tubing to end of feeding tube. Set rate by adjusting roller clamp on tubing or by placing on a feeding pump.

Prevents excessive air from entering patient's stomach and leakage of gastric contents.

(2) Allow bag to empty slowly over 30 to 45 minutes (the length of time of a comfortable meal) (see illustration).

Gradual emptying of tube feeding by gravity reduces risk for abdominal discomfort, vomiting, and diarrhea induced by bolus or too-rapid infusion of tube feeding.

(3) Immediately follow feeding with water (per health care provider's orders) to clean bag and feeding tube, prevent tube from clogging, and provide patient with adequate water. Cover end of bag with cap. Keep bag as clean as possible, and change bag every 24 hours.

Helps decrease bacterial growth.

b. Continuous-infusion feeding:

(1) Remove cap and connect feeding tube to distal end of administration set tubing.

Prevents excessive air from entering patient's stomach and leakage of gastric contents.

(2) Thread tubing through infusion pump for enteral feedings, set rate on pump, and turn on.

Delivers continuous feeding at steady rate and pressure. Pump alarms sound when there is increased resistance.

> **SAFE PATIENT CARE** Maximum hang time for formula is 12 hours in an open system and 24 to 48 hours in closed, ready-to-hang system (if it remains closed). Refer to manufacturer's guidelines.

STEPS	**RATIONALE**

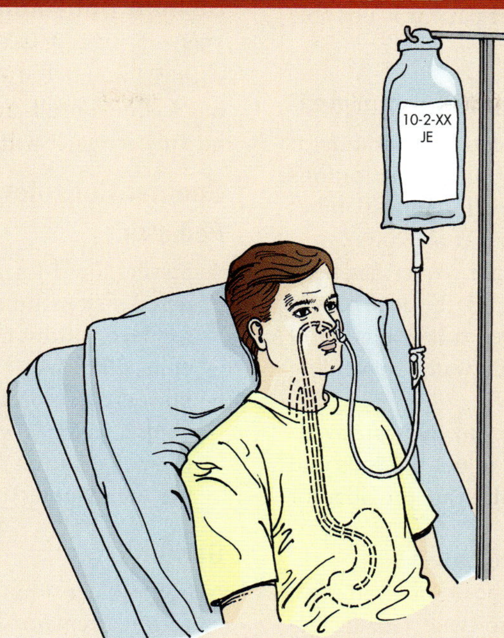

STEP 9a(2) Administer intermittent feeding.

STEPS	**RATIONALE**
10. Advance rate of feeding and concentration of tube feeding gradually per health care provider's orders.	Feedings may be advanced slowly for patients who are at risk for refeeding syndrome or intolerance. Gradual advancement helps prevent diarrhea intolerance (Bankhead et al., 2009).
11. Flush feeding tube with 30 mL of water every 4 hours during continuous feedings and after an intermittent feeding (check facility policy) (see Skill 12.4). Collaborate with the RD and health care provider regarding recommended total free water requirements per day and obtain order.	Clears tubing of formula and prevents clogging (Bankhead et al., 2009). Provides patient with a source of water to maintain fluid and electrolyte balance.
12. When patient is receiving intermittent tube feeding, cap or clamp proximal end of feeding tube when not in use.	Prevents air from entering stomach between feedings.
13. Rinse bag and tubing with warm water whenever feedings are interrupted. Use a new open administration set every 24 hours.	Prevents bacterial contamination of feeding solution.
14. For abdominally placed tubes, clean insertion site daily and as needed. A small breathable dressing may be used to protect the insertion site. The site is usually left open to air.	Decreases risk for infection.
15. **See Completion Protocol (inside front cover).**	

EVALUATION

1. Measure GRV per facility policy, usually every 4 to 6 hours, and ask if nausea or abdominal cramping is present.
2. Monitor fingerstick blood glucose level (Chapter 8) as ordered, especially in patients at risk (e.g., diabetes, renal failure).
3. Monitor I&O at least every 8 hours, and calculate daily totals every 24 hours.
4. Weigh patient daily until maximum tube feeding rate is reached and maintained for 24 hours and then weigh patient 3 times per week.
5. Monitor laboratory values.
6. Observe patient's respiratory status.
7. Examine abdomen and auscultate bowel sounds.
8. Observe nasoenteral tube insertion site for skin integrity. For tubes placed through the abdominal wall, observe insertion site for skin integrity and symptoms of infection, injury, or tightness of tube.
9. Use **Teach Back:** State to the patient, "We talked about the likelihood of your being on tube feedings when you go home. Tell me what you remember about why it is important to flush the tube regularly." Evaluates what the patient is able to explain or demonstrate. Revise your instruction

now or develop plan for revised patient teaching to be implemented at an appropriate time if patient is not able to teach back correctly.

Unexpected Outcomes and Related Interventions

1. The feeding tube becomes clogged. Frequent aspiration of gastric contents, frequent administration of medications without adequate flushing, and small-diameter tubes increase the risk of clogging (Bankhead et al., 2009).
   a. Attempt to flush the tube with water. Water has been shown to be the most effective and the least costly method to prevent and treat clogged tubes (Bankhead et al., 2009). Use clean tap or sterile water, depending on the patient's immune status.
   b. Special products, such as pancreatic enzymes, are available for unclogging feeding tubes; do not use soda and juice. Obtain an order from the health care provider for the product.
   c. Hold feeding and notify health care provider.
   d. Maintain patient in semi-Fowler's position.
2. GRV exceeds 500 mL once or 250 mL twice (see facility policy).
   a. Hold feeding and notify health care provider.
3. Patient aspirates formula.
   a. See Unexpected Outcomes and Related Interventions in Skill 12.2.
4. Patient develops large amount of diarrhea (more than three loose stools in 24 hours).
   a. Notify health care provider. Meet with RD to determine if need to change formula to provide fiber.
   b. Consider other causes (e.g., intolerance or bacterial contamination of the feeding).
   c. Provide skin care.
   d. Determine if patient is receiving medications (e.g., containing sorbitol) that induce diarrhea.

Recording and Reporting

- Record amount and type of feeding, GRV, infusion rate (continuous feeding), patient's response to tube feeding, patency of tube, and condition of skin at tube site.
- Document your evaluation of patient learning.
- Record volume of formula and any additional water on I&O form.
- Report type of feeding, infusion rate (continuous feeding) status of feeding tube, patient's tolerance, and adverse outcomes.

Sample Documentation

1500   NG Dobhoff feeding tube in place, position confirmed with pH of 4.0. GRV 80 mL, returned to stomach. Continuous feeding of full-strength Isosource HN infusing at 55 mL/hr. Tube irrigates without difficulty. No nasal irritation noted.

Special Considerations
Pediatric

- Sterile liquid formulas for infants are preferred to powdered, reconstituted formulas. Sterile water must be used for reconstitution and all flushes for infants (Bankhead et al., 2009).
- Powdered, reconstituted formula, human breast milk, and enteral feedings with additives cannot hang longer than 4 hours. Formulas for closed systems can hang 24 hours or per the manufacturers' guidelines (Bankhead et al., 2009).

Geriatric

- Some older adults have decreased gastric emptying and formula remains in the stomach longer than for younger patients. GRV checks are of special importance in patients with impaired cognition to decrease the risk for aspiration during gastric feeding.

Hospitalized Adults with Diabetes

- Adult patients with diabetes who receive enteral nutrition should have a target blood glucose of 140 to 180 mg/dL (ASPEN, 2013).
- Interruption of tube feeding can lead to hypoglycemia (blood glucose <70 mg/dL). Carbohydrate replacement, such as with dextrose IV fluids, should replace tube feedings when the patient is on basal insulin and the tube feeding is interrupted (Jacobi et al., 2012).

Home Care

- Instruct family caregiver and patient on:
  - How to administer feedings and monitor for symptoms of discomfort, diarrhea, and aspiration.
  - How to monitor I&O using household measuring devices.
  - How to provide skin care around tube insertion sites (see Procedural Guideline 12.1).

PROCEDURAL GUIDELINE 12.1
Site Care of Enteral Feeding Tubes

The exit site for feeding tubes, including the nose and abdominal surface, can easily become irritated from rubbing of a tube against the skin. Patients develop small ulcers of the nasal mucosa when feeding tubes have been in place a prolonged period and when adequate site care has not been provided. Although gastrostomy and jejunostomy tubes often have small dressings in place around the tube insertion site, irritation and erosion of the skin can lead to infection. Routine assessment and provision of site care make patients more comfortable and reduce the incidence of skin complications.

PROCEDURAL GUIDELINE 12.1
Site Care of Enteral Feeding Tubes—cont'd

Delegation Considerations

Care of an enteral feeding tube site cannot be delegated to nursing assistive personnel (NAP). The nurse instructs the NAP to:

- Inform the nurse of any patient complaints of discomfort at the insertion site.
- Inform the nurse of any drainage on the insertion site dressing.

Equipment

- Normal saline, dated and initialed container at patient's bedside
- 4 × 4–inch gauze dressings
- Tube fixation device; hypoallergenic tape, or transparent dressing (for NG tube)
- Prepared drain-gauze dressing (for gastrostomy and jejunostomy tubes)
- Tape, tincture of benzoin, skin barrier protectant
- Clean gloves

Procedural Steps

1. Identify patient using two identifiers (e.g., name and birthday or name and account number) according to facility policy. *Rationale: Ensures correct patient. Complies with The Joint Commission standards and improves patient safety (TJC, 2014b).*
2. Inspect the condition of the skin at the tube exit site, looking for inflammation, bleeding, excoriation, drainage, and tenderness. In the case of gastrostomy and jejunostomy tubes, if a dressing is in place, defer inspection until dressing is removed. *Rationale: Provides baseline for condition of exit site.*
3. For an NG tube, note the position of the ink mark at exit site indicating tube location. *Rationale: Provides reference point to prevent accidental pulling or advancement of tube.*
4. Determine whether gastrostomy or jejunostomy exit site is to be left open to air or covered with a dressing. Check health care provider's order or verify facility policy.

5. See Standard Protocol (inside front cover).
6. 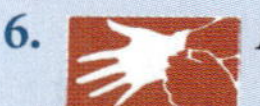 Apply clean gloves.
7. *Care of NG tube site:*
    a. Use your nondominant hand to anchor the NG tube as you remove the old tape, commercial fixation device, or transparent dressing that anchors the tube.
    b. With tape or fixation device removed, inspect again the condition of the skin and naris.
    c. Take a 4 × 4–gauze dressing moistened in normal saline and gently cleanse around the exit site. Remove any tape residue.
    d. Replace the old fixation device with new tape, transparent dressing, or commercial fixation device (see Skill 12.3).
8. *Care of gastrostomy and jejunostomy site:*
    a. Remove old dressing (if present) and discard in appropriate container.
    b. Assess exit site for evidence of excoriation, drainage, infection, or bleeding.
    c. Cleanse skin around site with warm water and mild soap using 4 × 4–inch gauzes.
    d. Rotate external bumper 90 degrees (see Fig. 12-3).
    e. Dry site completely. Apply thin layer of protective skin barrier to exit site if indicated (e.g., site excoriated).
    f. If dressing is ordered, place drain-gauze dressing over external bar. Note: Do not place dressing under external bar; this can cause gastric tissue erosion or internal abdominal wall pressure.
    g. Secure dressing with tape.
    h. Place date, time, and initials on new dressing.
9. See Completion Protocol (inside front cover).
10. Document in nurses' notes appearance of exit site, drainage noted, and dressing application.
11. Report to health care provider any exit site complications.
12. Routinely evaluate condition of exit site every shift.

CRITICAL THINKING EXERCISES

Case Study

The nurse is caring for a patient with a closed head injury admitted after a motor vehicle accident. A small-bore feeding tube has been placed in the small bowel for short-term nutritional needs until the patient is able to eat. The patient is receiving a continuous infusion of tube-feeding formula. The patient weighed 84.1 kg (185 pounds) before feedings were initiated.

1. When the nurse checks the position of the tube, which of the following pH values and aspirate descriptions should be expected?
    1. 8.0 and watery, blood-tinged aspirate
    2. 6.0 and bile-stained, brownish green aspirate
    3. 4.0 and grassy green aspirate
    4. 2.0 and colorless aspirate

2. The nurse prepares to irrigate the feeding tube to prevent clogging. In which clinical scenario should the nurse use sterile water for irrigation?
   1. When the pH of gastric aspirate is <5
   2. During routine irrigation every 4 hours
   3. Before administering crushed time-released medications
   4. When the patient receiving a tube feeding is immunocompromised

Review Questions

1. A nurse is assigned to a patient with the diagnosis of stroke, which is affecting the left side of his body. Which of the following suggest that the patient is at risk for aspiration? Select all that apply.
   1. Wet voice
   2. Difficulty smiling
   3. Coughing on food
   4. Aversion to food
   5. Change in taste
2. When feeding a patient who is known to have dysphagia, which of the following interventions prevents gastric reflux?
   1. Monitoring pulse oximetry readings
   2. Providing patient oral hygiene before feeding
   3. Positioning patient upright in a chair
   4. Adding thickener to thin liquids
3. A nurse observes a student nurse performing an irrigation of a feeding tube for a patient receiving a continuous tube feeding. Which of the following observations by the nurse suggests teaching has been successful?
   1. At 4 hours after the last irrigation, the student draws up 30 mL of air into an irrigating syringe, instills the air into the feeding tube, withdraws fluid to verify placement, kinks tubing, draws up 30 mL of water into irrigating syringe, inserts syringe tip into end of feeding tube, and irrigates tube.
   2. At 8 hours after the last irrigation, the student draws up 30 mL of air into an irrigating syringe, instills the air into the feeding tube, withdraws fluid to verify placement, kinks tubing, draws up 30 mL of water into irrigating syringe, inserts syringe tip into end of feeding tube, and irrigates tube.
   3. At 4 hours after the last irrigation, the student draws up 30 mL of air into an irrigating syringe, instills it into the feeding tube, draws up 30 mL of water into irrigating syringe, inserts syringe into end of feeding tube, and irrigates tube.
   4. At 8 hours after the last irrigation, the student draws up 30 mL of air into an irrigating syringe, instills it into the feeding tube, draws up 30 mL of water into irrigating syringe, inserts syringe into end of feeding tube, and irrigates tube.
4. A patient on a medical oncology unit has been receiving continuous tube feedings for the last 2 days. During a morning assessment, the nurse gathers information about the patient's tolerance and response to NG feedings. Which of the following are unexpected outcomes of the feedings? Select all that apply.
   1. The patient shows signs of aspiration.
   2. The patient develops symptoms of constipation.
   3. The patient's tube yields a gastric residual volume of 300 mL.
   4. The patient's tube cannot be irrigated.
   5. The patient has a small ulcer on the inner naris.
5. When a nurse educates patients and families about their nutritional needs, food safety is an important topic. Which of the following precautions ensure that it is safe to eat prepared foods? Select all that apply.
   1. Wash hands with warm soapy water before touching food.
   2. Encourage intake of unpasteurized milk.
   3. Keep foods properly refrigerated at 4.4° C (40° F).
   4. Do not save leftovers for more than 1 week in the refrigerator.
6. A patient is 2 days postoperative and has normal GI function but is unable to chew because of facial surgery. This patient would most likely receive which of the following for his nutritional needs:
   1. Clear-liquid diet
   2. High-fiber diet
   3. Mechanical diet
   4. Pureed diet
7. The nurse caring for a patient in a nursing home notices that the patient routinely has a bowel movement every 3 to 4 days and sometimes the stool is reportedly hard in consistency. The patient is alert and able to tolerate solid foods. The patient wears dentures. The best diet selection for this patient would be:
   1. Pureed diet
   2. High-fiber diet
   3. Fat-modified diet
   4. Low-residue diet
8. A patient on the neurosurgery unit is recovering from a traumatic injury resulting in an unstable vertebral fracture. The patient is ordered to remain supine and is on an air fluidized bed to prevent pressure ulcers. Which of the following positions does the nurse have the patient assume before a tube feeding?
   1. Head of bed elevated 90 degrees
   2. Reverse Trendelenburg's position
   3. Side-lying position
   4. Trendelenburg's position

9. When caring for a patient on continuous tube feedings, the nurse should take what action?
   1. Stop tube feedings 30 minutes before and after medication administration.
   2. Change the closed feeding system every week.
   3. Mix all of the medications together in 30 mL of water before administration.
   4. Place the head of bed up to at least 30 to 45 degrees.

10. A nurse is preparing to administer an intermittent tube feeding via a closed system. Place the following steps for this procedure in the correct order.
    a. Check for gastric residual volume (GRV).
    b. Connect distal end of administration set tubing to end of feeding tube. Set rate by placing on a feeding pump.
    c. Flush feeding tube.
    d. Verify tube placement.
    e. Connect administration tubing to prepared feeding container.
    f. Place patient in high-Fowler's position.
    g. Pinch proximal end of feeding tube and remove cap.

REFERENCES

Academy of Nutrition and Dietetics: *Nutrition care manual*, 2012. http://www.nutritioncaremanual.org. Accessed August 24, 2012.

American Academy of Pediatrics (AAP): *Infant food and feeding*, 2012. http://www.aap.org/en-us/advocacy-and-policy/aap-health-initiatives/HALF-Implementation-Guide/Age-Specific-Content/Pages/Infant-Food-and-Feeding.aspx. Accessed January 2014.

American Association of Critical Care Nurses (AACN): *Verification of feeding tube placement (blindly inserted), AACN Practice Alert 2010*, 2010. http://www.aacn.org/WD/Practice/Docs/PracticeAlerts/Verification_of_Feeding_Tube_Placement_05-2005.pdf. Accessed June 21, 2014.

American Association of Critical Care Nurses (AACN): AACN practice alerts: prevention of aspiration, *Crit Care Nurse* 32(3):71, 2012.

American Society for Parenteral and Enteral Nutrition (ASPEN): Clinical guidelines: nutrition support of adult patients with hyperglycemia, *JPEN J Parenter Enteral Nutr* 37(1):23, 2013.

Bankhead R, et al: ASPEN Enteral nutrition practice recommendations, *JPEN J Parenter Enteral Nutr* 33(2):122, 2009.

Chang C, Roberts B: Strategies for feeding patients with dementia, *Am J Nurs* 111(4):36, 2011.

Choban P, et al: A.S.P.E.N. clinical guidelines: nutrition support of hospitalized adult patients with obesity, *JPEN J Parenter Enteral Nutr* 37(6):714, 2013.

Dandeles LM, Lodolce AE: Efficacy of agents to prevent and treat enteral feeding tube clogs, *Ann Pharmacother* 45(5):676, 2011.

DeLegge MH: Managing gastric residual volumes in the critically ill patient: an update, *Curr Opin Nutr Metab Care* 14(2):193, 2011.

Gilbert RT, Burns SM: Increasing the safety of blind gastric tube placement in pediatric patients: the design and testing of a procedure using a carbon dioxide detection device, *J Pediatr Nurs* 27(5):528, 2012.

Gilbertson HR, et al: Determination of practical pH cutoff level for reliable confirmation of nasogastric tube placement, *JPEN J Parenter Enteral Nutr* 35(4):540, 2011.

Grodner M, et al: *Nutritional foundations and clinical applications: a nursing approach*, ed 5, St Louis, 2013, Mosby.

Hammond K, Litchford M: Dietary and clinical assessment. In Mahan LK, Escott Stump S, Raymond JL, editors: *Krause's food nutrition and the nutrient care process*, ed 13, Philadelphia, 2012, Saunders.

Hines S, et al: Identification and nursing management of dysphagia in individuals with acute neurological impairment (update), *Int J Evid Based Healthc* 9(2):148, 2011.

Jacobi J, et al: Guidelines for the use of an insulin infusion for the management of hyperglycemia in critically ill patients, *Crit Care Med* 40(12):3251, 2012.

Kitler P, et al: *Food and culture*, Belmont, CA, 2012, Wadsworth, Cengage Learning.

Krenitsky J: Blind bedside placement of feeding tubes: treatment or threat? *Pract Gastroenterol* XXXV(3):32, 2011.

Lalla RV, et al: Oral complications of cancer therapy. In Yagiela JA, et al, editors: *Pharmacology and therapeutics for dentistry*, ed 6, St Louis, 2011, Elsevier.

Mahan LK, et al, editors: *Krause's food nutrition and the nutrient care process*, ed 13, Philadelphia, 2012, Saunders.

Makic MB, et al: Evidence-based practice habits: putting more sacred cows out to pasture, *Crit Care Nurse* 31(2):38, 2011.

McClave SA, et al: Guidelines for the provision and assessment of nutrition support therapy in the adult critically ill patient: Society of Critical Care Medicine (SCCM) and American Society for Parenteral and Enteral Nutrition (A.S.P.E.N), *JPEN J Parenter Enteral Nutr* 33(3):277, 2009.

McGinnis C: The feeding tube bridle: one inexpensive, safe, and effective method to prevent inadvertent feeding tube dislodgement, *Nutr Clin Pract* 26(1):70, 2011.

Meals on Wheels Association of America: *FAQ*, 2013. http://www.mowaa.org/index.asp. Accessed August 2013.

Metheny NA: *Preventing aspiration in older adults with dysphagia, Best Practices in Nursing Care to Older Adults*, 2012, The Hartford Institute for Geriatric Nursing, New York University, College of Nursing. http://consultgerirn.org/uploads/File/trythis/try_this_20.pdf. Accessed June 2014.

Metheny NA, Frantz RA: Head-of-bed elevation in critically ill patients: a review, *Crit Care Nurse* 33(3):53, 2013.

Metheny NA, Meert KL: A review of published case reports of inadvertent pulmonary placement of nasogastric tubes in children, *J Pediatr Nurs* 29(1):e7, 2013.

Metheny NA, et al: Effectiveness of an aspiration risk-reduction protocol, *Nurs Res* 59(1):18, 2010.

Miles A, et al: Comparison of cough reflex test against instrumental assessment of aspiration, *Physiol Behav* 118(13):25, 2013.

National Cancer Institute (NCI): Oral Mucositis, Available at: http://www.cancer.gov/cancertopics/pdq/supportivecare/oralcomplications/HealthProfessional/page5. Accessed 6/20/14.

National Dysphagia Diet Task Force (NDDTF): *National dysphagia diet: standardization for optimal care*, Chicago, 2002, American Dietetic Association.

National Stroke Association: *Dysphagia symptoms*, 2013. http://www.stroke.org. Retrieved August 2013.

Nix S: *Williams' basic nutrition and diet therapy*, ed 14, St Louis, 2013, Mosby.

Proehl JA, et al: Emergency nursing resource: gastric tube placement verification, *J Emerg Nurs* 37(4):357, 2011.

Remig V, Weeden A: Medical nutrition therapy for neurologic disorders. In Mahan LK, Escott Stump S, Raymond JL, editors: *Krause's food nutrition and the nutrient care process*, ed 13, Philadelphia, 2012, Saunders.

Simons SR, Abdallah LM: Bedside assessment of enteral tube placement: aligning practice with evidence, *Am J Nurs* 112(2):40, 2012.

Simmons D, et al: Tubing misconnections: normalization of deviance, *Nutr Clin Pract* 26(3):286, 2011.

Stepter CR: Maintaining placement of temporary enteral feeding tubes in adults: a critical appraisal of the evidence, *Medsurg Nurs* 21(2):61, 2012.

Tada A, Miura H: Prevention of aspiration pneumonia (AP) with oral care, *Arch Gerontol Geriatr* 55(1):16, 2011.

Tanner DC: Lessons from nursing home dysphagia malpractice litigation, *J Gerontol Nurs* 36(3):41, 2010.

Taylor SJ, et al: Treating delayed gastric emptying in critical illness: metoclopramide, erythromycin, and bedside (Cortrak)

nasointestinal tube placement, *JPEN J Parenter Enteral Nutr* 34(3):289, 2010.

Terre R, Mearin F: Effectiveness of chin-down posture to prevent tracheal aspiration in dysphagia secondary to acquired brain injury. A videofluoroscopy study, *Neurogastroenterol Motil* 24(5):414, 2012.

The Joint Commission (TJC): *2014 Hospital Accreditation Standards*, Oakbrook Terrace, IL, 2014a.

The Joint Commission (TJC): *National Patient Safety Goals*, Oakbrook Terrace, IL, 2014b, The Commission. Available at: http://www.jointcommission.org/standards_information/npsgs.aspx.

Tho PC, et al: Implementation of the evidence review on best practice for confirming the correct placement of nasogastric tube in patients in an acute care hospital, *Int J Evid Based Healthc* 9(1):51, 2011.

Touhy T, Jett K: *Ebersole and Hess' gerontological nursing & healthy aging*, ed 4, St Louis, 2014, Elsevier.

Tutor JD, Gosa MM: Dysphagia and aspiration in children, *Pediatr Pulmonol* 47(4):321, 2012.

U.S. Food and Drug Administration (FDA): *Safety information: Simplythick: public health notification—risk of life-threatening bowel condition*, 2011. http://www.fda.gov/Safety/MedWatch/SafetyInformation/SafetyAlertsforHumanMedicalProducts/ucm256257.htm. Accessed February 2014.

Pain Management

Pain is the most common reason a person seeks health care. Patients experience various forms of stress, undergo painful procedures, and experience painful illnesses. Also, the experience of staying in a health care environment and the symptoms of diseases disrupt a patient's comfort level. Assisting patients with achieving comfort is a challenge. Your responsibilities as a nurse include creating a safe, comfortable environment and consistently applying principles of pain management. A key measure of the Hospital Consumer Assessment of Healthcare Providers and Systems (HCAHPS) satisfaction survey is patients' perceptions of pain control and health care providers' efforts to control pain. A study of surgical patients showed that their satisfaction was more strongly correlated with the perception that caregivers did everything possible to control pain than with pain actually being well controlled (Hanna et al., 2012).

Adequate pain management is a priority for health care facilities. Patients expect health care providers to provide good pain control. The Joint Commission (2014a) has set standards requiring that patients' reports of pain are to be addressed and appropriately treated. Optimal pain management is every patient's right. Many people receive inadequate pain relief for conditions that could be treated or managed (IOM, 2011; Pasero and McCaffery, 2011). The Agency for Healthcare Research and Quality, the American Pain Society,

and the World Health Organization have written guidelines for pain management. The pain management skills in this text are for use alone or in combination, depending on a patient's needs.

One approach to pain management included in this chapter is the use of hot and cold therapies. Local application of moderate heat and cold to a body part provides comfort and pain relief, reduces muscle spasm, improves mobility, and can promote healing of local tissues. The therapeutic effects of heat and cold result from changes in blood flow to an area. Many heat and cold therapies can be used in the home, and you are required to instruct patients and family caregivers thoroughly on safe and proper use.

PATIENT-CENTERED CARE

Pain is unique to each individual. Cultural differences in response to pain add to the challenges of assessing pain correctly. Effective pain management begins with a complete patient assessment, which includes a person's coping style, physical status, past experiences with pain and how it was managed, cultural habits and beliefs, and emotional health. Although people experience pain sensations similarly, research shows that there are important differences in the way people express their pain and expect others to respond to their discomfort (Carteret, 2011). Culturally based attitudes and beliefs exist about using medications and other treatments for pain. Members of some cultural minority groups frequently receive suboptimal pain management because of their difficulty in communicating their pain experience and are at risk for poor pain outcomes (Narayan, 2010).

Culture influences how people experience and respond to pain, including when and how to ask for treatment (Narayan, 2010). Patients' culturally based responses to pain are divided into two categories: stoic and emotive. Stoic patients are less expressive of their pain and often withdraw socially, whereas emotive patients are more likely to verbalize their expressions of pain and prefer to have people around them to listen (Carteret, 2011). Nurses must be aware of the cultural beliefs, values, and attitudes that influence their own response to pain and not stereotype patients by assuming that all patients will adhere to their particular culture's pain pattern (Narayan, 2010). Making such generalizations masks your ability to assess a patient's true pain experience accurately. Instead, it is critical that you approach each patient individually and not assess his or her needs in light of your own cultural norms or attitudes.

A factual, timely, and accurate pain assessment requires you to work closely with patients and their families and to explore the pain experience through the eyes of patients. Remain objective, listen, and explore thoroughly any symptoms that a patient expresses. Effective therapeutic communication is key to diagnosing a patient's pain accurately and subsequently intervening appropriately. Nurses often do not use interpreters when interviewing patients who are not proficient in English. When patients are nonverbal, remember that their expressions and activity level can vary by culture, and accurate assessment tools are needed. The following principles of patient-centered care offer a foundation for meeting patients' cultural needs and preferences (Pasero and McCaffery, 2011):

- Understand a patient as a unique person.
- Explore the patient's experiences of illness and pain.
- Observe and perceive pain management from a patient's perspective.
- Promote shared decision making and adapt care to meet a patient's needs and expectations.

SAFETY

Safe pain management begins with trying the least invasive therapy first along with previously used successful pain relief techniques. For example, a home health nurse might learn that repositioning a patient, controlling room noise, and giving a patient a cup of herbal tea helps the patient relax and fall asleep even while experiencing chronic back pain. Do not undertreat pain. Patients who receive opioids for chronic pain often require higher doses of analgesics to alleviate new or increased pain; this is tolerance, not an early sign of addiction. Drug-drug interactions, including enhanced or reduced effects or side effects, often occur with the multiple drug use

required by people with chronic pain. The use of multiple drugs to manage chronic pain is called rational polypharmacy (Pasero and McCaffery, 2011). Although 0 is an ideal goal for a pain level, it is often unrealistic for patients with chronic or persistent pain. Many people are able to do most of the things they desire at low pain intensity, such as 1, 2, or even 3 on a 0 to 10 pain scale. Always know a patient's goal for pain relief.

Protect a patient's skin from injury when using therapeutic heat or cold applications. Normally, when the skin is exposed to a warm or cold application, sensory adaptation occurs quickly. Although a patient may initially feel a temperature extreme, once the sensory receptors adapt, the patient may become unaware of any temperature variation. Excessive heat eventually causes a burning sensation, whereas excessive cold causes a numbing sensation before pain is sensed. Because the body adapts quickly to a temperature extreme, there is a high risk for tissue injury. Certain patients, such as patients with diabetes and conditions causing circulatory insufficiency, are at risk for skin injury. Precautions are also needed in patients with reduced sensation from spinal cord injuries or the ability to perceive sensation as in dementia.

EVIDENCE-BASED PRACTICE

Abdulla A et al: Guidance on the management of pain in older people, *Age Ageing* 42(Suppl 1):i1, 2013.

A literature review of studies involving management of pain in older adults has resulted in a set of best practices (Abdulla et al., 2013). There is inconsistent evidence as to whether pain increases or decreases in older adults and whether it is influenced by gender. However, the prevalence of pain is higher in patients who live in residential care settings. The three most common pain sites in older people are the back; leg, knee, or hip; and "other joints." Research offers best practice guidelines for the management of pain in older adults:

- Consider acetaminophen (Tylenol) a first-line treatment for management of acute and persistent pain, particularly musculoskeletal pain, because of its efficacy and good safety profile.
- Use nonselective nonsteroidal antiinflammatory drugs (NSAIDs) with caution in older patients after other, safer treatments have been used. Give the lowest dose provided, for the shortest duration.
- Opioids may be considered for patients with moderate or severe pain, especially if the pain causes functional impairment or reduced quality of life. However, patients should simultaneously receive appropriate laxatives (e.g., stool softener and stimulant laxative).
- Older adults often use assistive devices to live actively with chronic pain. However, the devices do not reduce pain and can increase pain if used incorrectly.
- Pain relief may be gained by increasing activity with exercise, including strengthening, flexibility, endurance and balance.

SKILL 13.1   NONPHARMACOLOGICAL PAIN MANAGEMENT

Effective pain management does not mean the elimination of pain. Many nonpharmacological interventions are available to lessen a patient's pain in any health care setting. Some of these interventions are classified as complementary or alternative therapies, and there is evidence to support pain relief (NIH, NCCAM, 2011). For example, massage therapy has been shown to significantly reduce pain, anxiety, and muscular tension while improving relaxation and satisfaction after cardiac surgery (Braun et al., 2012). Use these interventions in combination with pharmacological measures, not in place of medications, unless the pain is minor. Nonpharmacological techniques diminish the physical effects of pain, alter a patient's perception of pain, and provide a patient with a greater sense of control (Box 13-1).

Many nonpharmacological techniques trigger a relaxation response by stimulating the parasympathetic nervous system. Because pain often causes muscle tension and anxiety, stimulation of the parasympathetic nervous system relieves these responses (Baird et al., 2010; Drew and St. Marie, 2011). Nonpharmacological interventions are appropriate for patients who find such interventions appealing, express anxiety or fear, may benefit from avoiding or reducing drug therapy, and have incomplete pain relief with pharmacological interventions alone.

ASSESSMENT

1. Assess patients' risk for pain (e.g., patients undergoing invasive procedures, anxious patients, patients unable to communicate). *Rationale: Allows you to anticipate occurrence of pain and need for pain control.*

BOX 13-1   NONPHARMACOLOGICAL MEASURES FOR PAIN*

Relaxation and Power of the Mind
- Progressive muscle relaxation
- Breathing exercises
- Music relaxation
- Visual imagery
- Yoga

Put Your Body to Work
- Exercise
- Pacing
- Conserving energy
- Body mechanics

Spirituality and Reflection
- Engaging in religious practices
- Humor
- Setting aside time to focus on what *is*
- Talking about your stress with others
- Journaling
- Praying

What to Do When Pain Flares
- Cold and hot therapies
- Hand and foot massage
- Herbals†

*Should be used with analgesics.
†Herbals could interact with prescribed analgesics; check with health care provider.

2. Assess the patient's language level, and use an interpreter if necessary. Identify descriptive terms that the patient is likely to use to describe pain. *Rationale: Ensures more accurate pain assessment. Patients often use different terms than the terms used by health care providers to describe their pain. Some languages have no equivalent for the English word "pain" (Narayan, 2010).*

3. Ask patients if they are in pain and if they are willing to receive nonpharmacological relief measures. *Rationale: There is no objective test to measure pain. Accept a patient's report of pain. Patient acceptance increases effectiveness of a therapy.*

4. Assess characteristics of the patient's pain. Follow facility policy regarding frequency. Use the *PQRSTU* of pain assessment:
   - *P—Precipitating/palliative factors* (e.g., "What makes your pain better or worse?" "What have you used to relieve pain?"). Consider patient's experience with over-the-counter (OTC) drugs (including herbals and topicals) that have reduced pain in the past. *Rationale: Identifies possible sources of pain and what the patient uses to reduce the discomfort.*
   - *Q—Quality.* Use open-ended questions such as, "Tell me what your pain feels like." *Rationale: Helps determine underlying pain mechanism (e.g., somatic versus neuropathic pain).*
   - *R—Region/radiation* (e.g., "Show me where your pain is"). Have patient use finger (if possible) to point out area or areas of pain.
   - *S—Severity.* Use a valid pain rating scale (Figs. 13-1, 13-2, and 13-3) appropriate to patient's age, developmental level, and comprehension. Have patients rate their pain before any intervention. Also assess pain when patient is moving, not just lying in bed or sitting in a chair. *Rationale: An appropriate pain rating scale is reliable, is easy to use and understand, and reflects changes in pain severity (Herr, 2011).*
   - *T—Timing.* Ask if pain is constant, intermittent, continuous, or a combination. Does pain increase during specific times of day or during certain activities?

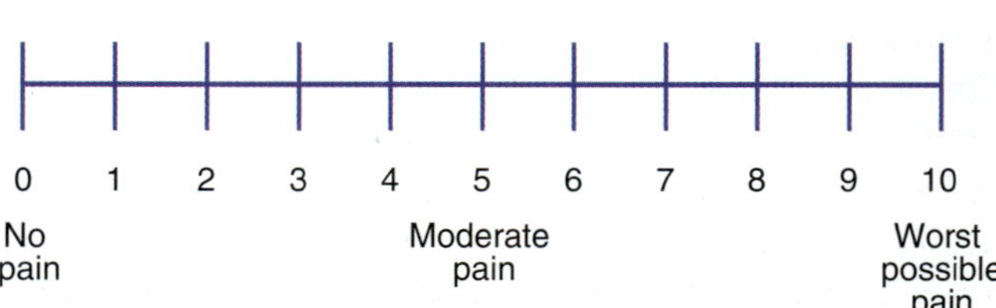

FIG 13-1 0-10 Numeric Pain Rating Scale. (From Pasero C, McCaffery M: *Pain assessment and pharmacologic management,* St Louis, 2011, Mosby.)

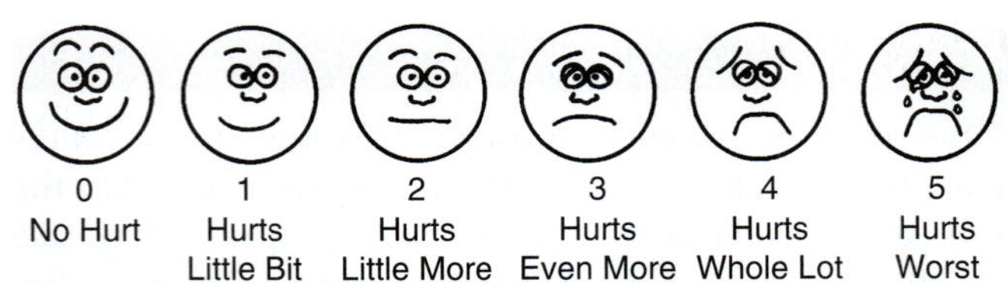

FIG 13-2 Wong-Baker FACES Pain Rating Scale. (From Hockenberry MJ, Wilson D: *Wong's essentials of pediatric nursing,* ed 9, St Louis, 2013, Mosby.)

OUCHER®

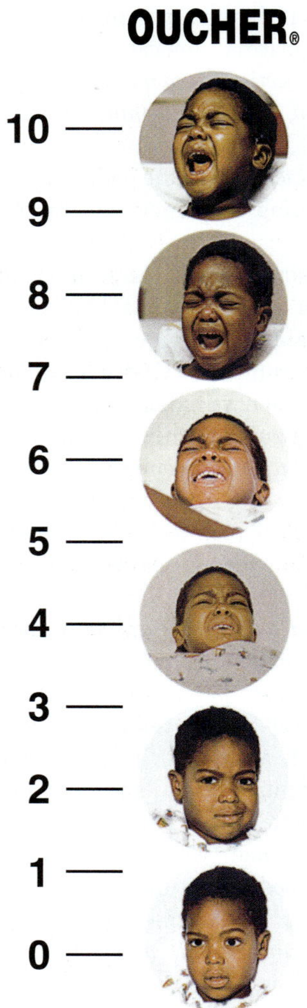

FIG 13-3 The Oucher Pain Scale. Hispanic and Caucasian versions are also available. (African-American version developed and copyrighted in 1990 by Mary J. Denyes, PhD, RN [Wayne State University], and Antonia M. Villarruel, PhD, RN [University of Michigan]. Cornelia P. Porter, PhD, RN, and Charlotta Marshall, RN, MSN, contributed to the development of the scale).

Rationale: Environmental stimuli, such as loud noises, bright lights, or temperature extremes, sometimes affect a patient's response to pain.

- *U*—U stands for the patient ("you") in "How is pain affecting *U* regarding activities of daily living (ADLs),

BOX 13-2 **PAIN ASSESSMENT IN A NONVERBAL PATIENT**

Recommended Assessment Approaches

- Attempt a self-report of pain using simple yes/no response or vocalizations; otherwise explain why self-report cannot be used.
- Search for the potential cause of pain through physical examination techniques (e.g., palpation).
- Assume that pain is present after ruling out other problems (infection, constipation) that cause it.
- Identify pathological conditions or procedures that may cause pain.
- Observe patient behaviors that indicate pain. These vary based on patient's developmental level.
- Ask family members, parents, and caregivers for a surrogate report.

Using a Behavioral Pain Assessment Tool

- Use reliable and valid tools to ensure that appropriate criteria are used in assessment (e.g., NOPPAIN for older adults).
- Select an appropriate scale for each patient (e.g., a visual analogue scale versus a FACES scale); no one scale is required for all specific groups of patients.
- Vital signs are not sensitive indicators for the presence of pain.

NOPPAIN, Non-Communicative Patient's Pain Assessment Instrument.
Adapted from Rose L et al: Behavioral pain assessment tool for critically ill adults unable to self-report pain, *Am J Crit Care 22(3):* 255, 2013.

work, relationships, and enjoyment of life?" *Rationale: Provides baseline to gauge effectiveness of interventions later.*

5. Examine site of patient's pain or discomfort. Inspect (discoloration or swelling) and palpate (change in temperature, area of altered sensation, painful area, and range of motion [ROM] of involved joints) the area. *Rationale: Reveals the nature of the pain and directs you toward appropriate interventions.*

6. Assess factors that influence perception of pain (e.g., past pain history and ability to cope, depression, fatigue, loneliness, anxiety, fear). *Rationale: Factors significantly reduce patients' ability to cope with pain.*

7. Assess patients' culturally determined beliefs about pain and pain treatment and how they express pain. *Rationale: Culture influences the meaning pain holds for a patient and how a patient reacts to discomfort.*

8. Assess physical, behavioral, and emotional signs and symptoms of pain. In cognitively impaired or nonverbal patients, use a behavioral pain assessment tool (Box 13-2). *Rationale: May reveal source and nature of pain. Nonverbal responses to pain are especially useful in assessing pain in patients who are cognitively impaired or nonverbal.*

a. Moaning, crying, whimpering, groaning, or vocalizations

b. Decreased activity

c. Facial expressions (e.g., frown, grimace, clenched teeth)

d. Change in usual behavior (e.g., less active, irritable)

e. Abnormal gait (e.g., shuffling) and posture (e.g., bent, leaning)

f. Guarding a body part (e.g., holding side)

g. Diaphoresis

h. Increased blood glucose level reflecting stress of unrelieved pain

i. Decreased gastrointestinal motility, nausea, and vomiting

j. Insomnia, anorexia, and fatigue

k. Depression, hopelessness, anger, fear, and social withdrawal

l. Concomitant symptoms—symptoms that often occur with pain (e.g., headache, nausea, constipation)

9. Assess for presence of noise, temperature, or bright lights when patient perceives pain. *Rationale: Environmental factors may intensify perception of discomfort.*

10. Review health care provider's orders for pain relief and activity or positioning restrictions. *Rationale: Affects choices used in positioning and massage.*

11. Assess patient's preferred activities for pain relief, including listening to music (determine preferences of vocal, instrumental, or both and classical, jazz, or other style), interactive activities (e.g., puzzles, board games), crocheting or knitting, and listening to relaxation tapes. *Rationale: Assists in selection of individualized method for relaxation.*

PLANNING

Expected Outcomes focus on attaining comfort and pain relief and improving patient's ability to participate in routine activities.

1. Patient verbalizes or expresses nonverbally full or partial pain relief.
2. Patient demonstrates and describes pain-relief measures.
3. Patient's function improves in sleep, appetite, physical activity (e.g., initiates hygiene, walking) and personal relationships.

DELEGATION AND COLLABORATION

Assessment of the patient's pain cannot be delegated to nursing assistive personnel (NAP). The skill of nonpharmacological pain management strategies may be delegated to NAP. The nurse instructs the NAP about:

- The type of nonpharmacological measures that may work best for the patient.
- Eliminating environmental conditions that enhance pain.
- Providing patient with appropriate rest periods.
- How to adapt interventions based on any positioning or ambulation restrictions.

Equipment

- Pain rating scale
- *Distraction:* Patient's preference (e.g., reading material, video game, puzzles)
- *Relaxation:* Patient's music preference for relaxation, using MP3 player, CD, or radio
- *Massage:* Lotion or oil (consider aroma therapy lotion), sheet, bath towel

IMPLEMENTATION *for* NONPHARMACOLOGICAL PAIN MANAGEMENT

STEPS	RATIONALE
1. **See Standard Protocol (inside front cover).**	

2. Prepare patient's environment.
  a. Temperature suited to patient
  b. Lighting
  c. Sound
  d. Minimize interruptions and coordinate care activities; allow for rest time.
	Temperature and sound extremes can enhance patient's perception of pain. Bright or very dim lighting can aggravate pain sensation. Fatigue increases pain perception.

3. Teach patient how to use pain rating scale (Box 13-3). Explain range of intensity scores and how they relate to measure of pain.	Accurate reporting by patient improves pain assessment and treatment.
4. Set mutual pain-intensity goal with patient (when able) for rest and during routine care activities.	Patient sets individual goal for tolerable pain severity.
5. Give pain-relieving medications as ordered (see Skill 13.2) at least 30 minutes before a nonpharmacological intervention.	When analgesics reach their peak effect, other pain relief measures may be more effective.
6. *Remove or reduce painful stimuli.* a. Assist patient into comfortable position within normal body alignment. Reposition underlying tubes or equipment.	Removes irritants.

Continued

STEPS	RATIONALE

b. Use pillows as needed for alignment and support and to position off of pressure areas (see illustration).

Repositioning reduces strain on muscles and pressure areas, resulting in less stimulation of pain receptors.

c. Smooth wrinkles in bed linens.

Reduces irritation to skin.

d. Loosen any constrictive bandage or device (e.g., blood pressure cuff, elastic bandages, band of elastic hose, intravenous (IV) dressing, and identification band).

Bandage or device encircling extremity may apply pressure and restrict circulation.

7. Reduce or eliminate emotional factors that increase the pain experience.

Fear or anxiety may cause muscle tension and vasoconstriction, which intensify the pain experience.

a. Offer information that reduces anxiety (e.g., explaining the cause of pain if known).

b. Offer patient opportunity to pray (if appropriate).

c. Accept patient, and acknowledge patient's report of pain.

d. Spend time to allow patient to talk about pain; answer questions and listen attentively. Ask, "What makes your pain feel better (or worse)?"

Conveys a sense of caring and interest in patient's welfare.

e. Answer call lights promptly.

Patients in pain expect caregivers to respond quickly when pain worsens.

8. Teach patient how to splint over the site of pain (e.g., using hand or pillow).

Splinting reduces pain by minimizing muscle movement around painful area.

a. Explain purpose of splinting.

Improves patient's ability to deep breathe, cough, and move.

b. Place pillow or a blanket over site of discomfort and assist patient to place hands firmly over area (see illustration).

Splinting immobilizes painful area.

c. Have patient hold area firmly while coughing, deep breathing, and turning.

Splinting decreases movement and subsequent pain during activity.

9. *Massage:*

a. Place patient in comfortable prone or side-lying position. Have patients with breathing difficulties lie on side with head of bed elevated.

Enhances relaxation and exposes area to be massaged.

b. Turn on soft, pleasing music of patient's preference.

Promotes relaxation.

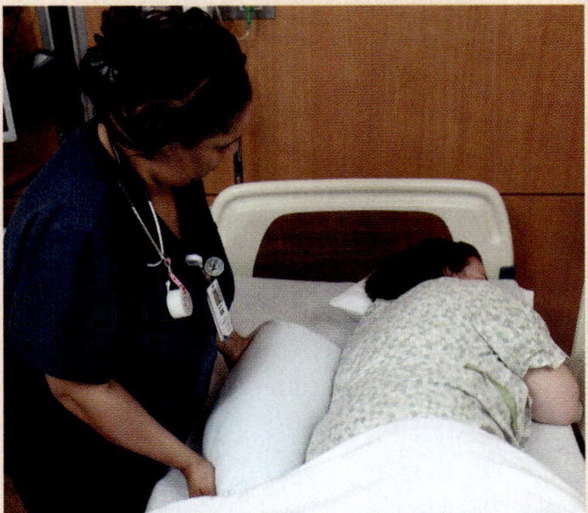

STEP 6b Positioning patient in side-lying lateral position for comfort.

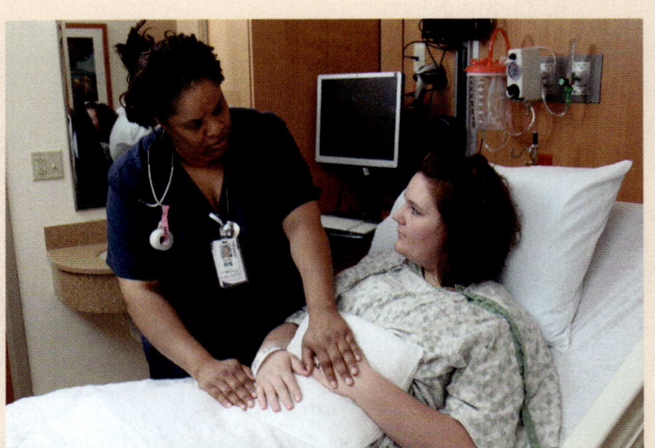

STEP 8b Patient splinting painful area.

STEPS	RATIONALE

c. Have bed in comfortable position for you; lower upper side rail on side where you are standing. Drape patient to expose only the area that you will massage.

Proper body mechanics lessens strain on back. Maintains patient's privacy and warmth.

d. Be sure that patient is not allergic to lotion, and then warm lotion in hands or basin of warm water. (Note: If you choose to massage head and scalp, defer use of lotion until completed.)

Warm lotion is soothing. Warmth helps to produce local muscle relaxation.

e. Choose stroke technique based on desired effect or body part.

Ensures fuller relaxation of body part.

> **SAFE PATIENT CARE** Use very gentle massage with patients who are heavily medicated or unable to communicate because they cannot tell you if massage becomes uncomfortable.

(1) Effleurage (see illustration): Massaging upward and outward from vertebral column and back again.

Gliding stroke, used without manipulating deep muscles. Smoothes and extends muscles, increases nutrient absorption, and improves lymphatic and venous circulation.

(2) Pétrissage (see illustration).

Kneading tense muscle groups promotes relaxation and stimulates local circulation.

(3) Friction.

Strong circular strokes bring blood to surface of skin. Increases local circulation and loosens tight muscles.

f. Ask patient to breathe slowly and deeply and relax during massage.

Potentiates effects of massage.

g. Standing behind patient, tell the patient as you touch the scalp and temples. Then use friction to rub muscles at base of head. Support patient's head.

Avoids startling the patient. Strong circular strokes stimulate local circulation and relaxation.

h. With patient in supine position, massage hands and arms for 5 minutes as appropriate:

Releases tension in hands and arms and promotes relaxation. Studies show that anxious behaviors may be significantly reduced with hand massage (Asadizker et al., 2011).

(1) Support hand and apply friction to palm using both thumbs.

(2) Support base of finger and work each finger in corkscrew-like motion.

(3) Complete hand massage using effleurage strokes from fingertips to wrist.

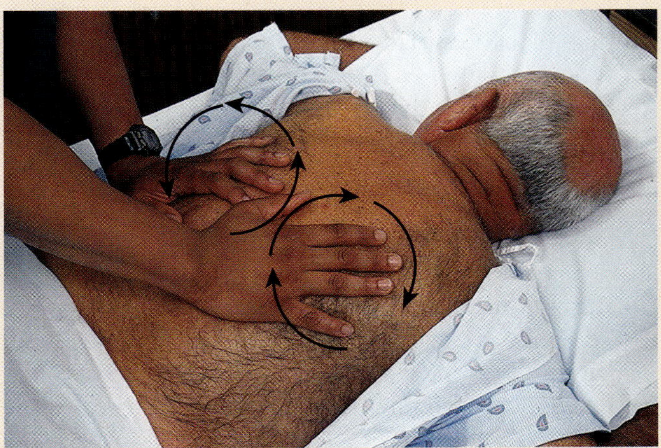

STEP 9e(1) Effleurage.

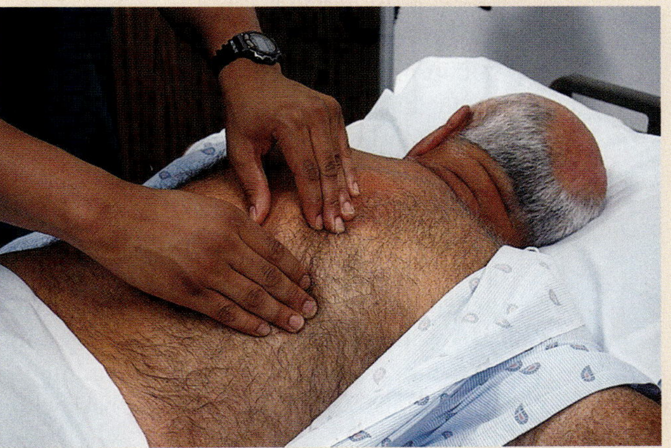

STEP 9e(2) Pétrissage.

Continued

STEPS	RATIONALE

(4) Knead muscles of forearm and upper arm between thumb and forefinger.

i. After determining that patient has no neck injury or condition that contraindicates neck manipulation, massage neck as appropriate.

Massage may be contraindicated after spinal cord injuries or surgery to head and neck because of risk of further injury.

(1) Place patient prone unless contraindicated.

Provides access to neck muscles.

(2) Knead each neck muscle gently between thumb and forefinger.

Reduces tension that often localizes in neck muscles.

j. Massage back as appropriate.

(1) Keep patient in prone position unless contraindicated; side-lying position is an option.

(2) Apply hands first to sacral area; massage in circular motion. Stroke upward from buttocks to shoulders. Massage over scapulas with smooth, firm stroke. Continue in one smooth stroke to upper arms and laterally along sides of back down to iliac crest (see illustration). Continue pattern for 3 minutes.

General firm pressure applied to all muscle groups promotes relaxation.

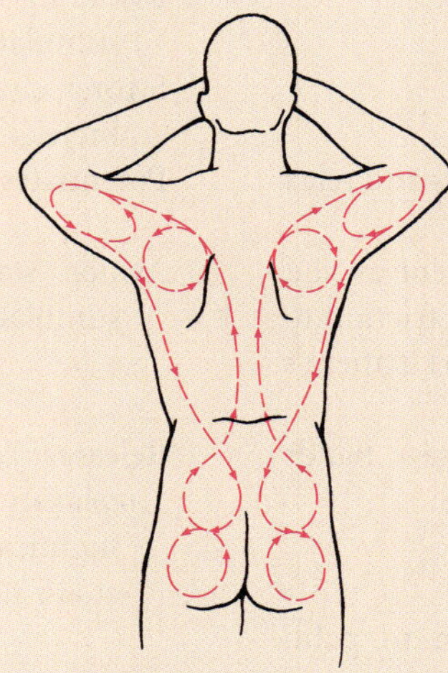

STEP 9j(2) Circular massage of the back.

(3) Use effleurage along muscles of spine in upward and outward motion.

Massage follows distribution of major muscle groups.

(4) Use pétrissage on muscles of each shoulder toward front of patient.

Area often tightens because of tension.

(5) Use palms in upward and outward circular motion from lower buttocks to neck.

Brings blood to surface of skin.

(6) Knead muscles of upper back and shoulder between thumb and forefinger.

These muscles are thick and can be massaged vigorously.

(7) Use both hands to knead muscles up one side of back and then the other side.

(8) End massage with long, stroking effleurage movements.

Most soothing of massage movements.

k. Tell patient that you are ending massage. Ask patient to inhale deeply and exhale. Caution patient to move slowly after resting a few minutes.

Returns patient to a more awake and alert state. When deeply relaxed, patient may experience dizziness on arising too rapidly from postural hypotension.

l. Wipe excess oil or lotion from patient's back with towel.

Excess lotion or oil can irritate skin and cause breakdown.

STEPS	RATIONALE
10. *Distraction:* Use a distraction technique preferred by patient. **a.** Ask patient to close eyes or to focus on single object in the room.	Redirection of attention alters emotional or cognitive aspects of pain (Allred et al., 2010). Allows patient to direct attention inward.
(1) *Music:* Play a music selection for approximately 30 minutes in a location where the patient spends most time. Set volume or loudness at a comfortable level. Emphasize listening to rhythm and adjust volume as pain increases or decreases. Offer earphones if desired.	Music has been shown to create positive psychological outcomes, including decreased anxiety and depression (Zhang et al., 2012).
(2) Prayer.	Helps minimize physical and psychological symptoms of distress.
(3) Describing pictures or discussing pleasant memories.	Reminiscing allows patient to focus on pleasant experiences that were pain-free.
11. See Completion Protocol (inside front cover).	

BOX 13-3   TEACHING PATIENT AND FAMILY HOW TO USE A PAIN RATING SCALE

- Show and briefly explain available pain rating scales and ask which one the patient prefers. Offer vertical and horizontal scales as options.
- Explain the purpose of the scale: "This scale allows us to know how much pain you have and how the pain changes over time as we try to make you more comfortable."
- Explain the range of the scale (e.g., "0 means no pain, whereas 10 means the worst pain you can imagine").
- Discuss pain as a broad concept that is not restricted to a severe or intolerable sensation. Discomfort, hurt, and ache are also pain sensations.
- Verify that patient understands the concept of pain. Ask patient to give an example of pain experienced in the past.
- Ask patient to practice using the pain rating scale with present pain or select one of patient's examples. Also ask to rate worst and average pain in past 24 hours.

implemented at an appropriate time if caregiver is not able to teach back correctly.

Unexpected Outcomes and Related Interventions

1. Patient reports pain intensity greater than desired or displays nonverbal behavior reflecting pain.
   a. Perform a complete pain reassessment.
   b. Implement alternative nonpharmacological pain-relief measures.
   c. Ask family caregivers what might be helpful.
   d. Consult with health care provider about type of analgesic to give, need to adjust dose, or trying different analgesic or coanalgesic.
2. Patient is unable to concentrate on pain-relief techniques.
   a. Administer analgesics before nonpharmacological measure.
   b. Ensure that environment is conducive to technique.

Recording and Reporting

- Record findings of assessment, interventions, and patient's response to interventions in nurses' notes.
- Document your evaluation of patient or family caregiver learning.
- Record patient response to instruction and feedback, and revise plan of care as needed.
- Report inadequate pain relief (not reaching goal), a reduction in patient function, or adverse effects from pain interventions. Box 13-4 lists suggestions for how to communicate with health care providers about pain.

Sample Documentation

0700   Patient rates pain in left shoulder at 6 (scale 0 to 10). Pain is intermittent and nonradiating. Grimaces during turning, holds shoulder when shifting position. Tylenol No. 3, 2 tablets po given. Repositioned to R side. Back massage provided, with soft jazz music played per request.
0730   Rates shoulder pain at 4. Repositions self more easily.

EVALUATION

1. Ask patient to use a pain rating scale (0 to 10) to rate comfort level after intervention. (Note: The Joint Commission [2014a] requires reassessment of pain based on criteria set by facility [e.g., 60 to 90 minutes after intervention].)
2. Observe patient's facial expression, body language, position, mobility, and relaxation.
3. Ask patient to describe ability to rest, sleep, eat, and participate in usual activities.
4. Use *Teach Back:* State to the family caregiver, "I want to know if you understand how to give your husband a massage; tell me what you have learned about massaging his back and feet." Evaluates what the learner is able to explain or demonstrate. Revise your instruction now or develop plan for revised patient teaching to be

BOX 13-4 **NURSE–HEALTH CARE PROVIDER PAIN COMMUNICATION (SBAR FORMAT)**

Situation: Give your name and where calling from; state patient by name; describe the general nature of the call (e.g., patient's pain severity increased following analgesic and use of positioning); report the most recent analgesic given, dose, and patient response.

Background: Summarize patient's medical diagnosis and condition pertinent to pain event (e.g., 1 day postoperative colon resection, up ambulating first time). Describe use of nonpharmacological measures and their effects.

Assessment: Report character of patient's pain, including current pain rating and effect of pain on patient's behavior and activities.

Recommendation: Suggest a solution on the basis of a clinical practice guideline or your expertise.

Special Considerations

Pediatric

- Adapt distraction strategies to a child's developmental level (e.g., use a pacifier for an infant, offer reading or playing a recording of a favorite story for a preschooler, provide music on a CD player with earphone for a teenager) (Allred et al., 2010; Hockenberry and Wilson, 2013).

- Parents are helpful in providing pain relief. They provide comfort by their presence, conversation, and holding a child.
- Infants and children respond to pain differently than adults based on their personality and development (Hockenberry and Wilson, 2013). For example, they may cry and thrash about, have a shortened attention span, suck or rock, or be quiet and withdrawn. Others may become active when they are in pain.

Geriatric

- Visual, hearing, cognitive, and motor impairments make it difficult for older adults to be able to use distraction. Ensure that glasses, hearing aids, and other assistive devices are in place. Do not assume that complementary or alternative techniques will work on older adults (NIH, NCCAM, 2011).
- Reminiscence (e.g., sharing stories from the past) is an effective form of distraction in older adults.

Home Care

- Consider patient's home living conditions, such as the type of bed and environmental stimuli. A supportive bed and quiet environment enhance sleep and promote pain management.
- Assess the pain management attitudes of family caregivers. Without participation of family caregivers, a patient may not achieve successful pain management.

PROCEDURAL GUIDELINE 13.1
Relaxation and Guided Imagery

Relaxation and guided imagery are often used for relief of pain (acute and chronic), anxiety, and depression. For example, relaxation exercises are effective in reducing postoperative pain for patients who have undergone upper abdominal surgery (Topcu and Findik, 2012). It is also effective in relieving labor pain (Jones et al., 2012). Deep, slow breathing associated with relaxation and guided imagery influences autonomic and pain processing, an essential feature in the modulation of sympathetic arousal and pain perception (Busch et al., 2012).

Relaxation techniques provide patients with self-control when pain occurs. Patients who use relaxation sometimes achieve physiological changes (e.g., decreased pulse, blood pressure, muscle tension) as well as behavioral changes. For effective relaxation, a patient needs to participate and cooperate. Teach relaxation only when a patient is not in acute discomfort or severe pain and is able to concentrate. Explain the techniques in detail. It often takes several coaching sessions before patients reduce pain effectively. A family caregiver can learn how to coach a patient through relaxation. Relaxation techniques have few side effects.

Guided imagery involves using focused concentration to gain relaxation and effectively reduce pain perception and reaction. In guided imagery, a patient draws on personal memories, dreams, and visions to create an image in the mind; concentrates on that image; and gradually becomes less aware of pain. The goal of imagery is to have the patient use one or several of the senses to create a desired image. This image creates a positive psychophysiological response. Use imagery with progressive relaxation or massage or as a distraction (see Skill 13.1). Certification in guided imagery is available nationally through the Academy for Guided Imagery (http://acadgi.com/certificationtraining/index.html).

Delegation and Collaboration

The assessment of the use of relaxation and guided imagery for patients cannot be delegated to nursing assistive personnel (NAP). The exercises of relaxation and guided imagery can be delegated to trained NAP. The nurse instructs the NAP by:

- Identifying and explaining which techniques work best for the patient.

PROCEDURAL GUIDELINE 13.1
Relaxation and Guided Imagery—cont'd

- Making clear the expected patient response.
- Instructing to report a worsening of patient's pain.

Equipment

- Relaxation tape on MP3 player, audiotape, or CD and DVD player

Procedural Steps

1. Assess patient's language level and identify descriptive terms that you will use when guiding patient through relaxation.
2. Assess character of patient's pain, including severity, to establish baseline (see Skill 13.1).
3. Assess facial expressions, nonverbal indications of discomfort (e.g., grimacing, frowning, tone of voice), and body position and movement (e.g., restlessness, muscle tension) to establish baseline.
4. Assess character of patient's respirations to establish baseline.
5. Assess site of pain and underlying probable cause of pain to determine if relaxation approaches are appropriate to use. Site of pain may indicate specific types of pain-relief measures.
6. Review health care provider orders (if required by facility).
7. Assess the type of image that patient would prefer to use in guided imagery to avoid using an image that could prove frightening.
8. Review any restrictions on patient's mobility or positioning.
9. Assess patient's willingness to receive nonpharmacological relief measure.
10. Administer an analgesic 30 minutes before implementing relaxation techniques so that patient can gain a level of comfort needed to practice noninvasive approaches.
11. **See Standard Protocol (inside front cover).**
12. Explain purpose of each technique and what will be expected of patient during activity.
13. Plan time to perform technique when patient is able to concentrate. Prepare patient's environment: control lighting and distractions (from visitors or staff), keep room temperature comfortable for patient, close curtains around patient's bed or close door.
14. *Progressive relaxation with deep breathing:*
    a. Have patient assume a comfortable sitting position: sit with feet uncrossed or lie in a supine position with small pillow under head.
    b. Instruct patient to take several slow, deep diaphragmatic breaths. It may help to have the patient close his or her eyes.
       (1) Explain as follows: "The air coming in through your nose should move downward into your lower belly. Let your belly expand fully. Now breathe out through your mouth or nose (whichever feels more natural). Alternate normal and deep breaths several times. Pay attention to how you feel when you breathe in and breathe out normally and when you breathe deeply. Shallow breathing feels tense, while deep breathing helps you relax."
       (2) Continue the exercise: "To practice, put one hand on your abdomen, just below your belly button. Feel your hand rise about an inch each time you breathe in and fall about an inch each time you breathe out. Your chest will rise slightly, too, along with your belly. Remember to relax your belly so that each time you breathe in, it expands fully. As you breathe out slowly, let yourself sigh out loud."
    c. Avoid hyperventilation.
    d. Coach patient to locate any area of muscle tension and alternate tightening and relaxing all muscle groups for 6 to 7 seconds, beginning at feet and working upward toward head.
       (1) Instruct patient to tighten muscles during inhalation and relax muscles during exhalation.
       (2) As each muscle group relaxes, ask patient to enjoy relaxed feeling and allow mind to drift and think how nice it is to be relaxed. Have patient breathe deeply.
       (3) Calmly explain during exercise that patient may feel sensations of tingling, heaviness, floating, or warmth as relaxation occurs.
       (4) Have patient continue slow deep breaths throughout exercise.
       (5) When finished, have patient inhale deeply, exhale, and then initially move about slowly after resting a few minutes.
15. *Guided imagery:*
    a. Direct patient through relaxation exercise while having him or her focus on an image.
       (1) Instruct patient to imagine that inhaled air is a ball of healing energy.
       (2) Have patient imagine that the inhaled air travels to his or her area of pain.
       (3) Alternatively select an image that patient would like to think about.
       (4) Have patient begin with slow deep breathing.
       (5) Suggest that patient think about going to a pleasant place (e.g., beach, field of flowers, top of mountain) to direct mental image toward a restful place.
       (6) Direct patient to experience all sensory aspects of the restful place (e.g., for beach—warm breeze, sound of surf hitting beach, smell of salt air).
       (7) Direct patient to continue deep, slow, rhythmic breathing to achieve relaxation.

Continued

PROCEDURAL GUIDELINE 13.1
Relaxation and Guided Imagery—cont'd

(8) Direct patient to count to three, inhale, and open eyes.

(9) End the experience. "Experience comfort and relaxation. When you open your eyes, you will feel alert and renewed. Breathe deeply. Be aware of where you are now; stretch gently; and, when you are ready, open your eyes." Suggest that patient move about slowly initially.

16. **See Completion Protocol (inside front cover).**

17. Observe character of patient's respirations, body position, facial expression, tone of voice, mood, mannerisms, and verbalization of discomfort.

18. Ask patient to rate pain on a pain rating scale of 0 to 10.

19. Use **_Teach Back:_** State to the patient, "I want to be sure you understand how to do the relaxation we practiced together when you get home." Observe and ask patient to demonstrate relaxation technique at a time of low stress. Encourage any questions. Evaluates what the patient is able to explain or demonstrate. Revise your instruction now or develop plan for revised patient teaching to be implemented at an appropriate time if patient is not able to teach back correctly.

20. Document in nurses' notes the relaxation strategies used and patient's response.

SKILL 13.2   PHARMACOLOGICAL PAIN MANAGEMENT

Analgesics are the most common and effective method of pain relief. However, undertreatment continues to be a problem because health care providers often do not assess pain thoroughly, may access incorrect drug information, and have concerns about addiction. Undertreatment is especially a problem in the care of older adults in long-term care settings (Alm and Norbergh, 2013) and when periodic prn ("as needed") medications predominate. Research shows nurses often feel very uncertain about pain in residents with dementia. Residents with dementia are often underassessed, experience delays in treatment for their pain, and are undertreated (Gilmore-Bykovskyi and Bowers, 2013). Nursing judgment is critical in the safe use and management of analgesics for all patients to ensure the best approach for pain management.

There are three types of analgesics: (1) nonopioids, including acetaminophen (Tylenol) and NSAIDs; (2) opioids (traditionally called narcotics); and (3) adjuvants or coanalgesics (e.g., anticonvulsants, sedatives, antidepressants, muscle relaxants) that enhance analgesics or have analgesic properties. Common nonopioids include acetaminophen (Tylenol) and ibuprofen (Advil). Acetaminophen (Tylenol) relieves mild pain and has no antiinflammatory or antiplatelet effects. It works peripherally on nerves and centrally on the brain. Its major side effect is liver toxicity. It is often combined with opioids (e.g., oxycodone [Percocet], hydrocodone [Vicodin]) for moderate pain relief because it reduces the dose of opioid needed for pain control. Nonselective NSAIDs such as ibuprofen relieve mild-to-moderate acute intermittent pain such as headache or muscle strain. NSAIDs are first-line treatment for mild-to-moderate postoperative pain unless contraindicated. NSAIDs do not depress the central nervous system (CNS) or interfere with bowel or bladder function.

Opioid or opioid-like analgesics are generally prescribed for moderate-to-severe pain. The term _opioid_ is preferred to the term _narcotic_ because narcotic generally infers illegal use of substances. Common opioids include codeine, morphine, hydromorphone (Dilaudid), fentanyl, and oxycodone.

Opioids work on higher centers of the brain and spinal cord by binding with opiate receptors to modify pain perception. Opioids may cause some respiratory depression. Sedation _always_ occurs before respiratory depression. Patients receiving opioids can also experience side effects such as nausea, vomiting, constipation, and altered mental processes. Except for constipation, these side effects usually stop once a patient has been receiving opioids around-the-clock (ATC) for 4 to 7 days.

Adjuvants or coanalgesics have analgesic properties to enhance pain control. For example, corticosteroids relieve pain associated with inflammation and bone metastasis. Adjuvants also relieve symptoms associated with pain, including nausea, anxiety, and depression. Although adjuvants enhance pain control, they have _no_ direct analgesic effect. Adjuvants are given alone or with analgesics, especially for treatment of chronic pain. Many adjuvants are more effective than opioids in relieving neuropathic pain. The drugs can cause drowsiness and impaired coordination. Do not automatically attribute these side effects to opioids. Always assess a patient carefully, and be alert for increased risk of sedation with the use of opioids and some classes of coanalgesics.

Effective pain management involves preventing pain and maintaining a pain rating that allows a patient to achieve functional or quality of life goals with relative ease (Lehne, 2013; Pasero and McCaffery, 2011). Timely administration of analgesics before a patient's pain becomes severe is crucial for optimal relief. Pain is easier to prevent than to treat. In many situations, administration of analgesics ATC rather than on a prn basis is preferable. ATC dosing regimens are designed to control baseline pain, the pain a patient reports as being the average pain intensity felt for 12 hours or more during a 24-hour period (Lehne, 2013; Pasero and McCaffery, 2011). It is best to use ATC dosing when pain is continuous or present for 12 or more hours each day; this applies to chronic cancer and noncancer pain and most postoperative pain for the first 24 hours after surgery. ATC administration ensures a more constant blood level of analgesic. Patients receiving ATC opioids have been shown to report lower pain intensity scores than patients receiving prn opioids, without added side effects (Paice, Noskin, and Vanagunas, 2005). Patients receiving ATC dosing also tend to be more adherent to their analgesic regimens (Lehne, 2013).

Dosing on a prn basis requires patients to request analgesics and to participate actively in their care (Lehne, 2013). Assess a patient's knowledge of prn dosing, provide appropriate usage instruction, and respond quickly to any patient request for a prn analgesic.

ASSESSMENT

1. Perform a complete pain assessment (see Skill 13.1) including patient's previous response to ordered analgesic. *Rationale: Provides baseline for pain condition, assists in selection of type of analgesic to administer, and assists in choosing amount of medication to give within a range order.*
2. Check the health care provider's orders against the medication administration record (MAR) for name of medication(s), dosage, route, and frequency of medication (e.g., one time, prn, range order). *Rationale: Ensures that right drug is administered to patient. This is the first check for accuracy.*
3. Assess the anticipated time of onset, time to peak effect, duration of action, and side effects of the analgesic to be administered (review pharmacology reference). For example, IV medications act quickly and can relieve severe acute pain within 1 hour; oral extended-release preparations may take 2 hours to be effective. *Rationale: Allows for planning pain-relief measures with patient activities, anticipating peak and duration of analgesic, and evaluating effectiveness of analgesic.*
4. Consider the type of activities patient is scheduled to undergo (e.g., rehabilitation, scheduled tests, ambulation). *Rationale: Allows you to time administration of analgesic early enough to gain maximal pain relief during the time of the activity.*
5. Check last time medication was administered (including dose and route) and degree of relief experienced. Verify the appropriateness of the dose and the dosing interval for the current situation. *Rationale: Determines if next dose can be administered and whether dose adjustment is necessary.*
6. Determine if patient has allergies to medications. *Rationale: Avoids possible allergic reaction to the analgesic.*
7. Assess patient's risk for using NSAIDs (e.g., history of gastrointestinal bleeding or renal insufficiency) or opioids (e.g., history of obstructive or central sleep apnea). *Rationale: Presence of risk factors contraindicates NSAID use.*
8. Know the comparative potencies of analgesics in oral and injectable form. Refer to an equianalgesic chart or

pharmacist. *Rationale: If nurses on succeeding shifts choose different routes for the same doses, a patient will not receive the same level of pain control.*
9. Assess patient's understanding of purpose and need for an analgesic, and discuss any fears or concerns. *Rationale: Allows for clarification of any misunderstanding and reinforces importance of analgesics in managing pain to improve patient's willingness to report pain.*
10. Talk with patient and determine a pain management strategy that is agreeable to the patient. Use the wipe-off board in patient's room to write the plan for administration times. Identify strategies such as staggering prn acetaminophen (Tylenol) between doses of prn opioids. *Rationale: Gives patient a sense of ownership and control of drug schedule without need to rely on memory. Also teaches patient how to make medication choices effectively after discharge or independently at home.*

PLANNING

Expected Outcomes focus on elimination or reduction of pain and return to optimal functioning with minimal side effects.

1. Patient sets mutually agreeable pain intensity goal with health care providers.
2. Patient achieves comfort with a self-report of pain intensity at or below pain intensity goal.
3. Patient achieves a reduction in pain behaviors (e.g., guarding, moaning, restlessness).
4. Patient is able to function adequately and perform ADLs (e.g., walking, working, eating, sleeping, interacting).
5. Patient does not experience intolerable or unmanageable adverse drug effects.
6. Patient understands the pain management plan and actively participates in the decision-making process.

Delegation and Collaboration

The skill of analgesic administration cannot be delegated to nursing assistive personnel (NAP). The nurse instructs the NAP by:

- Explaining the behaviors and physical changes associated with pain and to report their occurrence immediately.
- Reviewing comfort measures to use to support pain relief.

Equipment

- Prescribed medication
- Pain scale (0 to 10 range)
- Necessary administration device (see Chapters 22 and 23)
- Medication administration record (MAR) or computer printout
- Controlled substance record (for opioids only)

IMPLEMENTATION *for* PHARMACOLOGICAL PAIN MANAGEMENT

STEPS	RATIONALE
1. See Standard Protocol (inside front cover).	
2. Prepare selected analgesic, following "six rights" for administration of medications (see Chapter 21).	Ensures safe and appropriate medication administration. *This is the second check for accuracy.*
3. Identify patient using two identifiers (e.g., name and birthday or name and account number) according to facility policy. Compare identifiers with information on the patient's MAR or medical record.	Ensures correct patient. Complies with The Joint Commission standards and improves patient safety (TJC, 2014b).
4. At the bedside, compare MAR or computer printout with the name of the medication on the medication label and patient name (armband).	Timely administration improves pain management. Final check of medication ensures that right patient receives right medication. *This is the third check for accuracy.*
5. Administer medication (see Chapters 22 and 23) following these guidelines:	

> **SAFE PATIENT CARE** If a patient is unable to swallow or has a gastrostomy or jejunostomy tube in place, remember that, with the exception of methadone, the extended-release opioid formulations may not be crushed for administration. Some capsules may be opened and the contents mixed in applesauce or other soft food, but they may not be crushed.

STEPS	RATIONALE
a. Administer as soon as pain occurs.	Pain is easier to prevent than to treat.
b. Administer before pain increases in severity.	Higher levels of pain may not respond to ordered analgesic.
c. Administer 30 to 60 minutes before pain-producing procedures or activities.	Reduces or blocks pain transmission in the CNS, allowing procedure to be completed with less discomfort.
d. Administer ATC routinely.	Maintains analgesic within therapeutic range ATC. The ATC schedule avoids the low plasma concentrations that permit breakthrough pain.
e. Awaken any opioid-naïve or opioid-tolerant patient with continuous pain in a hospital setting after surgery to take pain medication (Lehne, 2013; Pasero and McCaffery, 2011). Reassess patient's sedation and respiratory status before administering the medication.	This is especially important the first 24 to 48 hours postoperatively to control pain. Avoid awakening in severe pain.
6. Provide nonpharmacological comfort measures in addition to analgesics (see Skill 13.1 and Procedure Guideline 13.1).	Increases effectiveness of pharmacological agents; treats nonphysiological aspects of pain.
7. Administer nursing care measures during times of peak effects of analgesics. Explain after giving medication (for example): "I will return in 30 minutes after the medicine reduces your pain to do the dressing change. That way you will feel less discomfort." Consider duration of action of analgesics when planning activities.	Effects vary depending on the type of medication used; allows for anticipation of next dose; permits evaluation of analgesic effects; maximizes effectiveness of nursing measures to prevent complications.

> **SAFE PATIENT CARE** Patients receiving ATC opioids should also receive stimulant laxatives. Opioids decrease intestinal propulsion (peristalsis) but not intestinal motility (churning) so that stool softeners alone are ineffective. Recommend stimulant laxatives.

8. See Completion Protocol (inside front cover).

EVALUATION

1. Ask patient to rate pain intensity using appropriate pain scale both at rest and with activity.

2. Monitor for adverse medication effects.

3. Evaluate PQRSTU aspects of pain; use nonverbal assessment if patient unable to respond (see Skill 13.1).

4. Observe patient's position; mobility; relaxation; and ability to rest, sleep, eat, and participate in usual activities.

5. When opioids are given, evaluate bowel function for constipation.

6. Use *Teach Back:* State to the patient, "I want to be sure you understand when to ask for medication to treat your pain. Can you give me an example?" Evaluates what the patient is able to explain or demonstrate. Revise your instruction now or develop plan for revised patient teaching to be implemented at an appropriate time if patient is not able to teach back correctly.

Unexpected Outcomes and Related Interventions

1. Patient reports that pain intensity is greater than desired or shows nonverbal behaviors reflecting pain.
   a. Discuss current pain-control regimen with the patient. Determine what has worked best to provide relief. If the medication has failed, document the result and inform the patient that you will notify the health care provider that the treatment is not effective and options will be discussed.
   b. Evaluate the dose of medication administered with the health care provider and consider an alternative dose or an adjuvant.
   c. Try alternative nonpharmacological interventions.
   d. *Reassure patient you will do everything you can to solve the problem of inadequate pain control.* Discomfort that is unrelieved or worse may indicate need for additional diagnostic, medical, or surgical intervention or a change in pain management.
2. Patient develops respiratory depression.
   a. Give no additional dose of analgesic. Stay with patient and protect airway.
   b. Call for help and ask for naloxone (Narcan) assistance. Administer naloxone IV push per health care provider's order.
   c. Continue to monitor vital signs, including pulse oximetry.

Recording and Reporting

- Record patient's pain rating (15 to 30 minutes after IV medication and 30 to 60 minutes after po medication), behavioral and physiological response to analgesic, and additional comfort measures given in nurses' notes. Incorporate pain-relief techniques in nursing care plan.
- Record medication, dose, route, and time given in MAR or computer printout.
- Document your evaluation of patient learning.
- Report unsuccessful or untoward patient response to analgesics to health care provider.

Sample Documentation

0800 Morphine 5 mg IV push administered over 3 minutes for c/o low back pain, pain rated 7 on 0 to 10 scale that increases when sitting. Positioned on L side with legs supported. Back massage given. States pain decreased to a rating of 4 within 5 minutes of IV push morphine.
0830 States, "I feel better now; the pain is still there but less than before." Rates pain 4 (0 to 10 scale).

Special Considerations
Pediatric
- Children (except infants <3 to 6 months old) metabolize drugs more rapidly than adults; younger children may require higher doses of opioids to achieve the same analgesic effect (Hockenberry and Wilson, 2013).
- Use the least traumatic route of medication administration for children.
- Offer a supportive attitude when giving analgesics to a child. Reinforce the cause and effect of the analgesic, involving the parents; then you can condition the child to expect pain relief (provided that the regimen is effective) (Hockenberry and Wilson, 2013).

Geriatric
- It is best for older adults to receive acetaminophen (Tylenol) as an initial and ongoing pharmacotherapy for mild-to-moderate musculoskeletal pain. Give nonselective NSAIDs and cyclooxygenase-2 selective inhibitors very cautiously and only in highly selected individuals (as identified by health care provider). All older adults with moderate-to-severe pain, pain-related functional impairment, or diminished quality of life should be considered for opioid therapy (Touhy and Jett, 2014).
- Avoid intramuscular analgesic administration in older adults because the injections hurt and analgesic uptake from the muscle into the cardiovascular system is unpredictable.
- Avoid administering a combination of opioids.
- Because of renal and liver decline, maximum daily dosages of acetaminophen (Tylenol) may need to be lower.
- If an older adult is cognitively impaired and had a procedure that usually causes pain, consult with the health care provider about ordering an appropriate analgesic ATC instead of prn.

Home Care
- Family caregivers need to know how to observe and recognize pain in the person they care for and to accept and acknowledge the patient's report of pain.
- Explain to family caregivers the importance of following ATC analgesic administration to maximize effect. Allay any anxieties about risk of addiction.
- Inform family caregivers how to access health care provider on a 24-hour basis.

SKILL 13.3   PATIENT-CONTROLLED ANALGESIA

Patient-controlled analgesia (PCA) is an interactive method of pain management. It gives patients control over pain through self-administration of analgesics. Routes for PCA administration include subcutaneous, IV (the most common), and epidural. PCA is a safe method of analgesic administration for acute and chronic pain, including postoperative, traumatic, labor and delivery, sickle cell crisis, myocardial infarction, cancer, and end-of-life pain. Patients receive analgesic doses as they need them by using a small, computerized pump to deliver a prescribed dose of medication with a push of a button. Patients prefer the PCA method because it is convenient and allows them some control over medication delivery. The three most common medications used in PCA are the opioids morphine, hydromorphone, and fentanyl.

The most important principle in administering PCA is patient safety. Risk factors for oversedation and respiratory depression when using PCA include opioid-naïve status; obesity; age (infants and small children or older adults); confused mental status; multiple comorbid conditions such as lung disease (asthma), obstructive sleep apnea, renal disease, and hepatic disease; and use of medications with sedating effects, such as antiemetics, muscle relaxants, and sleeping medications (Craft, 2010; D'Arcy, 2012; Lehne, 2013). Safe patient monitoring requires assessing a patient's level of sedation using a valid sedation scale. Assessment of sedation level is a more reliable way of detecting early opioid-induced respiratory depression than a decreased respiratory rate because hypoxemic episodes may occur in the absence of a low respiratory rate (Craft, 2010). The use of both continuous pulse oximetry and capnography is recommended during monitoring (D'Arcy, 2012). If a patient is receiving supplemental oxygen, the results of pulse oximetry are skewed reading higher saturations than the blood oxygenation. The use of end-tidal carbon dioxide detects developing oversedation as retained carbon dioxide levels increase and respiratory efforts decrease (D'Arcy, 2012).

Because patients depress a button on a PCA device to deliver a regulated dose of analgesic, they must be able to understand how, why, and when to self-administer medication and be able to depress the device physically. Family members must understand the purpose of PCA and why they cannot push the PCA button for a patient. The exception is in the care of children, where some hospitals allow parents to press the device; this is called Authorized Agent Controlled Analgesia (AACA) (ASPMN, 2006; Hockenberry and Wilson, 2013). A facility must have a policy describing clear guidelines for the use of AACA. Nurses must advise patients, family, and other visitors that PCA is for patient use only. PCA is not recommended in situations in which oral analgesics could easily manage pain.

A PCA device is individually programmed to deliver automatically a specific health care provider–prescribed continuous infusion (basal rate) of medication, a bolus dose (patient initiated), or both. PCA prevents overdosing by having a preprogrammed delay time or "lockout" (usually 6 to 16 minutes) between patient-initiated doses. A health care provider usually limits the total amount of opioid that a patient receives over 1 hour. The device consists of an infusion device, a prefilled drug reservoir, and tubing that delivers the medication from the infuser through the patient-control module to tubing connected to the patient's catheter (IV, epidural, or subcutaneous). To achieve maximum comfort, patients

should receive loading doses with the initiation of the PCA and subsequently should be able to maintain comfort with PCA bolus doses (D'Arcy, 2012).

Concerns involving PCA use are patient-related, pump failure, and operator errors. Patients may not understand how PCA therapy works, mistake the PCA button for a nurse call button, or have family members operate the demand button. A pump may fail to deliver drug on demand, have a faulty alarm or low battery, or lack free-flow protection. Operators may program the dose, concentration, or rate incorrectly. They also may fail to clamp or unclamp tubing, load the syringe or cartridge improperly, fail to monitor for side effects or overdose, or fail to respond to alarms. PCA requires careful, ongoing monitoring. Never try to operate a PCA without fully understanding the particular model in use.

ASSESSMENT

1. Check the health care provider's order against the medication administration record for name of medication, dosage, route, frequency of medication (continuous, demand, or both), and lockout settings. Verify that patient is not allergic to prescribed medication. *Rationale: Ensures that right drug is administered to patient. This is the first check for accuracy.*

> **SAFE PATIENT CARE** Nausea is not an allergic reaction and can be treated. Itching alone is not an allergic reaction but is a common side effect of opioids. Itching is treatable and should not preclude use of PCA.

2. Assess patient's cognitive and physical ability to press device button. *Rationale: Determines appropriateness of PCA for pain management based on patient's ability to use the device.*
3. Assess character of patient's pain (see Skill 13.1). *Rationale: Establishes baseline to determine patient's response to analgesia.*
4. Obtain a pulse oximetry or capnography reading (see facility policy). *Rationale: Provides baseline measure of oxygenation status.*
5. Assess environment for factors that heighten pain (e.g., noise, temperature of room). *Rationale: Elimination of irritating stimuli may further reduce pain perception.*
6. If patient has had surgery, apply clean gloves and inspect incision. Palpate gently around the area for tenderness. **Apply sterile gloves** if placing hand on incision. *Rationale: Reveals nature of pain and provides a baseline to determine response to analgesia.*
7. When administering IV medication, assess existing IV infusion line (peripheral or central) for patency and condition of venipuncture site for infiltration or inflammation. Check for IV compatibility if PCA is inserted into Y-port of an existing IV line. *Rationale: IV line must be patent with fluid infusing for medication to reach venous circulation safely and effectively. Never attach a PCA to an*

IV line with blood running or to IV lines with cardiovascular drugs infusing. If necessary, start another IV site.

> **SAFE PATIENT CARE** Do not give medication IV push through a line with a PCA infusion. Best practice is to have a designated IV site for a PCA.

8. Assess if patient has history of sleep apnea. *Rationale: Opioid analgesia contributes significantly to risk of respiratory depression and airway obstruction in sleep apnea (Lehne, 2013).*
9. Assess patient's knowledge and effectiveness of previous pain strategies. *Rationale: Helps to identify learning needs.*

PLANNING

Expected Outcomes focus on proper use of the PCA device and adequate pain control without oversedation and with no or manageable adverse effects.
1. Patient reports pain relief.
2. Patient exhibits relaxed facial expression and body position.
3. Patient correctly operates PCA device.
4. Patient remains alert and oriented.
5. Patient increasingly participates in self-care activities.

Delegation and Collaboration

The skill of PCA administration cannot be delegated to nursing assistive personnel (NAP). The nurse instructs the NAP about:
- The signs of sedation and unrelieved pain to report to the nurse when they occur.
- Reporting to the nurse any new symptom or change in patient status (e.g., drowsiness).
- *Never* administering a PCA dose for the patient (ASPMN, 2006).
- The patient being at a higher risk for a fall, which requires increased monitoring and reminding the patient to use the call light for assistance when getting up.

Equipment
- PCA system and tubing
- Identification label and time tape (may already be attached and completed by pharmacy)
- Needleless connector
- Alcohol swab
- Adhesive tape
- Clean gloves (when applicable)
- Opioid reversal agent (e.g., naloxone)
- Equipment for vital signs, pulse oximetry, and capnography
- MAR

IMPLEMENTATION *for* PATIENT-CONTROLLED ANALGESIA

STEPS	RATIONALE
1. **See Standard Protocol (inside front cover).**	
2. Check the prepared analgesic, following "six rights" for administration of medications (see Chapter 21). Note: Pharmacy prepares cartridge.	Ensures safe and appropriate medication administration. *This is the second check for accuracy.*
3. Identify patient using two identifiers (e.g., name and birthday or name and account number) according to facility policy. Compare identifiers with information on the patient's MAR or medical record.	*Ensures correct patient. Complies with The Joint Commission standards and improves patient safety (TJC, 2014b).*
4. At the bedside, compare MAR or computer printout with the name of medication on the drug cartridge and patient name (armband). Have a second registered nurse (RN) confirm health care provider's order and the correct setup of the PCA. The second RN should check the health care provider's order and the device independently and not just simply look at the first RN's setup.	*This is the third check for accuracy* and ensures that right patient receives right medication. Two nurses should independently double-check the patient's identification, drug selected and concentration, PCA pump settings, and line attachment.
5. Before initiating analgesia, explain purpose of PCA and benefits and demonstrate function of PCA to patient and family, as follows: **a.** Explain type of medication in PCA device.	Promotes patient participation in care and independence in pain control. PCA allows more constant serum levels of an opioid and avoids the peaks and troughs of a large bolus. Patients receive better pain relief and fewer side effects from opioids because blood levels are maintained at a level of minimum effective analgesia concentration for an individual. When used after surgery, fewer complications arise because earlier and easier ambulation occurs as a result of effective pain relief.

Continued

STEPS	RATIONALE

b. Explain that device safely administers self-initiated small but frequent amounts of medication prn for comfort and minimizes side effects from analgesia. Tell patient that self-dosing before repositioning, walking, or coughing and deep breathing helps in performing activities more easily.

Helps patient to understand the value of controlling pain. Small, frequent dosing with PCA produces constant serum drug levels with minimal fluctuation rather than peaks and troughs associated with prn analgesics (Lehne, 2013).

c. Explain that device is programmed to deliver ordered type and dose of pain medication, lockout interval, and 1-hour dosage limits. Explain how lockout time prevents overdose.

Confirms with patient the safety of a PCA device.

d. Demonstrate to patient how to push medication demand button on PCA unit. Explain that pressing the PCA button delivers a small dose of medication into the IV, eliminating the need to wait for a nurse to prepare medication for injection.

Gives patient control of pain. Because PCA provides medication on demand as soon as a patient feels the need, the total amount of opioid use can be reduced. PCA allows a patient to manage pain with minimal nursing intervention.

e. Instruct patient to notify you for possible side effects (be specific as to possible effects), problems in attaining pain relief, changes in severity or location of pain, alarm sounding, or questions that arise.

Ensures that you respond in a more timely way for developing problems. Because patients must be awake to push the device button to receive a dose, overdosing is less likely.

6. Check infuser and patient-control module for accurate labeling or evidence of leaking.

Avoids medication error and injury to patient.

7. Position patient to ensure that venipuncture or central line site is accessible.

Ensures unimpeded flow of infusion.

8. Apply clean gloves. Insert drug cartridge into infusion device (see illustration). Attach needleless adapter to tubing adapter and prime infusion tubing.

Locks system and prevents air from infusing into IV tubing.

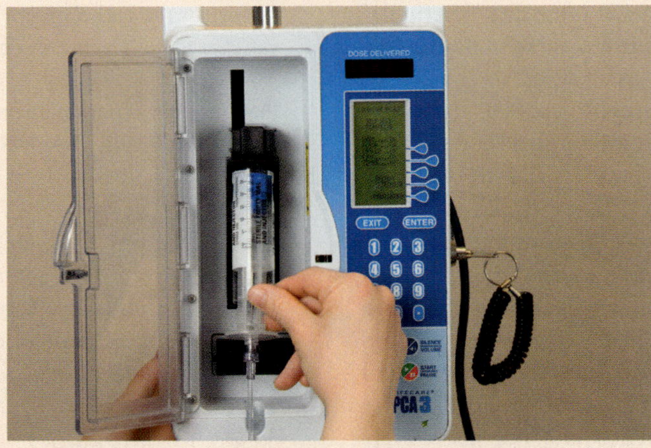

STEP 8 Nurse inserting drug cartridge into patient-controlled analgesia device.

9. Wipe injection port of main IV line vigorously with alcohol or antiseptic for 15 seconds and allow to dry.

Minimizes entry of microorganisms during needle insertion, reducing risk of catheter-related bloodstream infection.

10. Connect PCA tubing using needleless adapter at Y-site of peripheral IV (nearest patient) or central line or connect to its own IV site. There should not be a chance to use the PCA tubing to administer an IV push with another drug through the PCA tubing or push a bolus through the tubing that is connected to a needleless port.

Establishes route for medication to enter main IV line. Prevents transmission of microorganisms. Prevents medication interaction and incompatibility.

STEPS	RATIONALE
11. Secure connection and anchor PCA tubing with tape. Label PCA tubing and remove gloves.	Prevents dislodging of needleless adapter from port. Facilitates patient's ability to ambulate. Label prevents error from connecting tubing from different device to PCA (TJC, 2014a).
12. Program computerized PCA pump as ordered to deliver prescribed dose and lockout interval. Have second nurse check setting. (**NOTE:** Recheck with oncoming RN during shift-to-shift handoff to ensure line reconciliation.)	Ensures safe, therapeutic drug administration.
13. Administer loading dose of analgesia as prescribed: manually give a one-time dose or turn on pump and program dose into pump.	Establishes initial level of analgesia.
14. If patient is having pain, demonstrate use of PCA system (see illustration); if not, have patient verbally repeat instructions given earlier.	Return demonstration reveals patient's understanding and ability to manipulate device.

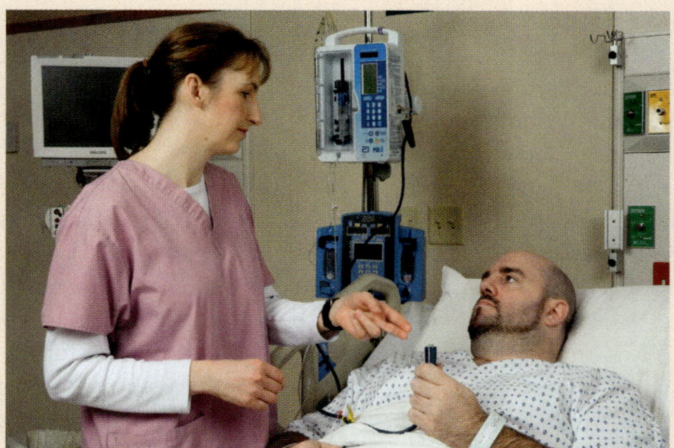

STEP 14 Patient learns how to press patient-controlled analgesia device button.

STEPS	RATIONALE
15. Be sure venipuncture or central line site is protected and recheck before leaving patient.	Ensures patency of line.
16. See Completion Protocol (inside front cover).	
17. To discontinue PCA:	
a. Check health care provider order for discontinuation. Obtain necessary PCA information from pump for documentation, including amount infused and amount to discard.	Ensures correct documentation of Schedule II drugs.
b. Perform hand hygiene.	Reduces transmission of infection.
c. Apply clean gloves. Turn pump off. Disconnect PCA tubing from primary IV line but maintain IV access (see Chapter 27).	Ensures continued IV therapy.
d. Dispose of empty cartridge according to facility policy.	Control and dispensation of opioids are regulated by the Controlled Substances Act.

> **SAFE PATIENT CARE** If PCA is discontinued before device is completely empty, record drug waste on PCA MAR per facility policy. Note date, time, amount of drug wasted, and reason for waste. Waste must be witnessed and the record signed by two RNs to comply with documentation of Schedule II drugs.

18. See Completion Protocol (inside front cover).

EVALUATION

1. Use pain rating scale to evaluate pain intensity after treatments and procedures.
2. Monitor patient's level of sedation, vital signs, and pulse oximetry or capnography every 1 to 2 hours for the first 12 hours (APS and AAPM, 2009). Monitor more frequently at the start, during first 24 hours, and at night when hypoventilation and hypoxia tend to occur (Ramachandran et al., 2011).
3. Observe patient for signs of adverse reactions, especially excessive sedation by using a sedation scale (see Chapter 11).
4. Evaluate number of attempts (number of times patient pushed the button) and delivery of demand doses (number of times drug actually given) and basal dose, if ordered, according to facility policy (usually every 4 to 8 hours). This maintains compliance with the Controlled Substances Act.
5. Observe patient initiate self-care activities.
6. Use **Teach Back:** State to the patient, "I want to be sure I explained to you when and how to use the PCA correctly. Tell me when you should press the PCA button." When patient is ready for a dose, ask patient to show you how to depress the button. Evaluates what the patient is able to explain or demonstrate. Revise your instruction now or develop plan for revised patient teaching to be implemented at an appropriate time if patient is not able to teach back correctly.

Unexpected Outcomes and Related Interventions

1. Patient verbalizes continued or worsening discomfort or displays nonverbal behaviors indicating pain.
   a. Perform complete pain reassessment.
   b. Check to see if patient manipulates PCA button correctly, and evaluate number of attempts and deliveries initiated by patient.
   c. Evaluate for possible complications other than pain.
   d. Inspect IV site for possible catheter occlusion or infiltration, and check tubing for possible kinking.
   e. Check that maintenance IV fluid is running continuously.
   f. Evaluate pump for operational problems.
   g. Use nonpharmacological comfort measures as appropriate.
   h. Contact health care provider to report unrelieved pain. Dose may have to be adjusted. A patient who is not opiate-naïve may need dose adjustments.

SAFE PATIENT CARE Do not increase demand or basal dose *and* decrease the interval time (e.g., from 10 to 5 minutes) simultaneously because this increases the risk for oversedation, respiratory depression, and other adverse effects.

---

2. Patient is sedated and not easily arousable.
   a. Stop PCA and elevate head of bed 30 degrees unless contraindicated.
   b. Instruct patient to take deep breaths.
   c. Stay with the patient and call for assistance. Notify health care provider. Prepare to administer oxygen as ordered.
   d. Delegate the measurement of vital signs, including pulse oximetry or capnography.
   e. Administer naloxone or reversal drug.
   f. Evaluate amount of opioid delivered within past 4 to 8 hours.
   g. Review MAR for other possible sedating drugs.
   h. Ask family caregivers if they depressed PCA button without patient's knowledge.
3. Patient is unable to manipulate PCA device.
   a. Consult with health care provider about alternative medication route and possible basal dose.
   b. Assess patient support system for family caregiver who can responsibly manipulate PCA device (check facility policy).

Recording and Reporting

- Record on appropriate MAR drug, concentration, dose (basal and demand), time started, lockout time, and amount of solution infused and remaining. Many facilities have a separate flow sheet for PCA documentation.
- Document your evaluation of patient learning.
- Record assessment of patient's response to analgesic on PCA medication form, narrative notes, or patient assessment flow sheet (see facility policy), including vital signs, oximetry and capnography results, sedation status, pain rating, and status of vascular access device.
- Calculate infused dose: add demand and continuous dose together. Follow facility policy.

Sample Documentation

1700   IV PCA with hydrocodone 0.5 mg/mL infusing at 5 mL/hr basal rate into L forearm. IV site without redness or swelling; dressing clean, dry, and occlusive. Dozing at intervals, arouses easily. Resp. 16/min, regular in rate, rhythm, and depth. Patient feels burning at abdominal incision and rates 4 on 0 to 10 scale when turning. Reports no pain when lying still.

Special Considerations
Pediatric

- PCA is safe and effective in children (beginning at 5 to 6 years) who can understand the concept (Hockenberry and Wilson, 2013). When a health care provider decides to order PCA for a child, the developmental and cognitive level and motor skills are considered.

Geriatric

- Older adults appear more sensitive to analgesics and experience more opioid side effects (Gloth, 2011; Touhy and Jett, 2014). Reduced renal function and reduced liver function slow opioid metabolism and excretion. Dosages should be started low and titrated upward slowly until pain relief is achieved (Gloth, 2011; Touhy and Jett, 2014).

- If an older adult becomes confused while using a PCA device, stop further infusions and call to get orders to discontinue, lower the dose, lengthen the lockout, or add a nonopioid analgesic to reduce opioid dose. Nurse-activated ATC dosing is another option (Pasero and McCaffery, 2011).

Home Care

- PCA should not be used in patients physically or cognitively unable to activate device. However, it is used commonly in patients under hospice care. Home care nurses should be available to patient and family caregivers through regular telephone contact and scheduled nursing visits.
- Provide instruction regarding appropriate dosage adjustment, potential errors, and when to notify health care provider if pain intensity remains unacceptable after dosage adjustments.

The administration of analgesics into the epidural space is an efficient intervention to manage acute pain during labor, after surgery, and for chronic pain such as cancer pain (D'Arcy, 2011). Studies show that patient-controlled epidural analgesia (PCEA) offers superior postoperative pain control after a variety of surgeries compared with IV PCA. Use of PCEA is safe and efficient, and complications of analgesia are rare. Epidural opioids reduce the total amount of opioids required to control pain, producing fewer opioid-related side effects.

The epidural space is a potential space that contains a network of vessels, nerves, and fat located between the vertebral column and the dura mater, the outermost meninges covering the spinal cord (Fig. 13-4). Analgesics delivered into this space are distributed (1) by diffusion through the dura mater into the cerebrospinal fluid (CSF), where they act directly on receptors in the dorsal horn of the spinal cord; (2) via blood vessels in the epidural space for systemic delivery; and (3) by absorption by fat in the epidural space, creating a

depot where the drug is slowly released systemically. The analgesic binds to opiate receptors in the dorsal horn of the spinal cord, blocking pain impulse transmission to the cerebral cortex.

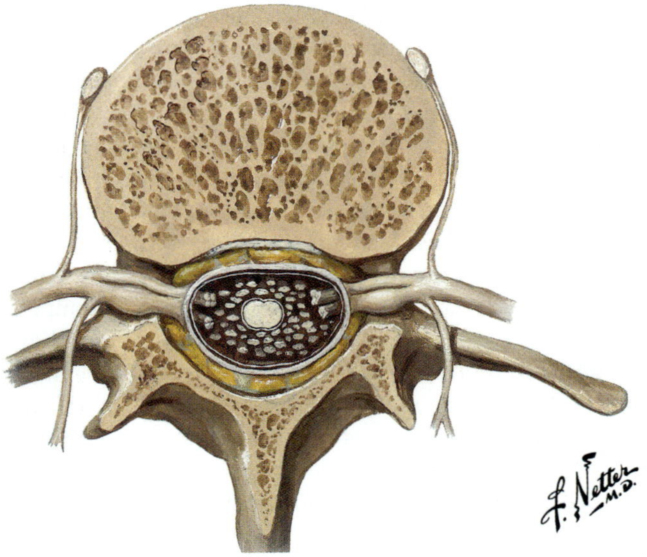

Opioids and local anesthetics, separately or in combination, are used in epidural analgesia. Opioids are delivered close to their site of action (CNS) and require much smaller doses to achieve the same pain relief (D'Arcy, 2011). Common opioids given epidurally include morphine, hydromorphone (Dilaudid), fentanyl, and sufentanil. These opioids differ by their lipophilic "fat-loving" and hydrophilic "water-loving" properties, which affect absorption rate and duration of action. Fentanyl and sufentanil are lipophilic, causing them to have a quicker onset and shorter duration of action (2 hours). Morphine and hydromorphone are hydrophilic, resulting in longer onset and duration of action (24 hours with a single bolus dose).

For an epidural catheter insertion, a patient is placed in the lateral side-lying or sitting position with shoulders and hips in alignment and hips and head flexed. An anesthesia provider places a catheter in the epidural space below the second lumbar vertebra, where the spinal cord ends (Fig. 13-5). Epidurals may also be placed at the thoracic level of the spinal cord. Catheters intended for temporary or short-term use exit from the insertion side on the back and are not sutured in place. A catheter intended for permanent or long-term use is "tunneled" subcutaneously, exits on the side of the body (Fig. 13-6) or on the abdomen, and is sutured in place. Tunneling reduces infection and catheter dislodgment. A sterile occlusive dressing covers the catheter exit site and is secured to the patient. An x-ray film is the only way to confirm placement of an epidural catheter.

A health care provider administers epidural medication intermittently via bolus or continuously (through an infusion pump), or a patient can inject intermittently on demand (PCEA) through a pump. The use of epidural opioids requires astute nursing observation and care. The anatomical location of the catheter tip, its potential to move through the dura mater, and its closeness to spinal nerves and blood vessels poses risks to patient safety (Pasero and McCaffery, 2011). If

FIG 13-4 Anatomical drawing of epidural space. (Reprinted from www.netterimages.com © Elsevier, Inc. All rights reserved.)

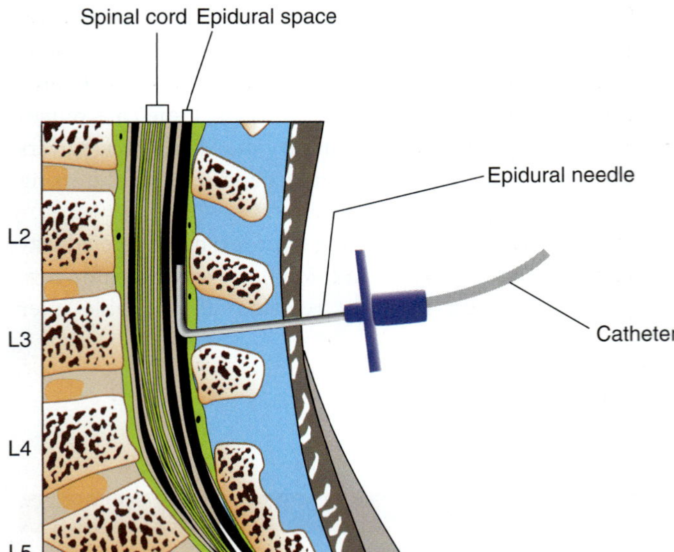

FIG 13-5 Placement of epidural catheter.

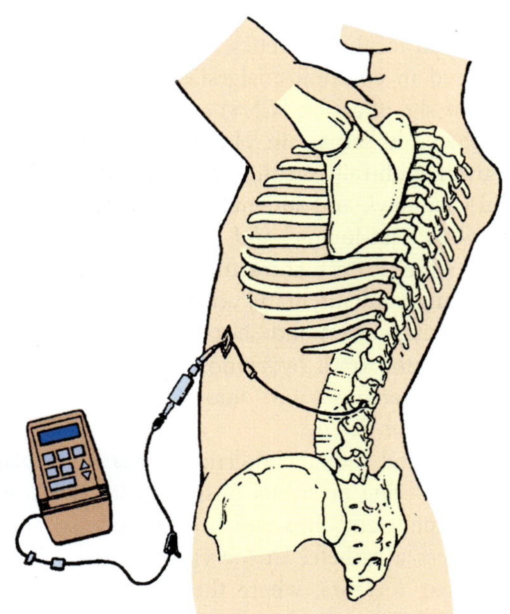

FIG 13-6 External epidural catheter attached to ambulatory infusion pump. (Courtesy SIMS Deltec, Inc., St Paul, Minnesota.)

a catheter reaches the subarachnoid space, dangerously high medication levels can result. Monitor a patient's motor and sensory function, including onset of urinary retention. Do not administer other supplemental opioids or sedatives when patients are receiving epidural analgesia. The combined effect can cause respiratory depression. Monitor a patient's vital signs, sedation score, pain intensity, and degree of motor and sensory block closely throughout the period of epidural analgesia (Rowbotham et al., 2010). Follow facility policy. Frequency of monitoring is determined by the nature of the surgery or need for analgesia and condition of a patient. More frequent observations are needed in the first 12 hours of an infusion, when changes of infusion rates are made, and when

a patient has cardiovascular or respiratory instability (Rowbotham et al., 2010). In many hospitals, anesthesia providers are the only health care professionals who may initiate an epidural opioid infusion or administer a bolus. Some hospitals allow nurses to become certified to begin an epidural opioid infusion or administer a bolus after a catheter has been placed (check facility policy).

ASSESSMENT

1. Assess if patient has completed informed consent and is aware of risk and benefits of epidural analgesia (see facility policy). *Rationale: Epidural analgesia is a significant procedure with specific and potentially serious complications, requiring informed consent (Rowbotham et al., 2010).*

2. Assess patient's comfort level and character of patient's pain (see Skill 13.1). *Rationale: Establishes baseline pain level.*

3. Confer with health care provider if you assess any presenting medical or surgical condition (e.g., major abdominal or thoracic surgery, trauma, advanced cancer, women in labor) where epidural analgesia may be the treatment of choice.

4. For cognitively impaired or non–English-speaking patients, assess nonverbal pain responses. *Rationale: Because patient cannot verbalize pain intensity, nonverbal responses help you to establish a baseline pain level.*

5. Check to see if patient takes anticoagulants. *Rationale: Anticoagulation may contraindicate placement of epidural catheter because of the inability to apply pressure at the epidural insertion site and risk of bleeding.*

6. Assess if patient takes herbal medicines and, if so, which ones. *Rationale: Some herbals (e.g., ginkgo biloba, ginseng, ginger) may interfere with clotting, but there is currently no contraindication to their use (NIH, NCCAM, 2011).*

7. Assess patient's history of drug allergies. *Rationale: Avoids possible allergic reaction to the analgesia.*

8. Assess patient's sedation level by assessing level of wakefulness or alertness, ability to follow commands, and drowsiness. *Rationale: Establishes a baseline before first dose. Assessment of sedation level is more reliable for detecting early opioid-induced respiratory depression than a decreased respiratory rate because hypoxemic episodes often occur in the absence of a low respiratory rate (Craft, 2010).*

9. Assess rate, pattern, and depth of respirations; pulse oximetry or capnography; blood pressure; and temperature. *Rationale: Establishes baseline circulatory and oxygenation status.*

10. Assess initial motor and sensory function (see Chapter 7). Test sensation in lower extremities. Have patient flex both feet and knees and raise each leg off the bed. Give special attention to patients with preexisting sensory or motor abnormalities. *Rationale: Establishes a baseline. Monitoring of motor and sensory function ensures that neural blockage does not affect function (D'Arcy, 2011).*

11. Verify that epidural catheter is secured to patient's skin from the back, side, or front. *Rationale: Prevents accidental catheter dislodgment.*

12. Assess catheter insertion site for redness, warmth, tenderness, swelling, and drainage. **Apply sterile gloves** if it is necessary to remove occlusive dressing. *Rationale: Establishes baseline. Catheter sites are at risk for local infection. Purulent drainage is a sign of infection. Clear drainage may indicate CSF leaking from punctured dura mater. Bloody drainage may indicate that catheter entered blood vessel.*

13. Check health care provider's orders against MAR for name of medication, dosage, route, infusion method (bolus, continuous, or demand), and lockout settings. Verify that patient is not allergic to prescribed medication. *Rationale: Ensures that right drug is administered to right patient. This is the first check for accuracy.*

14. Check patency of infusion tubing, and check infusion pump for proper calibration and operation. *Rationale: Ensures that patient will obtain prescribed analgesic dose. Kinked tubing interrupts analgesic infusion.*

❙ PLANNING

Expected Outcomes focus on elimination or reduction of pain and prevention of complications of epidural analgesia.

1. Patient verbalizes pain relief within 30 to 60 minutes of initiation of epidural infusion.

2. Patient has no headache during epidural analgesia or for 72 hours after discontinuation.

3. Patient experiences no redness, warmth, exudate, tenderness, or swelling at catheter insertion site during time epidural catheter is in place. The patient is afebrile.

4. Patient's respirations are regular, adequate depth, and equal to or greater than 8 breaths per minute; pulse oximetry SpO_2 95% or greater; capnography end-tidal carbon dioxide is 5% or 35 to 37 mm Hg.

5. Patient remains normotensive. Heart rate remains at or above patient's baseline.

6. Patient is easily awakened; alert; and oriented to person, place, and time.

7. Patient voids without difficulty; averages 30 to 60 mL per hour.

8. Patient has no or minimal pruritus and no paresthesias of lower extremities.

9. Epidural infusion system remains intact and functioning.

Delegation and Collaboration

The skill of epidural analgesia administration cannot be delegated to nursing assistive personnel (NAP). The nurse instructs the NAP to:

- Observe the insertion site and catheter location when repositioning or ambulating patients to prevent catheter disruption.
- Report any disconnection along the infusion system immediately to the nurse.
- Report any loss of sensation, movement, or bowel and bladder function immediately to nurse.

Equipment

- Clean gloves
- Sterile gloves (if removing epidural dressing)
- Prediluted preservative-free opioid as prescribed by health care provider for use in IV infusion pump (prepared by pharmacy)
- Infusion pump and compatible tubing. (Do not use Y-ports for infusions; some infusion pumps have color-coded tubing for intraspinal use.)
- Antibacterial filter
- Tape
- Label (for injection port)
- Equipment for vital signs and pulse oximetry or capnography (see facility policy)
- MAR or computer printout

IMPLEMENTATION *for* EPIDURAL ANALGESIA

STEPS	RATIONALE
1. **See Standard Protocol (inside front cover).**	
2. Place patients receiving epidural analgesia close to the nurses' station.	Ensures close supervision during infusion (Rowbotham et al., 2010).
3. Prepare analgesic, following "six rights" for administration of medications (see Chapter 21). Note: Pharmacy prepares medication for pump. In the case of a bolus injection, draw up prediluted, preservative-free opioid solution through filter needle into syringe.	Ensures safe and appropriate medication administration. *This is the second check for accuracy.*
4. At the bedside, identify patient using two identifiers (e.g., name and birthday or name and account number) according to facility policy. Compare identifiers with information on the patient's MAR or medical record. Compare MAR or computer printout with the name of medication on the drug container.	Ensures correct patient. Complies with The Joint Commission standards and improves patient safety (TJC, 2014b). *This is the third check for accuracy* and ensures that the right patient receives the right medication.

Continued

STEPS	RATIONALE
5. Explain purpose and function of epidural analgesia and expectations of patient during procedure (e.g., having patient call for assistance to get out of bed). Demonstrate to patient how to use pump on demand. Note: Explanation is also provided by analgesia provider.	Proper explanation of therapy enhances patient cooperation.
6. When receiving the patient during hand-offs or when assisting during insertion by anesthesia provider attach an "epidural line" label to the epidural infusion tubing. Be sure that there are *no* Y-*ports* on the tubing. Epidural infusions should be labeled "For Epidural Use Only."	Labeling helps to ensure that analgesic is administered into correct line and the epidural space. Labeling of high-risk catheters prevents connection with an inappropriate tube or catheter (TJC, 2014a). The epidural infusion system between pump and patient should be considered as closed, with no injection or Y-ports (Rowbotham et al, 2010).
7. **Apply clean gloves. Administer infusion: Anesthesia provider typically starts or administers first dose. Thereafter RN maintains infusion.**	Only certified RNs can initiate a PCEA.
a. *Continuous infusion:*	
(1) Be sure container of diluted preservative-free medication is attached to infusion pump tubing and prime the tubing (see Chapter 23).	Tubing filled with solution and free of air bubbles avoids an air embolus.
(2) Insert tubing into infusion pump (see Chapter 23), and attach distal end of tubing to antibacterial filter. Have ready for connection to epidural catheter (Rowbotham et al., 2010).	Pump propels fluid through tubing. Filter reduces entrance of microorganisms into infusion line.
(3) Check infusion pump for proper calibration, setting, and operation. Many facilities have two nurses check settings or nurse checks with anesthesia provider.	Ensures that patient is receiving proper dosing.
(4) Tape all connections. Anesthesia provider starts infusion.	Taping maintains a secure closed system to prevent infection.
b. *Bolus dose of analgesic via infusion pump.*	
(1) While assisting anesthesia provider, perform Steps 7a(1)-(4). Adjust infusion pump setting for preset limit (as ordered) for maximum bolus size. Initiate pump to deliver ordered bolus.	Prevents accidental infusion of an overdose.
c. *Administer dose on demand.*	Gives patient control over administration of analgesic.
(1) While assisting anesthesia provider, perform Steps 7a(1)-(4). Set pump for lockout time (as ordered).	
(2) Have patient initiate demand dose as needed.	
8. Explain that nurses will monitor patient's response to epidural analgesic routinely. Also instruct patient on signs or problems to report to nurses.	Builds trust to encourage patient to be a partner in care.
9. **See Completion Protocol (inside front cover).**	
10. Before health care provider removes epidural catheter, check for presence of therapeutic coagulation. Check facility policy.	Removal of catheter while a patient is anticoagulated increases the risk for spinal hematoma because of anticoagulation and inability to compress blood vessels.

EVALUATION

1. Evaluate patient's comfort level; use pain rating scale at rest and on movement.
2. Evaluate sedation level; respiratory rate, rhythm, depth, and pattern; and pulse oximetry or capnography based on patient's clinical condition. Measure more frequently in the first 12 hours of infusion (e.g., hourly) (see facility policy), after bolus infusions or changes in infusion rate, and in periods of cardiovascular or respiratory instability (Rowbotham et al., 2010).

> **SAFE PATIENT CARE** Be prepared to deliver an ampule of naloxone IV push per health care provider's order if respirations fall below 8 breaths per minute and are shallow. Goal is to increase respirations, not reverse analgesia. Rapid reversal can cause serious side effects.

3. Monitor blood pressure and pulse (see facility policy). Assist patient when changing positions to avoid postural hypotension.
4. Evaluate catheter insertion site every 2 to 4 hours for redness, warmth, tenderness, swelling, or drainage (note character of drainage [e.g., purulent, clear, or bloody]). Monitor body temperature for early sign of infection.
5. Inspect epidural site for disruption or displacement of catheter.
6. Evaluate for presence of headache and observe for non-verbal signs of headache (grimacing, massaging head).
7. Monitor intake and output. Evaluate for bladder distention (see Chapter 7). Assess for frequency or urgency. Consider consulting with health care provider or anesthesia provider to order intermittent catheterization.
8. Observe for pruritus, especially of face, head, neck, and torso. Inform the patient that this is a side effect but is not an allergic response. Itching is most common side effect.
9. Assess patient for pharmacological side effects: nausea, vomiting, presence of tinnitus, or mouth numbness. Nausea may worsen by movement.
10. Use *Teach Back:* State to the patient, "I want to be sure you understand what the epidural analgesia catheter is for and what to expect from it. Can you give me an example?" Evaluates what the patient is able to explain or demonstrate. Revise your instruction now or develop plan for revised patient teaching to be implemented at an appropriate time if patient is not able to teach back correctly.

Unexpected Outcomes and Related Interventions

1. Patient states that pain is still present or has increased.
   a. Check all tubing, connections, and pump settings for dosing.
   b. Confer with health care provider regarding adequacy of medication dose.

2. Patient is sedated or not easily arousable.
   a. Stop epidural infusion and elevate patient's head of bed 30 degrees (unless contraindicated). *Stay with patient and call for help.*
   b. Notify health care provider and prepare to give naloxone per health care provider's order.
   c. Monitor vital signs and sedation level continuously until patient is easily arousable.
3. Patient develops apnea, or respirations are less than 8 breaths per minute, shallow, or irregular.
   a. Instruct patient to take deep breaths.
   b. Stop epidural infusion. *Stay with patient and call for help.* Notify health care provider.
   c. Prepare to give naloxone per health care provider's order.
   d. Monitor every 30 minutes until respirations are 8 or more and of adequate depth; continue for 2 hours, observing for return of respiratory depression. Naloxone has a shorter half-life than immediate-release opioids.
4. Patient reports sudden headache. Clear drainage is present on epidural dressing.
   a. Stop infusion or bolus dosing. Stay with patient and call for help.
   b. Notify health care provider.
5. Blood is present on epidural dressing.
   a. Stop infusion. Stay with patient and call for help
   b. Notify health care provider.
6. Redness, warmth, tenderness, swelling, or exudate is noted at catheter insertion site. Patient is febrile.
   a. Notify health care provider.
7. Patient experiences minimal urinary output, urinary frequency or urgency, bladder distention, pruritus, or nausea and vomiting.
   a. Consult with health care provider about reducing opioid dose and discuss treatment for side effects.

Recording and Reporting

- Record drug, dose, method (bolus, demand, or continuous), and time given (if bolus) or time begun and ended (if continuous or demand infusion) on appropriate MAR. Specify concentration and diluent.
- With continuous or demand infusion, obtain and record pump readout hourly for first 24 hours after infusion begins and then every 4 hours. Review pump settings and usage with staff on next shift.
- Record regular periodic assessments of patient's status in nurses' notes or flow sheet, including vital signs, SpO_2 or end-tidal carbon dioxide, intake and output, sedation level, pain severity score, neurological status, appearance of epidural site, presence or absence of adverse reactions to medication, and presence or absence of complications resulting from placement and maintenance of epidural catheter.
- Document your evaluation of patient learning.
- Report any adverse reactions or complications to health care provider.

Sample Documentation

0800 Fentanyl 2000 µg in 500 mL 0.9 NS infusing at 15 mL/hr into epidural catheter via infusion pump. Respiratory rate 10 with moderate depth and regular pattern. States abdominal surgical pain is 5 compared with previous 7 at 0700.

1000 Respiratory rate 6 with shallow depth and periods of apnea, O_2 saturation 90%, HR 70, BP 110/70. Arouses with verbal stimulation. Epidural infusion stopped, anesthesia notified and Narcan 0.2 mg IV push given in titrated doses per Dr. Arnold's order.

1005 Respiratory rate 8, shallow depth, regular pattern, O_2 saturation 94%, HR 78, BP 118/72. Alert, awake, oriented ×3.

1020 Respiratory rate 12, moderate depth, regular pattern. HR 82, BP 124/78, O_2 saturation 95%. Rates abdominal surgical incision pain 4 on 0 to 10 scale.

Special Considerations

Pediatric

- Apply EMLA cream to an epidural site a minimum of 60 minutes before catheter insertion to minimize discomfort from procedure.
- Epidural analgesia may be used in all pediatric age groups; dose of analgesic is by milligram or microgram per kilogram.
- Infants and children require continuous cardiac, respiratory, and SpO_2 monitoring.

Geriatric

- Because older adults often receive medications for hypertension, evaluating for hypotension during epidural analgesia is essential.

Home Care

- Patients who need home therapy are discharged with a tunneled catheter. Before considering catheter placement and care in the home, assess patient's fine motor skills, cognitive ability, stage of disease and prognosis, and family caregiver's willingness and ability to assist.
- Teach patient and family caregiver the proper dosage and technique for administering medication. Assess their technique for catheter care and administering medication. Reinforce instructions.
- Explain how to assess pain using a pain scale. Observe family member assess patient.
- Teach patient and family caregiver aseptic technique for medication administration and for all catheter care procedures, including dressing changes. Instruct them to change dressing every week (see home health facility policy). Teach signs and symptoms of infection and what to report and when to nurse or health care provider.
- Provide a list of all supplies needed for procedures, where to purchase, and phone numbers of health care providers to contact in emergency.
- Teach about signs and symptoms of adverse reactions to medications and interventions used to treat side effects.
- *Pruritus:* Advise patient to wear clean, lightweight cotton clothing; keep room cool; use cool moist compresses; and lubricate skin.

SKILL 13.5 LOCAL ANESTHETIC INFUSION PUMP FOR ANALGESIA

The insertion of a small one-way catheter into a surgical wound bed (e.g., open hernia repair, knee joint) for delivering a local anesthetic (e.g., bupivacaine [Marcaine], lidocaine, ropivacaine [Naropin]) has been shown to relieve pain effectively and reduce use of other analgesics. Patients may still require oral analgesics, but the total dosage is often reduced. The catheter is usually secured to the skin with a surgical dressing such as Tegaderm and then attached to a portable infusion system (Fig. 13-7). The infusion system holds a limited amount of local anesthetic (e.g., 2 or 3 day supply) and is supplied with a carrying pouch that attaches to a patient's clothing. Devices vary, but most offer a demand bolus or a continuous slow infusion (2 to 4 mL/hr) feature. Use of local anesthetic pumps can significantly decrease the amount of early postoperative pain. Local infusion pumps are for one-time use only and left in for about 48 hours. Rarely is the pump removed during hospitalization. Patients learn how to remove the catheter at home. Nursing care involves assessment of catheter connections, evaluation of local anesthetic side effects, and patient teaching.

ASSESSMENT

1. Identify patient using two identifiers (e.g., name and birthday or name and account number) according to facility policy. Compare identifiers with information on the patient's MAR or medical record. *Rationale: Ensures correct patient. Complies with The Joint Commission standards and improves patient safety (TJC, 2014b).*
2. Patient arrives at recovery area or nursing unit with pump in place. Assess surgical dressing and site of catheter insertion. Dressing should be dry and intact. *Rationale: Determines if catheter is placed properly.*
3. Assess catheter connections. If connections become detached, do *not* reattach; notify surgeon immediately. *Rationale: Reattachment could lead to infection. Misconnection could lead to infusion of inappropriate agent into joint site.*
4. Perform complete pain assessment (see Skill 13.1), including type of activities influenced by pain (e.g., sleeping, eating, moving affected extremity). *Rationale: Provides baseline for evaluation.*

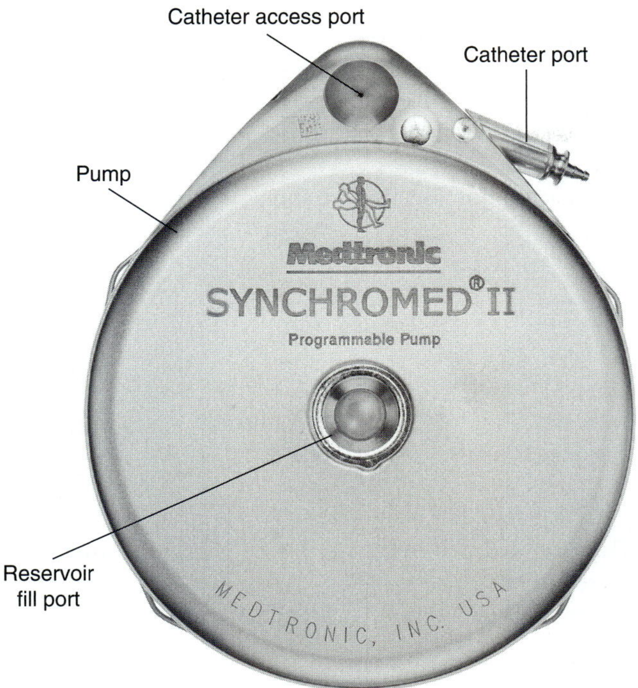

FIG 13-7 Local anesthetic infusion pump. (Used with permission from Medtronic, Columbia Heights, Minnesota.)

5. Review surgeon's operative report for position of catheter. Read label on infusion device. Label should show total dosage in mg/24 hours, the volume and concentration being delivered, and date and time prepared. Compare with health care provider's order. *Rationale: Confirms catheter location. Ensures proper medication delivery.*

6. Assess for blood backing up in tubing. If present, stop infusion and notify health care provider. *Rationale: Indicates possible displacement of catheter into blood vessel.*

7. Determine the level of extremity activity patient can perform per health care provider's order. *Rationale: Excessive activity may displace catheter.*

8. Assess for signs of local anesthetic toxicity: hypotension, dizziness, tremor, severe itching, swelling of the skin or throat, irregular heartbeat, palpitations, confusion, ringing in the ears, metallic taste, and seizures. *Rationale: Early identification of toxicity prevents or lessens the chance of complications. Local anesthetics can have serious systemic effects (ISMP, 2011)*

9. Assess patient's and family caregiver's knowledge and purpose of infusion pump and willingness to remove catheter at home. *Rationale: Determines level of teaching and support required by the patient and caregiver.*

▌PLANNING

Expected Outcomes focus on pain relief and improvement in patient's ability to resume activity.
1. Patient verbalizes full or partial pain relief at operative site.
2. Patient displays fewer nonverbal pain behaviors.
3. Patient is free of adverse drug reactions.
4. Patient moves about in bed, sleeps and eats, is active, and communicates easily with family and friends.
5. Catheter is removed correctly without injury to patient.

Delegation and Collaboration
The skill of managing local infusion pump analgesia cannot be delegated to nursing assistive personnel (NAP). The nurse instructs the NAP to:
- Pay close attention to the insertion site when providing care to avoid dislocation.
- Report any catheter disconnection to the nurse immediately.
- Notify the nurse immediately of a change in patient's status or level of comfort.

Equipment
- Pump in place from surgery

Home Catheter Removal
- Clean gloves
- Sterile 4 × 4–inch gauze pads
- Tape
- Plastic bag

IMPLEMENTATION for LOCAL ANESTHETIC INFUSION PUMP FOR ANALGESIA

STEPS	RATIONALE
1. **See Standard Protocol (inside front cover).**	
2. Use caution when repositioning or ambulating patient.	Avoids catheter dislodgment.
3. Encourage movement of operative joint per physician's order.	Maintains joint mobility.
4. Apply clean gloves. Teach patient or family caregiver how to remove catheter when appropriate (may also be done by home health nurse).	Prevents exposure to body fluids. RN can remove catheter during future clinic visit.
a. Instruct patient or family caregiver to perform hand hygiene and apply clean gloves.	Reduces transmission of infection.
b. Have patient assume a relaxed position in bed or chair. If catheter in leg, position extremity in normal alignment.	Relaxes joint muscles, reducing traction from muscle tension, and provides distraction.

Continued

STEPS	RATIONALE
c. Remove tape gently, followed by surgical dressing.	Provides access to infusion catheter.
d. Explain to patient what he or she will feel (slight burning and pulling sensation) when removing catheter.	Helping patient to anticipate nature of discomfort can relieve anxiety.
e. Place 4 × 4–inch gauze pad over site. Grasp catheter firmly and pull outward from skin with steady motion. If resistance occurs, stop pulling. Reposition extremity and try again. If tubing continues to stretch and shows resistance, stop pulling, cover area with sterile 4 × 4–inch gauze pad and notify health care provider.	Approach minimizes tissue trauma.
f. Look for mark on end of catheter tip.	Indicates complete removal of catheter.
g. After removing the catheter, place a new sterile gauze dressing over the area and apply pressure for at least 2 minutes.	Prevents hematoma formation.
h. Place catheter in plastic bag using standard precautions. Bring to health care provider's office.	Catheter will be inspected by surgeon to ensure all removed.
5. Remind patient of follow-up appointment with surgeon.	Improves likelihood of patient adherence.
6. See Completion Protocol (inside front cover).	

EVALUATION

1. Ask patient to rate pain intensity using a pain scale both at rest and with activity.
2. Observe patient's position; mobility; relaxation; and ability to rest, sleep, eat, and participate in usual activities.
3. Observe for signs of adverse drug reaction.
4. Inspect condition of surgical dressing.
5. Have patient or family caregiver describe steps to take to remove catheter.
6. Inspect catheter exit site during home visit.
7. Use *Teach Back:* State to the patient, "I want to be sure you understand what to do after the infusion pump has been removed. Can you give me an example?" Evaluates what the patient is able to explain or demonstrate. Revise your instruction now or develop plan for revised patient teaching to be implemented at an appropriate time if patient is not able to teach back correctly.

Unexpected Outcomes and Related Interventions

1. Dressing is moist and intact.
   a. Stop infusion and notify health care provider. Catheter may not be placed properly or has been displaced.
2. Patient verbalizes pain intensity greater than previously determined goal or demonstrates nonverbal behaviors indicative of pain. Catheter may be displaced or clogged, or surgical site may be developing complications.
   a. Check reservoir for presence of medication.
   b. Check patency of tubing.
   c. Notify health care provider.
3. Patient reports symptoms of local anesthetic adverse reaction.
   a. Stop pump and call surgeon immediately (ISMP, 2011).

Recording and Reporting

- Record drug, concentration, date catheter inserted, and type of demand feature (continuous or demand) in medication record. Record additional analgesics needed to control pain.
- Record location of catheter, patient's pain rating, response to anesthetic, and additional comfort measures given in nurses' notes.
- Record any adverse reactions to local anesthetic.
- Document your evaluation of patient learning.
- Report damp dressing or displaced catheter to surgeon.

Sample Documentation

1000   Returns from OR after right total knee replacement. Dressing dry and intact. Local anesthetic pump in place, catheter connections intact, receiving continuous 0.125% Marcaine infusion at 3 mL/hr. Patient currently rates knee pain as 3 (0 to 10 scale).

Special Considerations
Pediatric

- Local infusion pumps have been used for children undergoing certain types of orthopedic surgery. Explain precautions to take to avoid dislodging catheter.

Geriatric

- Continuous dosing is sometimes administered, but demand doses require a mentally competent adult.

Home Care

- If infusion is on demand, instruct patient on frequency to depress button.
- Instruct patient to notify home health nurse or surgeon if pain exceeds pain intensity goal and if excessive fluid or bleeding develops on the dressing.
- Provide written instructions regarding possible adverse reactions to bupivacaine (Marcaine) that patient should report to surgeon immediately: hypotension, dizziness, tremor, severe itching, swelling of the skin or throat, irregular heartbeat, palpitations, confusion, tinnitus, muscle twitching, numbness around the mouth, metallic taste, and seizures.
- Provide instructions regarding extremity movement.

SKILL 13.6   MOIST AND DRY HEAT

Heat and cold are the two common types of noninvasive and nonaddictive pain-relief therapies. Warm compresses, sitz baths, and commercial heat packs are examples of moist heat applications. A water flow pad such as an aquathermia pad, electrical heating pad, and a commercial heat wrap are forms of dry heat therapy.

External heat applications deliver heat through conduction. Heat transfers from the heat source (e.g., heat pack) directly to the skin. Typically, direct contact takes place between the heat source and the target tissues (e.g., an inflamed body part). Heat applications promote circulation to a treated area, reduce edema and inflammation, relieve pain, and promote muscle relaxation. In addition, moist heat can be used to débride wounds and apply medicated solutions. Patients typically receive heat applications for painful muscle spasms, joint stiffness, swollen rectal and perineal tissues following childbirth or surgery, abdominal muscle cramping, menstrual cramps, and superficial thrombophlebitis.

When preparing a moist heat application, remember that the heated solution is in direct contact with a patient's skin. Check the water temperature frequently to prevent burns. Keep the solution temperature constant to enhance the therapeutic effects of moist heat. Dry heat applications are also placed over the skin and can cause burns. Use a cotton cloth or towel to enclose a dry application to protect a patient's skin.

ASSESSMENT

1. Identify patient using two identifiers (e.g., name and birthday or name and account number) according to facility policy. *Rationale: Ensures correct patient. Complies with The Joint Commission standards and improves patient safety (TJC, 2014b).*
2. Refer to health care provider's order for type of heat application, location and duration of application, and desired temperature (when appropriate). *Rationale: Ensures safe and correct application. An order is required for any heat application.*
3. Assess skin around area to be treated for integrity, color, temperature, and sensitivity to touch (see Chapter 7). *Rationale: Establishes baseline for skin condition.*
4. If treating a wound, assess wound for size, color, drainage volume and character, presence of pain (using a pain scale), and odor. *Rationale: Provides a baseline to determine changes in wound after heat application.*
5. Assess patient's level of comfort (see Skill 13.1). *Rationale: Provides baseline measure.*
6. Measure joint ROM to any affected joint that is to be treated (see Chapter 16). *Rationale: Provides baseline to determine change in joint mobility.*
7. Refer to patient's medical record for contraindications to heat application (e.g., open wounds, certain cardiovascular conditions, certain medications that may result in sudden change in blood pressure and blood flow from vasodilation). *Rationale: May necessitate different form of therapy.*
8. Assess patient's level of consciousness and responsiveness (e.g., dementia). *Rationale: Patients with reduced level of consciousness are unable to sense or report reduced sensation or discomfort.*
9. Assess blood pressure and heart rate for patient receiving moist heat. *Rationale: Provides baseline for determining if patient becomes hypotensive during procedure.*
10. Determine patient's or family caregiver's knowledge of procedure, related safety factors, and whether heat has been used in the past. *Rationale: Determines health teaching needs.*

PLANNING

Expected Outcomes focus on promoting wound healing, increasing mobility, decreasing pain, and preventing burns.

1. After multiple applications, wound healing demonstrated by improved tissue granulation and reduced edema, inflammation, and drainage.
2. Patient's skin remains intact, pink, warm, and sensitive to touch immediately after heat application.
3. Patient denies any burning sensation during and after application.
4. Patient reports decrease in pain.
5. Patient's blood pressure and pulse are within his or her normal range.
6. Patient's joint mobility improves.

Delegation and Collaboration

Assessment of the patient's condition may not be delegated to nursing assistive personnel (NAP), however, the skill of

TABLE 13-1	TEMPERATURE RANGES FOR HOT AND COLD APPLICATIONS	
TEMPERATURE	**CELSIUS RANGE**	**FAHRENHEIT RANGE**
Warm	34°-37°	93°-98°
Tepid	26°-34°	80°-92°
Cool	18°-26°	65°-79°
Cold	10°-18°	50°-64°

applying moist or dry heat may be delegated. The nurse instructs the NAP about:

- Proper temperature of the application (Table 13-1)
- Skin changes (e.g., excess redness, blistering) or changes in patient's condition (e.g., dizziness) to report immediately to the nurse.
- Specific positioning and application time requirements (based on health care provider order or facility policy).
- Reporting when treatment is complete so that an evaluation of patient's response can be made.

Equipment

All Moist Heat Applications

- Bath blanket, dry bath towel
- Warmed prescribed solution (i.e., normal saline) or commercially prepared compress
- Biohazard waste bag
- Clean gloves
- Compress
- Clean basin
- Waterproof pad
- Ties or cloth tape
- Aquathermia pad (optional)
- Clean gauze or towel
- Options for sterile compress—sterile basin, sterile gauze, and sterile gloves
- Disposable sitz bath basin

Dry Heat Applications

- Aquathermia pad and control unit or commercial chemical heat pack
- Distilled water (for aquathermia pad)
- Bath towel or pillowcase
- Ties, tape, or roller gauze

IMPLEMENTATION *for* MOIST AND DRY HEAT

STEPS	RATIONALE
1. **See Standard Protocol (inside front cover).**	
2. Explain to patient the sensations he or she will feel, such as decreasing warmth over time and wetness. Explain precautions being taken to prevent burning.	Minimizes anxiety and promotes cooperation.
3. For moist application: Place a waterproof pad under patient (exception: sitz bath).	Prevents soiling of bed linen.
4. Help position patient in bed, keeping affected body part in proper alignment. Expose body part to be covered with heat application and drape patient with bath blanket as needed.	Limited mobility in an uncomfortable position causes muscular stress. Draping prevents cooling.
5. *Apply moist warm compress.*	
a. Heat prescribed solution to desired temperature by immersing closed bottle of solution in basin of very warm water for 10 minutes.	Proper warming reduces risk of patient incurring a burn.
b. Prepare aquathermia pad if needed. Temperature is usually set by bioengineering.	Prevents burns by ensuring proper temperature.
c. Apply clean gloves. Remove existing dressing (if present). Inspect wound and surrounding skin. Inflamed wound appears reddened, but surrounding skin is less red in color. Dispose of old dressing and gloves in biohazard bag.	Reduces transmission of microorganisms. Provides baseline to measure wound healing.

> **SAFE PATIENT CARE** If skin surrounding wound is inflamed or reddened or has active drainage, moist heat application may be contraindicated

d. Perform hand hygiene.	Reduces transmission of microorganisms.

STEPS	RATIONALE

  e. Prepare compress:

   (1) Pour warmed solution into container (use sterile technique if pouring into sterile basin).

   (2) Open gauze. If applying a sterile compress open supplies using sterile technique (see Chapter 5).

   (3) Add gauze to container of solution to immerse gauze; use proper aseptic technique.

   (4) If using a commercially prepared compress, follow manufacturer instructions for warming.

Use of appropriate aseptic technique keeps gauze compress clean or sterile. A sterile compress is needed when applied to an open wound.

  f. 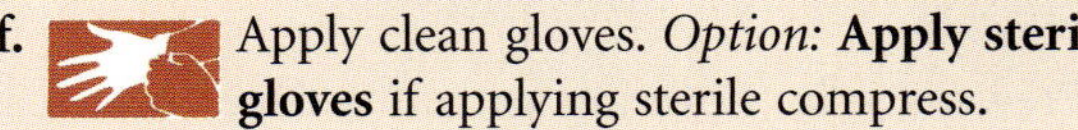 Apply clean gloves. *Option:* **Apply sterile gloves** if applying sterile compress.

Sterile gloves allow for manipulation of gauze without contamination.

> **SAFE PATIENT CARE** To avoid injury to a patient, test temperature of sterile solution by applying a drop to your forearm (without contaminating solution or gloves). It should feel warm to skin without burning.

  g. Pick up one layer of immersed gauze, wring out excess solution, and apply it lightly to wound. Avoid exposing unaffected skin as much as possible. *Option:* Apply commercial compress or heat pack over wound (clean wound only).

Provides therapeutic heat to injured tissues. Excess moisture on normal skin can cause maceration.

  h. After a few seconds, ask patient if he or she feels any burning and lift edge of gauze or compress to assess for redness.

Increased redness indicates burn. Burns and injuries from hot therapies are preventable events (NQF, 2011).

  i. If patient tolerates compress, pack gauze or compress snugly against wound. Cover all wound surfaces.

Packing compress prevents rapid cooling from underlying air currents.

  j. Cover moist compress with dry gauze (clean or sterile as appropriate) and then bath towel. If necessary, pin or tie in place. Cover commercial compress or heat pack with bath towel. Remove and dispose of gloves.

Dry dressing prevents transfer of microorganisms to wound via capillary action caused by moist compress. Towel insulates from heat loss.

  k. *Option:* When using a gauze compress, apply an aquathermia or waterproof heating pad over towel. Keep in place for duration of application.

Maintains constant temperature of compress.

  l. Leave compress in place for 20 minutes or less (per order or facility policy). If an aquathermia pad is not used, change warm compress using proper aseptic technique every 5 to 10 minutes. Dispose of gloves; perform hand hygiene.

Maintains constant temperature for best therapeutic benefit. Time limit prevents risk of overexposure and burning of skin.

  m. Apply clean gloves. After prescribed time, remove pad or external gauze, towel, and compress. Evaluate wound and condition of skin, and replace the type of dressing ordered for patient (see Chapter 26).

Continued exposure to moisture macerates skin. New dressing prevents entrance of microorganisms into wound site.

6. *Sitz bath:*

  a. Apply clean gloves. Remove any existing dressing covering wound. Dispose of dressing in proper receptacle. Inspect condition of wound and surrounding skin. Pay close attention to the suture line. Dispose of gloves and perform hand hygiene.

Reduces transmission of microorganisms.

Continued

STEPS	RATIONALE

b. When exudate or drainage is present, apply clean gloves and clean the intact skin around area of open wound with clean cloth and soap and water. Sterile gloves and gauze may be needed to cleanse open wound; check facility policy. Dispose of gloves and perform hand hygiene.

Cleansing removes organisms so that bath solution does not spread infection.

c. If using bag of normal saline, warm per facility policy. Otherwise pour warmed solution into disposable sitz bath in bathroom (see illustration). Check temperature (see facility policy).

Ensures proper temperature and reduces risk for burns.

d. Assist patient to bathroom to sit and immerse body part in bath. Cover patient with bath blanket. Assess heart rate and ask if patient feels dizzy. Stay with patient or place call light at side and instruct not to try to sit up unattended. Explain risk of orthostatic hypotension.

Prevents falls. Covering patient reduces heat loss from evaporation. Vasodilation from heat may alter cardiovascular dynamics and predispose patient to orthostatic hypotension when standing.

e. Maintain constant temperature of bath solution throughout 15- to 20-minute soak by draining used fluid and carefully adding additional warm solution.

Ensures proper therapeutic effect.

f. After 15 to 20 minutes, remove patient from basin, and dry body parts thoroughly. Inspect area treated. Wear clean gloves if drainage present.

Avoids chilling. Reduces transmission of infection.

g. Drain solution from basin. Clean and store properly.

7. *Applying dry heat:*

a. Prepare aquathermia pad. Check temperature, which is usually set by bioengineering. *Option:* Prepare commercial heat pack following package directions.

b. Cover or wrap affected area with bath towel or enclose aquathermia pad or commercial heat pack in pillowcase (see illustration).

Prevents heated surface from touching patient's skin directly and increasing risk for injury to skin.

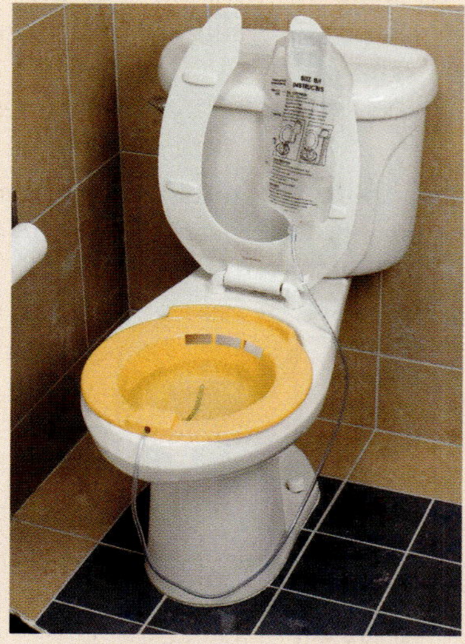

STEP 6c Disposable sitz bath. (Used with permission from Briggs Corporation, West Des Moines, Iowa.)

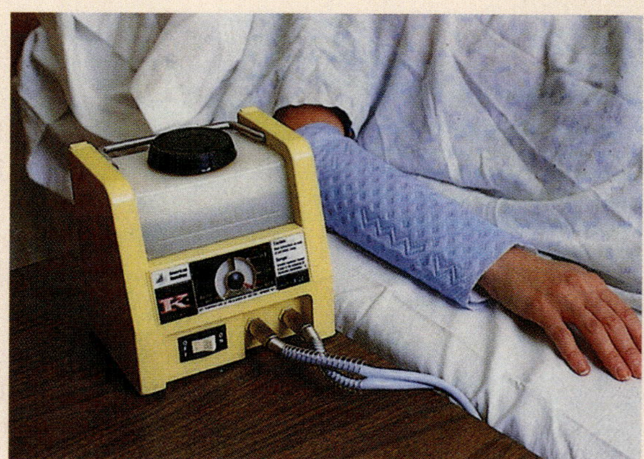

STEP 7b Aquathermia pad.

STEPS	RATIONALE
c. Place pad or pack over affected area and secure with tape, tie, or roller gauze.	Pad delivers warm heat to injured area and should not slip onto different body part.

> **SAFE PATIENT CARE** Never position patient so that he or she is lying directly on pad. This position prevents dissipation of heat and increases risk for burns.

STEPS	RATIONALE
d. Double check temperature setting on aquathermia pad.	Ensures patient safety.
e. Monitor condition of skin over treatment site every 5 minutes and ask patient about sensation of burning.	Determines if heat exposure is causing any burn, blistering, or injury to skin.
f. After 20 minutes (or time ordered by health care provider), remove pad and store.	Continued exposure can result in burns.

8. See Completion Protocol **(inside front cover).**

EVALUATION

1. Inspect patient's wound for size, appearance, and evidence of healing.
2. Inspect skin for integrity, color, temperature, dryness, and blistering. Evaluate again 30 minutes after procedure.
3. Ask patient to rate level of comfort on scale of 0 to 10.
4. Measure patient's ROM.
5. In the case of a warm compress or sitz bath, measure blood pressure and heart rate.
6. Use *Teach Back:* State to the patient, "I have talked about ways to avoid burns when using heat. I want to be sure I explained everything clearly to you. Can you tell me how to use a heat compress or pad at home without the risk of being burned?" Evaluates what the patient is able to explain or demonstrate. Revise your instruction now or develop plan for revised patient teaching to be implemented at an appropriate time if patient is not able to teach back correctly.

Unexpected Outcomes and Related Interventions

1. Patient's skin is reddened and sensitive to touch (either during treatment or 30 minutes after) or patient complains of burning.
   a. Stop treatment if still in place and notify health care provider.
   b. Ensure proper temperatures or check equipment for proper functioning before repeating treatment later.
   c. If there is a burn to the skin, complete an incident or adverse event report (see facility policy).
2. Body part is painful to move.
   a. Discontinue treatment.
   b. Assess affected area for edema.
   c. Notify health care provider.

Recording and Reporting

- Record and report procedure, noting type of application (solution, pad, or pack); location and duration of application; condition of body part, wound, or skin before and after treatment; and patient's response to therapy.
- Document your evaluation of patient learning.

Sample Documentation

1000   Warm moist compress applied for phlebitis at discontinued IV site in L forearm. Patient reports pain at a 5 on a scale of 0 to 10. Area red, edematous, 5 cm (2 inches) long, 2.5 cm (1 inch) wide, slightly raised, tender to touch, and warm.

1030   Compress removed, discontinued IV site remains reddened as at baseline. Patient states warmth is soothing to area. Rates pain at a 4.

Special Considerations
Pediatric

- The skin of infants and children is thin and fragile and easily damaged. Use special caution with heat applications (Hockenberry and Wilson, 2013). Remain with children during procedure for safety (include parents).

Geriatric

- An older adult who is receiving long-term steroid therapy or is malnourished can have thin, fragile skin that is more easily damaged. Older adults also may have impaired circulation to a given skin region or impaired sensation for pain or temperature (Touhy and Jett, 2014).
- If an older adult is frail and has a cardiac condition, monitor vital signs throughout a heat application.

Home Care

- Assess availability of family caregiver to help patient in application of heat therapy as well as his or her willingness to remain with patient. Provide instruction and evaluate understanding of procedure.
- Assess physical environment of the home (condition of electrical outlets) to determine adequacy of facilities for use of heat therapy.

SKILL 13.7   COLD APPLICATION

A variety of cold (cryotherapy) therapies are available, such as ice packs, chemical cold packs, and continuous flow cooling devices (ranging from gravity-fed devices that are manually filled with ice water to motorized units that both cool and circulate chilled water). Cold therapy treats localized inflammatory responses that lead to edema, hemorrhage, muscle spasm, and pain. Cold therapy most commonly is used immediately after soft tissue and musculoskeletal injuries such as sprains or strains. Cold is one step in the PRICE principle—the acronym used in treating sprains and strains (ACSM, 2011):

- *P—Protect* from further injury
- *R—Restrict* activity
- *I*—Apply *Ice*
- *C*—Apply *Compression*
- *E—Elevate* the injured area

Cold applications are common after orthopedic joint replacement surgery (shoulders and knees) for reducing inflammation, pain, and swelling. More recent research on cryotherapy reports that patients who undergo total knee replacement may experience a slight reduction in the amount of blood loss and pain postoperatively and have improved ROM at the knee in the first 1 to 2 weeks after surgery. However, the evidence is weak and more research is needed (Adie et al., 2012).

Cryotherapy is generally safe when applied correctly. The basic physiological effects include decreased local metabolism and vasoconstriction. The vasoconstriction reduces blood flow to an injured part and reduces fluid accumulation and slows bleeding and hematoma formation from trauma. In addition, cold produces analgesia secondary to impaired neuromuscular transmission. Cold also reduces the pain of muscle spasm.

Patients at risk for injury from cold applications have the same risks as patients at risk from heat therapy (see Skill 13.6) and patients with compromised circulation. When the skin is exposed to cold, over time it adapts, and a patient can be unaware of any temperature variation. Excessive cold causes a numbing sensation before pain is sensed. An order for a cold application is always needed, and it should include the duration of the treatment and the desired temperature to be used when settings can be controlled.

ASSESSMENT

1. Identify patient using two identifiers (e.g., name and birthday or name and account number) according to facility policy. *Rationale: Ensures correct patient. Complies with The Joint Commission standards and improves patient safety (TJC, 2014b).*
2. Refer to health care provider's order for type, location, and duration of cold application. Temperature of a cold flow device is ordered or preset. *Rationale: An order is required for all cold applications.*

3. Inspect condition of injured or affected body part. Gently palpate for area of edema. *Rationale: Provides baseline for determining change in condition after therapy.*

> **SAFE PATIENT CARE** If in an emergent situation, keep injured part in alignment and immobilized. Movement can cause further injury to strains, sprains, or fractures.

4. Consider time in which any injury occurred. *Rationale: Apply cold as soon as possible after injury to reduce bleeding and edema (Gottschalk, 2011).*
5. Ask patient to describe character of pain and rate on scale of 0 to 10. *Rationale: Provides baseline for determining pain relief after therapy.*
6. Perform a neurovascular check, and inspect surrounding skin for integrity, circulation and skin temperature, color of skin, and sensitivity to touch (see Chapter 7). *Rationale: Determines condition of skin and if patient is insensitive to cold extremes.*
7. Review medical history for conditions that contraindicate use of cold therapy: hypertension (owing to secondary vasoconstriction), Raynaud's disease, rheumatoid arthritis, local limb ischemia, history of vascular impairment such as frostbite or severe arteriosclerosis, cold allergy, and paroxysmal cold hemoglobinuria. *Rationale: Conditions that increase risk of skin injury when cold is applied.*
8. Assess patient's level of consciousness and responsiveness. *Rationale: Patients with reduced level of consciousness are unable to sense or report reduced sensation or discomfort.*
9. Assess patient's and family caregiver's understanding of use of cold therapy and ability to apply in the home. *Rationale: Determines level of instruction necessary.*

PLANNING

Expected Outcomes focus on achieving comfort and healing of injury site while preventing injury to skin.
1. Patient reports decreased pain.
2. Patient has decreased edema and bleeding at site of tissue injury.
3. Surrounding skin is slightly pale and cool to touch.
4. Patient or family caregiver correctly states how to apply cold therapy.

Delegation Considerations

Assessment of the condition of the patient's skin cannot be delegated. The skill of applying cold applications can be delegated to nursing assistive personnel (NAP). The nurse instructs the NAP about:
- Keeping the application in place for only the length of time specified in health care provider's order.
- Immediately reporting to the nurse any excessive redness on the skin, increase in pain, or decreased sensation.
- Reporting when the treatment is complete so that nurse can assess skin.

Equipment
All compresses, bags, and packs
- Soft cloth covering, stockinette, towel, or pillowcase
- Cloth ties or tape
- Waterproof absorbent pad
- Bath blanket for warmth
- Waterproof pad

Ice bag or gel pack
- Ice bag; ice chips and water for ice bag
- Reusable commercial gel pack (cold pack)
- Disposable commercial chemical cold pack

Electronically controlled cooling device
- Gauze roll or elastic wrap
- Cool-water flow pad or cooling pad and electrical pump

IMPLEMENTATION *for* COLD APPLICATION

STEPS	RATIONALE
1. **See Standard Protocol (inside front cover).**	
2. Explain to patient sensations he or she might feel such as coldness or numbness. Explain precautions being taken to prevent injury to skin.	Minimizes anxiety and promotes cooperation.
3. Position patient carefully, keeping body part in proper alignment and exposing only area to be treated. Drape patient with blanket.	Prevents further injury to body part. Avoids unnecessary exposure and maintains patient's comfort and privacy.
4. Apply clean gloves. Place a waterproof pad under patient	Prevents soiling of bed linen.

> **SAFE PATIENT CARE** In case of strains, sprains, or fractures, align extremity or body part following health care provider's orders. You might also be ordered to keep body part elevated to help lessen swelling.

STEPS	RATIONALE
5. *Apply ice pack or bag:*	
a. Fill ice bag with water, secure cap, and invert. For commercial cold pack, remove from freezer or package container.	Checks bag for leaks. Prepares device for application.
b. For the ice bag, empty water and fill it two-thirds full with small ice chips and water.	Bag is easier to mold over body part when not full.
c. Express excess air from ice bag, secure bag closure, and wipe bag dry.	Excess air interferes with cold conduction. Allows bag to conform to treatment area and promotes maximum contact.
d. Squeeze or knead commercial cold pack.	Releases alcohol-based solution to create cold temperature.
e. Enclose bag or pack in towel, pillowcase, or stockinette. Apply over injury (see illustration). Secure with cloth ties or tape. Note: Some commercial packs can be secured with attached Velcro straps.	Cover protects patient's tissues, absorbs condensation, and prevents direct exposure of cold against patient's skin. Securing the cold pack ensures cold applied to injured area.

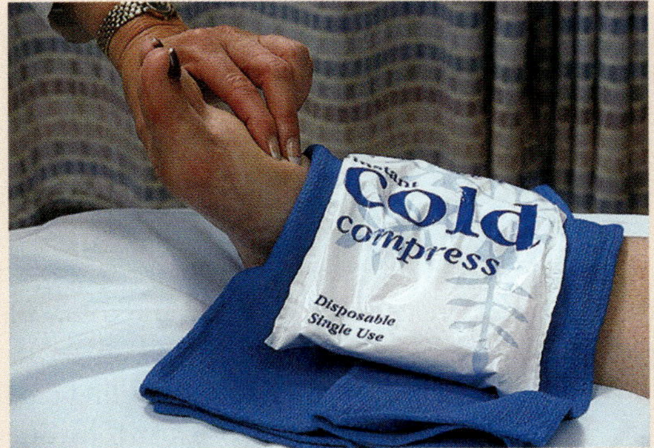

STEP 5e Commercial ice pack.

Continued

STEPS	RATIONALE

6. *Apply electrically controlled cooling device:*

a. Prepare device following product directions. Some devices are gravity-fed devices that require you to fill manually with iced water. Motorized units circulate chilled water enclosed in cooling coils connected to a pump.

Devices provide continuous flow of cold water through pad applied to the skin. Some devices also apply compression at the same time.

b. Ensure all connections are intact and that the device is set at correct temperature. Most are preset by bioengineering (see facility policy or health care provider order).

Preset temperature ensures safe temperature application.

c. Wrap the cooling pad in towel or pillowcase.

Prevents direct contact of cold against skin, preventing burn or frostbite.

d. Wrap cooling pad around body part.

Ensures even application of temperature to treatment site.

e. Turn device on and recheck temperature.

Prevents patient injury.

f. Secure with elastic wrap bandage, gauze roll or ties (see illustration).

Ensures cold is applied to injured area.

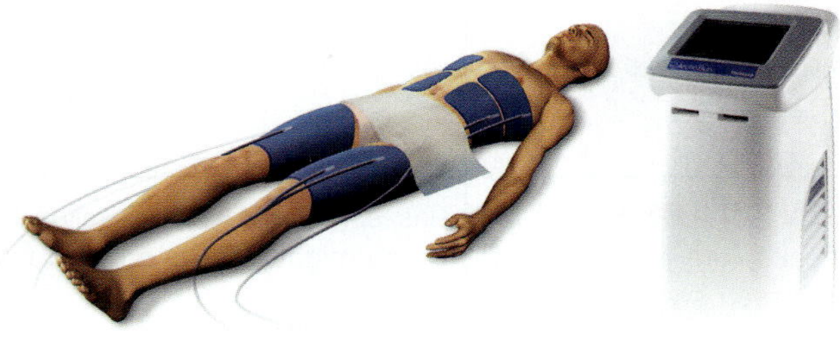

STEP 6f Electrical cooling device.

7. Remove and dispose of gloves in proper container.

Reduces transmission of microorganisms.

8. Check condition of skin every 5 minutes for duration of application. Look for mottling, redness, burning, blistering, and numbness.

Determines if there are adverse reactions to cold.

When applying cold, skin initially feels cold, followed by relief of pain. As cryotherapy continues, patient feels burning sensation, pain in skin, and then numbness.

a. If area is swollen, sensation may be reduced; use extra caution in checking patient's response.

b. Numbness and tingling are common sensations with cold applications and indicate adverse reactions only when severe and coupled with other symptoms. Stop application when patient displays adverse symptoms.

9. After 15 to 20 minutes (or as ordered by health care provider), apply clean gloves, remove ice bag/pack or cooling device, and gently dry off any moisture.

Drying prevents skin maceration.

10. **See Completion Protocol (inside front cover).**

EVALUATION

1. Reevaluate 30 minutes after procedure. Inspect treated area and surrounding skin for integrity, color, temperature, and sensitivity to touch.

2. Palpate tissue or wound for edema.

3. Ask patient to report pain level on scale of 0 to 10.

4. Use *Teach Back:* State to the patient, "We have discussed quite a bit about how to apply a cold pack. I want to be sure you know what to do to avoid injuring your skin from the cold. Tell me how your skin will feel if you keep the cold on for too long, and tell me what you should do if that feeling develops." Evaluates what the patient is able to explain or demonstrate. Revise your instruction now or develop plan for revised patient teaching to be implemented at an appropriate time if patient is not able to teach back correctly.

Unexpected Outcomes and Related Interventions

1. Skin appears mottled, reddened, or bluish purple, and patient complains of burning-type pain and numbness.
   a. Stop treatment; symptoms indicate prolonged exposure to cold and possible ischemia.
   b. Report to health care provider if signs persist for more than 30 minutes.
2. Patient or family caregiver is unable to describe how to apply cold pack or demonstrate its use.
   a. Provide reinstruction and clarification.
   b. Consider home health referral if patient is eligible.

Recording and Reporting

- Record procedure, including type, location, and duration of application and patient's response (including appearance of site and pain level).
- Document your evaluation of patient learning.

Sample Documentation

1030   Patient in supine position with left shoulder in arm sling and continuous cooling pack applied. Patient rates current pain at a 4 on a 0 to 10 scale, pain goes to level of 5 when turning or sitting up. Inspected surgical wound area; skin is pink, nontender, minimal swelling, no drainage. 1045   Administered hydrocodone 100 mg po, scheduled for PT at 1130.

Special Considerations

Pediatric

- Infants have an unstable temperature control mechanism; mottling of extremities is common and does not always indicate an adverse reaction. Monitor any cold application carefully every 5 minutes (Hockenberry and Wilson, 2013).

Geriatric

- Older adults are more at risk for tissue damage because of altered responses to change in body temperature (Touhy and Jett, 2014). Check site frequently during treatment.

Home Care

- See Skill 13.6 for considerations as they apply to cold therapy.

CRITICAL THINKING EXERCISES

Case Study

A 68-year-old woman has had chronic arthritis for more than 5 years. When her pain reaches a level affecting her ability to perform ADLs such as cooking and grooming, she takes an NSAID for pain relief. Her joint pain usually involves a deep ache, and it limits her ROM. She does not always get complete relief from taking an analgesic, but it "lessens my pain so I can get around." She tries to avoid taking analgesics as much as she can because she worries about the side effects of NSAIDs.

1. What factors make this patient a good candidate for nonpharmacological pain therapy?
2. A nurse who sees the patient in the pain clinic recommends distraction and relaxation to relieve her pain further. When the patient returns to the clinic, the nurse notices she is grimacing more than usual, and the patient's pain severity is reported as a 5 on a pain scale compared with a 3 on her last visit. What should be some of the nurse's next steps?

Review Questions

1. Which of the following statements are true about cultural influence on the pain experience? Select all that apply.
   1. There are differences in the way people express pain.
   2. A patient is likely to have culturally based beliefs about using pain medicines.
   3. Culture affects how people ask for pain relief.
   4. Patients from minority groups are at the same risk for pain outcomes as patients in majority groups.
2. A nurse has been assigned to care for a 72-year-old woman who has returned from surgery for a hip replacement. When providing the patient an analgesic, which of the following medications should be given with caution in the lowest dose possible?
   1. Morphine
   2. Dilantin
   3. Acetaminophen
   4. Ibuprofen
3. When assessing a patient's pain, the PQRSTU acronym is a useful guide to determine the character of the pain. Match the letter from the acronym on the left with the assessment question on the right.

   P = __   1. "Tell me what your pain feels like."
   Q = __   2. "Show me where the pain is."
   R = __   3. "Does your pain bother you all the time or just when you move about?
   S = __
   T = __   4. "Tell me what worsens your pain."
   U = __   5. "On a scale from 0 to 10, with 10 being the worst pain ever, how would you rate your pain?"
             6. "Tell me how your pain affects the way you bathe and dress each morning."
4. When providing patients pain relief, which of the following measures would you *not* consider implementing in all situations?
   1. Adjusting the level of lighting and noise in a room
   2. Giving an oral analgesic 15 minutes before any therapy
   3. Explaining to a patient how to use a pain scale
   4. Setting a pain intensity goal with a patient

5. The use of SBAR is a good way of communicating to a health care provider the situation when a patient is not receiving adequate pain relief. Match the letters from the acronym SBAR on the left with the appropriate approach described on the right.

   S = __
   B = __
   A = __
   R = __

   1. The patient is 24 hours postoperative following a knee replacement. She has been receiving morphine via PCA routinely. She was able to get up into a chair last night.
   2. Is it possible to change the dose of her morphine or add another medication? She has taken muscle relaxants in the past with good results.
   3. My name is Sarah Williams, RN; I am calling to consider changing pain medicines for Mrs. S., who is reporting an increase in her pain severity.
   4. The patient is having incisional pain, most recently rated at 6 compared with 4 consistently reported last night. She is refusing to get out of bed or do her therapy exercises.

6. A patient has expressed interest in trying relaxation to help relieve his chronic back pain. Which of the following explanations about relaxation is the most accurate?
   1. The use of relaxation gives you some self-control over the pain. I will teach and coach you through the exercise when you feel the most discomfort.
   2. Relaxation combined with your medication can relieve pain more effectively, but it often takes several coaching sessions for it to work well.
   3. It is important for you to know that relaxation techniques have several side effects.
   4. For relaxation to be effective, it works best for people having acute episodic pain.

7. A nurse is preparing to administer morphine to a patient who has chronic bone pain from cancer. Which of the following statements apply to morphine?
   1. The drug is chosen for its antiinflammatory effects on a tumor.
   2. The drug works on higher centers of the brain and spinal cord to modify pain perception for moderate to severe pain.
   3. The drug works peripherally on nerves and centrally on the brain.
   4. The drug is more effective than adjuvants for relief of neuropathic pain.

8. The nurse is explaining to a patient when it is best to give an analgesic. Which of the following is not correct?
   1. About 30 minutes after pain occurs
   2. Before pain increases in severity
   3. About 30 minutes before any pain-producing procedures, such as ambulating to a chair
   4. Around the clock

9. Which patient is the BEST candidate for use of a PCA pump?
   1. A very confused older adult having minor surgery
   2. An obese adult with sleep apnea
   3. An older teenager having an appendectomy
   4. A middle-aged adult who is having major surgery and requires an interpreter

10. Which patient is the WORST candidate for use of a PCA pump?
    1. A very confused older adult having minor surgery
    2. An obese adult with sleep apnea
    3. An older teenager having an appendectomy
    4. A middle-aged adult who is having major surgery and requires an interpreter

REFERENCES

Adie S, et al: Cryotherapy following total knee replacement, *Cochrane Database Syst Rev* (9):CD007911, 2012. doi: 10.1002/14651858.CD007911.pub2.

Allred K, et al: The effect of music on postoperative pain and anxiety, *Pain Manage Nurs* 11(1):15, 2010.

Alm AK, Norbergh KG: Nurses' opinions of pain and the assessed need for pain medication for the elderly, *Pain Manage Nurs* 14(2):e31, 2013.

American College of Sports Medicine (ACSM): *Sprains, strains and tears*, 2011. http://www.acsm.org/docs/brochures/sprains-strains-and-tears.pdf. Accessed December 31, 2013.

American Society for Pain Management Nursing (ASPMN): *Authorized and unauthorized ("PCA by proxy") dosing of analgesic infusion pumps*, June 2006. http://www.aspmn.org/organization/documents/PCAbyProxy-final-EW_004.pdf. Accessed December 30, 2013.

American Pain Society (APS) and American Association of Pain Medicine (AAPM): Opioids guideline panel—Part 1, *J Pain* 10(2):113.e22, 2009.

Asadizker M, et al: The effect of foot and hand massage on postoperative cardiac surgery pain, *Int J Nurs Midwifery* 3(10):165, 2011.

Baird C, et al: Efficacy of guided imagery with relaxation for osteoarthritis symptoms and medication intake, *Pain Manage Nurs* 11(1):56, 2010.

Braun LA, et al: Massage therapy for cardiac surgery patients: a randomized trial, *J Thorac Cardiovasc Surg* 144(6):1453, 2012.

Busch V, et al: The effect of deep and slow breathing on pain perception, autonomic activity, and mood processing—an experimental study, *Pain Med* 13(2):215, 2012.

Carteret M: *Cultural aspects of pain management, dimensions of culture*, 2011. http://www.dimensionsofculture.com/2010/11/cultural-aspects-of-pain-management/. Accessed June 17, 2013.

Craft J: Patient-controlled analgesia: is it worth the painful prescribing process?, *Proc (Bayl Univ Med Cent)* 23(4):434, 2010.

D'Arcy Y: New thinking about postoperative pain management, *OR Nurse* 5(6):29, 2011.

D'Arcy Y: Treating acute pain in the hospitalized patient, *Nurse Pract* 37(8):22, 2012.

Drew DJ, St Marie BJ: Pain in critically ill patients with substance abuse disorder or long-term opioid use for chronic pain, *AACN Adv Crit Care* 22(3):238, 2011.

Gilmore-Bykovskyi AL, Bowers BJ: Understanding nurses' decisions to treat pain in nursing home residents with dementia, *Res Gerontol Nurs* 6(2):127, 2013.

Gloth M: Pharmacological management of persistent pain in older persons: focus on opioids and nonopioids, *J Pain* 12(3 Suppl):S14, 2011.

Gottschalk AW: Ice and cold application for musculoskeletal soft-tissue trauma, *Evid Based Pract* 14(5):13, 2011.

Hanna MN, et al: Does patient perception of pain control affect patient satisfaction across surgical units in a tertiary teaching hospital?, *Am J Med Qual* 27(5):411, 2012.

Herr K: Pain assessment strategies in older patients, *J Pain* 12 (Suppl 3):S3, 2011.

Hockenberry MJ, Wilson D: *Essentials of pediatric nursing*, ed 9, St Louis, 2013, Mosby.

Institute of Medicine (IOM): *Relieving pain in America: a blueprint for transforming prevention, care, education and research*, Washington, D.C., 2011, National Academic Press.

Institute for Safe Medication Practices (ISMP): Medication safety alert: process for handling elastomere pain relief balls (On-Q Painbuster and others) requires safety improvements, *ISMP Acute Care Quarterly Action Agenda* 2011. http://www.ismp.org/Newsletters/acutecare/articles/20090716.asp. Accessed July 3, 2013.

Jones L, et al: Pain management for women in labour: an overview of systematic reviews, *Cochrane Database Syst Rev* (3):CD009234, 2012. doi: 10.1002/14651858.CD009234.pub2.

Lehne RA: *Pharmacology for nursing care*, ed 8, St Louis, 2013, Saunders.

Narayan MC: Culture's effects on pain assessment and management, *AJN* 110(4):38, 2010.

National Institutes of Health (NIH), National Center for Complementary and Alternative Medicine (NCCAM): *Selected results of NCCAM funded research on CAM*, 2011. http://nccam.nih.gov/research. Accessed December 29, 2013.

National Quality Forum (NQF): *National voluntary consensus standards for public reporting of patient safety event information*, 2011. http://www.qualityforum.org/Publications/2011/02/National_Voluntary_Consensus_Standards_for_Public_Reporting_of_Patient_Safety_Event_Information.aspx. Accessed December 30, 2013.

Paice JA, Noskin GA, Vanagunas A: Efficacy and safety of scheduled dosing of opioid analgesics: a quality improvement study, *J Pain* 6(10):639, 2005.

Pasero C, McCaffery M: *Pain assessment and pharmacologic management*, St Louis, 2011, Mosby.

Ramachandran SK, et al: Life-threatening critical respiratory events: a retrospective study of patients found unresponsive during analgesic therapy, *J Clin Anesth* 23(3):207, 2011.

Rowbotham D, et al: *Best practice in the management of epidural analgesia in the hospital setting*, London, Nov 2010, Faculty of Pain Medicine of The Royal College of Anaesthetists.

The Joint Commission (TJC): *Comprehensive accreditation manual for hospitals: the official handbook*, Oak Brook Terrace, IL, 2014a, The Commission.

The Joint Commission (TJC): *National Patient Safety Goals*, Oakbrook Terrace, IL, 2014b, The Commission. Available at: http://www.jointcommission.org/standards_information/npsgs.aspx. Accessed December 29, 2013.

Topcu SY, Findik UY: Effect of relaxation exercises on controlling postoperative pain, *Pain Manage Nurs* 13(1):11, 2012.

Touhy TT, Jett T: *Ebersole and Hess's gerontological nursing and healthy aging*, ed 5, St Louis, 2014, Mosby.

Zhang JM, et al: Music interventions for psychological and physical outcomes in cancer: a systematic review and meta-analysis, *Support Care Cancer* 20(12):3043, 2012.

Promoting Oxygenation

The need for air is one of the basic physiological needs found on Maslow's hierarchy of human needs. Respirations are effective when the body receives sufficient oxygen at the cellular level and removes cellular waste and carbon dioxide via the bloodstream and lungs. When this system is interrupted by lung tissue damage, obstruction of airways by inflammation and excess mucus, or impairment of the mechanics of ventilation, interventions are required to achieve adequate oxygenation. If interventions are untimely or inadequate, the person may experience dyspnea, which is a subjective feeling of being smothered or suffocated (Campbell, 2011).

pen boards are examples of common communication tools. Use positive verbal and nonverbal communication with direct eye contact, and ask questions one at a time that require only "yes" or "no" responses. Be sure that lighting is adequate and background noise is at a minimum when communicating. Assess for any visual or hearing impairment, if the person has adequate hand strength to use a communication board, and which hand is dominant. Be sure to include a clear communication plan so that all health care providers use a consistent method (Grossbach et al., 2011).

PATIENT-CENTERED CARE

When a person requires respiratory support, an artificial airway (e.g., endotracheal tube [ETT], tracheal tube [TT]) may be necessary. However, when an artificial airway is present, the patient is unable to speak. Many patients become stressed and have feelings of depression, anxiety, fear, and anger when they are unable to communicate with their health care providers and family members (Khalaila et al., 2011). Alphabet charts, pen and paper, slates, or magnetic

SAFETY

Patients with impaired oxygenation require supplemental oxygen (see Skill 14.1). When oxygen levels are low, patients have diminished cognitive skills and are at risk for confusion and falls (Campbell, 2011). Orienting a patient and instituting fall precautions are a must when impaired oxygenation occurs. In addition, there are other safety risks when oxygen is in use in any health care setting or in the home (Table 14-1).

TABLE 14-1   OXYGEN SAFETY GUIDELINES

GUIDELINE	EXPLANATION
"Oxygen in use" sign is on patient's door.	Notifies all personnel of oxygen in patient's room.
Ensure that oxygen is set at prescribed rate.	Oxygen is a medication, and you should not adjust it without a health care provider's order.
Smoking is not permitted. Avoid electrical equipment that may result in sparks.	Oxygen supports combustion. Delivery systems and cylinders must be kept 10 feet from open flames and at least 5 feet from electrical equipment or heat source.
Store oxygen cylinders upright. Secure with chain or holder.	Prevents tipping and falling while stationary or when patient is being transported.
Check oxygen available in portable cylinders before transporting or ambulating patients.	Gauge on cylinder should register in green range, indicating that oxygen is available. Have backup supply available if level is low.
Tubing extensions should not be added if patient is ambulatory.	Added tubing length increases fall hazard and also decreases amount of delivered oxygen.
Check for tight seal when delivering oxygen via mask.	When using a mask, a tight seal around the mouth is necessary to prevent room air from entering and decreasing the FiO_2. If a tight seal is required, a nasal cannula cannot be added.

FiO₂, Fraction of inspired oxygen concentration.

BOX 14-1   CARE BUNDLE FOR VENTILATOR-ASSOCIATED PNEUMONIA

- Practice good hand hygiene
- Check internal endotracheal cuff pressure at 25 to 30 cm H_2O every 2 hours
- Maintain head of bed at 30 to 45 degrees
- Prophylaxis for deep vein thrombosis and peptic ulcer disease
- Daily interruptions of sedation to assess accurately for readiness to extubate
- Oral care with chlorhexidine 0.12% every 12 hours and general oral care every 2 hours secondary to microbial colonization within the mouth
- Complete subglottal suctioning to decrease risk of oral fluid aspiration
- Maintain accurate and timely documentation
- Maintain timely ventilator circuit changes and removal of condensation
- Provide for mobility through turning and repositioning every 2 hours

Data from Sedwick M et al: Using evidence-based practice to prevent ventilator-associated pneumonia, *Crit Care Nurse* 32(4): 41, 2012.

are unable to remove these secretions. The frequency for suctioning depends on the patient assessment; some patients require suctioning every 1 or 2 hours, but oropharyngeal suction should be completed at least every 4 hours (Sole et al., 2011).

EVIDENCE-BASED PRACTICE

Morinec J, Iacaboni J, McNett M: Risk factors and interventions for ventilator-associated pneumonia in pediatric patients, *J Pediatr Nurs* 27(5):435, 2012.

Ramirez P, Baorres A: Measures to prevent nosocomial infections during mechanical ventilation, *Curr Opin Crit Care* 18(1):86, 2012.

Sedwick M et al: Using evidence-based practice to prevent ventilator-associated pneumonia, *Crit Care Nurse* 32(4):41, 2012.

When several EBPs are combined into one protocol, it is called a care bundle. Care bundles are a mechanism to provide evidence-based practice interventions for a specific problem. One such bundle is the ventilator bundle, which was developed to decrease the incidence of ventilator-associated pneumonia (VAP) (Box 14-1). The incidence of VAP ranges from 9% to 27% with a mortality rate of 46% and cost of $40,000 to $57,000 per occurrence (Ramirez and Baorres, 2012; Sedwick et al., 2012). "Modifiable risk factors include mechanical ventilation longer than 48 hours, high gastric residuals, supine position, use of antibiotics, frequent changes in ventilator circuits, presence of nasogastric tubes, and use of paralytic agents or continuous sedation" (Morinec et al., 2012).

Artificial airways require airway suctioning, which poses risks such as cardiac dysrhythmias; laryngeal spasm; and bradycardia, which is associated with stimulation of the vagus nerve. Additional risks related to insertion of a suction catheter include nasal trauma and bleeding (Sole et al., 2011).

The oropharynx and trachea are suctioned in most cases. Differences between oropharyngeal and tracheal airway suctioning include the depth of suctioning, sterile versus clean procedure, and the potential for complications. Oropharyngeal suctioning removes secretions from the back of the throat. When the secretions are in only the nose and mouth, only the oropharynx requires suctioning.

In a health care setting, sterile procedures are necessary when suctioning extends into the lower airways. Tracheal airway suctioning removes respiratory secretions and maintains optimum ventilation and oxygenation in patients who

SKILL 14.1   OXYGEN ADMINISTRATION

• **Nursing Skills Online: Airway Management, Lesson 1**

Oxygen therapy supplies supplemental oxygen to prevent or relieve hypoxia. Hypoxia results from hypoxemia, which is a deficiency of oxygen in the arterial blood. Hypoxia occurs when there is insufficient oxygen to meet the metabolic needs of tissues and cells. Normal partial pressure of oxygen (PaO_2) for an adult is 80 to 100 mm Hg. Supplemental oxygen is indicated when the PaO_2 is less than 60 mm Hg or oxygen saturation (SpO_2) is less than 95% (Pagana and Pagana, 2013). Supplemental oxygen is used for temporary relief of hypoxia or is used long-term when it is required for a chronic condition.

Room air has an oxygen concentration, or fraction of inspired oxygen (FiO_2), of 21%. Supplemental oxygen delivery is based on the FiO_2 required to maintain adequate oxygenation (Table 14-2), whether hospital or home use, and the portability desired.

ASSESSMENT

1. Identify patient using two identifiers (e.g., name and birthday or name and account number) according to facility policy. Compare identifiers with information on the

TABLE 14-2   OXYGEN DELIVERY SYSTEMS

DELIVERY SYSTEM	FiO₂ DELIVERED*	ADVANTAGES	DISADVANTAGES
Low-Flow Delivery Devices			
Nasal cannula	1-6 L/min: 24%-44%	Safe and simple Easily tolerated Effective for low concentrations Does not impede eating or talking Inexpensive, disposable	Unable to use with nasal obstruction Drying to mucous membranes Can dislodge easily May cause skin irritation or breakdown around ears or nares Patient's breathing pattern (mouth or nasal) affects exact FiO_2
Simple face mask	6-12 L/min: 35%-50%	Useful for short periods such as patient transportation	Contraindicated for patients who retain CO_2 May induce feelings of claustrophobia Therapy interrupted with eating and drinking Increased risk of aspiration
Partial and nonrebreather masks	10-15 L/min: 60%-90%	Useful for short periods Delivers increased FiO_2 Easily humidifies O_2 Does not dry mucous membranes	Hot and confining; may irritate skin; tight seal necessary Interferes with eating and talking Bag may twist or kink; should not totally deflate
Oxygen-conserving cannula (Oxymizer)	8 L/min: up to 30%-50%	Indicated for long-term O_2 use in the home Allows increased O_2 concentration and lower flow	Cannula cannot be cleaned More expensive than standard cannula
High-Flow Delivery Devices			
Venturi mask	24%-50%	Provides specific amount of O_2 with humidity added Administers low, constant O_2	Mask and added humidity may irritate skin Therapy interrupted with eating and drinking Specific flow rate must be followed

CO_2, Carbon dioxide; FiO_2, fraction of inspired oxygen concentration.
*FiO_2 delivered may differ by manufacturer. Check manufacturer's guidelines.

patient's MAR or medical record. *Rationale: Ensures correct patient. Complies with The Joint Commission standards and improves patient safety (TJC, 2014).*

2. Perform respiratory assessment (see Chapter 7). Assess for impaired gas exchange (hypoxia or hypercapnia) during both rest and activity, including the following:
   a. Observe for behavioral changes (e.g., apprehension, anxiety, confusion, decreased ability to concentrate, decreased level of consciousness, fatigue, and dizziness). *Rationale: Decreased levels of oxygen (hypoxia) or increased levels of carbon dioxide (hypercapnia) affect a person's cognitive abilities, interpersonal interactions, and mood (Campbell, 2011).*
   b. Obtain vital signs, including rate, rhythm, and depth of respirations and SpO_2 via pulse oximetry. *Rationale: Provides baseline of oxygenation status and enables early detection of hypoxia. In the presence of hypoxemia, the percent of hemoglobin saturated with oxygen declines, and the patient's pulse oximetry level declines.*
   c. Observe skin and mucosa for changes in color: pallor, cyanosis, or flushing. *Rationale: Pallor may occur when patient's oxygen levels decline. Cyanosis is a late sign of hypoxia. Flushing may be noted when hypercapnia is present.*
3. When available, check arterial blood gas (ABG) or pulse oximetry results (SpO_2). *Rationale: ABGs and SpO_2 objectively quantify changes in oxygen and carbon dioxide that affect acid-base balance.*
4. Observe for patent airway. *Rationale: Secretions obstruct airway and decrease the amount of oxygen that is available for gas exchange.*

▌PLANNING

Expected Outcomes focus on optimum oxygenation, safe application of oxygen therapy, and an understanding of and compliance with the oxygen prescription.

1. Patient's oxygen saturation (SpO_2) and/or ABGs return to or remain within normal limits or baseline levels.
2. Patient verbalizes improved comfort; subjective experiences of anxiety, fatigue, and breathlessness return to normal.
3. Patient's pulse, respirations, and color return to normal.
4. Patient is able to state the reasons for supplemental oxygen by discharge.
5. Patient follows safety guidelines for supplemental oxygen therapy by discharge.
6. Patient uses supplemental oxygen as prescribed by discharge.

Delegation and Collaboration

The nurse is responsible for assessment of the patient's condition, setup and administration of proper oxygen concentration, and patient response to oxygen therapy. The skill of nasal cannula or mask placement may be delegated to nursing assistive personnel (NAP). The nurse instructs the NAP about:
- How to safely place or adjust the oxygen delivery device for a specific patient.
- Reporting immediately to the nurse any changes in vital signs or pulse oximetry, changes in patient's anxiety or behavior, confusion, or changes in skin color.
- Providing skin care around patient's nose, ears, and other areas where pressure from the oxygen device occurs.

Equipment
- Delivery device ordered by health care provider
- Oxygen tubing
- Humidifier if indicated
- Sterile water for humidifier
- Oxygen source
- Oxygen flowmeter
- "Oxygen in use" sign

▌IMPLEMENTATION *for* OXYGEN ADMINISTRATION

STEPS	RATIONALE
1. **See Standard Protocol (inside front cover).**	
2. Attach oxygen delivery device (e.g., cannula, mask) to oxygen tubing.	
3. Attach end of tubing to appropriate flowmeter and humidified oxygen source (see illustration).	Humidity prevents nasal drying. Flowmeters with smaller calibrations may be safer for patients requiring low-dose oxygen when larger doses may be harmful, as in patients with chronic obstructive pulmonary disease (COPD) (AARC, 2012).
4. Apply oxygen device: a. Place tips of cannula into patient's nares. If tips are curved, they should point downward inside the nostrils. Loop the cannula tubing up and over patient's ears. Adjust the lanyard until cannula fits snugly and comfortably.	Directs flow of oxygen into patient's upper respiratory tract. Patient is more likely to keep device in place if it fits comfortably.

Continued

STEPS	RATIONALE

b. Apply a mask by placing it over patient's mouth and nose. Bring the straps over patient's head and adjust to form a comfortable but tight seal.

5. Observe for proper function of oxygen delivery device.

Ensures patency of delivery device and accuracy of prescribed oxygen flow rate.

   a. *Nasal cannula:* Cannula is positioned properly in nares; oxygen flows through tips (see illustration).

Provides prescribed oxygen rate and reduces pressure on tips of nares.

   b. *Partial or nonrebreather mask:* Mask seals tightly around mouth. Reservoir fills on exhalation and almost collapses on inspiration. The reservoir should not collapse completely (see illustration).

Easily humidifies oxygen and does not dry mucous membranes. Useful for short-term therapy of 24 hours or less (AARC, 2012).

   c. *Oxygen-conserving cannula (Oxymizer):* Fit as for nasal cannula. Reservoir is located under patient's nose or worn as a pendant.

Delivers higher flow of oxygen with nasal cannula without changing to a mask, which is claustrophobic for some patients. Delivers a 2 : 1 ratio (e.g., 6-L/min nasal cannula is approximately equivalent to 3.5-L/min with Oxymizer).

   d. *Nonrebreathing mask:* Apply as a regular mask. Contains one-way valves with a reservoir; exhaled air does not enter reservoir bag. Can be combined with a nasal cannula to provide higher FiO_2.

Device of choice for short-term high FiO_2 delivery.

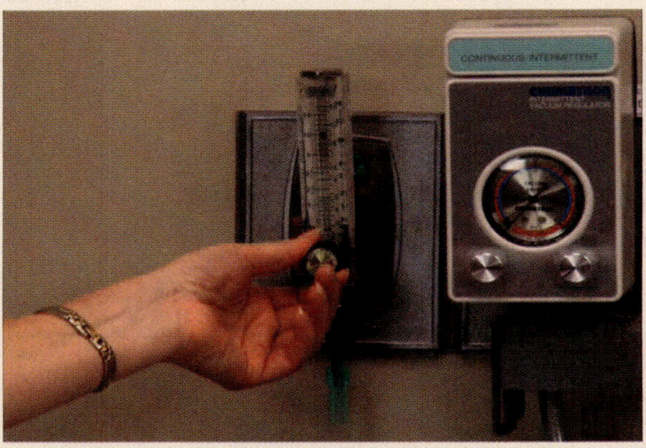

STEP 3 Flowmeter attached to oxygen source.

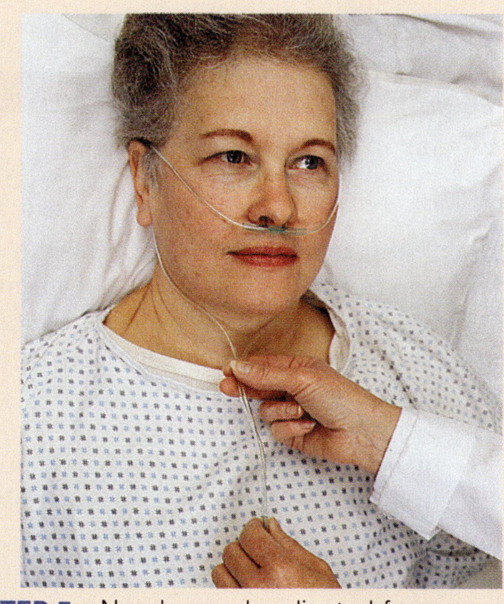

STEP 5a Nasal cannula adjusted for proper fit.

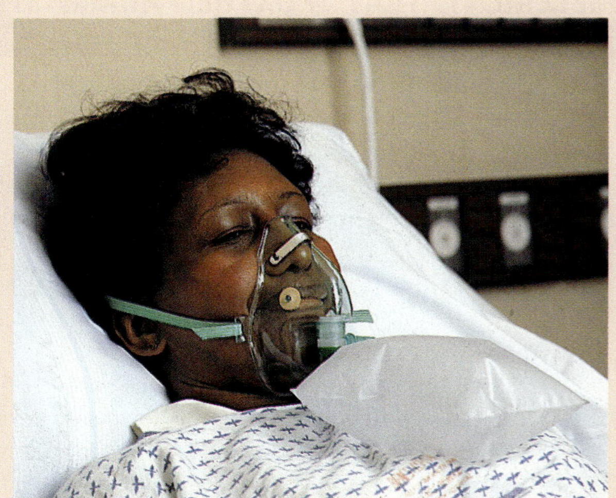

STEP 5b Partial or nonrebreather mask.

STEPS	RATIONALE

   e. *Simple face mask:* Select appropriate flow rate (see illustration).

Used for short-term oxygen therapy.

   f. *Venturi mask:* Apply as a regular mask. Select appropriate flow rate (see illustrations).

Used when a high-flow device is desired.

6. Verify settings on flowmeter and oxygen source for proper setup and prescribed flow rate.

Ensures delivery of prescribed oxygen therapy in conjunction with specific cannula or mask.

7. Maintain sufficient slack on oxygen tubing and secure to patient's clothing.

Allows patient to turn head without causing mask to shift or dislodge nasal cannula.

8. Check cannula or mask every 8 hours. Keep humidification container filled at all times.

Ensures patency of cannula and oxygen flow. Oxygen is a dry gas; when administered via nasal cannula of 4 L/min or more, you must add humidification so that patient inhales humidified oxygen (ATS, 2012).

9. Place "Oxygen in use" signs on wall behind bed and at entrance to room.

Alerts visitors and care providers that oxygen is in use.

10. Consult with health care provider regarding the need for continuous pulse oximetry if patient's oxygen level is unstable.

Oximetry provides objective data regarding blood oxygenation and is used for trending.

11. **See Completion Protocol (inside front cover).**

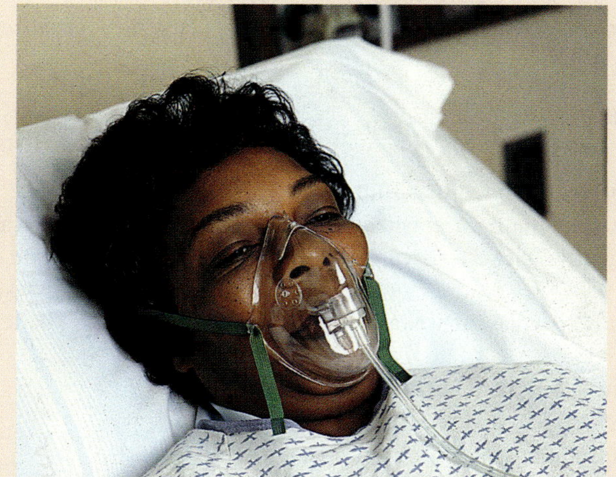

STEP 5e Simple face mask. Covers patient's face and nose.

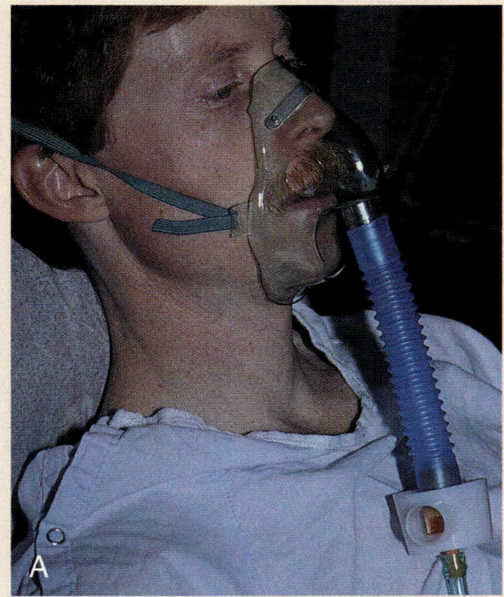

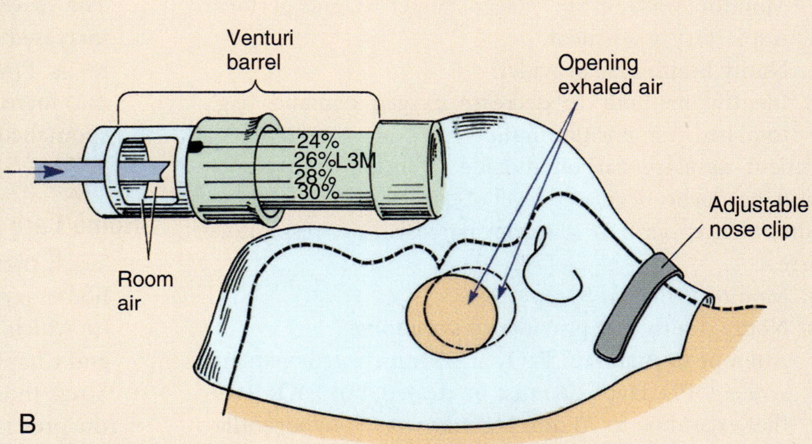

STEP 5f A, Venturi mask. **B,** Oxygen is delivered by turning barrel to preset intervals.

EVALUATION

1. Obtain repeat ABG values or SpO_2 for objective measurement of improvement. Whenever possible, obtain values both at rest and with activity.
2. Observe patient for decreased anxiety, improved level of consciousness and cognitive abilities, decreased fatigue, and absence of dizziness.
3. Monitor vital signs and pulse oximetry, if ordered; review ABG results. Expect a decreased pulse with regular rhythm, decreased respiratory rate, and improved color. Observe use of thoracic accessory muscles.
4. Ask patient to verbalize indications for supplemental oxygen.
5. Use **Teach Back:** State to the patient, "I want to make sure that I explained the importance of keeping your oxygen mask on in order to provide adequate oxygen. Can you explain to me why this is important?" Evaluates what the patient is able to explain or demonstrate. Revise your instruction now or develop plan for revised patient teaching to be implemented at an appropriate time if patient is not able to teach back correctly.

Unexpected Outcomes and Related Interventions

1. Patient experiences skin and nasal irritation from cannula or mask, drying of nasal mucosa, sinus pain, or epistaxis.
   a. Remove delivery system; gently cleanse area of secretions.
   b. Apply a water-soluble lubricant to areas of irritation around nares.
   c. Recommend use of an isotonic saline nasal spray.
   d. Determine if a reservoir cannula is appropriate (decreased liter flow without reducing FiO_2, oxygen delivery on inspiration only); if so, obtain order from health care provider.
   e. Consider humidification.
2. Patient has continued hypoxia: increased or irregular heart rate, SpO_2 declines, complaint of dyspnea.
   a. Monitor ABGs or SpO_2 (see Chapter 6), and perform respiratory assessment.
   b. Notify health care provider.
   c. Identify methods to decrease oxygen demand (e.g., total bed rest, positioning).
3. Patient develops carbon dioxide retention with confusion, headache, decreased level of consciousness, flushing, somnolence, carbon dioxide narcosis, or respiratory arrest.
   a. Monitor ABGs or SpO_2.
   b. Notify health care provider of symptoms.
   c. Attempt to maintain PaO_2 at 55 mm Hg for patients with COPD. Hypoxia must be treated, but PaO_2 levels that exceed 60 to 70 mm Hg may worsen hypoventilation in patients with obstructive airway diseases (Campbell, 2011).

Recording and Reporting

- Record the respiratory assessment findings, method of oxygen delivery, and flow rate.
- Record and report patient's response and any adverse reactions.
- Document your evaluation of patient learning.

Sample Documentation

0800   Alert and oriented. Respirations 20, regular rate, rhythm and depth noted and nonlabored. Lungs clear to auscultation. Mucous membranes pink and moist. Skin pink and dry. O_2 4 L/min nasal cannula. SpO_2 90%. Cough productive of small amount yellow sputum; no blood noted. Fluids encouraged as tolerated. Water within reach at bedside.
1000   Patient complains of tenderness behind right ear. Reddened area noted behind right ear. Foam ear protector added to nasal cannula tubing. Patient verbalized understanding that the nasal cannula must remain in place to help with respiratory status.
1230   Patient verbalized decreased tenderness behind right ear.

Special Considerations
Pediatric

- Oxygen hoods are transparent enclosures that surround the head of a neonate or small infant and deliver continuous humidified oxygen. Larger "tents" are available for larger children (Bailey, 2013; Hockenberry and Wilson 2013).

Geriatric

- Decrease in PaO_2 that occurs with aging is about 0.3% per year. After age 75, healthy nonsmokers do not show a noticeable decline. The decrease in oxygen is related to the loss of elasticity in the lungs and the increase in physiological dead space (Touhy and Jett, 2013).
- The drive to breathe in patients who have chronically increased carbon dioxide levels is based on their oxygen levels. Providing oxygen flow rates greater than 2 L/min may increase oxygen levels to a degree that would decrease spontaneous respirations.

Home Care

- Teach patient and family caregiver about the hazards of home oxygen and how to administer oxygen safely based on which system is selected for home use (see Table 14-1 and Chapter 31).
- Stress the dangers of changing the oxygen flow rate from the prescribed flow.
- Teach patient and family caregiver signs and symptoms of hypoxia.

SKILL 14.2 AIRWAY MANAGEMENT: NONINVASIVE INTERVENTIONS

Airways must remain open and free of obstruction to decrease resistance of airflow to and from the lung. Positioning enhances airway patency in all patients. A high-Fowler's or semi-Fowler's position promotes chest expansion with the least amount of effort. A patient with COPD who is short of breath may gain relief by sitting with the back against a chair and rolling the head and shoulders forward or leaning over a bedside table while in bed. Other interventions include balancing rest and activity and spacing out nursing care (Campbell, 2011).

Deep-breathing and coughing techniques help patients clear their airways effectively while maintaining their oxygen levels. Teach controlled coughing techniques described in this skill to assist patients to cough effectively and efficiently. Devices are available to assist with secretion clearance, such as vests that inflate with large volumes of air and vibrate the chest wall and handheld devices that assist in providing positive expiratory pressure to prevent airway collapse in exhalation (Restrepo et al., 2011). Usefulness of these therapies depends on the individual patient situation and preference of both the patient and the health care provider.

Pharmacological management is essential for patients with respiratory disease. Medications such as bronchodilators effectively relax smooth muscles and open airways in certain disease processes such as asthma. Glucocorticoids relieve inflammation and assist in opening air passages. Mucolytics and adequate hydration decrease the thickness of pulmonary secretions so that they are easily expectorated (Lehne, 2013).

Patients with obstructive sleep apnea (OSA) are often unable to maintain a patent airway. In OSA, nasopharyngeal abnormalities that cause narrowing of the upper airway produce repetitive airway obstruction during sleep, with the potential for periods of apnea, carbon dioxide retention, and hypoxemia. People at risk for OSA are obese (BMI of ≥30), are older, have hypothyroidism, are men or postmenopausal women, and have neck circumference of more than 43 cm (17 inches) (in men) and 41 cm (16 inches) (in women). Continuous positive airway pressure (CPAP) or bi-level positive airway pressure (BiPAP) delivers pressurized oxygen by mask to reduce carbon dioxide levels. The mask delivers pressure during the inspiratory and expiratory phases of the respiratory cycle to maintain airway patency. The use of this device is individualized and requires assessment of each patient's ability to use the equipment as instructed (Carlucci et al, 2013).

ASSESSMENT

1. Identify patient using two identifiers (e.g., name and birthday or name and account number) according to facility policy. *Rationale: Ensures correct patient. Complies with The Joint Commission standards and improves patient safety (TJC, 2014).*

2. Assess patient's respiratory effort, sense of breathlessness, and ability to clear copious or tenacious secretions by coughing. *Rationale: Indicates risk for impaired airway clearance. Secretions can plug the airway, decreasing the amount of oxygen available for gas exchange in the lung.*

3. Auscultate lung sounds for adventitious sounds (see Chapter 7). *Rationale: Decreased lung sounds can indicate plugging of the airway from mucus. Adventitious sounds indicate obstructed airflow; these sounds result from bronchospasm, laryngospasm, or mucus.*

4. Observe for dyspnea, use of accessory muscles of respiration, pallor, diaphoresis, or cyanosis. *Rationale: Indicators of respiratory distress from decreased oxygenation levels* (Campbell, 2011).

5. Monitor patient's vital signs and SpO_2 with oximetry or collect ABGs. *Rationale: Establishes baseline for determining response to therapy.*

6. Ask about interrupted sleep and snoring respirations. Ask patient about history of sleep apnea. *Rationale: Indications for use of CPAP/BiPAP. Refer patient for evaluation* (Carlucci et al., 2013).

PLANNING

Expected Outcomes focus on patient's airway patency, comfort, and self-care maintenance.

- Patient maintains a position that promotes maximum lung expansion and comfort.
- Patient's airways are clear of retained secretions.
- Patient's periods of sleep apnea are reduced to fewer than two episodes in 6 hours.
- Patient's ABGs and SpO_2 readings improve or remain normal.
- Patient and family demonstrate correct use of CPAP/BiPAP and express comfort using equipment by discharge.

Delegation and Collaboration

The nurse is responsible for assessment of the patient's condition and response to therapy. The skills of positioning, therapeutic coughing, and CPAP/BiPAP mask application can be delegated to nursing assistive personnel (NAP). The nurse instructs the NAP to:

- Report immediately to the nurse the patient's complaint or observed difficulty breathing or any change in vital signs, skin color, respiratory effort, or behavior.

Equipment

- CPAP or BiPAP mask (Fig. 14-1) (Note: Several types of masks are available because of the difficulties in achieving a comfortable fit.)
- Mask straps (face or nasal)
- Valve (CPAP or BiPAP)
- Oxygen source and tubing
- Generator (CPAP or BiPAP)
- Clean gloves
- Appropriate signs

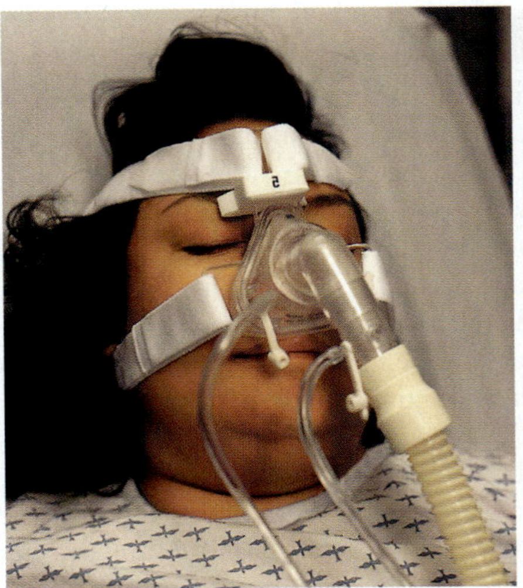

FIG 14-1 CPAP mask/BiPAP mask.

IMPLEMENTATION *for* AIRWAY MANAGEMENT: NONINVASIVE INTERVENTIONS

STEPS	RATIONALE
1. **See Standard Protocol (inside front cover).**	
2. Explain to patient that you are aware of the discomfort he or she is experiencing (e.g., breathlessness, pain) and that correct positioning is necessary.	Helps to allay patient anxiety.
a. *Sitting:* Assist to semi-Fowler's or high Fowler's, sitting on side of bed or in chair with elbows resting on knees. Patients with COPD may benefit from leaning over table with arms propped up (see illustrations).	Promotes optimum lung expansion and maximizes use of accessory muscles. Decreases patient's work of breathing (Campbell, 2011).
b. *Leaning:* Have patient lean forward over the back of a chair or against the wall.	Leaning forward allows the lungs to expand with less transdiaphragmatic pressure.

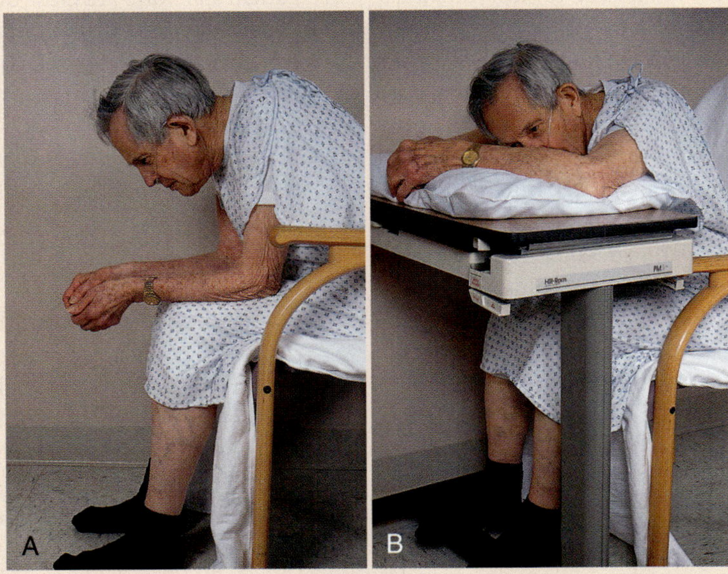

STEP 2a A, Positioning optimizes chest expansion and reduces the work of breathing. **B,** Leaning position allows lungs to expand.

STEPS	RATIONALE
c. *30-degree head-of-bed elevation:* Most patients are more comfortable supported by two pillows or with the head of the bed up at least 30 degrees.	Decreases orthopnea. Obese patients may experience increased abdominal pressure, which may inhibit full lung expansion when lying flat.
d. *Turning:* Turn at least every 2 hours. Turn to drain areas of lungs with retained secretions by gravity if tolerated by patient. If unilateral reexpansion is needed (e.g., after general surgery), have patient lie with side requiring expansion up: "good side down, affected lung up."	Encourages drainage of secretions and promotes lung expansion on the affected side. Promotes gas exchange by increasing blood flow to area of greater surface area available for gas exchange.
3. Teach controlled coughing:	
a. Place patient in upright position, high-Fowler's, leaning forward, or with knees bent and a small pillow or hand to support the abdomen.	Facilitates inhalation and lung expansion during coughing maneuver. May augment expiratory pressure.
b. Instruct patient to take two slow, deep breaths, inhaling through the nose and exhaling through the mouth.	Control of respiratory rate facilitates coughing and minimizes risk of paroxysms of coughing.
c. Instruct patient to inhale deeply a third time, hold this breath, and count to three and then to cough deeply for two or three consecutive coughs without inhaling between coughs. Instruct patient to push air forcefully out of the lungs.	Ensures full, effective cough. Explain to patient that controlled coughing clears secretions that may obstruct the airway by allowing air behind the mucus to move during the cough.
d. Have patients with difficulty coughing use a "huff" cough by taking a medium breath and making a sound like "ha" to push the air out fast with the mouth slightly open. Repeat three or four times, and then instruct patient to cough.	Assists patients to generate more pressure to force secretions through airways.
e. Repeat coughing to ensure airway is clear. Do not continue past patient's tolerance.	Continued coughing may cause breathlessness and decreased SaO_2.
4. CPAP/BiPAP administration:	
a. Position patient comfortably with head elevated.	Allows for maximum lung expansion.
b. Determine correct mask size. Use a masking chart to determine the correct size (S, M, L, XL). *Note: It is imperative that the mask have quick-release straps.* Position face mask or nasal mask tightly and adjust head strap until seal is maintained and tolerable to patient (see Fig. 14-1).	In case of emergency (e.g., vomiting, respiratory arrest), quick-release straps allow mask to be removed quickly. Patient may experience claustrophobic sensations and feel discomfort from continuous pressure (Simmons and Pruitt, 2012).
c. Connect CPAP/BiPAP device delivery tubing to pressure generator.	
d. Connect patient to pulse oximetry.	Oxygenation levels need constant monitoring.
e. Set CPAP/BiPAP initial settings:	
(1) CPAP: 4 to 8 cm H_2O	CPAP provides single positive pressure throughout the breathing cycle, which helps to keep the alveoli open at end expiration.
(2) BiPAP: Inspiratory pressure usually set at 10 to 15 cm H_2O; expiratory pressure usually set at 4 to 10 cm H_2O.	BiPAP supplies pressure at both inhalation and exhalation. The inhalation pressure is set per the health care provider's order and helps prevent airway closure. The expiratory pressure is set per the health care provider's order and keeps the alveoli open at end expiration.
5. Perform frequent skin assessment to determine presence of pressure, skin irritation, or skin breakdown from the mask.	Mask that is too tight increases risk of skin breakdown over bridge of nose.
6. **See Completion Protocol (inside front cover).**	

EVALUATION

1. Observe patient's body alignment and position whenever in visual contact with patient.
2. Auscultate lung fields for adventitious lung sounds.
3. Observe patient's respiratory status during sleep to determine response to CPAP/BiPAP.
4. Observe vital signs and pulse oximetry. Review ABGs when available.
5. Observe patient and family caregiver's use of CPAP/BiPAP mask and compliance with therapy (Carlucci et al., 2013).
6. Use *Teach Back:* State to the patient, "I want to make sure that I explained to you the purpose and benefits of positioning and CPAP/BiPAP correctly. Can you explain the benefits of using the CPAP/BiPAP?" Evaluates what the patient is able to explain or demonstrate. Revise your instruction now or develop plan for revised patient teaching to be implemented at an appropriate time if patient is not able to teach back correctly.

Unexpected Outcomes and Related Interventions

1. Patient is unable to maintain a patent airway.
   a. Evaluate positioning. Consider suctioning and use of artificial airway (see Skill 14.4).
   b. Monitor ABGs/pulse oximetry (SpO$_2$).
2. Patient experiences worsening dyspnea with bronchospasm and hypoxemia.
   a. Notify health care provider.
   b. Monitor ABGs/pulse oximetry (SpO$_2$).
   c. Medicate as ordered.
   d. Evaluate for methods to decrease oxygen demand (e.g., bed rest, positioning).
3. Patient is unable to tolerate CPAP/BiPAP.
   a. *Carbon dioxide retention:* Notify health care provider.
   b. *Mask fit:* Check fit of device. Consider alternative if difficulties continue. If skin breakdown occurs across bridge of nose, apply porous tape until skin becomes adjusted to the pressure. If generalized breakdown occurs, consider a reaction to the mask material (e.g., latex) (Carlucci et al., 2013; Simmons and Pruitt, 2012).
   c. *Pressure:* Feelings of suffocation, shortness of breath, and discomfort related to pressure from CPAP/BiPAP. Determine if another pressure setting will give similar results with more comfort or if BiPAP is required (Carlucci et al., 2013; Simmons and Pruitt, 2012).

Recording and Reporting

- Record activity level, including assistance needed with positioning, coughing effectiveness, and respiratory assessment.
- For CPAP/BiPAP, record patient adherence and tolerance, mask fit and skin assessment beneath mask, effectiveness of therapy, witnessed periods of apnea, and status of daytime hypersomnolence.
- Document your evaluation of patient learning.

Sample Documentation

2400   Observed sleeping. Respirations 18; regular in rate, rhythm, and depth without snoring. SpO$_2$ 93%, Skin is pink, warm, and dry. No jerking movements noted. CPAP continues per face mask with good seal at 7.5 cm H$_2$O. Patient opted to use normal saline nose spray to assist with dry nares.

Special Considerations
Home Care

- Frequent follow-up may be necessary to enhance CPAP/BiPAP compliance and address unexpected outcomes promptly (Carlucci et al., 2013; Simmons and Pruitt, 2012).

PROCEDURAL GUIDELINE 14.1
Use of a Peak Flowmeter

For patients who have measurable changes in airflow through their airways, such as patients with asthma or reactive airways disease, peak expiratory flow rate (PEFR) measurements are useful except in children younger than 5 years old (Callahan et al., 2010; Hockenberry and Wilson, 2013). PEFR is the maximum flow that a patient forces out during one quick, forced expiration and is measured in liters. Use these measurements as an objective indicator of a patient's current status or the effectiveness of treatment. Decreased PEFR may indicate the need for further interventions, such as increased doses of bronchodilators or antiinflammatory medications. Normal values vary according to a person's age, sex, and size. Use a "traffic light" pattern to help the patient know what to do when the peak flow number changes (Callahan et al., 2010). For example, if a patient's peak flow value is in the green zone, no action is necessary. However, if the value is in the yellow (caution) zone, the health care provider might instruct the patient to use a different type of inhaler (NIH, 2010).

Delegation and Collaboration

Initial assessment of a patient's condition is a nursing responsibility and cannot be delegated. The skills of follow-up PEFR measurements in a stable patient can be delegated to nursing assistive personnel (NAP). The nurse instructs the NAP to:

PROCEDURAL GUIDELINE 14.1
Use of a Peak Flowmeter—cont'd

- Report immediately to the nurse patient's difficulty breathing or decrease in PEFR measurement.

Equipment

- Peak flowmeter
- Patient diary/action plan, if appropriate

Procedural Steps

1. **See Standard Protocol (inside front cover).**
2. Review medical record for patient's baseline PEFR (if available).
3. Assist patient to high-Fowler's position, which promotes optimum lung expansion.
4. Assess patient's baseline knowledge of when and how to use PEFR and correct response to results.
5. Slide clean mouthpiece into base of the numbered scale.
6. Instruct patient to take a deep breath through nose and slowly blow out through mouth. Take second deep breath.
7. Have patient place meter mouthpiece in mouth and close lips, making a firm seal.
8. Have patient blow out as hard and fast as possible through mouth only.
9. Monitor PEFR results and assess if patient is in expected range.
10. Inform patient of his or her individualized acceptable range and mark on meter.
11. If patient is to record PEFR at home, have him or her demonstrate PEFR technique independently and assess

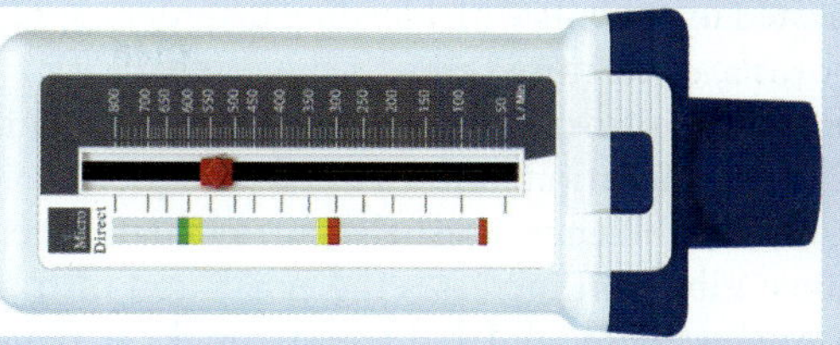

STEP 11 A typical peak flowmeter shows faster exhalation rates in green, reduced rates in yellow, and seriously reduced rates in red. (asmaPLAN+ Peak Flow Meter image courtesy of MD Spiro, a Micro Direct Company. All rights reserved.)

ability to record PEFR accurately on chart using "traffic light" pattern (see illustration).

12. Use **Teach Back:** State to the patient, "I want to make sure that I showed you how to correctly measure your PEFR. Can you demonstrate to me how you would use this PEFR device?" Evaluates what the patient is able to explain or demonstrate. Revise your instruction now or develop plan for revised patient teaching to be implemented at an appropriate time if patient is not able to teach back correctly.
13. Determine patient's PEFR and compare with his or her personal best.
14. Record PEFR measurement before and after therapy and patient's ability and effort to perform PEFR.
15. Instruct patient to clean unit weekly following manufacturer's instructions.
16. **See Completion Protocol (inside front cover).**

SKILL 14.3 CHEST PHYSIOTHERAPY

Chest physiotherapy (CPT) is used to mobilize pulmonary secretions. CPT includes postural drainage, chest percussion, and vibration, followed by productive coughing or suctioning. CPT is for patients who produce more than 30 mL of sputum per day; have evidence of atelectasis, pneumonia, or lung abscesses by chest x-ray film; or cystic fibrosis (CF) or certain neuromuscular diseases. It is imperative that patients with cystic fibrosis have routine chest physiotherapy to promote lung expansion and reduce risks for pulmonary infections (CFF, 2012).

Chest percussion involves striking the chest wall over the area being drained. Position the hand so that your fingers and thumb touch, cupping the hand. Percussion on the surface of the chest wall sends waves of varying amplitude and frequency through the chest, changing the consistency and location of the sputum. Perform chest percussion by alternating hand motion against the chest wall over a single layer of clothing, not over buttons, snaps, or zippers (Fig. 14-2).

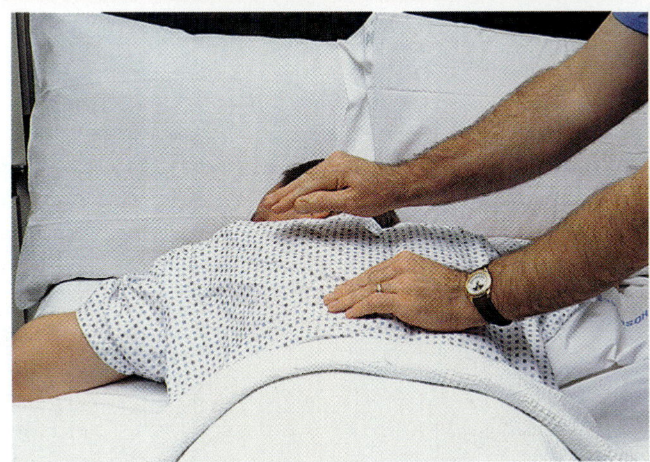

FIG 14-2 Chest wall percussion, alternating hand motion against the patient's chest wall.

Use caution and do not percuss on the scapular area, breasts, or below ribs because trauma will occur to the skin and underlying musculoskeletal structures. Percussion is contraindicated in patients with bleeding disorders, spinal injury, osteoporosis, or fractured ribs.

Vibration is a fine, shaking pressure applied to the chest wall during exhalation only. This technique increases the velocity and turbulence of exhaled air, facilitating removal of secretions. Vibration increases the exhalation of trapped air, shakes mucus loose, and induces a cough. It is used with patients with CF or conditions causing thick secretions.

Postural drainage is the use of positioning techniques that drain secretions from specific segments of the lungs and bronchi into the trachea. Each position drains a specific corresponding section of the tracheobronchial tree, from the upper, middle, or lower lung field, into the trachea. The procedure for postural drainage includes most lung segments (Table 14-3). Use patient history and clinical assessment findings to determine which lung segments require postural drainage. For example, some patients with left lower lobe bronchiectasis or pneumonia require postural drainage of the affected region, whereas a child with CF requires postural drainage of all segments.

Health care providers select areas for drainage based on (1) knowledge of the patient's condition and disease process, (2) physical assessment of the chest, (3) chest x-ray film results, and (4) the extent of the pathological condition and lobe involvement based on the physical examination and chest x-ray film findings. Treatments should be completed four times per day before meals and bedtime.

TABLE 14-3	POSITIONS AND PROCEDURES FOR DRAINAGE, PERCUSSION, VIBRATION, AND SHAKING	
AREA AND PROCEDURE	**ANATOMICAL AREA**	**POSITION OF PATIENT**
Left and Right Upper Lobe Anterior Apical Bronchi Position patient in chair, or high-Fowler's, leaning back. Percuss and vibrate with heel of hands at shoulders and fingers over collarbones (clavicles) in front; do both sides at same time. Note body posture and arm position of nurse. Nurse's back is kept straight, and elbows and knees are slightly flexed. Direction of mucus flow through upper lobe anterior apical bronchi.	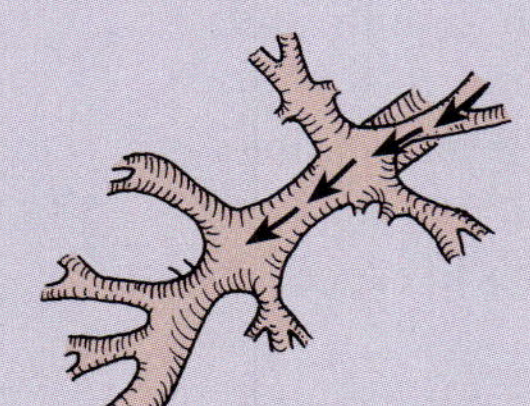	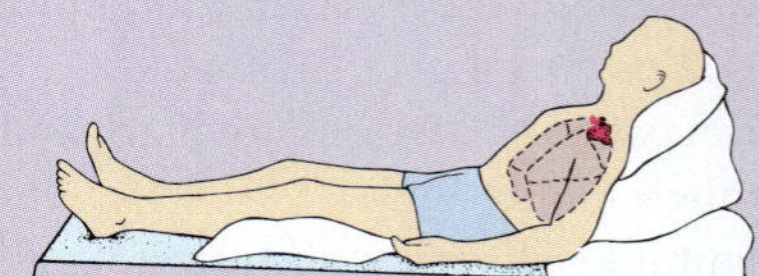 Anterior apical segments Position hands for chest physiotherapy over left and right upper anterior apical bronchi.
Left and Right Upper Lobe Posterior Apical Bronchi Position patient in chair, leaning forward on pillow or table. Percuss and vibrate with hands on either side of upper spine. Do both sides at same time. Direction of mucus flow through upper lobe posterior apical bronchi.	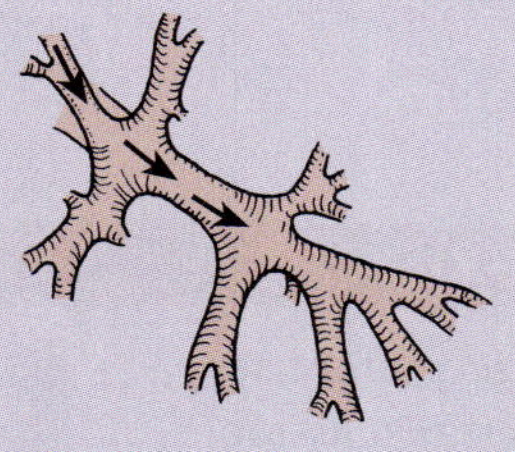	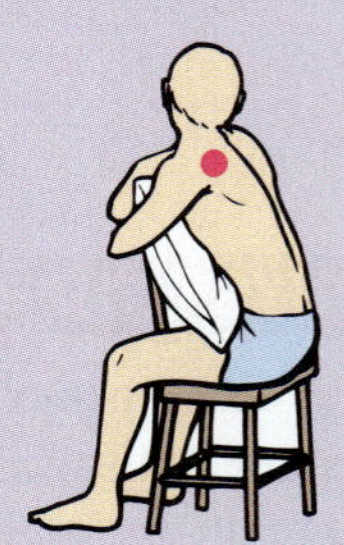 Posterior apical segments Position hands for chest physiotherapy over left and right upper lobe posterior apical bronchi.
Right and Left Anterior Upper Lobe Bronchi Position patient flat on back with small pillow under knees. Percuss and vibrate just below clavicle on either side of sternum. Direction of mucus flow through anterior upper bronchi.	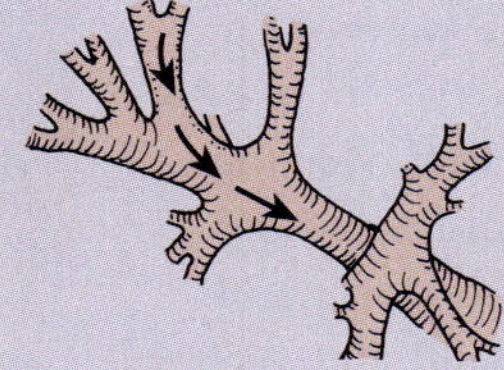	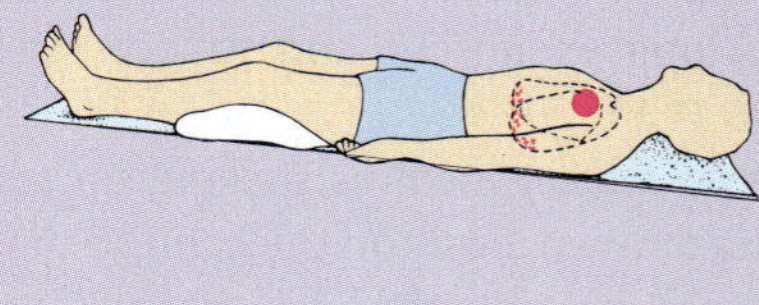 Left and right anterior upper lobe segments Position hands for chest physiotherapy over right and left anterior upper lobe bronchi.

TABLE 14-3   POSITIONS AND PROCEDURES FOR DRAINAGE, PERCUSSION, VIBRATION, AND SHAKING—cont'd

AREA AND PROCEDURE	ANATOMICAL AREA	POSITION OF PATIENT

Left Upper Lobe Lingular Bronchus

Position patient on right side with arm overhead in Trendelenburg's position, with foot of bed raised 30 cm (12 inches), as tolerated.* Place pillow behind back, and roll patient one-quarter turn onto pillow. Percuss and vibrate lateral to left nipple below axilla.

Direction of mucus flow through left upper lobe lingular bronchus.

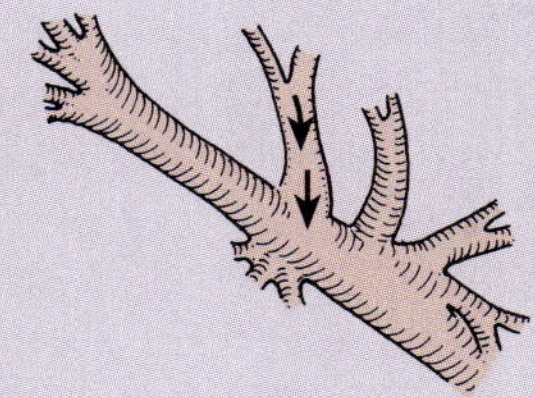
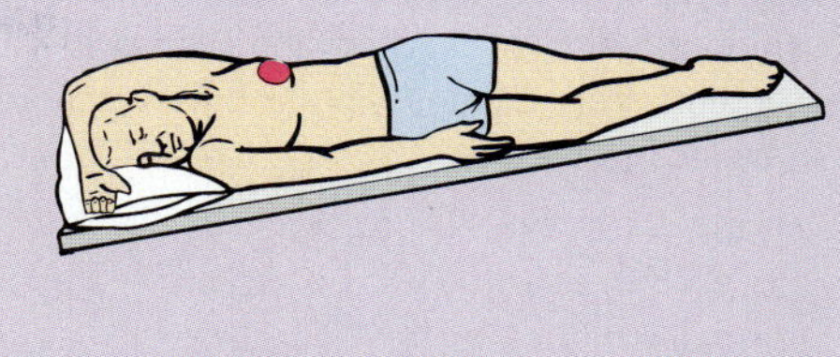

Left upper lobe lingular segment
Position hands for chest physiotherapy over left upper lobe lingular bronchus.

Right Middle Lobe Bronchus

Position patient on left side or abdomen. Place pillow behind back, and roll patient one-quarter turn onto pillow. Percuss and vibrate to right nipple below axilla.

Direction of mucus flow through right middle lobe bronchus.

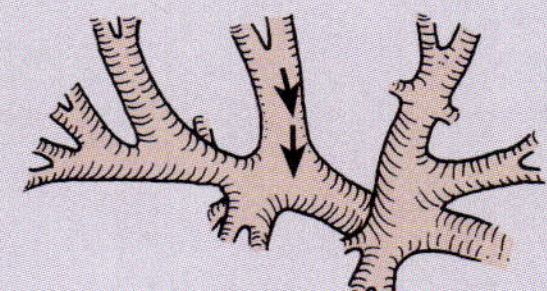
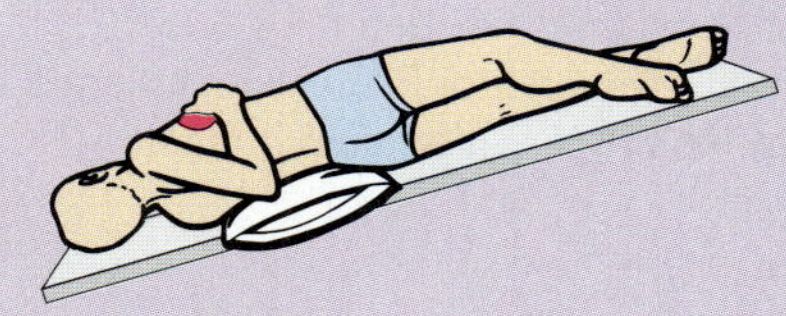

Right middle lobe segment
Position hands for chest physiotherapy over right middle lobe bronchus.

Left and Right Anterior Lower Lobe Bronchi

Position patient on back, with foot of bed elevated to 45-50 cm (18-20 inches). Have knees bent on pillow. Percuss and vibrate over lower anterior ribs on both sides.

Direction of mucus flow through anterior lower lobe bronchi.

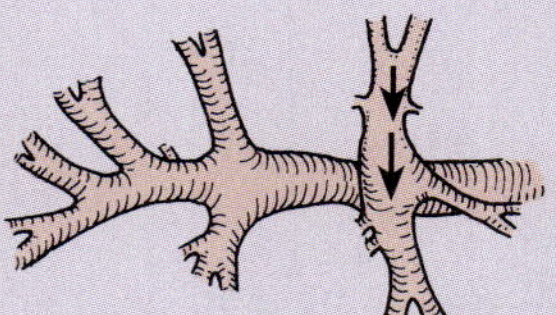
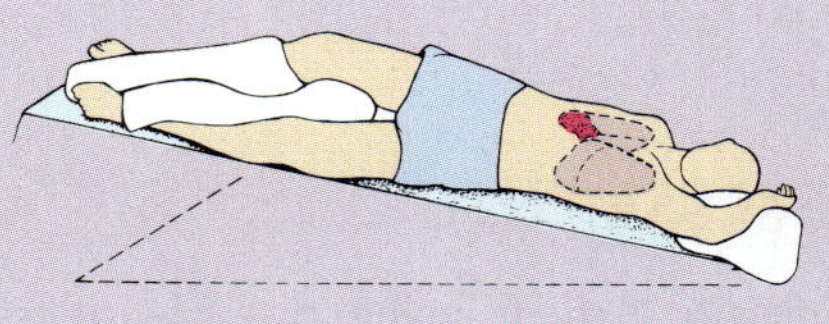

Left and right anterior lower lobe segments
Position hands for chest physiotherapy over left and right anterior lower lobe bronchi.

Right Lower Lobe Lateral Bronchus

Position patient on abdomen in Trendelenburg's position with foot of bed raised 45-50 cm (18-20 inches), as tolerated. Percuss and vibrate on left and right sides of chest below shoulder blades (scapulas) posterior to midaxillary line.

Direction of mucus flow through right lower lobe lateral bronchus.

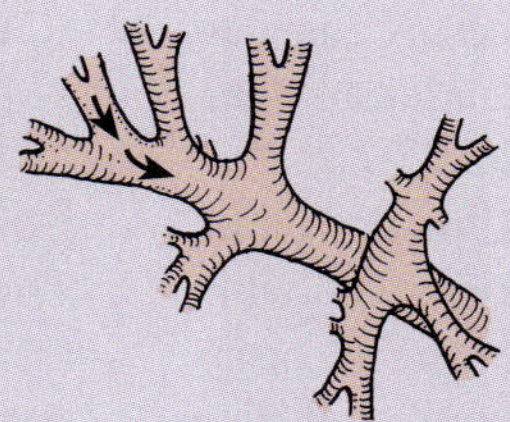
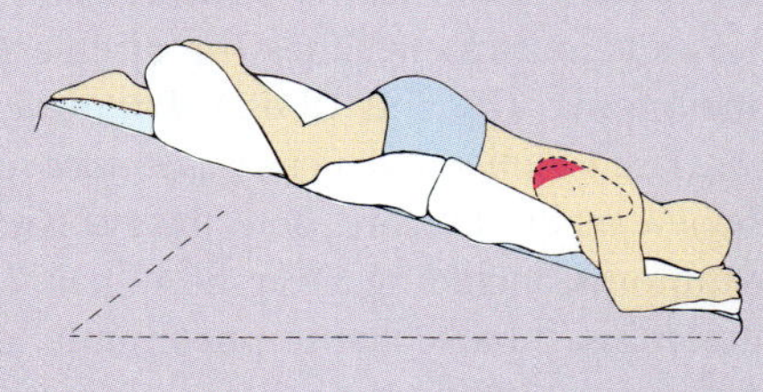

Right lower lateral lobe segment
Position hands for chest physiotherapy over right lower lobe lateral bronchus.

Left Lower Lobe Lateral Bronchus

Position patient on right side in Trendelenburg's position with foot of bed raised 45-50 cm (18-20 inches), as tolerated. Percuss and vibrate on left side of chest below scapulas posterior to midaxillary line.

Direction of mucus flow through left lower lobe lateral bronchus.

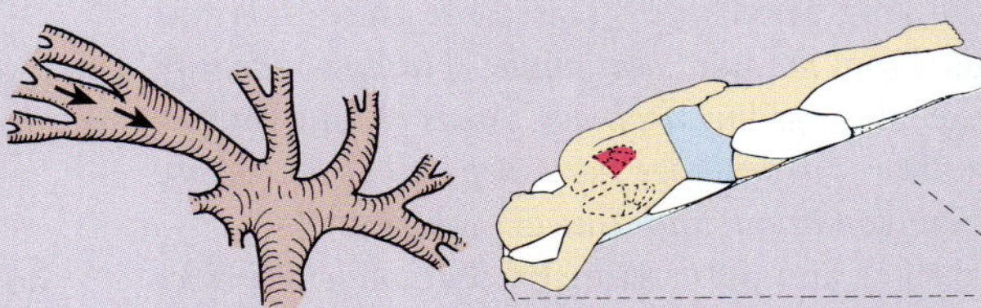

Left lower lobe lateral segment
Position hands for chest physiotherapy over left lower lobe lateral bronchus.

Continued

TABLE 14-3   POSITIONS AND PROCEDURES FOR DRAINAGE, PERCUSSION, VIBRATION, AND SHAKING—cont'd

AREA AND PROCEDURE	ANATOMICAL AREA	POSITION OF PATIENT
Right and Left Lower Lobe Superior Bronchi Position patient flat on stomach with pillow under stomach. Percuss and vibrate below scapula on either side of spine. Direction of mucus flow through lower lobe superior bronchi.	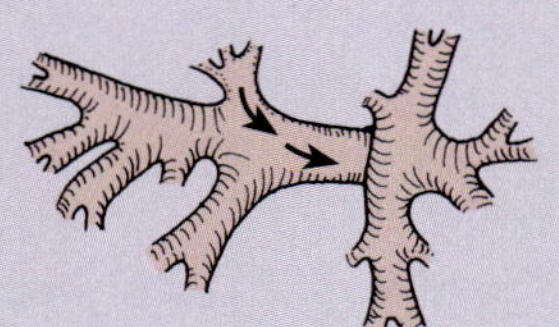 Right and left lower lobe superior segments	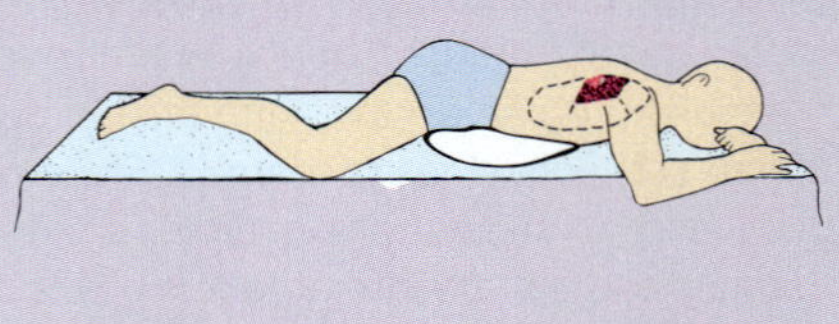 Position hands for chest physiotherapy over right and left lower lobe superior bronchi.
Right and Left Posterior Basal Bronchi Position patient on stomach in Trendelenburg's position with foot of bed raised 45-50 cm (18-20 inches), as tolerated. Percuss and vibrate over low posterior ribs on either side of spine. Direction of mucus flow through posterior basal bronchi.	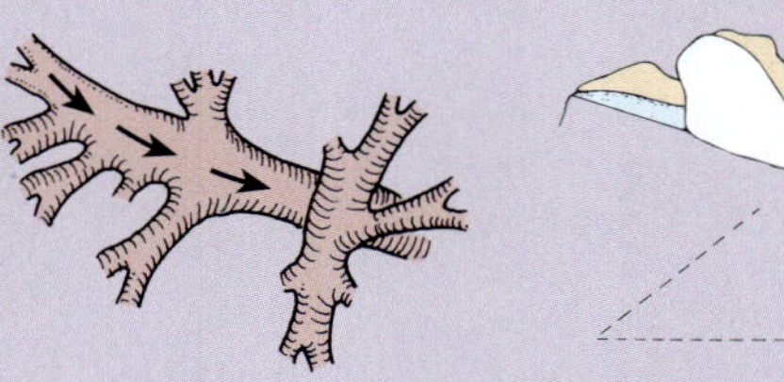 Right and left posterior segments	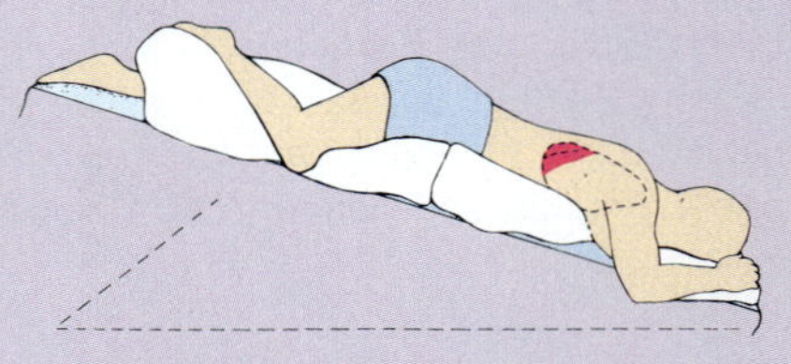 Position hands for chest physiotherapy over right and left posterior lower lobe bronchi.

*In adult settings, Trendelenburg's position is not used as frequently. Verify use with facility policy and health care provider's order.

ASSESSMENT

1. Identify patient using two identifiers (e.g., name and birthday or name and account number) according to facility policy. *Rationale: Ensures correct patient. Complies with The Joint Commission standards and improves patient safety (TJC, 2014).*
2. Assess patient for history of decreased level of consciousness and muscle weakness or disease processes such as pneumonia, CF, and COPD. *Rationale: Conditions that pose risk for impaired airway clearance require CPT.*
3. Review medical record, and observe patient for signs and symptoms, including x-ray film changes consistent with atelectasis, lobar collapse pneumonia, or bronchiectasis; ineffective coughing; or thick, sticky, tenacious, and discolored secretions that are difficult to cough up. *Rationale: Indicates need to perform postural drainage. X-ray film data and signs and symptoms indicate accumulation of pulmonary secretions and ineffective airway clearance.*
4. Auscultate all lung fields for decreased breath sounds and adventitious lung sounds. *Rationale: Findings identify bronchial segments needing drainage. Areas of lung congestion and postures for drainage vary, depending on disease process, patient condition, and clinical problems.*
5. Obtain vital signs and pulse oximetry. *Rationale: Provides baseline to evaluate patient's response to therapy.*
6. Determine patient's understanding of and ability to perform home postural drainage. *Rationale: Identifies potential areas for instruction.*

PLANNING

Expected Outcomes focus on airway clearance.
- Lung sounds improve or become clear.
- Sputum is more easily expectorated or suctioned out.
- Secretions appear more normal in color and consistency.
- Dyspnea decreases
- Chest x-ray shows improvements.
- Patient is able to relax and breathes more deeply.

Delegation and Collaboration

The skill of CPT can be delegated to properly trained nursing assistive personnel (NAP) in special situations. It is the nurse's responsibility to assess the patient, review laboratory and x-ray results, determine that the patient is stable and able to tolerate the procedure, and evaluate patient response to CPT. The nurse instructs the NAP about:
- The need to immediately report changes in patient's comfort level, tolerance of the procedure, or changes in breathing pattern.
- Specific patient precautions related to disease, mobility status, positioning restrictions, or treatment.

Equipment
- Stethoscope
- Pulse oximeter
- Trendelenburg's hospital bed or tilt table (more common in pediatric facilities)

- Water in pitcher and glass
- Chair (for draining upper lobes)
- Extra pillows
- Tissues and paper bag
- Clear graduated screw-top container

- Clean gloves (if there is a risk of exposure to patient's respiratory secretions)
- Oral hygiene care products
- Suction equipment (if patient is unable to cough and clear own secretions)

IMPLEMENTATION *for* CHEST PHYSIOTHERAPY

STEPS	RATIONALE
1. **See Standard Protocol (inside front cover).**	
2. Prepare patient for procedure.	
a. If patient's pain rating is 4 or greater on assessment, administer analgesia 20 minutes before CPT.	Pain control is essential for patient to participate actively in CPT and cough forcefully to clear airways.
b. Explain purpose and rationale for procedure. Explain positioning, sensations, how long it will take, and any discomforts or side effects.	
c. Encourage high fluid–intake program (minimum 1500 mL) unless contraindicated by other diseases with approval from health care providers. Maintain a record of fluid intake and output.	Fluid thins secretions and makes them easier to cough up. Patients need close monitoring and encouragement when first starting high fluid–intake program.
d. Coordinate therapy at appropriate times (e.g., 20 minutes after bronchodilator therapy). Plan treatments so that they do not overlap with meals or tube feeding. Avoid postural drainage 1 to 2 hours before a meal or 1 to 2 hours after meals or bolus tube feedings. Stop all continuous gastric tube feedings for 30 to 45 minutes before postural drainage. Check for residual feeding in patient's stomach; if greater than 100 mL, hold treatment.	Scheduling after bronchodilator enhances movement of secretions out of airways. Scheduling of CPT should avoid conflict with other interventions or diagnostic testing. Performing postural drainage when patient's stomach is empty helps avoid gastric reflux or vomiting and aspiration of stomach contents.
e. Have patient remove any tight or restrictive clothing.	
3. Identify selected lung segments for draining based on assessment findings.	Individualized treatment helps relieve specific areas of congestion identified during patient assessment.
4. Position patient to drain the first lung segment (see Table 14-3). Assist patient to assume position as needed. Place pillows for support and comfort. Drape patient appropriately.	Proper patient positioning promotes drainage of pulmonary secretions.
5. For each selected segment, perform chest percussion, vibration, and shaking in that order.	Provides mechanical forces to help move airway secretions.
6. After each 10 to 15 minutes of drainage, have patient sit up and cough, using controlled coughing (see Skill 14.2). If patient cannot cough, suctioning is necessary (see Skill 14.4). Any secretions moved to the central airways are removed by cough or suctioning before placing patient into next drainage position.	Coughing is most effective when patient is sitting up and leaning forward.

> **SAFE PATIENT CARE** Sometimes patients experience transient dyspnea and fatigue because of airway irritation and bronchospasm from the secretions. These patients often benefit from an oscillating or vibrating device such as an Acapella device (Fig. 14-3).

7. Have patient rest briefly if necessary.	Short rest periods between postures help prevent fatigue and increase tolerance for the therapy.

Continued

STEPS	RATIONALE
8. Repeat Steps 5 through 7 until all congested areas selected are drained. Make sure that each treatment does not exceed 30 to 60 minutes (3 to 15 minutes for each position).	Postural drainage is used only in the involved areas and is based on individual assessment.
9. Offer or assist patient with oral hygiene. Have patient take sips of water.	Promotes comfort and reduces bad breath. Keeping mouth moist aids in expectoration of secretions.
10. **See Completion Protocol (inside front cover).**	

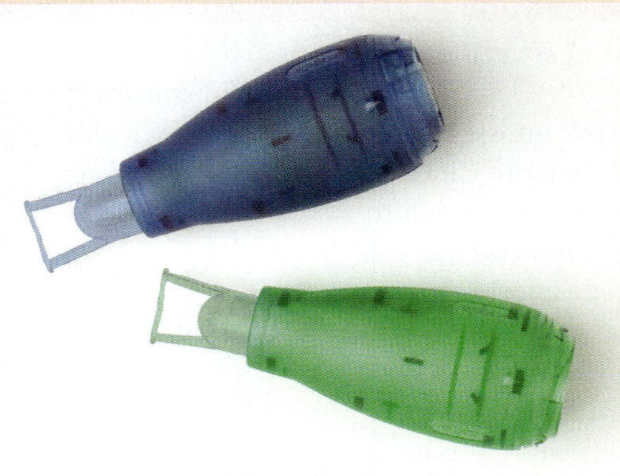

FIG 14-3 Acapella device.

EVALUATION

1. Auscultate lung fields.
2. Inspect character and amount of sputum.
3. Review diagnostic reports, including sputum collections and cultures, chest x-ray films, and ABG levels, with health care provider.
4. Obtain vital signs, pulse oximetry.
5. Use *Teach Back:* State to the patient, "I want to be sure that I explained CPT correctly. Can you explain the steps and benefits of this treatment?" Evaluates what the patient is able to explain or demonstrate. Revise your instruction now or develop plan for revised patient teaching to be implemented at an appropriate time if patient is not able to teach back correctly.

Unexpected Outcomes and Related Interventions

1. Patient experiences severe dyspnea, bronchospasm, hypoxemia, or hypercarbia or is unable to tolerate treatment.
   a. Discontinue, modify, or shorten treatments.
   b. Administer bronchodilator or nebulizer therapy 20 minutes before CPT.
   c. Suction and ventilate with bag-valve-mask as needed and monitor ABG levels, O_2 saturation, and vital signs closely.
2. No improvement occurs in respiratory condition, assessment, or chest x-ray film results.
   a. Initially increase treatments and encourage coughing exercises.
   b. Notify health care provider because patient may need sputum culture, change in antibiotics, mucolytics, or a bronchoscopy to remove thick mucus plugs.
   c. Increase hydration as appropriate.
3. Hemoptysis occurs, or patient develops acute hypotension, severe chest pain, vomiting, aspiration, or dysrhythmias.
   a. Stop therapy, place patient in high-Fowler's position, and obtain vital signs.
   b. Notify health care provider.
   c. Obtain vital signs and remain with patient, call for help, and keep patient calm.
   d. If patient vomits or aspirates, suction airway and place patient on his or her side.

Recording and Reporting

- Record assessment of chest findings before and after therapy; frequency and duration of treatment; postures used and bronchial segments drained; cough effectiveness; need for suctioning; color, amount, and consistency of sputum; hemoptysis or other unexpected outcomes; and patient's tolerance and reactions.
- Document your evaluation of patient learning.

Sample Documentation

1340   Patient complaining of shortness of breath. Noted respirations elevated at 20 but regular in rate, rhythm, and depth. Crackles noted in right lower lobe and diminished in left. Patient asked to cough and deep breathe. Minimal sputum noted with weak cough. CPT completed in lower lobes. Patient stated that he did not understand the benefit of CPT. Additional education and handouts provided. Noted moderate amount yellow sputum when patient asked to cough. Patient states, "Breathing better" and "Now I know why I need CPT." Lung sounds are now clear.

Special Considerations
Pediatric

- In a child with CF, CPT is usually performed at least twice daily, on rising in the morning and in the evening (Hockenberry and Wilson, 2013). Many patients with CF use the chest vest when at home so they are independent.

Geriatric

- Take extra care and assessment when using postural drainage in older adults. Change positions more slowly, and closely assess for any changes in oxygen saturation or vital signs with position changes.
- Older adults with chronic cardiac and pulmonary conditions do not always tolerate a supine or side-lying position for CPT. In these positions, patients experience decline in forced vital capacity and subsequent decline in oxygen saturation.

Home Care Considerations

- Refer patient to pulmonary nurse specialist, pulmonary rehabilitation team, or home care personnel.
- Home care CPT is indicated in patients with chronic inability to clear lung secretions adequately, such as patients with CF, chronic bronchitis, asthma, or bronchiectasis.
- Obtain foam wedge or multiple pillows for correct positioning.

SKILL 14.4   AIRWAY MANAGEMENT: SUCTIONING

• **Nursing Skills Online: Airway Management, Lessons 3-5**

For some patients, noninvasive techniques and medications are insufficient to maintain a patent airway and improve oxygenation. Suctioning is appropriate in these cases. Apply patient assessment findings, the presence of an artificial airway, and the thickness and volume of the airway secretions to determine the best method of suctioning. Suction the oropharyngeal cavity by using a rigid plastic catheter (called a *Yankauer*) with one large and several small eyelets to remove mucus (Fig. 14-4). The catheter supplies continuous suction when you connect it to a suction source. Teach patients or family caregivers how to use this catheter to clear secretions from the oral cavity. For patients with an ETT, continuous subglottic suctioning is advocated to minimize pooling of oral secretions above the ETT cuff. Subglottic suctioning was found to decrease the risk of VAP by decreasing aspiration (Scherzer, 2010; Sedwick et al., 2012; Speroni et al., 2011). Suctioning of the lower airway is needed when patients cannot cough forcefully enough to clear secretions. Suctioning of the lower airway requires sterile technique. ETTs (Fig. 14-5) and tracheostomy tubes (Fig. 14-6) allow direct access to the lower airways for suctioning. Certified health care providers insert these artificial airways to create a route for mechanical ventilation, relieve mechanical airway obstruction, or protect the airway from aspiration because of impaired cough or gag reflexes.

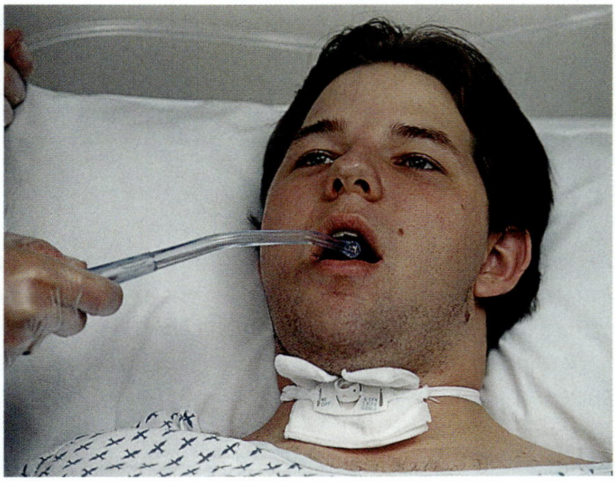

ASSESSMENT

1. Identify patient using two identifiers (e.g., name and birthday or name and account number) according to facility policy. *Rationale: Ensures correct patient. Complies with The Joint Commission standards and improves patient safety (TJC, 2014).*
2. Assess for risk factors for upper and lower airway obstruction, pulmonary disease, impaired mobility, decreased level of consciousness, nasal feeding tube, decreased cough or gag reflex, and decreased swallowing ability. *Rationale: These risk factors can impair patient's ability to clear secretions from airway, increase risk for retaining secretions, and necessitate nasopharyngeal or nasotracheal suctioning.*
3. Perform respiratory assessment, auscultating for adventitious breath sounds. *Rationale: Provides baseline to determine effects of suctioning.*
4. Assess pulse, respirations, and blood pressure. Observe for an increase or decrease from baseline; prolonged expiratory breath sounds; and decreased lung expansion. Secretions in the airway, decreased oxygen saturations (SpO_2) or level of consciousness, anxiety, lethargy, unilateral breath sounds, and cyanosis may also indicate a need for

FIG 14-4 Oropharyngeal suctioning with a Yankauer catheter.

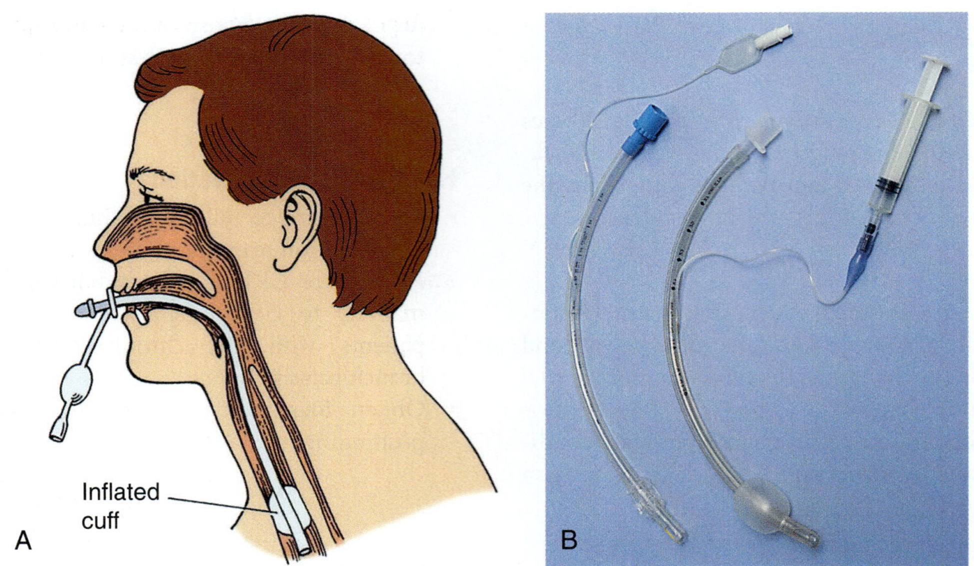

FIG 14-5 A, Endotracheal tube with inflated cuff. **B,** Endotracheal tubes with uninflated and inflated cuffs with syringe for inflation.

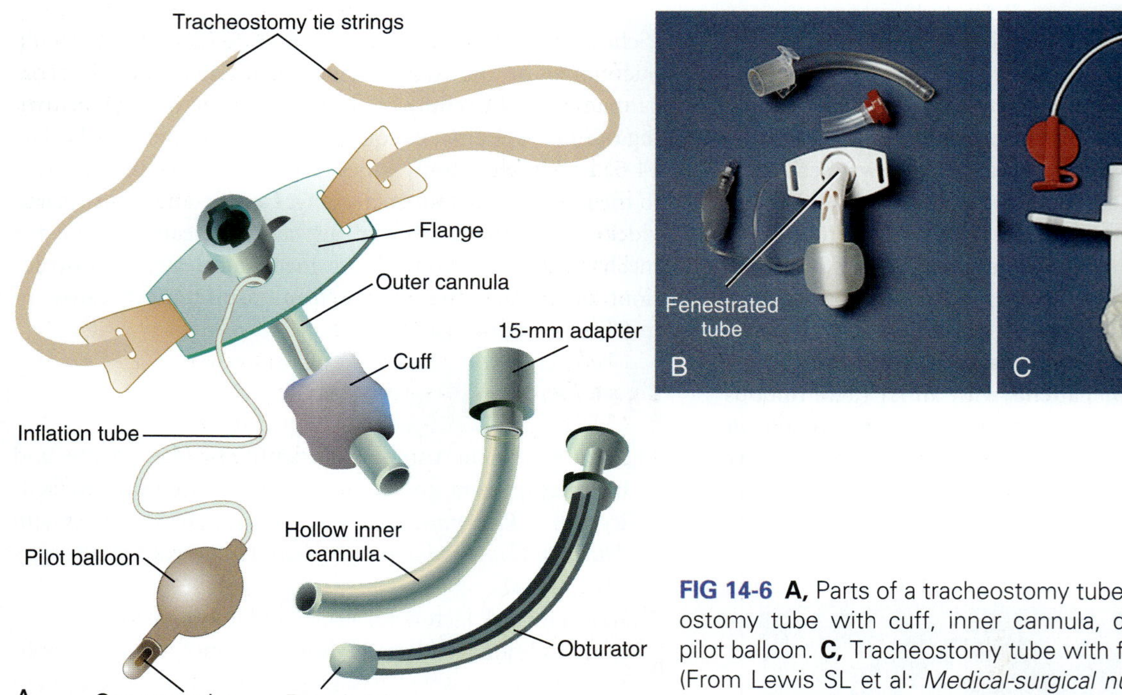

FIG 14-6 A, Parts of a tracheostomy tube. **B,** Fenestrated tracheostomy tube with cuff, inner cannula, decannulation plug, and pilot balloon. **C,** Tracheostomy tube with foam cuff and obturator. (From Lewis SL et al: *Medical-surgical nursing: assessment and management of clinical problems,* ed 9, St Louis, 2014, Mosby.)

suctioning. *Rationale: Physical signs and symptoms result from airway obstruction and decreased oxygen to tissues.*

5. Observe and assess nasal and oral cavity for nasal or oral secretions, drooling, gastric secretions, or vomitus in mouth. *Rationale: Removal of oral secretions prevents aspiration pneumonia.*

6. Identify patients with an increased risk for ineffective airway clearance (e.g., patients with a decreased level of consciousness or other neuromuscular or neurological impairment, dehydration, thick pulmonary secretions). *Rationale: Changes in neurological status and neuromuscular impairment increase the likelihood that the patient may need to be suctioned. Thick pulmonary secretions impede the patient's ability to effectively clear the airway through the cough mechanism.*

7. Identify contraindications to nasotracheal suctioning: facial or neck trauma or surgery, acute head injuries, bleeding disorder, nasal bleeding, epiglottitis or croup,

laryngospasm, and irritable airway (AARC, 2010). *Rationale: Passage of catheter can cause additional trauma, increased bleeding, or severe bronchospasm.*

8. Determine patient's understanding of procedure. *Rationale: Procedure can be distressing.*
9. Assess patency of ETT with capnography. *Rationale: The ETT may become displaced or blocked by secretions. The carbon dioxide detector is pH sensitive and can identify changes in respiratory gas (Walsh et al., 2011).*

▌PLANNING

Expected Outcomes focus on airway patency, avoidance of infection, and patient's comfort and understanding.

1. Adventitious breath sounds are decreased or cleared.
2. Patient reports easier breathing.
3. SpO$_2$ improves or remains the same.
4. Patient demonstrates correct oropharyngeal suctioning technique.
5. Indication of aspiration is absent.

Delegation and Collaboration

The skill of deep tracheal suctioning in acutely ill patients cannot be delegated to nursing assistive personnel (NAP). Oropharyngeal suctioning can be delegated to NAP. When a new tracheostomy is present, the skill of performing tracheostomy tube suctioning cannot be delegated. However, the skill can be delegated in stable, chronically ill patients with permanent tracheostomy tubes. The nurse instructs the NAP about:

- Any modifications of the skill (e.g., the use of supplemental oxygen before suctioning or clean versus sterile technique).
- Appropriate suction limits and risk of applying excessive or inadequate suction pressure.
- Reporting changes in vital signs or pulse oximetry, bloody sputum, difficulty breathing, or discomfort during or after the procedure.
- Reporting any change in secretion quality, quantity, and color.

Equipment

- Stethoscope
- Pulse oximeter
- Portable or wall suction machine
- Connecting tubing (6 feet)

Oropharyngeal (Nonsterile) and Nasotracheal (Sterile) Suctioning

- *Nasotracheal:* Sterile suction catheter (12 to 16 Fr) (smallest diameter that effectively removes secretions)
- *Oropharyngeal:* Clean, nonsterile suction catheter or Yankauer suction tip catheter
- Two sterile gloves or one sterile and one clean glove
- Sterile basin (e.g., sterile disposable cup)
- Sterile water or normal saline (about 100 mL)
- Clean towel or paper drape
- Mask, goggles, or face shield if indicated

Endotracheal or Tracheostomy Suctioning

- 12- to 16-Fr catheter (approximate; size of the suction catheter in an adult patient should be no more than half of the internal diameter of the artificial airway to minimize decrease in PaO$_2$) (AARC, 2010). Formula for suction tracheostomy catheter size: divide internal diameter of the tube by 2 and multiply by 3 (Freeman, 2011).
- Bedside table
- Two sterile gloves or one sterile and one clean glove
- Sterile basin
- Sterile normal saline (about 100 mL)
- Clean towel or sterile drape
- Mask, goggles, or face shield, if indicated

Closed-System or In-Line Suctioning

- Closed-system or in-line suction catheter
- 5- to 10-mL normal saline in syringe or vials
- Two clean gloves

IMPLEMENTATION *for* AIRWAY MANAGEMENT: SUCTIONING

STEPS	RATIONALE
1. **See Standard Protocol (inside front cover).**	
2. Position patient in semi-Fowler's or high-Fowler's position.	Aligns the airway and aids in maximal lung expansion.
3. Preparation for all types of suctioning:	
a. Open suction kit or catheter using aseptic technique. If sterile drape is available, place it across patient's chest. Do not allow suction catheter to touch any nonsterile surfaces.	Prepares catheter and prevents transmission of microorganisms.
b. Fill basin or cup with approximately 100 mL of sterile water or normal saline.	Sterile water or saline lubricates the suction catheter and helps check the patency of the tube.
c. If performing nasotracheal suctioning, open packet of lubricant.	

Continued

STEPS	RATIONALE

d. Connect one end of connecting tubing to suction machine or port. Check that suction is functioning properly by suctioning a small amount of water or saline from basin.

Always check for proper functioning of equipment before starting procedure.

e. Increase oxygen flow rate via oxygen delivery device or ventilator as ordered by health care provider.

Hyperoxygenation is recommended, especially for patients who are hypoxemic or prone to hypoxia (AARC, 2010).

f. Set suction regulator to appropriate negative pressure: suggested wall suction, 100 to 150 mm Hg for adults, 40 to 60 mm Hg for infants, and 60 to 100 mm Hg for children (AARC, 2010; Hockenberry and Wilson, 2013).

Elevated pressure settings increase risk of trauma to mucosa. The best practice is to use the lowest suction pressure. Follow facility guidelines and clinical judgment.

4. *Oropharyngeal suctioning:*

a. Apply clean gloves. Apply mask, goggles, or face shield if risk of spray. Attach suction catheter to connecting tubing. Remove oxygen mask if present, but keep near patient's face.

Suction may cause splashing of body fluids. The CDC (2013) guidelines suggest using masks or shields whenever there is the risk of airborne body fluids. Reduces chance of hypoxia.

b. With suction not applied, insert catheter into patient's mouth along gum line to pharynx. Then apply suction and move catheter around mouth until secretions are cleared.

If catheter does not have a suction control to apply intermittent suction, take care not to allow suction tip to damage oral mucosal surfaces with continuous suction.

c. Encourage patient to cough and repeat suctioning if needed. Replace oxygen mask if used.

Coughing moves secretions from lower and upper airways into mouth.

d. Suction water or saline from basin through catheter until catheter is cleared of secretions.

Clearing secretions before they dry reduces probability of transmission of microorganisms and clears catheter.

e. Place catheter in a clean, dry area for reuse with suction turned off. If patient is capable of self-suction, place it within reach.

Facilitates prompt removal of airway secretions when suctioning is needed in the future.

5. *Nasotracheal suctioning:*

a. Apply mask, goggles, or face shield if risk of spray. **Apply sterile gloves** or clean glove to nondominant hand and sterile glove to dominant hand. Attach nonsterile suction tubing to sterile catheter, keeping hand holding catheter sterile.

Suction may cause splashing of body fluids. The CDC (2013) guidelines suggest using masks or shields whenever there is the risk of airborne body fluids. Gloving reduces transmission of microorganisms and allows you to maintain sterility of suction catheter.

b. Secure catheter to suction tubing aseptically. Coat distal 6 to 8 cm (2.4 to 3.2 inches) of catheter with water-soluble lubricant from suction kit.

Eases passage of catheter and reduces mucosal surface trauma.

c. If indicated, increase supplemental oxygen therapy as ordered by health care provider. Have patient deep breathe with oxygen delivery device in place. If patient is unable to take deep breaths, hyperoxygenate with ventilation bag with mask attached.

Hyperoxygenation before suctioning can minimize hypoxemia after suctioning (AARC, 2010).

d. Remove oxygen delivery device, if present, with nondominant hand. Insert catheter into nares during inspiration without applying suction. Do not force catheter through nares. Have patient extend neck slightly (if not contraindicated) and breathe in.

Forcing the catheter causes trauma to the airway tissues. Extending patient's neck may facilitate passage of the catheter.

SAFE PATIENT CARE Keep oxygen delivery device readily available in case patient exhibits symptoms of hypoxemia.

STEPS	**RATIONALE**

e. As patient takes deep breath, advance catheter to just above entrance into trachea, without applying suction. Quickly insert catheter (approximately 20 cm [8 inches] in adults; in older children, about 16 to 20 cm [6 to 8 inches]; and in young children and infants, 8 to 14 cm [3 to 5½ inches]) into trachea until resistance is met or patient coughs; then pull back 1 to 2 cm (½ inch).

Ensures proper placement of catheter in airway to remove secretions. Pulling back on catheter before initiating suction prevents invagination of the tracheal membrane (AARC, 2010).

f. Apply intermittent or continuous suction no longer than 10 seconds. Apply intermittent suction by placing and releasing nondominant thumb over vent of catheter and slowly withdrawing catheter while rotating it back and forth between dominant thumb and forefinger (AARC, 2010; Lewis et al., 2014). Encourage patient to cough. Replace oxygen device if applicable.

Both intermittent and continuous suction can cause tracheal tissue damage (Lynn-McHale and Weigand, 2011). Suctioning longer than 10 seconds causes cardiopulmonary compromise, usually from hypoxemia or vagal overload (AARC, 2010).

g. Rinse catheter and connecting tubing by suctioning water or normal saline from the basin until tubing is clear.

Clearing secretions before they dry reduces probability of transmission of microorganisms and clears catheter.

h. Assess need to repeat suction procedure. Observe for alterations in cardiopulmonary status. Allow adequate time (1 to 2 minutes) between suction passes.

Suctioning may cause an increase in heart rate.

6. *Artificial airway suctioning:*

a. Apply mask or face shield if risk of spray. **Apply sterile gloves** or clean glove to nondominant hand and sterile glove to dominant hand. Attach nonsterile suction tubing to sterile catheter, keeping hand holding catheter sterile (see illustration).

Suction may cause splashing of body fluids. Wearing a mask or shield when there is risk of airborne body fluids is recommended (CDC, 2013). Reduces transmission of microorganisms and allows you to maintain sterility of suction catheter (Freeman, 2011).

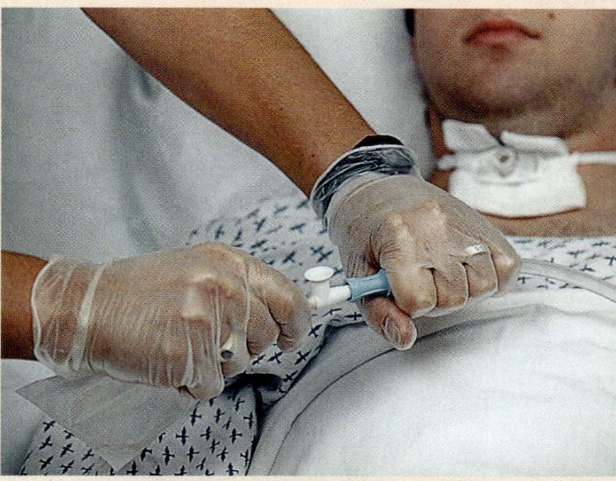

STEP 6a Attaching catheter to suction.

b. Check that equipment is functioning properly by suctioning small amounts of saline from basin.

Lubricates catheter and tubing.

> **SAFE PATIENT CARE** If mucus is visible at tracheostomy or endotracheal opening, suction to remove secretions *before* hyperoxygenation; this prevents secretions from being pushed back into the trachea. If this occurs, change suction catheter after removing mucus.

Continued

STEPS	RATIONALE

c. Hyperoxygenate patient before suctioning, using manual resuscitation bag and increasing FiO_2 for several minutes; or, if mechanically ventilated, use the ventilator to provide additional breaths without increasing tidal volume. Up to 5 minutes may be necessary to provide for time for the increased oxygen to reach the mechanically ventilated patient (Ignatavicius and Workman, 2013).

Hyperoxygenation for 30 to 60 seconds before suctioning decreases suctioning-induced hypoxemia (AARC, 2010). Most sources recommend hyperoxygenating with 100% FiO_2 for adult and pediatric patients. Neonates should receive 10% increase above current baseline (AARC, 2010).

d. Advise the patient that you are beginning to suction and that the patient may feel like breath is being taken away.

Prepares patient for discomfort and reduces anxiety.

e. Open swivel adapter on tracheostomy or ETT or, if necessary, remove oxygen or humidity delivery device with nondominant hand.

Exposes artificial airway.

f. Without applying suction and using dominant thumb and forefinger, gently but quickly insert catheter into artificial airway (time catheter insertion with patient's inspiration) until resistance is met or patient coughs; then pull back 1 cm (½ inch) (Ozden and Gorgulu, 2012).

Application of suction pressure (80 to 120 mm Hg) while introducing catheter into trachea increases risk of damage to tracheal mucosa. Pulling back on catheter 1 cm before initiating suction prevents invagination of the tracheal membrane (Ozden and Gorgulu, 2012).

> **SAFE PATIENT CARE** Be sure to insert catheter during inspiration, especially when performing tracheal suctioning. The patient will cough. Never apply suction during catheter insertion. Do not insert catheter when the patient is swallowing because the catheter will most likely enter the esophagus. If patient gags or becomes nauseated, the catheter is most likely in the esophagus, and you will need to remove it.

g. Apply intermittent or continuous suction no longer than 10 seconds (Ozden and Gorgulu, 2012). Apply intermittent suction by placing and releasing nondominant thumb over vent of catheter (see illustration) and slowly withdrawing catheter while rotating it back and forth between dominant thumb and forefinger (AARC, 2010). Encourage patient to cough.

No more than two passes with the suction catheter are recommended during any one suctioning session to decrease the risk of hypoxia.

> **SAFE PATIENT CARE** Use nursing judgment to determine whether to use intermittent or continuous suctioning. Newer research suggests continuous suctioning on withdrawal may reduce the risk of mucosal injury (AACN, 2010; Lewis et al., 2014; Lynn-McHale Weigand, 2011; Ozden and Gorgulu, 2012).

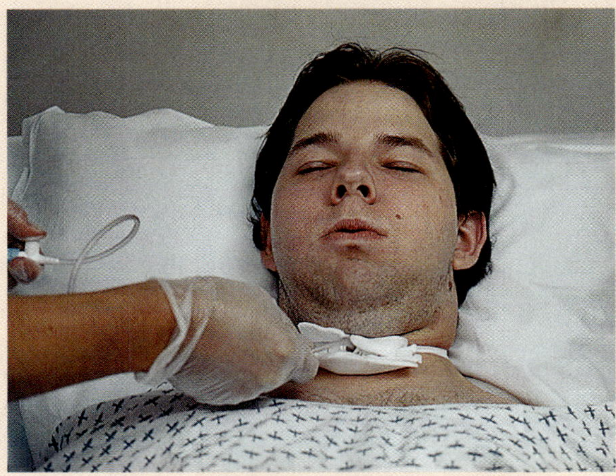

STEP 6g Suctioning tracheostomy.

STEPS	**RATIONALE**

h. Close swivel adapter or replace oxygen delivery device. Encourage patient to deep breathe. Some patients respond well to several manual breaths from the mechanical ventilator or resuscitation bag.

Reoxygenates and reexpands alveoli. Suctioning can cause hypoxemia and atelectasis. Monitor patient for signs of distress after suctioning.

> **SAFE PATIENT CARE** If the patient is on a ventilator, readjust the ventilator settings to preprocedural levels to avoid the risk of oxygen toxicity, carbon dioxide retention, and atelectasis.

i. Rinse catheter and connecting tube with sterile water or normal saline until clear. Use continuous suction.

Removes catheter secretions. Secretions left in tubing decrease suction efficiency and provide environment for growth of microorganisms.

j. Evaluate patient's cardiopulmonary, neurological, and hemodynamic status. Repeat Steps 6e through 6i three times if you determine that secretion clearance was inadequate. Allow adequate time (up to 5 minutes) between suction passes to reestablish baseline oxygenation (Ignatavicius and Workman, 2013).

The effects of hypoxia from suctioning can cause dysrhythmias, hemodynamic instability, and increased intracranial pressure, among other complications. A maximum of three suction passes is recommended to minimize effects of hypoxemia (Freeman, 2011; Ignatavicius and Workman, 2013; Ozden and Gorgulu, 2012).

k. Perform nasopharyngeal and oropharyngeal suctioning to clear upper airway of secretions. After suctioning upper airway, the catheter is contaminated, and you should not reinsert it into the lower airway.

Removes upper airway secretions. Upper airway is considered "clean," whereas lower airway is considered "sterile." You can use the same catheter suction from sterile to clean areas but not from clean to sterile areas.

l. Disconnect catheter from connecting tubing. Roll catheter around fingers of dominant hand. Pull glove off inside out so that catheter remains in glove. Pull off other glove in same way. Discard into appropriate receptacle. Perform hand hygiene. Turn off suction device.

Reduces transmission of microorganisms. Do not touch clean equipment with contaminated gloves.

m. Place new, unopened suction kit at bedside.

7. *Closed-system (in-line) suction catheter* (see illustration):

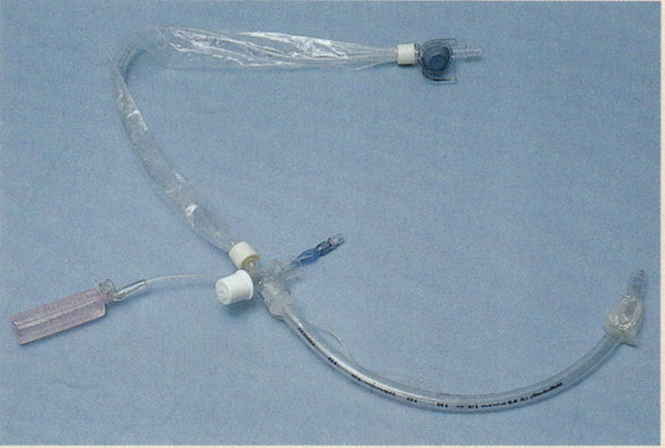

STEP 7 Closed-system suction catheter attached to an ETT.

Continued

STEPS	RATIONALE

a. Apply clean gloves. Apply face shield.

b. Attach suction.

  (1) In many facilities, a respiratory therapist attaches the catheter to the mechanical ventilator circuit. If not already in place, open suction catheter package using aseptic technique. Attach closed-system suction catheter to ventilator circuit by removing swivel adapter and placing closed-system catheter apparatus on ETT or tracheostomy tube. Connect Y on mechanical ventilator circuit to closed-system catheter with flex tubing.

  Catheter becomes part of the circuit and is often changed by respiratory therapist with each circuit change, when contaminated, or according to facility policy.

  (2) Connect one end of connecting tube to suction machine. Connect other end to end of closed-system or in-line suction catheter if not already done. Turn suction device on and set vacuum regulator to appropriate negative pressure (80 to 120 mm Hg for adults) (Ozden and Gorgulu, 2012).

  Prepares suction apparatus. Excessive negative pressure damages tracheal mucosa and can induce greater hypoxia.

c. Hyperoxygenate (increase FiO_2) patient using resuscitation bag or manual breathing mechanism on mechanical ventilator according to facility protocol and clinical status (100% oxygen usually recommended).

  Decreases atelectasis caused by negative pressure and increases oxygen available to tissues during suctioning. Both hyperinflation and hyperoxygenation are recommended before and after suctioning (Ozden and Gorgulu, 2012).

d. Unlock suction control mechanism if required by manufacturer. Open saline port and attach saline syringe or vial.

e. Pick up suction catheter enclosed in plastic sleeve with dominant hand.

  Plastic sheath provides catheter sterility and secretion containment.

f. Wait until patient inhales to insert catheter, while repeatedly pushing catheter and sliding (or pulling) plastic back between thumb and forefinger until you feel resistance or if patient coughs. Pull back 1 cm ($\frac{1}{2}$ inch) before applying suction to avoid tissue damage to the carina (Ozden and Gorgulu, 2012). (Note: Some catheters contain depth markings that are useful in positioning catheter.)

  Mechanical ventilator breaths, oxygen, and positive end-expiratory pressure are not interrupted during suctioning. Catheter slides within plastic sheath. Coughing occurs or resistance is felt when catheter touches carina.

g. Encourage patient to cough and then apply suction while withdrawing.

  Removes secretions from airway.

h. Evaluate cardiopulmonary status, including pulse oximetry, to determine need for subsequent suctioning or complications. If cardiac monitoring is available, observe rhythm during suctioning. Repeat Steps 7c through 7g one or two more times to clear secretions. Allow adequate time (at least 1 full minute) between suction passes for ventilation and reoxygenation.

  Repeated passes clear airway of secretions to promote ventilation and oxygenation. Suctioning can cause complications such as irregular heartbeats, hypoxia, and bronchospasm.

i. When airway is clear, withdraw catheter completely into sheath. Be sure that black line on catheter is visible in sheath. Squeeze vial or push syringe while applying suction to rinse inner lumen of catheter. Use at least 5 to 10 mL of normal saline to clear catheter of retained secretions. Lock suction mechanism, if applicable, and turn off suction.

  Black line is reference point to determine correct position of catheter when not in use. Inability to see black line suggests that catheter is in airway and may be impeding airflow. Rinsing interior of catheter prevents bacterial growth.

STEPS	RATIONALE
j. Patient may require suctioning of oral cavity (see Step 4).	Separate suction catheter is necessary for oral cavity.
k. Place new, unopened suction kit on suction machine or at head of bed.	Provides immediate access to suction catheter when needed.
8. See Completion Protocol (inside front cover).	

EVALUATION

1. Auscultate lungs and compare patient's respiratory assessments before and after suctioning.
2. Ask patient if breathing is easier and if congestion is decreased.
3. Observe the amount, color, and consistency of suctioned content.
4. Observe patient's respirations and color; measure pulse oximetry (SpO_2).
5. Observe patient's oropharyngeal suctioning technique.
6. Use **Teach Back:** State to the patient, "I want to be sure that I explained the suctioning procedure correctly. Squeeze my hand if you understand each of the steps that we discussed." (You can also use the communication board for a patient with an ETT.) Evaluates what the patient is able to explain or demonstrate. Revise your instruction now or develop plan for revised patient teaching to be implemented at an appropriate time if patient is not able to teach back correctly.

Unexpected Outcomes and Related Interventions

1. Patient becomes cyanotic or restless or develops tachycardia, bradycardia, or other abnormal heart rhythm.
   a. Discontinue attempt at suctioning until stabilized unless patient's condition is deteriorating because of secretions in airway.
   b. Provide supplemental oxygen.
   c. Monitor vital signs and pulse oximetry.
   d. Assess patient with capnography to confirm placement of ETT.
2. Bloody secretions are returned, which may indicate trauma.
   a. Evaluate technique and frequency of suctioning.
   b. If bleeding continues, notify health care provider of potential hemorrhage and monitor vital signs.
3. Thick secretions are present and difficult to suction.
   a. Monitor patient's hydration status. Dehydration contributes to thick secretions.
   b. Increase fluids if not contraindicated.

Recording and Reporting

- Record respiratory assessments before and after suctioning; size of catheter used; route; amount, consistency, and color of secretions obtained; and frequency of suctioning.
- Report patient's intolerance to procedure or worsening of oxygenation status.
- Document your evaluation of patient learning.

Sample Documentation

1200   Noted crackles in bilateral bases. Requires hourly suctioning per ETT. Patient complained of feeling short of breath with suctioning. Discussed plan to add more time to hyperoxygenation before suctioning. Patient then verbalized decrease in dyspnea. Moderate amount (≤ 5 mL) of thick yellow sputum. Patient able to use Yankauer catheter to suction mouth with good technique. Lungs clear after suctioning. SpO_2 92% to 94%. Respirations regular in rate, rhythm, and depth after suctioning, 14 per minute.

Special Considerations
Pediatric

- Diameter of suction catheter should be no more than one half the internal diameter of the child's tracheostomy or other artificial airway (Hockenberry and Wilson, 2013).
- Unless secretions are thick, lower range of vacuum pressure is recommended (Hockenberry and Wilson, 2013).
- Closed suction systems are used only on older children. Use care so that the weight of the closed system does not displace the child's ETT.

Geriatric

- Older adults with ischemic cardiac or obstructive pulmonary disease may benefit from maintenance of oxygen supply during suctioning to reduce the risk of irregular heartbeats.
- Because of increased tissue fragility, older adults may have bloody secretions on suctioning. Monitor the suction return for clearing and avoid unnecessary suctioning.

Home Care

- In the home, patients should follow best practices for infection control while weighing the necessity of cost-effectiveness in a chronic situation. For example, clean suctioning techniques are acceptable, and the patient cleans the secretion collection container and disinfects it every 24 hours.

SKILL 14.5   AIRWAY MANAGEMENT: ENDOTRACHEAL TUBE AND TRACHEOSTOMY CARE

• **Nursing Skills Online: Airway Management, Lessons 7 and 8**

ETTs are short-term artificial airways used to administer mechanical ventilation, relieve upper airway obstruction, protect against aspiration, or clear secretions (see Fig. 14-5, *A*). After insertion of an ETT, the cuff is inflated. Preventing cuff-related problems is a critical component of nursing care and depends on securing the tube and inflating the cuff properly. Allowing an ETT to slip lower into the airway can prevent ventilation of a lung, usually the left lung. Allowing an ETT to slide too far up the tracheobronchial tree can allow air to escape through or damage the vocal cords. Properly securing the ETT prevents accidental extubation from coughing or pulling on the tube. Capnography, a noninvasive monitoring device, is recommended to validate the correct placement of the ETT by analyzing the exhaled gas for carbon dioxide levels (Walsh et al., 2011).

If a patient requires continued assistance from an artificial airway, a tracheostomy is considered for long-term use (see Fig. 14-6). A tracheostomy offers advantages over long-term ETT placement, such as decreased laryngeal and tracheal tissue injury, ease of breathing, and access for better oral hygiene (White et al., 2010). Some patients with a tracheostomy tube are able to cough secretions out of the tracheostomy tube completely, whereas others are able only to cough secretions up into the tracheostomy tube.

ASSESSMENT

1. Identify patient using two identifiers (e.g., name and birthday or name and account number) according to facility policy. *Rationale: Ensures correct patient. Complies with The Joint Commission standards and improves patient safety (TJC, 2014).*
2. Apply clean gloves. Observe condition of tube, and inspect mouth and surrounding skin. ETT: soiled or loose tape; pressure sores on nares, lip, or corner of mouth; unstable tube; excessive secretions. Tracheostomy tube: soiled or loose ties or dressing; unstable tube; excessive secretions. *Rationale: A patient with an artificial airway is at risk for impaired skin integrity and infection because of difficulty controlling secretions and pressure points of the artificial airway (Zaratkiewicz et al., 2012).*
3. Identify factors that increase risk of complications from ETT and tracheal tubes: type and size of tube, movement of tube up and down trachea, amount of inflation of tube cuff, pressure from artificial airways to adjacent skin tissue, and duration of placement. *Rationale: ETT moving up and down trachea predisposes patient to tracheal trauma or dislodgment. Cuff underinflation may allow aspiration, whereas overinflation may cause ischemia or necrosis of tracheal tissue. Use of tubes for longer periods increases the risk of lower airway complications such as pneumonia.*

4. Auscultate lungs. *Rationale: Provides baseline confirming bilateral lung inflation, presence of adventitious sounds.*
5. Determine proper ETT depth as noted by the number of centimeters at lip or gum line. This line is marked and recorded in patient's chart at time of intubation. *Rationale: Ensures that tube is at proper depth to ventilate lungs adequately.*
6. Assess patient's knowledge and comfort with procedure. *Rationale: Facilitates patient's learning and participation in care and may help to decrease anxiety.*
7. If applicable, assess patient's understanding of and ability to perform own tracheostomy care. *Rationale: Increases patient's feeling of autonomy and determines need for instruction.*

PLANNING

Expected Outcomes focus on preventing infection, preventing breakdown of skin and mucosa around the artificial airway, and promoting patient's self-care.
1. Patient maintains or improves SaO_2 readings.
2. Patient's artificial airway or tube is in correct position and properly secured.
3. Patient remains afebrile without signs and symptoms of infection.
4. Patient's oral mucous membrane or stoma remains free of breakdown or accumulation of secretions.
5. Patient's artificial airway is intact and free of secretions.
6. Patient is able to demonstrate correct technique of tracheostomy care when appropriate.

Delegation and Collaboration

The skill of ETT care cannot be delegated to nursing assistive personnel (NAP). The skill of tracheostomy care can be delegated to NAP when a permanent or long-term tracheostomy is in place in stable, chronically ill patients. The nurse instructs the NAP about:
• Reporting any signs of respiratory problems or increased airway secretions.
• Reporting if the ETT appears to have moved or becomes dislodged or obstructed.
• Reporting changes in patient's level of consciousness, irritability, vital signs, or decreased pulse oximetry.

Equipment
• Stethoscope
• Face shield

Endotracheal Tube Care
• Towel
• ETT and oropharyngeal suction equipment
• 1- to 1½-inch adhesive or waterproof tape (not paper tape) or commercial ETT stabilizer (follow manufacturer's instructions for securing)

- Two pairs of clean gloves
- Adhesive remover swab
- Mouth care supplies (e.g., pediatric-size toothbrush, sponge toothette for edentulous patients, toothpaste, and nonalcohol-based mouthwash)
- Face cleanser (e.g., wet washcloth, towel, soap, shaving supplies)
- Clean 2 × 2–inch gauze
- Tincture of benzoin or liquid adhesive
- Oral airway or bite block

Tracheostomy Care
- Bedside table
- Towel

- Tracheostomy suction supplies
- Sterile tracheostomy care kit if available or:
  - Three sterile 4 × 4–inch gauze pads
  - Sterile cotton-tipped applicators
  - Sterile tracheostomy dressing
  - Sterile basin
  - Small sterile brush (or disposable cannula)
  - Tracheostomy ties (e.g., twill tape, manufactured tracheostomy ties, Velcro tracheostomy ties)
- Normal saline
- Scissors
- Pair of sterile and clean gloves

IMPLEMENTATION *for* AIRWAY MANAGEMENT: ENDOTRACHEAL TUBE AND TRACHEOSTOMY CARE

STEPS	RATIONALE
1. **See Standard Protocol (inside front cover).**	
2. *ETT care*	
a. Apply clean gloves. Apply face shield. Suction ETT (see Skill 14.4). Remove gloves and perform hand hygiene.	Removes secretions. Diminishes patient's need to cough during procedure.

> **SAFE PATIENT CARE** Keep an oral airway or bite-block immediately accessible in the event that patient bites down and obstructs the ETT. A bite-block also assists in stabilizing the ETT.

STEPS	RATIONALE
b. Connect oral suction catheter to suction source. Help patient to comfortable position.	Prepares patient for oropharyngeal suctioning.
c. Prepare ETT securement option.	
(1) *Tape method:* Cut piece of tape long enough to go completely around patient's head from nares to nares plus 15 cm (6 inches): total length for adult, about 30 to 60 cm (1 to 2 feet). Lay the tape adhesive side up on bedside table. Cut and lay an 8- to 15-cm (3- to 6-inch) strip of tape in center of long strip, adhesive sides together.	Adhesive tape must be placed around head from cheek to cheek below ears. Placing adhesive sides together in center of strip prevents the tape from adhering to hair. Cotton tape ties may also be used.
(2) *Commercially available ETT holder:* Open package and set device aside with the head guard in place and Velcro strips open.	
d. Have an assistant apply a pair of gloves and hold ETT firmly so that tube does not move throughout procedure. Note the number marking once again on the ETT at the lip line.	Reduces transmission of microorganisms. Maintains proper tube position and prevents accidental extubation.
e. Remove old tape or commercial tube holder.	Provides access to skin under tape for assessment and hygiene. Reduces transmission of microorganisms.
(1) *Tape:* Carefully remove tape from ETT and patient's face. If tape is difficult to remove, moisten with water or adhesive tape remover. Discard in receptacle.	Adhesive can cause damage to skin and prevent adhesion of new tape.
(2) *Commercial tube holder:* Remove Velcro strips from ETT and remove tube holder.	Devices are latex-free, fast, and convenient.

Continued

STEPS	RATIONALE
f. Remove oral airway or bite-block if present and place in towel. (Do not remove oral airway if patient is actively biting ETT. This may result in occlusion of the airway.)	Provides access to and complete observation of patient's oral cavity.
g. Keep ETT cuff inflated. As assistant continues to hold tube, clean mouth, gums, and teeth opposite ETT with nonalcohol-based mouthwash solution (e.g., chlorhexidine 0.12%) (Zurmehly, 2013) as needed or up to every 4 hours (Prendergast et al., 2013). Oral care with a soft toothbrush should be completed every 12 hours (Prendergast et al., 2013). Suction fluid from oral cavity with Yankauer catheter or use toothbrush made to be connected to suction. Use sponge-tipped applicators to apply moisture to gums and buccal mucosa.	Inflated cuff on the ETT reduces risks for aspiration and accidental extubation. Alcohol-based mouthwashes dry oral mucosa (Lewis et al., 2014).
h. *Oral ETT only:* Note "cm" ETT marking at lips. With help of assistant, move ETT to opposite side or center of mouth. Do not change tube depth.	Prevents pressure-sore formation at sides of patient's mouth. Ensures correct position of tube (Zaratkiewicz et al., 2012).
i. Repeat oral cleaning as in Step 2g on opposite side of mouth. Complete every 12 hours.	Removes secretions from oropharynx; removes plaque from teeth (Sedwick et al., 2012).
j. Clean face and neck with soapy washcloth; rinse and dry. Shave male patient after ETT is secured.	Moisture and beard growth prevent adhesive tape adherence.
k. Secure ETT (assistant continues holding tube). **(1)** Tape method:	Positions tape to secure ETT in proper position. Protects and makes it easier for tape to adhere to skin.
(a) Pour small amount of tincture of benzoin on clean 2 × 2–inch gauze or swab and dot on skin above upper lip (oral ETT) or across nose (nasal ETT) and cheeks to ear. Allow to dry completely.	
(b) Slip prepared tape under patient's head and neck, adhesive side up. Take care not to twist tape or catch hair. Do not allow tape to stick to itself. Stick end of tape gently to tongue blade, which serves as a guide while sliding under neck. Center the strip of tape so that double-faced tape extends around back of neck from ear to ear.	
(c) On one side of face secure tape from ear to nares (nasal ETT) or edge of mouth (oral ETT). Tear remaining tape in half lengthwise, forming two pieces that are $\frac{1}{2}$ to $\frac{3}{4}$ inch wide. Secure bottom half of tape across upper lip (oral ETT) or across top of nose (nasal ETT) (see illustration *A*). Wrap top half of tape around tube and up from bottom. Tape should encircle tube at least two times for security (see illustration *B*).	Secures tape to face. Using top tape to wrap prevents downward drag on ETT.
(d) On other side of face, gently pull tape firmly to pick up slack and secure to remaining side of face (see illustration). Assistant can release hold when tube is secure. You may want assistant to help reinsert oral airway.	Secures tape to face and tube. ETT should be at same depth at the lips. Check earlier assessment for verification of tube depth in centimeters.

STEPS	RATIONALE

(2) Commercial tube holder:

(a) Thread ETT through opening designed to secure it. Be sure that the pilot balloon is accessible. Place strips of ETT holder under patient's head at the occiput.

Commercial holders have a slit in the front of the holder designed to secure the ETT.

(b) Verify that ETT is at the established depth, using the lip line marker as a guide. Attach Velcro strips at the base of the patient's head. Leave 1-cm (½-inch) slack in strips. Verify that tube is secure.

Ensures that ETT remains at correct depth as determined during assessment.

l. Clean oral airway in warm water and rinse well. Shake excess water from oral airway.

Promotes hygiene. Reduces transmission of microorganisms.

m. Reinsert oral airway without pushing tongue into oropharynx by initially inserting upside down until the tip is beyond the end of the tongue and then rotating 180 degrees into place (see Skill 29.1).

Prevents patient from biting ETT and allows access for oropharyngeal suctioning by sliding catheter along outer edge.

3. *Tracheostomy care:*

a. Apply clean gloves. Apply face shield. Suction tracheostomy (see Skill 14.4). Remove soiled tracheostomy dressing (discard in glove with coiled catheter), remove gloves, and perform hand hygiene.

Removes secretions so as not to occlude outer cannula while inner cannula is removed.

b. Provide preoxygenation for a minimum of 30 seconds by asking the patient to take 5 to 6 deep breaths or by using a reservoir-equipped manual resuscitation bag (MRB) connected to 100% O_2. Prepare equipment on bedside table.

Replenishes oxygen lost in suctioning of tracheostomy (Lewis et al., 2014).

(1) Open sterile tracheostomy kit. Open three 4 × 4–inch gauze packages using aseptic technique and pour normal saline on the gauze in two packages. Leave gauze in third package dry.

Preparation and organization of equipment allows you to complete procedure efficiently and reconnect patient to oxygen source in a timely manner.

(2) Open two packages of cotton-tipped swabs and pour normal saline on the tip of swabs, keeping packages sterile. Do not recap bottles.

(3) Open sterile tracheostomy dressing package.

(4) Unwrap sterile basin and pour about 2 cm (¾ inch) of normal saline. Open small sterile brush package and place aseptically into sterile basin.

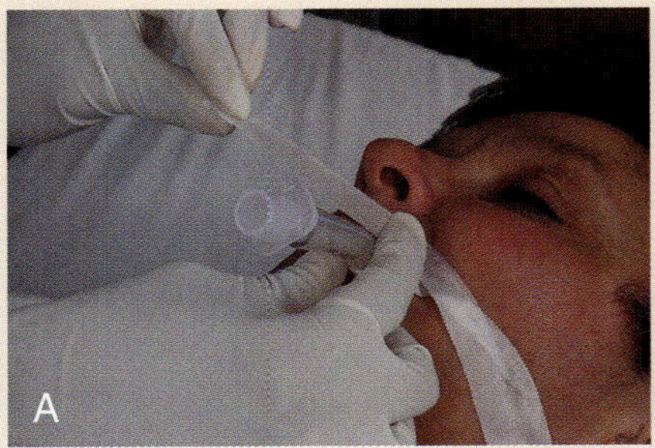 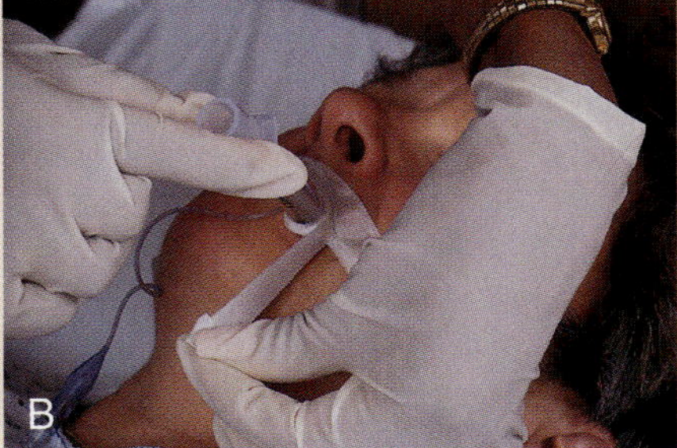 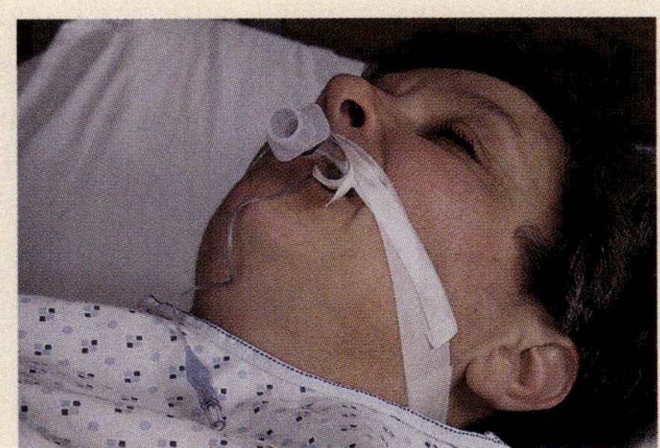

STEP 2k(1)(c) A, Securing bottom half of tape across patient's upper lip. **B,** Securing top half of tape around tube.

STEP 2k(1)(d) Tape securing ETT.

Continued

STEPS	RATIONALE
(5) Prepare length of twill tape long enough to circle around patient's neck twice (about 60 to 75 cm or 24 to 30 inches for an adult). Cut ends on diagonal.	Diagonal cut ends allow for easy threading through the tracheostomy device.
(6) If using commercial tracheostomy tube holder, open package.	
c. Apply sterile gloves. Keep dominant hand sterile throughout procedure.	Reduces transmission of microorganisms.
d. Remove oxygen source (if present).	
e. If a nondisposable inner cannula is used (see Fig. 14-6, *A*):	
(1) While touching only the outer aspect of the tube, remove the inner cannula with nondominant hand. Drop inner cannula into basin with normal saline or hydrogen peroxide (full or half strength) (Morris et al., 2013).	Normal saline or hydrogen peroxide loosens crusted secretions from inner cannula.
(2) Place tracheostomy collar or T tube and ventilator oxygen source over or near tracheostomy opening. Note: T tube and ventilator oxygen devices cannot be attached to most outer cannulas when inner cannula is removed. You may insert a new inner cannula quickly so the oxygen source can be maintained. Clean the old inner cannula in normal saline or hydrogen peroxide and store it in a sterile container for use the next time the tracheostomy is cleaned (two cannulas on hand at all times).	Maintains supply of oxygen to patient to prevent desaturation. Allows quick reconnection to oxygen source.
(3) To prevent oxygen desaturation in affected patients, quickly pick up inner cannula and use small brush to remove secretions inside and outside cannula (see illustration).	Brush removes thick or dried secretions.
(4) Hold inner cannula over basin and rinse with normal saline, using nondominant hand to pour.	Removes secretions from inner cannula.
(5) Replace inner cannula and secure "locking" mechanism (see illustration). Reapply ventilator or oxygen sources when inner cannula is in place.	
f. If a disposable inner cannula is used:	
(1) Remove new cannula from manufacturer's packaging.	
(2) While touching only the outer aspect of the tracheostomy tube, withdraw old inner cannula and replace with new cannula. Lock into position.	Maintains sterility of the inner aspect of the new cannula.
(3) Dispose of contaminated cannula in appropriate receptacle.	

STEPS	RATIONALE

g. Using normal saline–saturated cotton-tipped swabs and 4 × 4–inch gauze, clean in circular motion from stoma site outward, using dominant hand to handle sterile supplies. Half-strength hydrogen peroxide can be used for dried or difficult-to-remove secretions, but the area must be rinsed well with normal saline (Morris et al., 2013). Clean exposed outer cannula surfaces and stoma under faceplate, extending 5 to 10 cm (2 to 4 inches) in all directions from stoma (see illustration).

h. Using dry 4 × 4–inch gauze, pat skin and exposed outer cannula surfaces lightly.

Dry surfaces decrease growth of microorganisms and skin excoriation.

i. Secure tracheostomy.

   (1) Instruct assistant, if available, to apply clean gloves and hold tracheostomy tube securely in place.

Reduces transmission of microorganisms, and secures airway.

> **SAFE PATIENT CARE** Assistant must not release hold on tracheostomy tube until new ties are firmly attached to reduce risk of injury, discomfort, or accidental extubation. If no assistant is present, do not remove old ties until you secure the new ones. (Follow manufacturer's guidelines for Velcro ties.)

   (2) Insert one end of prepared tie through faceplate eyelet (see illustration) and pull ends of tie even.

   (3) Slide both ends of tie behind head and around neck to other eyelet and insert one tie through second eyelet. Cut old ties and remove.

   (4) Pull new ties snugly.

Prevents tube displacement.

   (5) Tie ends securely in double square knot, allowing space for only one finger between neck and the tie.

One-finger slack prevents ties from being too tight. Knot should be to the side of the neck. Foam and Velcro tracheostomy holders are also commonly used.

   (6) Insert fresh tracheostomy dressing under clean ties and faceplate (see illustration).

Absorbs drainage. Dressing prevents pressure on clavicle heads.

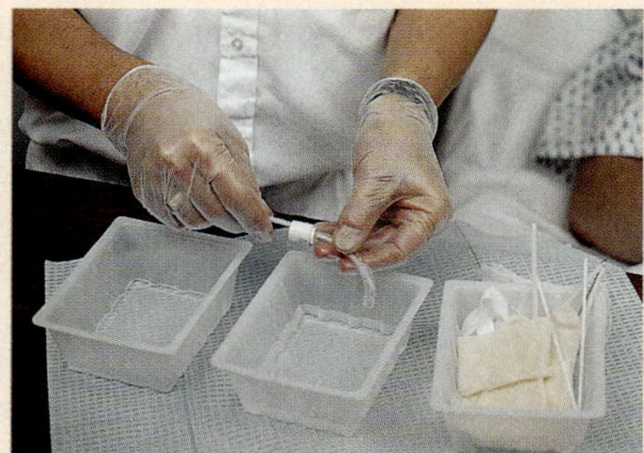

STEP 3e(3) Cleaning tracheostomy inner cannula.

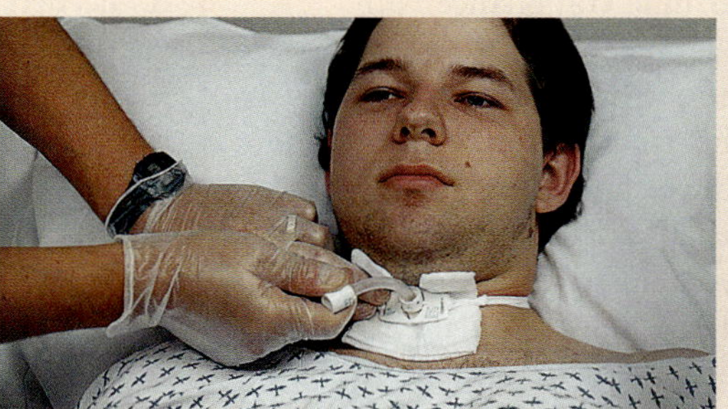

STEP 3e(5) Reinserting inner cannula.

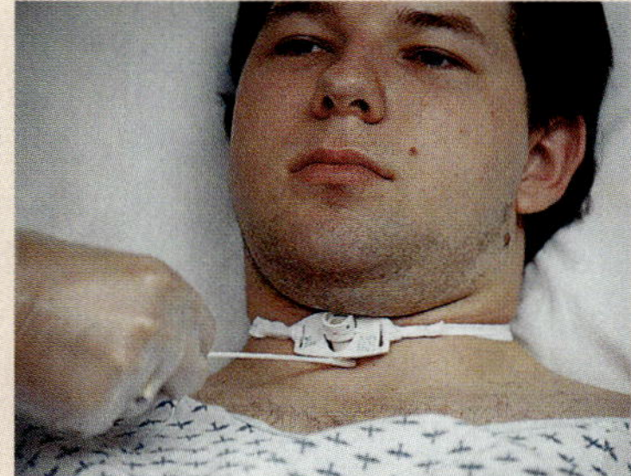

STEP 3g Cleaning around stoma.

Continued

STEPS	RATIONALE
j. Position patient comfortably and assess respiratory status.	Promotes relaxation. Some patients may require post–tracheostomy care suctioning.

> **SAFE PATIENT CARE** For accidental extubation, call for assistance and manually ventilate patient with resuscitation bag if necessary. Keep tracheostomy obturator at bedside with a fresh tracheostomy to facilitate reinsertion of the outer cannula if dislodged. Keep an additional tracheostomy tube of the same size and shape on hand for emergency replacement (McGrath et al., 2012).

4. See Completion Protocol (inside front cover).

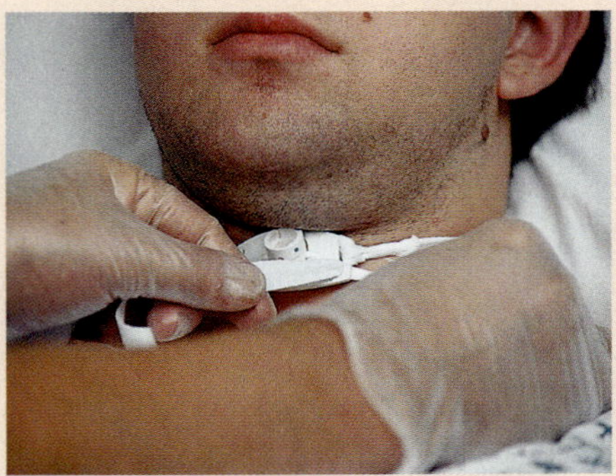

STEP 3i(2) Replacing tracheostomy ties.

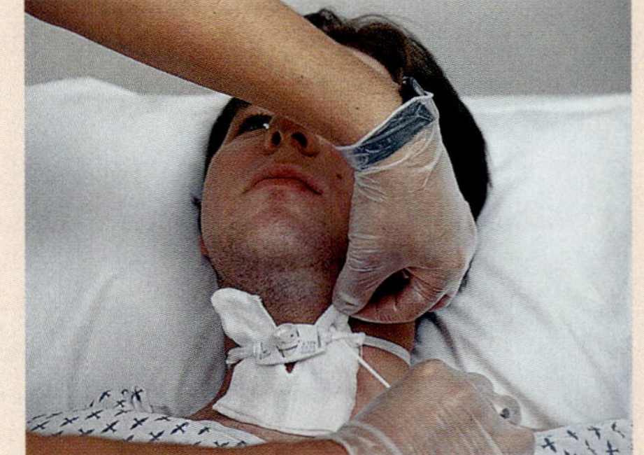

STEP 3i(6) Applying tracheostomy dressing.

EVALUATION

1. Auscultate lungs and observe that airway is in proper position with tape or ties secure and comfortable for patient. ETT should be at the same depth as before care (as per health care provider order), with the same centimeter marking at lips and equal bilateral breath sounds.
2. Observe stoma for signs of infection.
3. Compare oral mucosa and airway assessments before and after artificial airway care. Observe for signs of tissue breakdown or persistent dried secretions.
4. Observe patient's actions to determine compliance with the procedure.
5. Use *Teach Back:* State to the patient, "I want to make sure that I explained how to do tracheostomy care correctly. Next time, can you demonstrate the technique for tracheostomy tube care?" Evaluates what the patient is able to explain or demonstrate. Revise your instruction now or develop plan for revised patient teaching to be implemented at an appropriate time if patient is not able to teach back correctly.

Unexpected Outcomes and Related Interventions

1. Tube is not secure. Artificial airway moves in or out or is coughed out by patient.
   a. Adjust or apply new ties.
2. Breath sounds not equal bilaterally with an ETT in place.
   a. Evaluate ETT for proper depth. If incorrect, arrange for ETT to be repositioned as allowed by facility.

   b. Obtain order for chest x-ray study to verify placement if applicable.
   c. Assess patient's respiratory status and observe for the presence of mucus plugs.
3. Breakdown, pressure areas, or stomatitis (tracheostomy tube) develop around tube.
   a. Increase frequency of tube care.
   b. Ensure that skin areas are clean and dry.
4. Accidental extubation.
   a. Call for assistance, monitor vital signs, keep head of bed elevated.
   b. If needed, insert oral airway and provide MRB ventilation.
   c. Maintain patent airway by replacing old tracheostomy tube with new tube for established tracheostomy. Use obturator to insert new tube and then remove obturator. Assess placement with capnography (McGrath et al., 2012).
   d. For a new tracheostomy, cover the site with gauze and ventilate via bag-valve-mask with 100% oxygen. Do not attempt to recannulate because of potential for damage to stoma or trachea. Call for assistance.

Recording and Reporting

- Record respiratory assessments before and after tube care, depth of ETT or type and size of tracheostomy tube, frequency and extent of care, patient tolerance, and any complications related to presence of the tube.

- Report signs of infection or displacement of ETT or tracheostomy tube immediately.
- Document your evaluation of patient learning.

Sample Documentation

0800   Routine tracheostomy tube care done. Patient indicated need for education related to care of the stoma. After allowing patient to visualize process in mirror, he successfully completed the cleaning of the stoma and inner cannula. No irritation or skin breakdown noted. Respirations regular in rate, rhythm, and depth at 16 breaths per minute. Clear breath sounds bilaterally. SaO_2 remains at 98%.

Special Considerations
Pediatric

- Monitor children with new tracheostomy for complications such as hemorrhage, edema, accidental decannulation, and airway obstruction (Hockenberry and Wilson, 2013).
- Because of infants' delicate skin, you do not always use skin preparation before securing ETT. ETT holders are best to use in infants.

Geriatric

- Older adult skin may be more fragile and prone to breakdown from secretions or pressure or tearing when removing tape.
- Additional communication difficulties may occur for older adults who have visual or auditory deficits. Ensure that glasses and hearing aids are available and working properly.

Home Care

- Family caregivers must know how to clean established tracheostomy tubes and recognize the signs and symptoms of respiratory and stoma infections.

SKILL 14.6 MANAGING CLOSED CHEST DRAINAGE SYSTEMS

• Nursing Skills Online: Chest Tubes, Lessons 1 to 3

Trauma, disease, or surgery can interrupt the closed negative-pressure system of the lungs, causing lung collapse. Air (pneumothorax), blood (hemothorax), or fluid may leak into the pleural cavity. A chest tube is inserted, and a closed chest drainage system is attached to promote drainage of air and fluid from the pleural space so the lung can reexpand. A one-way valve prevents the air or fluid from flowing back into the pleural cavity. This type of tube is also called a thoracostomy tube or thoracic catheter. Suction may be added to assist gravity in draining fluid (Kane et al., 2013).

In an emergent situation, a catheter is inserted through the chest wall, and a rubber flutter one-way valve (e.g., a Heimlich valve) is attached to the catheter (Fig. 14-7). As a patient exhales, the positive pressure generated by the air leaving the chest enters the tubing, causing the valve to open so air is released. During inspiration the tube collapses on itself, preventing air from reentering the chest. No drainage chamber is used with this device. This device is contraindicated when patient needs fluid drained, such as when a hemothorax or plural effusion is present.

The placement of a chest tube depends on the type of drainage that is present. Because air rises, apical and anterior chest tube placement promotes removal of air. Chest tubes are placed low and posterior or lateral to drain fluid (Fig. 14-8). Mediastinal chest tubes are placed just below the sternum (Fig. 14-9) and drain blood or fluid, preventing its accumulation around the heart (e.g., after open-heart surgery) (Durai et al., 2010; Kane et al., 2013).

Although single-bottle systems are available, single-unit water-seal or waterless systems are most often used. The water-seal system contains two or three compartments or chambers (Fig. 14-10). Fluid drains into the first chamber. The second chamber contains the water seal, which allows air to escape because of the force of expiration but not to reenter on inspiration. If suction is needed, a third chamber is used. The suction pressure should not exceed 20 cm H_2O because lung tissue damage may occur (Kane et al., 2013).

The principles that a waterless system follows are similar to those of a water seal system except that sterile water is not required for suction. The suction control chamber is replaced by a one-way valve located near the top of the system. The drainage chamber takes up most of the space in the drainage unit. The suction control chamber contains a suction control float ball that is set by a suction control dial (between 10 and 40 cm H_2O after the suction is connected and turned on) (Kane et al., 2013).

ASSESSMENT

1. Identify patient using two identifiers (e.g., name and birthday or name and account number) according to facility policy. *Rationale: Ensures correct patient. Complies with The Joint Commission standards and improves patient safety (TJC, 2014).*

2. Perform a complete respiratory assessment, baseline vital signs, and oximetry (see Chapters 6 and 7). *Rationale: Baseline vital signs are essential for any invasive procedure. Chest tube insertion often causes respiratory distress.*

3. Assess patient for known allergies. Ask patient about any problems with medications, latex, or anything applied to

the skin. *Rationale: Antiseptic skin preps, such as chlorhexidine, are used to clean the skin before tube insertion. Lidocaine is a local anesthetic administered to reduce pain. These, along with the tape used to secure the tube, can cause allergic reactions.*

4. Assess patient's comfort level on a scale of 0 to 10. Provide pain medication before procedure per health care provider's order. *Rationale: Determines need for and level of pain management.*

5. Assess if patient is able to breathe deeply and comfortably. *Rationale: Detects early signs and symptoms of complications. Promotes reexpansion of the lung.*

6. Review patient's hemoglobin and hematocrit levels. *Rationale: Parameters reflect if blood loss is occurring, which may affect oxygenation.*

7. Review patient's medications for anticoagulant therapy, use of nonsteroidal antiinflammatory medications, and any platelet aggregation inhibitors, such as ticlopidine (TicLid). *Rationale: May contribute to blood loss during and after procedure.*

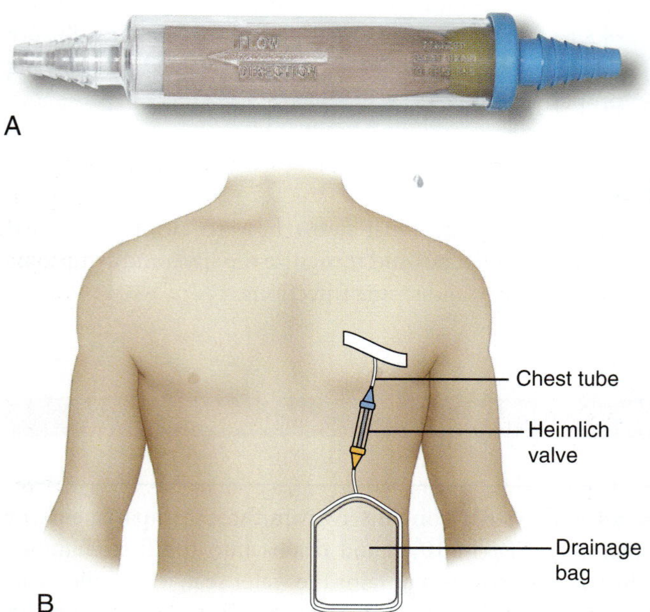

FIG 14-7 A, Heimlich chest drain valve is a specially designed flutter valve that is used in place of a chest drainage unit for a small uncomplicated pneumothorax with little or no drainage and no need for suction. The valve allows for escape of air but prevents reentry of air into the pleural space. **B,** Placement of the valve between chest tube and drainage bag, which can be worn under clothing.

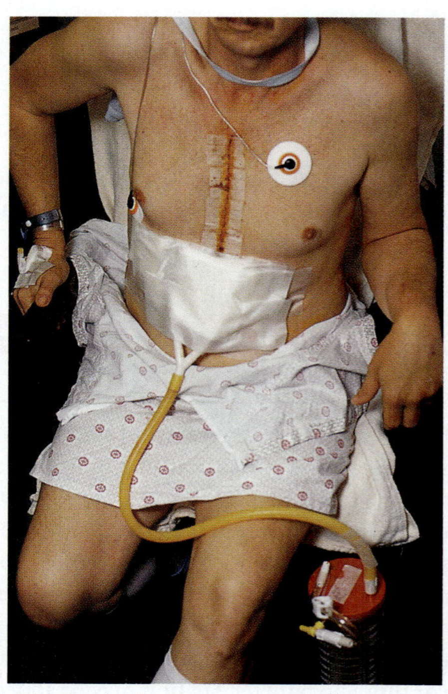

FIG 14-9 Mediastinal chest tube following open heart surgery.

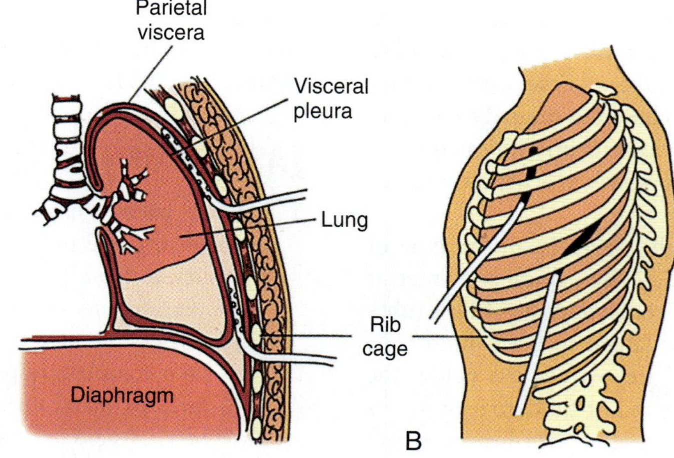

FIG 14-8 Diagram of sites for chest tube placement. **A,** Anatomical drawing showing upper tube placement (for air) and lower tube placement (for blood and fluid). **B,** View of tubes exiting through intracostal sites.

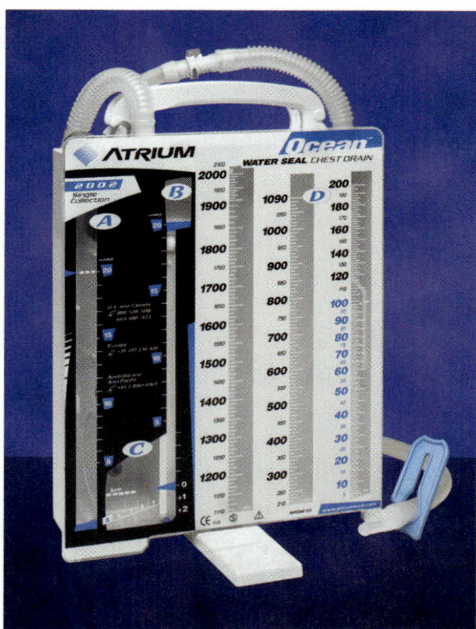

FIG 14-10 Disposable water-seal chest drainage system with suction. (Courtesy Atrium Medical.)

4. Patient's vital signs, oxygenation saturation (SpO_2), hemoglobin level, and hematocrit improve or are within normal ranges by discharge.
5. Patient performs breathing exercises correctly.
6. Patient reports improved comfort on a scale of 0 to 10.
7. Chest tube and drainage system remains intact and functioning properly.

Delegation and Collaboration

The skill of chest tube management cannot be delegated to nursing assistive personnel (NAP). The nurse instructs the NAP about:

- Proper positioning of a patient with chest tubes to facilitate chest tube drainage.
- How to ambulate and transfer patient with chest drainage.
- Reporting changes in vital signs, complaints of chest pain or sudden shortness of breath, or excessive bubbling in water-seal chamber.
- Danger of any disconnection of drainage system, change in color and/or amount of drainage, sudden sensation of bubbling.

Equipment

- Local anesthetic, if not an emergent procedure
- Prescribed chest drainage system
- Water-seal system versus waterless system: sterile water or normal saline per manufacturer's directions
- Clean gloves
- Suction source and setup
- Sterile skin preparation solution (povidone-iodine or chlorhexidine solutions)
- Chest tube tray (all items are sterile), typically: knife handle, clamps, small sponge forceps, needle holder, knife blade No. 10, 3-0 silk sutures, sterile drape, two clamps, 4 × 4–inch sponges, suture scissors, and sterile gloves
- Dressings: Petroleum or Xeroform gauze, large dressing of choice, split chest tube dressing, additional 4 × 4–inch dressings, 4-inch tape or elastic bandage
- Two rubber-tipped hemostats (shodded) for each chest tube
- 1-inch waterproof adhesive tape for taping connections
- Face mask, face shield, or head cover
- Sterile gloves
- 1-inch adhesive tape or zip tie for securing connections
- Stethoscope, sphygmomanometer, and pulse oximeter

8. For patients who have chest tubes, observe integrity of chest tube dressing, drainage tubing (kinks, dependent loops, or clots), and drainage system. *Rationale: Observation verifies that (1) chest tube dressing is intact and occlusive seal remains without fluid or air leaks. The drainage tube must be patent to facilitate drainage, and functional drainage system is essential to facilitate lung expansion and drainage (Briggs, 2010).*
9. Determine patient's knowledge of the procedure. *Rationale: Encourages patient cooperation, minimizes risks and anxiety. Identifies teaching needs.*

PLANNING

Expected Outcomes focus on removal of air and fluid from the pleural space and reexpansion of the lung with maximum patient comfort.

1. Patient's respirations are nonlabored.
2. Patient's breath sounds are present in all lobes.
3. Patient's lung expansion is symmetrical.

IMPLEMENTATION *for* MANAGING CLOSED CHEST DRAINAGE SYSTEMS

STEPS	RATIONALE
1. **See Standard Protocol (inside front cover).**	
2. Check facility policy to determine if informed consent is needed. Complete "Time Out" procedure.	Invasive medical procedures typically require informed consent. "Time Out" is completed to determine right patient, procedure, and location of insertion (Kane et al., 2013).

Continued

STEPS	RATIONALE

3. Set up water-seal or dry system. (See manufacturer's guidelines).

   a. Obtain a chest drainage system. Remove wrappers and prepare to set up as a two- or three-chamber system.

Maintains sterility of system for use under sterile operating room conditions.

   b. While maintaining sterility of the drainage tubing, stand system upright, and add sterile water or normal saline to appropriate compartments.

Reduces possibility of contamination (Kane et al., 2013).

     (1) *Two-chamber system (without suction):* Add sterile solution to water-seal chamber (second chamber), bringing fluid to the required level as indicated.

Water-seal chamber acts as a one-way valve so air cannot enter pleural space (Briggs, 2010).

     (2) *Three-chamber system (with suction):* Add sterile solution to water-seal chamber (second chamber). Add amount of sterile solution prescribed by health care provider to suction control chamber (third chamber), usually 20 cm H_2O pressure. Connect tubing from suction control chamber to suction source. Tailor length of drainage tube to patient. **Note: Suction control chamber vent must not be occluded when using suction.**

Depth of float below fluid level dictates highest amount of negative pressure that can be present within system. For example, 20 cm H_2O is approximately 20 cm of water pressure. Any additional negative pressure applied to system is vented into the atmosphere through suction control vent. This safety device prevents damage to pleural tissues from an unexpected surge of negative pressure from suction source. Excessively long drainage tube may result in occlusions. Provides safety factor of releasing excess negative pressure into the air through suction control vent.

4. Set up waterless system (see manufacturer's guidelines).

   a. Remove sterile wrappers and prepare to set up.

Maintains sterility of system for use under sterile operating room conditions.

   b. For two-chamber system (without suction), nothing is added or needs to be done to system.

Waterless two-chamber system is ready for connecting to patient's chest tube after opening wrappers.

   c. For three-chamber system with suction, connect tubing from suction control chamber to suction source.

Suction source provides additional negative pressure to system.

   d. Instill 15 mL of sterile water or normal saline into diagnostic indicator injection port located on top of system.

Allows for observation of a rise and fall in water in diagnostic air leak window. This is not necessary for mediastinal drainage because there is no tidaling. In an emergency, system *does not* require water for setup.

5. Secure all tubing connections in a double-spiral fashion using 2.5-cm (1-inch) adhesive tape. Then check the system for patency by:

   a. Clamping the drainage tubing that will connect to the patient's chest tube.

   b. Connecting tubing from float ball chamber to suction source.

   c. Turning on suction to prescribed level.

Prevents atmospheric air from leaking into system and patient's intrapleural space. Provides chance to ensure airtight system before connecting it to patient. Allows correction or replacement of system if it is defective before connecting it to patient.

6. Turn off suction source and unclamp drainage tubing before connecting patient to system. Make a second check to be sure drainage tubing is not excessively long. Suction source is turned on again after patient is connected (Step 9).

Having patient connected to suction when it is initiated could damage pleural tissues from sudden increase in negative pressure. Tubing that is coiled or looped may become clotted, impeding drainage while draining a hemothorax, and may potentially cause a tension pneumothorax (Kane et al., 2013).

7. Apply clean gloves. Position patient for tube insertion so that the side in which the chest tube will be placed is accessible to the health care provider.

For a pneumothorax, place patient in a lateral supine position. For a hemothorax, place the patient in a semi-Fowler's position (Kane et al., 2013).

STEPS	RATIONALE
8. Assist health care provider with chest tube insertion by providing needed equipment and local analgesic and offering patient support and instruction. Health care provider inserts and clamps tube, sutures it in place, and applies occlusive dressing.	
9. Help health care provider attach drainage tube to chest tube while maintaining sterility; remove clamp. Turn on suction to prescribed level.	Connects drainage system and suction (if ordered) to chest tube.
10. Tape tube connection between chest tube and drainage tube. One method: One long strip of tape on each side with an overlapping tape wrapped spirally enables connections to be observed and remain secure.	Secures chest tube to drainage system and reduces risk of air leaks that cause breaks in airtight system.
11. Check system for proper functioning. Health care provider orders a chest x-ray film.	Verifies intrapleural placement of tube.
12. After tube placement, position patient:	
a. Using semi-Fowler's to high-Fowler's position to evacuate air (pneumothorax).	Permits optimum drainage of fluid or air. Air rises to highest point in the chest.
b. Using high-Fowler's position to drain fluid (hemothorax).	Permits optimum drainage of fluid.
13. Check patency of air vents in system.	
a. Water-seal vent must have no occlusion.	Permits displaced air to pass into atmosphere.
b. Suction control chamber vent must not be occluded when using suction.	Provides safety factor of releasing excess negative pressure into atmosphere.
c. Waterless systems have relief valves without caps.	
14. Position tubing on mattress next to patient. Secure to linen with the clamp provided so that it does not obstruct tubing.	Excess tubing hanging over the edge of mattress may form a dependent loop where drainage could pool, causing a blockage (Kane et al., 2013).
15. Adjust tubing to hang in a straight line from top of mattress to drainage chamber.	Promotes drainage.
16. Place two rubber-tipped hemostats (for each chest tube) in an easily accessible position such as taped to the top of patient's headboard. These should remain with patient if ambulating.	Chest tubes are double clamped under specific circumstances: (1) to assess for an air leak (Table 14-4), (2) to empty or quickly change disposable systems, or (3) to assess if patient ready to have tube removed (Kane et al., 2013).
17. Care of patient after chest tube insertion:	
a. Assess vital signs; oxygen saturation; skin color; breath sounds; and rate, depth, and ease of respirations every 15 minutes for first 2 hours, then at least every shift (see facility policy).	Provides data to compare with baseline and information about procedure-related complications.
b. Monitor color, consistency, and amount of drainage every 15 minutes for the first 2 hours. Indicate level of drainage fluid, date, and time on chamber's write-on surface.	Provides baseline for continuous assessment of type and quantity of drainage. Ensures early detection of complications.
(1) From a mediastinal tube, less than 100 mL/hr immediately after surgery is expected and no more than 800 mL in first 24 hours.	Sudden gush of drainage may result from coughing or changing patient's position, releasing pooled/collected blood rather than indicating active bleeding.
(2) From a postoperative chest tube, 100 to 300 mL is expected during first 3 hours after insertion, with 500 to 1000 mL expected in the first 24 hours. Drainage is grossly bloody during the first several hours after surgery and then changes to serous (Kane et al., 2013).	Acute bleeding indicates hemorrhage. Notify health care provider.

Continued

STEPS	RATIONALE

(3) From an anterior chest tube that is inserted for a pneumothorax, there should be little or no output (Kane et al., 2013).

c. Observe chest dressing for drainage.

d. Apply clean gloves. Palpate around tube for swelling and crepitus (subcutaneous emphysema) as evidenced by crackling.

e. Check tubing to ensure that it is free of kinks and dependent loops.

f. Observe for fluctuation of drainage in the tubing and water-seal chamber during inspiration and expiration. Observe for clots or debris in tubing.

g. Keep drainage system upright and below level of the patient's chest.

h. Check for air leaks by monitoring the bubbling in water-seal chamber. Intermittent bubbling is normal during expiration when air is being evacuated from the pleural cavity, but continuous bubbling during both inspiration and expiration indicates a leak in the system (Kane et al., 2013).

Rationale:

Drainage around tube may indicate blockage.

Indicates presence of air trapping in subcutaneous tissues. Small amounts are commonly absorbed. Large amounts are potentially dangerous (Kane et al., 2013).

Promotes drainage.

If fluctuation or tidaling stops, it means that either the lung is fully expanded or the system is obstructed (Kane et al., 2013).

Promotes gravity drainage and prevents backflow of fluid and air into the pleural space.

Absence of bubbling may indicate that the lung has fully expanded if patient had pneumothorax. Bubbling occurs at first because there is air in tubing and system. This should stop after a few minutes unless other sources of air are entering system. If bubbling continues, check connections and locate source of air leak as described in Table 14-4.

> **SAFE PATIENT CARE** Stripping the chest tube is controversial and generally not recommended because it greatly increases negative pressure within the tube, causing lung injury. Also, milking of a chest tube by squeezing and releasing one hand at a time is sometimes performed on tubes with high volumes of bloody drainage but is discouraged. (Crawford, 2011; Kane et al., 2013).

---

18. *Assist in chest tube removal:*

a. Administer prescribed medication for pain relief about 30 minutes before procedure (Kane et al., 2013).

b. Assist patient with sitting on edge of bed or lying on side without chest tubes.

c. Health care provider prepares an occlusive dressing of petroleum gauze on a pressure dressing and sets it aside on a sterile field. Sutures are removed.

d. Health care provider asks patient to take a deep breath and hold it or exhale completely and hold it.

e. Health care provider holds prepared dressing at point of tube insertion and quickly pulls out chest tube (Kane et al., 2013).

f. Health care provider quickly and firmly secures dressing in position with elastic bandage (Elastoplast) or wide tape. Health care provider sometimes uses skin clips or draws purse-string sutures together before applying dressing.

19. See Completion Protocol (inside front cover).

Rationale:

Reduces discomfort and relaxes patient by allowing time for medication to take effect.

Health care provider prescribes patient's position to facilitate tube removal.

Essential to prepare in advance for quick application to wound during tube withdrawal.

Prevents air from being sucked into chest as tube is removed.

Prevents entry of air through chest wound.

Keeps wound aseptic. Prevents entry of air into chest. Wound closure occurs spontaneously. Clips or sutures aid in skin closure (Kane et al., 2013).

TABLE 14-4	PROBLEM SOLVING WITH CHEST TUBES
ASSESSMENT	**INTERVENTION**
1. Air leak can occur at insertion site, connection between tube and drainage device, or within drainage device itself. Continuous bubbling is noted in water-seal chamber that is attached to suction (Briggs, 2010). If a water-seal unit is not attached to suction, a total absence of bubbling and drainage would indicate a leak.	Locate leak by quickly clamping tube at different intervals. Leaks are corrected when constant bubbling stops.
2. Assess for location of leak by clamping chest tube with two rubber-shod or toothless clamps close to the chest wall. If bubbling stops, air leak is inside patient's thorax or at chest insertion site.	Unclamp tube, reinforce chest dressing, and notify health care provider immediately. *Rationale:* Leaving chest tube clamped can cause collapse of lung, mediastinal shift, and eventual collapse of other lung from buildup of air pressure within the pleural cavity (Crawford, 2011).
3. If bubbling continues with clamps near the chest wall, gradually move one clamp at a time down drainage tubing away from patient and toward suction control chamber. When bubbling stops, leak is in section of tubing or connection between clamps (Kane et al., 2013).	Replace tubing, or secure connection and release clamps.
4. If bubbling still continues, this indicates that leak is in the drainage system.	Change the drainage system.
5. Assess for tension pneumothorax: • Severe respiratory distress • Low oxygen saturation • Chest pain • Absence of breath sounds on affected side • Tracheal shift toward unaffected side • Hypotension and signs of shock • Tachycardia	Ensure that chest tubes are patent: remove clamps, eliminate kinks, or eliminate occlusion. Notify health care provider and rapid response team immediately and prepare for another chest tube insertion. You may use a flutter (Heimlich) valve or large-gauge needle for short-term emergency release of pressure in the intrapleural space. Have emergency equipment, oxygen, and code cart available because condition is life-threatening (Briggs, 2010).
6. Water-seal tube is no longer submerged in sterile fluid because of evaporation.	Add sterile water to water-seal chamber until distal tip is 2 cm (1 inch) under surface level.

▌EVALUATION

1. Assess patient for decreased respiratory distress.
2. Auscultate patient's lungs and observe chest expansion.
3. Monitor vital signs, hematocrit, hemoglobin level, and oxygen saturation.
4. Evaluate patient's ability to use deep-breathing exercises while maintaining comfort.
5. Reassess patient level of comfort (on a scale of 0 to 10), comparing level with comfort before chest tube insertion.
6. Monitor continued functioning of system as indicated by reduction in the amount of drainage, resolution of the air leak, and complete reexpansion of the lung (Kane et al., 2013).
7. Use **Teach Back:** State to the patient, "I want to make sure that I explained how important it is to deep breathe. Can you explain to me how deep breaths help? Then show me a deep breath." Evaluates what the patient is able to explain or demonstrate. Revise your instruction now or develop plan for revised patient teaching to be implemented at an appropriate time if patient is not able to teach back correctly.

Unexpected Outcomes and Related Interventions

1. Air leak is unrelated to patient's respiration.
   a. See Table 14-4 for determining the source of an air leak and problem solving.
2. Chest tubes become obstructed by a clot or kinked tube.
   a. Observe patient for mediastinal shift or respiratory distress, which may constitute a medical emergency.
   b. Determine source of obstruction, as noted by lack of flow through tube or clot detected in system. If kinked, reposition patient, and straighten tubing and adjust to prevent continued problems.
   c. If clot is identified, notify health care provider.
3. Chest tube becomes dislodged.
   a. Immediately apply pressure over chest tube site with anything that is within immediate reach (e.g., several layers of patient's hospital gown, bed sheet, towel, gauze dressings).
   b. Have assistant obtain a sterile petroleum dressing. Apply as patient exhales. Secure dressing with a tight seal.
   c. Notify health care provider and remain with patient.

4. Substantial increase in bright red drainage is observed.
   a. Observe for tachycardia and hypotension.
   b. Report to health care provider because this may indicate that patient is actively bleeding.

Recording and Reporting

- Record respiratory assessment; amount of suction, if used; amount of drainage since the previous assessment; type of drainage in chest tubing; and presence or absence of an air leak, including amount if present.
- Record integrity of dressing and presence of drainage on dressing.
- Record patient comfort and tolerance.
- Document your evaluation of patient learning.

Sample Documentation

0800   Resting comfortably, denies complaint after chest tube insertion. Patient was unable to verbalize understanding of deep breathing. After further education, patient was able to demonstrate a deep breath. Respirations regular in rate, rhythm, and depth at 16 breaths/min. Lungs generally clear with breath sounds heard over right and left upper lung fields. Left posterior lung sounds diminished. Left posterior chest tube and dressing intact with tidaling present in water-seal chamber. No air leak noted. 50 mL serous drainage collected in past 8 hours. Patient taking deep breaths as instructed without complaints of discomfort.

▊ CRITICAL THINKING EXERCISES

Case Study

A newly admitted patient has a 25-year history of smoking. He had a recent fall and while in the emergency department he had a right chest tube placed for a pneumothorax. He is now on the orthopedic floor for a fractured right femur. He is receiving oxygen via a nasal cannula with the oxygen regulator set at 2 L/min. The chest tube with a three-chamber system is set on suction at 20 cm. Bubbling is noted during expiration.

1. The nurse performs a respiratory assessment on this patient, who is complaining of shortness of breath. Which of the following are appropriate when assessing respiratory status? Select all that apply.
   1. Inspect the patient for rate, rhythm, and depth of breathing.
   2. Auscultate posterior lung sounds while he is flat.
   3. Obtain a pulse oximeter reading to assess oxygenation.
   4. Evaluate the chest tube for bubbling.
2. The nurse caring for this patient assesses that he is becoming anxious and has a decreased level of consciousness. What actions should the nurse take based on this information? Select all that apply.
   1. Apply nasal cannula at 6 L/min
   2. Notify health care provider
   3. Apply nonrebreathing mask at 15 L/min
   4. Apply partial rebreathing mask at 6 L/min
   5. Ask the NAP to stay with the patient while the nurse continues assessing other patients
3. The nurse notices that the patient's chest tube is bubbling continuously. Which of the following steps are appropriate for the nurse to complete? Select all that apply.
   1. Check to ensure that all connections are secure.
   2. Determine that no kinks are affecting the tubing from the chest tube to the drainage system.
   3. Disconnect the chest tube from the drainage tube to assess for adequate suction.
   4. Assess for location of leak by clamping chest tube with two rubber-shod or toothless clamps close to the chest wall.

Review Questions

1. You are acting as preceptor to a student nurse in the intensive care unit. The student is caring for a patient who has an ETT. You discuss the assessment needs for this patient related to the ETT. You know that further teaching is needed when the student:
   1. Observes the lips and oral tissue for any breakdown from the position of the ETT.
   2. Assesses the level of the ETT at the lip or gum line based on the markings on the tube.
   3. Determines the patient's level of consciousness by asking the patient to blink for a "yes" response.
   4. Assesses for proper cuff inflation.
2. Which activities could a nurse delegate to nursing assistive personnel (NAP)? Select all that apply.
   1. Suctioning an ETT
   2. Tracheostomy care for a chronically ill patient on humidified oxygen
   3. Application of functioning nasal cannula
   4. Tracheostomy care on an acutely ill mechanically ventilated patient
3. Patients are unable to speak when they have an ETT. What are some recommended ways to communicate with these patients? Select all that apply.
   1. Talk to patients as if they have a hearing loss by speaking very loudly.
   2. Leave a pen and paper within reach of the patient so that he or she can write comments to health care providers and family members.
   3. Provide an alphabet board for family and friends to communicate with the patient.
   4. Ask family members to explain the plan of care to the patient.

4. Several of your assigned patients are on oxygen therapy. Which of the following is *not* an oxygen safety guideline?
   1. Place a sign on the patient's door that reads "Oxygen in use" to inform visitors and other health care providers.
   2. Be sure to store oxygen cylinders upright to prevent them from falling over.
   3. Maintain the oxygen rate at the prescribed rate.
   4. If a visitor asks if he can smoke in the room, state that he must stay at least 6 feet away from the patient.

5. VAP is a hospital-acquired illness that nurses can help prevent based on evidence-based interventions. Which of the following interventions do not decrease the risk of VAP? Select all that apply.
   1. Maintaining internal cuff pressures at 50 cm H_2O
   2. Elevating the head of the bed at 30 to 45 degrees to prevent aspiration
   3. Practicing good hand hygiene
   4. Providing oral care with a toothette daily to remove dental plaque organisms
   5. Limiting patient mobility to promote rest and conserve oxygen
   6. Providing daily sedation interruptions to assess readiness to extubate.

6. A patient has a nasal cannula that is causing irritation to her nares and ears. What interventions should be completed to provide comfort for this patient before replacing the device? Select all that apply.
   1. Cleanse the nares of any secretions with mild soap and water.
   2. Thoroughly dry the area around the nares.
   3. Consider adding humidification.
   4. Apply alcohol to tops of the ears and allow to dry.

7. A patient has been diagnosed with OSA. The nurse can determine that he understands the importance of wearing the CPAP machine at night because the patient states:
   1. "I can take the machine off after getting a couple of hours of sleep each night."
   2. "I only need to wear this machine for a couple of weeks and then the problem will be better."
   3. "I will use the machine every night when I go to bed and leave it in place so I will feel more rested in the mornings."
   4. "If I feel like I am suffocating in this machine, I will not use it any longer."

8. A 10-year-old asthmatic patient is using the PEFR measure for the first time. What is the proper sequence of steps the nurse needs to explain to the patient?
   a. Slide clean mouthpiece into base of the numbered scale.
   b. Have patient place meter mouthpiece in mouth and close lips, making a firm seal.
   c. Instruct patient regarding his or her individualized acceptable range and mark on meter.
   d. Determine patient's PEFR and compare with his or her personal best.
   e. Have patient blow out as hard and fast as possible through mouth only.
   f. Assist patient to high-Fowler's position, which promotes optimum lung expansion.
   g. Assess patient's baseline knowledge of when and how to use PEFR and correct response to results.
   h. Instruct patient to take a deep breath through nose and slowly blow out through mouth. Take second deep breath.
   1. a, h, d, f, g, c, b, e
   2. d, g, f, h, a, b, e, c
   3. c, f, a, d, b, e, h, g
   4. f, g, a, h, b, e, c, d

9. Which of the following assessment findings should the nurse document after CPT is complete?
   1. Frequency and duration of ambulation
   2. Color, amount, and consistency of sputum
   3. Need for an antibiotic
   4. The oxygen flow rate

10. An understanding of general preparation for suctioning of all types is necessary for the nurse. Place the following steps for ETT suctioning in the correct sequence.
    a. Connect one end of connecting tubing to suction machine or port.
    b. Fill basin or cup with approximately 100 mL of sterile water or normal saline.
    c. Open suction kit or catheter using aseptic technique.
    d. Set regulator to appropriate negative pressure.
    e. Check that suction is functioning properly by suctioning a small amount of water or saline from basin.
    1. a, b, c, d, e
    2. b, d, a, e, c
    3. c, e, a, d, b
    4. c, b, a, e, d

REFERENCES

American Association for Respiratory Care (AARC): AARC Clinical Practice Guidelines. Endotracheal suctioning of mechanically ventilated patients with artificial airways: 2010, *Respir Care* 55(6):758, 2010.

American Association for Respiratory Care (AARC), Restrepo RD, Walsh BK: Humidification during invasive and noninvasive mechanical ventilation: 2012, *Respir Care* 57(5):782, 2012.

American Thoracic Society (ATS): Home oxygen use, 2012. http://www.thoracic.org.clinical/copd-guideline/for-healthprofessionals/management-of-stable-copd/long-term-oxygen-therapy.home-oxygen-therapy.php. Accessed November 13, 2013.

Bailey P: Continuous oxygen delivery systems for infants, children, and adults, 2013. http://www.uptodate.com/contents/continuous-oxygen-delivery-systems-for-infants-children-and-adults. Accessed June 27, 2014.

Briggs D: Nursing care and management of patients with interpleural drains, *Nurs Stand* 24(21):47, 2010.

Callahan K, et al: Peak flow monitoring in pediatric asthma management: a clinical practice column submission, *J Pediatr Nurs* 25(1):12, 2010.

Campbell M: Dyspnea, *Adv Crit Care* 22(3):257, 2011.

Carlucci M, et al: Poor sleep, hazardous breathing: an overview of obstructive sleep apnea, *Nurs Pract* 38(3):20, 2013.

Centers for Disease Control and Prevention (CDC): Precautions to prevent the spread of MRSA in healthcare settings, 2013. http://www.cdc.gov/mrsa/index.html. Accessed June 27, 2014.

Crawford D: Care and nursing management of a child with a chest drain, *Nurs Child Young People* 23(10):27, 2011.

Cystic Fibrosis Foundation (CFF): An introduction to postural drainage and percussion, 2012. http://www.cff.org/UploadedFiles/treatments/Therapies/Respiratory/PosturalDrainage/An-Introduction-to-Postural-Drainage-and-Pecussion-03-2012.pdf. Accessed June 27, 2014.

Durai R, et al: Managing a chest tube and drainage system, *Nurs Stand* 91(2):275, 2010.

Freeman S: Care of adult patients with a temporary tracheostomy, *Nurs Stand* 26(20):49, 2011.

Grossbach I, et al: Promoting effective communication for patients receiving mechanical ventilation, *Crit Care Nurs* 31(3):46, 2011.

Hockenberry MJ, Wilson D: *Wong's essentials of pediatric nursing*, ed 9, St Louis, 2013, Mosby.

Ignatavicius D, Workman ML: *Medical-surgical nursing: patient centered collaborative care*, ed 7, St Louis, 2013, Saunders.

Kane C, et al: Chest tubes in the critically ill patient, *Dimens Crit Care Nurs* 32(3):112, 2013.

Khalaila R, et al: Communication difficulties and psychoemotional distress in patients receiving mechanical ventilation, *Am J Crit Care* 20(6):470, 2011.

Lehne RA: *Pharmacology for nursing care*, ed 8, St Louis, 2013, Saunders.

Lewis SL, et al: *Medical surgical nursing, assessment and management of clinical problems*, ed 9, St Louis, 2014, Mosby.

Lynn-McHale Weigand DJ: *AACN procedure manual for critical care*, ed 6, St Louis, 2011, Saunders.

McGrath B, et al: Multidisciplinary guidelines for the management of tracheostomy and laryngectomy airway emergencies, *Anesthesia* 67(9):1025, 2012.

Morris LL, Whitmer A, McIntosh E: Tracheostomy care and complications in the intensive care unit, *Crit Care Nurse* 33(5):18, 2013.

National Institutes of Health (NIH): *National Asthma Control Initiative*, 2010. http://www.nhlbi.nih.gov/health/prof/lung/asthma/naci/pubs/naci-factsheet.pdf. Accessed June 27, 2014.

Ozden D, Gorgulu S: Development of standard of practice guidelines for open and closed system suctioning, *J Clin Nurs* 21(9–10):1327, 2012.

Pagana K, Pagana T: *Mosby's diagnostic and laboratory test reference*, ed 11, St Louis, 2013, Mosby.

Prendergast V, et al: The bedside oral exam and the Barrow oral care protocol: translating evidence-based oral care into practice, *Intensive Crit Care Nurs* 29(5):282, 2013.

Restrepo RD, et al: Incentive spirometry: 2011, *Respir Care* 56(10):1600, 2011.

Scherzer R: Subglottic secretion aspiration in the prevention of ventilator-associated pneumonia, *Dimens Crit Care Nurs* 29(6):276, 2010.

Sedwick M, et al: Using evidence-based practice to prevent ventilator-associated pneumonia, *Crit Care Nurse* 32(4):41, 2012.

Simmons S, Pruitt B: Sounding the alarm for patients with obstructive sleep apnea, *Nursing* 42(4):34, 2012.

Sole M, et al: Oropharyngeal secretion volume in intubated patients: the importance of oral suctioning, *Am J Crit Care* 20(6):e141, 2011.

Speroni K, et al: Comparative effectiveness of standard endotracheal tubes vs. endotracheal tubes with continuous subglottic suctioning on ventilator-associated pneumonia rates, *Nurs Econ* 29(1):15, 2011.

The Joint Commission (TJC): *National Patient Safety Goals*, Oakbrook Terrace, IL, 2014, The Commission. Available at: http://www.jointcommission.org/standards_information/npsgs.aspx. Accessed June 27, 2014.

Touhy TA, Jett K: *Ebersole & Hess' gerontological nursing and healthy aging*, ed 4, St Louis, 2013, Elsevier.

Walsh BK, et al: Capnography/capnometry during mechanical ventilation: 2011, *Respir Care* 56(4):503, 2011.

White AC, et al: When to change a tracheostomy tube, *Respir Care* 55(8):1069, 2010.

Zaratkiewicz S, et al: Retrospective review of the reduction of oral pressure ulcers in mechanically ventilated patients: a change in practice, *Crit Care Nurs Q* 35(3):247, 2012.

Zurmehly J: Oral care education in the prevention of ventilator-associated pneumonia: quality patient outcomes in the intensive care unit, *J Contin Educ Nurs* 44(2):67, 2013.

Safe Patient Handling, Transfer, and Positioning

 **EVOLVE WEBSITE/EVOLVE RESOURCES LIST**

http://evolve.elsevier.com/Perry/nursinginterventions
Audio Glossary • Checklists • Review Questions

Rates of musculoskeletal injuries in health care occupations are among the highest of all U.S. industries. Data show that in 2012, the rate of overexertion injuries averaged across all industries was 112 per 10,000 full-time workers. By comparison, the overexertion injury rate for hospital workers accounted for 25% of all injuries (BLS, 2012). The greatest risk factor for overexertion injuries in health care workers is the manual lifting, moving, and repositioning of patients. Most of the patient handling that occurs in health care settings is performed by nurses and support staff. More recent data show that within the health care industry, workers in these occupations suffered the most lost-time cases of general musculoskeletal pain and back pain (13,000) (BLS, 2012). The rising obesity rates in the United States contribute to the problem by increasing the physical demands on caregivers (Flegal et al., 2010).

To date, no federal safe patient handling law has yet been enacted. The most recently introduced federal bill is the Nurse and Health Care Worker Protection Act of 2013 (H.R. 2480). However, health care providers are required to provide employees with safety information and training to use when transferring, positioning, and lifting patients. Injuries are not only related to lifting. Nurses spend time in many activities involving bending and twisting that also can cause injury. Examples of such activities include lifting and carrying supplies and equipment and pushing and pulling equipment (Waters et al., 2011b, 2011c).

If you need help, assess if a second person is adequate or if you need mechanical assistance. Once you determine the amount of assistance needed, use the following steps for proper body mechanics:
- Keep the weight (patient) to be lifted as close to the body as possible; this action places the weight in the same plane as the lifter and close to the center of gravity for balance.
- Bend at the knees to help maintain your center of gravity. Let the strong muscles of the legs do the lifting.
- Avoid twisting. Twisting your spine can lead to serious injury.
- Before lifting, tighten stomach muscles and tuck the pelvis to provide balance and protect the back.
- Maintain the trunk erect and knees bent so that multiple muscle groups work together in a synchronized manner.
- The best height for lifting vertically is approximately 2 feet off the ground and close to the lifter's center of gravity.

Body mechanics are the coordinated effort of the musculoskeletal and nervous systems to maintain balance, posture, and body alignment during lifting, bending, moving, and performing activities of daily living (ADLs). Body mechanics also facilitate body movement so that a person can carry out a physical activity without using excessive muscle energy.

PATIENT-CENTERED CARE

Ultimately it is the patients' choice to increase their mobility and activity level. When developing a plan of care, consider the patient's knowledge, cultural beliefs, and circumstances surrounding the loss of independent activity. Care planned with the patient motivates and encourages the patient to participate. For example, taking a few minutes to assess a patient's knowledge and providing information about the complications of immobility may be all that is needed to elicit their cooperation in ambulating after surgery. It is also important to assess the patient's cultural and ethnic beliefs to incorporate appropriate interventions that match individual beliefs. For instance, some patients have a fear of becoming addicted to a narcotic (opioid) after one dose. Pain prevents them from increasing their mobility. Knowing that the patient has a fear of opioids, individualize the plan of care and explain the safe and proper use of opioids for pain control. In addition, taking into consideration the circumstances surrounding the loss of independent activity and mobility is crucial in developing a plan of care that is realistic and attainable. Consider the example of a patient who has recently undergone surgery and who is expected to ambulate a prescribed number of feet on the second postoperative day. The nurse knows that this patient has a long history of pulmonary disease. This information prompts the nurse to alter the patient's plan of care based on this activity limitation to achieve a reasonable level of mobility and activity.

SAFETY

Professional standards and guidelines, such as those from the American Nurses Association (2013a, 2013b), U.S. Department of Health and Human Resources (2010), and Quality and Safety Education for Nurses (Sherwood and Barnsteiner, 2012), concerning the use of assistive equipment and devices to transfer and position patients safely, provide valuable information for the safety of you and your patient. In addition, these standards help you promote the patient's independence while safely adhering to the prescribed rehabilitation plan.

To ensure patient safety, communicate clearly with members of the health care team, assess and incorporate the patient's priorities of care and preferences, and use the best evidence when making decisions about your patient's care. When performing the skills in this chapter, remember the following points to ensure safe, individualized patient care:

- Mentally review the transfer steps before beginning to ensure both the patient's safety and your safety.
- Assess the patient's mobility and strength to determine the assistance he or she is able to offer during transfer. Stand on the patient's weak side when assisting (Pierson and Fairchild, 2013).
- Determine the amount and type of assistance you require. This includes determining the type of transfer equipment and the number of personnel it will take to transfer the patient safely and prevent harm to the patient and yourself.
- Explain the procedure, and describe what you expect of the patient.

- Raise the side rail on the side of the bed opposite of where you are standing to prevent the patient from falling out of bed on that side.
- Position the level of the bed to a comfortable and safe height.
- Arrange equipment (e.g., intravenous lines, feeding tube, Foley catheter) so that it will not interfere with the transfer.
- Evaluate the patient for correct body alignment and pressure areas after the transfer.

Some patients are at higher risk for complications from improper positioning and have increased risk of injury during transfer. Patients with alterations in bone formation or joint mobility, impaired muscle development, and central nervous system (CNS) damage may experience motor impairment, proprioceptive loss, or cognitive dysfunction, all of which affect mobility. The application of proper body mechanics, alignment, and the use of transfer and positioning techniques assist the patient in achieving an optimal level of independence without resultant injury to the health care provider.

EVIDENCE-BASED PRACTICE

Krill C, Staffileno BA, Raven C: Empowering staff nurses to use research to change practice for safe patient handling, *Nurs Outlook* 60(3):152, 2012.

Occupational Health and Safety Administration (OSHA): *Technical manual,* revised August 16, 2010, http://www.osha.gov/dts/osta/otm/otm_toc.html. Accessed March 20, 2014.

Pelczarski KM: Back in action, *Health Facil Manage* 25(8):21, 2012.

Waters T et al: AORN ergonomic tool 2: positioning and repositioning the supine patient on the OR bed, *AORN J* 93(4):445,2011a.

Waters T et al: AORN ergonomic tool 6: lifting and carrying supplies and equipment in the perioperative setting, *AORN J* 94(2):173, 2011b.

Waters T et al: AORN ergonomic tool 7: pushing, pulling, and moving equipment on wheels, *AORN J* 93(3):254, 2011c.

Using principles of body mechanics during routine activities helps to prevent injury. However, body mechanics alone are insufficient to prevent musculoskeletal injuries when positioning or transferring patients. Teaching the use of patient-handling equipment in combination with proper body mechanics is more effective than either one in isolation (Krill, et al., 2012; Pelczarski, 2012; Waters et al., 2011a).

The U.S. National Institute of Occupational Safety and Health Administration released federal ergonomic guidelines to prevent musculoskeletal injuries in the workplace (OSHA, 2010). Half of all back pain is associated with manual lifting tasks. The most common back injury is strain on the lumbar muscle group, which includes the muscles around the lumbar vertebrae. Injury to these areas affects the ability to bend forward, backward, and from side to side. The ability to rotate the hips and lower back is also decreased. Manual lifting is the last resort, and it is used only when it does not involve lifting most or all of the patient's weight (Pelczarski, 2012;

Waters et al., 2011a, 2011b, 2011c). Before lifting, assess the weight to be lifted and determine the assistance needed and the resources available. Use safe patient-handling equipment in conjunction with facility lift teams to reduce the risk of injury to the patient and members of the health care team.

- Use patient-handling equipment and devices, such as height-adjustable beds, ceiling-mounted lifts, friction-reducing slide sheets, and air-assisted devices.

- Perform manual lifting as a last resort and only if it does not involve lifting most or all of a patient's weight.
- Slide patient toward yourself using a pull sheet or slide board. When transferring a patient onto a stretcher or bed, a slide board is more appropriate.

SKILL 15.1 TRANSFER TECHNIQUES

• Nursing Skills Online: Safety Module, Lesson 3

Transferring is a nursing skill that helps a dependent patient or a patient with restricted mobility attain positions to regain optimal independence as quickly and safely as possible. Physical activity maintains and improves joint motion, increases strength, promotes circulation, relieves pressure on skin, and improves urinary and respiratory functions. It also benefits the patient psychologically by increasing social activity and mental stimulation and providing a change in environment (Huether and McCance, 2012). Mobilization plays a crucial role in the patient's rehabilitation.

A major concern during transfer is the safety of the patient and the nurse. The nurse prevents self-injury by using correct posture, minimal muscle strength, and effective body mechanics and lifting techniques. You must consider any special problems during a patient's transfer to avoid injury such as in a fall. For example, a patient who has been immobile for several days or longer may be weak or dizzy or may develop orthostatic hypotension (a decrease in blood pressure) when transferred (Freeman et al., 2011). As a rule of thumb, if there is any doubt about safe transfer, use a transfer belt and obtain assistance when transferring patients.

ASSESSMENT

1. Review medical records to assess physiological capacity of a patient to transfer and need for special adaptive techniques. Assess the following:
   a. Muscle strength (legs and upper arms). *Rationale: Immobile patients have decreased muscle strength, tone, and mass, which affects the ability to bear weight or raise the body.*
   b. Joint mobility and contracture formation. *Rationale: Immobility or inflammatory processes (e.g., arthritis) may lead to contracture formation and impaired joint mobility.*
   c. Paralysis or paresis (spastic or flaccid). *Rationale: Patient with CNS damage may have bilateral paralysis (requiring transfer by swivel bar, sliding bar, or mechanical lift) or unilateral paralysis, which requires belt transfer to strong side. Weakness (paresis) requires stabilization of knee while transferring. Support flaccid arm with sling during transfer.*

   d. Bone continuity. *Rationale: Patients with trauma to one leg or hip may be non–weight-bearing during a transfer. Amputees may use slide board to transfer.*
2. Assess for presence of weakness, dizziness, or orthostatic (postural) hypotension. *Rationale: Determines patient's risk of fainting or falling during transfer. The move from a supine to a vertical position redistributes about 500 mL of blood; immobile patients may have decreased ability for autonomic nervous system to equalize blood supply, resulting in orthostatic hypotension (Lagro et al., 2012).*
3. Assess activity level by noting level of fatigue during activity and measuring vital signs. *Rationale: Estimates patient's ability to participate in transfer. Vital sign changes, such as increased pulse and respiration, may indicate activity intolerance (see Chapter 6).*
4. Assess patient's proprioceptive function (awareness of posture and changes in equilibrium), including ability to maintain balance while sitting in bed or on side of bed and tendency to sway or position self to one side. *Rationale: Determines stability of patient's balance for transfer and risk of falling.*
5. Assess sensory status, including central and peripheral vision, adequacy of hearing, and presence of peripheral sensation loss. *Rationale: Determines influence of sensory loss on ability to make transfer. Visual field loss decreases patient's ability to see in direction of transfer. Peripheral sensation loss decreases proprioception. Patients with visual and hearing losses need transfer techniques adapted to their deficits.*

SAFE PATIENT CARE Patients with hemiplegia may "neglect" one side of the body (inattention to or unawareness of one side of the body or environment), which distorts perceptions of the visual field.

6. Assess patient for pain (e.g., joint discomfort, muscle spasm) and measure level of pain using a scale from 0 to 10. Offer prescribed analgesic 30 minutes before transfer. *Rationale: Pain reduces patient's motivation and ability to be mobile. Pain relief before transfer enhances patient participation (Christo et al., 2011).*
7. Assess patient's cognitive status, including ability to follow verbal instructions, short-term memory,

and recognition of physical deficits and limitations to movement. *Rationale: Determines patient's ability to follow directions and learn transfer techniques.*

> **SAFE PATIENT CARE** Patients with head trauma or cerebrovascular accident (CVA) may have perceptual cognitive deficits that create safety risks. If the patient has difficulty in comprehension, simplify instructions by providing one step at a time, and maintain consistency.

8. Assess patient's level of motivation such as eagerness versus unwillingness to be mobile. *Rationale: Altered psychological states reduce patient's desire to engage in activity.*

9. Assess patient's specific risk for falling or being injured when transferred (e.g., neuromuscular deficits, visual loss, motor weakness, fear of falling, or calcium loss from long bones). *Rationale: Increases patient's risk of falling and incurring injury.*

10. Assess special transfer equipment needed for home setting and previous mode of transfer (if applicable). *Rationale: Prior teaching to family and support people and determination of previous modes of transfer and assistance facilitate continuity of care when transitioning between care settings.*

PLANNING

Expected Outcomes focus on maintaining body alignment and achieving safe transfer without injury.

1. Patient dangles legs or sits without dizziness, weakness, or orthostatic hypotension.
2. Patient transfers with minimal or no assistance.
3. Patient transfers without injury.
4. Patient tolerates increased activity.
5. Patient can bear more weight with increased endurance.
6. Patient is more motivated to be mobile.

Delegation and Collaboration

The skill of transfer techniques can be delegated to nursing assistive personnel (NAP). Patients whom you are transferring for the first time after prolonged bed rest, extensive surgery, critical illness, or spinal cord traumas require supervision by professional nurses. Before delegation, the nurse instructs the NAP about:

- Seeking assistance when moving or lifting a patient (e.g., overweight patient, confused patient).
- Patient limitations (e.g., changes in blood pressure, mobility restrictions) that impact transfer techniques.

Equipment

- Transfer belt, sling, or lap board (as needed)
- Nonskid shoes, pillow, bath blanket
- Slide board (friction-reducing board)
- Stretcher
- *Option:* Mechanical/hydraulic lift, stand-assist lift device
- Chair with arms or wheelchair

IMPLEMENTATION *for* TRANSFER TECHNIQUES

STEPS	RATIONALE
1. **See Standard Protocol (inside front cover).**	
2. *Assist patient to sitting position on side of bed.*	Reduces the risk of developing hypotension before transfer.
a. With bed flat at waist level, turn patient onto side facing you on side of bed on which patient will be sitting.	Prepares patient to move to side of bed and protects from falling.
b. With patient in supine position, raise head of bed 30 degrees and place bed in low position.	Decreases amount of work needed by patient and nurse to raise patient to sitting position. Low bed position prevents fall while sitting.
c. Stand opposite patient's hips. Turn diagonally to face patient and far corner of foot of bed.	Places nurse's center of gravity nearer patient. Reduces twisting of nurse's body because nurse is facing direction of movement.
d. Place feet apart in a wide base of support with foot closer to head of bed in front of other foot (see illustration).	Increases balance and allows nurse to transfer weight as patient is brought to sitting position on side of bed.
e. Place arm nearer head of bed under patient's shoulders, supporting head and neck.	Maintains alignment of head and neck as nurse brings patient to sitting position.
f. Place other arm over and around patient's thighs (see illustration).	Supports hip and prevents patient from falling backward during procedure.
g. Move patient's lower legs and feet over side of bed. Pivot toward rear leg, allowing patient's upper legs to swing downward (see illustration). At same time, shift weight to rear leg and elevate patient.	Weight of patient's legs when off bed allows gravity to lower legs, and weight of legs assists in pulling upper body into sitting position. Allows nurse to transfer weight in direction of motion.

STEPS	RATIONALE

3. *Transferring patient from bed to chair:*
   a. Determine if patient can bear weight.

   (1) Full weight bearing, nurse assistance not needed: Nurse stands by to assist.

   (2) Partial weight bearing and patient is cooperative: Use the bariatric transfer or pivot techniques that follow.

Determines degree of risk during transfer and technique required to assist patient safely.

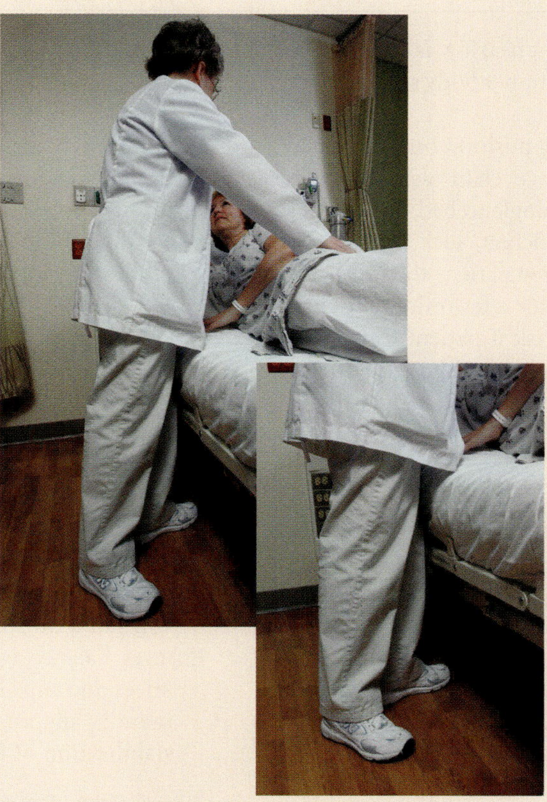

STEP 2d Proper foot placement.

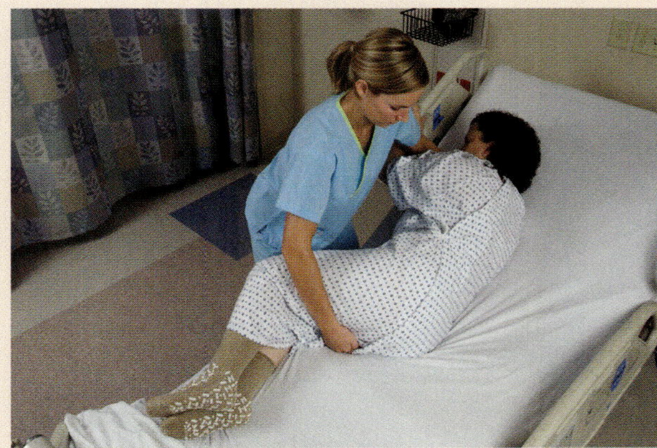

STEP 2f Nurse places arm over patient's thighs.

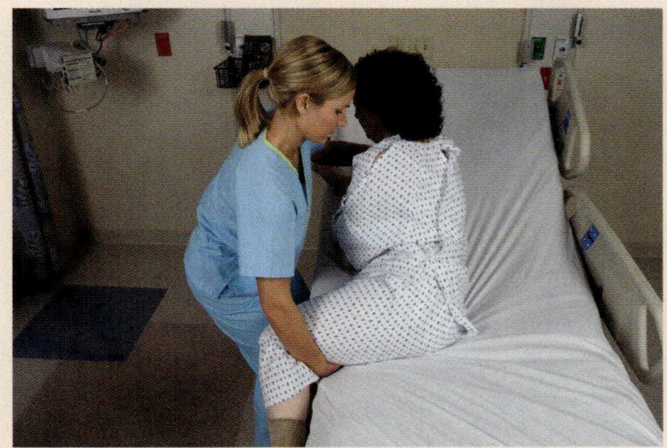

STEP 2g Nurse shifts weight to rear leg and elevates patient.

Continued

STEPS	RATIONALE

b. If patient has partial weight bearing with upper body strength and caregiver must lift more than 15.9 kg (35 pounds) of patient's weight, use a bariatric transfer aid with minimum of two or three caregivers (see illustration).

The use of mechanical lift devices is strongly recommended to transfer a patient to reduce risk of musculoskeletal injury (Pelczarski, 2012; Waters et al., 2011a, 2011b).

> **SAFE PATIENT CARE** If patient demonstrates weakness or paralysis of one side of the body, place chair on patient's strong side.

c. If patient has partial weight bearing, is cooperative and able to stand, and has upper body strength, use stand-and-pivot technique.

(1) Assist patient to sitting position on side of bed (see Steps 2a-2g). Place chair with arms in position at 45-degree angle to bed on patient's strong side. For wheelchair, lock brakes and remove foot rests. Allow patient to sit on side of the bed (dangling) for a few minutes before transferring to chair. Ask if patient feels dizzy. Do not leave patient unattended during dangling. Provide patient his or her glasses.

Positioning chair on patient's strong side allows for patient to assist with transfer. Dangling or allowing a patient to sit on the side of the bed before transfer helps equilibrate blood pressure, reducing the risk of dizziness or fainting when standing (Thompson et al., 2011).

(2) Apply transfer belt or other transfer aids. Patient's arm should be in sling if flaccid paralysis is present.

Transfer belt allows nurse to maintain stability of patient during transfer and reduces risk of falling (OSHA, 2011).

(3) Assist patient in applying stable nonskid shoes. Have patient place weight-bearing or strong leg forward, with weak foot back.

Nonskid soles decrease risk of slipping during transfer. Always have patient wear shoes during transfer; bare feet or wearing only socks increases risk of falls. Patient will stand on stronger, or weight-bearing, leg.

(4) Spread your feet apart, flex hips and knees, and align your knees with patient's knees (see illustration).

Ensures balance with wide base of support. Flexion of knees and hips lowers center of gravity to object to be raised; aligning knees with patients allows for stabilization of knees when patient stands.

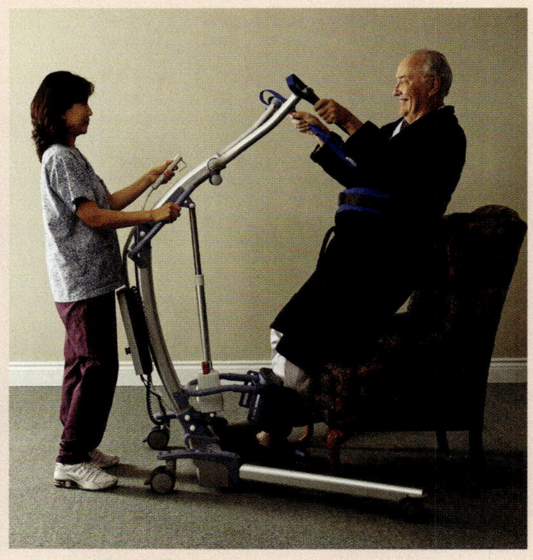

STEP 3b Stand-assist lift device.

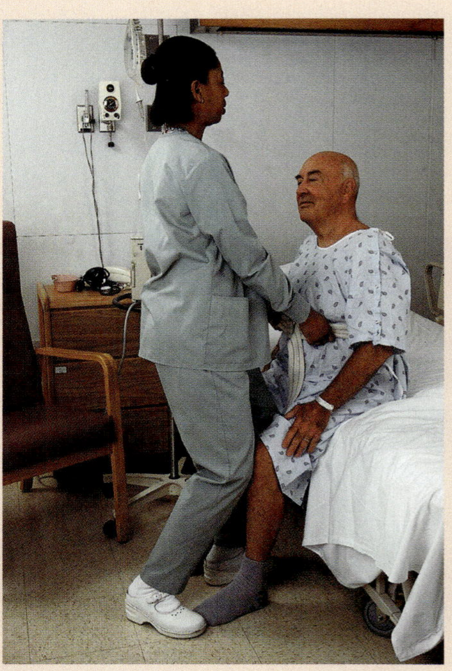

STEP 3c(4) Nurse flexes hips and knees, aligns knees with patient's knee, and grasps transfer belt.

STEPS	RATIONALE

(5) Grasp transfer belt from underneath along patient's side.

Provides movement of patient at center of gravity.

> **SAFE PATIENT CARE** Always use transfer belt. Never lift patients by or under arms. This method has been found to be physically stressful for the nurse and uncomfortable for patients (Pierson and Fairchild, 2013).

(6) Rock patient up to standing position on count of three while straightening hips and legs and keeping knees slightly flexed. Have patient push up with hands and knees (see illustration). While rocking the patient back and forth, make sure that your body weight is moving in the same direction as the patient's to ensure that you and the patient are moving in the same direction simultaneously.

Rocking motion gives patient's body momentum and requires less muscular effort to lift patient.

(7) Support the paralyzed or weak limb with your knee to stabilize the patient.

Maintains stability of patient's weak or paralyzed leg.

(8) Pivot and turn patient toward chair; pivot on your foot farther from chair. (See right foot in illustration for Step 3c(6).)

Maintains support of patient while allowing adequate space for patient to move.

(9) Instruct patient to feel back of chair against legs and to use armrests on chair for support. Have patient ease into chair (see illustration).

Increases patient stability.

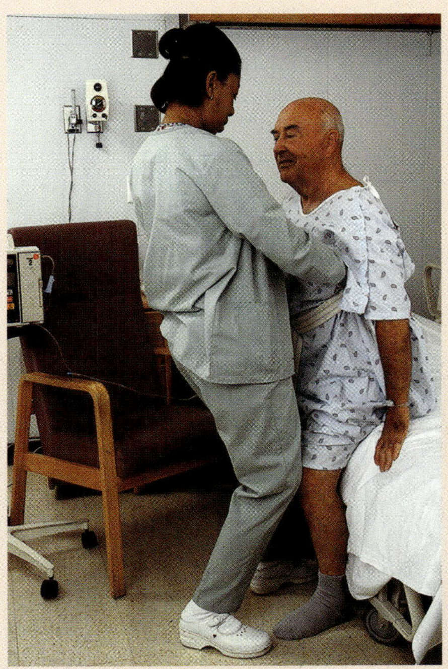

STEP 3c(6) Nurse rocks patient to standing position.

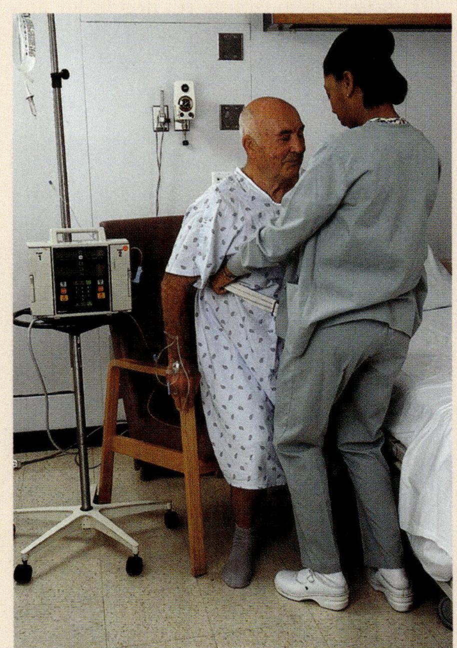

STEP 3c(9) Patient uses armrests for support.

Continued

STEPS	RATIONALE
(10) Flex hips and knees while lowering patient into chair (see illustration).	Prevents injury to nurse from poor body mechanics.
(11) Help patient shift to back of chair. Assess patient for proper alignment for sitting position. Provide support for paralyzed extremities. Support flaccid arm with lap board or sling. Stabilize leg with bath blanket or pillow.	Prevents injury to patient from poor body alignment.
(12) Proper alignment for sitting position: Head is erect, and vertebrae are in straight alignment. Body weight is evenly distributed on buttocks and thighs. Thighs are parallel and in horizontal plane. Both feet are supported on floor, and ankles are comfortably flexed. A 2.5- to 5-cm (1- to 2-inch) space is maintained between edge of seat and popliteal space on posterior surface of knee.	Prevents stress on intravertebral joints. Prevents increased pressure over bony prominences and reduces damage to underlying musculoskeletal system.
(13) Praise patient's progress, effort, and performance. Place call light in reach.	Support and encouragement provide incentive for patient perseverance. Patient needs call light to ask for assistance as needed.
4. *Perform lateral transfer from bed to stretcher using slide board or friction-reducing board* **(see illustration).**	The three-person lift for horizontal transfer from bed to stretcher is not recommended (OSHA, 2011). Physical stress can be decreased significantly by the use of a slide board or friction-reducing board. The patient is more comfortable with this method.
a. Determine if patient can assist.	Determines degree of risk during transfer and technique required to assist patient safely.
(1) Patient is able to assist by moving laterally, nurse assistance not needed; nurse stands by to assist.	
(2) Patient is partially or not at all able to move laterally; requires uses of a friction-reducing device.	

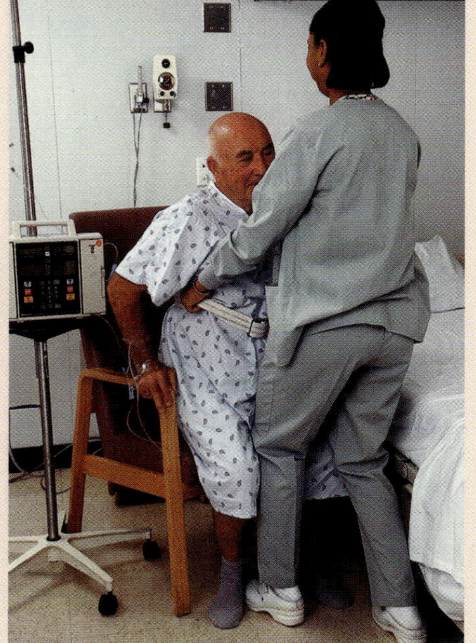

STEP 3c(10) Nurse eases patient into chair.

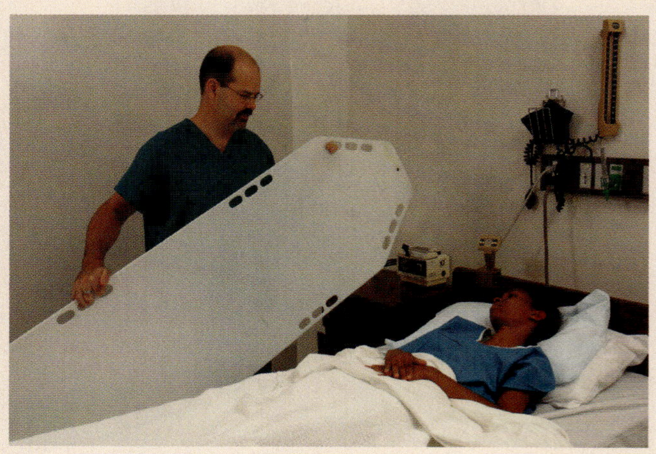

STEP 4 Slide board.

STEPS	RATIONALE

b. Determine number of staff required for safe lateral transfer of patient: patient less than 90.9 kg (200 pounds), nurse can transfer using friction-reducing device; patient more than 90.9 kg (200 pounds), use device with three caregivers.

During lateral transfer of a patient who has limited ability to assist, a caregiver should use a lift team when the patient weighs more than 90.9 kg (200 pounds). If any caregiver is required to lift more than 15.9 kg (35 pounds) of a patient's weight, the patient is considered fully dependent, and an assist device is used (OSHA, 2011).

c. Place bed at working height. Ensure that bed's wheel breaks are on. Lower head of bed as much as patient can tolerate.

Maintains alignment of spinal column.

d. Cross patient's arms on chest.

Prevents injury to arms during transfer.

e. To place slide board under patient, lower side rails and position two nurses on side of bed to which patient will be turned. Position third nurse on the other side of bed.

Reduces overstretching by caregivers and distributes weight equally among nurses.

f. Fanfold the drawsheet on both sides of patient.

Provides strong handles to grip the drawsheet without slipping.

g. On the count of three, turn patient onto side toward the two nurses. Turn patient as one unit with a smooth, continuous motion.

Maintains body in alignment, preventing stress on any part of the body.

h. Place slide board under drawsheet (see illustration).

Prevents friction from contact of skin with board.

i. Gently roll patient back onto slide board.

j. Line up stretcher with bed. Lock brakes on stretcher and bed.

Ensures that stretcher or bed does not move during transfer.

k. Two nurses position themselves on the side of the stretcher, while the third nurse positions self on the side of the bed without the stretcher.

> **SAFE PATIENT CARE** A nurse may also be positioned at the head of patient's bed to protect and support patient's head and neck if he or she is weak or unable to assist.

l. Fanfold drawsheet; on the count of three, the two nurses pull drawsheet with patient onto stretcher, while the third nurse holds slide board in place (see illustration).

The slide board remains stationary, provides a slippery surface to reduce friction, and allows patient to transfer easily to the stretcher.

m. Position patient in center of stretcher. Apply safety restraint on patient, and raise head of stretcher if not contraindicated. Raise side rails of stretcher. Cover patient with blanket or sheet.

Provides for patient comfort and safety.

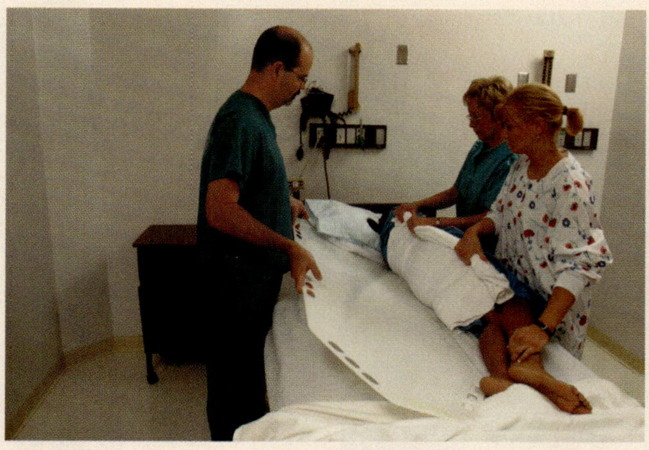

STEP 4h Placing slide board under drawsheet.

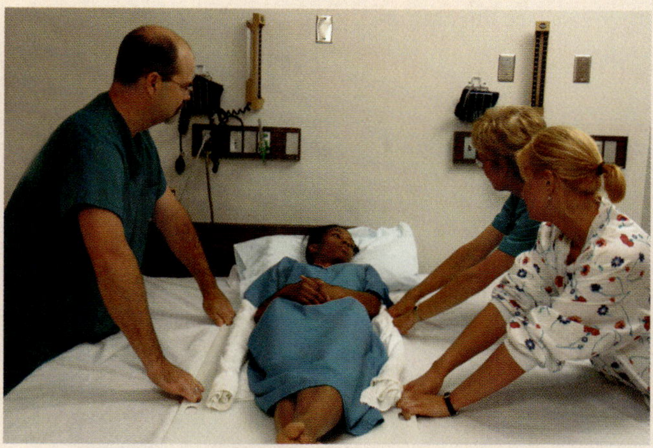

STEP 4l Transfer of patient to stretcher using slide board.

Continued

STEPS	RATIONALE
5. *Use mechanical/hydraulic lift to transfer patient from bed to chair.*	Research supports the use of mechanical lifts to prevent musculoskeletal injuries (Pelczarski, 2012; Waters et al., 2011a, 2011b). The use of ceiling-mounted lifts is becoming a more popular choice because of the availability of the lift in each patient's room.
a. Determine if patient can bear weight and is cooperative.	Determines degree of risk during transfer and technique required to assist patient.
(1) Unable to bear weight and uncooperative patient requires use of full body sling lift and two caregivers.	
b. Position lift at bedside. (Before using lift, be thoroughly familiar with its operation.)	Ensures safe elevation of patient off bed.
c. Position chair near bed and allow adequate space to maneuver lift.	Prepares environment for safe use of lift and subsequent transfer.
d. Raise bed to high position with mattress flat. Lower side rail. Have a nurse stand on each side of patient's bed. Keep side rails on opposite side of the bed in the up position.	Allows nurses to use proper body mechanics. Maintains patient safety.
e. Roll patient onto opposite side.	Positions patient for use of lift sling.
f. Place sling under patient. Place lower edge under patient's knees (wide piece) and upper edge under patient's shoulders (narrow piece). Hooks should face away from patient's skin. Place sling under patient's center of gravity and greatest portion of body weight.	Two types of seats are supplied with mechanical/hydraulic lift: Hammock style is better for patients who are flaccid, weak, and need support; canvas strips can be used for patients with normal muscle tone.
g. Roll patient to opposite side and pull body sling through.	Completes positioning of patient on mechanical/hydraulic sling.
h. Roll patient supine onto canvas seat.	Sling should extend from shoulders to knees (hammock) to support patient's body weight equally.
i. Remove patient's glasses if appropriate.	Swivel bar is close to patient's head and could break eyeglasses.
j. If using portable Hoyer lift, place horseshoe-shaped base of lift under side of bed (on side with chair).	Positions lift efficiently and promotes smooth transfer.
k. Lower horizontal bar to sling level by releasing hydraulic valve. Lock valve.	Positions hydraulic lift close to patient. Locking valve prevents injury to patient.
l. Attach hooks on strap to holes in sling. Short chains or straps hook to top holes of sling; longer chains hook to bottom of sling.	Secures hydraulic lift to sling.
m. Elevate head of bed. Fold patient's arms over chest (see illustration).	Positions patient in sitting position. Prevents injury to patient's arms.

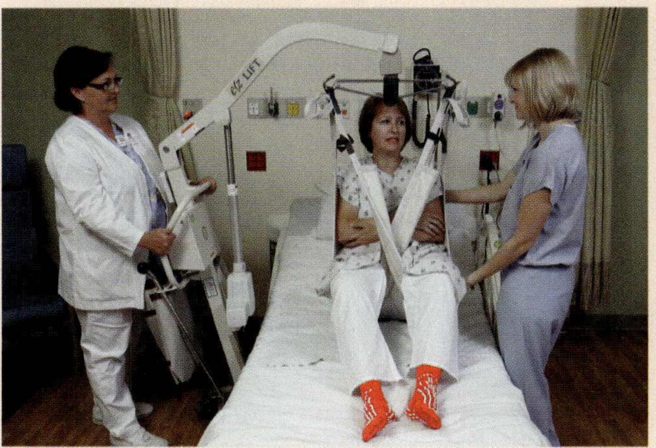

STEP 5m Patient lifted in hydraulic lift above bed.

STEPS	RATIONALE

n. Use lift to raise patient off bed and use steering handle to pull lift from bed and maneuver to chair. Have a nurse move on each side of patient.

Lifts patient off the bed. Moves patient from bed to chair. Nurses' positions reduce risk of fall from sling.

o. Roll base of lift around chair.

Positions lift in front of chair in which patient is to be transferred.

p. Release check valve slowly (turn to left), and lower patient into chair (see illustration).

Safely guides patient into back of chair as seat descends.

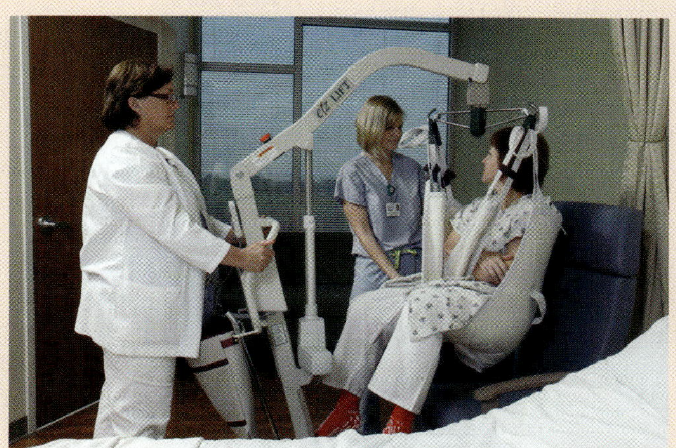

STEP 5p Use of hydraulic lift to lower patient into chair.

q. Close check valve as soon as patient is down and straps can be released.

If valve is left open, boom may continue to lower and injure patient.

r. Remove straps and mechanical/hydraulic lift.

Prevents damage to skin and underlying tissues from canvas or hooks.

s. Check patient's sitting alignment and correct if necessary.

Prevents injury from poor posture.

6. See Completion Protocol (inside front cover).

EVALUATION

1. Monitor vital signs. Ask if patient feels dizzy or fatigued.
2. Note patient's behavioral response to transfer.
3. Ask if patient experienced pain during transfer.
4. Observe patient's body alignment after transfer.
5. Use **Teach Back:** State to the patient, "I want to be sure I explained the steps we are going to use to transfer you to the chair. Can you repeat the steps back to me?" Evaluates what the patient is able to explain or demonstrate. Revise your instruction now or develop plan for revised patient teaching to be implemented at an appropriate time if patient is not able to teach back correctly.

Unexpected Outcomes and Related Interventions

1. Patient is unable to comprehend and follow directions for transfer.
   a. Reassess continuity and simplicity of instruction.
   b. Add family caregivers in transfer technique.

2. Patient sustains injury on transfer.
   a. Stay with patient and notify health care provider immediately.
   b. Provide necessary supportive care until patient is stable.
   c. Evaluate incident that caused injury (e.g., assessment inadequate, change in patient status, improper use of equipment, insufficient number of caregivers to assist).
   d. Complete occurrence report according to facility policy.
3. Patient's level of weakness does not permit active transfer (e.g., unable to stand for time required to move to chair).
   a. Increase number of nursing personnel to assist during transfer.
   b. Increase bed activity and exercise to heighten tolerance.

Recording and Reporting

- Record procedure, including pertinent observations: weakness, ability to follow directions, weight-bearing ability, balance, ability to pivot, number of personnel needed to assist, and amount of assistance (muscle strength) required.
- Document your evaluation of patient learning.

- Report transfer ability and assistance needed to next shift or other caregivers. Report progress or remission to rehabilitation staff (physical therapist, occupational therapist).

Sample Documentation

0800 Patient able to teach back transfer technique. Transferred patient from bed to chair with gait belt and assistance of one. Cooperative and able to stand erect with encouragement.

0815 Requested to return to bed. Stated, "I'm so tired; I just can't sit up any longer." Used stand-assist lift device to transfer back to bed. Vital signs remained within patient's baseline.

Special Considerations
Pediatric

- Whenever possible, transporting child by stretcher, stroller, or wheelchair outside confines of room increases environmental stimuli and provides social contact with others (Hockenberry and Wilson, 2013).

Geriatric

- A major health concern that threatens the function of the older adult is the risk of falls. Concern increases when the older adult is admitted to the hospital. Assess patient for the risk for falls on admission, and implement a protocol to prevent falls (Touhy and Jett, 2014) (see Chapter 4).

Home Care

- Assess special transfer equipment needed for home setting. Assess home environment for hazards.
- Family caregiver should practice transfer in hospital to achieve success before taking patient home. Alternatively, patient (if living alone) should practice transfer skills in bed that will be used at home. Patient should learn to transfer to chair with arms for ease of rising and sitting.
- Home should be free of hazards (e.g., throw rugs, electric cords, slippery floors). If wheelchair is used, access must be possible through all doors, and space for transfer must be available in bedroom and bathroom.

PROCEDURAL GUIDELINE 15.1
Wheelchair Transfer Techniques

Transferring a patient from a bed to a wheelchair encompasses many of the same principles discussed in Skill 15.1. The following procedural guideline focuses on the safety precautions that need to be considered when using a wheelchair. Several additional steps must be taken to maintain safety of the patient and nurse to prevent injury when transferring from or to a wheelchair (Pierson and Fairchild, 2013). Check wheelchair locks, footplates, and wheels for proper functioning before use.

Delegation and Collaboration

The skill of transferring a patient to or from a wheelchair can be delegated to nursing assistive personnel (NAP). The nurse instructs the NAP by:

- Assisting and supervising when moving patients who are transferring for the first time after prolonged bed rest, extensive surgery, critical illness, or spinal cord trauma.
- Explaining the patient's mobility restrictions, changes in blood pressure, or sensory alterations that may affect safe transfer.
- Reminding NAP to back a wheelchair into or out of an elevator to avoid tipping.

Equipment

- Transfer belt
- Nonskid shoes
- Wheelchair

Procedural Steps

1. **See Standard Protocol (inside front cover).**
2. *Transfer a patient from a bed to a wheelchair (patient is weight bearing and able to cooperate (Pierson and Fairchild, 2013).*
   a. Adjust the height of the bed to the level of the seat of the wheelchair if possible.
   b. Position the wheelchair at a 45-degree angle next to the same side of the bed as the patient's strong side.
   c. Face the wheelchair toward the foot of the bed midway between the head and foot of the bed.
   d. Lock the wheelchair. Locks are located above the rims of the wheels. Push handle forward to lock. Raise the footplates.
   e. Sit patient up on side of the bed (see Skill 15.1).
   f. Place transfer belt on patient, and assist patient to move to the edge of the mattress.
   g. Position yourself slightly in front of patient to guard and protect patient throughout the transfer.
   h. Coordinate transfer to chair with patient by counting to three (see Skill 15.1, Steps 3c(1-13).
   i. Lower footplates and place patient's feet on them.
   j. Unlock wheelchair. Pull lock toward you to release.
   k. Ensure that patient is positioned well back in the seat and ready to use wheelchair.
3. *Transfer a patient from a wheelchair to bed*
   a. Adjust the height of the bed to the level of the seat of the wheelchair if possible.

PROCEDURAL GUIDELINE 15.1
Wheelchair Transfer Techniques—cont'd

  b. Position the wheelchair at a 45-degree angle next to the bed.

  c. Face the wheelchair toward the foot of the bed midway between the head and foot of the bed.

  d. Lock the wheelchair. Locks are located above the rims of the wheels. Push handle forward to lock.

  e. Raise the footplates, and place the transfer belt on patient (if not already in place).

  f. Assist patient to move to the front of the wheelchair.

  g. Position yourself slightly in front of patient to guard and protect patient throughout the transfer. If patient has sufficient upper body strength, use a slide board during transfer (see illustration).

  h. Coordinate transfer to the bed by having patient stand and then pivot to the side of the bed. Then have patient sit on the side of the mattress (see Skill 15.1).

  i. With patient sitting on side of the bed, place your arm nearer the head of the bed under the person's shoulders while supporting the head and neck. Take your other arm and place it under the person's knees. Bend your knees and keep your back straight.

  j. Tell patient to help lift the legs when you begin to move. On a count of three, standing with a wide base of support, raise patient's legs as you pivot his or her

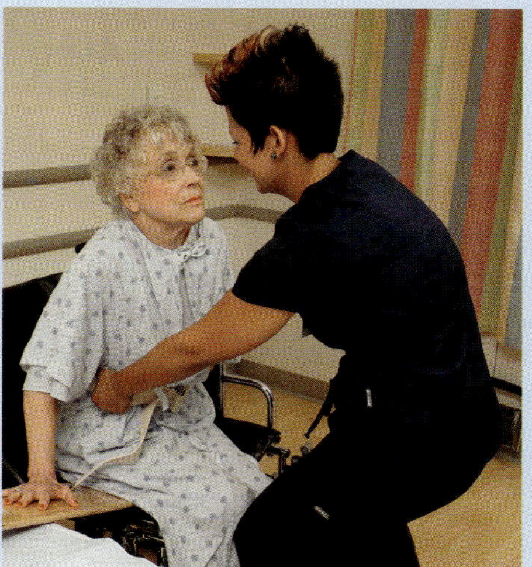

STEP 3g Transfer from wheelchair to bed using a slide board.

body and lower the shoulders onto the bed. Remember to keep your back straight.

4. **See Completion Protocol (inside front cover).**

5. Monitor vital signs as needed. Ask if patient feels dizzy or fatigued.

6. Note patient's behavioral response to transfer.

SKILL 15.2 MOVING AND POSITIONING PATIENTS IN BED

• **Nursing Skills Online: Safety Module, Lesson 3**

Correct positioning of patients is crucial for maintaining body alignment and comfort; preventing injury to the musculoskeletal and integumentary systems; and providing sensory, motor, and cognitive stimulation. A patient with impaired mobility, decreased sensation, impaired circulation, or lack of voluntary muscle control can develop damage to the musculoskeletal and integumentary systems while lying down. You must minimize this risk by promoting circulation and correct body alignment while moving, turning, or positioning patients. The term *body alignment* refers to the conditions of the joints, tendons, ligaments, and muscles in various body positions. When the body is aligned, whether standing, sitting, or lying, no excessive strain is placed on these structures. Body alignment means that the body is in line with the pull of gravity and contributes to body balance. Without this balance, the center of gravity is displaced, which increases the force of gravity and predisposes the patient to falls and injuries. You achieve body balance when a wide base of support exists, the center of gravity falls within the base of support, and you can draw a vertical line from the center of gravity through the base of support (Fig. 15-1).

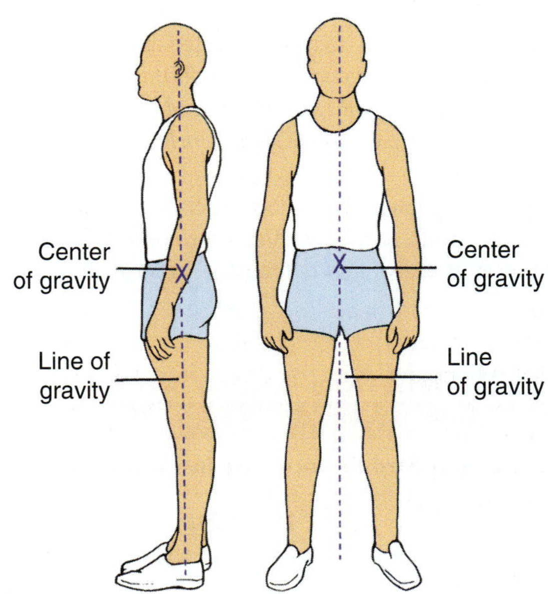

FIG 15-1 Body alignment when standing.

ASSESSMENT

1. Identify patient using two identifiers (e.g., name and birthday or name and account number) according to facility policy. *Rationale: Ensures correct patient. Complies with The Joint Commission standards and improves patient safety (TJC, 2014).*
2. Assess patient's body alignment and level of comfort while patient is lying down. *Rationale: Provides baseline for later comparisons. Determines ways to improve position and alignment.*
3. Assess for risk factors that may contribute to complications of immobility:
   a. Paralysis: Hemiparesis resulting from CVA. *Rationale: Paralysis impairs movement and muscle tone.*
   b. Impaired mobility: Traction, arthritis, hip fracture, joint surgery, or other contributing disease processes. *Rationale: Conditions result in decreased range of motion (ROM).*
   c. Impaired circulation: Arterial insufficiency. *Rationale: Decreased circulation predisposes patient to pressure ulcers.*
   d. Age: Very young or older adult. *Rationale: Premature and young infants require frequent turning because their skin is fragile. Normal physiological changes associated with aging predispose older adults to greater risks for developing complications of immobility.*
   e. Sensation: Decreased from CVA, paralysis, or neuropathy. *Rationale: Because of poor awareness of body part or reduced sensation, patient is unable to protect and position body part from pressure.*
4. Assess patient's level of consciousness. *Rationale: Determines need for special aids or devices. Patients with altered levels of consciousness may not understand instructions or be able to help during positioning.*
5. Assess patient's physical ability to help with moving and positioning, which may be affected by disease process, strength, ROM, and coordination. *Rationale: Enables nurse to use patient's mobility, strength, and coordination. Determines need for additional help, which ensures patient and nurse safety.*
6. Assess for presence of tubes, incisions, and equipment (e.g., traction). *Rationale: Alters positioning procedure, type of positions to use, and approach used for instruction.*
7. Assess motivation of patient and ability of family members to participate in moving and positioning patient in bed in anticipation of discharge to home. *Rationale: Indicates if instruction is needed.*
8. Check health care provider's orders before positioning patient. Clarify whether patient's condition contradicts any positions (e.g., spinal cord injury; hip fracture; respiratory difficulties; certain neurological conditions; presence of incisions, drains, or tubing). *Rationale: Some positions may be contraindicated in certain situations and can cause further harm if used.*

PLANNING

Expected Outcomes focus on safe mobility, self-care, and prevention of complications.
1. Patient retains ROM
2. Patient's skin shows no evidence of breakdown (see Chapter 25).
3. Patient experiences increased comfort.
4. Patient experiences increased level of independence in completing ADLs.

Delegation and Collaboration

The skills of moving and positioning patients in bed and maintaining correct body alignment can be delegated to nursing assistive personnel (NAP). The nurse instructs the NAP by:
- Explaining any moving and positioning restrictions unique to patient (e.g., avoid prone position, patient has one-sided weakness).
- Designating specific times throughout the shift that NAP must reposition patient.
- Providing information about patient's individual needs for body alignment (e.g., patient with spinal cord injury).

Equipment

- Pillows, drawsheet
- Friction-reducing device
- Therapeutic boots/splints (optional)
- Trochanter rolls
- Hand rolls

IMPLEMENTATION *for* MOVING AND POSITIONING PATIENTS IN BED

STEPS	RATIONALE
1. See Standard Protocol (see inside front cover).	

> **SAFE PATIENT CARE** Before placing bed in flat position, account for all tubing drains and equipment to prevent dislodgment or spillage if caught in mattress or bedframe as bed is lowered.

STEPS	RATIONALE
2. Assist patient in moving up in bed.	This task is not a one-person task unless patient can fully assist (OSHA, 2011).

STEPS	RATIONALE
a. Can patient assist?	Determines degree of risk in repositioning patient and technique required to assist patient safely.
(1) Fully able to assist, nurse assistance not needed; nurse stands by to assist.	
(2) Partially able to assist; patient can assist using positioning cues or aids (e.g., drawsheet or friction-reducing device).	
b. *Assist moving up in bed using a drawsheet (two to three nurses assist).*	
(1) Place patient supine with head of bed flat. A nurse stands on each side of bed.	Enables nurse to assess body alignment. Reduces pull of gravity on patient's upper body.
(2) Remove pillow from under head and shoulders and place it at head of bed.	Prevents striking patient's head against head of bed.
(3) Turn patient side to side to place drawsheet under patient, extending from shoulders to thighs.	Supports patient's body weight and reduces friction during movement.
(4) Return patient to supine position.	Even distribution of weight makes lift easier.
(5) Fanfold drawsheet on both sides, with each nurse grasping firmly near patient.	Provides strong handles to grip drawsheet without slipping.

> **SAFE PATIENT CARE** Protect patient's heels from shearing force by having a third nurse lift heels while moving patient up in bed.

STEPS	RATIONALE
(6) Nurses place their feet apart with forward-backward stance. Flex knees and hips. On the count of three, shift weight from front to back leg and move patient and drawsheet to desired position in bed (see illustration).	Facing direction of movement ensures proper balance. Shifting weight reduces force needed to move load. Flexing knees lowers nurses' center of gravity and uses thighs instead of back muscles.
c. *Assist moving up in bed using a friction-reducing device (three nurses assist).*	Patients weighing less than 90.9 kg (200 pounds) require at least three nurses; patients weighing more than 90.9 kg (200 pounds) require mechanical assist device.
(1) Position patient as in Steps 2b(1-3).	Supine position on drawsheet prepares patient for placement of friction-reducing device.
(2) Place friction-reducing device under drawsheet by having patient turn side to side.	Prevents friction from contact of skin with board.
(3) Move patient up in bed by having two nurses grasp drawsheet and one hold onto friction-reducing device. Follow Steps 2b(5 and 6), moving patient up in bed.	The slide board remains stationary, provides a slippery surface to reduce friction, and allows the patient to move easily up in bed.

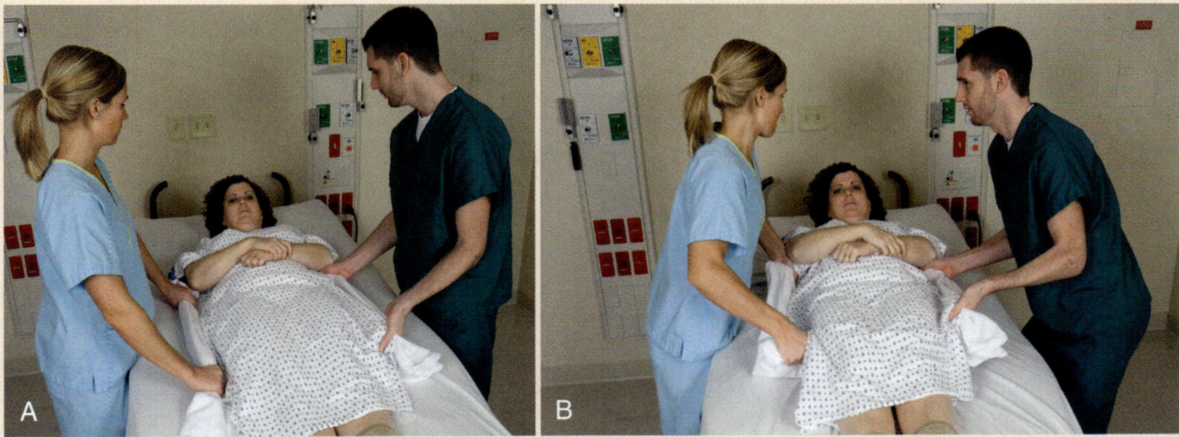

STEP 2b(6) A and **B,** Moving immobile patient up in bed with drawsheet.

Continued

STEPS	RATIONALE

3. Position patient in one of the following positions using correct body alignment to protect pressure areas. Begin with patient lying supine and move up in bed following either Steps 2b or 2c.

Prevents injury to musculoskeletal system.

 a. Position patient in supported Fowler's position (see illustration).

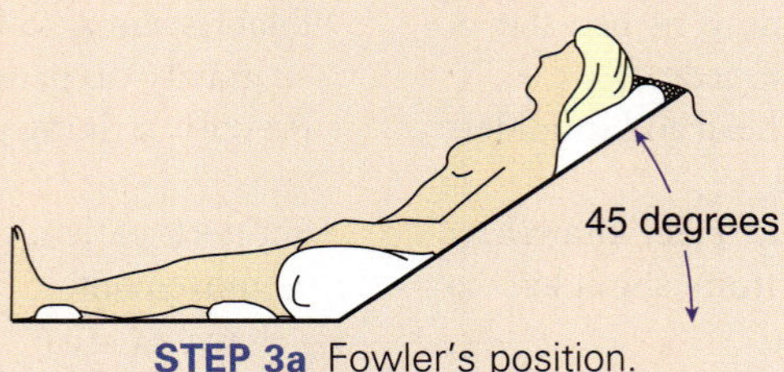

STEP 3a Fowler's position.

 (1) With patient lying supine, elevate head of bed 45 to 60 degrees if not contraindicated.

Increases comfort, improves ventilation, and increases patient's opportunity to socialize or relax.

 (2) Rest head against mattress or on small pillow.

Prevents flexion contractures of cervical vertebrae.

 (3) Use pillows to support arms and hands if patient does not have voluntary control or use of hands and arms.

Prevents shoulder dislocation from effect of downward pull of unsupported arms, promotes circulation by preventing venous pooling, and prevents flexion contractures of arms and wrists.

 (4) Position small pillow at lower back.

Supports lumbar vertebrae and decreases flexion of vertebrae.

 (5) Place small pillow or roll under thighs. Support calves with pillows.

Prevents hyperextension of knee and occlusion of popliteal artery from pressure from body weight. Heels should not be in contact with bed to prevent prolonged pressure of mattress on heels. This is sometimes referred to as "floating" heels.

 b. *Position hemiplegic patient in supported Fowler's position.*

 (1) Elevate head of bed 45 to 60 degrees. Adjust head of bed according to patient's condition. For example, patients with increased risk of pressure ulcers remain at 30-degree angle (semi-Fowler's) (see Chapter 25).

Increases comfort, improves ventilation, and increases patient's opportunity to relax.

 (2) Position patient in Fowler's position as straight as possible.

Counteracts tendency to slump toward affected side. Improves ventilation and cardiac output; decreases intracranial pressure. Improves patient's ability to swallow and helps to prevent aspiration of food, liquids, and gastric secretions.

 (3) Position head on small pillow with chin slightly forward. If patient is totally unable to control head movement, avoid hyperextension of the neck.

Prevents hyperextension of neck. Too many pillows under head may cause or worsen neck flexion contracture.

 (4) Provide support for involved arm and hand by placing arm away from patient's side and supporting elbow with pillow.

Paralyzed muscles do not automatically resist pull of gravity as they do normally. As a result, shoulder subluxation, pain, and edema may occur.

 (5) Take a rolled blanket (trochanter roll) and place firmly alongside patient's legs.

Ensures proper alignment. Prevents external rotation of hips, which contributes to contractures.

STEPS	RATIONALE

(6) Support feet in dorsiflexion with therapeutic boots or splints (see illustration).

Prevents plantar flexion contractures or footdrop by positioning patient's ankle in neutral dorsiflexion. Foot is positioned so heel is aligned in the opening of the splint to prevent pressure. Other therapeutic boots or splints are manufactured with thick padding to cushion the heel and prevent pressure ulcers.

c. *Position patient in supported supine position.*

(1) Place small rolled towel under lumbar area of back.

Provides support for lumbar spine.

(2) Place pillow under upper shoulders, neck, or head.

Maintains correct alignment and prevents flexion contractures of cervical vertebrae.

(3) Place trochanter rolls parallel to lateral surface of patient's thighs.

Reduces external rotation of hip.

(4) Place patient's feet in therapeutic boots or splints.

Maintains feet in dorsiflexion. Prevents plantar flexion contractures or footdrop.

(5) Place pillows under pronated forearms, keeping upper arms parallel to patient's body (see illustration).

Reduces internal rotation of shoulder and prevents extension of elbows. Maintains correct body alignment.

(6) Place hand rolls in patient's hands. Consider physical therapy referral for use of hand splints.

Reduces extension of fingers and abduction of thumb. Maintains thumb slightly adducted and in opposition to fingers.

d. *Position hemiplegic patient in supine position.*

(1) Place folded towel or small pillow under shoulder or affected side.

Decreases possibility of pain, joint contracture, and subluxation. Maintains mobility in muscles around shoulder to permit normal movement patterns.

(2) Keep affected arm away from body with elbow extended and palm up. Position affected hand in one of recommended positions for either flaccid or spastic hand. (Alternative is to place arm out to side, with elbow bent and hand toward head of bed.)

Maintains mobility in arm, joints, and shoulder to permit normal movement patterns. (Alternative position counteracts limitation of ability of arm to rotate outward at shoulder [external rotation]. External rotation must be present to raise arm over head without pain.)

(3) Place folded towel under hip of involved side.

Diminishes effect of spasticity in entire leg by controlling hip position.

(4) Flex affected knee 30 degrees by supporting it on pillow or folded blanket.

Slight flexion breaks up abnormal extension pattern of leg. Extensor spasticity is most severe when patient is supine.

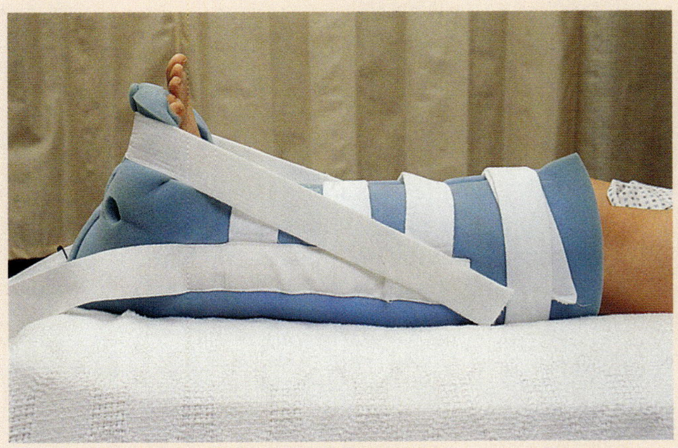

STEP 3b(6) Foot boot with lower leg extension

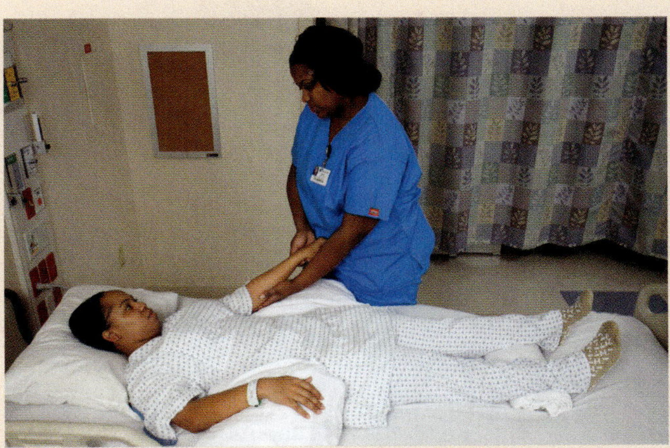

STEP 3c(5) Supported supine position with pillows in place.

Continued

STEPS	RATIONALE
(5) Support feet with soft pillows at right angle to leg.	Maintains foot in dorsiflexion and prevents footdrop. Pillows prevent stimulation to ball of foot by hard surface, which has tendency to increase muscle tone in patient with extensor spasticity of lower extremity.
e. Position patient in prone position, using two nurses.	In certain patients with pulmonary conditions such as acute respiratory distress syndrome, the use of the prone position can help improve oxygenation.
(1) With head of bed flat and one nurse standing on each side of bed, roll patient to one side while placing arm on side to be turned alongside of body.	Prepares patient for positioning.
(2) Roll patient over arm positioned close to body, with elbow straight and hand under hip. Position on abdomen in center of bed.	Positions patient correctly so that alignment can be maintained.
(3) Turn patient's head to one side and support head with small pillow.	Reduces flexion or hyperextension of cervical vertebrae.
(4) Place small pillow under patient's abdomen below level of diaphragm.	Reduces pressure on breasts of some female patients and decreases hyperextension of lumbar vertebrae and strain on lower back. Improves breathing by reducing mattress pressure on diaphragm.
(5) Support arms in flexed position level at shoulders.	Maintains proper body alignment. Support reduces risk of joint dislocation.
(6) Support lower legs with pillow to elevate toes (see illustration).	Prevents footdrop. Reduces external rotation of legs. Reduces mattress pressure on toes.

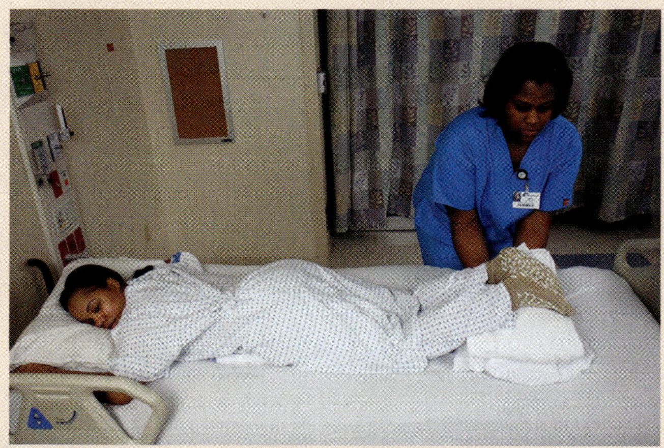

STEP 3e(6) Prone position with pillows supporting lower legs.

STEPS	RATIONALE
f. Position patient in 30-degree lateral (side-lying) position (one nurse).	
(1) Lower head of bed completely or as low as patient can tolerate.	Provides position of comfort for patient, and removes pressure from bony prominences on back.
(2) Position patient in supine position on side of bed opposite direction toward which patient is to be turned. Move upper trunk first, supporting shoulders, followed by lower trunk, supporting hips. Raise side rails and move to opposite side of bed.	Provides room for patient to turn to side.

STEPS	RATIONALE
(3) Prepare to turn patient onto side. Flex patient's knee that will not be next to mattress. Place one hand on patient's knee and one hand on patient's shoulder.	Use of leverage makes turning to side easy.
(4) Roll patient onto side toward you.	Rolling decreases trauma to tissues. In addition, patient is positioned so that leverage on hip makes turning easy.
(5) Place pillow under patient's head and neck.	Maintains alignment. Reduces lateral neck flexion. Decreases strain on sternocleidomastoid muscle.
(6) Bring dependent shoulder blade forward.	Prevents patient's weight from resting directly on shoulder joint.
(7) Position both arms in slightly flexed position. Support upper arm by pillow level with shoulder; support the other arm with mattress.	Decreases internal rotation and adduction of shoulder. Supporting both arms in slightly flexed position protects joint and improves ventilation because chest is able to expand more easily.
(8) Place your hands under patient's hips and bring dependent hip slightly forward so that angle from hip to mattress is approximately 30 degrees.	The 30-degree lateral position reduces pressure on trochanter.
(9) Place small tuck-back pillow behind patient's back. (Make by folding pillow lengthwise. Smooth area is slightly tucked under patient's back.)	Provides support to maintain patient on side.
(10) Place pillow under semiflexed upper leg level at hip from groin to foot (see illustration).	Flexion prevents hyperextension of leg. Maintains leg in correct alignment. Prevents pressure on bony prominences.

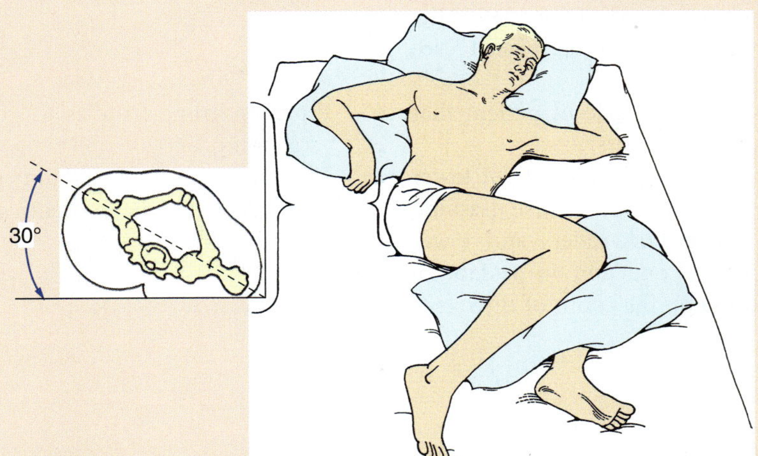

STEP 3f(10) 30-degree lateral position with pillows in place.

(11) Place sandbags parallel to plantar surface of dependent foot.	Maintains dorsiflexion of foot.
g. Position patient in Sims' (semi-prone) position (one nurse).	
(1) Position patient in supine position on side of bed opposite direction toward which patient is to be turned. Move upper trunk first, supporting shoulders; move lower trunk, supporting hips. Raise side rails and move to opposite side of bed.	Prepares patient for position.

Continued

STEPS	RATIONALE
(2) Move to other side of bed, and turn patient on side. Position in lateral position, lying partially on abdomen, with dependent shoulder lifted out and arm placed at patient's side.	Patient is rolled only partially on abdomen.
(3) Place small pillow under patient's head.	Maintains proper alignment and prevents lateral neck flexion.
(4) Place pillow under flexed upper arm, supporting arm level with shoulder.	Prevents internal rotation of shoulder. Maintains alignment.
(5) Place pillow under flexed upper legs, supporting leg level with hip.	Prevents internal rotation of hip and adduction of leg. Flexion prevents hyperextension of leg. Reduces mattress pressure on knees and ankles.
(6) Place sandbags parallel to plantar surface of foot.	Maintains foot in dorsiflexion. Prevents plantar flexion contractures or footdrop.

h. Logroll the patient (three nurses).

> **SAFE PATIENT CARE** A nurse supervises and aids the NAP when there is an order to logroll a patient. Patients who have sustained a spinal cord injury or are recovering from neck, back, or spinal surgery often need to keep the spinal column in straight alignment to prevent further injury.

STEPS	RATIONALE
(1) Place patient in supine position on side of bed opposite direction to be turned.	Prepares patient for turning onto side.
(2) Place small pillow between patient's knees.	Prevents tension on spinal column and adduction of hip.
(3) Cross patient's arms on chest.	Prevents injury to arms.
(4) Position two nurses on the side toward which patient is to be turned and one nurse on the side where pillows are to be placed (see illustration).	Distributes weight equally between nurses during turning.
(5) Fanfold drawsheet along side of patient that will be turning.	Provides strong handles to grip the drawsheet without slipping.
(6) With one nurse grasping drawsheet at lower hips and thighs and the other nurse grasping drawsheet at patient's shoulders and lower back, roll patient as one unit in a smooth, continuous motion on the count of three (see illustration).	This maintains proper alignment by moving all body parts at the same time, preventing tension or twisting of the spinal column.

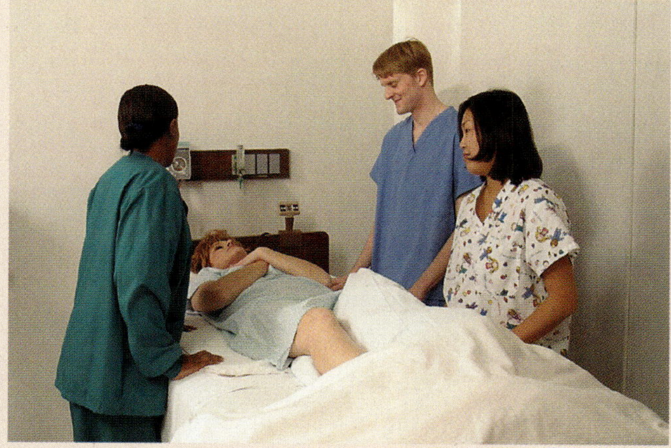

STEP 3h(4) Preparing patient for logroll.

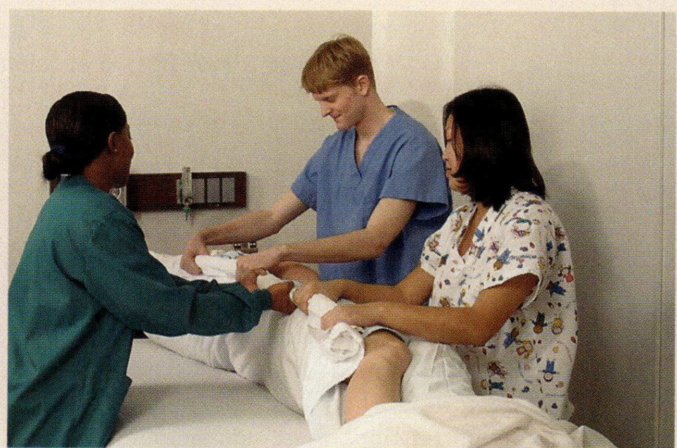

STEP 3h(6) Logrolling patient onto side.

STEPS	RATIONALE
(7) Nurse on opposite side of the bed places pillows along length of patient for support (see illustration).	Maintains patient in side-lying position.

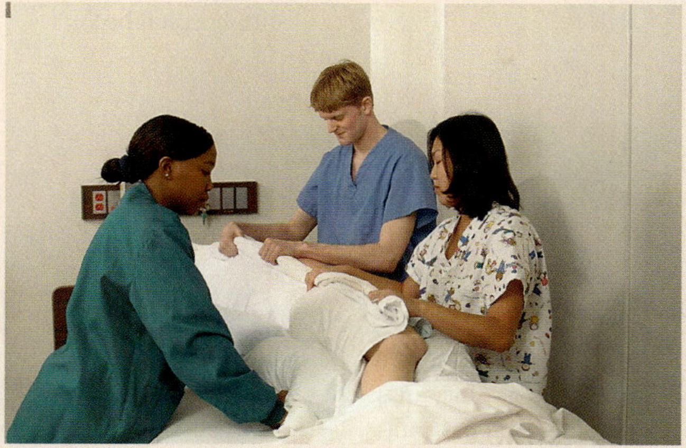

STEP 3h(7) Place pillows along patient's back for support.

STEPS	RATIONALE
(8) Gently lean patient as a unit back toward the pillows for support.	Ensures continued straight alignment of spinal column, preventing injury.
4. See Completion Protocol (inside front cover).	

EVALUATION

1. Evaluate patient's body alignment and position. Patient's body should be supported by adequate mattress, and vertebral column is without observable curves.
2. Evaluate patient's level of comfort. (Pain scale is an option.)
3. Measure ROM (see Chapter 7).
4. Observe for areas of erythema or breakdown involving skin.
5. Observe patient attempt self-care activities (e.g., bathing, eating).
6. Use **Teach Back:** State to the patient, "I want to be sure I explained the reason for turning you to the prone position and the steps we are using to make sure you are comfortable. Will you repeat the reason and the steps back to me in your own words?" Evaluates what the patient is able to explain or demonstrate. Revise your instruction now or develop plan for revised patient teaching to be implemented at an appropriate time if patient is not able to teach back correctly.

Unexpected Outcomes and Related Interventions

1. Joint contractures develop or worsen.
   a. Offer ROM exercises to affected and immobilized areas (see Chapter 16).
2. Skin shows localized areas of erythema and breakdown.
   a. Increase frequency of repositioning.
   b. Place a turning schedule in location easily visible for all care providers.
3. Patient avoids moving.
   a. Medicate with analgesia as ordered by health care provider to ensure patient's comfort before moving.
   b. Allow pain medication to take effect before proceeding.

Recording and Reporting

- Record transfer or positioning change and observations (e.g., condition of skin, joint movement, patient's ability to assist with positioning) in flow sheet or nurses' notes.
- Document your evaluation of patient learning.
- Report observations at change of shift.
- Report skin or joint complications to health care provider.

Sample Documentation

0900 Patient reports feeling of pressure over coccyx area. Coccyx slightly reddened. Patient able to teach back purpose of prone position. Positioned prone with assist of three caregivers. Pillows placed to support lower legs; small pillow positioned under head and below diaphragm. Patient denies discomfort or pain.

1000 Patient turned to left-lateral position. No further redness noted on coccyx area. Patient resting comfortably without report of pain or discomfort.

Special Considerations
Pediatric

- Encourage children to be as active as their condition and restrictive devices allow. Use developmentally appropriate toys or items that stimulate activity and participation in care.

- Children who are unable to move need passive exercise and movement (see Chapter 16).

Geriatric

- Reposition older adult patients at least every 1 to 2 hours, and maintain a regular program of ROM exercises (Touhy and Jett, 2014).

Home Care

- Assess ability and motivation of patient and family caregivers to participate in moving and positioning patient in bed.
- Assess home to determine compatibility of environment with assistive devices (e.g., over-bed trapeze, mechanical lift, hospital bed).

CRITICAL THINKING EXERCISES

Case Study

A 37-year-old man who sustained a spinal cord injury in a motor vehicle accident has just been admitted. He has multiple deep lacerations on his face and trunk and facial fractures of maxillary and zygomatic bones. He rates his pain at 9 on a scale of 0 to 10.

1. The patient is scheduled for a computed tomography (CT) scan of the head and spine. He now reports pain at a level of 7 on a 0 to 10 scale. He weighs 95.45 kg (210 pounds) and refuses to allow the nurse to move him onto the stretcher. What interventions would the nurse select to get the patient successfully to the procedure? Select all that apply.
   1. Administer pain medication as ordered.
   2. Use two nurses to move patient to stretcher.
   3. Prepare to have three nurses assist with transfer.
   4. Tell him that it is the health care provider's order and must be carried out.
   5. Explain the procedure to him and allow time for the pain medication to take effect.
2. The patient has returned from the CT scan. The health care provider has ordered him to be turned and positioned every 1 to 2 hours until he is taken to surgery to stabilize his spinal fracture. What is the safest technique to use to move him from side to side? Fill in the blank and provide a rationale: ________________________________.
3. The transporter has returned the patient to his room and requests assistance to move him to the bed. The NAP tells you, "I do not need your assistance; the transporter and I are able to move him." The most appropriate action is:
   1. Allow the transporter and NAP to transfer the patient to the bed.
   2. Instruct the NAP on the appropriate transfer technique to move this patient.
   3. Accompany the NAP to the patient's room and supervise the transfer.
   4. Tell the NAP to allow the patient to transfer to the bed with minimal assistance.

Review Questions

1. Before transferring a patient from the bed to a stretcher, which assessment data does the nurse need to gather? Select all that apply.
   1. Patient's weight
   2. Patient's level of cooperation
   3. Patient's ability to assist
   4. Presence of medical equipment
   5. 24-hour calorie intake
2. Which of the following is a principle of proper body mechanics when lifting or carrying objects?
   1. Keep the knees in a locked position.
   2. Bend at the waist to maintain a center of gravity.
   3. Maintain a narrow base of support.
   4. Hold objects away from the body for improved leverage.
3. Which of the following indicates that additional assistance is needed to transfer a patient from the bed to the stretcher?
   1. The patient is 5 feet 6 inches (165 cm) and weighs 90.9 kg (200 pounds).
   2. The patient speaks and understands English.
   3. The patient has agreed to assist.
   4. You feel comfortable handling a patient of his size and with his level of cooperation.
4. A patient has been on bed rest for several days. When he tries to sit on the side of the bed, he becomes dizzy and nauseated. These are most likely symptoms of which of the following?
   1. Rebound hypertension
   2. Orthostatic hypotension
   3. Dysfunctional proprioception
   4. CNS rebound hypotension
5. A patient who weighs 104.5 kg (230 pounds) is being transferred from his bed to a chair. The patient is on partial weight bearing as a result of bilateral reconstructive knee surgery. Which of the following is the best technique for transfer?
   1. Friction-reducing device
   2. Bariatric transfer aid
   3. Three-person carry
   4. Stand-and-pivot using two nurses

6. An adolescent has been admitted with an unstable spinal cord injury sustained from a motor vehicle accident. The patient needs to be taken to the operating room. What is the most appropriate method to move this patient to a stretcher for transport?
   1. Use a step-by-step method: move the trunk, the hips, and finally the legs.
   2. Logroll the patient, place a slide board, and slide the patient to the stretcher as one unit maintaining body alignment.
   3. Allow the patient to stand and transfer to the stretcher.
   4. Use a mechanical lift device to transfer to the stretcher.

7. A patient is 1 day status post abdominal surgery. He is refusing to move from the bed to the chair. What should the nurse assess first in determining appropriateness of transfer?
   1. Level of pain
   2. Any equipment connected to his body
   3. Patient's weight
   4. Patient's ability to follow directions

8. The nurse is transferring a patient from bed to chair. The patient has been on prolonged bed rest. Which one of the following should the nurse do first?
   1. Apply a transfer belt.
   2. Use the under-axilla method to assist the patient to a sitting position.
   3. Provide the patient with his or her glasses.
   4. Allow the patient to dangle his or her feet at the side of the bed for a few minutes.

9. Two NAPs ask for the nurse's assistance to transfer a 56.8-kg (125-pound) patient from the bed to the stretcher. The patient is unable to assist. What is the best response?
   1. "As long as we use proper body mechanics, no one will get hurt."
   2. "The patient only weighs 56.8 kg (125 pounds). You do not need my assistance."
   3. "The three-man lift technique is recommended to ensure your safety and that of the patient."
   4. "Use the slide board; it's more comfortable for the patient and will lessen the chance of injury to us."

10. Place the following steps in sequence that promotes safe transfer of a patient from a wheelchair to a bed.
    1. Position wheelchair at a 45-degree angle next to the bed.
    2. Assist patient to move to the front of wheelchair.
    3. Raise the footplates and apply transfer belt.
    4. Lock the wheelchair. Push forward to lock.
    5. Position yourself slightly in front of the patient to guard and protect the patient throughout the transfer.
    6. Have patient stand and pivot to side of bed.
    7. Adjust the height of the bed to the level of the seat of the wheelchair.

REFERENCES

American Nurses Association (ANA): *Safe patient handling and mobility interprofessional national standards*, Silver Spring, MD, 2013a, The American Nurses Association.

American Nurses Association (ANA): *ANA leads initiative to develop national safe patient handling standards*, Silver Spring, MD, 2013b, The American Nurses Association.

Bureau of Labor Statistics (BLS): *Incidence rates for nonfatal occupational injuries and illnesses involving days away from work per 10,000 full-time workers by industry and selected events or exposures leading to injury or illness, private industry*, 2012. http://www.bls.gov/news.release/osh2.nr0.htm.

Christo P, et al: Effective treatments for pain in the older patient, *Curr Pain Headache Rep* 15(1):22, 2011.

Flegal KM, et al: Prevalence and trends in obesity among US adults, 1999-2008, *JAMA* 303(3):235, 2010.

Freeman R, et al: Consensus statement on the definition of orthostatic hypotension, neutrally mediate syncope and the postural tachycardia syndrome, *Auton Neurosci* 161(1–2):46, 2011.

Hockenberry MJ, Wilson D: *Wong's essentials of pediatric nursing*, ed 9, St Louis, 2013, Elsevier.

Huether SE, McCance KL: *Understanding pathophysiology*, ed 5, St Louis, 2012, Mosby.

Lagro J, et al: Diastolic blood pressure drop after standing as a clinical sign for increased mortality in older falls clinic patients, *J Hypertens* 30(6):1195, 2012.

Occupational Health and Safety Administration (OSHA): *Activity 6—everyone benefits from an ergonomic program*, 2011. http:// www.osha.gov/SLTC/healthcarefacilities/training/ activity_6.html. Accessed March 20, 2014.

Pelczarski KM: Back in action, *Health Facil Manage* 25(8):21, 2012.

Pierson F, Fairchild S: *Principles and techniques of patient care*, ed 5, St Louis, 2013, Saunders.

Sherwood G, Barnsteiner J: *Quality and safety in nursing*, Oxford, UK, 2012, Wiley-Blackwell.

The Joint Commission (TJC): *National Patient Safety Goals*, Oakbrook Terrace, IL, 2014, The Commission. Available at: http://www.jointcommission.org/standards_information/ npsgs.aspx.

Thompson P, et al: Non-pharmacological treatments for orthostatic hypotension, *Age Ageing* 40(3):292, 2011.

Touhy T, Jett K: *Ebersole and Hess's gerontological nursing and healthy aging*, ed 4, St Louis, 2014, Mosby.

U.S. Department of Health and Human Services (HHS): *Safe patient handling and lifting standards for a safer American workforce*, 2010. http://www.help.senate.gov/imo/media/doc/ Collins4.pdf. Accessed March 20, 2014.

Waters T, et al: AORN ergonomic tool 2: positioning and repositioning the supine patient on the OR bed, *AORN J* 93(4):445, 2011a.

Waters T, et al: AORN ergonomic tool 6: lifting and carrying supplies and equipment in the perioperative setting, *AORN J* 94(2):173, 2011b.

Waters T, et al: AORN ergonomic tool 7: pushing, pulling, and moving equipment on wheels, *AORN J* 93(3):254, 2011c.

16

Exercise and Mobility

EVOLVE WEBSITE/EVOLVE RESOURCES LIST

http://evolve.elsevier.com/Perry/nursinginterventions
Audio Glossary • Checklists • Review Questions

Mobility is one's capacity for movement and is a means for people to explore their surroundings and engage in personal contact (Touhy and Jett, 2012). Patients achieve enhanced mobility through simple activities, such as walking, and with the aid of assistive devices. The benefits of physical activity have been well documented and include weight loss, improvement in mental health and mood, improved ability to perform activities of daily living (ADLs), prevention of falls, and strengthening of bones and muscles (CDC, 2011). It is useful to incorporate active exercise into ADLs whenever possible (see Table 16-1). Nurses make every effort to promote and maintain patients' functional mobility and are in a unique position to influence patients' participation in these health-promoting activities.

Three elements essential for mobility include (1) the ability to move based on adequate muscle strength, control, coordination, and range of motion (ROM); (2) the motivation to move; and (3) the absence of barriers in the environment. As a nurse, you are responsible for helping to keep patients active by promoting mobility within their abilities. Bed rest is a medical intervention in which a patient is restricted to bed for one of the following purposes: (1) to decrease oxygen requirements of the body, (2) to reduce pain, or (3) to promote rest and recovery. Bed rest requires a nurse to keep patients active by performing what they can in self-care and doing range-of-motion exercises. Inactivity in older adults can result from functional loss; however, maintaining activity such as frequent walking is important to aid in recovering health and wellness (Meiner, 2011). Consider all of the mobility elements when incorporating activity into a patient's plan of care.

PATIENT-CENTERED CARE

Patients in pain are less mobile if they fear that activity will increase their pain or if the pain is limiting their ROM. When assessing a patient's level of pain, be aware that culture and gender can affect a patient's response. Members of some cultures believe that suffering must be endured, which contributes to a high pain tolerance (Spencer and Burke, 2011). Other cultures often try herbal remedies first, so education about pain medication alternatives may be needed. Respect the beliefs of your patients, while being careful to examine verbal and nonverbal cues of all patients in assessing and evaluating pain (see Chapter 13). You must understand how to communicate effectively with patients so that you can explain the benefits of mobility and the increased risks of complications to patients if they are immobile. Include family members in any discussions so that they can reinforce the importance of activity.

SAFETY

There is a complex circulatory response that occurs when a patient stands upright (Valbusa et al., 2012). Caution patients about the risk for orthostatic hypotension during exercise. Signs and symptoms of orthostatic hypotension include dizziness, light-headedness, nausea, tachycardia, pallor, and fainting. In these patients, moving to the dangling position (see Skill 16.1) may cause a gravity-induced decrease in blood pressure, creating a risk for falling. When a patient stands, blood shifts from the thorax to the pelvis and lower extremities because of gravity. To aid in managing and preventing orthostatic hypotension, instruct the patient to keep hydrated, exercise calf muscles before sitting up, sit on the edge of the bed for 1 minute before standing, and avoid bending at the waist when standing (Mayo Clinic, 2011).

To prevent injury to both the patient and the caregiver, use of safe patient handling techniques is essential. Programs exist that protect nurses and other health care providers from musculoskeletal injuries that commonly occur when nurses lift and handle patients (Campo et al., 2013). Use your clinical judgment when making decisions about patient handling. Take into account the patient's comfort, preferences, size, and overall physical and mental condition as well as communication barriers and environmental issues to determine the best approach (de Ruiter and Liaschenko, 2011). Nurses must work together with patients and members of the health care team to develop safe practices. When nurses and patients work together to plan the best transfer approach, all parties are empowered to participate and ensure that the care provided is acceptable and appropriate for the patient. When lifting a patient, arrange for adequate help. If your facility has a lift team, use it as a resource. When necessary, plan to use patient-handling equipment and devices (e.g., adjustable-height beds, ceiling-mounted lifts, friction-reducing slide sheets, air-assisted devices). Safe patient handling practices are essential in health care; these practices protect both nurses and patients (see Chapter 15).

Immobility and lack of physical exercise have profound effects on patients and their quality of life. Approach a plan for a patient's physical activity from a holistic perspective, which considers cardiorespiratory health, musculoskeletal health, and body awareness (Chui et al., 2013). Obesity has become an epidemic in the United States, with women of all ages and people of lower income reported to be the least active groups (Chui et al., 2013). Instruct your patients to incorporate physical activity gradually into their daily lives and to limit sedentary activities (e.g., watching TV). In addition, discuss the importance of collateral issues of fluid intake, heart monitoring, risk factors, and rest periods to ensure safety in exercise.

EVIDENCE-BASED PRACTICE

Nitz JC, Josephson DL: Enhancing functional balance and mobility among older people living in long-term care facilities, *Geriatr Nurs* 32(2):106, 2011.

A balance strategy training program (BSTP) is designed to improve a patient's balance. When balance is improved, patients have the potential to be more active, to improve functional abilities, and in some situations to be more independent. This training is best delivered over time, such as twice weekly for 12 weeks, and is often effective with long-term care residents (Nitz and Josephson, 2011). In a study of 47 residents enrolled in a BSTP, 34 individuals (12 men, 35 women; average age, 85.4 years) completed all assessments (Nitz and Josephson, 2011). The study investigated the effectiveness of a BSTP in improving functional mobility and reducing falls. At the end of the training period, the BSTP improved the participants' functional ability; for example, participants were able to reach 15% further. The use of this BSTP or other balance-improving programs has implications for older adults in long-term care and other practice settings:

- Increase in functional ability allows for more independence as patients become more stable and are able to reach clothing and personal care items and perform ADLs.
- The enhanced ability to reach could have an impact on fall rates because patients are more stable in reaching for items.
- The BSTP activities (e.g., tossing small beanbags and kicking a beach ball) are easily integrated into care facilities and daily care routines.
- Encourage patients to practice balance techniques several times a day.

PROCEDURAL GUIDELINE 16.1
Range of Motion

Range of motion (ROM) refers to the amount of rotating, bending, or twisting that a joint allows (Edlin and Golanty, 2010). ROM exercises may be active, passive, or active assisted. An active exercise is one a patient is able to perform independently, and a passive exercise is one performed for a patient by a caregiver. Continuous passive motion machines (CPMs) have been used to exercise different joints postoperatively. With the addition of computer-assisted surgery, the question has been raised about the benefits of CPM. Recent studies indicate there is no significant benefit to the patient when using CPM (Harvey et al., 2014; Martin, 2014). In every aspect of ADL, you must encourage a patient to be as independent as possible. The nurse encourages and supervises active and passive ROM exercises for patients daily. Active ROM exercises can be incorporated into the patient's ADLs (Table 16-1). You can easily incorporate passive ROM exercises into bathing and feeding activities. Always collaborate with a patient to develop a schedule for ROM activities.

Continued

PROCEDURAL GUIDELINE 16.1
Range of Motion—cont'd

Delegation and Collaboration

The skill of performing ROM exercises can be delegated to nursing assistive personnel (NAP). However, patients with spinal cord or orthopedic trauma usually require exercise to be performed by nurses or physical therapists. The nurse instructs the NAP to:

- Adapt the skill for specific patients, such as which joints need passive versus active ROM.
- Observe and report back to the nurse patient responses, such as pain or fatigue during ROM.

Equipment

- No mechanical or physical equipment needed; clean gloves (if drainage or skin lesions present)

Procedural Steps

1. Review patient's medical record for physical assessment findings, health care provider orders, medical diagnosis, medical history, and progress.
2. Obtain data on patient's baseline joint function while observing patient's ability to perform ROM exercises during ADLs. Observe for limitations in joint mobility, redness or warmth over joints, joint tenderness, deformities, or crepitus produced by joint motion.
3. Determine patient's or family caregiver's readiness to learn. Explain all rationales for ROM exercises, and describe and demonstrate exercises to be performed.
4. Assess patient's level of comfort (on a pain scale of 0 to 10) before exercises.

> **SAFE PATIENT CARE** Consider premedicating patient 30 minutes before ROM exercises begin if necessary.

5. **See Standard Protocol (inside front cover).**
6. Apply clean gloves if wound drainage or skin lesions are present.
7. Assist the patient to a comfortable position, preferably sitting or lying down.
8. When performing active-assisted or passive ROM exercises (Table 16-2), support joint by holding distal and proximal areas adjacent to joint, cradling distal portion of extremity, or using cupped hand to support joint (see illustrations).
9. Complete exercises in head-to-toe sequence. Repeat each movement five times during exercise period. Inform patient how these exercises are performed and how they can be incorporated into ADLs (see Table 16-1).

> **SAFE PATIENT CARE** If new resistance is noted within a joint, do not force joint motion. Consult with health care provider or physical therapist.

10. Observe patient as he or she performs ROM activities.
11. Measure joint motion as needed.
12. Reassess patient during exercise, ask patient to rate any discomfort on a pain scale of 0 to 10.
13. Use *Teach Back:* State to the patient, "I want to be sure I explained why I want you to move your arms throughout the day. Can you tell me why this is important?" Evaluates what the patient is able to explain or demonstrate. Revise your instruction now or develop plan for revised patient teaching to be implemented at an appropriate time if patient is not able to teach back correctly.
14. **See Completion Protocol (inside front cover).**

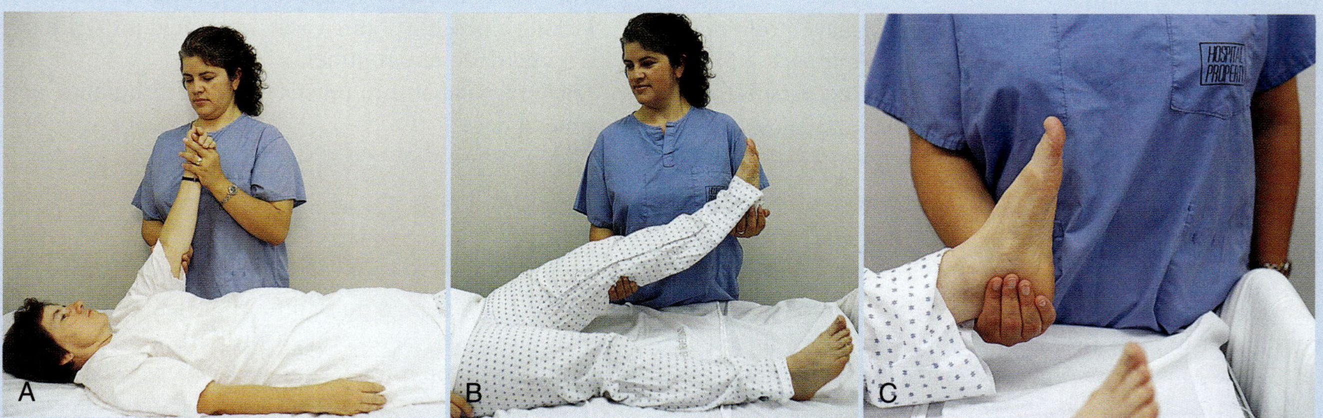

STEP 8 A, Support joint by holding distal and proximal areas adjacent to joint. **B,** Support joint by cradling distal portion of extremity. **C,** Use cupped hand to support joint.

TABLE 16-1 — INCORPORATING ACTIVE RANGE-OF-MOTION EXERCISES INTO ACTIVITIES OF DAILY LIVING

JOINT EXERCISED	ACTIVITY OF DAILY LIVING	MOVEMENT
Neck	Nodding head "yes"	Flexion
	Shaking head "no"	Rotation
	Moving right ear to right shoulder	Lateral flexion
	Moving left ear to left shoulder	Lateral flexion
Shoulder	Reaching to turn on overhead light	Flexion, extension
	Reaching to bedside stand for book	Extension
	Applying deodorant	Abduction
	Combing hair	Flexion
	Scratching back; brushing or combing hair	Hyperextension
Elbow	Eating, bathing, shaving, grooming	Flexion, extension
Wrist	Eating, bathing, shaving, grooming	Flexion, extension, abduction, adduction
Fingers and thumb	All activities requiring fine motor coordination (e.g., writing, eating, hobbies)	Flexion, extension, abduction, adduction, opposition
Hip	Walking	Flexion, extension, hyperextension
	Moving to side-lying position	Flexion, extension, abduction
	Moving from side-lying position	Extension, adduction
	Rolling feet inward	Internal rotation
	Rolling feet outward	External rotation
Knee	Walking	Flexion, extension
	Moving to and from side-lying position	Flexion, extension
Ankle	Walking	Dorsiflexion, plantar flexion
	Moving toe toward head of bed	Dorsiflexion
	Moving toe toward foot of bed	Plantar flexion
Toes	Walking	Extension, flexion
	Wiggling toes	Abduction, adduction, extension, flexion

TABLE 16-2 — RANGE-OF-MOTION EXERCISES

BODY PART	TYPE OF JOINT	TYPE OF MOVEMENT	RANGE (DEGREES)	PRIMARY MUSCLES
Neck, cervical spine	Pivotal	*Flexion:* Bring chin to rest on chest.	45	Sternocleidomastoid
		Extension: Return head to erect position.	45	Trapezius
		Hyperextension: Bend head back as far as possible.	10	Trapezius
		Lateral flexion: Slowly tilt head as far as possible toward each shoulder.	40-45	Sternocleidomastoid
		Rotation: Slowly turn head as far as possible in circular movement.	180	Sternocleidomastoid, trapezius
Shoulder	Ball-and-socket	*Flexion:* Raise arm from side position forward to position above head.	45-60	Coracobrachialis, deltoid, pectoralis major
		Extension: Return arm to position at side of body.	180	Latissimus dorsi, teres major, triceps brachii
		Hyperextension: Move arm behind body, keeping elbow straight.	45-60	Latissimus dorsi, teres major, deltoid
		Abduction: Raise arm from side to position above head with palm away from head.	180	Deltoid, supraspinatus
		Adduction: Lower arm sideways and across body as far as possible.	320	Pectoralis major
		Internal rotation: With elbow flexed, rotate shoulder by moving arm until thumb is turned inward and toward back.	90	Pectoralis major, latissimus dorsi, teres major, subscapularis

Continued

TABLE 16-2		RANGE-OF-MOTION EXERCISES—cont'd		
BODY PART	**TYPE OF JOINT**	**TYPE OF MOVEMENT**	**RANGE (DEGREES)**	**PRIMARY MUSCLES**
		External rotation: With elbow flexed, move arm until thumb is upward and lateral to head.	90	Infraspinatus, teres major, deltoid
		Circumduction: Move arm in full circle (circumduction is combination of all movements of ball-and-socket joint).	360	Deltoid, coracobrachialis, latissimus dorsi, teres major
Elbow	Hinge	*Flexion:* Bend elbow so that lower arm moves toward its shoulder joint and hand is level with shoulder.	150	Biceps brachii, brachialis, brachioradialis
		Extension: Straighten elbow by lowering hand.	150	Triceps brachii
Forearm	Pivotal	*Supination:* Turn lower arm and hand so that palm is up.	70-90	Supinator, biceps brachii
		Pronation: Turn lower arm so that palm is down.	70-90	Pronator teres, pronator quadratus
Wrist	Condyloid	*Flexion:* Move palm toward inner aspect of forearm.	80-90	Flexor carpi ulnaris, flexor carpi radialis
		Extension: Move fingers and hand posterior to midline.	80-90	Extensor carpi radialis brevis, extensor carpi radialis longus, extensor carpi ulnaris
		Hyperextension: Bring dorsal surface of hand back as far as possible.	80-90	Extensor carpi radialis brevis, extensor carpi radialis longus, extensor carpi ulnaris
		Abduction (ulnar deviation): Bend wrist laterally toward fifth finger.	30-50	Flexor carpi ulnaris, extensor carpi ulnaris
		Adduction (radial deviation): Bend wrist medially toward thumb.	Up to 30	Flexor carpi radialis, extensor carpi radialis brevis, extensor carpi radialis longus
Fingers	Condyloid hinge	*Flexion:* Make fist.	90	Lumbricales, interosseus volaris, interosseus dorsalis
		Extension: Straighten fingers.	90	Extensor digiti quinti proprius, extensor digitorum communis, extensor indicis proprius
		Hyperextension: Bend fingers back as far as possible.	30-60	Extensor digitorum
		Abduction: Spread fingers apart.	30	Interosseus dorsalis
		Adduction: Bring fingers together.	30	Interosseus volaris
Thumb	Saddle	*Flexion:* Move thumb across palmar surface of hand.	90	Flexor pollicis brevis
		Extension: Move thumb straight away from hand.	90	Extensor pollicis longus, extensor pollicis brevis
		Abduction: Extend thumb laterally (usually done when placing fingers in abduction and adduction).	30	Abductor pollicis brevis and longus
		Adduction: Move thumb back toward hand.	30	Adductor pollicis obliquus, adductor pollicis transversus
		Opposition: Touch thumb to each finger of same hand.	—	Opponens pollicis, opponens digiti minimi
Hip	Ball-and-socket	*Flexion:* Move leg forward and up.	90-120	Psoas major, iliacus, sartorius
		Extension: Move leg back, beside other leg.	90-120	Gluteus maximus, semitendinosus, semimembranosus
		Hyperextension: Move leg behind body as far as possible.	30-50	Gluteus maximus, semitendinosus, semimembranosus
		Abduction: Move leg laterally away from body.	30-50	Gluteus medius, gluteus minimus

TABLE 16-2   RANGE-OF-MOTION EXERCISES—cont'd

BODY PART	TYPE OF JOINT	TYPE OF MOVEMENT	RANGE (DEGREES)	PRIMARY MUSCLES
		Adduction: Move leg back toward medial position and beyond if possible.	30-50	Adductor longus, adductor brevis, adductor magnus
		Internal rotation: Turn foot and leg toward other leg.	90	Gluteus medius, gluteus minimus, tensor fasciae latae
		External rotation: Turn foot and leg away from other leg.	90	Obturatorius internus, obturatorius externus, quadratus femoris, piriformis, gemellus superior and inferior, gluteus maximus
		Circumduction: Move leg in circle.	120-130	Psoas major, gluteus maximus, gluteus medius, adductor magnus
Knee	Hinge	*Flexion:* Bring heel back toward back of thigh.	120-130	Biceps femoris, semitendinosus, semimembranosus, sartorius
		Extension: Return leg to floor.	120-130	Rectus femoris, vastus lateralis, vastus medialis, vastus intermedius
Ankle	Hinge	*Dorsiflexion:* Move foot so toes are pointed upward.	20-30	Tibialis anterior
		Plantar flexion: Move foot so toes are pointed downward.	45-50	Gastrocnemius, soleus
Foot	Gliding	*Inversion:* Turn sole of foot medially.	≤10	Tibialis anterior, tibialis posterior
		Eversion: Turn sole of foot laterally.	≤10	Peroneus longus, peroneus brevis
Toes	Condyloid	*Flexion:* Curl toes downward.	30-60	Flexor digitorum, lumbricalis pedis, flexor hallucis brevis
		Extension: Straighten toes.	30-60	Extensor digitorum longus, extensor digitorum brevis, extensor hallucis longus
		Abduction: Spread toes apart.	≤15	Abductor hallucis, interosseus dorsalis
		Adduction: Bring toes together.	≤15	Adductor hallucis, interosseus plantaris

PROCEDURAL GUIDELINE 16.2
Applying Elastic Stockings and Sequential Compression Device

Prolonged immobilization related to surgery or hospitalization, trauma, malignancy, hormone therapy, pregnancy, advanced age, and dehydration can lead to a deep vein thrombosis (DVT), a blood clot that forms in a vein deep in the body (Anthony, 2013). DVTs can be the cause of pulmonary embolisms. DVTs are caused by conditions of venous stasis, blood hypercoagulability, or endovascular damage; these conditions are collectively referred to as Virchow's triad (Andrews and Habashi, 2010). Prevention is the best approach for DVTs and includes anticoagulant medications such as warfarin (Coumadin) and low-molecular-weight heparin; however, movement of the extremities and wearing elastic stockings, foot pumps, or sequential compression devices (SCDs) are equally important. Elastic stockings help reduce blood stasis and venous wall injury by promoting venous return and limiting venous stasis and dilation, which decreases the risk of endothelial tears. SCDs pump blood into deep veins, removing pooled blood and preventing venous stasis. Another device, venous plexus foot pumps, promotes circulation by mimicking the natural action of walking (Fig. 16-1).

Delegation

The skill of applying elastic stockings and SCDs can be delegated to nursing assistive personnel (NAP). The nurse initially determines the size of elastic stockings and assesses the patient's lower extremities for any signs and symptoms of DVTs or impaired circulation. The nurse instructs the NAP to:

- Remove the SCD sleeves before allowing the patient to get out of bed.

Equipment

- Tape measure
- Powder or cornstarch (optional)
- Elastic or compression stockings
- SCD motor, disposable SCD sleeve(s), tubing assembly

Continued

PROCEDURAL GUIDELINE 16.2
Applying Elastic Stockings and Sequential Compression Device—cont'd

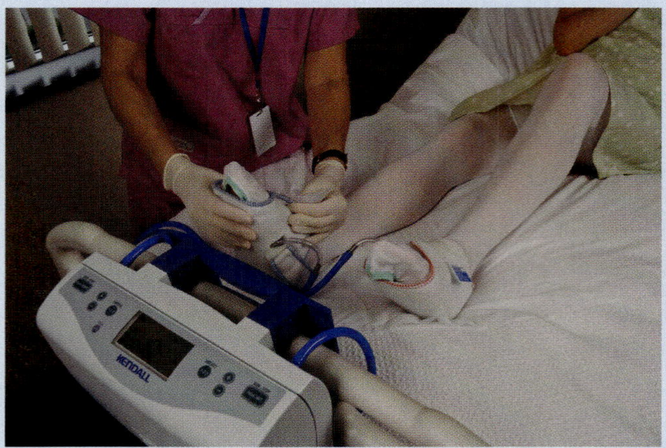

FIG 16-1 Venous plexus foot pump with bedside controls. (Courtesy Tyco Healthcare Group LP.)

Procedural Steps

1. Identify patient using two identifiers (e.g., name and birthday or name and account number), according to facility policy.
2. Assess patient for risk factors in Virchow's triad:
   a. Hypercoagulability (i.e., clotting disorders [laboratory test results], fever, dehydration)
   b. Venous wall abnormalities (i.e., history of orthopedic surgery, varicose veins, atherosclerosis)
   c. Blood stasis (i.e., immobility, obesity, pregnancy)
3. Observe for contraindications for use of elastic stockings or SCDs:
   a. Dermatitis or open skin lesions
   b. Recent skin graft
   c. Decreased arterial circulation in lower extremities as evidenced by cyanotic, cool extremities or gangrenous conditions affecting the lower limbs
4. Assess condition of patient's skin and circulation to the legs (i.e., presence of pedal pulses, edema, discoloration of skin, skin temperature, capillary refill, lesions, cuts).
5. Obtain health care provider order.
6. **See Standard Protocol (inside front cover).**
7. Explain procedure and reason for applying elastic stockings and SCDs.
8. Position patient in supine position. Elevate head of bed to comfortable level. Use tape measure to measure patient's leg to determine proper elastic stocking length/size, and SCD size.
9. *Option:* Apply a small amount of powder or cornstarch to legs provided that patient does not have sensitivity to either.
10. Apply elastic stocking:
    a. Turn elastic stocking inside out by placing one hand into the sock, holding toe of sock with other hand, and pulling. Pull until reaching the heel (see illustration).

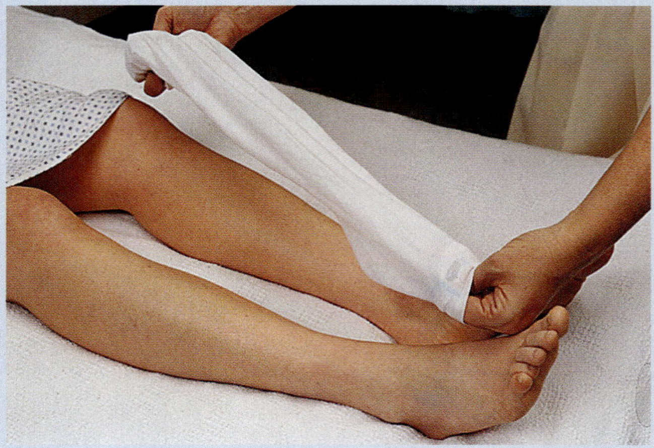

STEP 10a Turn stocking inside out; hold toe and pull through.

b. Place patient's toes into foot of elastic stocking, making sure that sock is smooth (see illustration).

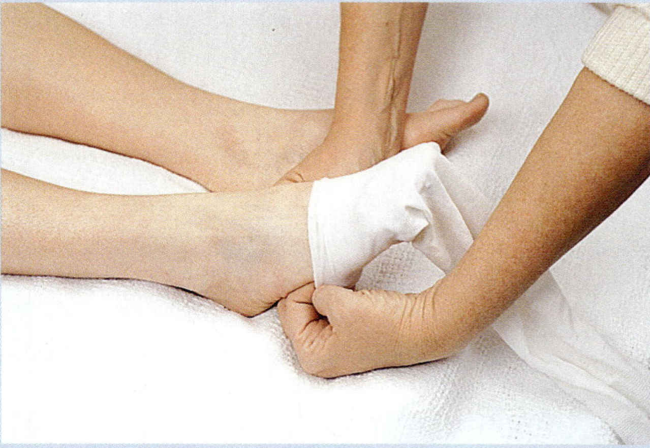

STEP 10b Place toes into foot of stocking.

c. Slide remaining portion of sock over patient's foot up to the heel, making sure that the toes are covered. Make sure that foot fits into the toe and heel position of the sock. Sock will now be right side out (see illustration).

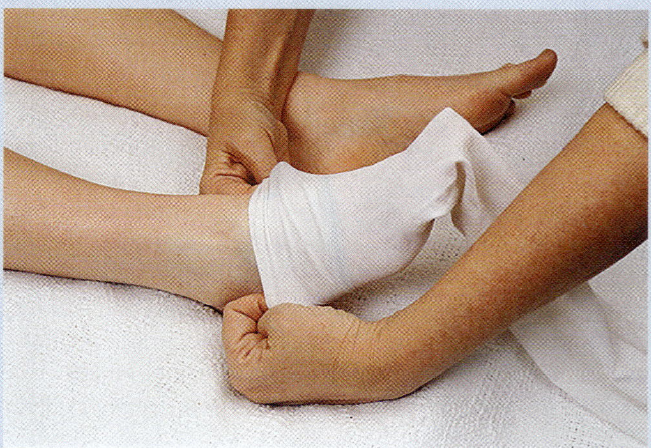

STEP 10c Slide remaining portion of sock over foot.

d. Slide sock up over patient's calf until sock is completely extended. Be sure that sock is smooth and that no ridges or wrinkles are present (see illustration).

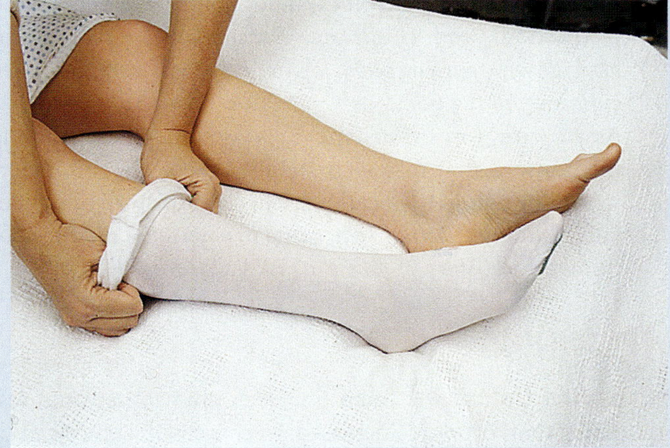

STEP 10d Slide sock up leg until completely extended.

e. Instruct patient not to roll socks partially down because constricting ring around leg can occlude circulation.

11. Apply SCD sleeve(s):
   a. Remove SCD sleeves from plastic cover; unfold and flatten.
   b. Arrange SCD sleeve under patient's leg according to leg position indicated on inner lining of sleeve.
   c. Place patient's leg on SCD sleeve. Back of ankle should line up with ankle marking on inner lining of sleeve.
   d. Position back of knee with popliteal opening on the sleeve (see illustration).

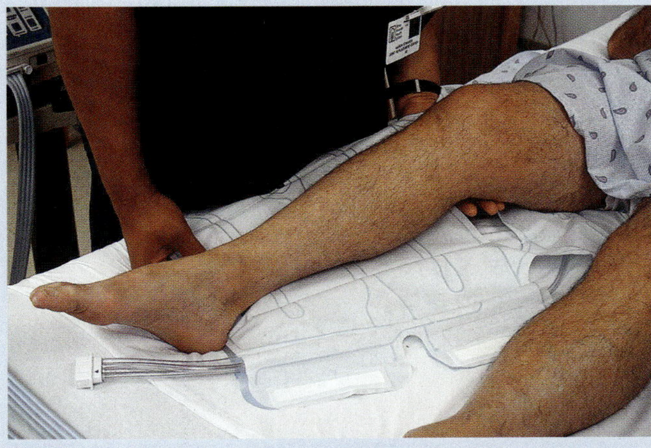

STEP 11d Position back of patient's knee with the popliteal opening.

e. Wrap SCD sleeve securely around patient's leg. Check fit of SCD sleeve by placing two fingers between patient's leg and sleeve (see illustration).

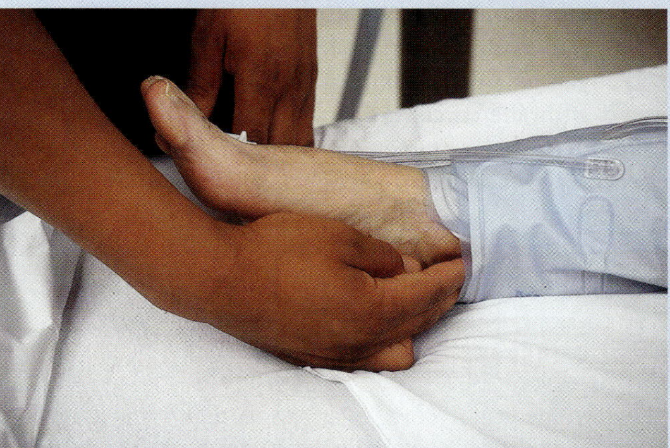

STEP 11e Check fit of sequential compression device sleeve.

f. Attach SCD sleeve connector to plug on mechanical unit. Arrows on connector line up with arrows on plug from mechanical unit (see illustration).

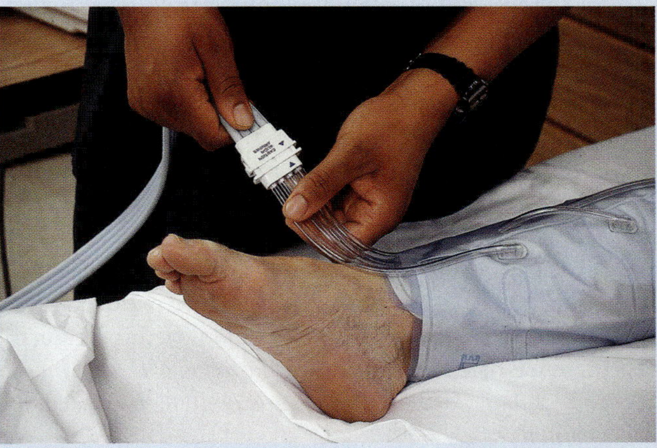

STEP 11f Align arrows when connecting to mechanical unit.

g. Turn mechanical unit on. Green light indicates that unit is functioning. Monitor functioning SCD through one full cycle of inflation and deflation.

12. **See Completion Protocol (inside front cover).**
13. Remove elastic stockings or SCD sleeves at least once per shift (e.g., long enough to inspect skin on leg and foot for irritation or breakdown).

SKILL 16.1   ASSISTING WITH AMBULATION

In the normal walking posture, the head is erect; the cervical, thoracic, and lumbar vertebrae are aligned; the hips and knees have slight flexion; and the arms swing freely. Illness, surgery, injury, advanced age, and prolonged bed rest can reduce activity tolerance and affect the ability to maintain a normal postural stance and balance, so assistance is required. Temporary or permanent damage to the musculoskeletal or nervous system may require use of an assistive device, such as a cane, crutches, or walker (see Skill 16.2). Patients with altered cardiovascular or respiratory function or prolonged bed rest may experience activity intolerance evidenced by chest pain, dizziness, diaphoresis, abnormal heart rate response, dyspnea, orthostatic hypotension, or fatigue. For this reason, it is important to monitor a patient during ambulation.

ASSESSMENT

1. Review medical record to assess patient's most recent activity experience, including distance ambulated, tolerance of activity, balance, and gait. *Rationale: This facilitates realistic planning and identifies degree of assistance needed.*
2. Determine the best time to ambulate, taking into consideration other scheduled activities such as bathing. *Rationale: Rest is necessary after activities that require exertion and after meals. Ambulating 30 minutes after analgesic administration improves patient's tolerance.*
3. Check the availability of handrails on the walls for patient's safety.
4. Assess patient's physical readiness:
   a. Assess baseline resting heart rate, blood pressure and respirations before beginning ambulation. *Rationale: Comparison of vital signs after ambulation with baseline values determines patient's activity tolerance and whether patient is experiencing orthostatic hypotension.*
   b. If patient's strength and endurance have been affected, assess range of motion (ROM) lower extremities, muscle strength, coordination and whether there is presence of foot deformities. *Rationale: Determine if patient has flexibility and muscle strength needed to ambulate safely.*
   c. Assess patient's comfort level (using pain scale 0 to 10). *Rationale: Patient may be in pain or fear pain resulting from exercise. If necessary, administer analgesic 30 to 60 minutes before exercise.*

   d. Review health care provider's order for mobility restrictions associated with condition. Also, determine if his or her weight is an issue in ambulation. *Rationale: Determines degree of assistance patient needs. For safety, another person may be needed initially to assist with patient ambulation.*
5. Assess patient's motivation and ability to understand instructions and cooperate. *Rationale: Comparing this activity with patient plans for the home environment often enhances motivation.*
6. Assess risk for orthostatic hypotension by identifying medications that may alter stability, including antihypertensive or opioid medications. Check for history of patient falls. *Rationale: Drugs may cause hypotension, dizziness, or instability. History of falls is a risk factor for falls.*

PLANNING

Expected Outcomes focus on developing activity and rest patterns that support increased tolerance of activity. It is essential that you individualize these to each patient's needs and abilities.

1. Patient ambulates without episode of injury.
2. Patient ambulates without excessive fatigue or dizziness.
3. Patient maintains respirations, pulse, and blood pressure within 10% of resting values.
4. Patient maintains erect posture while standing and walking.

Delegation and Collaboration

The skill of assisting the patient with ambulation can be delegated to nursing assistive personnel (NAP). The nurse instructs the NAP to:

- Adapt skill for specific patient such as obtaining an intravenous (IV) pole for a patient with continuous IV fluids and use of visual aid (e.g., glasses).
- Observe and report back to nurse (e.g., the distance patient was able to ambulate without fatigue).

Equipment

- Robe or suitable clothing
- Nonskid footwear
- Portable IV pole (if needed)
- Transfer (gait) belt

IMPLEMENTATION *for* ASSISTING WITH AMBULATION

STEPS	RATIONALE
1. See Standard Protocol (inside front cover).	
2. Remove SCD if present.	Prevents patient from becoming tangled in cord.
3. Encourage patient to move slowly at own pace, maintain erect posture, and look straight ahead.	Reduces risk of losing balance, tripping, or falling.

> **SAFE PATIENT CARE** If patient is overweight, unstable, or fearful, determine the need for additional help or use a sit-to-stand assistive device before beginning.

4. Follow Skill 15.1, Step 2, for assisting patient to side of bed. With patient sitting, wait a few minutes and ask if he or she feels dizzy. Have patient dangle legs on side of bed and take a few deep breaths until dizziness subsides and balance is gained. Have patient move legs and feet while dangling (see illustration).

Allows a few minutes for circulation to equilibrate. Prevents orthostatic hypotension and potential injuries (Mayo Clinic, 2011). Pumping feet plantar flexion/dorsiflexion increases venous return to the heart and brain.

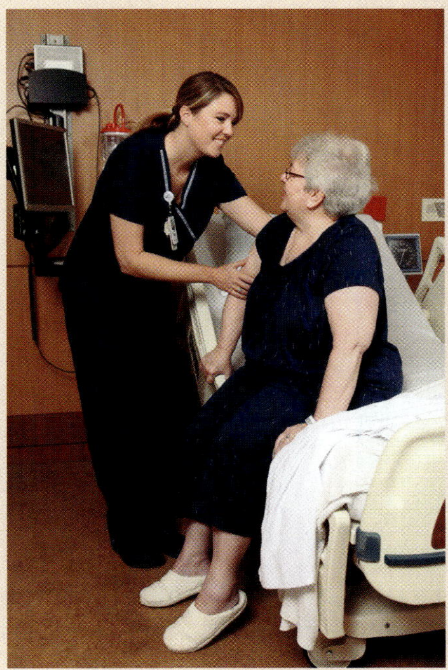

STEP 4 Patient dangling.

5. Decide with patient how far to ambulate. Assist patient with putting on shoes or slippers with nonskid soles.

Determines mutual goal. Shoes or slippers provide stable walking support.

6. Ask if patient feels dizzy or light-headed. If patient appears light-headed, have patient lie back down and recheck blood pressure.

Allows you to detect orthostatic hypotension before ambulation begins and determine if there is a need to postpone ambulation.

7. Apply transfer (gait) belt around patient's waist. Be sure belt is snug but not too tight.

Transfer belt allows you to maintain stability of patient during ambulation and reduces risk of falling.

8. Assist patient to stand at the bedside. Encourage patient to stand fully erect with shoulders back and looking ahead (not at the floor).

Standing at bedside allows patient opportunity to stabilize before ambulating.

9. If patient is unstable, seat him or her in chair or return to bed immediately. May need use of mechanical lift.

Provides added stability. Lift provides maximum safety for both patient and caregiver if patient is unstable.

10. If patient has an IV line, place the IV pole on the same side as the site of infusion and instruct patient where to hold and push the pole while ambulating.

Prevents accidental pulling on IV catheter.

11. If a Foley catheter is present, patient or nurse carries the bag below the level of the bladder and prevents tension on the tubing.

Prevents reflux of urine from the bag back into bladder.

12. Stand on patient's strong side. Take a few steps, supporting patient with one arm grasping the gait belt and the other under the elbow of the flexed arm (see illustration). *Option:* Use ambulation lift or ceiling lift with gait harness for more dependent patients who are now walking for first time after being in bed.

This provides balance and facilitates lowering patient to the floor if he or she is unable to continue because of weakness or dizziness.

Continued

STEPS	RATIONALE

13. When ambulating in a hallway, position patient between yourself and the wall. Encourage patient to use handrails if available (see illustration).

14. See Completion Protocol (inside front cover).

The wall provides stable support for patients who start to fall away from nurse.

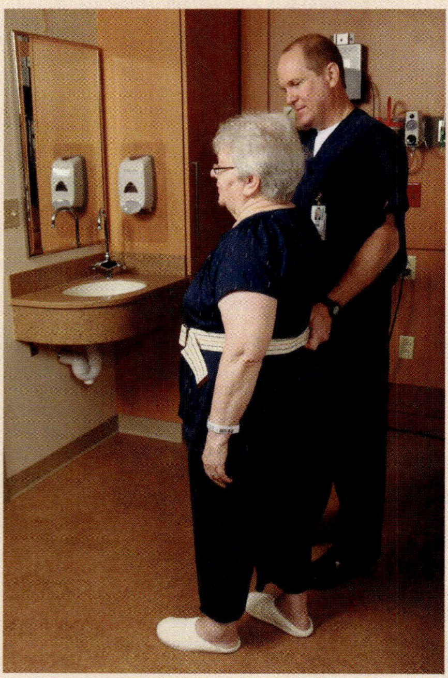

STEP 12 Nurse grasps transfer belt firmly.

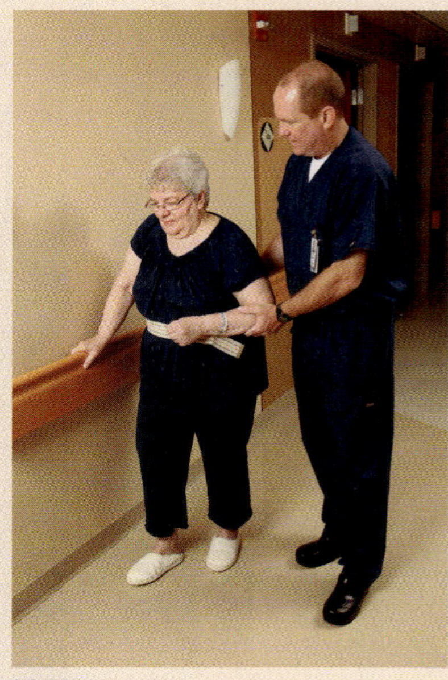

STEP 13 Nurse positions patient for use of hand rail.

EVALUATION

1. Observe ambulation and tolerance of ambulation, noting the frequency of rest periods.
2. Compare patient's heart rate, respiratory rate, and blood pressure with baseline values immediately after ambulation and again after 5 minutes of rest.
3. Observe patient's body alignment, posture, and balance while standing and walking.

Unexpected Outcomes and Related Interventions

1. Vital signs are altered: pulse more than 10% to 20% over resting rate or greater than 120 beats/min; systolic blood pressure shows orthostatic changes; or dyspnea, labored breathing, and wheezing are present. Patient reports feelings of excessive fatigue or weakness.
   a. Plan activity after adequate rest period.
   b. Pace activity to proceed more slowly and allow time to stop and rest at regular intervals. Sitting periodically may be helpful.
   c. Assistive devices such as a cane or walker may decrease energy required (see Skill 16.2).
2. Patient starts to fall.
   a. Call for help.
   b. Put both arms around patient's waist or grasp gait belt tightly (Fig. 16-2, *A*).
   c. Stand with feet apart for a broad base of support (see Fig. 16-2, *B*).
   d. Extend one leg and let patient slide against it to the floor. *Caution:* If patient is heavy, do not risk personal injury.
   e. Bend knees and lower your body as patient slides to the floor (see Fig. 16-2, *C*).
   f. Stay with patient until assistance arrives to help lift patient to wheelchair.

Recording and Reporting

- Record and report distance ambulated, patient's tolerance, any changes in vital signs, and onset of pain.

Sample Documentation

1300   Ambulated 100 feet in hall with assistance of one. Gait steady. States, "I am so tired. I don't know if I can make it back to my room." BP 160/82, HR 120, RR 20. Placed in wheelchair.

1305   Back in bed with assistance. BP 145/78, HR 92, RR 12. Denies dizziness.

Special Considerations
Geriatric

- Older patients are often fearful of falling when ambulatory, especially if they have fallen previously. This fear

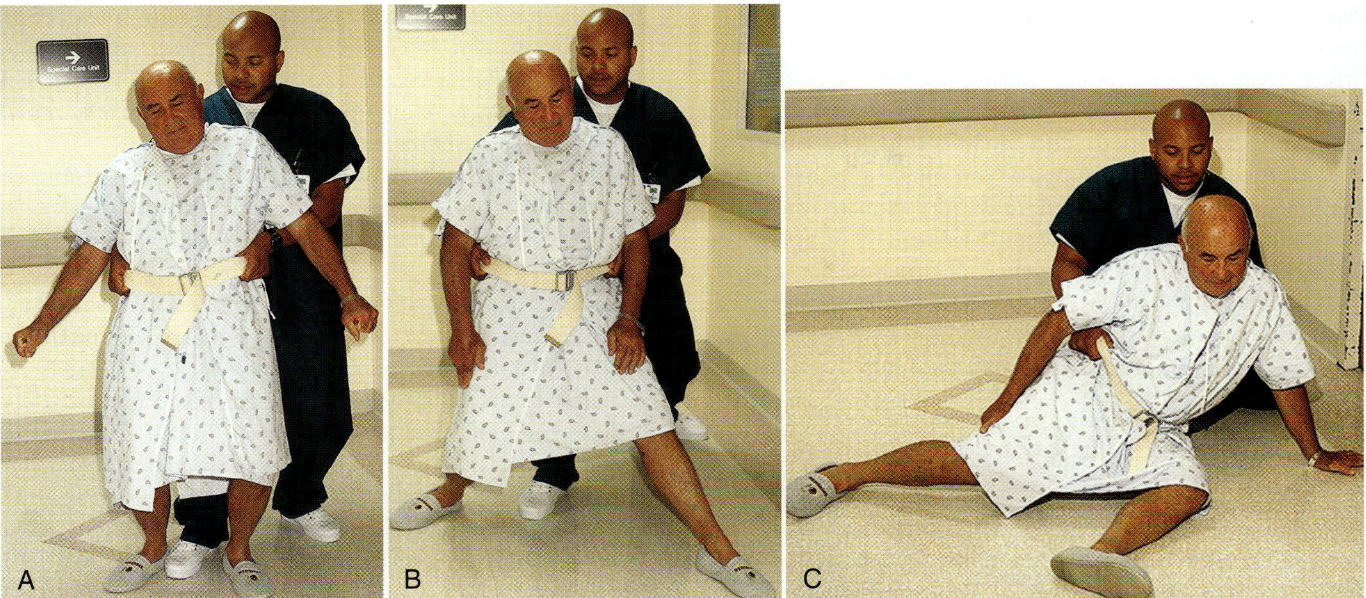

FIG 16-2 A, Stand with feet apart to provide broad base of support. **B,** Extend one leg and let patient slide against it to the floor. **C,** Bend knees to lower body as patient slides to floor.

causes a person to move less often, which causes greater problems with gait. Encouragement, reassurance, and assistance from family or caregiver decrease anxiety. Older adults may need more time in the morning to resume activity.

Pediatric

For children, immobility is one of the most difficult aspects of an illness. Physical activity is essential for physical growth and development (Hockenberry and Wilson, 2013).

SKILL 16.2 TEACHING USE OF CANES, CRUTCHES, AND WALKERS

Assistive devices such as canes, crutches, and walkers are recommended for patients who cannot bear full weight on one or more joints of the lower extremities. Other indications for use are instability, poor balance, or pain in weight bearing. The benefits of using an assistive device include reduction in risk of falling (Touhy and Jett, 2012). However, an assistive device can be a risk for falling if the device is not used correctly. It is important to know a patient's weight-bearing status, any specific movement precautions, and the type of device ordered by the health care provider. The nurse collaborates with the physical therapist to help the patient use the assistive device correctly and safely.

Non–weight-bearing status requires a patient to support weight on the assistive device and the unaffected limb. The affected leg is kept off the floor at all times. Partial or touch-down weight bearing is similar to that for non–weight bearing status, but either limb can be advanced initially. Partial weight bearing more closely approximates normal walking except that less weight is placed on the affected limb. Total weight bearing allows a patient to distribute equal weight between each limb with minimal weight on the assistive device. Muscle-strengthening exercises such as knee-and-foot extension (kicking leg straight out while sitting in a chair) or hip flexion (marching while sitting in a chair) and walking in parallel bars help a patient increase strength and confidence before using an assistive device.

An assistive device should be kept in good working condition. Often patients bring assistive devices with them to the hospital. As a home health nurse, you need to teach patients and family caregivers how to check the condition of their devices routinely. Rubber tips on the ends of assistive devices prevent slipping. Be sure that the tips are not cracked; otherwise they need replacing. Examine the condition of an assistive device to be sure that there are no bent parts, missing screws, or worn hand grips.

Teach the patient to lift rather than slide a device to reduce the possibility of catching the tips, which could cause the user to lose balance, trip, or fall. Personnel should attend to a patient when using an assistive device until they are assured that the patient's understanding and strength are sufficient for safe solo ambulation. Observing unaccompanied patients on their walks may reveal a need for additional or continued reminders about the proper way to stand, the amount of weight permitted, or the distance covered. Talk to the patient about risks for falls. Let patients who have a fear of falling know that they can regain confidence with practice.

CANES

Canes are lightweight, easily movable devices designed to increase a person's security and balance by broadening the base of support. Use of a cane eases the strain on weight-bearing joints. Canes also absorb or take the body weight when necessary for mobility during partial weight-bearing periods. Three types of commonly used canes are the standard crook, tripod, and quad cane. The standard crook provides the least support, and quad canes are useful for patients who have a partial or complete paralysis. Selection of the proper cane requires assessment of a patient's balance, strength, and confidence. Instruction for use of cane-assisted ambulation is essential. When canes are used unilaterally, they are most often used on a person's strong side and are advanced forward with the injured or affected limb.

CRUTCHES

Crutches are wooden or metal staffs that reach from the ground almost to the axilla. They remove weight from one or both legs. Persons will use one or two crutches as aids for ambulation. Crutches are used when a person needs to transfer more weight to their arms than is possible with a cane. The user's proficiency varies with factors such as age, condition, degree or extent of injury, and musculoskeletal functions. Crutches may be a temporary aid for persons with sprains, in a cast, or following surgical treatments. Crutches may be used routinely and continuously by patients with congenital or acquired musculoskeletal anomalies, neuromuscular weakness, or paralysis. There are three types of crutches: axillary (the most common), Lofstrand, and platform. Lofstrand crutches have a handgrip and a metal band that fits around a patient's forearm. Patients who are unable to bear weight on their wrists use a platform crutch, which has a horizontal trough for resting the forearm and wrist and a vertical hand grip.

WALKERS

A walker is an extremely lightweight, movable device that stands about waist high. It consists of an aluminum or metal alloy frame with handgrips, four widely placed sturdy legs, and one open side. Because it has a wide base of support, a walker provides great stability and security. Heights and weights are adjustable for individual needs. Other versions are available in addition to a standard walker: a foldable version, a version with a fold-down seat, and a version with wheels on the front legs. Before using a walker, a patient should understand the correct way to stand and advance the walker, the specific amount of weight bearing permitted, and how to use and care for the walker.

ASSESSMENT

1. Review patient's medical record, including medical history, previous activity level, and current activity order, including type of gait. *Rationale: Reveals patient's current and previous health status and limitations.*

2. Assess patient's physical readiness: vital signs; presence of confusion; and orientation to time, place, and person. *Rationale: Baseline vital signs offer a means of comparison after exercise. Level of orientation or confusion may reveal risk for fall or ability to cooperate.*

3. Assess ability to bear weight, ROM, balance, and muscle strength or the presence of foot deformities. *Rationale: Determines if assistance is needed for patient to ambulate safely.*

4. Assess patient for any visual, perceptual, or sensory deficits. *Rationale: Determines if patient can use assistive device safely and how much direction is needed.*

5. Assess environment for potential threats to patient safety (e.g., bed brake, bed position, objects in pathway). Ensure that floor is dry and area is well lit. *Rationale: Provides for a safe, clutter-free environment.*

6. Assess patient for discomfort. *Rationale: Determines if patient needs prescribed analgesic before exercise.*

7. Assess patient's understanding of technique of ambulation to be used. *Rationale: Allows patient to verbalize concerns and assesses need for direction.*

8. Assess patient's fall risks (e.g., vision, elimination problems, gait problems, or loss of sensation) (see Chapter 4). *Rationale: Determines if patient has other conditions that need to be addressed before attempting ambulation.*

PLANNING

Expected Outcomes focus on improving mobility, minimizing activity intolerance, preventing risk for injury, minimizing fatigue, and improving patient's knowledge.

1. Patient demonstrates correct use of assistive device, gait pattern, and weight-bearing status.
2. Patient rates discomfort or fatigue as 4 or less on a scale of 0 to 10 during ambulation.
3. Patient performs activities with return of vital signs to baseline 3 to 5 minutes after rest.
4. Patient independently performs all ADLs using assistive device safely.

Delegation and Collaboration

Teaching the patient the use of assistive devices may not be delegated to nursing assistive personnel (NAP). The skill of accompanying patients while ambulating with assistive devices can be delegated to NAP. The nurse instructs the NAP to:

- Adapt skill for specific patients such as weight-bearing status.
- Observe and report back to nurse episodes of dizziness or fatigue.

Equipment

- Ambulation device (cane, crutches, walker)
- Well-fitting, nonskid flat shoes or slippers
- Robe; well-fitting pants or dress
- Transfer (gait) belt

IMPLEMENTATION *for* TEACHING USE OF CANES, CRUTCHES, AND WALKERS

STEPS	RATIONALE

1. See Standard Protocol (inside front cover).

> **SAFE PATIENT CARE** Ensure that surface patient will walk on is flat, clean, dry, and well lit. Remove objects that obstruct the pathway.

2. Prepare patient for procedure.

   a. Explain reasons for exercise, and demonstrate specific gait technique to patient or family caregiver.

> Teaching and demonstration enhance learning, reduce anxiety, and encourage cooperation.
> Combination of assistive walking and conversation may reduce decline in functional ability and improve mood (Touhy and Jett, 2012).

> **SAFE PATIENT CARE** Be extremely cautious if the patient has IV tubing or a Foley catheter. Obtain an IV pole with wheels that can be pushed as the patient walks. Urinary catheter drainage bags must stay below the level of the bladder; a second person may be needed to assist with IV pole or drainage bag.

   b. Decide with patient how far to ambulate.

> Determines mutual goal.

   c. Schedule ambulation around patient's other activities. Apply patient's glasses (if worn). Provide analgesic 30 to 60 minutes before ambulating if patient is experiencing pain. **Caution:** Do not administer an analgesic that makes patient feel dizzy.

> Helps minimize patient fatigue. Ensures patient can see walking path. Minimizes pain during ambulation.

   d. Begin from side of bed with bed in low position or with patient in a chair. Follow steps in Skill 16.1 to be sure patient is not dizzy before rising to a standing position. Help patient put on well-fitting, flat shoes or nonskid slippers.

> Reduces risk of injury from orthostatic hypotension.

3. Apply transfer (gait) belt. Gait belt encircles patient's waist. Assist patient to standing position and observe balance and check for dizziness.

> Providing constant contact by nurse reduces risk of fall or injury.

4. While standing next to patient's side, have patient take a few steps. When using a cane, stand next to patient's weak side with the device on the strong side. In the case of a walker and crutches, grasp the gait belt and stand behind and to the side of patient. If patient has weakness or paralysis, stand on his or her strong side.

> Position of the nurse offers stability. Nurse can pull patient toward strong side in case of a loss of balance.

5. Take a few steps forward with patient standing straight and looking straight ahead. Assess patient's strength and balance.

> Ensures that patient has satisfactory strength and balance to continue.

6. If patient becomes weak or dizzy, return him or her to bed or chair, whichever is closer.

> Prevents patient from falling to floor.

7. Recheck that assistive device is the appropriate height and has rubber tips.

> Rubber tips increase surface tension and reduce the risk of the device slipping.

8. *Cane (same steps are taught for standard, tripod, or quad cane):*

   a. Have patient hold cane on strong side 10 to 15 cm (4 to 6 inches) to side of foot. Cane extends from greater trochanter to floor while cane is held 15 cm (6 inches) from foot. Allow approximately 15- to 30-degree elbow flexion.

> Offers most support when on stronger side of body. Cane and weaker leg work together with each step. If cane is too short, patient has difficulty supporting weight and is bent over and uncomfortable. As weight is taken on by hands and affected leg is lifted off floor, complete extension of elbow is necessary. Cane handle should fit comfortably in palm of hand, similar to a tight shoe (Touhy and Jett, 2012).

Continued

STEPS	RATIONALE

b. To begin, direct patient to place cane forward 15 to 25 cm (6 to 10 inches), keeping body weight on both legs.

Distributes body weight equally.

c. Move involved leg forward, even with the cane (see illustration). The cane and injured leg swing and strike the ground at the same time.

Body weight is supported by cane and strong leg.

d. Advance strong leg 15 to 25 cm (6 to 10 inches) past cane.

Aligns patient's center of gravity. Returns patient body weight to equal distribution.

e. Move involved leg forward, even with strong leg.

f. Repeat steps. Once comfortable, have patient advance cane and weak leg together.

9. *Crutches:*

a. Crutch measurement includes three areas: patient's height, distance between crutch pad and axilla, and angle of elbow flexion. Measurements may be taken with patient standing or lying down. Make sure shoes are on before performing measurements.

Measurement promotes optimal support and stability. Radial nerves that pass under axilla are superficial. If crutch is too long, it places pressure on axilla. Injury to nerve causes paralysis of elbow and wrist extensors, commonly called crutch palsy. If crutch is too long, shoulders are forced upward, and patient cannot push body off the ground. If ambulation device is too short, patient is bent over and uncomfortable and less stable.

> **SAFE PATIENT CARE** Instruct patient to report any tingling or numbness in upper torso. This may mean that crutches are being used incorrectly or that they are the wrong size.

(1) *Standing:* Position crutches with crutch tips at point 15 cm (6 inches) to side and 15 cm (6 inches) in front of patient's feet. Position crutch pads 5 cm (2 inches) below axilla. Two or three fingers should fit between top of crutch and axilla (see illustration).

Provides broad base of support.

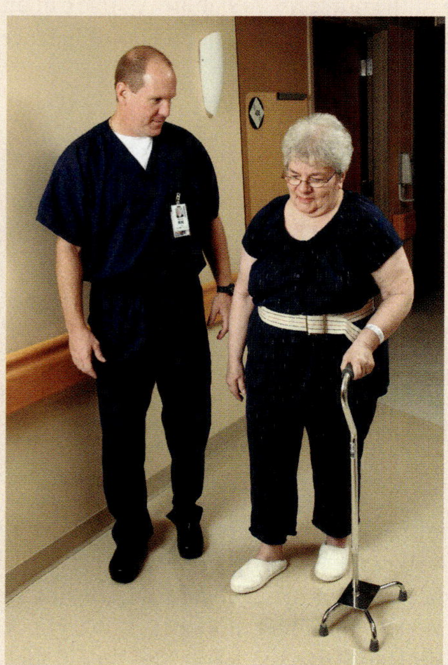

STEP 8c Patient moves involved leg forward even with the cane.

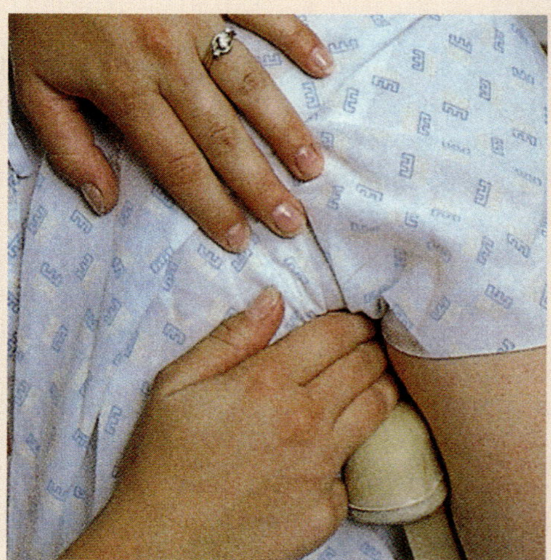

STEP 9a(1) Crutch pad is 2 to 3 finger widths under axilla.

STEPS	RATIONALE

(2) *Supine:* Crutch pad is approximately 5 cm (2 inches) or 2 to 3 finger widths under axilla, with crutch tips positioned 15 cm (6 inches) lateral to patient's heel (see illustration).

(3) Verify elbow flexion with a goniometer (see illustration). Adjust the handgrip so that patient's elbow is flexed 15 to 20 degrees.

Low handgrips cause radial nerve damage. High handgrips cause patient's elbow to be sharply flexed, decreasing strength and stability of arms.

b. To use crutches, patient supports self with hands and arms. Strength in arm and shoulder muscles, ability to balance body in upright position, and stamina are necessary. Type of crutch gait depends on amount of weight patient is able to support with one or both legs.

c. Have patient stand up from a sitting position.

(1) Move to edge of chair, with strong leg slightly under chair seat.

(2) Place both crutches in the hand on the involved side. If chair has armrests and is heavy and solid enough to avoid tipping, patient uses one armrest and both crutches for bracing while rising. (If the chair is lightweight, patient should use both armrests for even bracing.)

Patients can lose balance or tip chairs with uneven or one-sided pressure.

(3) Push down on the crutch hand rests while raising the body to a standing position. Switch one crutch to strong side.

d. Assist patient to walk with prescribed crutch gait (darkened areas in illustrations indicate moving foot).

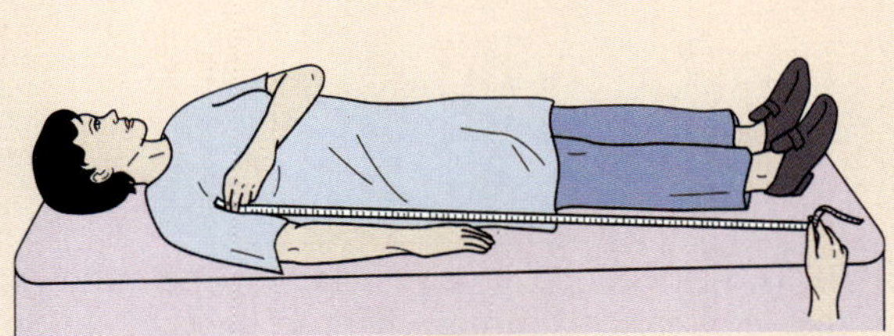

STEP 9a(2) Measuring length of crutch.

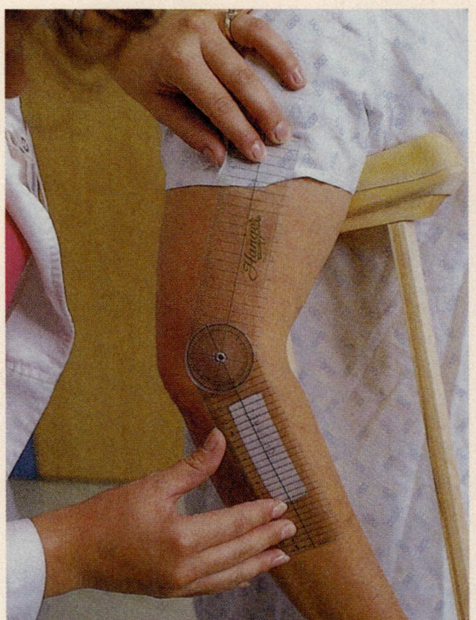

STEP 9a(3) Goniometer determines elbow flexion.

Continued

<table>
<tr><td>**STEPS**</td><td>**RATIONALE**</td></tr>
</table>

(1) Four-point gait:

   (a) Begin in tripod position (see illustration) with crutches placed 15 cm (6 inches) in front and 15 cm (6 inches) to side of each foot. Posture should be erect head and neck, straight vertebrae, and extended hips and knees.

   (b) Move right crutch forward 10 to 15 cm (4 to 6 inches) (see illustration).

   (c) Move left foot forward to level of left crutch (see illustration).

   (d) Move left crutch forward 10 to 15 cm (4 to 6 inches) (see illustration).

   (e) Move right foot forward to level of right crutch (see illustration).

   (f) Repeat sequence.

Most stable of crutch gaits, provides at least three points of support at all times. Requires weight bearing on both legs. Often used for paralysis, as in spastic children with cerebral palsy (Hockenberry and Wilson, 2013). May also be used for arthritic patients. Tripod position improves balance by providing wider base of support.

Crutch and foot position are similar to arm and foot position during normal walking.

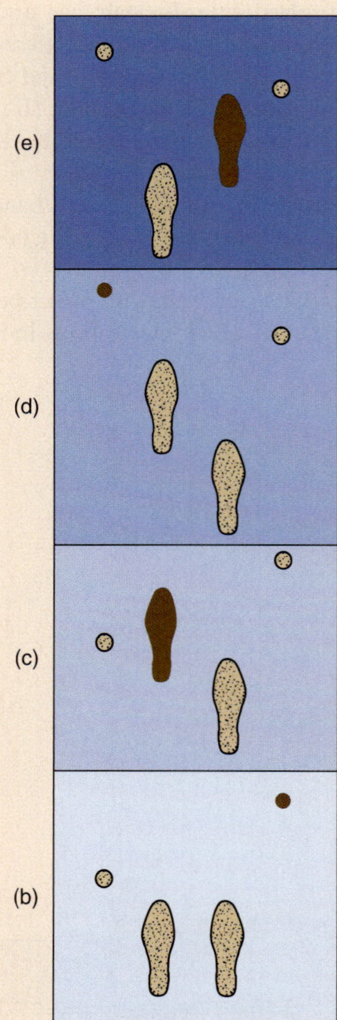

STEP 9d(1)(b-e) Four-point gait. Solid feet and crutch tips show foot and crutch tip movement in each of the four phases (read from bottom to top). Right tip moves forward *(b)*. Left foot moves toward left crutch *(c)*. Left crutch tip moves forward *(d)*. Right foot moves toward right crutch *(e)*.

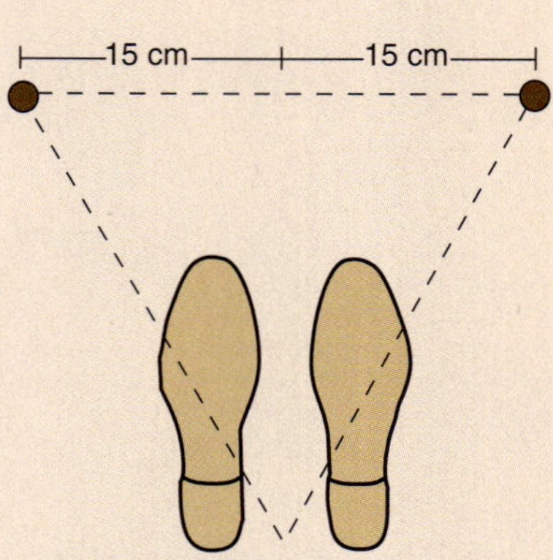

STEP 9d(1)(a) Tripod position.

STEPS	RATIONALE

(2) Three-point gait:

   (a) Begin in tripod position with weight placed on strong leg (see illustration).

   (b) Advance both crutches and involved leg (see illustration).

   (c) Move stronger leg forward (see illustration).

   (d) Repeat sequence.

Requires patient to bear all weight on one foot. Weight is placed on strong leg and then on both crutches. Involved leg does not touch ground during early phase of three-point gait. Useful for patients with broken leg or sprained ankle. Tripod position provides wide base of support.

(3) Two-point gait:

   (a) Begin in tripod position (see illustration) with partial weight bearing on both feet.

   (b) Move left crutch and right foot forward (see illustration).

   (c) Move right crutch and left foot forward (see illustration).

   (d) Repeat sequence.

Requires at least partial weight bearing on each foot. Is faster than four-point gait. Requires more balance because only two points support body at one time. Tripod position provides wide base of support.

Crutch movements are similar to arm movement during normal walking.

(4) Swing-to gait:

   (a) Begin in tripod position with partial weight bearing on both feet.

   (b) Move both crutches forward.

   (c) Lift and swing legs to crutches, letting crutches support body weight.

   (d) Repeat two previous steps.

Frequently used by patients whose lower extremities are paralyzed or who wear weight-supporting braces on their legs. This is the easier of the two swinging gaits. It requires the ability to bear body weight partially on both legs.

(5) Swing-through gait:

   (a) Start in tripod position with partial weight bearing on both feet.

   (b) Move both crutches forward.

Requires that patient have the ability to sustain partial weight bearing on both feet.

Increases base of support so that when the body swings forward, patient is moving the center of gravity toward the additional support provided by crutches.

   (c) Lift and swing legs through and beyond crutches. Repeat sequence.

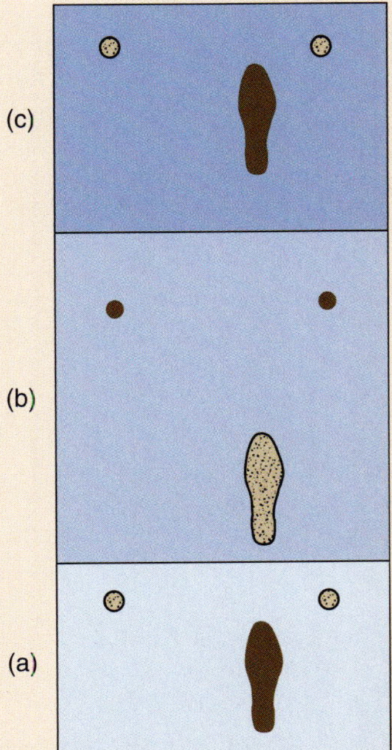

STEP 9d(2)(a-c) Three-point gait with weight borne on unaffected right leg. Solid foot and crutch tips show weight bearing in each phase (read bottom to top).

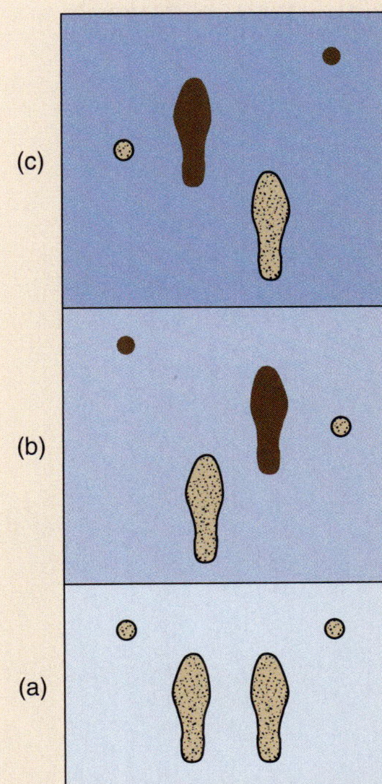

STEP 9d(3)(a-c) Two-point gait. Solid areas indicate weight-bearing leg and crutch tips (read bottom to top).

Continued

(6) *Climbing stairs with crutches, non–weight-bearing, one leg:*

(a) Begin in tripod position.

Improves patient's balance by providing wider base of support.

(b) Patient transfers body weight to crutches (see illustration).

Prepares patient to transfer weight to unaffected leg when ascending first stair.

(c) Advance strong leg onto the step (see illustration).

Crutch adds support to affected leg. Patient then shifts weight from crutches to unaffected leg.

(d) Align both crutches with the strong leg on the step (see illustration).

Maintains balance and provides wide base of support.

(e) Repeat sequence until patient reaches top of stairs.

Improves patient's balance by providing wider base of support.

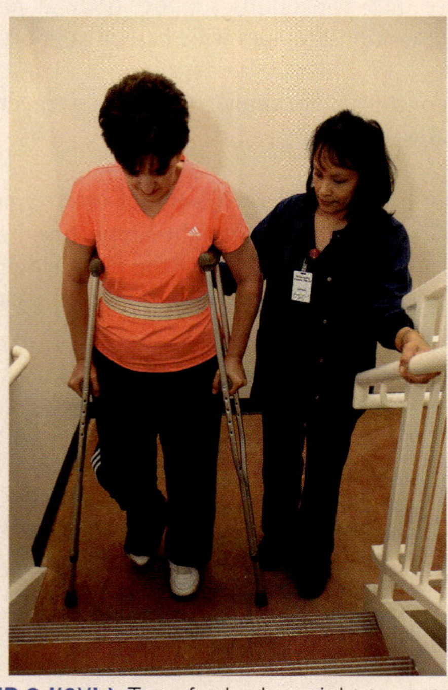

STEP 9d(6)(b) Transfer body weight to crutches.

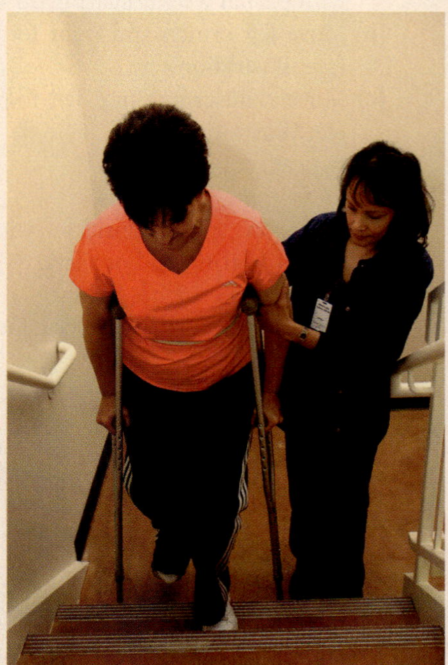

STEP 9d(6)(c) Advance unaffected leg to stair.

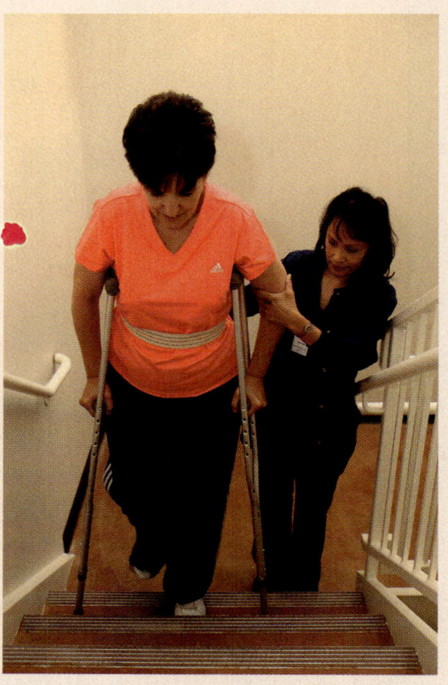

STEP 9d(6)(d) Align crutches with unaffected leg.

STEPS	RATIONALE

(7) Descending stairs with crutches, non–weight-bearing, one leg:

    (a) Begin in tripod position.

Prepares patient to release support of body weight maintained by crutches.

    (b) Transfer body weight to strong leg.

Maintains patient's balance and base of support.

    (c) Move crutches to stair below and instruct patient to transfer body weight to crutches and move involved leg forward.

    (d) Move strong leg to stair below and align with crutches.

    (e) Repeat sequence until patient reaches bottom step.

Non–weight-bearing patient should be able to balance on one leg before transferring both crutches to the same hand.

(8) Sitting in a chair:

    (a) Transfer both crutches to the same hand and transfer weight to crutches and unaffected leg. Feel back of chair against legs.

Provides stable base of support.

    (b) Grasp arm of chair with free hand and extend affected leg out while lowering into chair (see illustration).

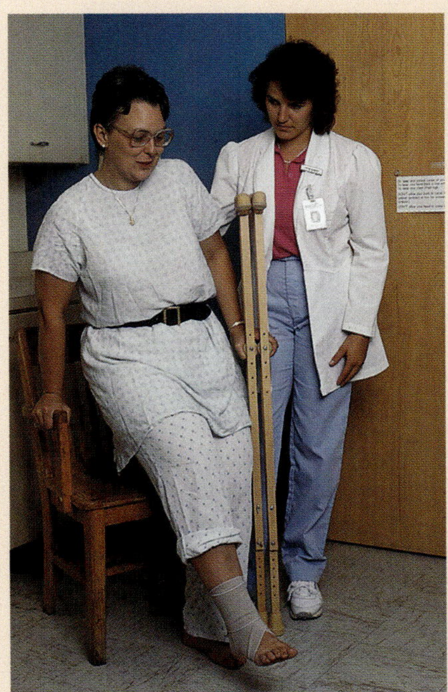

STEP 9d(8)(b) Grasp arm of chair with free hand.

10. Walker:

    a. When patient relaxes the arms at the side of the body, the top of the walker should line up with the crease on the inside of the wrist. Elbows should be flexed about 15 to 30 degrees when standing with walker, with hands on handgrips.

Walkers without wheels must be picked up and moved forward. Patient must have sufficient strength to be able to move walker. A walker with wheels, which does not need to be picked up, is not as stable and may cause injury.

Continued

STEPS	RATIONALE

b. Assist patient in ambulating.

(**1**) Have patient stand in center of walker and grasp handgrips on upper bars.

Patient balances self before attempting to walk. Position provides broad base of support between walker and patient. Patient then moves center of gravity toward the walker. It is necessary to keep all four feet of the walker on the floor to prevent tipping the walker.

(**2**) Have patient lift walker, moving it 15 to 20 cm (6 to 8 inches) forward, making sure that all four feet of walker stay on the floor. Take a step forward with either foot. Follow through with the other foot (see illustration). *If patient has one-sided weakness:* After patient advances the walker, instruct him or her to step forward with the weaker leg, support self with the arms, and follow through with the strong leg. *If patient is unable to bear full weight on the involved leg:* After patient advances walker, have him or her step forward with the stronger leg while supporting weight on hands. Instruct patient not to advance the lower extremity past the front bar of the walker. Instruct the patient not to climb stairs with the walker (Touhy and Jett, 2012).

Moving 15 to 20 cm (6 to 8 inches) simulates normal distance of steps. Providing constant contact of all four walker feet with the floor reduces the risk of injury or fall. Advancing with weaker extremity allows patient to have maximal support of walker.

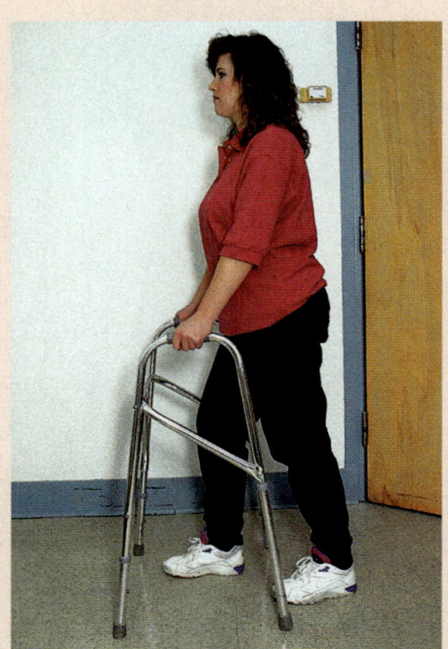

STEP 10b(2) Lift walker, move it 15 to 20 cm (6 to 8 inches), and take step forward.

11. Have patient take a few steps with the assistive device being used. If patient is hemiplegic (one-sided paralysis) or has hemiparesis (one-sided weakness), stand next to his or her strong side. Support patient by placing arm closest to patient on gait belt.

Ensures that patient has satisfactory strength and balance to continue.

12. Take a few steps forward with patient. Assess for strength and balance.

Allows patient to rest.

13. If patient becomes weak or dizzy, return to bed or chair, whichever is closer.

14. See Completion Protocol (inside front cover).

EVALUATION

1. Observe patient using assistive device.
2. Inspect hands and axillae for redness, swelling, or skin irritation caused by using assistive device.
3. Ask patient to rate level of discomfort or fatigue if present after ambulating.
4. Monitor patient for postural hypotension, increased heart rate, decreased blood pressure, increased respirations, or shortness of breath during and after ambulation.
5. Ask patient and family about the ease with which ADLs are performed using assistive device.
6. Use *Teach Back:* State to the patient: "I want to be sure you are comfortable using the assistive device. Can you demonstrate for me how you ambulate using your cane/walker/crutches?" Evaluates what the patient is able to explain or demonstrate. Revise your instruction now or develop plan for revised patient teaching to be implemented at an appropriate time if patient is not able to teach back correctly.

Unexpected Outcomes and Related Interventions

1. Patient is unable to ambulate correctly.
   a. Reassess patient for correct fit of assistive device.
   b. Review correct procedure for ambulation.
   c. Have added assistance nearby to ensure safety.
   d. Reassess comfort level.
   e. Reassess muscle strength in uninvolved extremities. Alternative device may be necessary.
   f. Obtain physical therapy referral for gait or additional strength training.
2. Patient becomes dizzy and light-headed when rising to sitting or standing position.
   a. Call for assistance.
   b. Have patient sit or lie down on nearest chair or bed.
   c. Assess patient's vital signs.
   d. Allow patient to rest thoroughly before resuming activity.
   e. Ask if patient is ready to continue.

Recording and Reporting

- Record type of gait patient used, weight-bearing status, amount of assistance required, tolerance of activity, and distance walked in progress notes. Document instructions given to patient and family.
- Record patient teaching and revise plan to ensure patient is ambulating correctly.
- Document your evaluation of patient learning.

- Immediately report any injury sustained during attempts to ambulate, alteration in vital signs, or inability to ambulate.

Sample Documentation

0900   Demonstrated correct use of cane. Ambulated 20 feet correctly using quad cane, standby assist of one, and partial weight bearing on right lower extremity. Requested pain pills. Rates pain in right knee at 6 (scale 0 to 10). Returned to bed. Administered Tylenol #2, 2 tablets PO.

0930   Resting quietly in bed. Rates pain in right knee at 2 (scale of 0 to 10).

Special Considerations
Pediatric

- If a child has been immobilized for a long time, perform upper body strengthening exercises to condition and strengthen arms and shoulders (Hockenberry and Wilson, 2013).
- For rehabilitation of a small child who has not yet learned to walk or who is unsteady, front-rolling or rear-rolling walkers are often used before progressing to special crutches (Hockenberry and Wilson, 2013).

Geriatric

- Assist the patient in obtaining a prescription for assistive devices; Medicare may cover up to 80% of the cost of the device (Touhy and Jett, 2012).
- Older adults with arthritis may require additional time in the morning before resuming activities.

Home Care

- Instruct patient on how to use the assistive device on various terrains (e.g., carpet, stairs, rough ground, inclines) and when it is unsafe to use the device.
- Instruct patient on how to maneuver around obstacles such as doors and how to use the aid when transferring (e.g., to and from a chair, toilet, tub, and car).
- Instruct patient and family caregiver in proper way to check that assistive device is functioning.
- Have family caregiver remove scatter rugs, electrical cords, and spills.
- Have patient use a backpack, fanny pack, or apron, or attach a "saddle bag" to patient's walker to carry objects. Caution patients not to overfill bag attached to walker to prevent forward tipping of walker.

CRITICAL THINKING EXERCISES

Case Study

A woman is preparing to be discharged the next day from the hospital after experiencing a heart attack. The patient lives in a single-family home with her husband and two cats. She gets short of breath and feels unsteady at times when walking and will require the use of an assistive device short-term for the first time in her life. During discharge planning with the nurse, the patient states that she wants to be as mobile as possible but has concerns about her ability to manage an assistive device.

1. It is determined that the patient will benefit from use of a cane. On what should initial teaching by the nurse focus? Select all that apply.
   1. Using the cane on her strong side
   2. Ensuring that walking surface is clean and dry
   3. Instructing patient to walk barefoot
   4. Avoiding flexion of elbow when ambulating
2. The patient's husband is concerned for his wife's safety during ambulation. The nurse gives him suggestions to help his wife be as mobile as possible in a safe manner. What should the nurse instruct the husband to do? Select all that apply.
   1. Give his wife an opioid analgesic just before ambulating.
   2. Encourage his wife to bend forward when walking.
   3. Schedule daily activities so there is time for rest between them.
   4. Have his wife dangle on side of bed before standing.
3. The NAP enters the room prepared to teach the patient how to ambulate with the cane. How should the nurse instruct the NAP?
   1. First demonstrate use of the cane for the NAP and leave the room.
   2. Tell the NAP the patient will practice alone first.
   3. Inform the NAP that the nurse must teach the patient how to use the cane.
   4. Watch the NAP as he teaches the patient to use the cane.

Review Questions

1. The nurse is presenting a health promotion program on exercise and mobility to a group of older adults who reside in single-family homes in their community. The older adults are on fixed incomes and are concerned that they have no options for exercise. Which activity should the nurse suggest?
   1. Join a local fitness club.
   2. Form a walking group.
   3. Organize a readers' club.
   4. Invest in home exercise equipment.
2. A patient has been experiencing difficulty with movement, loss of balance, and lack of muscle control. Which gait does the nurse instruct the patient to use for crutch walking?
   1. Four-point
   2. Three-point
   3. Two-point
   4. Swing-to

3. The nurse is assisting a patient to the side of the bed and recognizes that the patient is experiencing orthostatic hypotension. Which of the following signs and symptoms alert the nurse to this condition? Select all that apply.
   1. Pallor
   2. Bradycardia
   3. Nausea
   4. Dizziness
   5. Irritability
4. The nurse teaches a patient ROM exercises for the shoulder. For abduction, how high is the patient taught to raise the arm?
   1. 120 degrees
   2. 140 degrees
   3. 180 degrees
   4. 220 degrees
5. An 85-year-old man lives in an assisted living community. His health care provider wants this gentleman to increase his exercise plan. The nurse assesses his daily activities and determines that he prefers to watch TV all day. What measures can the nurse use to assist this patient to increase his activity? Select all that apply.
   1. Teach patient to increase range-of-motion exercises when he showers or dresses.
   2. Obtain a listing of exercise activities in the assisted living community.
   3. Work with the facility's fitness coordinator to identify other men in the same age-group who are exercising.
   4. Refer the man to the psychologist for counseling.
6. Which of the following activities may be delegated to nursing assistive personnel (NAP) related to assisting patients with ambulation?
   1. Checking a patient's medications to determine if they may influence the ability to ambulate independently.
   2. Instructing a patient about the correct use of a walker.
   3. Inspecting the environment for potential threats to patient safety.
   4. Evaluating a patient's ability to perform crutch walking.
7. Which situation is a contraindication for the use of elastic stockings?
   1. Prior use of stockings within 3 months
   2. Recent skin graft to the lower leg
   3. Increased circulation of lower extremities
   4. Immobility for more than 1 week
8. Place the following steps for climbing stairs with crutches in correct order.
   1. Align both crutches with unaffected leg on step.
   2. Stand in tripod position.
   3. Advance unaffected leg forward onto step.
   4. Transfer body weight to crutches.

9. The nurse has been given the responsibility to develop a safe patient handling program on her acute care unit. Which of the following factors should the nurse consider when developing this program? Select all that apply.
   1. Individual patient preferences
   2. Available assistive equipment
   3. Physical conditions of the unit's patients
   4. Potential communication barriers between care providers and patients

10. A 45-year-old woman is required to lay flat in bed following a surgical eye procedure. She complains to the nurse that her hips are not comfortable in this position. What ROM exercise can the nurse suggest the patient try?
    1. Reach her arm above her head
    2. Comb her hair
    3. Reach to her side
    4. Roll her feet inward

REFERENCES

Andrews PL, Habashi NM: Detecting, managing, and preventing pulmonary embolism, *American Nurse Today*, 2010. http://www.americannursetoday.com/assets/0/434/436/440/10986/10988/10992/11044/baddec9dfb494b93b8555ab20925cb8e.pdf. Accessed July 14, 2014.

Anthony M: Nursing assessment of deep vein thrombosis, *Medsurg Nurs* 22(2):95, 2013.

Campo M, et al: Effects of a safe patient handling program on rehabilitation outcomes, *Arch Phys Med Rehabil* 94(1):17, 2013.

Centers for Disease Control and Prevention (CDC): *Physical activity and health*, 2011. http://www.cdc.gov/physicalactivity/everyone/health/index.html. Accessed July 12, 2014.

Chui K, et al: Exercise. In Edelman CL, Mandle CL, Kudzma EC, editors: *Health promotion throughout the lifespan*, ed 8, St Louis, 2013, Mosby.

de Ruiter HP, Liaschenko J: To lift or not to lift: patient-handling practices, *AAOHN J* 59(8):337, 2011.

Edlin G, Golanty E: *Health and wellness*, ed 10, Sudbury, MA, 2010, Jones & Bartlett.

Harvey L, et al: Continuous passive motion following total knee arthroplasty in people with arthritis. *Cochrane Database of Systematic Reviews* 2:20134, 2014. DOI: 10.1002/1465188. CD004260.pub3.

Hockenberry MJ, Wilson D: *Essentials of pediatric nursing*, ed 9, St Louis, 2013, Mosby.

Martin G: *Patient information: Total knee replacement (arthroplasty) (beyond the basics)*, 2014. http://www.uptodate.com/contents/total-knee-replacement-arthroplasty-beyond-the-basics.

Mayo Clinic: *Orthostatic hypotension (postural hypotension): lifestyle and home remedies*, 2011. http://www.mayoclinic.com/health/orthostatic-hypotension/DS00997/DSECTION=lifestyle-and-home-remedies. Accessed July 12, 2014.

Meiner SE: *Gerontologic nursing*, ed 4, St Louis, 2011, Mosby.

Spencer C, Burke P: The impact of culture on pain management, *MedSurg Matters* 20(4):13, 2011.

The Joint Commission (TJC): *National Patient Safety Goals*, Oakbrook Terrace, IL, 2014, The Commission. Available at: http://www.jointcommission.org/standards_information/npsgs.aspx. Accessed July 12, 2014.

Touhy TA, Jett K: Mobility. In Ebersole P, et al, editors: *Toward healthy aging: human needs and nursing response*, ed 8, St Louis, 2012, Mosby.

Valbusa F, et al: Orthostatic hypotension in very old individuals living in nursing homes: the PARTAGE study, *J Hypertens* 30(1):53, 2012.

Trauma or disease affecting the musculoskeletal system requires immobilization, stabilization, and support to the affected body part. Traction, casts, and immobilization devices are used to accomplish these purposes and enhance the healing process.

Traction, casts, and immobilization devices are prescribed to correct or improve deformities or joint contractures. They are also used to treat a joint dislocation; reduce, immobilize, and align a fracture (Box 17-1); and prevent and manage muscle spasms. By controlling spasms and fractured bones, these devices prevent further soft tissue damage. Finally, preoperative and postoperative positioning and alignment, skeletal lengthening, and rest of a damaged joint can be managed using one or more of these devices.

Traction involves a pulling force applied through weights to a part of the body, while a second force, called countertraction, pulls in the opposite direction. Age, condition of the patient, and purpose of the traction determine the amount of weight on the pulling force. In straight or running traction, the force pulls against the long axis of the body, while the patient's body supplies countertraction. In balanced-suspension skeletal traction (BSST), the amount of force in the traction is equal to the amount of force in the countertraction. A sling or hammock and a system of weights attached to an over-bed frame support the affected part, while weight is attached to the pin or wire traversing the femoral bone.

Although there are many types of traction, there are six general principles of traction care (Brooker and Nicol, 2013), as follows:

1. Maintain the established line of pull
2. Maintain traction equipment
3. Maintain countertraction
4. Maintain continuous traction unless otherwise ordered
5. Maintain correct body alignment
6. Prevent friction and pressure on the skin

A second treatment method for immobilization involves the use of a cast. Applied externally, a cast immobilizes injured or deformed musculoskeletal tissues in proper position to promote healing. Tissue structures must be in an optimal position for healing when the cast is applied. An advantage of using a cast is that it permits early ambulation and in some cases partial weight bearing on the injured extremity.

A third treatment device used with a musculoskeletal injury or disorder is an orthotic device. These devices immobilize a body part, prevent deformity, protect against injury, relieve pain and muscle spasm, maintain position until healing is complete, and assist with function. Immobilization devices are applied externally to the body and are available in many variations ranging from arm slings to back braces and finger splints. They are made from various materials such as rubber, leather, metal, and plastics. Walker boots are a device that can be used to manage soft tissue injury, sprains, and stable toe and ankle fractures and promote early postoperative weight bearing for internal fixation with ligament tears. They provide musculoskeletal stabilization and support through the use of pneumatics. Research has demonstrated that there is no loss of stability when a walker boot is used (Hashim et al., 2012; Hyer et al., 2010).

BOX 17-1 TYPES OF FRACTURES

Closed fracture	Skin intact over fracture
Open or compound fracture	Skin punctured by bone ends
Comminuted	Having three or more bone fragments
Compression	Bone that is crushed (e.g., vertebra)
Depressed	Bone fragments pushed inward
Displaced	Two parts of fracture that have moved out of alignment
Impacted	Bone ends pushed into each other
Longitudinal	Fracture that runs parallel with bone
Oblique	Fracture that slants across bone
Pathologic	Results from minor stress applied to pathologically weakened bone
Segmental	Segment of bone fractured and detached
Spiral	Twisting around the bone
Transverse	Across the bone

PATIENT-CENTERED CARE

When a patient has had a musculoskeletal injury, patient-centered care focuses on minimizing pain, managing stabilization and immobilization devices to minimize tissue injury, and recognizing how the injury affects the patient's well-being. Routine assessment ensures that you can identify pain early and find the most appropriate comfort measures.

When traction or other orthopedic devices are applied, it is normal for patients to feel anxious about whether the procedure will be painful. Explaining procedures helps to minimize a patient's anxiety and fear. With many orthopedic injuries, some degree of immobility and restriction occurs. Lack of ability to function in a normal role may lead to feelings of frustration and depression.

It is also important to understand a patient's cultural beliefs and values related to issues of immobility and possible pain. Maintain privacy of a patient in a cast or in traction by providing adequate draping and closing the bedside curtain. Female modesty is valued in many cultures.

SAFETY

Proper and timely monitoring of all immobilization and stabilization devices helps to prevent the occurrence of skin and nerve damage. Skin traction noninvasively applies pull to an affected body structure by straps attached to the skin around the structure. However, there is a risk for pressure from the traction itself. It is important to monitor the patient's skin and underlying tissues for signs of pressure.

The swelling from soft tissue trauma of a fracture creates pressure that affects circulation and neurological function. In addition, pressure exerted from tightly applied circumferential bandages, casts, or braces may result in neurovascular deficits. Cool skin temperature, pale skin color, diminished pulses, and prolonged capillary refill are evidence of decreased perfusion. Ashen-gray appearance of skin and nail beds in African-American patients may indicate a deficit instead of the pallor seen in Caucasian patients. Sensory complaints such as pain, numbness, and tingling and motor changes such as weakness or inability to move the extremity distal to the pressure may indicate a developing neurovascular problem. Assess a patient's neurovascular status frequently to identify early impairment of any sensory changes. It is essential to monitor the five *P*'s (*pain, pallor, paralysis, paresthesia,* and *pulselessness*) of neurovascular status because permanent damage results if circulation is not restored and maintained. Pain on passive motion is often the first clinical manifestation when a neurovascular deficit is developing. Report the development of compromised neurovascular status promptly to the patient's health care provider.

Pin-site infection with skeletal traction can occur at the entry point through the skin. The pin site provides a point of entry for microorganisms to enter the soft tissues and bone. Meticulous skin care prevents the development of pin-site infection.

EVIDENCE-BASED PRACTICE

Lagerquist D et al: Care of external fixator pin sites, *Am J Crit Care* 21(4):288, 2012.

Timms A, Pugh H: Pin site care: guidance and key recommendations, *Nursing Standard* 27(1):50, 2012.

Voda S: Bad breaks: a nurse's guide to distal radius fractures, *Nursing 2011* 41(8):37, 2011.

The treatment of complicated fractures often includes the use of pins and plates to stabilize bones and promote healing. The use of external fixation devices allows for early mobilization, increased comfort and compliance, and discharge to home. There is no debate on the need for daily assessment of pin sites, but the approach to pin-site care has been the center of debate for years (Timms and Pugh, 2012). Many factors may affect the pin site, including loosening of the pin site, diameter of the pins and wires, preoperative skin preparation, postoperative dressings, and type of compression to prevent bleeding (Timms and Pugh, 2012). The level of evidence for pin-site care is low, but guidelines and reports from an integrative review of the literature provide recommendations for clinical practice (Lagerquist et al., 2012; Timms and Pugh, 2012; Voda, 2011):

- Perform pin care daily or weekly after the first 48 to 72 hours. Weekly pin care is supported for noninfected pins.
- Clean pin sites with chlorhexidine 2 mg/mL solution.
- Dressings using 5% chlorhexidine/1% silver sulfadiazine or Xeroform have shown a reduction in rates of pin-site infection.
- Wrap pin sites loosely with gauze until sites are dry.

SKILL 17.1 ASSISTING WITH CAST APPLICATION AND REMOVAL

A cast immobilizes an injured extremity to protect it from further injury, provides alignment of a fracture by holding the bone fragments in reduction and alignment during the healing process, and promotes comfort. In addition, a cast maintains a limb in alignment to prevent or correct deformity. Casts are used in many different ways (Fig. 17-1). The use and type of application materials required depend on the anatomic area of injury.

Cast materials are natural (plaster of Paris), synthetic acrylic, fiberglass-free, latex-free polymer, or a combination of materials. Today the preferred casting material is synthetic, but plaster of Paris is still the first choice when serial casting is required.

Plaster of Paris is composed of several layers of open-weave cotton roll or strips covered with calcium sulfate crystals. When moistened with water, this material molds easily during application; however, drying may take 24 to 72 hours, depending on the size of the cast. During drying, the cast must be exposed to air, well supported on a firm surface, handled with palms (not fingertips) to avoid indentations, and turned regularly so that it dries evenly. Weight bearing is delayed until the cast is completely dry. Lifting the cast by supporting the joints above and below the casted area prevents injury to underlying soft tissues. This type of cast is heavier than a synthetic cast.

Synthetic casting materials are composed of open-weave fiberglass tape covered with a polyurethane resin that is activated by water. This cast sets very quickly, in approximately 15 minutes, and can withstand pressure or weight bearing after 20 minutes. It forms a lightweight, sturdy cast that is both radiolucent and waterproof. Different colors of this casting material are also available, ranging from fluorescent pink and green to navy blue and purple. Colors are often more appealing to children and aid in maintaining the appearance of the cast. These casts are more expensive than plaster casts.

When caring for patients with casts, it is also important to understand the techniques for cast removal, which consist of removing the cast and padding, followed by skin care to the affected area. The cast is removed with a noisy cast saw, but the procedure is painless because the saw vibrates and does not cut the skin. However, it is necessary to prepare the patient adequately for cast removal. A small child or confused adult may require gentle restraint during removal to prevent any injury. A vibrating saw, specifically designed for synthetic casts, is used to remove the cast. Careful removal of a synthetic cast (with GORE® PROCEL® Cast Liner) is important to prevent burns from the heat generated by the vibrating saw. However, sometimes a synthetic cast is removed in the home by a parent. This process is less stressful and is often used with children. After cast removal, the patient may experience some tenderness, soreness, muscle weakness, and atrophy as well as a buildup of dead skin cells.

This skill includes frequent assessment before, during, and after cast application and removal, including peripheral neurovascular status. In addition, optimal skin care is important, including removal of dirt and debris before cast application and removal of any plaster crumbs after application.

ASSESSMENT

1. Identify patient using two identifiers (e.g., name and birthday or name and account number) according to facility policy. *Rationale: Ensures correct patient. Complies with The Joint Commission standards and improves patient safety (TJC, 2014).*
2. Assess patient's ability to cooperate and level of understanding concerning the casting procedure. *Rationale: Sudden movement during procedure could cause injury.*
3. Inspect condition of the skin that will be under the cast. Specifically note any areas of skin breakdown, rashes, bruising, or incisional wound. *Rationale: Provides baseline for skin condition. Open lesions may prohibit casting.*
4. Assess neurovascular status of the area to be casted. Specifically note alteration of motor and sensory function, skin color, temperature, and capillary refill. Compare with opposite extremity or surrounding tissues. Pay particular attention to tissues distal to cast. *Rationale: Changes in neurovascular status may occur after casting, possibly further compromising already injured tissues. It is important to note the baseline neurovascular status so that these changes, if they occur, are accurately assessed and compared with the baseline data.*
5. Assess patient's pain status using a scale of 0 to 10. *Rationale: Using a pain rating scale provides baseline data to determine efficacy of comfort measures.*

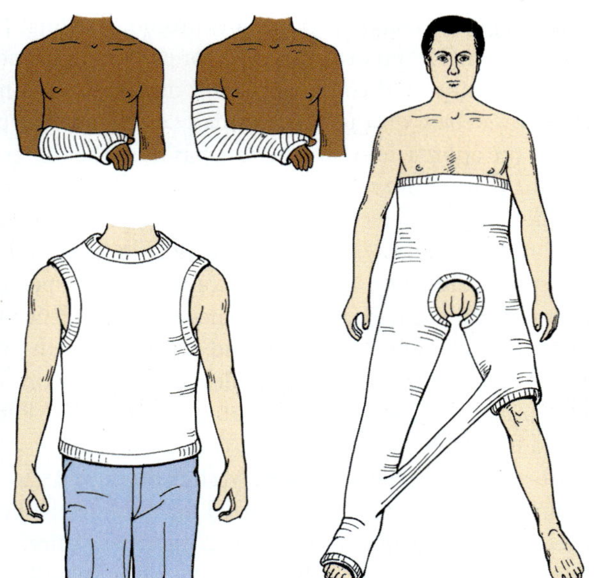

FIG 17-1 Common types of casts. *Top left,* Short arm cast. *Top center,* Long arm cast. *Bottom left,* Plaster body jacket cast. *Far right,* One and one-half hip spica cast.

6. Determine extent to which patient will be able to use the casted extremity. *Rationale: Predicts degree of assistance needed for self-care and/or ambulation.*
7. Assess patient's understanding of the bone healing process and potential mobility restrictions. *Rationale: Serves as a baseline for teaching patients how to care for casted extremity at home.*

PLANNING

Expected Outcomes focus on skin integrity, comfort, self-care, mobility, prevention of neurovascular complications, and maintenance of cast integrity.

1. Patient's skin below cast is warm and pink, with capillary refill less than 2 seconds. Pulses distal to the cast are palpable, strong, and regular.
2. Patient has edema of 1+ or less, mild pain, and some limitation in range of motion (ROM) but less than 25% decrease in active range of motion (ROM) of affected extremity after cast application.
3. Patient verbalizes no abnormal or unusual sensation in extremity and is able to move fingers or toes below casted part.
4. Cast remains clean, without indentations or fraying, until removal.
5. Patient verbalizes pain of 4 or less (scale of 0 to 10) after cast has been applied.
6. Patient requires minimal assistance with activities of daily living (ADLs) after extremity is casted.
7. Patient verbalizes cast care procedures.

Delegation and Collaboration

A complete assessment of the patient before or after cast application or removal cannot be delegated to nursing assistive personnel (NAP). However, the skill of assisting with cast application and removal can be delegated to NAP. The nurse instructs the NAP about:

- How to assist in positioning for specific patient with mobility restrictions.
- The proper skin care required after cast removal.

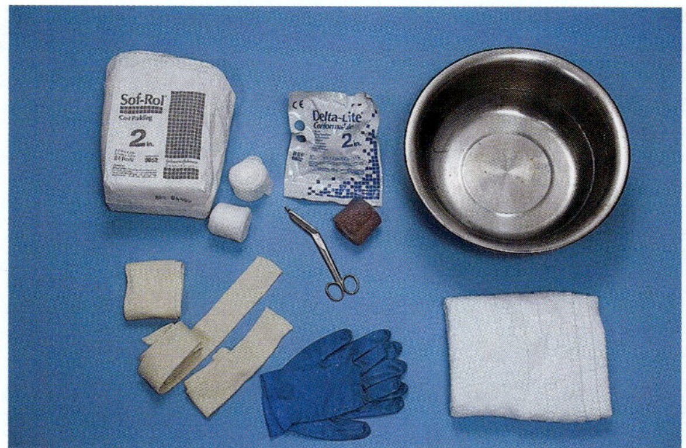

FIG 17-2 Casting materials.

Equipment

Equipment for Cast Application (May Be on Cast Cart) (Fig. 17-2)

- Plaster rolls (sizes include 2-, 3-, 4-, and 6-inch rolls) or cast materials such as fiberglass, casting tape, or plastic depending on purpose of cast or specific patient condition
- Padding material (felt, Webril, stockinette, GORE® PROCEL® Cast Liner, or any other cast specific lining)
- Plastic-lined bucket or basin filled three-fourths full with warm water
- Clean gloves, apron, or protective cover
- Cart, chair, and fracture table scissors
- Paper or plastic sheets
- Cast cutter (to trim edge of cast or remove old cast)
- Clean cast saw blades

Equipment for Cast Removal

- Cast saw
- Plastic sheets or paper
- Cold water enzyme wash
- Skin lotion
- Basin, water, washcloths, and towels
- Scissors
- Clean gloves
- Eye protection for health care provider and patient

IMPLEMENTATION *for* ASSISTING WITH CAST APPLICATION AND REMOVAL

STEPS	RATIONALE
1. **See Standard Protocol (inside front cover).**	
2. Discuss procedure with patient.	Decreases patient anxiety.
3. *Cast Application*	
a. Administer analgesic before cast application: oral (po), 30 to 40 minutes before; intramuscular, 20 to 30 minutes before; intravenous (IV), 2 to 5 minutes before. If patient has a patient-controlled analgesia (PCA) pump, instruct to administer a dose 2 to 5 minutes before cast application.	Reduces pain during cast application. Provides optimal analgesic effect.
b. Apply clean gloves. Note: Use latex-free gloves if there is risk of an allergic reaction.	Reduces transmission of infection. Synthetic cast can leave glue-like resin on hands. Prevents exposure to allergen.

Continued

STEPS	RATIONALE

c. Assist health care provider or certified technician position patient and injured extremity as desired, depending on type of cast to be used and area to be casted.

The parts to be casted must be supported and in optimal alignment.

d. Prepare skin that will be enclosed in the cast. Clean the skin with mild soap and water and change any dressing (if present). Skin must be completely dry before application of cast.

Assists in maintaining skin integrity.

> **SAFE PATIENT CARE** Patients with skin damage or skin lesions may not be candidates for casting.

e. Assist with application of padding material around body part to be casted (see illustration). Apply a minimum of four layers of padding. Avoid wrinkles or uneven thickness.

Prevents pressure points under the cast. Four layers of padding have been shown to decrease incidence of burning when cast is removed (Satryb et al., 2011).

f. Hold body part or parts to be casted or assist with preparation of casting materials.

Support of body part may require application of slight manual traction.

  (1) *Plaster cast:* Mark the end of the roll by folding one corner of the material under itself. With your thumb under outer edge, submerge the plaster roll under water in casting bucket or plastic basin until bubbles stop; squeeze slightly, and hand roll to person applying the cast.

When dampened, the end of the casting tape is sometimes difficult to find. Dampened plaster rolls are unrolled and molded to fit the extremity or body part to be casted.

  (2) *Synthetic cast:* Submerge cast roll in lukewarm water for 10 to 15 seconds. Squeeze to remove excess water. You can use a water bottle to apply water to the casting material.

The polyurethane prepolymer is activated by the application of water.

g. Continue to hold the body part as necessary as the cast is applied (see illustration) or supply additional rolls of casting tape as needed.

Support of body part involves applying slight manual traction, if desired, to maintain optimal position of the casted extremity. Thickness of the cast determines strength.

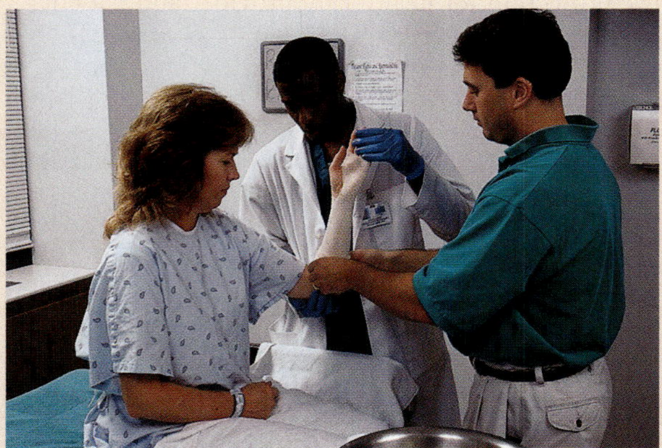

STEP 3e Padding under cast is smooth.

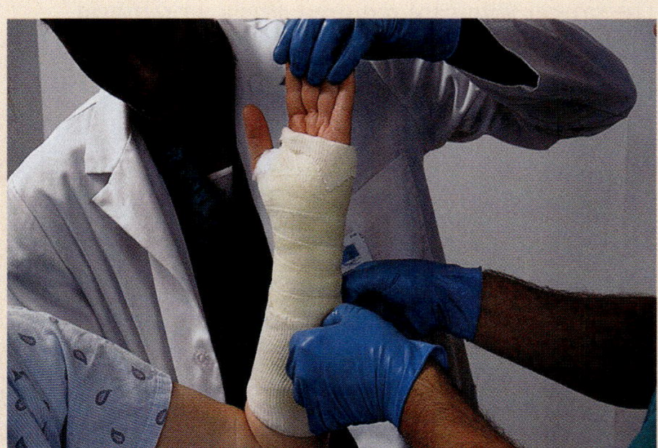

STEP 3g Support extremity during cast application.

STEPS	RATIONALE

h. Hold body part while casting tape is applied and molded. Synthetic tape is applied with slight tension. When wrapping is complete, gently compress with hands (see illustration).

Casting tape has synthetic adhesive or glass-fiber materials that dry quickly and are lightweight. Compression promotes bonding of cast layers. Plaster casts are smoothed at the end to finish outside of cast and ensure that plaster has bonded to other layers.

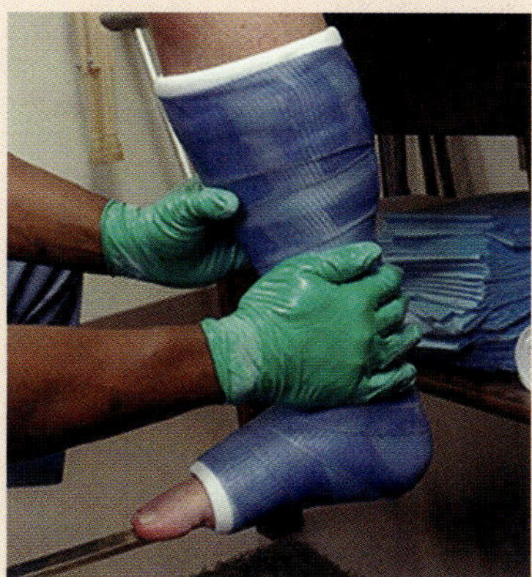

STEP 3h Applying synthetic cast roll.

i. Provide walking heel, cast brace, bar, or other cast stabilization material as ordered by the health care provider.

Ambulation may be permitted with partial weight bearing on the affected extremity after cast has dried. Bars stabilize spica cast, or "posts" (metal poles) stabilize four-poster cast. Braces incorporated into a cast assist in joint motion and mobility.

> **SAFE PATIENT CARE** Do not use abduction bar on spica cast as a handle for positioning the patient.

j. Assist with "finishing" the cast by folding edge of the stockinette down over the cast to provide a smooth edge. Unroll dampened plaster roll over the stockinette to hold it in place. Cushion any rough edges of cast with tape or moleskin.

Smooth edges decrease the chance for skin irritation or tissue injury.

k. Using scissors, trim the cast around fingers, toes, or the thumb as necessary. Remove and discard gloves and perform hand hygiene.

Cast should be snug but not constrict uninvolved joint movement or circulation.

l. Depending on the tissue to be casted:

(1) Elevate casted tissue to heart level on two to three cloth-covered pillows or in a sling. Avoid complete encasing of the cast. Air dry. If ice is ordered, place to side of cast to prevent indentation to top.

Pillows prevent indentations, which could harden and cause underlying pressure. Elevation enhances venous return and decreases edema. Covering the cast delays drying.

(2) When applying a sling, ensure that the sling supports but does not encase the cast.

Covering impedes air movement and delays drying.

m. Using the palms of your hands to support casted areas, assist patient with transfer to stretcher or wheelchair for return to nursing unit or preparation for discharge. Use additional personnel to transfer patient safely, especially with a patient in a spica or other body cast.

Safe transfer may require additional personnel, use of pillows to support cast, and side rails.

> **SAFE PATIENT CARE** Synthetic casts dry or set in 7 to 15 minutes. Soft tissues around affected area may swell from processes of "reducing" or manipulating before cast was applied.

Continued

STEPS	RATIONALE

n. Reposition patient every 2 to 3 hours. Do not rest heel of cast on bed or pillow.

Avoids indentation and prevents continuous pressure to one area.

o. Inform patient to notify health care provider of any alteration in sensation, numbness, tingling, burning, pain on passive motion, or inability to move fingers or toes in affected extremity (Voda, 2011).

Edema within a casted extremity causes pressure on nerves, blood vessels, and muscle tissues. This leads to neurovascular deficit, compartment syndrome, and necrosis of tissues.

4. *Cast Removal*

a. Assess patient's understanding of and response to upcoming cast removal.

Provides baseline for teaching.

b. Assist with positioning patient.

Assists with proper alignment of extremity and protects limb during cast removal.

c. Describe the physical sensations to expect during cast removal (vibration of cast saw and generation of heat) (see illustration).

Allows patient to know what to expect and eases anxiety during cast removal.

d. Describe the expected appearance of the extremity. Skin under cast is often scaly with dead cells that slough off. Muscle atrophy occurs from disuse.

Allows patient to know what to expect and eases anxiety after cast removal.

e. Describe and demonstrate the loud noise of the cast saw.

Eases anxiety during cast removal and allows patient to know what to expect.

f. Apply clean gloves. Apply eye goggles or protective glasses to self and patient.

Reduces transmission of microorganisms and protects eyes of patient and nurse.

g. Stay with patient and explain progress of procedure as cast and underlying padding are removed (see illustration).

Reduces anxiety and promotes cooperation.

h. Inspect tissues underlying the cast after removal. If skin is intact, apply cold water enzyme wash (if available) to skin and leave on for 15 to 20 minutes. Use oil or mild soap and water to soften crust. Do not scrub skin.

Protects fragile skin and promotes removal of dead skin cells.

i. Gently wash off enzyme wash or soap and water. If possible, immerse tissues in basin or tub to assist in dead cell removal.

Removes excess soap or enzyme wash to avoid further drying of skin.

j. Pat extremity dry. Apply generous coat of lotion to patient's skin. After cast removal, explain and provide written skin care procedures for patient before discharge.

Educates patient on how to care for skin after cast removal.

k. Obtain health care provider order to perform active and passive ROM, and clarify level of activity permitted.

Clarifies expected ROM needed after cast removal.

5. **See Completion Protocol (inside front cover).**

STEP 4c Vibration of cast cutter generates heat.

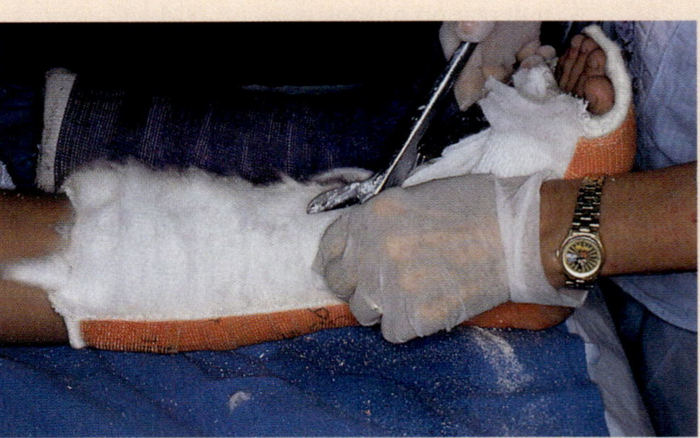

STEP 4g Removing padding beneath cast with scissors.

EVALUATION

1. Perform neurovascular assessment every 1 to 2 hours for first 24 hours. Assess for pain, pallor, pulselessness, paresthesia, and paralysis. Compare findings with neurovascular assessment performed before casting application (Fig. 17-3).
2. Palpate the temperature of tissues around the casted area for warmth, and assess for hot spots, which could indicate underlying localized infection.
3. Observe condition of cast, and assess for edema of tissues distal to the cast.
4. Inspect alignment of the limb and condition of the cast.
5. Observe patient for signs of pain or anxiety: ask patient to rate pain on a scale of 0 to 10, observe for discolored or pale fingers or nail beds, inability to move body parts distal to cast, pain on passive motion of distal body part, hyperventilation, tachycardia, blood pressure elevation, and nausea or vomiting.
6. Ask patient to perform ADLs and ROM within limitations of cast. Compare ROM in noncasted extremity.
7. **For Cast Application.** Use *Teach Back:* State to the patient or family caregiver, "I want to be sure I explained how to take care of the cast. Can you tell me how to care for your cast?" Evaluates what the patient is able to explain or demonstrate. Revise your instruction now or develop plan for revised patient teaching to be implemented at an appropriate time if patient is not able to teach back correctly.
8. **For Cast Removal.** Use *Teach Back:* State to the patient, "I want to be sure I clearly explained what to do after the cast is removed. Can you explain to me how to observe for swelling and what you are supposed to do at home after the cast is removed?" Evaluates what the patient is able to explain or demonstrate. Revise your instruction now or develop plan for revised patient teaching to be implemented at an appropriate time if patient is not able to teach back correctly.

Unexpected Outcomes and Related Interventions

1. Patient experiences impaired physical mobility related to the cast.
   a. Assist patient with ROM exercises every 3 to 4 hours.
   b. Teach isometric exercises.

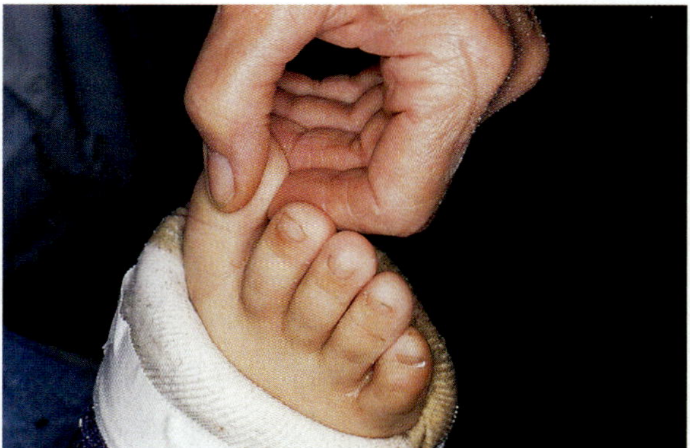

FIG 17-3 Inspecting toe to assess capillary refill.

2. Patient reports increased severity in pain after application of the cast.
   a. Reposition casted extremity or the patient. Adjust elevation of pillows as necessary.
   b. Apply ice bags along sides of cast. Do not place heavy ice bags on top of damp cast because of risk of indentation.
   c. Administer analgesics as ordered to maintain patient's comfort level.
   d. Increase frequency of neurovascular checks.
   e. Assess tightness of the cast by checking with two fingers around the edges and checking with patient. Cast should be snug but not tight.
   f. If pain continues, notify health care provider before administering additional analgesics (analgesics do not relieve edema and could mask these symptoms).
3. Patient develops compartment syndrome with severe pain unrelieved by analgesics; change in neurovascular status such as numbness, tingling, pain on passive motion, or decreased movement in distal skin and tissues; bluish color to distal parts; marked edema; diminished or absent pulse in area distal to casted extremity (pulselessness develops late in the syndrome); or capillary refill greater than 3 seconds.
   a. Elevate cast.
   b. Notify health care provider immediately.
   c. Prepare to bivalve cast using a cast cutter. Cut through underlying wadding and padding.
4. Patient or family caregiver could not provide an explanation of how to care for cast after application or removal.
   a. Provide additional education using teach back technique.
   b. Allow patient or family caregiver to explain cast care after application or removal.

Recording and Reporting

- Record cast application, condition of skin, status of circulation (before and after application or removal), and motion of distal part.
- Record instructions given to patient and family caregiver.
- Document your evaluation of patient learning.
- Report abnormal findings from neurovascular assessments; report signs and symptoms of compartment syndrome immediately.
- Record odor and drainage from cast. Report to health care provider.

Sample Documentation

0900   Left long-arm synthetic cast applied, and left arm placed in shoulder sling by health care provider. Capillary refill of left index finger is 2 seconds. Skin warm, dry, and intact. Able to move all fingers of left hand, fingers warm to touch, nail beds pink, no swelling noted. Complains of pain at 5 (scale of 0 to 10).
0910   Tylox 1 tab administered po. Left long-arm cast and sling readjusted.
0945   Left long-arm cast intact with sling. Capillary refill of left index finger unchanged. Moves all fingers of left hand,

denies any numbness or tingling present, fingers warm to touch. No edema noted. Reports pain decreased to 1 (scale of 0 to 10).

Special Considerations

Pediatric

- Teach family caregivers to protect plaster cast from moisture or unnecessary wear. Plastic wrap placed around perineal area during urination or defecation prevents soiling. Protect cast with plastic bag or plastic wrap when the child bathes or showers. With a spica cast, tuck the ends of a small disposable diaper around the edges of the casted area to cover and protect the perineum in infants (Hockenberry and Wilson, 2013).

- Monitor children closely to ensure that they do not place objects beneath the cast to scratch. Use antihistamine, ice pack, or a hair dryer set to cool setting to control itching (Hockenberry and Wilson, 2013).

Geriatric

- Synthetic casts are less restrictive and have the advantage of lighter weight for older adults, helping them maintain better balance.
- Older adults with age-related decreases in muscle strength may have difficulty ambulating with a cast.

Home Care

- See Boxes 17-2 and 17-3.

BOX 17-2 CAST CARE INSTRUCTIONS

First 24 Hours

- Follow health care provider's instructions.
- Keep the cast and extremity above the level of the heart for at least 48 hours by propping your cast up on firm pillows. Elevation reduces swelling.
- Put ice next to the fractured area for 24 hours, but be sure to enclose the ice in a plastic bag to keep the cast dry. Do not place ice on the top of a damp cast.
- Move the parts of your body above and below the cast regularly to aid circulation and relieve stiffness. Massaging the joints and extremities gently around the cast also improves circulation.
- Your cast needs at least 24 hours to dry completely if it is plaster and possibly 72 hours for a large cast. Avoid handling it as much as possible. When you do have to move the cast, such as when you change your body position, use only the palms of your hands and support the cast under your joints. You want to avoid putting indentations in the cast that will put pressure on the skin inside.
- Use a fan placed 46 to 61 cm (18 to 24 inches) from the cast to aid its drying in the first 24 hours. Be sure to expose the whole cast for drying, and do not cover it with linen for the first 24 hours.
- Never insert any object into your cast for any purpose (e.g., do not try to scratch under cast when it itches).

How to Care for Your Cast

Plaster

- Do not get the cast wet because it will lose its strength. If cast does become wet, dry immediately. Use a towel to blot moisture off the cast and then dry it with a hair dryer set on low. When your cast does not feel cold and damp, it is dry.
- To keep the cast clean and dry, cover it with plastic when bathing, using the toilet (if it is a spica cast), or going out in rain or snow.
- Use a damp cloth and scouring powder to clean soiled spots on the cast. Be sure to brush away plaster crumbs or other objects from the edges of the cast, but do not remove or rearrange any padding. Do not break off or trim cast edges.

Synthetic

- If you have a fiberglass cast without wounds or incisions under it, you may be able to continue a more normal lifestyle (e.g., bathing) if your health care provider approves. A fiberglass cast can become wet.
- Washing or rinsing inside your fiberglass cast may reduce odor and irritation and improve the overall skin condition of the cast area. You may use a spray nozzle at a sink or a flexible shower head to rinse inside your cast with warm water.
- You must dry the cast thoroughly after wetting. Lightly towel off excess water and use a hair dryer on cool or low setting to dry inside cast. Do not cover the cast while it is drying.

Skin Care

- Skin care is very important during the time a cast is worn. Routinely look at the skin condition around the cast each day for signs of redness or friction. Also, look for areas of cracks in the cast.
- Do not insert objects under the cast because you could scrape the skin or add pressure and cause an infection or sore under the cast.
- You may use powders and lotions only outside the cast so the skin stays clean and soft. Powder inside a cast can cake and cause sore areas.

Activity

- Do not walk on a leg cast for the first 48 hours. If you are allowed to walk on it, be sure to walk on the walking heel.
- If your arm is in a cast, be sure to use your sling for support and comfort.

Contact Your Health Care Provider if:

- You have pain, burning, or swelling.
- You feel a blister or sore developing inside the cast.
- You experience numbness or persistent tingling.
- Your cast becomes badly soiled.
- Your cast breaks, cracks, or develops soft spots.
- Your cast becomes too loose.
- You develop skin problems at the cast edges.
- You develop a fever or foul odor under the cast.
- You have any questions regarding your treatment.

> ### BOX 17-3   CARE AFTER CAST REMOVAL
>
> **Skin Care**
> - Apply enzyme wash solution such as Woolite or Delicare and leave in place for at least 20 minutes. The enzymes in the solution loosen dead cells and help emulsify fatty or crusty lesions but cause no skin irritation.
> - After 20 minutes, immerse the area in warm water and gently wash away the debris. Do not rub or scrub the skin areas; gently swab them with a soft cloth.
> - Rinse with clear warm water and pat dry.
> - Apply a moisturizing skin lotion or a little oil, gently massaging it in to help maintain the integrity of the tissues.
> - Repeat these steps in 24 to 48 hours, after which the area should need no special care.
>
> **Relieving Edema**
> - Apply cloth-covered ice bags if there is significant edema. Do not place ice directly on skin.
> - Elevate the affected tissues no higher than the heart for the next 24 hours or when swelling occurs.
>
> **Managing Tenderness, Weakness, and Discomfort**
> - Take prescribed analgesic every 3 to 4 hours to develop a therapeutic blood level, and continue the medication for 24 to 48 hours.
> - Immerse the part or the entire body in warm water and gently exercise muscles under water.
> - Begin to reuse affected tissues and muscles slowly to avoid pain. It usually takes twice as long as the part was in a cast to regain full function.
> - Perform prescribed muscle exercises with 5 to 10 repetitions every 4 hours while awake to aid in regaining muscle strength. If muscle soreness persists, continue to take a nonnarcotic analgesic and soak in warm water before exercise. Soreness should lessen as muscle regains strength. The health care provider may prescribe a consultation with a physical therapist for appropriate exercises to increase mobility and strength.

SKILL 17.2   CARE OF A PATIENT IN SKIN TRACTION

Skin traction is the application of a pulling force directly to the skin and soft tissue that indirectly pulls on the skeletal system. Use of continuous traction immobilizes a fracture and relieves muscle spasms and pain. Skin traction usually provides temporary immobilization until the fracture can be repaired surgically by open reduction and internal fixation or skeletal traction (Wheeless, 2011). With current advances in orthopedic surgery and technology, traction is rarely used as the primary management for fractures (Handoll, Queally, and Parker, 2011). Skin traction maintains alignment and reduces contractures and dislocations. The health care provider provides specific orders for traction weights, bed position, and turning regimen. Skin traction is applied by skilled practitioners with specialized knowledge (Jester et al., 2011).

There are several types of skin traction. The most common type of adult skin traction is Buck's extension. It is applied to one or both legs using straps or a commercially prepared foam boot with Velcro straps (Fig. 17-4). The straps or boot are then attached to a spreader bar, and no more than 7 pounds of weight are attached at the end of the extremity. Dunlop's traction is another form of skin traction that is applied to an upper limb for treatment of contractures or fractures of the humerus or elbow (Fig. 17-5). Russell's traction is used on the lower leg with a padded sling under the knee. There are two lines of pulling force: one is along the longitudinal plane and the lower leg, and one is perpendicular to the leg (Fig. 17-6).

Cervical traction uses a head halter with a cutout for the ears and face (Fig. 17-7). The halter cradles the chin and has straps leading to a bar attached to ropes, pulleys, and weights. Between 7 and 10 pounds of weight are applied. Cervical traction immobilizes conditions of the cervical vertebrae, not fractures, and can be removed periodically.

The more weight applied to the traction, the greater the risk of skin breakdown. Contraindications to skin traction include pressure ulcers, dermatitis, burns, or abrasions. Older patients with tissue perfusion problems are at increased risk of skin breakdown.

When caring for patients in skin traction, initially and regularly monitor patients for correct maintenance of the traction device and proper musculoskeletal alignment. Facility policy may specify the frequency of assessment, which should be at least every 4 hours. Traction maintenance involves monitoring the weights, the direction of pull, the ropes and pulleys, and all connections (Box 17-4).

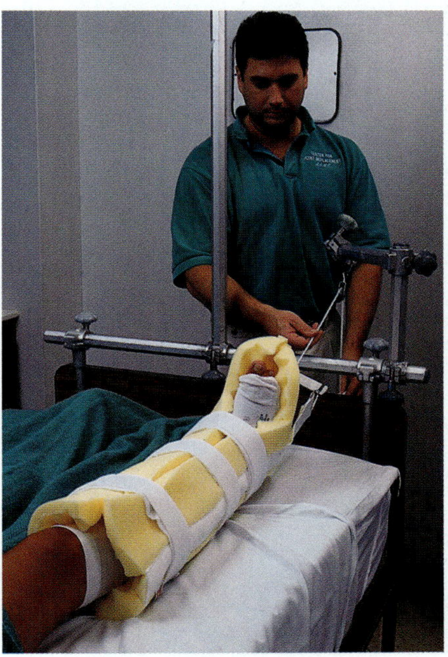

FIG 17-4 Buck's extension.

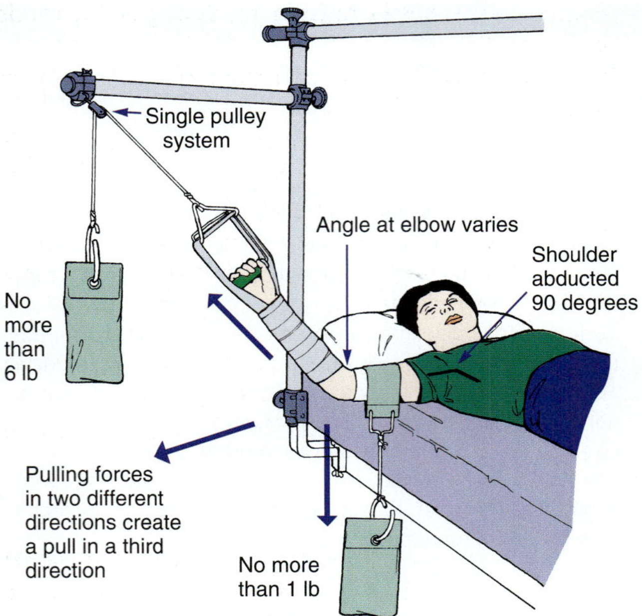

FIG 17-5 Dunlop's traction.

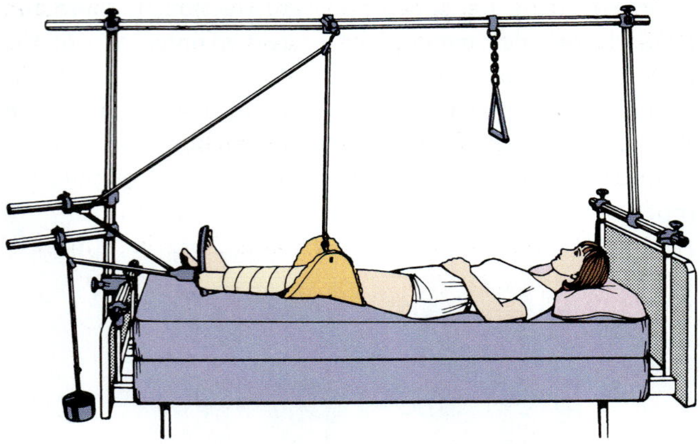

FIG 17-6 Russell's traction.

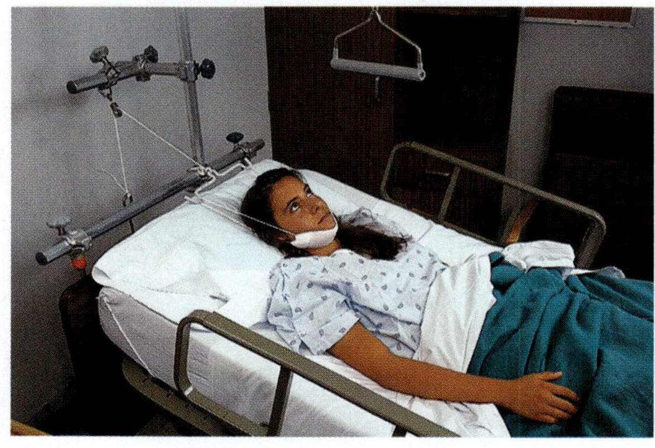

FIG 17-7 Cervical traction.

BOX 17-4   TRACTION ASSESSMENT

1. Maintain Established Line of Pull
The direction of pull should be along the long axis of the bone. Weights will hang freely, not hitting the bed or resting on the floor. Recheck the position of the weights if the level of the bed is altered. Avoid bumping against the weights when walking near the bed and allowing the weights to sway; both movements can cause pain for the patient in traction. It is preferred that the weights not hang over the patient; if this is necessary, tape the ropes so the weights will not fall on the patient.

2. Maintain Traction Equipment
Traction rope rests in the groove of the pulley and moves easily. Monitor the rope for fraying. Securely tie the knots in the traction rope, and tape the rope ends. Ensure the rope knots are not lodged against the pulley because this will interfere with the line of pull. Ensure that the pulley, spreader bar, and footplate do not rest against the foot of the bed.

3. Maintain Countertraction
To provide traction, ensure that countertraction is maintained by the weight of the patient's body, the pull of the weights in the opposite direction, or elevation of the bed. For instance, the feet of a patient in Buck's traction will not touch the foot of the bed; or if the patient is in cervical traction, the head will not touch the head of the bed.

4. Maintain Continuous Traction Unless Ordered Otherwise
Maintain continuous traction unless the health care provider orders intermittent traction. To change the patient's position in bed, do not lift or adjust the weights if traction is continuous. Ensure the correct amount of weight is used. For intermittent traction, gently place and slowly remove the weights, avoiding jerking or suddenly moving the weights because these could jar the patient.

5. Maintain Correct Body Alignment
Be sure the patient has correct body alignment while lying centered in the bed. Instruct the patient regarding any restricted positions. The nurse must ensure that the patient does not angle the body or lean off the side of the bed because the line of traction pull would be changed or interrupted.

6. Prevent Friction to the Skin
Remove skin traction and reapply daily. The usual amount of weight used for skin traction in adult patients is 5 to 8 pounds. With any traction, monitor the skin for evidence of redness, bruising, or skin breakdown. Avoid friction or pressure from the equipment.

Modified from Jester R et al: *Oxford handbook of orthopaedic nursing*, New York, 2011, Oxford University Press.

ASSESSMENT

1. Identify patient using two identifiers (e.g., name and birthday or name and account number) according to facility policy. *Rationale: Ensures correct patient. Complies with The Joint Commission standards and improves patient safety (TJC, 2014).*
2. Assess patient's knowledge of the reason for traction. *Rationale: Determines patient's concerns and fears and need for further teaching.*
3. Assess integrity and condition of skin before traction application. *Rationale: Establishes baseline for skin integrity. Intact skin and local tissue have increased ability to tolerate the pulling forces of traction.*
4. Assess patient's overall health condition, including degree of mobility, ability to perform ADLs, and current medical conditions. *Rationale: Determines patient's ability to tolerate traction, self-care ability, and anticipated need for assistance.*
5. Assess patient's position in bed: supine, perpendicular to the ends of the bed, with the affected limb in proper body alignment. *Rationale: Ensures that the pull of the traction is at the proper angle in relation to the patient's body.*
6. Assess patient's level of pain using a scale of 0 to 10 and determine need for analgesics before application of traction. *Rationale: Analgesics decrease patient's discomfort while skin traction is being applied, and assessment serves as the baseline for later comparison.*
7. Assess neurovascular status of extremity distal to the traction, including skin color, temperature, capillary refill, presence of distal pulses, sensation, and patient's ability to move digits. *Rationale: Provides necessary baseline information for early detection of neurovascular deficit.*
8. Review medical record for amount of weight to be used in traction. *Ensures appropriate weight is applied at all times.*

PLANNING

Expected Outcomes focus on improving patient's mental status, skin integrity, comfort level, neurovascular status, and mobility.

1. Patient participates in ADLs as much as possible within limitations.
2. Skin under traction boot or elastic wrap remains intact, without redness or breakdown.
3. Patient verbalizes increase in comfort after traction application and rates pain as 4 or lower on a scale of 0 to 10 after repositioning and administration of analgesics.
4. Neurovascular status remains stable. Distal skin tissue remains warm and pink, with capillary refill of 2 seconds or less. Patient is able to move fingers or toes distal to fracture site.
5. Patient verbalizes understanding of procedure, including traction setup and mobility restrictions.
6. Patient moves all extremities independently by date of discharge.

Delegation and Collaboration

Neurovascular assessment of the patient's condition cannot be delegated. The assessment of the traction placement, traction weights, and the integrity of the traction system cannot be delegated. The skill of assisting with application of skin traction can be delegated to nursing assistive personnel (NAP) who have had specific training. The nurse instructs the NAP to:

- Adapt hygiene and other skills for specific patients.
- Inform the nurse if patient demonstrates any change in skin condition or complains of discomfort.

Equipment

- Overhead frame for attachment of traction
- Traction bar
- Cross clamp and pulley
- Buck's extension boot or moleskin and elastic bandages
- 1- to 7-pound weights
- Spreader bar

IMPLEMENTATION *for* CARE OF A PATIENT IN SKIN TRACTION

STEPS	RATIONALE
1. **See Standard Protocol (inside front cover).**	
2. Discuss procedure with patient.	Assists with decreasing anxiety.
3. Administer analgesic for acute pain and muscle relaxant for spasms in advance of traction application.	Allows drugs to reach peak effect at time of traction application, reducing pain and resultant muscle spasm. Analgesics do not effectively reduce muscle spasm pain.
4. Position patient. *Buck's extension:* Position patient supine and nearly flat with no more than 30 degrees of elevation, with the affected leg halfway between the edge and the middle of the bed.	Maintains pull of traction at the proper angle in relation to the patient's body.
5. Apply clean gloves. Wash affected extremity gently and pat dry. Do not shave extremity.	Shaving may nick skin, which could become inflamed and infected under traction straps.

Continued

STEPS	RATIONALE
6. Apply foam boot, moleskin, or elastic bandages to affected extremity, proceeding from distal to proximal. For *Buck's extension:*	Applying in distal-to-proximal pattern prevents trapping of blood in distal region.
a. Before placing foam boot, wrap leg in soft roll. Ensure that boot fits snugly.	Boot that is too tight applies pressure to skin, peroneal nerve, and vasculature structures. Too loose leads to slipping and lack of traction force.
b. Seat heel properly in traction boot. Do not pad at heel.	Prevents pressure on patient's heel.
c. Do not apply traction boot over sequential pneumatic compression devices. Use foot pumps instead.	Causes pressure on tissues and does not allow compression device to function.
7. Attach weight to boot gradually and gently at the end of the bed. Health care provider determines exact amount of weight to be applied and position to be maintained.	Traction is applied slowly to avoid involuntary muscle spasms or pain for patient. Weight should create enough pull to overcome muscle spasms but not cause marked increase in pain.

> **SAFE PATIENT CARE** When applying *Buck's extension,* avoid pressure to the peroneal nerve at the neck of the fibula. Decreased sensation in the web space between the great and second toes and an inability to dorsiflex the foot and extend the toes may indicate pressure to the nerve.

STEPS	RATIONALE
8. Inspect traction equipment, making sure that: • Knots are secure. • Ropes are in pulleys and not frayed. • Weights are hanging freely, not caught on bed or resting on floor. • Bed linens and bedclothes are not interfering with traction equipment. • Check the four *P*'s of traction maintenance: *pounds, pressure, pull,* and *pulleys.*	Routine observation of these checkpoints is necessary to maintain appropriate amount of traction and effective immobilization.
9. Before health care provider leaves, assess patient's position and ask about additional permissible positions for patient and bed.	Ensures patient's safety and position for effective traction.
a. *Buck's extension:* Patient is primarily on back but may be allowed to turn to unaffected side for brief periods (10 to 15 minutes).	Positioning on side allows for back care and relief of pressure to tissues.
b. *Dunlop's traction:* Patient must lie on back. Bed may be tilted on low shock blocks toward side opposite traction. Head of bed is flat.	Tilting uses body for some countertraction.
c. *Russell's traction:* Patient lies on back; head of bed may be elevated 30 to 45 degrees, depending on injury.	Low-Fowler's position creates most effective traction pull.

> **SAFE PATIENT CARE** If tissues distal to skin traction are cold or cool or if capillary refill is greater than 2 seconds, compare with unaffected extremity. If deficit is related to traction, wrap extremity, remove traction, and report neurovascular compromise.

STEPS	RATIONALE
10. Release and reapply traction and provide skin care according to health care provider's orders.	Permits visualization of skin and opportunity to provide skin care.
11. See Completion Protocol (inside front cover).	

EVALUATION

1. Evaluate patient's ability to perform ADLs.
2. Assess condition of skin around traction straps or bandages frequently for signs of pressure, color changes, edema, or tenderness.
3. Observe patient for correct alignment.
4. Ask patient to rate discomfort on a scale of 0 to 10 and to report muscle spasms.
5. Evaluate neurovascular status of extremity every 30 minutes after application of skin traction twice, then every 2 hours for 24 hours, and every 4 hours thereafter (see facility policy). Check skin temperature, capillary refill, presence of distal pulses, sensation, and patient's ability to move digits.
6. Observe patient's use of trapeze and unaffected limbs to reposition self correctly.
7. Use **Teach Back:** State to the patient, "I want to be sure I explained clearly the need for traction, how to maintain the traction, and the limitations related to the traction. Can you tell me how you will use this traction safely?" Evaluates what the patient is able to explain or demonstrate. Revise your instruction now or develop plan for revised patient teaching to be implemented at an appropriate time if patient is not able to teach back correctly.

Unexpected Outcomes and Related Interventions

1. Patient complains of increased pain, soreness, or stiffness after traction is applied.
   a. Remove traction (if permitted by health care provider), reposition patient, and reapply the traction.
   b. Administer analgesics as prescribed.
   c. Realign body or extremity.
   d. If pain is unrelieved or occurs on passive motion, notify health care provider of possible neurovascular deficit.
2. Patient experiences reddened areas on extremity under traction.
   a. Obtain health care provider order to remove foam boot for 1 hour to relieve pressure.
   b. Apply foam boot securely (you should be able to insert one finger between patient's skin and foam boot). Recheck correct tightness frequently.
   c. Increase frequency of skin assessment.
   d. Apply protective barrier agent (e.g., Aloe Vesta or Sween cream) to affected extremity.
   e. Ensure that heels do not rest on bed or pillow.

Recording and Reporting

- Record pain assessment and assessment of skin integrity beneath traction, nursing interventions, and length of time patient is in or out of specific traction in nurses' notes.
- Document your evaluation of patient learning.
- Record neurovascular assessments on flow sheet or nurses' notes.
- Report any neurovascular deficits to health care provider immediately.

Sample Documentation

0900   Buck's traction boot applied to patient's left leg and attached to a 5-pound weight. No complaints of pain, tingling, or numbness. Bilateral pedal pulses strong, equal, and regular. Capillary refill 2 seconds in nail beds of toes bilaterally; able to move or flex toes; skin warm, dry, and pink to lower left leg. Side rails up, bed down, brakes locked, call light within reach, and weights hanging freely. Knots tied, rope in pulley. In supine position with left leg in proper alignment.

Special Considerations
Pediatric

- Infants and young children are unable to remain still and in alignment.

Geriatric

- Some older adults may have keratoses, rashes, or other lesions that could become irritated in skin traction.
- The presence of long-standing conditions of musculoskeletal tissues such as arthritis or gout can increase the risk for inflamed tissues and skin breakdown.
- Older patients and patients with chronic illness have increased need for position changes as a result of limitations from osteoporosis, osteomalacia, weakened muscles, or increased risk of skin breakdown.
- Skin of older adults heals more slowly and is more fragile, less elastic, and thinner than skin of younger adults (Touhy and Jett, 2014). Use pressure-relief devices to reduce the risk of impaired skin integrity (see Chapter 25).

Home Care

- Before discharge home, teach family caregivers how to manage home traction, including positioning, level of mobility, rest, and nutritional considerations.
- Teach family caregivers how to maintain integrity of traction by inspecting at least daily: weights hang freely; traction ropes rest in groove of pulley and hang freely, not caught on bed or resting on floor.

SKILL 17.3　CARE OF A PATIENT IN SKELETAL TRACTION AND PIN-SITE CARE

Skeletal traction immobilizes fractures of the cervical spine, fractures of the femur below the trochanter, and some fractures of the bones of the arm or ankle. It also immobilizes the femoral head when there is an acetabular fracture. Skeletal traction is being used less frequently because of newer surgical repair procedures (Brooker and Nicol, 2013: Handoll et al., 2011).

A common form of skeletal traction is balanced-suspension skeletal traction (BSST), which is usually used for a fractured femur (Fig. 17-8). BSST relieves muscle spasms, realigns

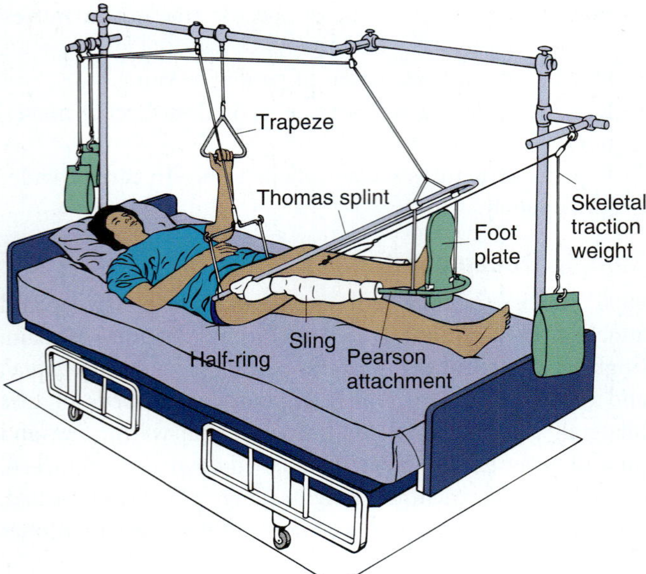

FIG 17-8 Balanced-suspension skeletal traction. Traction in long axis of right thigh is applied by means of a Kirschner wire through proximal portion of tibia. Limb is supported by a Thomas splint beneath thigh and Pearson attachment beneath leg. Footplate attachment prevents footdrop. Weights apply countertraction to upper end of Thomas splint and suspend its lower end. By using the left arm and leg as shown, the patient can shift position of the hips without change in amount of traction.

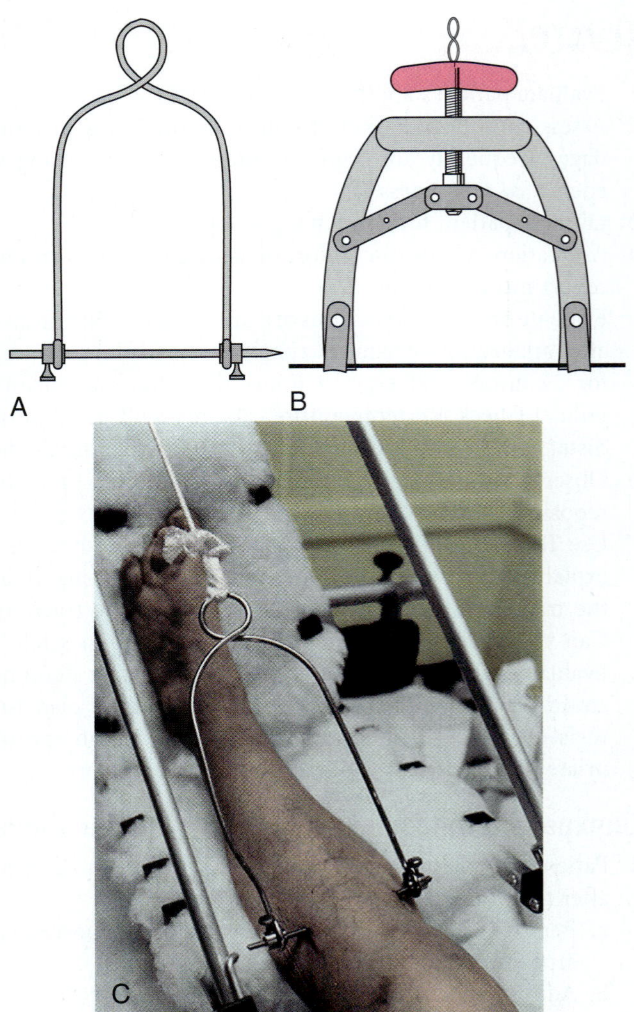

FIG 17-9 A, Steinmann pin and holder. **B,** Kirschner wire and tractor. **C,** Steinmann pin placed in tibial plateau for treatment of distal femoral fracture.

fracture fragments, and promotes callus formation. Callus formation is the development of new supportive bone around the injured site. BSST temporarily stabilizes the patient's condition while waiting for surgical insertion of an internal fixation device such as a plate, screw, or nail. Balanced suspension involves a sling attached to splints around the leg and a Steinmann pin or Kirschner wire supplying the traction (Fig. 17-9). Sufficient weight to overcome the quadriceps and hamstring muscle spasms ranges from 30 to 40 pounds.

Other common forms of skeletal traction are sidearm traction (with a pin drilled through the lower humerus) and external fixation (used for comminuted fractures with soft tissue injury, skull and facial fractures, and pelvic fractures). For cervical spine fractures, Crutchfield or Gardner-Wells tongs are inserted into the skull. Halo traction is frequently used for neurologically intact patients, stabilizing the spinal vertebra and preventing further injury to the spinal cord (Fig. 17-10).

External fixation is a form of skeletal traction that consists of a frame or apparatus to hold pins placed into or through bones above and below a fracture site. External fixation devices promote early ambulation and use of other joints while maintaining immobilization of affected bones. Various external fixation frames are used for skull and facial fractures, ribs, bones of the extremities, and pelvic bones (Fig. 17-11).

Skeletal traction involves piercing the skin at the site where the pin enters and exits. In the case of external fixation or halo traction, the device attaches to the bone through the skin. Slow healing requires longer periods of traction (6 to 8 weeks) to promote bone repair. This prolonged immobilization influences nursing care, which focuses on supporting ADLs, maintaining traction, and preventing fat embolism and complications of immobility (e.g., skin breakdown and pulmonary emboli).

Because skeletal traction involves placement of a pin, meticulous pin-site care reduces the risk of pin-tract infections. Pin-site care reduces the risk of infection and must be implemented using current evidence-based practice guidelines. Some facilities have policies outlining pin-site care. Chlorhexidine 2 mg/mL solution is recommended for stable pins (Lagerquist et al., 2012; Timms and Pugh, 2012; Voda, 2011). Some facilities require specific health care provider's orders to specify frequency of pin-site care and the cleansing agent to be used. Skeletal pin-site care guidelines were established by a panel of experts (see Evidence-Based Practice).

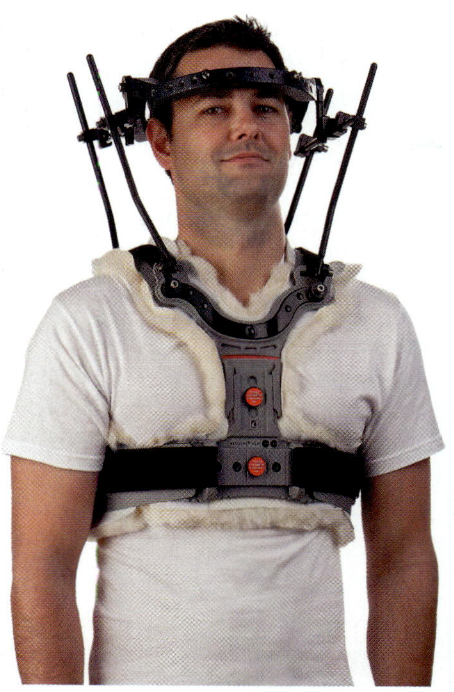

FIG 17-10 Halo traction with vest. (Image used with permission, Össur Americas. All rights reserved.)

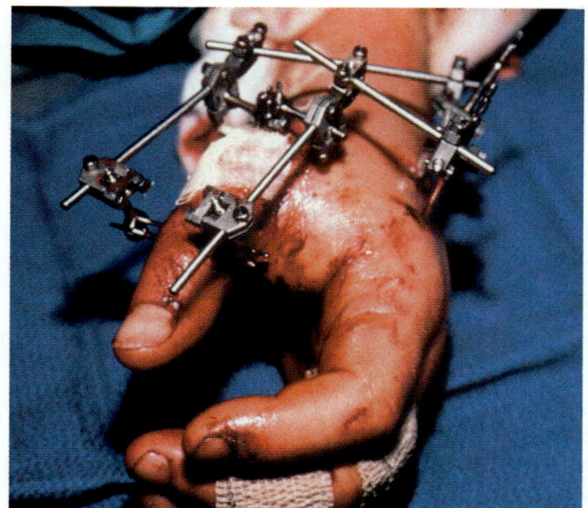

FIG 17-11 External fixator.

ASSESSMENT

1. Identify patient using two identifiers (e.g., name and birthday or name and account number) according to facility policy. *Rationale: Ensures correct patient. Complies with The Joint Commission standards and improves patient safety (TJC, 2014).*
2. Assess patient's knowledge of the reason for traction, including nonverbal behavior and responses. *Rationale: Determines concerns, anxiety, and need for further teaching.*
3. Inspect integrity and condition of skin over bony prominences (e.g., use Braden Scale to assess risk for pressure ulcers) and under devices in use. Consider need for special bed or mattress (see Chapter 25). *Rationale: Provides baseline status of dependent tissues at risk for pressure ulcer formation.*
4. Assess for proper alignment of extremity. *Rationale: Ensures that the pull of the traction is at the proper angle in relation to the patient's body.*
5. Assess patient's degree of mobility, ability to reposition and perform ADLs, and current medical conditions. *Rationale: Determines patient's health state as a baseline for future reference.*
6. Assess patient's level of pain using a scale of 0 to 10 and determine the need for analgesics before procedure begins. *Rationale: Decreases patient's discomfort while applying traction and serves as a baseline for later comparison.*
7. Before application, assess neurovascular status of extremity distal to the traction, including skin color, temperature, capillary refill, presence of distal pulses, sensation, and patient's ability to move digits. *Rationale: Provides necessary baseline information and detects neurovascular deficits.*
8. Following application, assess traction equipment: weights hanging freely, ordered amount of weight applied, ropes moving freely through pulleys, all knots tight in ropes and away from pulleys. *Rationale: Ensures accurate function of traction.*
9. Following pin insertion, assess pin sites for redness, edema, discharge, or odor. *Rationale: Establishes baseline for condition of pin insertion sites and identifies signs and symptoms associated with infection.*
10. Assess respiratory rate, rhythm, depth, and chest expansion. *Rationale: Pulmonary embolus can occur in a patient who has associated spinal cord injury or who is on prolonged bed rest. Fat embolus syndrome (FES) can occur with long-bone fracture.*

PLANNING

Expected Outcomes focus on patient's anxiety level, skin integrity, self-care abilities, comfort and mobility level, neurovascular status, infection risks, and pulmonary status.

1. Skeletal deformity is reduced, alignment is maintained, and injury is healed.
2. Patient verbalizes decreased anxiety and performs ADLs independently to all unaffected areas.
3. Skin remains intact, without redness, inflammation, or purulent drainage, especially over pressure points.
4. Patient verbalizes a sense of comfort and rates pain as 4 or lower on a scale of 0 to 10 after repositioning and administration of analgesics.
5. Patient is free of neurovascular deficit after application of skeletal traction. Patient verbalizes no abnormal sensations and is able to move digits below fracture site.
6. Patient performs ROM in unaffected extremities.
7. Patient describes purpose of skeletal traction and demonstrates correct use of trapeze.

Delegation and Collaboration

Skeletal traction is applied by the health care provider. Ongoing assessment of the complete traction set up and for complications, including infection or inflammation at pin insertion site, may not be delegated to nursing assistive personnel (NAP). The skill of assisting with insertion of skeletal pins and pin-site care may be delegated to NAP who are adequately trained in principles of surgical asepsis. The nurse instructs the NAP to:

- Report any signs and symptoms of inflammation or infection at the pin insertion site.

Equipment
Balanced-Suspension Skeletal Traction
- Ropes, pulleys, weights, weight holders
- Thomas splint
- Pearson attachment with sheepskin padding
- Footplate
- Trapeze bar
- Clean gloves

Halo Traction
- Halo ring with four pins
- Molded vest jacket
- Vertical metal bars connecting ring to jacket
- Tracheostomy tray (for emergency resuscitation)
- Allen wrench (allows for the removal of screws for resuscitation)

Pin-Site Care Supplies
- Sterile cotton-tipped applicators
- Prescribed cleansing agent. Preferred agent chlorhexidine 2 mg/mL solution (check facility policy)
- Topical antibiotic ointment (check facility policy)
- Split 2 × 2–inch gauze dressings (optional)
- Clean gloves

IMPLEMENTATION *for* CARE OF A PATIENT IN SKELETAL TRACTION AND PIN-SITE CARE

STEPS	RATIONALE
1. **See Standard Protocol (inside front cover).**	
2. Discuss procedure with patient.	Decreases patient anxiety.
3. Apply clean gloves.	Reduces transmission of infection.
4. Initial traction setup:	
a. Position patient per health care provider's order. Support limb at joint above or below fracture to be placed in traction. Do not move distal portion unnecessarily. Patient will likely be placed in supine position with head of bed slightly elevated.	Ensures proper alignment during and after traction application. Movement can cause severe pain or additional trauma.
b. Health care provider wears sterile gloves and gown while cleaning skin over pin site and injecting local anesthetic.	Anesthetic desensitizes area where pin site will be made. Patient feels pressure during drilling but should feel no pain. Procedure requires surgical asepsis.
c. Assist (usually by holding spreader bar, splint, or Pearson attachment) while health care provider continues to use drill to insert number of pins needed for traction. Support area of joints not at injury site. Do not move distal portion unnecessarily.	Movement can cause severe pain and additional trauma.
d. After traction setup is completed, attach weights and gently lower until rope is taut.	Reduces spasms and discomfort.

e. Inspect traction setup; ensure that:
   • Knots are secure and footplate is in place.
   • Ropes and pulleys are not frayed.
   • Weights are hanging freely, not caught on bed or resting on floor.
   • Bedclothes are not interfering with traction apparatus.
	Ensures that traction and immobilization are effective. Footplate prevents footdrop.

5. Provide pin-site care according to facility policy or health care provider's orders.	
a. Apply clean gloves. Remove gauze dressings from around pins and discard in receptacle.	
b. Inspect pin sites for redness, edema, or purulent drainage. Note: Clear drainage and crusting are expected findings. Remove and discard gloves. Perform hand hygiene.	Signs indicate infection. Reduces transmission of infection.

STEPS	RATIONALE

   c. Prepare supplies.

   d. Apply clean gloves. Clean each pin site with prescribed cleaning solution by placing tip of moistened sterile applicator close to the pin and cleaning away from the insertion site. Dispose of applicator. Use a clean applicator for each swipe. — *Removes infectious material without contaminating pin site.*

   e. Repeat the process for each pin site.

   f. Using a sterile applicator, apply a small amount of topical antibiotic ointment to pin site (see health care provider's order or according to facility policy). — *May reduce development of infection.*

   g. Cover with a sterile 2 × 2–inch split gauze dressing or leave site open to air (see health care provider's order or according to facility policy).

6. Provide routine traction care. — *Massage to compromised tissues increases tissue breakdown.*

   a. Inspect skin (bony prominences, heels, elbows, sacrum, and areas under appliances) for signs of pressure. Use pressure relief devices as appropriate (see Chapter 25). Try to reposition any areas under pressure, if possible. Do not massage areas of pressure if there is tenderness, reactive hyperemia (see Chapter 25), or areas of skin breakdown.

7. Provide nonpharmacological and pharmacological pain relief as indicated (see Chapter 13). — *Pain relief improves patient's ability to remain active within mobility limitations.*

8. Encourage the use of unaffected extremities for ADLs and active and passive exercises (see Chapter 16). Encourage use of trapeze bar for repositioning in bed. — *Prevents muscle atrophy and maintains muscle tone for later ambulation.*

9. For elimination provide a fracture pan if necessary (see Chapter 19). — *Smaller bedpan is more comfortable for and easier to place under patient.*

10. **See Completion Protocol (inside front cover).**

EVALUATION

1. Inspect body part that is in traction for alignment.
2. Monitor neurovascular status and peripheral tissue perfusion every 2 hours for the first 24 hours and every 4 hours thereafter (see facility policy). This includes inspecting color and temperature of distal area, observation for edema, and measurement of capillary refill.
3. Observe behaviors reflecting patient's anxiety level in response to traction and immobilization.
4. Evaluate for presence of pain and muscle spasm on a scale of 0 to 10.
5. Monitor respiratory status for FES, atelectasis, and pulmonary embolism every shift.
6. Observe for local and systemic indications of infection, including purulent drainage and inflammation at pin sites; fever; elevated white blood cell count; and continuous dull aching pain, redness, or warmth in extremity (possible osteomyelitis [i.e., bone infection]).
7. Use **Teach Back:** State to the patient, "I want to be sure you clearly understand the reasons for the external fixator on your wrist, pin-site care, and how to care for the device at home. Can you explain to me how you will care for the pin sites?" Evaluates what the patient is able to explain or demonstrate. Revise your instruction now or develop plan for revised patient teaching to be implemented at an appropriate time if patient is not able to teach back correctly.

Unexpected Outcomes and Related Interventions

1. Patient has severe edema, marked increase in pain, or inability to move joint actively or increased pain on passive movement, indicating compartment syndrome.
   - **a.** Prompt management is critical. Notify health care provider immediately.
   - **b.** Elevate extremity.
   - **c.** Reduce or eliminate compression caused by therapeutic devices.
2. Patient develops signs of infection or osteomyelitis, including fever, elevated white blood cell count, and general malaise. This is especially a concern with open fractures and extensive soft tissue injury.
   - **a.** Cultures of drainage may be indicated to identify infecting organism (health care provider's order is required; see facility policy) (see Chapter 8).

   b. Notify health care provider.

   c. Be prepared to administer ordered IV antibiotics or irrigate the site with antibiotic solution or both.

   d. Encourage fluid intake, and provide comfort measures for fever.

3. Patient experiences nerve damage:

   • Peroneal nerve: Foot drop may develop with inability to evert and dorsiflex foot.

   • Radial or median nerve at wrist: inability to approximate thumb and fingers (radial) and numbness and tingling of thumb, index, and middle fingers (medial) with wrist drop.

   a. Eliminate pressure if possible according to type of traction in place.

   b. Notify health care provider immediately.

4. FES (more common in fractures of pelvic and long bones) develops with symptoms of hypoxia, restlessness, mental changes, tachycardia, tachypnea, dyspnea, low blood pressure, and occasionally petechial rash over upper chest and neck.

   a. FES is a life-threatening emergency.

   b. Notify health care provider, and initiate resuscitation efforts if indicated.

Recording and Reporting

• Record in nurses' notes type of traction, site to which traction is applied, time of application, amount of weights, and patient's response.

• Document your evaluation of patient learning.

• Record in nurses' notes pin-site care performed and appearance of sites.

• Record on flow sheet specific routine assessments and frequency of assessment.

Sample Documentation

0700   BSST in place with 20-pound weight to left femur. Knots secure, ropes in pulleys, weights hanging freely. Neurovascular assessment to left foot—color pink, temperature warm, no numbness or tingling, wiggles toes on command, capillary refill 2 seconds. Reports pain at 2 on scale of 0 to 10. Lateral pin site dry, medial pin site draining small amount clear fluid (0.5-cm [¼-inch] diameter circle). No odor. No redness.

0900   Medial pin-site drainage changed to yellow drainage (1-cm [½-inch] diameter circle). Pin site cultured. Reports pain of 6 on scale of 0 to 10. Health care provider notified of pin-site drainage.

Special Considerations
Pediatric

• Blood loss from a fracture in a child poses a greater danger because the blood volume in a child is 70% to 85% of total body weight compared with only about 60% in an adult (Hockenberry and Wilson, 2013).

• Reassure children that someone will be there to assist them while they are in traction.

Geriatric

• Older adults are at increased risk for impaired skin integrity when they are immobilized and not repositioned frequently. This risk results from a decreased amount of subcutaneous fat and skin that is less elastic, thinner, drier, and more fragile than skin of a younger adult (Touhy and Jett, 2014).

Home Care

• After removal of skeletal traction, teach patient to ambulate slowly within medical guidelines, gradually increasing length of time out of bed and distance walked.

• Teach patient and family caregiver proper pin care.

• Teach patient to notify health care provider of signs such as marked increase in pain, muscle spasms, and increased numbness, indicating reinjury or insufficient healing.

• Teach family caregivers how to apply skin traction correctly if it is prescribed for home use after removal of the skeletal traction.

SKILL 17.4   **CARE OF A PATIENT WITH AN IMMOBILIZATION DEVICE**

Immobilization devices increase stability, support an extremity, or reduce the load on weight-bearing structures such as hips, knees, or ankles. A splint immobilizes and protects a body part. Temporary splints reduce pain and prevent tissue damage from further motion immediately after an injury such as a fracture or sprain. Air splints, Thomas splints, and improvised splints from material on hand are examples of temporary splints applied in emergency situations. Upper extremity fractures are sometimes managed using splints such as hand and digital splints or sugar-tong splints. Slings support splints, casts, or injured upper extremities. They are available commercially or can be made for almost any body part. Velcro or buckle closures permit these devices to be adjusted to fit a body part of almost any size and shape.

An abduction splint or pillow (Fig. 17-12), used after hip replacement surgery, maintains the patient's legs in an abducted position. This permits a patient to be turned without changing the position of the healing limb and prevents dislocation of the hip prosthesis. The splint is easily removed for nursing care (e.g., skin care, dressing changes, and neurovascular assessments). A posterior splint with elastic wraps is sometimes used to support an extremity.

Cloth and foam splints, known as *immobilizers,* provide long-term immobilization (Fig. 17-13). Immobilizers treat sprains and dislocations that do not require complete and continuous immobilization in a cast or traction. Other common types of immobilizers include cervical collars (soft or hard), belt-type shoulder immobilizers, and knee immobilizers. Molded splints made of plastic provide support to patients with chronic injuries or diseases such as arthritis. They maintain the body part in a functional position to prevent contractures and muscle atrophy during the period

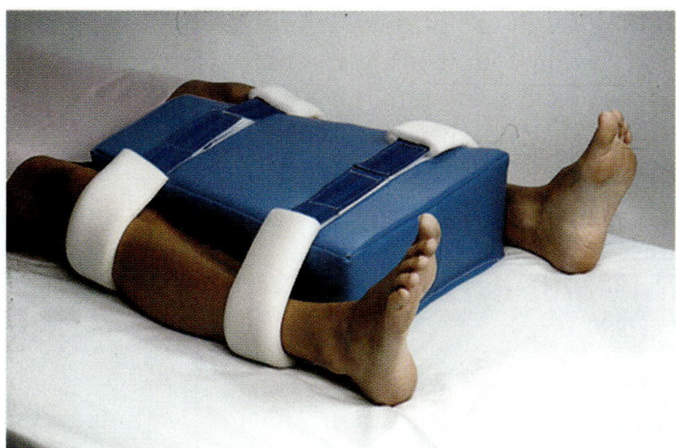

FIG 17-12 Abduction pillow.

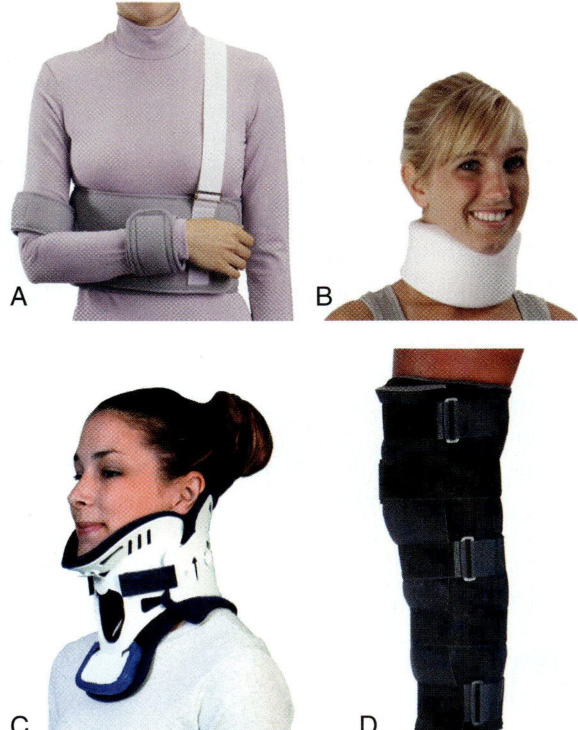

FIG 17-13 Examples of immobilizers. **A,** Shoulder immobilizer. **B,** Soft cervical collar. **C,** Hard cervical collar. **D,** Knee immobilizer. (Used with permission from **A,** ProCare, and **B-D,** Össur Americas. All rights reserved.)

of disuse. Splints and immobilizers can be removed quickly for assessment of the skin or a wound.

Braces support weakened structures during weight bearing. For this reason, they are made of sturdy materials such as leather, metal, and molded plastic. Chest and abdominal braces such as the Boston brace immobilize the thoracic and lumbar vertebral column to treat scoliosis (curvature of the spine). The brace does not correct the curve but instead attempts to prevent its progression. Lumbar braces support lumbar and sacral tissues after spinal surgery. Leg braces hold the thigh, leg, and foot in functional positions for weight bearing and ambulation. Both short-leg and long-leg braces

support weak leg muscles, aid in control of involuntary muscle movement, and maintain surgical correction during the postoperative healing process.

ASSESSMENT

1. Identify patient using two identifiers (e.g., name and birthday or name and account number) according to facility policy. *Rationale: Ensures correct patient. Complies with The Joint Commission standards and improves patient safety (TJC, 2014).*
2. Review patient's medical history, previous and current activity level, and description of the condition requiring immobilization. *Rationale: Reveals patient's current and previous health status and purpose for immobilization.*
3. Determine patient's previous experience with braces/splints/slings. *Rationale: Reveals patient's baseline knowledge and need for instruction.*
4. Assess patient's understanding of reason for brace/splint/sling and its care, application, and schedule of wear. *Rationale: Determines need for further teaching.*
5. Inspect area of skin to be in contact with support device. *Rationale: Provides baseline to monitor patient for skin breakdown. Immobile and older patients are particularly vulnerable.*
6. Assess patient's level of pain on a scale of 0 to 10. *Rationale: Provides baseline to determine if immobilization device affects comfort.*
7. Refer to occupational or physical therapy consultation to determine type of brace to be used, desired position, and amount of activity and movement permitted. *Rationale: Provides direction in proper use of brace.*
8. Assess patient's additional need for an assistive device, such as a cane, walker, or crutches (see Chapter 16). *Rationale: Patient may need an assistive device to provide support and promote balance during ambulation.*

PLANNING

Expected Outcomes focus on maintaining skin integrity, improving patient's knowledge, and preventing risk for injury.
1. Patient's skin remains intact, warm, without signs of pressure, and with normal sensation.
2. Patient and family caregiver verbalize purpose, correct application, and care of the device.
3. Patient reports a temporary increase in pain on a scale of 0 to 10 during device application.
4. Patient uses the device correctly, including schedule of wear, activity limitations, and positioning.

Delegation and Collaboration

The skill of caring for a patient wearing a brace/splint/sling can be delegated to nursing assistive personnel (NAP). The nurse instructs the NAP by:
- Reviewing correct application of the brace/splint/sling and positioning of any ties or straps.

- Reviewing prescribed schedule of wear and activities permitted while in the brace/splint/sling.
- Instructing to inform the nurse if patient complains of pain, rubbing, or pressure from the brace/splint/sling or if a change occurs in patient's skin condition.

Equipment

- Brace/splint/commercially prepared sling or triangular bandage and safety pin
- Cotton shirt or gown
- Clean gloves

IMPLEMENTATION *for* CARE OF A PATIENT WITH AN IMMOBILIZATION DEVICE

STEPS	RATIONALE
1. **See Standard Protocol (inside front cover).**	
2. Explain reasons for brace/splint/sling, and demonstrate how device works.	Teaching and demonstration enhance learning, reduce anxiety, and encourage cooperation.
3. Perform hand hygiene. Assist patient to a comfortable position: apply upper extremity brace/splint/sling with patient sitting upright; apply lower extremity brace with patient lying down.	Facilitates correct, aligned placement of brace/splint/sling.
4. Apply clean gloves. Prepare skin that will be enclosed in brace/splint/sling by cleaning skin with soap and water; rinse, pat dry, and change any dressings (if present). If applying a back brace, put a thin cotton shirt or gown on patient. Ensure that there are no wrinkles to cause pressure.	This protects skin and keeps brace clean. Smooth cotton clothing between the brace and skin protects skin from irritation and absorbs moisture.
5. Inspect device for wear, damage, or rough edges.	Decreases potential for skin breakdown and maintains correct alignment.
6. Apply brace/splint/sling as directed by health care provider, orthotist, physical therapist, or occupational therapist.	Proper application of the brace/splint/sling is important to avoid skin breakdown, pressure ulcers, neurovascular compromise, calluses, or worsening of deformity.
a. Apply even tension as bandage is wrapped from distal to proximal.	Prevents trapping of blood and fluid distal to immobilization device.
b. Prevent padding from gathering or bunching.	Prevents irritation to underlying tissues.
c. Support joints when brace/splint/sling is placed.	Reduces risk of musculoskeletal injury during application.
7. Apply sling using triangular bandage:	
a. Position one end of the bandage over the shoulder of the unaffected arm (see illustration).	Commercially available slings secure arm to chest for added support and have padding on strap for comfort.

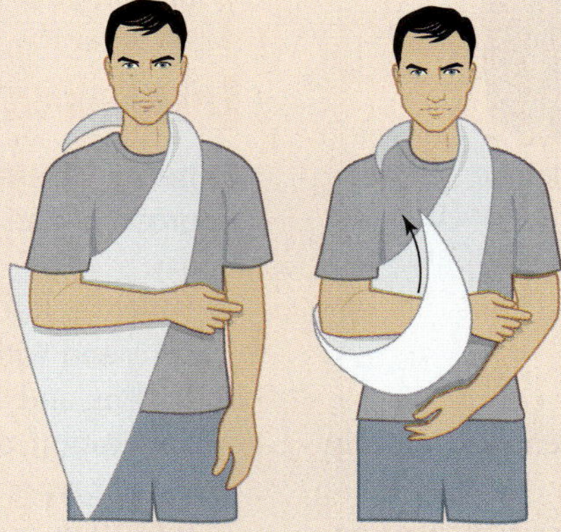

STEP 7a Applying a sling.

b. Take remaining bandage and place the material against the chest, then under and over the affected arm, cradling the arm.	Position supports the arm.
c. Position the pointed end of the triangle toward the elbow.	Position supports arm.
d. Tie the two ends of the triangle at the side of the neck.	Avoids placing knot over cervical spine, causing pressure and discomfort.

STEPS	RATIONALE
e. Fold the pointed end of the sling at the elbow in the front and secure with a safety pin, closing the end of the sling.	
f. Be sure the sling supports the limb comfortably without interfering with circulation.	Prevents skin irritation and pressure to back of neck.
8. Remove and dispose of gloves. Perform hand hygiene.	Reduces transmission of microorganisms.
9. Teach patient prescribed schedule of wear and activities while in brace/splint/sling as directed by health care provider, physical therapist, or occupational therapist.	Proper use of brace/splint/sling facilitates healing and mobility and reduces pain and stress.
10. Reinforce instruction regarding signs of skin breakdown, pressure, or rubbing to report.	Brace/splint/sling may need to be adjusted. Changes may also be required because of growth or atrophy, when muscles regain or lose strength, or after reconstructive surgery.
11. Teach patient how to care for brace/splint/sling:	To maintain integrity of brace/splint/sling.
a. When not in use, store metal braces upright in a safe but easily accessible location.	To prevent deformity or bending of brace.
b. Store splints of molded materials away from heat.	To prevent melting and deformation of splint.
c. Treat any leather material with leather preservative.	To prevent drying or cracking.
d. Keep brace clean, dry, and in good working order.	Plastic parts are cleaned with a damp cloth and thoroughly dried. Metal joints are cleaned with a pipe cleaner and oiled weekly. Remove rust with steel wool and clean metal parts with a solvent.
12. Assist patient in ambulating with brace/splint/sling in place.	Determines if patient is able to ambulate safely.
13. Have patient or family caregiver apply and remove brace/splint/sling.	Promotes patient independence; demonstration confirms level of learning skill.
14. **See Completion Protocol (inside front cover).**	

EVALUATION

1. Inspect area of skin underneath brace/splint/sling for signs of pressure including redness or breakdown.
2. Palpate temperature, pulse, and sensation of extremity distal to brace/splint/sling. Check capillary refill by pressing on toe or finger.
3. Inspect alignment of the limb after application of brace/splint/sling.
4. Ask patient to rate level of pain on a scale of 0 to 10 after brace/splint/sling application.
5. Use *Teach Back:* State to the patient, "I want to be sure I explained clearly the need for the brace/splint/sling, how to maintain the device, and the limitations related to the device. Can you tell me how you will use this brace/splint/sling safely?" Evaluates what the patient is able to explain or demonstrate. Revise your instruction now or develop plan for revised patient teaching to be implemented at an appropriate time if patient is not able to teach back correctly.

Unexpected Outcomes and Related Interventions

1. Patient reports increased severity in pain after application of the device.

   a. Reposition extremity.
   b. Administer analgesics as ordered to maintain patient's comfort level.
   c. Increase frequency of neurovascular checks.
   d. Inform health care provider.
2. Patient develops areas of pressure, redness, or skin breakdown.

   a. Inspect device for proper fit and positioning and for areas of damage, wear, or rough edges.
   b. Inform health care provider.
   c. Inform orthotist, physical therapist, or occupational therapist so that adjustments to brace/splint/sling can be made.

Recording and Reporting

- Record assessments of skin integrity, neurovascular status, application of and type of brace/splint/sling, schedule of wear, activity level, movement permitted, patient's tolerance of procedure, and instructions given to patient and family caregiver in nurses' notes.
- Record observations about patient's ability to apply brace/splint/sling, ambulate, and remove brace/splint/sling.
- Document your evaluation of patient learning.

Sample Documentation

0900   Splint applied to left wrist. Skin warm, dry, and intact. Able to move all fingers of left hand, fingers warm to touch, nail beds pink, no swelling noted. Complains of pain at 3 (scale of 0 to 10).

Special Considerations
Pediatric

- Monitor children closely to ensure that they do not remove immobilization device.
- Recognize that bracing in adolescents affects body image and self-esteem.

Geriatric

- Lightweight immobilization devices are less restrictive.
- Older adults may have decreased sensation (Touhy and Jett, 2014).

Home Care

- Remind patient to inspect skin daily for pressure or areas of breakdown.
- Remind patient to inspect and clean brace/splint/sling weekly.

CRITICAL THINKING EXERCISES

Case Study

A 5-year-old child is seen in the emergency department after falling off the swings while playing after school. She has broken her left radius and ulna. A fiberglass cast is going to be placed on her left arm.

1. To assist in caring for her short-arm fiberglass cast, the nurse recommends to the mother that she do which of the following?
   1. Completely cover the cast with plastic wrap to keep it clean.
   2. Cushion any sharp edges of the cast with tape or moleskin.
   3. Scrape rough edges off the cast with a blunt knife.
   4. Blow dry the cast using low setting following a shower.
2. After 12 hours, the fingers of the left hand are becoming swollen. The mother states that she has elevated the cast and applied ice packs on either side. The child's pain continues to increase despite these interventions. What should you advise the mother to do at this point?
   1. Try applying heat around the cast where the pain is located.
   2. Contact the health care provider possibly to bivalve the cast.
   3. Apply ice on the top and bottom of the cast.
   4. Do nothing because this is an expected finding at this point.
3. After 6 weeks, it is time to remove the cast. The nurse is assisting with the removal of the cast. Place the following steps in the correct order for removal of the cast.
   a. Describe the vibration of the cast saw and the feeling of warmth that the saw causes.
   b. Assist with positioning during removal.
   c. Inspect the tissues underlying the cast.
   d. Gently wash intact skin with cold water enzyme.
   1. a, b, c, d
   2. b, a, c, d
   3. a, b, d, c
   4. b, a, d, c

Review Questions

1. The health care provider has ordered Buck's extension skin traction to a patient's right leg for a fractured right hip until surgery can be performed. The nurse gathers the traction boot and equipment to set up the traction. When applying the traction boot, the nurse performs the following nursing actions. Select all that apply.
   1. Shave the affected leg.
   2. Ensure that the boot fits snugly.
   3. Pad the heel of the traction boot.
   4. Attach weight to the boot gradually and gently at the end of the bed.
   5. Reassess neurovascular status of the extremity proximal to the traction.
2. Which of the following describes the correct method to position a fiberglass casted arm?
   1. Carefully with the palms of the hands to prevent any indentations.
   2. On a plastic-covered pillow to keep the linens dry.
   3. On several pillows with the hand above the elbow to decrease swelling.
   4. With a bed cradle over it to maintain adequate air flow for proper drying.
3. A patient develops severe pain and swelling in the tissues beneath the cast with the toes on the casted foot cold, and capillary refill to the toes is more than 6 seconds. Place the following nursing actions in the correct order.
   1. Assess tightness of cast.
   2. Elevate casted extremity on pillows.
   3. Increase the frequency of neurovascular checks.
   4. Lower the casted extremity.
   5. Notify health care provider before administering analgesics.
   6. Apply warm compresses to the sides of the cast.
   7. Apply ice bags along the sides of the cast.

4. The nurse is teaching a patient how to use and care for a back brace. What instructions should the nurse provide the patient?
   1. Place no clothing between the brace and the skin.
   2. Inspect the brace for wear, damage, or rough edges daily.
   3. Clean the metal joints with a small steel brush and apply emollient cream to the joints weekly.
   4. Clean the plastic parts of the brace with ammonia and dry thoroughly weekly.

5. Which of the following might indicate an infection at a pin site inserted for skeletal traction?
   1. Crusting
   2. Ashen skin color
   3. Clear drainage from pin sites
   4. Erythema at pin sites

6. Which of the following nursing actions are included when inspecting the patient's BSST setup?
   1. Add weight to the traction if it does not seem to be exerting enough force.
   2. Adjust position of the weights if the weights are not hanging freely at the end of the bed.
   3. Alter the line of pull of the ropes to ensure that they are at a 45-degree angle.
   4. Reinsert a slipped Steinmann pin back into place.

7. Which precautions should the nurse include in the plan of care for a patient in skeletal traction?
   1. Avoid using an overhead trapeze.
   2. Remove weights when moving the patient in bed.
   3. Maintain alignment of the injured limb with the trunk.
   4. Release the traction for 15 minutes every 8 hours.

8. What instructions should the nurse provide for a patient who complains of severe itching under the cast?
   1. "The health care provider can provide medication for the itching."
   2. "Go ahead and scratch if you are able to reach your fingers down the cast."
   3. "Itching is part of the healing process and you should not interfere with it."
   4. "I'll get you a tongue blade to use to scratch. Do not use your fingernails."

9. A patient in traction is using a PCA pump for pain control after a fracture of the femur. The patient has been using the pump correctly but complains of increased pain and a jumping, squeezing sensation in the thigh. As the nurse, you would first:
   1. Massage the thigh to relax the muscles.
   2. Medicate the patient with a muscle relaxant to decrease the muscle spasms.
   3. Medicate the patient with a bolus of the pain medication for breakthrough pain.
   4. Release the traction briefly to decrease the pain.

10. A patient has presented in the emergency department with a dislocated shoulder, and the nurse is assisting with the placement of a temporary sling. Place the steps of applying a sling in the correct order.
   1. Tie two ends of triangle at side of neck.
   2. Take remaining bandage and place material against chest and under and over affected arm, cradling arm.
   3. Position one end of the bandage over shoulder of unaffected arm.
   4. Position pointed end of triangle toward elbow.
   5. Fold pointed end of sling at elbow in front and secure with safety pin, closing end of sling.

REFERENCES

Brooker C, Nicol M: *Alexander's nursing practice*, ed 4, St Louis, 2013, Elsevier.

Handoll H, Queally J, Parker M: Pre-operative traction for hip fractures in adults, *Cochrane Database Syst Rev* (12):CD000168, 2011.

Hashim Z, et al: Bilateral simultaneous Achilles tendon rupture in the absence of risk factors: a case report, *Foot Ankle Spec* 5(1):68, 2012.

Hockenberry MJ, Wilson D: *Wong's essentials of pediatric nursing*, ed 9, St Louis, 2013, Mosby.

Hyer C, et al: Early weight bearing of calcaneal fractures fixated with locked plates, *Foot Ankle Spec* 3(6):320, 2010.

Jester R, et al: *Oxford handbook of orthopaedic nursing*, New York, 2011, Oxford University Press.

Lagerquist D, et al: Care of external fixator pin sites, *Am J Crit Care* 21(4):288, 2012.

Satryb S, et al: Casting: all wrapped up, *Orthop Nurs* 30(1):37, 2011.

The Joint Commission (TJC): *National Patient Safety Goals*, Oakbrook Terrace, IL, 2014, The Commission. Available at: http://www.jointcommission.org/standards_information/npsgs.aspx. Last accessed July 30, 2014.

Timms A, Pugh H: Pin site care: guidance and key recommendations, *Nurs Stand* 27(1):50, 2012.

Touhy T, Jett K: *Ebersole and Hess' gerontological nursing and healthy aging*, St Louis, 2014, Elsevier.

Voda S: Bad breaks: a nurse's guide to distal radius fractures, *Nursing* 41(8):37, 2011.

Wheeless C: *Wheeless' textbook of orthopaedics*, Durham, NC, 2011, Data Trace Publishing.

CHAPTER

18

Urinary Elimination

 **EVOLVE WEBSITE/EVOLVE RESOURCES LIST**

http://evolve.elsevier.com/Perry/nursinginterventions
Audio Glossary • Checklists • Review Questions

A basic human function is urinary elimination, a function that can be compromised by a wide variety of illnesses and conditions. It is the role of a nurse to support bladder emptying by assisting patients as needed in toileting, which may include use of a commode, urinal, or bedpan. During acute illness, a patient may require urinary catheterization for close monitoring of urine output or to facilitate bladder emptying when bladder function is compromised. Some patients require long-term indwelling catheters, urethral or suprapubic, when the bladder fails to empty effectively. A nurse also implements measures to minimize risk for infection when bladder function is impaired or urinary drainage tubes are required.

PATIENT-CENTERED CARE

When a patient is no longer able to access a toilet independently or the bladder empties inadequately, nursing intervention is required. Urinary elimination is a private human activity. You need to incorporate sensitivity and awareness of factors that affect your care of patients. Patients may experience embarrassment, fear, or apprehension associated with meeting their elimination needs. It is essential that you acknowledge these feelings and respect patient privacy and dignity as much as possible.

SAFETY

The use of indwelling urinary catheters is associated with numerous complications, including catheter-associated urinary tract infection (CAUTI), discomfort, bladder pain and spasms, genitourinary trauma, formation of bladder calculi, blood in the urine (hematuria), and squamous cell carcinoma of the bladder (Geng et al., 2012). Catheter-related complications such as urinary tract infection (UTI) and trauma to the genitourinary tract have been recognized as a cause for prolonged catheterization, increased use of diagnostic procedures, and increased length of hospital stay (Aaronson et al., 2011; Leuck et al., 2012; Tiwari et al., 2012). The risk for life-threatening infection increases whenever the urinary tract is compromised such as during catheterization. Nursing care must include measures to minimize catheter-related complications and infection, such as using aseptic technique when inserting urinary catheters; maintaining a closed urinary drainage system; providing catheter care that uses principles of asepsis; anchoring catheters; and, above all, removing urinary catheters as soon as medically indicated.

EVIDENCE-BASED PRACTICE

Bernard MS et al: Decrease the duration of indwelling urethral catheters and potentially reduce the incidence of catheter-associated urinary tract infections, *Urol Nurs* 32(1):29, 2012.

Chen Y et al: Using a criteria-based reminder to reduce use of indwelling urinary catheters and decrease urinary tract infections, *Am J Crit Care* 22(2):105, 2013.

Knoll BM et al: Reduction of inappropriate urinary catheter use at a veterans affairs hospital through a multifaceted quality improvement project, *Clin Infect Dis* 52(11):1283, 2011.

Meddings J et al: Reducing unnecessary urinary catheter use and other strategies to prevent catheter-associated urinary tract infections: brief update review. In: *Making Health Care Safer II: An Updated Critical Analysis of the Evidence for Patient Safety Practices,* Rockville, MD, 2013, Agency for Healthcare Research and Quality. Available at http://www.ahrq.gov/research/findings/evidence-based-reports/ptsafetyuptp.html. Accessed August 28, 2013.

Major recommendations in evidence-based guidelines to reduce catheter-related problems and infection include reducing inappropriate catheter use and removing catheters as soon as possible (Meddings et al., 2013). Nurses are recognized as key members of the health care team in initiatives to reduce catheter-related complications and CAUTI (Bernard et al., 2012). Evidence has shown that using some kind of a reminder system such as cues for daily catheter re-evaluation reduces the inappropriate use of indwelling catheters and CAUTI (Meddings et al., 2013; Chen et al., 2013; Knoll et al., 2011). In some systems, the nurse is empowered to evaluate and remove the catheter based on a removal protocol (Meddings et al., 2013). Evidenced-based interventions for the prevention of CAUTI include the following:

- Use aseptic catheter insertion using sterile equipment.
- Secure indwelling catheters to prevent movement and pulling on the catheter.
- Maintain a closed urinary drainage system.
- Maintain an unobstructed flow of urine through the catheter, drainage tubing, and drainage bag.
- Keep the urinary drainage bag below the level of the bladder at all times.
- When emptying the urinary drainage bag, use a separate measuring receptacle for each patient. Do not let the drainage spigot touch the receptacle.
- Perform routine perineal hygiene daily and after soiling.
- Quality improvement/surveillance programs should be in place that alert providers that a catheter is in place and include regular educational programming about catheter care.

PROCEDURAL GUIDELINE 18.1
Assisting with Use of a Urinal

A urinal is a container that collects and holds urine when access to a toilet is restricted. Patients who may need a urinal include those who have compromised mobility, severe dyspnea, or other illnesses that prevent access to a toilet. Although men more typically use urinals, specially designed urinals are available for women. The female urinal has a larger opening at the top with a defined rim that helps position the urinal close against the genitalia (Fig. 18-1).

Delegation and Collaboration

The skill of assisting a patient with a urinal can be delegated to nursing assistive personnel (NAP). The nurse instructs the NAP to:

- Assist the patient with special needs or adaptations related to positioning or holding the urinal.
- Provide personal hygiene as necessary after urination.
- Report immediately any changes in urine color, clarity, and odor; development of incontinence (involuntary loss of urine); patient reports of dysuria, which could indicate an infection; and any changes in the frequency and amount of urine output.

Equipment

- Urinal
- Clean gloves

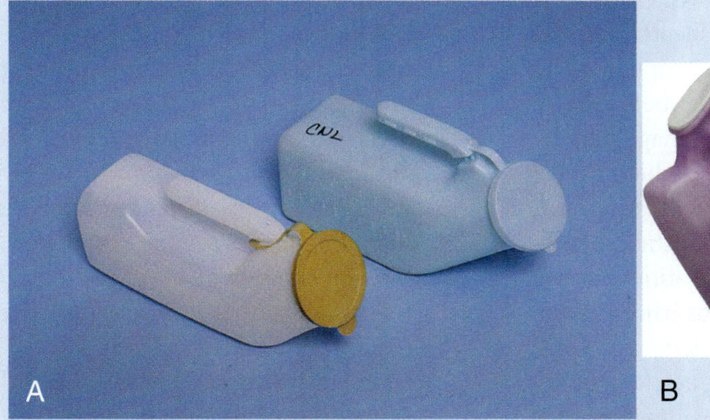
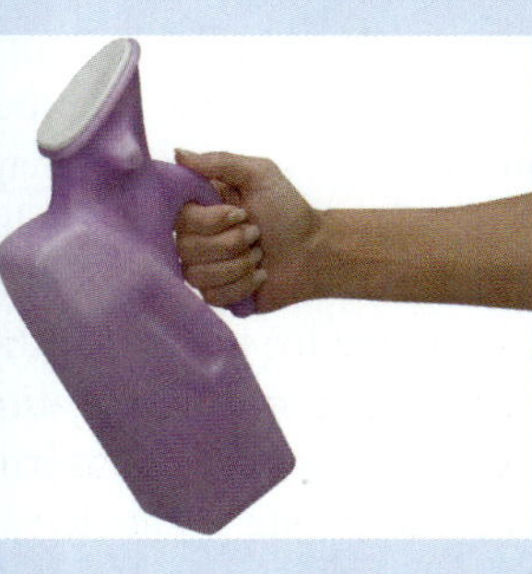

FIG 18-1 Male **(A)** and female **(B)** urinals. (Courtesy Briggs Medical Service Company.)

Continued

PROCEDURAL GUIDELINE 18.1
Assisting with Use of a Urinal—cont'd

- Graduated container (used for measuring volume if on intake and output [I&O])
- Toilet tissue (women)
- Supplies for diagnostic urine tests and specimen collection (see Chapter 8)
- Washbasin
- Washcloths, towels, and soap (as needed for patient hand and perineal hygiene)

Procedural Steps

1. **See Standard Protocol (inside front cover).**
2. Assess patient's normal urinary elimination habits, including any episodes of incontinence.
3. Determine patient's ability to place and remove the urinal.
4. Determine if a urine specimen is to be collected.
5. Provide privacy by closing curtains around bed and door of room.
6. Apply clean gloves. Assist patient into appropriate position. Position male patients on their side or back, sitting with head of bed elevated, or a standing position. Position female patients supine. Place an absorbent pad under the patient's buttocks to protect bed linens from accidental spills. Always determine mobility status and risk for orthostatic hypotension before having a patient stand to void.
7. If possible, patient should hold urinal. If a male patient needs assistance, position penis completely in urinal and hold urinal in place or assist patient in holding urinal. Ensure that the urinal is placed dependent of the flow of urine. Assist a female patient in positioning the urinal against the genitalia.
8. Give the patient privacy by covering the genitalia with the bed linens. If possible, give the patient further privacy by leaving the bedside after ensuring that the patient is in a safe and comfortable position. Place the call device within reach.
9. After the patient has finished voiding, remove urinal and assess characteristics of the urine for color, clarity, odor, and amount. Collect and label specimen if ordered. Assist patient with washing and drying penis or genitalia and with hand hygiene.
10. Empty and cleanse urinal. Return urinal to patient for future use.
11. **See Completion Protocol (inside front cover).**

SKILL 18.1   APPLYING A CONDOM-TYPE EXTERNAL CATHETER

• Nursing Skills Online: Urinary Catheterization Module, Lessons 1 and 3

The external catheter, also called a *condom catheter* or *penile sheath*, is a soft, pliable condom-like sheath that fits over the penis, providing a safe and noninvasive way to contain urine for men who have complete and spontaneous bladder emptying. Most external catheters are made of soft silicone that reduces friction and are clear to allow for easy visualization of skin under the catheter. Latex catheters are still available and used by some patients. It is important to verify that a patient does not have a latex allergy before applying this type of catheter.

Condom-type external catheters are held in place by an adhesive coating on the internal lining of the sheath, a double-sided self-adhesive strip, brush-on adhesive applied to the penile shaft, or an external strap or tape. A catheter may be attached to a small-volume (leg) urinary drainage bag or a large-volume (bedside) drainage bag, both of which need to be kept lower than the level of the bladder. Various styles and sizes are available, so it is important to refer to the manufacturer's guidelines for fitting and correct application. For men who cannot be fitted for a condom-type external catheter, other externally applied catheters are available.

ASSESSMENT

1. Identify patient using two identifiers (e.g., name and birthday or name and account number) according to facility policy. *Rationale: Ensures correct patient. Complies with The Joint Commission standards and improves patient safety (TJC, 2014).*
2. Review health care provider's order for size and type of condom-type external catheter. *Rationale: Ensures safe and correct application of the device.*
3. Assess urinary elimination patterns, ability to empty the bladder effectively, and degree of incontinence. *Rationale: Incontinent patients are at risk for skin breakdown and are candidates for condom catheters. However, if the patient is unable to empty the bladder effectively, an indwelling catheter may be needed.*
4. Assess mental status of patient and patient's knowledge of the purpose of an external catheter. *Rationale: Reveals need for patient instruction. Teaching can include self-application.*
5. Assess condition of penis. *Rationale: Provides a baseline to compare changes in condition of skin after application of the condom catheter.*
6. Use manufacturer's measuring guide to measure the diameter of the penis in a flaccid state. The penile shaft should be at least 2 cm (0.8 inch) in length. *Rationale: Measurement of the penile shaft aids in determining appropriate catheter size.*
7. Assess for latex allergy. *Rationale: Influences choice of condom material.*

PLANNING

Expected Outcomes focus on promoting dryness and preventing continual exposure of skin to urine.

1. Patient's skin is free from urine wetness.
2. Penile shaft is free of skin irritation, breakdown, or swelling.
3. Patient can explain the purpose of the procedure and what to expect.

Delegation and Collaboration

The skill of applying a condom catheter can be delegated to nursing assistive personnel (NAP), depending on facility policy. The nurse instructs the NAP to:

- Follow manufacturer's guidelines for applying and securing the condom catheter.

- Measure and record urine output and I&O if applicable.
- Report immediately pain, swelling, redness, skin irritation, or breakdown of the glans penis or penile shaft.

Equipment

- Condom catheter kit—condom sheath of appropriate size, securing device (internal adhesive, strap, or tape), skin preparation solution (per manufacturer's recommendations)
- Urinary collection bag with drainage tubing or leg bag and straps
- Basin with warm water and soap
- Towels and washcloth
- Bath blanket
- Clean gloves
- Scissors, hair guard, or paper towel

IMPLEMENTATION *for* APPLYING A CONDOM-TYPE EXTERNAL CATHETER

STEPS	RATIONALE
1. **See Standard Protocol (inside front cover).**	
2. Verify patient's size and type of condom catheter on the plan of care.	Ensures that the patient receives the correct size and type of condom catheter. If too small, the condom catheter may fall off, compress the urethra stopping urine flow, or cause local tissue trauma; if too big, it may leak or fall off (Kyle, 2011).
3. Prepare urinary drainage collection bag and tubing (large-volume drainage bag or leg bag). Clamp off drainage bag port. Place nearby ready to attach to condom catheter after catheter has been applied.	Provides easy access to drainage equipment after applying catheter.
4. Assist patient into supine position, thighs slightly apart, with a bath blanket over upper torso and sheets folded over the lower extremities; expose only genitalia for procedure.	Promotes comfort; draping prevents unnecessary exposure of body parts.
5. Apply clean gloves. Provide perineal care (see Procedural Guideline 10.1). Dry thoroughly before applying device. In a uncircumcised male patient, ensure that the foreskin has been replaced before applying the condom catheter. Do not apply barrier cream.	Prevents skin breakdown from exposure to secretions. Removes any residual adhesives. Minimizes skin irritation and promotes adhesion of the new external catheter. If the foreskin is not replaced to the normal down position, dangerous swelling and pain can occur. Barrier creams prevent the sheath from adhering to the penile shaft.

> **SAFE PATIENT CARE** Before application of the external condom catheter, reassess the skin carefully for erythema, open areas, and rashes. The catheter can be applied only to intact skin (Kyle, 2011).

STEPS	RATIONALE
6. If prescribed, apply skin protectant to penis and allow to dry.	Reduces risk of skin irritation from catheter adhesives and moisture. The protectant increases the adherence of the condom catheter to the skin.
7. Clip hair at base of penis, as necessary, before application of the condom catheter. Some manufacturers provide a hair guard that is placed over the penis before applying the device. The hair guard is removed after application. An alternative to a hair guard is to tear a hole in a paper towel, place it over the penis, and remove after application of the device.	Hair adheres to condom and is pulled during condom removal or may get caught in the adhesive as external catheter is applied.

Continued

STEPS	RATIONALE

> **SAFE PATIENT CARE** The pubic area should not be shaved because it may increase risk for skin irritation, and infection can develop in the micro abrasions.

8. Apply condom catheter. With nondominant hand, grasp penis along shaft. With dominant hand, hold rolled condom sheath at tip of penis with the head of the penis in the cone. Smoothly roll sheath onto penis. Allow 2.5 to 5 cm (1 to 2 inches) of space between tip of glans penis and end of condom catheter (see illustration).

Excessive wrinkles or creases in an external catheter sheath after application may mean that the patient needs a smaller size.

9. Apply appropriate securing device (see Manufacturer's Guidelines).
   a. Self-adhesive condom catheters: Apply gentle pressure on penile shaft for 10 to 15 seconds to secure catheter.
   b. Spiral wrap penile shaft with supplied strip of elastic adhesive. Strip should be spiral wrapped and not overlap itself (see illustration). The elastic strip should be snug, not tight.

Condom must be secured firmly so that it is snug and stays on but not tight enough to cause constriction of blood flow. Application of gentle pressure ensures adherence of adhesive with penile skin.

> **SAFE PATIENT CARE** Do not apply standard adhesive tape, Velcro, or elastic strips around the penis; this could interfere with circulation and cause necrosis of the penis (Kawoosa, 2011).

10. Connect drainage tubing to end of condom catheter. Be sure that condom is not twisted. Catheter can be connected to a large-volume bag or leg bag. Teach patient to keep the condom and catheter kink-free. If a leg bag is used, ensure that the straps are not too tight. Teach patient to check for straps that are too tight.

Allows urine to be collected and measured. Keeps patient dry. Twisted condom obstructs urine flow, causing urine pooling, skin irritation, and catheter to come off.

11. If using a large drainage bag, place excess coiling of tubing on bed and secure to bottom sheet. Empty drainage bags frequently.

Prevents looping of tubing and promotes free drainage of urine. Emptying drainage bags when half full avoids unnecessary tension on the catheter, which prevents accidental dislodgment.

12. **See Completion Protocol (inside front cover).**

13. Remove and reapply daily following the listed steps, unless an extended wear device is used. Apply clean gloves. For removal, wash the penis with warm, soapy water, and gently roll the sheath off the penile shaft.

Helps prevent trauma and irritation.

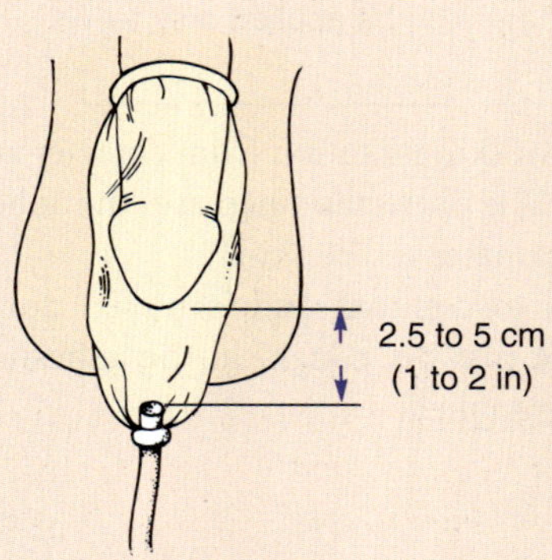

STEP 8 Condom catheter.

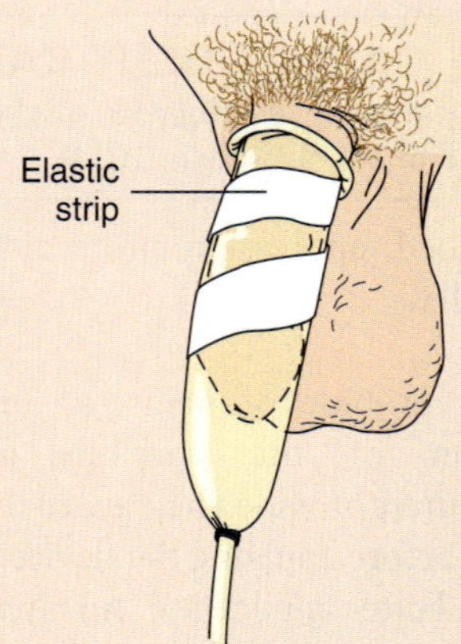

STEP 9b Tape applied in spiral fashion.

EVALUATION

1. Observe urinary drainage.
2. Inspect penis with condom catheter in place within 30 minutes after application. Assess for swelling and discoloration. Ask patient if there is any discomfort.
3. Inspect skin on penile shaft for signs of breakdown or irritation at least daily when removing condom catheter, providing perineal care and before reapplying condom catheter.
4. Use **Teach Back:** State to the patient, "I want to be sure I explained clearly about your external condom catheter and some things you can do to prevent it from accidentally falling off. Can you tell me some of those things?" Evaluates what the patient is able to explain or demonstrate. Revise your instructions now or develop plan for revised patient teaching to be implemented at an appropriate time if the patient is not able to teach back correctly.

Unexpected Outcomes and Related Interventions

1. Urination is reduced in amount or frequency.
   a. Check for bladder distention.
   b. Observe whether urine is pooling at tip of condom, bathing the penis in urine; if so, reapply as necessary.
   c. Check for kinks in tubing or condom catheter.
2. Skin on penis is reddened, ulcerated, or denuded.
   a. Reassess for possible latex allergy.
   b. Remove condom catheter and notify health care provider.
   c. Do not reapply until penis and surrounding skin are free from irritation.
3. Condom catheter does not stay on.
   a. Ensure that catheter tubing is anchored and that patient understands not to pull or tug on catheter.
   b. Reassess condom catheter size. Refer to manufacturer's guidelines for sizing.
   c. Observe whether condom catheter outlet is kinked and urine is pooling at tip of condom, bathing the penis in urine; reapply as necessary and avoid catheter obstruction.
   d. Assess need for another brand of condom catheter (i.e., self-adhesive versus one with spiral wrap).

4. Penile swelling or discoloration occurs.
   a. Remove condom catheter.
   b. Notify health care provider.
   c. Reassess current condom catheter size and type.

Recording and Reporting

- Record condom application; condition of penis, skin, and scrotum; urinary output and voiding pattern; and patient response to external catheter application.
- Report penile erythema, rashes, or skin breakdown.
- Document your evaluation of patient learning.

Sample Documentation

0900   Incontinent of small volumes of urine multiple times. Skin of penis intact without erythema or edema. Scrotum and groin without erythema, breakdown, or rash. Applied self-adhesive size large condom catheter and attached to leg drainage bag. Patient tolerated procedure well. Patient identifies measures he can use to prevent accidental catheter removal.
1300   Condom catheter intact. No erythema or skin breakdown. 400 mL of clear yellow urine in drainage bag.

Special Considerations
Pediatric

- Condom catheters are uncommon in children. When used in adolescents, take precautions to minimize embarrassment.

Geriatric

- Evaluate patients with neuropathy carefully before application of a condom catheter, and assess penile skin at more frequent intervals, at least twice daily.
- Condom catheters are not recommended in patients with prostatic obstruction.

Home Care

- Teach patient and family caregivers appropriate assessments, such as signs and symptoms of UTI, signs of skin irritation, or poor-fitting catheter sheath.
- Loose-fitting clothing may be needed to accommodate the catheter and drainage system.
- Ensure that patient and caregiver understand correct steps in applying the condom catheter and how to empty the drainage bag. Manufacturers often supply educational materials for patients.

PROCEDURAL GUIDELINE 18.2
Bladder Scan

A bladder scanner is a noninvasive device that measures the volume of urine in the bladder by creating an ultrasound image of the bladder from which calculations are made to report urine volumes. The bladder scanner can be used to assess bladder volume whenever inadequate bladder emptying is suspected such as after the removal of indwelling urinary catheters, in the evaluation of new-onset incontinence, when bladder distention is suspected, and to assess voiding after urologic surgery. The most common use for the bladder scan is to measure postvoid residual (PVR).

Continued

PROCEDURAL GUIDELINE 18.2
Bladder Scan—cont'd

PVR is the volume of urine in the bladder after a normal voiding. To be most accurate, PVR must be measured within 5 to 15 minutes of voiding (Huether and McCance, 2012). If a bladder scanner is unavailable, obtain a PVR by measuring urine emptied from the bladder using straight catheterization (see Skill 18.2).

Delegation and Collaboration

The use of the bladder scanner can be delegated to nursing assistive personnel (NAP) (see facility policy). The nurse, in collaboration with the health care provider, determines the timing and frequency of bladder scan measurement, assesses the patient's ability to toilet before measurement of PVR, assesses the abdomen for distention if urinary retention is suspected, and interprets the measurements obtained. The nurse instructs the NAP to:

* Follow the manufacturer's recommendations for the use of the device.
* Measure PVR volumes within 5 to 15 minutes after assisting patient to void.
* Report and record bladder scan volumes.

Equipment

* Bladder scanner (Fig. 18-2)
* Ultrasound gel
* Cleaning agent for scanner head such as an alcohol pad
* Paper towels

Procedural Steps

1. **See Standard Protocol (inside front cover).**
2. Identify patient using two identifiers (e.g., name and birthday or name and account number) according to facility policy.
3. Assess I&O record to determine urine output trends, and check the plan of care to verify correct timing of the bladder scan measurement.
4. Apply clean gloves. If the measurement is for PVR, ask patient to void first and then use scanner to measure voided urine volume.
5. Assist patient to the supine position with the head slightly elevated. Raise bed to appropriate working height. If side rails are raised, lower side rail on working side.
6. Expose patient's lower abdomen.
7. Turn on the scanner per manufacturer's guidelines.
8. Set the gender designation per manufacturer's guidelines. Women who have had a hysterectomy should be designated as male on the scanner.

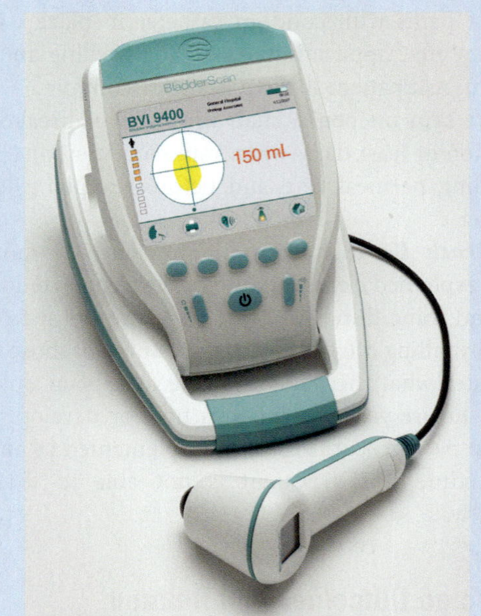

FIG 18-2 Bladder scan image. (Courtesy Verathon, Inc.)

9. Wipe the scanner head with an alcohol pad and allow to air dry.
10. Palpate the patient's symphysis pubis (pubic bone). Apply a generous amount of ultrasound gel (or, if available, a bladder scan gel pad) to the midline abdomen 2.5 to 4 cm (1 to 1.5 inches) above the symphysis pubis. The ultrasound gel ensures adequate transmission and accurate measurement.
11. Place the scanner head on the gel, ensuring that the scanner head is oriented per the manufacturer's guidelines.
12. Apply light pressure, keep the scanner head steady, and point the scanner head slightly downward toward the bladder. Press and release the scan button.
13. Verify accurate aim (refer to manufacturer's guidelines). Repeat scan as needed to ensure accurate volume measurement. Complete the scan and print the image (if needed).
14. Remove ultrasound gel from patient's abdomen with a paper towel.
15. Remove ultrasound gel from scanner head and wipe with alcohol pad; let air dry.
16. **See Completion Protocol (inside front cover).**

• **Nursing Skills Online: Urinary Catheterization, Lessons 1 and 2**

Urinary catheterization is the placement of a tube into the bladder to remove urine. This is an invasive procedure that requires a medical order and sterile technique (Hooton et al., 2010). Urinary catheterization may be short-term (≤2 weeks) or long-term (>14 days) (Geng et al., 2012). Conditions that require use of urinary catheters include the need to monitor urine output, relief of urinary obstruction, postoperative care until a patient can void independently, or a bladder that inadequately empties as a result of a neurological condition. Excessive accumulation of urine in the bladder increases the risk for UTI and can cause backward flow of urine up the ureters to the kidneys, causing kidney infection or damage or both. Urinary incontinence, an involuntary leakage of urine, may require indwelling catheterization if the leaking urine interferes with wound healing. Intermittent catheterization is used to measure postvoid residual (PVR) when a bladder scanner is unavailable or as a way to manage chronic urinary retention.

The steps for inserting an indwelling and a single-use straight catheter are the same. The difference lies in the inflation of a balloon to keep the indwelling catheter in place and the presence of a closed drainage system. Urinary catheters are made with one to three lumens (Fig. 18-3). Single-lumen catheters (see Fig. 18-3, *A*) are used for intermittent catheterization (i.e., the insertion of a catheter for one-time bladder emptying). Double-lumen catheters, designed for indwelling catheters, provide one lumen for urinary drainage and a second lumen for balloon inflation to keep the catheter in

place (see Figure 18-3, *B*). Triple-lumen catheters (see Fig. 18-3, *C*) are used for continuous bladder irrigation (CBI) or to instill medications into the bladder. One lumen drains the bladder, a second lumen is used to inflate the balloon, and a third lumen delivers fluid from an irrigation bag into the bladder.

A health care provider chooses a catheter on the basis of factors such as latex allergy, history of catheter incrustation, and susceptibility for infection. Indwelling catheters are made of latex or silicone. Some have special coatings that reduce urethral irritation and incrustation. Silver-coated catheters have been used as a measure to reduce infection, but efficacy data have been inconsistent, and silver-coated catheter use is uncommon because of the increased cost of the catheters (Beattie and Taylor, 2010; Muzzi-Bjornson and Macera, 2011). Straight or intermittent catheters are made of rubber (softer and more flexible) or polyvinyl chloride. A large selection of catheters is available for patients who self-catheterize: some with special coatings that do not require lubrication and others that are self-contained systems consisting of a lubricated catheter and packaged with a connected drainage bag.

The size of a urinary catheter is based on the French (Fr) scale, which reflects the internal diameter of the catheter. Most adults with an indwelling catheter should have a size 14 to 16 Fr to minimize trauma and risk for infection. Older women or older men with an enlarged prostate may need a smaller size (12 to 14 Fr). Larger catheter diameters increase

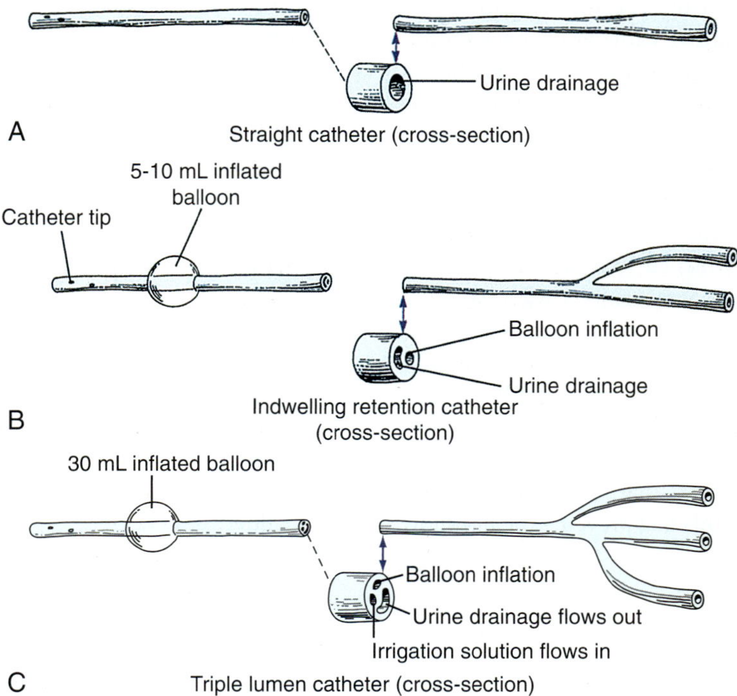

FIG 18-3 A, Single-lumen or straight catheter (cross section). **B,** Double-lumen or indwelling retention catheter (cross section). **C,** Triple-lumen catheter (cross section).

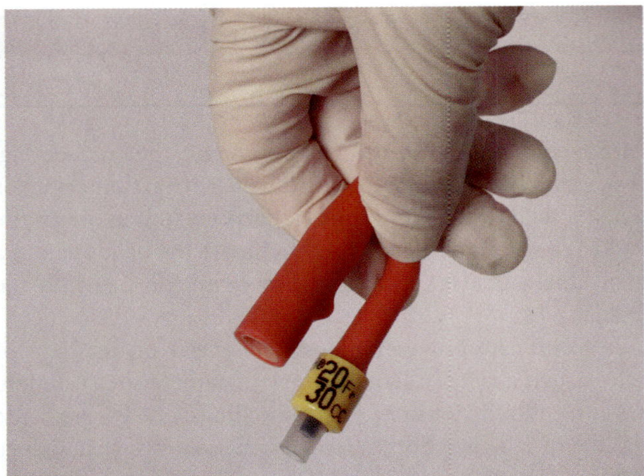

FIG 18-4 Size of catheter and balloon printed on catheter.

the risk for trauma to the bladder neck and urethra (Geng et al., 2012). However, larger sizes such as 20 to 22 Fr are needed in special circumstances, such as after urological surgery or in the presence of gross hematuria. Smaller sizes are needed for infants (5 to 6 Fr) and children (8 to 10 Fr).

Indwelling catheters come in a variety of balloon sizes ranging from 3 mL (for a child) to 30 mL for CBI. The size of the catheter and balloon is usually printed on the catheter port (Fig. 18-4). The recommended balloon size for an adult is a 5-mL balloon (filled with 10 mL). Long-term use of larger balloons (30 mL) has been associated with increased patient discomfort, irritation and trauma, increased risk of catheter expulsion, and incomplete emptying of the bladder resulting from urine that pools below the level of the catheter drainage eyelets or balloon occlusion of the drainage eyelets (Geng et al., 2012; Hooton et al., 2010).

For patients requiring long-term catheterization (i.e., urinary retention or critical illness), catheter changes should be individualized, not routine (Geng et al., 2012). Catheters should be changed for leaking or blockage and before obtaining a sterile specimen for urine culture (Geng et al., 2012). Long-term catheterization should be avoided because of its association with UTIs. Every effort should be made to remove a catheter as soon as a patient can void.

An indwelling catheter is attached to a urinary drainage bag to collect the continuous flow of urine. Always hang the bag below the level of the bladder on the bedframe or a chair so that urine drains down, out of the bladder. The bag should never touch the floor. Have the patient carry the bag below the level of the bladder during ambulation. The only exception to this rule is when a catheter is attached to a specially designed drainage bag (belly bag) that is worn across the abdomen. A one-way valve on this bag prevents the backflow of urine into the bladder.

ASSESSMENT

1. Identify patient using two identifiers (e.g., name and birthday or name and account number) according to facility policy. *Rationale: Ensures correct patient. Complies with The Joint Commission standards and improves patient safety (TJC, 2014).*
2. Review health care provider's order and nurses' notes. Note previous catheterization, including catheter size, response of patient, and time of last catheterization. *Rationale: Identifies purpose of inserting catheter such as for measurement of residual urine or specimen collection, previous catheter size, and potential difficulty with catheter insertion.*
3. Assess patient's knowledge and prior experience with catheterization. *Rationale: Reveals need for patient instruction or support or both.*
4. Review the medical record for any pathological conditions that may impair passage of catheter (e.g., enlarged prostate gland in men, urethral strictures). *Rationale: Obstruction of the urethra may prevent passage of the catheter into the bladder.*
5. Ask patient about and check medical record for allergies. *Rationale: Identifies allergy to antiseptic, tape, latex, and lubricant.*
6. Assess patient's weight, level of consciousness, developmental level, ability to cooperate, and mobility. *Rationale: Determines positioning for catheterization and indicates how much assistance is needed to position patient properly, ability of patient to cooperate during the procedure, and level of explanation needed.*
7. Assess patient's gender and age. *Rationale: Determines catheter size.*
8. Ask patient the time of last voiding or check I&O flow sheet. *Rationale: Determines time of last void and indicates if urinary retention is likely.*
9. Assess the bladder for fullness by palpating it over the symphysis pubis or by using the bladder scanner (see Procedural Guideline 18.2). *Rationale: A full bladder with an inability to void or voiding small amounts frequently indicates a need to insert a catheter. Palpation of a full or overfull bladder causes pain or urge to void or both.*
10. Perform hand hygiene. Apply clean gloves. Inspect perineal region, observing for perineal landmarks, erythema, drainage, or discharge and odor. *Rationale: Determines the visibility of the urethra and need for cleansing the perineum.*

PLANNING

Expected Outcomes focus on emptying the bladder and promoting patient comfort.
1. Patient's bladder is not palpable.
2. Patient verbalizes absence of a sensation of discomfort or bladder fullness.
3. Patient has a urine output of at least 30 mL/hr of clear, light yellow urine in urinary drainage bag.

Delegation and Collaboration

The skill of inserting an indwelling or straight urinary catheter cannot be delegated to nursing assistive personnel (NAP). The nurse instructs the NAP to:

- Assist the nurse with patient positioning, focus lighting for the procedure, maintain patient privacy, empty urine from the collection bag, and assist with perineal care.
- Report any changes in the color, amount, and odor of the urine and if the indwelling catheter leaks or causes pain.

Equipment
- Catheter kit containing sterile items (NOTE: Catheter kits vary)
  - Straight catheterization kit: single-lumen catheter (12 to 14 Fr), drapes (one fenestrated—has an opening in the center), sterile gloves, lubricant, cleansing solution incorporated in an applicator or to be added to cotton balls, and specimen container and label.
  - Indwelling catheterization kit: Double lumen catheter, drapes (one fenestrated—has an opening in the center), sterile gloves, lubricant, antiseptic cleansing solution incorporated in an applicator or to be added to cotton balls, specimen container and label, and a prefilled syringe with sterile water (to inflate balloon). NOTE: Some kits contain a catheter with attached drainage bag; others contain only a catheter; others have no catheter.
- Sterile drainage tubing and bag (if not included in indwelling catheter insertion kit)
- Device to secure catheter (catheter strap or other device)
- Extra sterile gloves and catheter (optional)
- Clean gloves
- Basin with warm water, washcloth, towel, and soap for perineal care
- Flashlight or other additional light source
- Bath blanket, waterproof absorbent pad
- Measuring container for urine

IMPLEMENTATION *for* INSERTION OF A STRAIGHT OR INDWELLING CATHETER

STEPS	RATIONALE
1. See Standard Protocol (inside front cover).	
2. Check patient's plan of care for size and type of catheter. Use smallest size catheter possible.	Ensures that patient receives the correct size and type of catheter.
3. Discuss procedure with patient.	Decreases patient anxiety.
4. Provide privacy by closing room door and bedside curtain.	Protects patient confidentiality.

> **SAFE PATIENT CARE** Obtain assistance to position and support weak, frail, obese, or confused patients.

STEPS	RATIONALE
5. Position and drape patient.	
a. *Position female* patient dorsal recumbent (on back with knees flexed) and ask patient to relax thighs. Drape with bath blanket so that only the perineum is exposed (see illustration).	Exposes perineum, allows hip joints to be rotated externally, and minimizes the risk for contamination by fecal material.
b. *Alternate female position*: position side-lying (Sims') with upper leg flexed at knee and hip. Ensure that rectal area is covered with drape to reduce risk of contamination. Support patient with pillows if necessary to maintain position.	Alternate position is more comfortable if patient cannot abduct leg at the hip joint (e.g., if patient has arthritic joints or contractures).
c. *Position male* patient supine with legs extended and thighs slightly abducted. Cover upper body with small sheet or towel. Cover legs with separate sheet so that only genitals are exposed (see illustration).	Aids in visualization of penis.
6. Apply clean gloves. Place waterproof pad under patient. Cleanse patient's perineal area with soap and water, rinse, and dry (see Procedural Guideline 10.1). Identify the urinary meatus. Remove and discard gloves. Perform hand hygiene.	Hygiene before initiating aseptic catheter insertion removes secretions, urine, and feces around meatus and perineum that could contaminate the sterile field and increase risk of introducing bacteria into the bladder, causing a CAUTI.
7. Position light to illuminate perineum or have assistant available to hold light source to visualize urinary meatus.	Adequate visualization of the urinary meatus helps with the speed and accuracy of catheter insertion.

Continued

STEPS	RATIONALE

8. Open outer wrapping of catheterization kit (some products have double wrapping that requires removal of outer wrapper or plastic covering; others require peeling back a paper top). Place inner wrapped catheter kit tray on clean surface such as a bedside table or between patients' open legs if possible. Patient size and positioning dictate exact placement.

Provides easy access to supplies during catheter insertion.

9. Open inner sterile wrap using sterile technique (see Chapter 5).

The sterile wrap serves as a sterile field.

    a. Indwelling catheterization open system: Open the separate package that contains the drainage system bag, check to ensure that clamp on drainage port is closed, and place drainage bag and tubing so they are easily accessible. Open outer package of catheter, maintaining sterility of inner wrapper.

An open drainage bag system will have separate sterile packaging for the sterile catheter, drainage bag and tubing, and insertion kit.

    b. Indwelling catheterization closed system: All supplies are in the sterile tray. Once sterile gloves are put on, check to ensure the clamp on the drainage bag is closed.

Closed drainage bag systems have catheter preattached to drainage tubing and bag.

    c. Straight catheterization: All needed supplies are in the sterile tray. Use the tray that contains supplies for urine collection.

10. Put on sterile gloves.

11. Drape perineum, keeping gloves sterile.

The sterile drapes provide a sterile field over which you work during catheterization.

    a. Drape female:

      (1) Pick up square drape and allow it to unfold without touching unsterile surfaces. Allow top edge of drape to form cuff over both hands. Place drape with the shiny side down on bed between patient's thighs. Slip cuffed edge just under buttocks as you ask patient to lift the hips. Take care not to touch contaminated surfaces with sterile gloves.

When creating the cuff over the sterile gloved hands, the sterility of gloves and workspace is maintained.

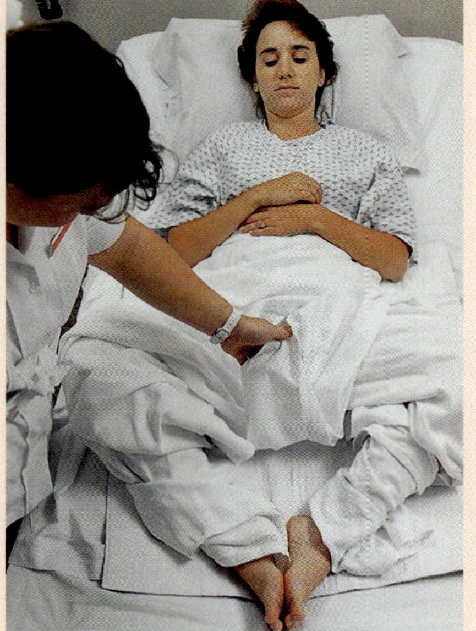

STEP 5a Draping female patient with blankets.

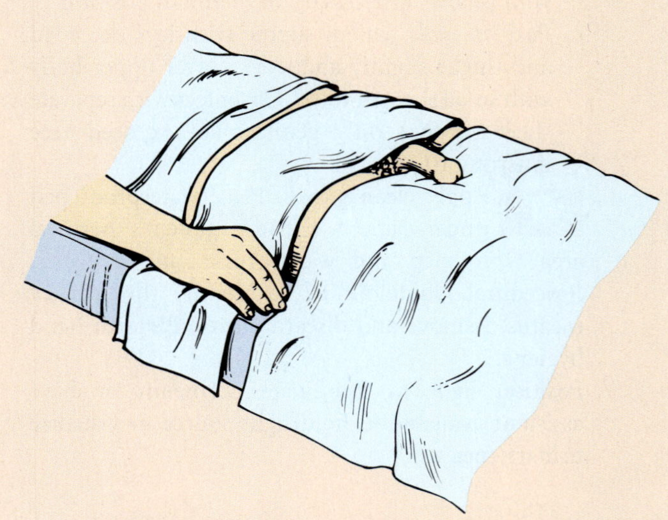

STEP 5c Draping male patient with blankets.

STEPS	RATIONALE

STEPS

    (2) Pick up fenestrated sterile drape. Allow drape to unfold without touching unsterile surfaces. Allow top edge of drape to form cuff over both hands. Drape over perineum, exposing the labia (see illustration).

   b. *Drape male:* Pick up square drape and allow it to unfold without touching unsterile surfaces; place over thighs with shiny side down, just below penis. Place fenestrated drape with opening centered over penis (see illustration).

   c. In some kits, the sterile gloves may be below the square sterile drape. In this case, you pick up the square drape from the tray by the edges and allow it to unfold without touching unsterile surfaces. Fold away the top edge (sterile side up, hands on shiny underside) to form a cuff over both hands, and carefully place the drape. Next, put on sterile gloves and place fenestrated drape (see Step 11a(2)).

12. Arrange supplies on sterile field, maintaining sterility of gloves. Place sterile tray with cleaning solution (premoistened swab sticks or cotton balls, forceps, and solution), lubricant, catheter, and prefilled balloon inflation syringe (indwelling catheterization only) on the sterile drape close to the perineum.

   a. Open package of sterile antiseptic solution. Pour solution over sterile cotton balls. Some kits may contain a package of premoistened swab sticks. Open the end of the package for easy access.

   b. Open sterile specimen container if specimen is required (see Skill 8.1).

   c. For indwelling catheterization, open inner sterile wrapper of catheter. If part of the kit, remove tray with catheter and attached drainage bag and place on sterile drape. Make sure that clamp on drainage port of the bag is closed.

RATIONALE

Opening in drape creates sterile field around labia.

The sequence of supplies in a kit varies. Use supplies in order of use to prevent contamination of underlying supplies.

Provides easy access to supplies during catheter insertion and helps to maintain aseptic technique. Appropriate placement is determined by size of patient and position during catheterization.

Use of sterile supplies and antiseptic solution reduces the risk of CAUTI (Geng et al., 2012; Gould et al., 2010).

Makes container accessible to receive urine from catheter if specimen is needed.

Indwelling catheterization trays vary. Some have preattached catheters, others need to be attached but are part of the sterile tray, and others do not have a catheter or drainage system as part of the tray. Closure of the drainage port on the bottom of the bag prevents urine from draining out of the bag after catheter insertion.

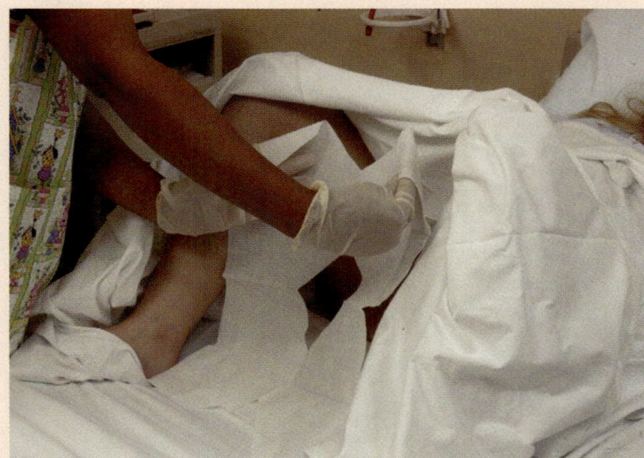

STEP 11a(2) Place sterile fenestrated drape (with opening in center) over perineum with labia exposed.

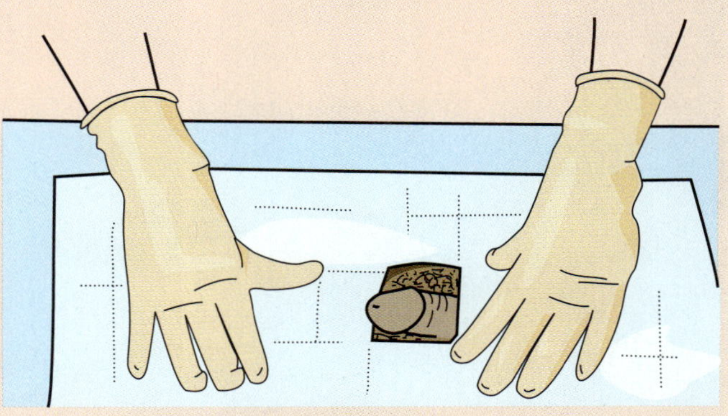

STEP 11b Draping male patient.

Continued

<table>
<tr><td>STEPS</td><td>RATIONALE</td></tr>
</table>

> **SAFE PATIENT CARE** It is essential to check the manufacturer's instructions before inserting an indwelling catheter. Some manufacturers do not recommend pretesting the inflation balloon. Pretesting by inflation and deflation of the balloon may lead to the formation of ridges in the balloon that could potentially cause trauma on insertion.

13. Open packet of lubricant and squeeze out on catheter tray or sterile field. Lubricate catheter by dipping catheter into water-soluble gel 2.5 to 5 cm (1 to 2 inches) for women and 12.5 to 17.5 cm (5 to 7 inches) for men (see illustration).

Lubrication minimizes trauma to the urethra and discomfort during catheter insertion (Geng et al., 2012). The male catheter needs enough lubricant to cover the length of the catheter inserted.

14. Cleanse urethral meatus.

a. *Female patient:*

(1) Separate labia with fingers of nondominant hand (**now contaminated**) to expose urinary meatus fully.

Optimal visualization of urethral meatus is possible.

(2) Maintain position of nondominant hand continuously until catheter has been inserted.

Closure of the labia during cleansing means the area is now contaminated and requires the cleansing procedure to be repeated.

(3) Use the forceps to hold one cotton ball or hold one swab stick at a time. Clean labia and urinary meatus from clitoris toward anus. Use a new cotton ball/swab stick for each area cleansed. Cleanse by wiping the far labial fold, the near labial fold, and directly over center of urethral meatus (see illustration).

Front-to-back cleansing is cleaning from area of least contamination toward highly contaminated area. Follows principles of medical asepsis. Dominant gloved hand remains sterile.

b. *Male patient:*

(1) With nondominant hand (**now contaminated**) retract foreskin (if uncircumcised) and gently grasp penis at shaft just below glans. Hold shaft of penis at right angle to body. This hand remains in this position for remainder of procedure.

When grasping shaft of penis, avoid pressure on dorsal surface to prevent compression of urethra.

(2) Using sterile dominant hand, cleanse meatus with cotton balls/swab sticks using circular strokes, beginning at the meatus and working outward in a spiral motion.

Circular cleansing pattern follows principles of medical asepsis (see Chapter 5).

(3) Repeat three times using clean cotton ball/swab stick each time (see illustration).

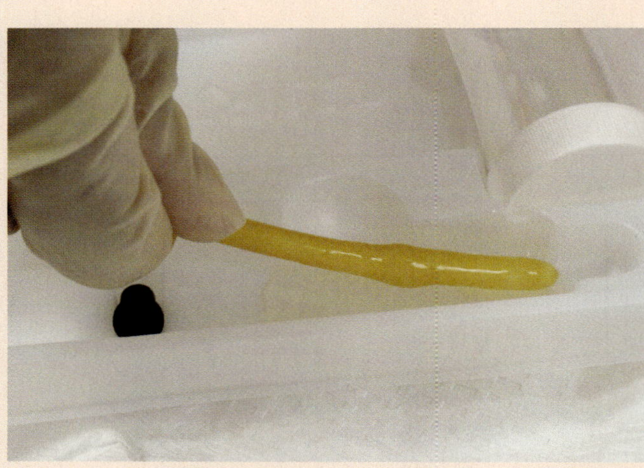

STEP 13 Lubricating catheter.

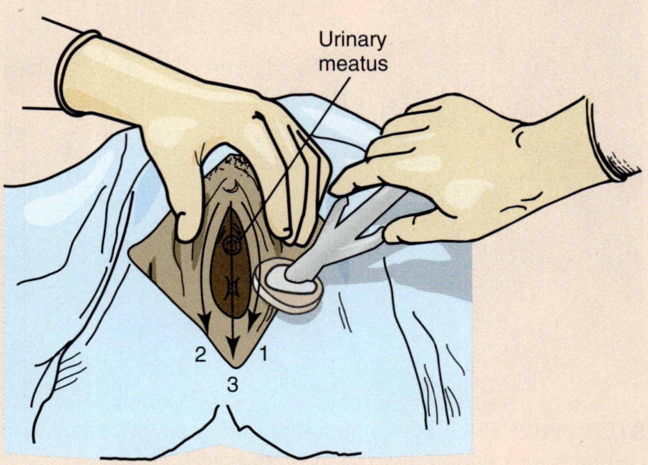

STEP 14a(3) Cleansing female perineum.

STEPS	**RATIONALE**

15. Pick up and hold catheter 7.5 to 10 cm (3 to 4 inches) from tip. Hold end of catheter loosely coiled in palm of sterile dominant hand. If catheter is not attached to a drainage bag, make sure to position urine tray so that end of catheter can be placed there when insertion begins.

Holding catheter near tip allows for easier manipulation during insertion. Coiling the catheter in the palm prevents distal end from striking a nonsterile surface.

16. Insert catheter. Explain to the patient that a feeling of burning, pinching, or pressure may be experienced when the catheter is inserted into the urethra. This sensation is normal and will go away.

   a. Female patient:

     (1) Ask patient to bear down gently and insert catheter through urethral meatus (see illustration).

Bearing down may make it easier to visualize urinary meatus and promotes relaxation of external urinary sphincter, aiding in catheter insertion.

     (2) Advance catheter slowly 5 to 7.5 cm (2 to 3 inches) or until urine flows out end of catheter. As soon as urine appears, advance catheter another 2.5 to 5 cm (1 to 2 inches). Do not force catheter if resistance is met.

Urine flow indicates that catheter tip is in bladder.

     (3) Release labia, but maintain secure hold of catheter with nondominant hand.

Prevents accidental dislodgment of catheter.

> **SAFE PATIENT CARE** If no urine appears, catheter may be in vagina. If misplaced, leave catheter in vagina as a landmark indicating where not to insert, and insert a new sterile catheter.

   b. Male patient:

     (1) Gently apply upward traction to penis as it is held in a 90-degree angle from body (see illustration).

Straightens urethra to ease catheter insertion.

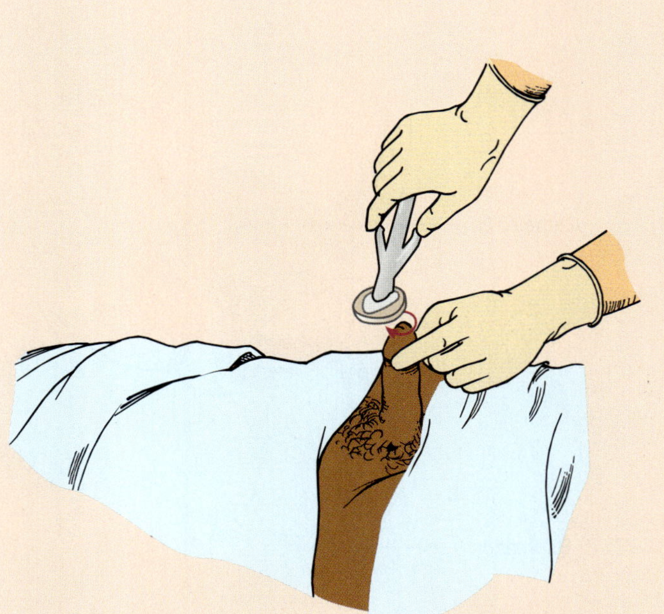

STEP 14b(3) Cleansing male urinary meatus.

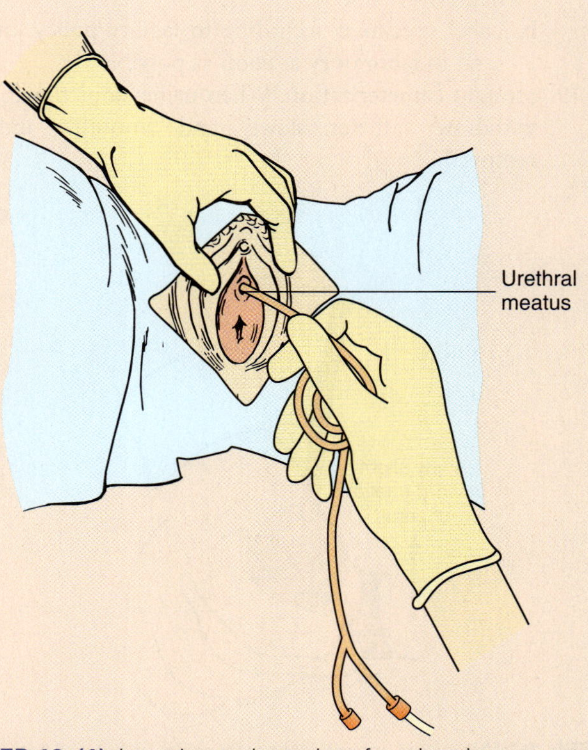

STEP 16a(1) Inserting catheter into female urinary meatus.

Continued

STEPS	RATIONALE

(2) Ask patient to bear down as if to void, and then slowly insert catheter through the meatus.

Bearing down relaxes the external sphincter and aids in catheter insertion.

(3) Advance catheter 17 to 22.5 cm (7 to 9 inches) or until urine flows out end of catheter. Stop advancing a straight catheter. When urine appears, advance indwelling catheter to bifurcation (inflation and deflation port exposed) (see illustration).

Length of male urethra varies. The flow of urine indicates that the tip of the catheter is in the bladder but not necessarily the balloon portion of an indwelling catheter. Further advancement of catheter to bifurcation of drainage and balloon inflation port ensures that the balloon portion of the catheter is not still in the prostatic urethra (Méndez-Probst et al., 2012).

(4) Lower penis, and hold catheter securely in nondominant hand.

Prevents accidental dislodgment of catheter.

> **SAFE PATIENT CARE** If there is resistance or pain when advancing the catheter, *do not use force* and stop catheter advancement. Ask the patient to take slow, deep breaths to promote relaxation. Hold catheter gently in place without forcing. After a few seconds, the sphincter may relax, and the catheter can be advanced. An inability to advance a catheter may mean an enlarged prostate or some other obstruction of the urethra.

17. Allow bladder to empty fully unless facility policy restricts maximum volume of urine drained (see facility policy).

There is no definitive evidence regarding whether limiting maximal volume drained is beneficial.

> **SAFE PATIENT CARE** In the case of acute urinary retention (rapid onset) when the volume of urine is known to be excessive (greater than 1 L) notify the health care provider for guidance about gradual bladder decompression to avoid decompression-induced hematuria (Mendez-Probst et al., 2012).

18. Collect urine specimen as needed.
  a. Fill specimen container to desired level (20 to 30 mL) by holding end of catheter in dominant hand over cup.

A sterile specimen for culture analysis can be obtained.

  b. Label specimen according to facility policy and send to laboratory as soon as possible.

Fresh urine specimen ensures more accurate findings.

19. Straight catheterization: When urine stops flowing, withdraw catheter slowly and smoothly until removed.

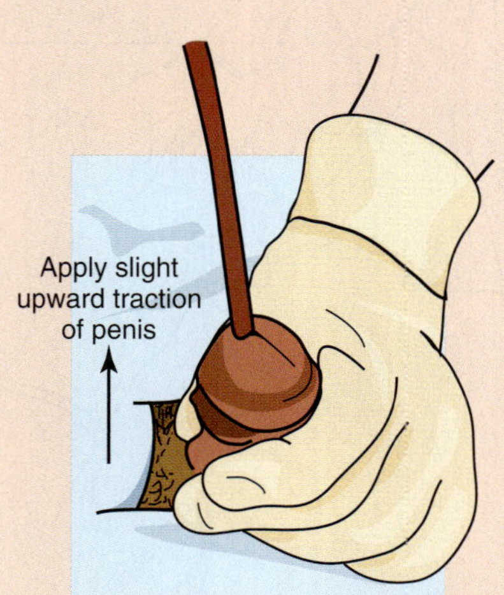

STEP 16b(1) Inserting catheter into male urinary meatus.

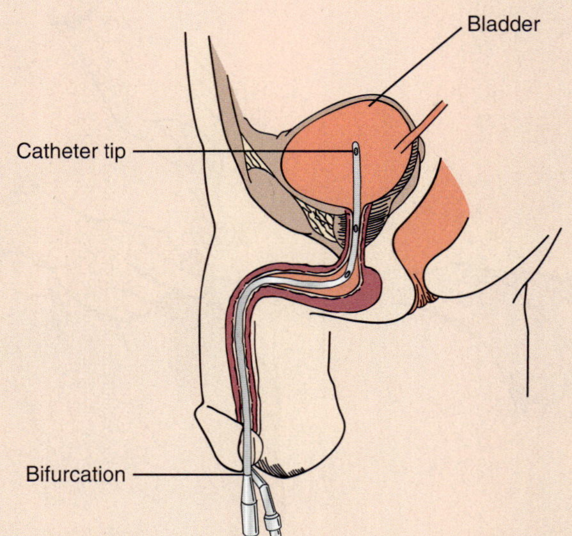

STEP 16b(3) Correct catheter insertion to the bifurcation of the drainage and balloon inflation port in male patient.

STEPS	RATIONALE

20. Balloon inflation for indwelling catheter: Use amount of fluid designated by manufacturer.

Indwelling catheter balloons should not be overinflated or underinflated owing to balloon distortion and potential bladder damage (Geng et al., 2012).

a. Continue to hold catheter with nondominant hand.

Holding on to catheter before inflating balloon prevents expulsion of catheter from urethra.

b. With free dominant hand, attach prefilled syringe in injection port at end of catheter.

c. Slowly inject total amount of fluid (see illustration).

d. After inflating catheter balloon, release catheter from nondominant hand. *Gently* pull catheter until resistance is felt. Then advance it slightly.

Withdrawing catheter places balloon at base of bladder; slight advancement reduces risk of pressure on bladder neck (Geng et al., 2012)

e. Connect drainage tubing to catheter if it is not already preconnected.

> **SAFE PATIENT CARE** If a patient complains of sudden pain during inflation of a catheter balloon, *stop injection,* allow the fluid from the balloon to flow back into the syringe, advance catheter further, and reinflate balloon. The balloon may be inflating in the urethra.

21. Secure indwelling catheter with catheter strap or other securement device. Leave enough slack to allow leg movement and avoid any traction on catheter. Attach the securement device at tubing above or below the catheter bifurcation as directed by the manufacturer.

Securing the catheter reduces the risk of urethral erosion, CAUTI, or accidental catheter removal (Geng et al., 2012; Gould et al., 2010). Attaching the device at the catheter bifurcation prevents catheter occlusions.

a. *Female:* Secure catheter to inner thigh, allowing enough slack to prevent tension (see illustration).

b. *Male:* Secure catheter tubing to upper thigh or lower abdomen (with penis directed toward chest). Allow slack in catheter so that movement does not create tension on catheter (see illustration). *If retracted, replace foreskin over the glans penis.*

Anchoring catheter to lower abdomen reduces traction on the urethra and urethral injury preventing trauma or necrosis (Geng et al., 2012). Leaving the foreskin retracted can cause discomfort and dangerous edema.

22. Clip drainage tubing to edge of mattress. Position drainage bag lower than bladder by attaching to bedframe. Do not attach to side rails of bed (see illustration).

Drainage bags that are below the level of the bladder ensure free flow of urine decreasing the risk for CAUTI (Geng et al., 2012; Gould et al., 2010). Bags attached to movable objects such as a side rail increase risk for urethral trauma secondary to pulling or accidental dislodgment.

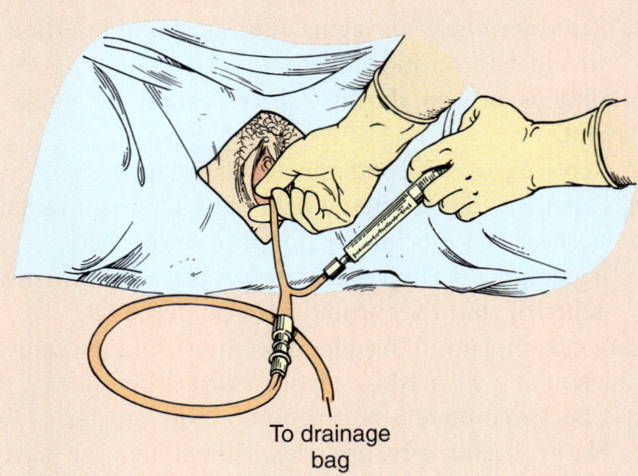

STEP 20 Inflating the balloon (indwelling catheter).

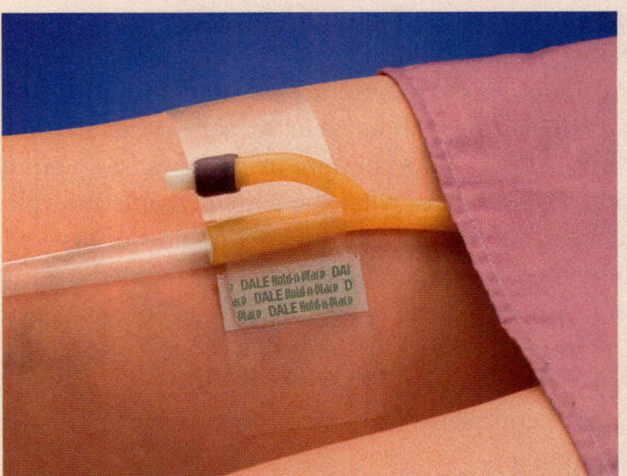

STEP 21a Securing female indwelling catheter.

Continued

STEPS	RATIONALE
23. Check to ensure there is no obstruction to urine flow. Coil excess tubing on bed and fasten to bottom sheet with clip or other securing device.	Obstruction to flow of urine increases the risk for CAUTI (Geng et al., 2012; Gould et al., 2010).
24. Provide hygiene as needed. Assist patient to a comfortable position.	
25. Measure urine volume and record.	Ensures accurate I&O.
26. Discuss with the patient routine care of the catheter and drainage system; this includes avoiding any kinking in the drainage tubing, keeping the drainage bag dependent, avoiding any pulling on the catheter, daily hygiene with soap and water, and maintaining an adequate fluid intake to prevent catheter blockage.	
27. **See Completion Protocol (inside front cover).**	

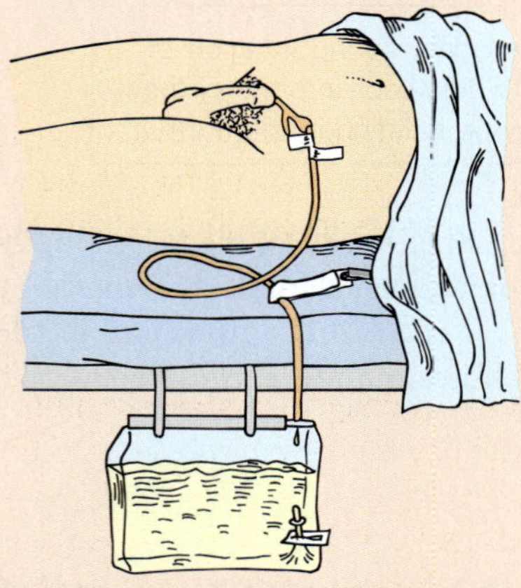

STEP 21b Securing male indwelling catheter.

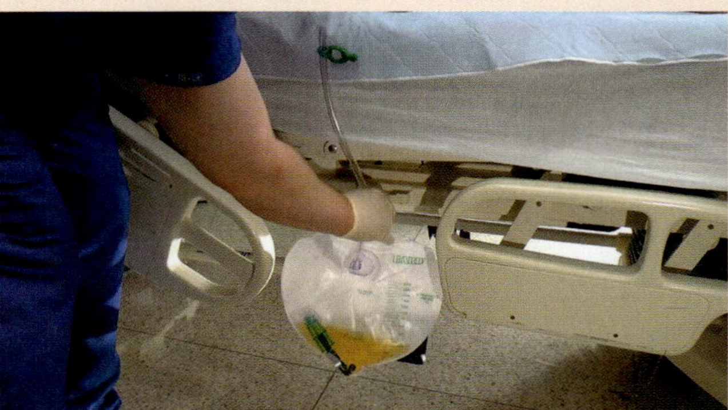

STEP 22 Drainage bag below level of bladder, connected to bedframe.

▌EVALUATION

1. Palpate bladder, and observe amount, color, and clarity of urine.
2. Ask the patient to describe level of comfort and if the sensation of discomfort or fullness has been relieved.
3. Indwelling catheter: Observe character and amount of urine in drainage tubing and bag and that there is no urine leaking from catheter or tubing connections.
4. Use *Teach Back:* State to the patient, "I want to be sure I explained clearly about your urinary catheter and some things you can do to be sure urine flows freely out of the catheter." Evaluates what the patient is able to explain or demonstrate. Revise your instruction now or develop plan for revised patient teaching to be implemented at an appropriate time if patient is not able to teach back correctly.

Unexpected Outcomes and Related Interventions

1. Patient complains of discomfort during inflation of balloon.
   a. Stop inflation immediately; allow inflation fluid to return to syringe.
   b. Advance another 2.5 cm (1 inch) and retry inflation.
   c. If patient still complains of pain, remove catheter and report to health care provider.
2. Catheter goes into vagina.
   a. Leave catheter in vagina. Replace gloves if contaminated and start over.
   b. Recleanse urinary meatus. Using another catheter kit or another sterile catheter, insert catheter into meatus.
   c. Remove catheter in vagina after successful insertion of second catheter in bladder.
3. Sterility is broken during catheterization by nurse or patient.
   a. Replace gloves if contaminated and start over.
   b. If patient touches sterile field but equipment remains sterile, avoid touching that part of sterile field.
   c. If equipment is contaminated, replace it with sterile items, or start over again with new sterile kit.
4. Patient complains of bladder discomfort, and the catheter is patent as evidenced by adequate urine flow.
   a. Check that there is no traction on the catheter.
   b. Notify health care provider. Patient may be having bladder spasms or symptoms of UTI.
   c. Monitor catheter output for color, clarity, odor, and amount.

Recording and Reporting

- Report and record reason for catheterization, type and size of catheter inserted, amount of fluid used to inflate balloon, specimen collection (if applicable), characteristics and amount of urine, patient's response to procedure, and any education.
- Record on I&O flow sheet record.
- Report persistent catheter-related pain and discomfort.
- Document your evaluation of patient learning.

Sample Documentation

0800   Patient c/o lower abdominal fullness and inability to void; lower abdomen tender and distended. Health care provider notified and 16-Fr/5-mL balloon catheter inserted without difficulty; 700 mL of clear yellow urine returned. Balloon inflated with 10 mL sterile solution. Specimen sent for urinalysis and culture. After catheterization patient denies discomfort or pain and lists measures to ensure free flow of urine in the catheter.

Special Considerations
Pediatric

- When caring for an infant or young child, explain procedures to parents. Describe procedure to child at level the child is able to understand (Hockenberry and Wilson, 2013).
- Catheterization in infants and children may be more comfortable with the use of an adequate amount of lubricant containing 2% lidocaine (Xylocaine) (Hockenberry and Wilson, 2013).

- Teaching young children to blow into a straw or pinwheel can aid in relaxing pelvic muscles (Hockenberry and Wilson, 2013).
- In uncircumcised infant boys, it is not possible to retract the foreskin fully.

Geriatric

- The urethral meatus of an older woman may be difficult to identify because of urogenital atrophy.
- Symptoms of UTI in an older adult may be difficult to recognize and may be indicated only by a change in mental status or fever (Caterino et al., 2012; Matthews and Lancaster, 2011).
- Older adults have an increased risk for UTI related to increased prevalence of chronic disease such as diabetes, prostatic hypertrophy in men, and a higher prevalence of incontinence (Caljouw et al., 2011).

Home Care

- Patients who are at home may use a leg bag during the day and switch to a larger volume bag at night. If a patient changes from a large-volume bag to a leg bag, instruct in the importance of handwashing and cleansing of the connection ports with alcohol before changing bags.
- Teach patients and family caregivers signs of UTI and how to position the drainage bag properly; empty the urinary drainage bag; and observe urine color, clarity, odor, and amount.
- Arrange for home delivery of catheter supplies, always ensuring that there is at least one extra catheter, insertion kit, and drainage bag in the home.

SKILL 18.3   REMOVAL OF AN INDWELLING CATHETER

• Nursing Skills Online: Urinary Catheterization, Lesson 5

Timely removal of indwelling catheters is important for reducing the risk of CAUTI (Gould et al., 2010; Meddings et al., 2013). When removing a catheter, it is important to ensure that the catheter balloon is fully deflated to minimize trauma to the urethra. Evidence is unclear that the practice of clamping a catheter before removal improves bladder function after removal (Geng et al., 2012; Gould et al., 2010; Nyman et al., 2010).

All patients should have their voiding monitored after catheter removal for at least 24 to 48 hours by using a voiding record or bladder diary to record the time and amount of each voiding, including any incontinence. A bladder scanner can be used to monitor bladder functioning by measuring PVR (see Procedural Guideline 18.2). Abdominal pain and distention, a sensation of incomplete emptying, incontinence, constant dribbling of urine, and voiding in very small amounts can indicate inadequate bladder emptying that requires intervention. Symptoms of infection can develop 2 or more days after catheter removal. Always inform patients about the risk for infection, prevention measures, and signs and symptoms that need to be reported to the primary health care provider.

▌ASSESSMENT

1. Identify patient using two identifiers (e.g., name and birthday or name and account number) according to facility policy. *Rationale: Ensures correct patient. Complies with The Joint Commission standards and improves patient safety (TJC, 2014).*
2. Review health care prescriber's order and nurses' notes. Note length of time catheter has been in place. *Rationale: Removal requires a health care provider order or approved protocol. Catheters in place for more than a few days are more likely to cause urethral irritation and buildup of incrustation.*
3. Assess patient's knowledge and prior experience with catheter removal. *Rationale: Reveals need for patient instruction or support or both.*
4. Assess urine color, clarity, odor, and amount. Note any urethral discharge or the presence of incrustation. *Rationale: May indicate inflammation or UTI and is a source of pain during catheter removal.*
5. Determine the size of catheter inflation balloon. *Rationale: Determines size of syringe required to deflate balloon.*

PLANNING

Expected Outcomes focus on patient comfort, adequate bladder emptying, and patient's learning about early detection of UTI.

1. Patient voids at least 150 mL with each voiding no more than 6 to 8 hours after catheter removal.
2. Patient verbalizes feeling of comfort after catheter is removed.
3. Patient identifies signs and symptoms of UTI.

Delegation and Collaboration

Assessment of the patient's condition cannot be delegated to nursing assistive personnel (NAP); however, the skill of removing a urinary catheter may be delegated as indicated by facility policy. The nurse instructs the NAP to:

- Report characteristics of urine (color, odor, and amount) before and after catheter removal and to record urine volume on I&O record.
- Report the condition of the patient's genital area (e.g., color, rashes, open areas, odor, soiling from fecal incontinence, and trauma to tissues around urinary meatus).
- If allowed to remove a catheter: check size of balloon and size of syringe needed to deflate balloon, report if balloon does not deflate and if there is bleeding after removal. Report time and amount of first voiding after catheter is removed.
- Report how the patient tolerated the procedure, the exact time the catheter was removed, and the time and amount of subsequent voiding.

Equipment

- Clean gloves
- Basin with warm water, washcloth, towel, and soap for perineal care
- 10-mL syringe or larger without a needle (size depends on volume of solution used to inflate the balloon)
- Waterproof pad
- Toilet, bedside commode, urine "hat," urinal, or bedpan

IMPLEMENTATION *for* REMOVAL OF AN INDWELLING CATHETER

STEPS	RATIONALE
1. **See Standard Protocol (inside front cover).**	
2. Apply clean gloves. Position patient supine and place waterproof pad under buttocks. For male patient, pad can lie on thighs. Cover with bath blanket, exposing only perineal area. If soiled, perform perineal hygiene (see Procedural Guideline 10.1).	Shows respect for patient dignity by exposing only the genital area and catheter.
3. Remove catheter-securing device and free drainage tubing.	
4. Remove gloves, perform hand hygiene, and apply new pair of clean gloves.	
5. Move syringe plunger up and down to loosen and then withdraw plunger 0.5 mL from end of syringe. Insert hub of syringe into inflation valve (balloon port). Allow all balloon fluid to drain into syringe by gravity; plunger will move farther out. Make sure that entire amount of fluid is removed by comparing removed amount with volume needed for inflation.	A partially inflated balloon can traumatize the urethral wall during removal. Passive drainage of the catheter balloon will prevent the formation of ridges in the balloon. These ridges can cause discomfort or trauma during removal (Geng et al., 2012).
6. Pull catheter out smoothly and slowly. Examine it to ensure that it is whole. Catheter should slide out very easily. Do not use force. If you note any resistance, repeat Step 5 to remove remaining water in balloon. Notify health care provider if balloon does not deflate completely.	A catheter that is not whole means that pieces of catheter may still be in bladder. Notify health care provider immediately.
7. Wrap contaminated catheter in waterproof pad. Unhook collection bag and drainage tubing from bed.	
8. Reposition patient as necessary. Provide perineal hygiene if needed.	Promotes patient comfort and safety.

STEPS	RATIONALE
9. Empty, measure, and record urine present in drainage bag.	Records urinary output.
10. See Completion Protocol (inside front cover).	
11. Teach patient to maintain or increase fluid intake (unless contraindicated).	Maintains normal urinary output.
12. Initiate voiding record or bladder diary. Instruct patient to tell you when the need to empty the bladder occurs and that all urine needs to be measured. Make sure that patient understands how to use the collection container.	Evaluates bladder function.
13. Explain that many patients experience mild burning, discomfort, or small-volume voiding with first voiding, which soon subsides.	Burning is result of urethral irritation from catheter.
14. Inform patient to report any signs of UTI.	Increases likelihood of timely treatment.
15. Ensure easy access to toilet, commode, bedpan, or urinal. Place urine "hat" on toilet seat if patient is using toilet. Place call bell within easy reach.	

▌EVALUATION

1. Inspect the catheter for any abnormalities.
2. Inspect the genital area for soiling, irritation, and skin breakdown. Ask patient about discomfort.
3. Observe time and amount of first voiding after catheter removal.
4. Evaluate the patient for signs and symptoms of UTI.
5. Use **Teach Back:** State to the patient, "I want to be sure I explained clearly the signs of a urinary tract infection and some things you should do to prevent infection. Can you tell me ways to prevent infection?" Evaluates what the patient is able to explain or demonstrate. Revise your instruction now or develop plan for revised patient teaching to be implemented at an appropriate time if patient is not able to teach back correctly.

Unexpected Outcomes and Related Interventions

1. Water from inflation balloon does not return into syringe.
   a. Reposition patient; ensure that catheter is not pinched or kinked.
   b. Remove syringe. Attach new syringe and allow enough time for passive emptying.
   c. Attempt to empty balloon by gently pulling back on the syringe plunger.
   d. If a catheter balloon does not deflate, do not cut balloon inflation valve to drain the water. Notify health care provider.
2. Patient exhibits one or more of the following after catheter removal: fever, chills, painful urination, cloudy or foul-smelling urine, abdominal pain, flank pain, frequent small-volume voiding, hematuria, change in mental status, lethargy (Hooton et al., 2010).
   a. Assess for bladder distention.
   b. Monitor vital signs and urine output.
   c. Report findings to health care provider; signs and symptoms may indicate UTI.
3. Patient is unable to void after catheter removal, has a sensation of not emptying the bladder, strains to void, or experiences small voiding amounts with increasing frequency.
   a. Assist to normal position for voiding.
   b. Provide privacy.
   c. Perform bladder ultrasound (see Procedural Guideline 18.2) to assess residual urine. Notify health care provider if volume is greater than 100 mL.

Recording and Reporting

- Record and report time catheter was removed; teaching related to increasing fluid intake and signs and symptoms of UTI; and time, amount, and characteristics of first voiding.
- Record intake and voiding times and amounts on voiding record or bladder diary as indicated.
- Report hematuria, dysuria, inability or difficulty voiding, and any new incontinence after a catheter is removed.
- Document your evaluation of patient learning.

Sample Documentation

0600 No. 16-Fr/5-mL balloon catheter removed without difficulty. Patient instructed to report any symptoms of UTI; encouraged to increase fluids and save urine for measurement. Patient can list symptoms of UTI.
0800 Voided 100 mL of clear yellow urine. No complaints of dysuria.

Special Considerations

Pediatric

- Do not force catheter out of bladder if resistance is met. When excessive length of catheter has been inserted in the bladder, there have been occurrences of knotting of the catheter (Hockenberry and Wilson, 2013).

Geriatric

- Older adults may exhibit atypical signs and symptoms of UTI such as a change in mental status, which is wrongly attributed to delirium. A change in mental status may include confusion, agitation, or lethargy (Matthews and Lancaster, 2011).

Home Care

- Include family caregivers in the plan of care. Some family caregivers may need extra support when learning how to take care of someone who now needs regular help with toileting.

PROCEDURAL GUIDELINE 18.3
Care of an Indwelling Catheter

- **Nursing Skills Online: Urinary Elimination, Lesson 5**

Indwelling urinary catheters are one of the most common sources for hospital-acquired infection, and CAUTI carries significant risk for chronic and life-threatening infection (Geng et al., 2012). If an indwelling catheter is required, you can take measures to reduce infection risk, such as maintaining a closed drainage system, ensuring a continuous flow of urine, and daily meatal care (Geng et al., 2012; Gould et al., 2010; Meddings et al., 2013).

Delegation and Collaboration

Routine catheter care can be delegated to nursing assistive personnel (NAP) and is often incorporated into perineal care during bathing. The nurse instructs the NAP to:
- Report characteristics of the urine (color, clarity, odor, and amount).
- Report the condition of the patient's genital area (e.g., color, rashes, open areas, odor, soiling from fecal incontinence, trauma to tissues around urinary meatus).
- Record urine output.

Equipment

- Soap
- Washcloth and towel
- Basin with warm water
- Clean gloves
- Bath blanket
- Waterproof pad

Procedural Steps

1. Identify patient using two identifiers (e.g., name and birthday or name and account number) according to facility policy.
2. Wash hands and apply gloves. Assess the urethral meatus and surrounding tissues for inflammation, swelling, secretions, and tissue trauma. Remove and dispose of gloves.
3. Assess color, clarity, and odor of urine.
4. Assess for presence of a CAUTI: fever, chills, burning, flank pain, back pain, blood in urine, lower abdominal pain, change in mental status or lethargy (Hooton et al., 2010).
5. Assess patient's understanding of catheter care.
6. **See Standard Protocol (inside front cover).**
7. Apply clean gloves. Position female patients in dorsal recumbent position and male patients supine. Place waterproof pad under buttocks. Cover with bath blanket, exposing only catheter and perineal area. Provide perineal care as needed (see Procedural Guideline 10.1).
8. Remove catheter tubing from the securing device.
9. With nondominant hand:
    a. *Female:* Gently retract labia to expose urethral meatus and catheter fully.
    b. *Male:* Retract foreskin if not circumcised and hold penis at shaft just below glans.
    c. Grasp catheter with two fingers to stabilize catheter near the meatus.
10. Using a clean washcloth, soap, and water, with your dominant hand wipe in a circular motion along the length of the catheter for about 10 cm (4 inches) starting at the meatus and moving away. Avoid placing tension on or pulling on the exposed catheter tubing. Make sure to remove all traces of soap. If applicable, return the foreskin to the down position.
11. Reapply the catheter securement device, and secure tubing above or below the bifurcation as directed by the manufacturer. Allow slack in the catheter so that movement does not create tension on the catheter causing trauma to the bladder, urethra, or meatus (Cipa-Tatum et al., 2011; Geng et al., 2012; Gould et al., 2010).
12. Check drainage tubing and bag to ensure that:
    a. Tubing is coiled and secured onto bed linen, not kinked or clamped.
    b. Drainage bag is positioned below the level of bladder.
    c. Drainage bag is positioned on lower bedframe with urine flowing freely from tubing.
    d. Drainage bag is not overfull. Empty drainage bag when $\frac{1}{2}$ full to prevent tension and pulling on the catheter (Cipa-Tatum et al., 2011).
13. **See Completion Protocol (inside front cover).**

SKILL 18.4 SUPRAPUBIC CATHETER CARE

A suprapubic catheter is a urinary drainage tube inserted surgically into the bladder through the abdominal wall above the symphysis pubis (Fig. 18-5). The catheter may be sutured to the skin, secured with an adhesive material, or retained in the bladder with a fluid-filled balloon similar to an indwelling catheter. Suprapubic catheters are placed when there is blockage of the urethra (e.g., enlarged prostate, urethral stricture, after urological surgery) and in situations when a long-term urethral catheter causes irritation or discomfort or interferes with sexual functioning.

ASSESSMENT

1. Identify patient using two identifiers (e.g., name and birthday or name and account number) according to facility policy. *Rationale: Ensures correct patient. Complies with The Joint Commission standards and improves patient safety (TJC, 2014).*
2. Review health care provider's order or facility policy for sterile versus clean technique needed for care. *Rationale: Ensures safe and correct site care.*
3. Assess urine in drainage bag for amount, clarity, color, odor, and sediment. *Rationale: Abnormal findings may indicate potential complications, such as infection, decreased urinary output, and catheter occlusion.*
4. During dressing removal assess catheter insertion site for inflammation, pain, erythema, edema, drainage, and growth of overgranulation tissue. Ask patient if there is any pain at site; if so, have patient rate on scale of 0 to 10. *Rationale: If insertion site is new, slight inflammation may be expected as part of normal wound healing, but it can also*

indicate infection. Overgranulation tissue can develop at the insertion site as a reaction to the catheter. In some instances, intervention may be needed (Geng et al., 2012).
5. Assess for elevated temperature and chills. *Rationale: May indicate UTI or site infection.*
6. Assess site where catheter is secured on abdomen for signs of irritation. *Rationale: Repeated taping can cause skin irritation and breakdown.*
7. Check for allergies. *Rationale: Patient may be sensitive to tape, latex, or antiseptic solution.*
8. Assess patient's and family caregiver's knowledge of purpose of catheter and its care. *Rationale: Determines level of instruction and support required.*

PLANNING

Expected Outcomes focus on maintaining flow of urine, patient comfort, and prevention of infection.
1. Catheter is patent, and output is 30 mL or greater per hour.
2. Catheter insertion site is free of signs of infection including erythema, edema, discharge, or tenderness.
3. Patient remains afebrile.
4. Patient verbalizes no pain or discomfort at insertion site.

Delegation and Collaboration

The skill of caring for a newly established suprapubic catheter cannot be delegated to nursing assistive personnel (NAP); however, care of an established suprapubic catheter can be delegated (refer to facility policy). The nurse instructs the NAP to:
- Report if the patient has any discomfort related to the suprapubic tube.
- Empty the drainage bag, document urinary output on I&O record, and report any change in the amount and character of the urine.
- Report any signs of redness, drainage, or foul odor around catheter insertion site.

Equipment
- Clean gloves (sterile gloves may be needed in some cases, see facility policy)
- Cleansing agent (sterile normal saline solution)
- Sterile cotton-tipped applicators
- Sterile surgical drainage sponge (split gauze)
- Sterile gauze dressing
- Washcloth, towel, soap, and water
- Tape
- Velcro tube holder or tube stabilizer (optional)

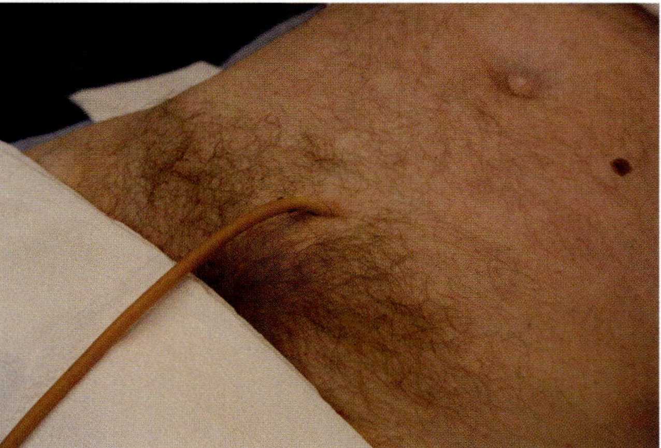
FIG 18-5 Suprapubic catheter without dressing.

IMPLEMENTATION *for* SUPRAPUBIC CATHETER CARE

STEPS	RATIONALE
1. **See Standard Protocol (inside front cover).**	
2. Prepare supplies in the same manner as for applying a dry dressing (see Skill 26.1). Explain procedure to patient.	

Continued

3. Apply clean gloves. Remove existing dressing. Note type and presence of drainage. Remove gloves and perform hand hygiene.

Provides baseline for condition of suprapubic wound.

4. Inspect insertion site and patency of catheter.

Reveals condition of catheter insertion site and how catheter is held in place. With newly established catheters, sutures should be clearly seen wrapped around catheter and secured to skin. Urine should be seen draining in tubing.

5. Perform site care.
   a. Newly established suprapubic catheter may need sterile technique as determined by facility policy or individual patient need.

   The catheter site is surgically made and is treated similarly to other incisions as designated by facility policy as using either aseptic or sterile technique.

      (1) Apply sterile gloves.
      (2) Without creating tension, hold catheter erect with nondominant hand while cleaning. Cleanse in circular motion, starting near catheter insertion site and continuing in outward widening circles for approximately 5 cm (2 inches) (see illustration).

   Moves from area of least contamination to area of most contamination. Tension on catheter may cause discomfort or damage to wall of bladder or cause catheter to slip out of place.

      (3) With fresh, moistened gauze, gently cleanse base and length of catheter without pulling; move up and away from site of insertion (proximal to distal).

   Removes microorganisms and any drainage that adheres to tubing.

      (4) With sterile gloved hand, apply drain dressing (split gauze) around catheter and tape in place (see illustration).

   b. Long-term/established catheters:
      (1) Apply clean gloves. Without creating tension, hold catheter erect with nondominant hand while cleansing. Cleanse with soap and water in circular motion, starting near catheter insertion site and continuing in outward widening circles for approximately 5 cm (2 inches).

   A clean and dry suprapubic insertion site requires general hygienic measures. Sterile technique and a dressing are not needed (Bullman, 2011).

      (2) With a fresh washcloth or gauze, gently cleanse base and length of catheter without pulling, moving up and away from site of insertion (proximal to distal).

   Removes microorganisms and any drainage that adheres to tubing.

      (3) If indicated, apply drain dressing (split gauze) around catheter and tape in place.

   An established suprapubic tube may need a dressing if there is drainage to contain.

6. Secure catheter to lateral abdomen with tape or Velcro multipurpose tube holder. Teach patient the need to avoid any tension on the tubing.

Secures catheter and reduces risk of excessive tension on suture or catheter.

7. Coil excess tubing on bed and secure it to dressing. Keep drainage bag below level of bladder at all times.

Maintains a free flow of urine decreasing risk for CAUTI (Geng et al., 2012; Gould et al., 2010).

8. **See Completion Protocol (inside front cover).**

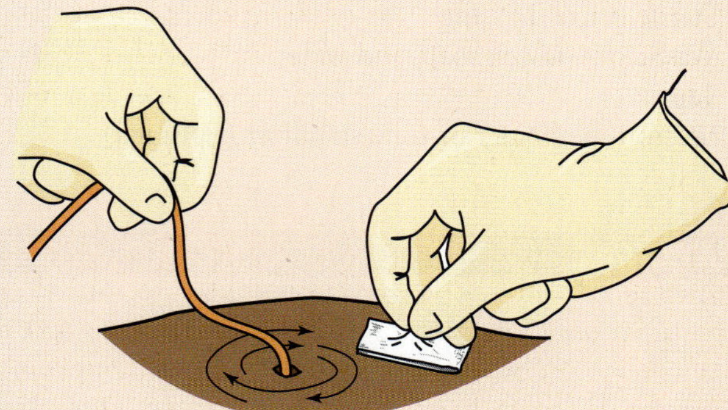

STEP 5a(2) Cleansing around suprapubic catheter in a circular pattern.

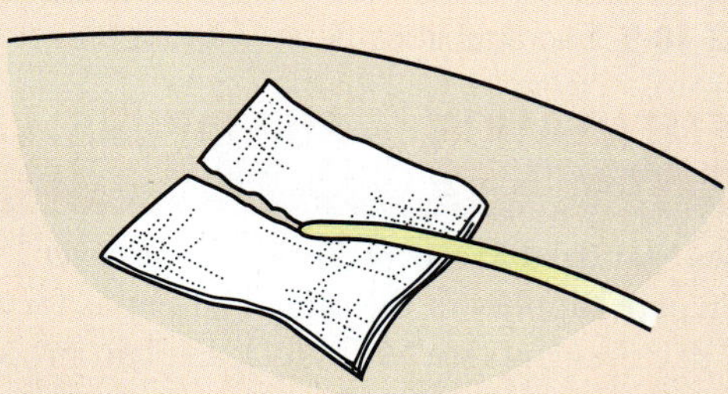

STEP 5a(4) Split drain dressing for suprapubic catheter.

EVALUATION

1. Monitor suprapubic catheter urine output.
2. Observe catheter insertion site for erythema, edema, discharge, or tenderness.
3. Monitor for signs of infection (e.g., fever, elevated white blood cell count), and observe patient's urine for clarity, sediment, or unusual odor.
4. Ask patient to rate any discomfort or pain related to the catheter on a scale of 0 to 10.
5. Use *Teach Back:* State to the patient, "I want to be sure I explained clearly about the care of your suprapubic catheter. Can you tell me about some of the things you need to do?" Evaluates what the patient is able to explain or demonstrate. Revise your instruction now or develop plan for revised patient teaching to be implemented at an appropriate time if patient is not able to teach back correctly.

Unexpected Outcomes and Related Interventions

1. Patient complains of lower abdominal pain or distention; urine flow slows or stops. Catheter suspected to be obstructed (blood clot or sediment formation; tip of catheter in bladder is positioned against bladder wall).
   a. Check catheter and drainage tubing for kinks.
   b. Ensure that the patient is not lying on the catheter or drainage tubing.
   c. Reposition the patient and observe for any increase in urine flow.
   d. Notify health care provider. In some cases, you may need to irrigate the catheter, which requires an order.
2. Patient develops symptoms of UTI or catheter site infection.
   a. Increase fluid intake.
   b. Monitor vital signs and I&O; observe amount, color, and consistency of urine; assess site.
   c. Notify health care provider.
3. Urine leaks around catheter.
   a. Check catheter and drainage tubing for kinks or for other causes of occlusion.

   b. Monitor vital signs; assess urine for signs of infection.
   c. Change dressing frequently; protect skin from moisture.
   d. Notify health care provider.
4. Catheter becomes dislodged.
   a. Cover site with a sterile dressing.
   b. Notify health care provider. If it is a newly established catheter, it will need to be reinserted immediately.

Recording and Reporting

- Record and report condition of insertion site, character of urine, type of dressing change, and patient's comfort level with the catheter and dressing change.
- Record urine output on I&O flow sheet. In a situation in which there is both a suprapubic and a urethral catheter, record outputs from each catheter separately.
- Document your evaluation of patient learning.

Sample Documentation

0800   Suprapubic catheter drained 100 mL of clear yellow urine. Dressing with small amount of dark brown drainage removed from suprapubic catheter site. No redness, edema, or drainage at the site. Insertion site cleansed and dressed with drain dressing. Denies any pain at insertion site. Describes accurately steps in suprapubic catheter site care.

Special Considerations
Home Care

- Patients and family caregivers should learn how to cleanse and apply a dressing (if applicable) using a clean technique.
- Caution patients and family caregivers to avoid the use of powders, creams, or ointments around the catheter unless specifically instructed to do so (Bullman, 2011).
- Teach patients and family caregivers how to position the drainage bag properly; how to empty the urinary drainage bag; signs of catheter obstruction, UTI, and wound infection; and to observe urine color, clarity, odor, and amount.

SKILL 18.5   PERFORMING CATHETER IRRIGATION

Following surgery on the bladder and other GU structures, it is common to have hematuria for several days. Intermittent or continuous urinary catheter irrigations maintain catheter patency by keeping the bladder clear and free of blood clots or sediment. There are two types of irrigation: closed catheter irrigation and open irrigation. Closed catheter irrigation provides intermittent or continuous irrigation of the urinary catheter without disrupting the sterile connection between the catheter and the drainage system (Fig. 18-6). Continuous bladder irrigation (CBI) is an example of a continuous infusion of a sterile solution into the bladder, usually using a three-way irrigation closed system with a triple-lumen catheter.

   Open catheter irrigation is used for intermittent irrigation of the catheter and bladder. The skill involves breaking or opening the closed drainage system at the connection between the catheter and the drainage system. Strict asepsis is required throughout the procedure to minimize contamination and subsequent development of a UTI. Both open and closed irrigation can be used to instill medication, such as antibiotics, into the bladder.

ASSESSMENT

1. Identify patient using two identifiers (e.g., name and birthday or name and account number) according to facility policy. *Rationale: Ensures correct patient. Complies with The Joint Commission standards and improves patient safety (TJC, 2014).*

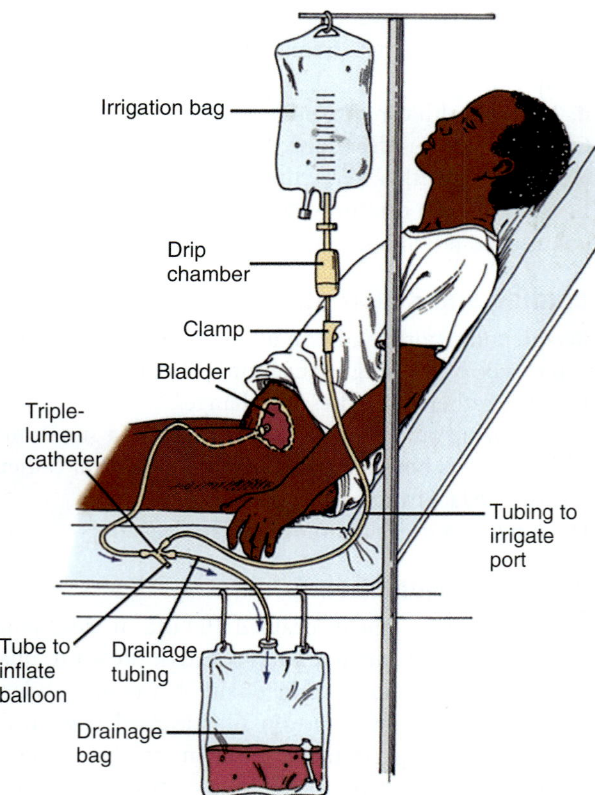

FIG 18-6 Continuous bladder irrigation setup.

2. Review health care provider's order for:
   a. The irrigation method (continuous or intermittent), type of solution (sterile saline or medicated solution) and amount of irrigant. *Rationale: A health care provider's order is required to initiate therapy. Frequency and volume of solution used for irrigation may be in the order or standardized as part of facility policy. Each type of irrigation requires different equipment.*
   b. Type of catheter in place. *Rationale: Single-lumen and double-lumen catheters are used with open irrigation. Triple-lumen catheters are used for both intermittent and continuous closed irrigation.*
3. Palpate bladder for distention and tenderness or use a Bladder Scan (see Procedural Guideline 18.2). *Rationale: Bladder distention indicates that flow of urine may be blocked from draining.*
4. Assess patient for abdominal pain or spasms, sensation of bladder fullness, or catheter bypassing (leaking). *Rationale: May indicate overdistention of the bladder caused by blockage of the catheter. Offers baseline to determine if therapy is successful.*
5. Observe urine for color; amount; clarity; and presence of mucus, clots, or sediment. *Rationale: Indicates if patient is bleeding or sloughing tissue, which would require increased irrigation rate or frequency of catheter irrigation.*
6. Monitor I&O. *Rationale: If CBI is being used, the amount of fluid draining from the bladder should exceed the amount of fluid infused into the bladder. If output does not exceed solution infused, catheter obstruction (i.e., blood clots, kinked*

tubing) should be suspected, the irrigation stopped, and the prescriber notified (Lewis et al., 2014).
7. Assess patient's knowledge regarding purpose of performing catheter irrigation. *Rationale: Reveals need for patient instruction and support.*

▌PLANNING

Expected Outcomes focus on continuous urine flow and patient comfort.
1. With CBI: Urine output is greater than volume of irrigating solution instilled.
2. Patient's urine output has decreased blood clots and sediment. (Note: Urine is bloody after bladder or urethral surgery, gradually becoming lighter and blood-tinged in 2 to 3 days.)
3. Patient reports relief of bladder pain or spasms.
4. Patient remains afebrile and free of lower abdominal pain and cloudy or foul-smelling urine.

Delegation and Collaboration
The skill of catheter irrigation cannot be delegated to nursing assistive personnel (NAP). The nurse instructs the NAP to:
- Report if the patient complains of pain or discomfort or leakage of fluid around the catheter.
- Watch and record I&O; report immediately any decrease in urine output.
- Report any change in the color of the urine, especially the presence of blood clots.

Equipment
Closed Intermittent Irrigation
- Antiseptic swabs
- Sterile irrigation solution at room temperature as prescribed
- Sterile container
- Syringe to access system: Luer-Lok syringe for needleless access port (per manufacturer's instructions)
- Screw clamp or rubber band (used to occlude catheter temporarily as irrigant is instilled)

Closed Continuous Irrigation
- Antiseptic swabs
- Sterile irrigation solution at room temperature as prescribed
- Irrigation tubing with clamp to regulate irrigation flow rate
- Y connector (optional) to connect irrigation tubing to double-lumen catheter
- Intravenous (IV) pole (closed continuous or intermittent)

Open Intermittent Irrigation
- Antiseptic swabs
- Sterile irrigation solution at room temperature as prescribed
- Disposable sterile irrigation kit that contains solution container, collection basin, drape, gloves, 30- to 60-mL irrigation syringe (piston type)
- Sterile catheter plug

IMPLEMENTATION *for* PERFORMING CATHETER IRRIGATION

STEPS	RATIONALE

1. **See Standard Protocol (inside front cover).**
2. Apply clean gloves. Position patient supine, and expose catheter junction (catheter and drainage tubing). Organize supplies according to type of irrigation prescribed. Explain procedure to patient.

   Position provides access to catheter and promotes patient dignity as much as possible.
3. Remove catheter securing device.
4. *Closed continuous irrigation:*
   a. Close clamp on new irrigation tubing.

      Closing the clamp on tubing allows the tubing drip chamber to fill after the (spike) tip of the tubing is inserted into the port of the irrigation solution bag.

   b. Hang bag of irrigating solution on IV pole.
   c. Insert (spike) tip of sterile irrigation tubing into designated port of irrigation solution bag using aseptic technique (see illustration).

      Prevents transmission of microorganisms.

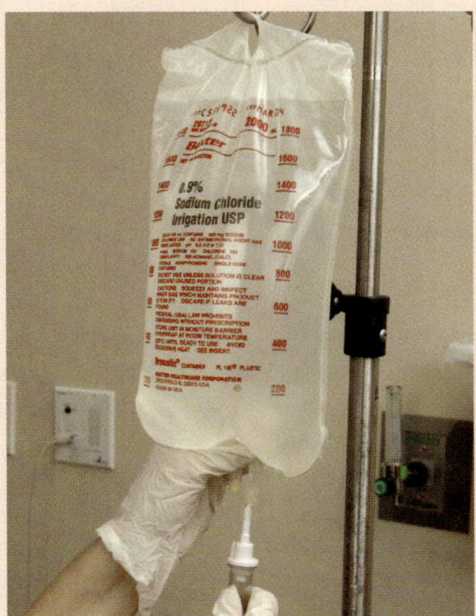

STEP 4c Spiking bag of sterile irrigation solution for continuous bladder irrigation.

   d. Fill drip chamber half full by squeezing chamber; then open tubing clamp and allow solution to flow (prime) through tubing, keeping end of tubing sterile. When fluid has completely filled the tubing, close the clamp and recap end of tubing.

      Priming the tubing with fluid prevents introduction of air into the bladder.

   e. Using aseptic technique, remove cap and connect tubing securely to drainage port of Y connector on double/triple–lumen catheter.

      Prevents transmission of microorganisms.

   f. Calculate drip rate and adjust rate at roller clamp. If urine is bright red or has clots, increase irrigation rate until drainage appears pink (according to ordered rate or facility protocol).

      Continuous drainage in the collection bag is normal and helps prevent catheter occlusion by flushing clots out of the bladder when active bleeding is present in bladder.

   g. Observe for outflow of fluid into the drainage bag. Empty catheter drainage bag as needed.

      Discomfort, bladder distention, and possibly injury can occur from overdistention of the bladder when bladder irrigant cannot flow from the bladder adequately. Bag fills rapidly and may need to be emptied every 1 to 2 hours.

Continued

STEPS	RATIONALE
h. Compare urine output with infusion of irrigation solution every hour.	Determines urinary output and ensures that irrigant is draining freely.
i. Inform patient that bleeding is common after many urological procedures and to expect bright red–tinged urine during the first 48 hours postoperatively, followed by a change in urine color ranging from pink-tinged to clear. If not contraindicated, encourage oral fluids.	Increasing oral fluids increases the volume of urine. Higher flow of urine helps maintain catheter patency.
5. Closed intermittent irrigation:	
a. Prepare sterile supplies (see Chapter 5) Pour prescribed sterile irrigation solution into sterile container.	Fluid is instilled through catheter in a bolus, flushing the system. Fluid drains out after irrigation is complete.
b. Draw prescribed volume of solution into syringe using aseptic technique (usually 30 to 50 mL).	
c. Place sterile cap on tip of needleless syringe.	
d. Clamp catheter tubing below soft injection port with screw clamp (or fold catheter tubing onto itself and secure with rubber band).	Occluding catheter tubing below the point of injection allows the irrigating solution to enter the catheter and flow upward toward the bladder.
e. Using circular motion, cleanse catheter port (specimen port) with antiseptic swab.	Prevents the transmission of microorganisms.
f. Insert tip of needleless syringe using twisting motion into port.	Ensures that syringe tip enters port.
g. Inject solution using slow, even pressure.	Gentle instillation of solution minimizes trauma to the bladder mucosa.
h. Withdraw syringe.	
i. Remove clamp (or rubber band) and observe outflow of solution. Some medicated solutions may need to dwell in the bladder for a prescribed period, requiring the catheter to be clamped temporarily.	Some irrigation solutions require time in the catheter and bladder to exert therapeutic effect. Clamped drainage tubing and bag should not be left unattended.
6. Open intermittent irrigation:	
a. Open sterile irrigation tray: Establish sterile field (see Chapter 5) and pour required amount of sterile solution into sterile solution container. Replace cap on large container of solution. Add sterile irrigation syringe (piston type) to field.	Maintains a sterile field.
b. Position sterile drape under catheter.	Creates sterile field on which you can work and prevents soiling of bed linen.
c. Aspirate prescribed volume of irrigation solution into irrigating syringe (usually 30 to 60 mL). Place syringe in sterile solution container until ready to use.	Maintains sterility of irrigating syringe.
d. Move sterile collection basin close to patient's thigh.	
e. Wipe connection point between catheter and drainage tubing with antiseptic wipe before disconnecting.	Reduces transmission of microorganisms.
f. Disconnect catheter from drainage tubing, allowing any urine to flow into sterile collection basin; cover open end of drainage tubing with sterile protective cap and position tubing so that it stays coiled on top of bed with the end on the sterile drape.	Maintains sterility of inner aspects of catheter lumen and drainage tubing. Reduces potential for infection via microorganism contamination.
g. Insert tip of syringe into lumen of catheter, and gently push plunger to instill solution (see illustration).	Gentle fluid instillation minimizes risk of trauma to bladder.

STEPS   RATIONALE

> **SAFE PATIENT CARE** When irrigating a catheter using the open method, do not force the irrigation. Catheter may be completely occluded and needs to be changed.

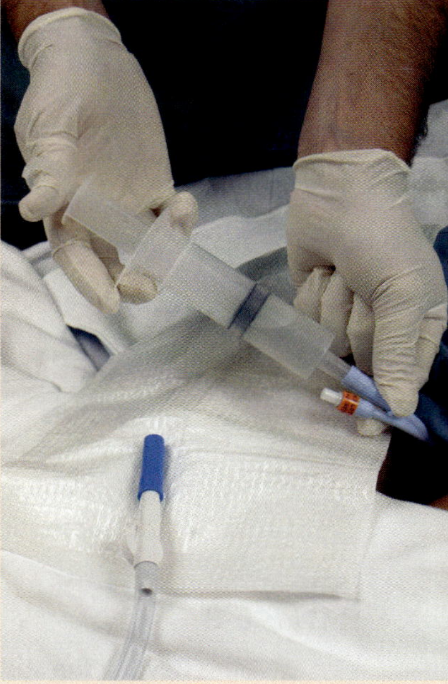

STEP 6g Gentle instillation of sterile irrigation solution irrigates catheter.

h. Remove syringe, lower catheter, and allow solution to drain into basin. Drainage solution amount should be equal to or greater than amount instilled. If ordered, repeat instilling solution and drain until drainage is clear of clots and sediment.

   If clot has been removed, solution drains freely into basin.

i. After irrigation is complete, remove protector cap from urinary drainage tubing adapter, cleanse adapter with antiseptic wipe, and reinsert adapter into lumen of catheter.

7. Anchor catheter with catheter securement device (see Skill 18.2).
8. **See Completion Protocol (inside front cover).**

EVALUATION

1. Measure actual urine output by subtracting total amount of irrigation fluid infused from total volume drained.
2. Review I&O flow sheet. Verify that hourly output into drainage bag is in appropriate proportion to irrigating solution entering bladder. Expect more output than fluid instilled because of urine production.
3. Observe for catheter patency; inspect urine for blood clots and sediment, and inspect tubing to ensure it is not kinked or occluded.
4. Assess patient comfort.
5. Assess for signs and symptoms of infection.
6. Use **Teach Back:** State to the patient, "I want to be sure I explained clearly about the irrigation of your catheter. Can you tell me some of the reasons why we are irrigating your bladder?" Evaluates what the patient is able to explain or demonstrate. Revise your instruction now or develop plan for revised patient teaching to be implemented at an appropriate time if patient is not able to teach back correctly.

Unexpected Outcomes and Related Interventions

1. Irrigation solution does not return (intermittent) or is not flowing at prescribed rate (CBI).
   a. Examine drainage tubing for clots, sediment, or kinks.
   b. Notify health care provider if solution is retained, patient complains of severe pain, or bladder is distended.

2. Drainage output is less than amount of irrigation solution infused.
   a. Examine drainage tubing for clots, sediment, or kinks.
   b. Inspect urine for presence of or increase in blood clots and sediment.
   c. Evaluate patient for pain and distended bladder.
   d. Notify health care provider.
3. Bright red bleeding noted with irrigation (CBI) drip wide open.
   a. Assess for hypovolemic shock (vital signs, skin color and moisture, anxiety level).
   b. Leave irrigation drip wide open, and notify health care provider.
4. Patient experiences pain with irrigation.
   a. Examine drainage tubing for clots, sediment, or kinks.
   b. Evaluate urine for presence of or increase in blood clots and sediment.
   c. Evaluate for distended bladder.
   d. Notify health care provider.

Recording and Reporting

- Record irrigation method, amount of and type of irrigation solution, amount returned as drainage, characteristics of output, and urine output.
- Report catheter occlusion, sudden bleeding, infection, or increased pain.
- Record I&O.
- Document your evaluation of patient learning.

Sample Documentation

0800   Lower abdomen soft and flat. CBI with normal saline infusing at 60 mL/hr. Catheter draining bright red urine with moderate-size dark bloody clots. Patient denies any pain. Patient can teach back and list reasons for CBI.

Special Considerations
Home Care

- Patient or family caregiver can learn to perform catheter irrigations with adequate support, demonstration/return demonstration, and written instructions.

CRITICAL THINKING EXERCISES

Case Study

A 78-year-old man who recently underwent bowel surgery had his urinary catheter removed yesterday and reports voiding frequently in small amounts. On assessment, his abdomen is distended and tender. The health care provider orders that an indwelling catheter be inserted.

1. What is a critical step when inserting an indwelling catheter into this patient?
   1. Quickly inflate the catheter balloon with sterile saline.
   2. Secure the catheter drainage tubing to the bedsheets.
   3. Advance to the bifurcation of the drainage and balloon ports.
   4. Advance until urine flows, then insert ¼ inch more.
2. What should be included in the patient's plan of care to prevent catheter-related trauma?
   1. Empty the catheter drainage bag when ½ full.
   2. Wash the catheter with soap and water.
   3. Keep the foreskin retracted while catheter is in.
   4. Secure the drainage bag to patient's bed side rail.
3. What should be included in the instructions given to the NAP caring for this patient and his indwelling urinary catheter? Select all that apply.
   1. Tape the catheter to the abdomen using a securement device.
   2. Attach the catheter per directions to the securement device.
   3. Tape the catheter drainage tubing securely to the lower abdomen avoiding traction.
   4. Secure the catheter drainage tubing to the upper inner thigh with slight traction.

Review Questions

1. What nursing interventions decrease the risk for CAUTI? Select all that apply.
   1. Cleansing the urinary meatus with antiseptic solution
   2. Hanging the urinary drainage bag below the level of the bladder
   3. Changing the urinary drainage bag daily
   4. Daily urinary catheter irrigations with sterile water
2. What size catheter and balloon for an indwelling catheter would the nurse anticipate to be ordered for an adult patient who needs a catheter inserted for urinary retention?
   1. 10 Fr, 3 mL
   2. 14 Fr, 30 mL
   3. 16 Fr, 10 mL
   4. 20 Fr, 10 mL
3. Place the following steps for open intermittent irrigation of an indwelling urinary catheter in the correct sequence.
   1. Insert tip of syringe into lumen of catheter and gently push plunger to instill solution.
   2. Aspirate prescribed volume of irrigation solution into irrigating syringe (usually 30 mL). Place syringe in sterile solution container until ready to use.
   3. Wipe connection point between catheter and drainage tubing with antiseptic wipe before disconnecting.
   4. Open sterile irrigation tray, establish sterile field, and pour required amount of sterile solution into sterile solution container.
   5. Position sterile drape under catheter.
   6. Disconnect catheter from drainage tubing, allowing any urine to flow into sterile collection basin.
   7. Remove syringe, lower catheter, and allow solution to drain into basin.

4. Which nursing interventions should the nurse implement when removing an indwelling urinary catheter in an adult patient? Select all that apply.
   1. Attach a 3-mL syringe to the inflation port
   2. Allow the balloon to drain into the syringe by gravity
   3. Initiate a voiding record or bladder diary
   4. Pull catheter quickly
   5. Clamp the catheter before removal

5. A patient with an indwelling urinary catheter complains of abdominal pain; on assessment, the nurse finds the abdomen tender and distended, and only a small volume of urine is in the drainage bag. What would be an initial nursing action?
   1. Check the drainage tubing for kinks
   2. Encourage patient to drink fluids
   3. Remove the catheter
   4. Notify the health care provider

6. Which nursing intervention helps minimize the risk for trauma and infection when applying an external catheter?
   1. Leave a gap of 7.5 to 12.5 cm (3 to 5 inches) between the tip of the penis and drainage tube.
   2. Shave the pubic area so that hair does not adhere.
   3. Provide hygiene before applying the condom-type catheter.
   4. Apply adhesive tape to the condom sheath to keep it securely in place.

7. Which nursing interventions apply to the care of a patient with a new suprapubic catheter? Select all that apply.
   1. Using sterile technique, cleanse the skin close to the catheter using a circular motion
   2. Wipe away any drainage on the catheter by wiping down the catheter toward the skin
   3. Inspect the insertion site for any sutures, erythema, edema, discharge, or tenderness
   4. Secure catheter to abdomen with tape or a tube holder device
   5. Apply upward tension to the catheter when cleansing the site and tubing

8. After insertion of an indwelling catheter approximately 1 inch into the urethra of a female patient, there is no urine flow. What should the nurse do next? Select all that apply.
   1. Remove the catheter and start all over with a new kit and catheter
   2. Check to see if catheter is in the vagina, leave it there and start over with a new catheter
   3. If misplaced, pull the catheter back and reinsert at a different angle
   4. Continue to insert the catheter further up to 2 to 3 inches

9. What instructions should the nurse give the NAP concerning an ambulatory patient who has had an indwelling urinary catheter removed that day?
   1. Limit oral fluid intake to avoid urinary incontinence
   2. Expect patient complaints of suprapubic fullness and discomfort
   3. Report the time and amount of first voiding
   4. Instruct patient to stay in bed and use a urinal or bedpan

10. What step when performing catheter care helps prevent trauma *and* CAUTI?
    1. Administer perineal care with soap and water
    2. Cleanse the catheter starting at the meatus
    3. Grasp the catheter with two fingers to stabilize catheter
    4. Retract the foreskin before cleansing

REFERENCES

Aaronson DS, et al: National incidence and impact of noninfectious urethral catheter related complications on the surgical care improvement project, *J Urol* 185(5):1756, 2011.

Beattie M, Taylor J: Silver alloy vs. uncoated urinary catheters: a systematic review of the literature, *J Clin Nurs* 20(15–16):2098, 2010.

Bullman S: Ins and outs of suprapubic catheters—a clinician's experience, *Urol Nurs* 31(5):259, 2011.

Caljouw MA, et al: Predictive factors of urinary tract infections among the oldest old in general population. A population-based prospective follow-up study, *BMC Med* 9:57, 2011.

Caterino JM, et al: Age, nursing home residence, and presentation of urinary tract infection in U.S. emergency departments, 2001-2008, *Acad Emerg Med* 19(10):1173, 2012.

Cipa-Tatum J, et al: Urethral erosion: a case for prevention, *J Wound Ostomy Continence Nurs* 38(5):581, 2011.

Geng V, et al; European Association of Urology Nurses: *Evidence-based guidelines for best practice in urological health care catheterisation indwelling catheters in adults urethral and supra pubic*, 2012. http://www.uroweb.org/fileadmin/EAUN/guidelines/EAUN_Paris_Guideline_2012_LR_online_file.pdf. Accessed August 28, 2013.

Gould CV, et al: Guideline for prevention of catheter-associated urinary tract infections, *Infect Control Hosp Epidemiol* 31(4):319, 2010.

Hockenberry MJ, Wilson D: *Wong's nursing care of infants and children*, ed 11, St Louis, 2013, Mosby.

Hooton TM, et al: Diagnosis, prevention, and treatment of catheter-associated urinary tract infection in adults: 2009 international clinical practice guidelines from the Infectious Diseases Society of America, *Clin Infect Dis* 50(5):625, 2010.

Huether SE, McKance KL: *Understanding pathophysiology*, ed 5, St Louis, 2012, Mosby.

Kawoosa N: Isolated gangrene of the penis in a paraplegic patient secondary to a condom catheter, *Indian J Surg* 73(4):304, 2011.

Kyle G: The use of urinary sheaths in male incontinence, *Br J Nurs* 20(6):338, 2011.

Leuck AM, et al: Complications of Foley catheters—is infection the greatest risk? *J Urol* 187(5):1662, 2012.

Lewis SL, et al: *Medical surgical nursing: assessment and management of clinical problems*, ed 9, St Louis, 2014, Mosby.

Matthews SJ, Lancaster JW: Urinary tract infections in the elderly population, *Am J Pharmacol* 9(5):286, 2011.

Meddings J, et al: Reducing unnecessary urinary catheter use and other strategies to prevent catheter-associated urinary tract infections: brief update review. In *Making Health Care Safer II: An Updated Critical Analysis of the Evidence for Patient Safety Practices*, Rockville, MD, 2013, Agency for Healthcare Research and Quality. Available at: http://www.ahrq.gov/research/findings/evidence-based-reports/ptsafetyuptp.html. Accessed August 28, 2013.

Meddings J, et al: Systematic review and meta-analysis: reminder systems to reduce catheter-associated urinary tract infections and urinary catheter use in hospitalized patients, *Clin Infect Dis* 51(5):550, 2010.

Méndez-Probst CE, et al: Fundamentals of instrumentation and urinary tract drainage. In Wein A, et al, editors: *Campbell-Walsh urology*, ed 10, Philadelphia, 2012, Saunders.

Muzzi-Bjornson L, Macera L: Preventing infection in elders with long-term indwelling urinary catheters, *J Am Acad Nurse Pract* 23(3):127, 2011.

Nyman MH, Johansson J, Gustafsson M: A randomized controlled trial on the effect of clamping the indwelling urinary catheter in patients with hip fracture, *J Clin Nurs* 19(3–4):405, 2010.

The Joint Commission (TJC): *National Patient Safety Goals*, Oakbrook Terrace, IL, 2014, The Commission. Available at: http://www.jointcommission.org/standards_information/npsgs.aspx.

Tiwari MM, et al: Inappropriate use of urinary catheters: a prospective observational study, *Am J Infect Control* 40(1):51, 2012.

Bowel Elimination and Gastric Intubation

 **EVOLVE WEBSITE/EVOLVE RESOURCES LIST**

http://evolve.elsevier.com/Perry/nursinginterventions
Audio Glossary • Checklists • Review Questions

Regular elimination of bowel waste products is essential for normal body functioning. Alterations in bowel elimination are often early signs or symptoms of problems either within the gastrointestinal (GI) system or other body systems. A patient's physical condition, psychological factors, fluid intake, lifestyle, and medications influence bowel function. When patients' functional status changes or they become ill, they may require assistance to maintain or regain their normal elimination habits. To manage patients' bowel elimination problems, you need to understand the factors that promote, impede, or alter normal elimination.

Disorders of the bowel requiring direct nursing intervention include diarrhea, constipation, and bowel incontinence. Left unrecognized or untreated, constipation progresses to fecal impaction, in which stool blocks the intestinal lumen. Stasis of bowel contents produces abdominal distention and pain. In some cases, liquid stool passes around an impaction, which is frequently misinterpreted as diarrhea. Fecal impaction can potentially result in bowel obstruction, causing aspiration, stercoral ulcers (loss of bowel integrity from the pressure effects of dried, thickened feces), and perforation.

When patients undergo surgery or experience an alteration in GI peristalsis, the insertion of a nasogastric (NG) tube is needed for gastric decompression. Gastric decompression reduces nausea and vomiting by keeping the stomach empty.

PATIENT-CENTERED CARE

Bowel elimination is a very private activity. It is important to show respect for a patient's privacy, provide necessary comfort and hygiene measures, and attend to each patient's emotional needs when performing required skills. Assist immobilized patients with the elimination process by helping them on and off bedpans. Provide patient-centered care by determining a patient's normal pattern of bowel elimination and accommodating that pattern in the health care setting.

Show respect and understanding. Emotional factors affect bowel elimination. Anxiety, fear, and anger may accelerate peristalsis, resulting in diarrhea and gaseous distention. Other emotional factors (e.g., depression) and physical factors (e.g., reduced mobility, changes in diet) often cause decreased peristalsis, resulting in increased reabsorption of water from the stool and subsequent constipation.

Be aware of a patient's cultural practices. Provide gender-congruent care for patients from cultures that emphasize separate gender roles and female modesty. Also be aware of patients' unique hygiene needs. For example, some patients have distinct hygiene practices, such as using the left hand for unclean procedures such as practices associated with bowel elimination (Giger, 2013). In this case, use the right hand to touch the patient first and assist with other aspects of care, and use the left for handling the bedpan and perineal cleansing after bowel elimination.

SAFETY

When assisting patients with bowel elimination or inserting an NG tube for gastric decompression, safe nursing practices are essential. Safe patient handling techniques when positioning a patient for removal of a fecal impaction or administering an enema are essential. It is important that a patient understand the need to maintain the position and try to relax. During an enema, sudden movement increases the risk of injury from the rectal tube.

There are additional safety issues when removing a fecal impaction. If the patient has a history of cardiac dysrhythmias, there is a risk for procedural-associated bradycardia because of stimulation of the sacral branch of the vagus nerve. This procedure is often contraindicated in patients with cardiac disease. However, if the procedure is absolutely necessary, monitor the patient's heart rate before and during the procedure.

Correct placement of an NG tube for gastric decompression reduces risks associated with aspiration. In addition, patient safety includes preventing injury from tube insertion or placement. For example, pressure of the tube against a patient's nares increases the risk for skin breakdown. Meticulous skin care around the nares and nose is needed. Frequent oral hygiene minimizes oral discomfort and the risk of damage to the oral mucosa.

EVIDENCE-BASED PRACTICE

Hodin R et al: Nasogastric and nasoenteric tubes, *UpToDate*, 2014, http://pmtwww.uptodate.com/contents/nasogastric -and-nasoenteric-tubes.

National Pressure Ulcer Advisory Panel (NPUAP): *Mucosal pressure ulcers: an NPUAP Position Statement*, 2012, http://www.npuap.org/wp-content/uploads/2012/03/ Mucosal_Pressure_Ulcer_Position_Statement_final.pdf. Accessed January 25, 2014.

National Pressure Ulcer Advisory Panel (NPUAP): *Best practices for prevention of medical device pressure ulcers*, 2013, http://www.npuap.org/wp-content/uploads/2013/04/ Medical-Device-Poster.pdf. Accessed January 25, 2014.

Pressure applied to mucous membranes lining the nasal passages can render the tissue ischemic and lead to ulceration (NPUAP, 2012). Mucosal tissues are especially vulnerable to pressure from medical devices such as NG and feeding tubes. These devices and their securement products cause pressure on the skin. Patients who cannot convey discomfort may have a higher risk for the development of pressure ulcers than an alert patient (Hodin et al., 2014). The National Pressure Ulcer Advisory Panel (2013) recommends these best practices for prevention of medical device–related pressure ulcers:

- Choose the correct size of medical device to fit the individual.
- Cushion and protect the skin (when possible) with dressings in high-risk areas (e.g., nasal bridge).
- Remove or move the device daily to assess skin.
- Avoid placement of device over sites of prior or existing pressure ulceration.
- Educate staff on correct use of devices and prevention of skin breakdown.
- Be aware of edema under device and potential for skin breakdown.
- Confirm that tubing of device is not placed directly under an individual who is bedridden or immobile.

PROCEDURAL GUIDELINE 19.1
Providing a Bedpan

A patient restricted to bed uses a bedpan for bowel elimination. Two types of bedpans are available (Fig. 19-1). The regular and most commonly used bedpan has a curved, smooth upper end and a tapered lower end. The upper end (wide end) of a regular bedpan fits under a patient's buttocks toward the sacrum, with the lower end (tapered end) fitting just under the upper thighs.

A fracture pan, designated for patients with body or leg casts or patients restricted from raising their hips (e.g., after a total joint replacement), slips easily under a patient. The shallow upper end of the pan with a flat, wide rim fits under a patient's buttocks toward the sacrum, with the deep lower open end aimed toward the foot of the bed.

Delegation and Collaboration

The skill of providing a bedpan can be delegated to nursing assistive personnel (NAP). The nurse instructs the NAP about the following:

- Correct positioning guidelines for patients with mobility restrictions or for patients who have therapeutic equipment such as wound drains, intravenous (IV) catheters, or traction.
- Providing perineal and hand hygiene for the patient as necessary after using the bedpan.

Equipment

- Clean gloves
- Bedpan (regular or fracture) (see Fig. 19-1) (optional: bedpan cover)
- Toilet tissue
- Specimen container (if necessary) or plastic specimen bag clearly labeled with date, patient's name, and identification number
- Washbasin, washcloths (regular or disposable), towels, and soap
- Skin cleansing wipes

PROCEDURAL GUIDELINE 19.1
Providing a Bedpan—cont'd

- Waterproof, absorbent pads (if necessary)
- Stethoscope
- Clean drawsheet (if necessary).

Procedural Steps

1. **See Standard Protocol (inside front cover).**
2. Assess patient's normal elimination habits: routine pattern, character of stool, effect of certain foods or fluids and eating habits on bowel elimination, effect of stress and level of activity on normal bowel elimination patterns, current medications, and normal fluid intake.
3. Auscultate for bowel sounds and palpate lower abdomen for distention.
4. Assess patient's level of mobility, including ability to sit upright and lift hips or turn.
5. Assess patient's level of comfort. Note presence of rectal or hemorrhoidal pain, abdominal pain, or skin irritation surrounding anus.
6. Apply clean gloves. Inspect condition of skin around rectal and perineal area. Repeated diarrheal stools can cause skin irritation and breakdown. Remove gloves and dispose in appropriate receptacle. Perform hand hygiene.
7. Determine if a stool specimen is needed.
8. For a patient's comfort, place metal bedpan under warm, running water for a few seconds and dry. Be careful that pan is not too hot.

9. Raise side rail on opposite side of bed.
10. Raise bed horizontally according to your height.
11. Have patient assume supine position.

> **SAFE PATIENT CARE** Observe for presence of drains, IV fluids, and traction ropes. These devices may impede a patient from assisting with the procedure and may require more staff to assist placing the patient on a bedpan.

12. *Place patient who can assist on bedpan.*
    a. Apply clean gloves. Raise head of patient's bed 30 to 60 degrees.
    b. Remove upper bed linens just enough so that they are out of the way but patient is not exposed. Place bedpan in accessible location.
    c. Instruct patient on how to flex knees and lift hips upward.
    d. Place hand closest to patient's head palm up under patient's sacrum to assist lifting. Ask patient to bend knees and raise hips. As patient raises hips, use other hand to slip regular bedpan under patient (see illustrations). Be sure that open rim of bedpan is facing toward foot of bed. Do not shove bedpan under patient's hips. (Optional: Have patient use overhead trapeze frame to raise hips.)

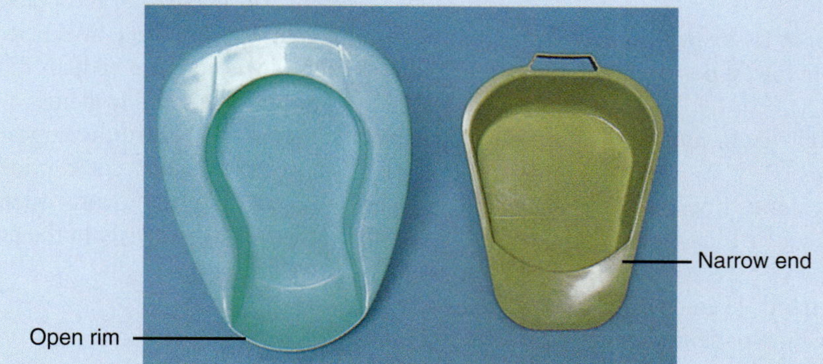

FIG 19-1 Types of bedpans. *Left,* Regular bedpan. *Right,* Fracture bedpan.

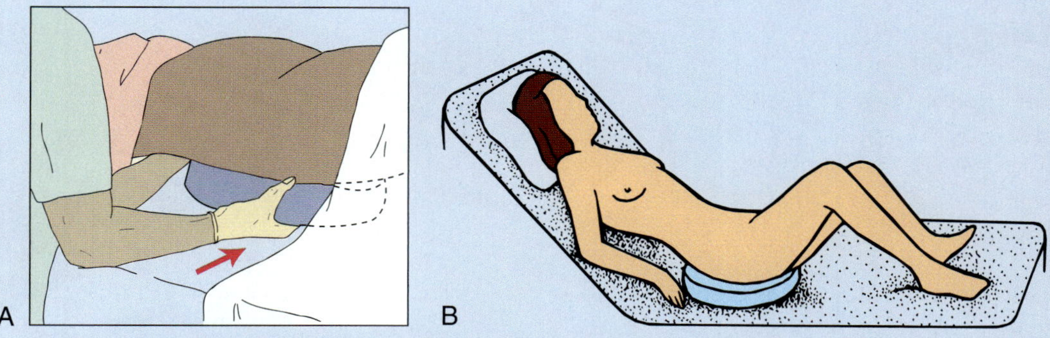

STEP 12d A, Placement of bedpan under patient's hips. **B,** Correct positioning for patient on bedpan.

PROCEDURAL GUIDELINE 19.1
Providing a Bedpan—cont'd

e. Optional: If using a fracture pan, slip it under patient as hips are raised. Be sure that narrow rim of bedpan is facing toward foot of bed.

> **SAFE PATIENT CARE** Use a fracture pan if the patient had a total hip replacement. An abduction pillow must be placed between the legs when turning to prevent dislocation of the new joint.

13. *Place patient who is immobile or has mobility restrictions on bedpan.*
    a. Apply clean gloves. Lower head of bed flat or raise head slightly (if tolerated by medical condition).
    b. Remove top linens as needed to turn patient while minimizing exposure.
    c. Assist patient with rolling onto one side, with buttocks facing toward you.
    d. Place regular bedpan firmly against patient's buttocks and down into mattress. Be sure open rim of bedpan is facing toward foot of bed (see illustrations).
    e. Keeping one hand against bedpan, place other hand around patient's far hip. Ask patient to roll back onto bedpan. Do not force bedpan under patient.
    f. Raise patient's head 30 degrees or to level of comfort (unless contraindicated). Have patient bend knees or raise knee gatch (unless contraindicated).
14. Maintain patient's comfort and safety. Cover patient for warmth.
15. Keep call bell and toilet tissue within easy reach for patient and place bed in lowest position with upper side rails raised.
16. Remove and discard gloves in appropriate receptacle. Perform hand hygiene.
17. Allow patient to be alone, but monitor status and respond promptly.
18. *Remove bedpan.*
    a. Perform hand hygiene and apply clean gloves. Position patient's bedside chair close to working side of bed.

b. Maintain privacy; determine if patient is able to wipe own perineal area. If you must wipe perineal area, use several layers of toilet tissue or disposable washcloths. For female patients, cleanse from mons pubis toward rectal area.
c. Deposit contaminated tissue in bedpan. However, if you need to measure intake and output (I&O) or need a specimen, discard contaminated tissue in the toilet.
d. *For mobile patient:* Ask patient to flex knees, placing body weight on lower legs, feet, and upper torso; lift buttocks up from bedpan. At same time, place hand farther from patient on side of bedpan and place other hand (closer to patient) under sacrum to assist in lifting. Have patient lift hips and remove bedpan. Place bedpan on draped bedside chair and cover.
e. *For immobile patient:* Lower head of bed. Assist patient with rolling onto side and off of bedpan. Hold bedpan flat and steady while patient is rolling off to avoid spillage. After patient is completely lifted off bedpan, place it on bedside chair and cover.
f. Allow patient to perform hand hygiene.
19. Change any soiled linens, cleanse skin with soap and water if soiled, or use cleansing wipes to minimize rubbing and irritation to skin.
20. **See Completion Protocol (inside front cover).**
21. Option: Apply clean gloves. Obtain specimen as ordered (see Chapter 8). Empty bedpan into toilet or in special receptacle in appropriate utility room. Spray faucet attached to most facility toilets allows you to rinse bedpan thoroughly. Remove gloves and perform hand hygiene.
22. Observe and record the appearance and characteristics of stool, including color, odor, consistency, frequency, amount, shape, and constituents in medical record.
23. Observe skin integrity in the perineal and perianal area.

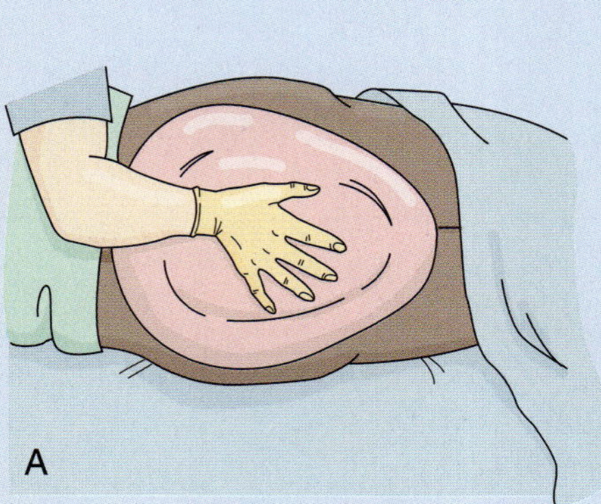

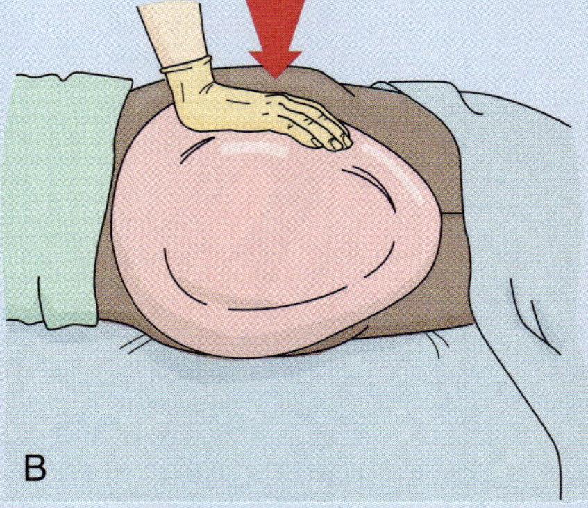

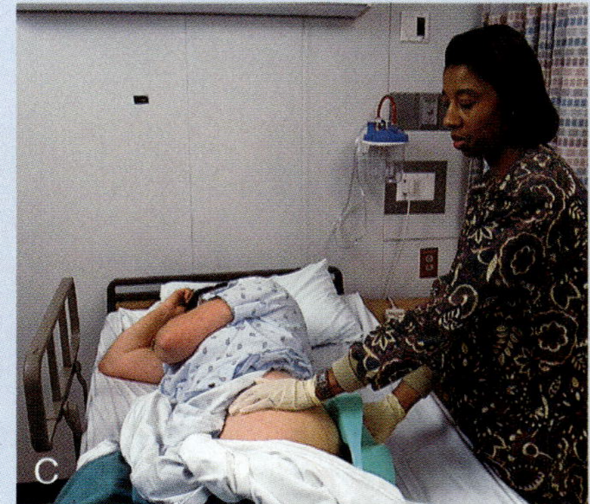

STEP 13d A, Position patient on one side and place bedpan firmly against buttocks. **B,** Push down on bedpan and toward patient. **C,** Nurse places the bedpan in position. (**A** and **B,** From Sorrentino SA: *Mosby's textbook for nursing assistants,* ed 7, St Louis, 2008, Mosby.)

SKILL 19.1 REMOVING A FECAL IMPACTION

Fecal impaction, the inability to pass a hard collection of stool commonly found in the lower colon and rectum, can occur in all age groups. Physically and mentally incapacitated persons and institutionalized older adults are at greatest risk. Patients with neurologic disorders affecting the nerves that innervate the muscles of the intestines are also at risk. Many of these patients receive regular laxatives and stool softeners, which alters their elimination patterns and contributes to impactions and ultimately fecal incontinence (McKay et al., 2012). Fecal impaction occurs when there is a history of constipation. Constipation is defined as infrequent stools. However, a consensus definition of functional constipation includes two or more of the following factors for at least 3 months: (1) straining with defecation at least one fourth of the time, (2) lumpy or hard stools (or both) at least one fourth of the time, (3) sensation of incomplete evacuation at least one fourth of the time, or (4) two or fewer bowel movements in a week (McKay et al., 2012). Varieties of interventions (e.g., diet and exercise) normally successfully relieve constipation and reduce the risk of impaction.

Symptoms of fecal impaction include constipation, rectal discomfort, anorexia, nausea, vomiting, abdominal pain, diarrhea (leaking around the impacted stool), and urinary frequency. Prevention is the key to managing fecal impaction. However, when impaction occurs, digital removal of the stool is a treatment option. Digital removal of an impaction is embarrassing and uncomfortable for patients. Excessive rectal manipulation may cause irritation to the mucosa and subsequent bleeding or vagus nerve stimulation, which can produce a reflex slowing of heart rate. Digital removal is performed when the administration of enemas (e.g., oil retention) or suppositories is unsuccessful at removing impacted stools.

The Royal College of Nursing (Ness and Hibberts, 2012) emphasizes some crucial points for nursing to practice when managing patients who need digital removal of feces. Before performing the invasive intervention, a nurse needs to do the following: assess each patient's risk factors, assess religious and cultural beliefs, and obtain informed consent (follow facility policy). Informed consent may be written, verbal, or implied (follow facility policy). Document the consent in the patient's chart.

▍ASSESSMENT

1. Identify patient using two identifiers (e.g., name and birthday or name and account number) according to facility policy. *Rationale: Ensures correct patient. Complies with The Joint Commission standards and improves patient safety (TJC, 2014).*
2. Ask patient about normal and current bowel elimination pattern, including frequency and characteristics of stool; use of laxatives, enemas, and other medications; level of regular exercise; urge to defecate but inability to do so; presence of hemorrhoids; abdominal discomfort, especially when attempting to defecate; feelings of incomplete emptying; and sensations of bloating, cramping, or excessive gas. *Rationale: This information is valuable in determining contributing factors and preventive measures.*
3. Inspect patient's abdomen for distention. *Rationale: Observation initially identifies any distended or asymmetrical areas, which are investigated further on auscultation or palpation.*
4. Auscultate all four quadrants for presence of bowel sounds. *Rationale: Hypoactive bowel sounds may result from partial obstruction of the GI tract as with constipation or masses. Hyperactive bowel sounds may be present as a result of intestinal irritation as with diarrhea, partial obstruction of GI tract, or before defecation.*
5. Palpate patient's abdomen for distention, discomfort, or masses. *Rationale: Symptoms are related to accumulation of feces in intestinal tract. When severe constipation occurs, a palpable mass may be felt.*
6. Measure patient's current heart rate and comfort level on a scale of 0 to 10. *Rationale: Establishes a baseline for detecting slowing in heart rate. Sacral branch of vagus nerve is stimulated during digital manipulation; this stimulation results in reflex bradycardia (Seidel et al., 2015).*
7. Perform hand hygiene and apply clean gloves. Observe the anal area for signs of irritation from passing stool or hemorrhoids. *Rationale: Indicates possible straining on defecation.* Observe consistency of stool, seepage of liquid stool, or continual passage of small amounts of hard stool. Remove gloves and perform hand hygiene. *Rationale: Seepage of stool is symptomatic of an impaction high in colon. Patient may be able to pass small pieces of hard stool or have episodes of passing small amounts of liquid stool.*
8. Determine if patient is receiving anticoagulant therapy. *Rationale: Procedure may be contraindicated. Irritation and manipulation of the rectum often cause rectal bleeding, which will be more prolonged with anticoagulation.*
9. Check patient's record for health care provider's order for digital removal of impaction. *Rationale: A health care provider's order is necessary because of possible vagus nerve stimulation.*

> **SAFE PATIENT CARE** Because of the potential to stimulate the vagus nerve, patients with a history of dysrhythmias or heart disease have a greater risk for changes in heart rhythm. Removal of an impaction is often contraindicated in these patients. Verify with health care provider.

▍PLANNING

Expected Outcomes focus on removal of the impaction and prevention of patient injury.

1. Patient's rectum is free of stool.
2. Patient's vital signs remain stable during and after procedure.

3. Patient is free of rectal or abdominal discomfort.
4. Anal area is free of tissue damage.

Delegation and Collaboration

The skill of removing an impaction cannot be delegated to nursing assistive personnel (NAP). The nurse instructs the NAP about the following:

- Assisting the nurse in positioning patient for the procedure.
- What to observe for (e.g., color and consistency of any evacuated stool, rectal bleeding, or bloody mucus) and report back to nurse.
- Providing frequent perineal care to patient.

Equipment

- Clean gloves
- Water-soluble local anesthetic lubricant (Note: Some facilities require use of water-soluble lubricant without anesthetic when nurse performs procedure.)
- Waterproof, absorbent pads
- Bedpan
- Bedpan cover (optional if available)
- Bath blanket
- Washbasin, washcloths, towels, and soap
- Sphygmomanometer

IMPLEMENTATION *for* REMOVING A FECAL IMPACTION

STEPS	RATIONALE
1. **See Standard Protocol (inside front cover).**	
2. Obtain assistance to help change patient's position if necessary.	Promotes safe patient handling and good body mechanics.
3. Lower side rail on patient's right side. Keeping far side rail raised, assist patient to left side-lying position with knees flexed and back toward you.	Promotes patient safety. Provides access to rectum.
4. Apply clean gloves. Drape patient's trunk and lower extremities with bath blanket, and place waterproof pad under patient's buttocks.	Maintains patient's sense of privacy and prevents unnecessary exposure of body parts.
5. Place bedpan next to patient.	
6. Lubricate gloved index and middle fingers of dominant hand with anesthetic lubricant.	Reduces discomfort and permits smooth insertion of finger into anus and rectum.
7. Instruct patient to take slow deep breaths during procedure; gradually and gently insert gloved index finger and feel anus relax around the finger. Then insert middle finger.	Slow deep breaths may help to relax patient. Gradual insertion of index finger helps to dilate anal sphincter.
8. Gradually advance fingers slowly along rectal wall in the direction toward the umbilicus.	Aiming toward rectal wall follows natural direction of colon allowing for access to impacted stool.
9. Gently loosen fecal mass by moving fingers in a scissors motion to fragment fecal mass. Work fingers into hardened mass.	Loosening and penetrating mass allows you to remove it in small pieces, resulting in less discomfort to patient.
10. Work stool downward toward end of rectum. Remove small sections of feces and discard into bedpan.	Prevents need to force finger up into rectum and minimizes trauma to mucosa.
11. Observe patient's response, and periodically assess heart rate and look for signs of fatigue.	Vagal stimulation slows heart rate and may cause dysrhythmias. Procedure may exhaust patient.

> **SAFE PATIENT CARE** Stop procedure if heart rate decreases, rhythm changes, or rectal bleeding occurs.

STEPS	RATIONALE
12. Continue to clear rectum of feces, allowing patient to rest at intervals.	Rest improves patient's tolerance of procedure.
13. After removal of impaction, provide perineal hygiene (see Chapter 10).	Promotes patient comfort and sense of cleanliness.
14. Remove bedpan and dispose of feces.	Reduces transmission of microorganisms.
15. If needed, assist patient to toilet or clean bedpan. (Procedure may be followed by enema or cathartic.)	Removal of impaction stimulates defecation reflex.
16. **See Completion Protocol (inside front cover).**	

EVALUATION

1. Perform rectal examination for stool, and observe anal and perianal area for irritation or skin breakdown.
2. Obtain heart rate and blood pressure and compare with baseline values. Continue to monitor patient for bradycardia for 1 hour after procedure.
3. Auscultate for bowel sounds.
4. Palpate abdomen to determine if it is soft and not tender.
5. Ask patient to rate comfort level on a scale of 0 to 10.

Unexpected Outcomes and Related Interventions

1. Patient experiences bradycardia, decrease in blood pressure, and decrease in level of consciousness as a result of vagus nerve stimulation.
   a. Stop procedure and measure vital signs.
   b. Notify health care provider immediately.
   c. Remain with patient, and monitor vital signs and level of consciousness.
2. Patient has seepage of liquid fecal material after removal of impaction.
   a. Assess patient for continuing impaction.
   b. Contact health care provider. A suppository or an enema is often needed to remove hardened feces higher in the rectum.
   c. Increase fluids (if allowed), fiber in diet, and activity level to increase peristaltic activity.
3. Patient has trauma to the rectal mucosa as evidenced by blood on the gloved finger.
   a. Stop procedure if bleeding is excessive.
   b. If bleeding continues, notify health care provider for further treatment measures.

Recording and Reporting

- Record patient's tolerance to procedure, amount and consistency of stool removed, vital signs, pain level on a scale of 0 to 10, and adverse effects.
- Report any changes in vital signs or adverse effects to nurse in charge or health care provider.

Sample Documentation

1600   Ten pieces, ranging from 1 to 2 cm, of hard, dark brown, lumpy stool removed from rectum without rectal bleeding. Pain rated at 4, stopped procedure, then continued after 2-3 minutes. Pulse 80 to 88 strong and regular. Normal bowel sounds present in all four quadrants. No abdominal distention or complaints of pain after procedure.

Special Considerations
Pediatric

- Digital removal of stool is not recommended in pediatric patients because of risk for anal fissures and pain, which triggers stool withholding (Hockenberry and Wilson, 2013).

Geriatric

- Many older adults are especially prone to dysrhythmias and other problems related to vagal stimulation; monitor heart rate and rhythm closely.
- Institute a diet adequate in dietary fiber to add bulk, weight, and form to stool and improve defecation: men age 51 or older, 30 grams/day; women age 51 or older, 21 grams/day (Mayo Clinic, 2012).
- Consider development of regular toileting routine that includes responding to the urge to defecate.

Home Care

- Consider having patient or family caregiver keep a diary for 1 week of meals and fluid intake. Determine if dietary pattern contributes to constipation.
- Have patient or family caregiver maintain a weekly bowel diary.

SKILL 19.2   ADMINISTERING AN ENEMA

- **Nursing Skills Online: Bowel Elimination Module, Lesson 2**

An enema is the instillation of a solution into the rectum and sigmoid colon to promote defecation by stimulating peristalsis. Enemas treat constipation or empty the bowel before diagnostic procedures or abdominal surgeries. Preoperative enemas are common for some GI surgeries. Teach your patients not to rely on enemas to maintain bowel regularity because they do not treat the cause of irregularity or constipation. Frequent enemas can disrupt normal defecation reflexes, resulting in dependence on them for elimination.

Cleansing enemas help to evacuate feces from the colon. The enemas act by stimulating peristalsis through infusion of a large volume of solution or through irritation of the colon mucosa. Each solution influences the movement of fluids in the colon. When "enemas until clear" is ordered in preparation for surgery or diagnostic testing, the water expelled may be colored but should not contain solid fecal material. When administering "enemas until clear," patients usually receive no more than three consecutive enemas to prevent fluid and electrolyte imbalance (check facility policy).

Enemas that are used less frequently include medicated enemas, such as sodium polystyrene sulfonate [Kayexalate] enema for high serum potassium levels and carminative enemas, such as the Harris or return-flow enema, for relieving accumulated flatus.

The enema volume or type of fluid that breaks up a fecal mass stretches the rectal wall and initiates the defecation reflex. Table 19-1 summarizes common types of enemas.

ASSESSMENT

1. Identify patient using two identifiers (e.g., name and birthday or name and account number) according to

TABLE 19-1   TYPES OF ENEMAS

TYPE OF ENEMA	DESCRIPTION AND IMPLICATIONS
Tap water (hypotonic) enema	Do not repeat after first installation because water toxicity or circulatory overload can develop.
Physiological normal saline	Safest enema to administer. Infants and children can tolerate only this type because of their predisposition to fluid imbalance.
Hypertonic solution (e.g., Fleet's enema)	Useful for patients who cannot tolerate large fluid volumes.
Harris flush enema	A return-flow enema that helps to expel intestinal gas. Administer a small amount (100 to 200 mL) of enema solution into patient's rectum and colon. Then lower the enema container to allow the total volume of solution to flow back. The repeated back-and-forth administration and return of the fluid reduces flatus and promotes return of peristalsis.
Soapsuds enema	Pure castile soap added to either tap water or normal saline. Use only pure castile soap. Recommended ratio of pure soap to solution is 5 mL (1 tsp) soap to 1000 mL (1 quart) warm water or saline. Add soap to enema bag after water to reduce suds.
Oil-retention	Oil-based solution. The colon absorbs a small volume, which softens stool for easier evacuation.
Carminative solution	Relieves gaseous distention. Example: MGW enema (30 mL magnesium, 60 mL glycerin, 90 mL water)

facility policy. *Rationale: Ensures correct patient. Complies with The Joint Commission standards and improves patient safety (TJC, 2014).*

2. Review health care provider's order for enema and clarify reason for enema administration. *Rationale: Order by health care provider is required for hospitalized patient. The order states the type of enema and how many enemas patient will receive.*

3. Determine patient's level of understanding of purpose of enema. *Rationale: Allows for planning appropriate instruction.*

4. Inspect abdomen for distention and auscultate for bowel sounds. *Rationale: Provides baseline to evaluate response to enema.*

5. Assess medical history for presence of undiagnosed GI disease or bleeding; cardiac disease; paralytic ileus or suspected intestinal obstruction; Hirschsprung's disease; symptoms of appendicitis or inflammatory bowel disease; dehydration; or recent abdominal, rectal, or prostate surgery. *Rationale: Conditions may contraindicate use of enemas.*

6. Assess patient for allergy to any active ingredients of a Fleet's enema. *Rationale: Prevents hypersensitivity or allergic reaction.*

7. Assess last bowel movement, normal versus most recent bowel elimination pattern, presence of hemorrhoids, mobility, and presence of abdominal pain or cramping. *Rationale: Determines factors indicating need for enema and influences type of enema used. Also establishes baseline for bowel function. Hemorrhoids may obscure the rectal opening and cause discomfort or bleeding with evacuation.*

PLANNING

Expected Outcomes focus on establishing a normal pattern of bowel elimination and normal consistency of stools.

1. Stool is evacuated.
2. Enema return is clear.
3. Abdomen is soft and nondistended.

Delegation and Collaboration

The skill of enema administration can be delegated to nursing assistive personnel (NAP). The nurse instructs the NAP about the following:

- How to position patients with therapeutic equipment such as drains, IV catheters, or traction properly.
- How to properly position patients with mobility restrictions.
- Informing the nurse immediately about the presence of blood in the stool or around rectal area; any change in vital signs; and abdominal pain, cramping, or distention.

Equipment

- Clean gloves
- Water-soluble lubricant
- Waterproof absorbent underpads
- Toilet tissue
- Bedpan, bedside commode, or access to toilet
- Washbasin, washcloths, towel, and soap
- Bath blanket

Enema Bag Administration

- Enema container (Fig. 19-2)
- IV pole
- Tubing and clamp (if not already attached to container)
- Appropriate-size rectal tube (adult, 22 to 30 Fr; child, 12 to 18 Fr)
- Correct volume of warmed (tepid) solution (adult, 750 to 1000 mL; adolescent, 500 to 700 mL; school-age child, 300 to 500 mL; toddler, 250 to 350 mL; infant, 150 to 250 mL)
- Prepackaged enema
- Prepackaged enema container with lubricated rectal tip (Fig. 19-3)

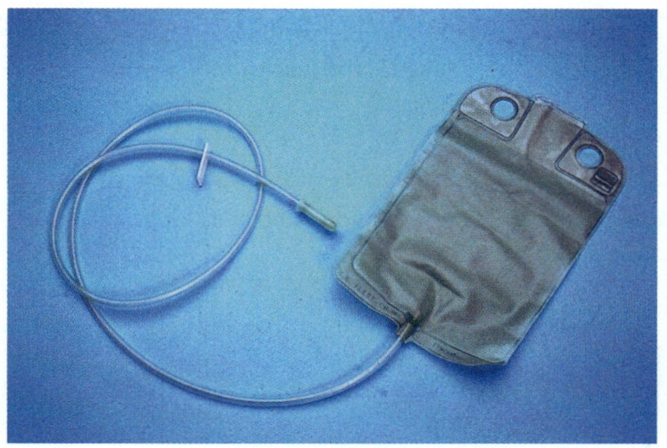

FIG 19-2 Enema bag with tubing.

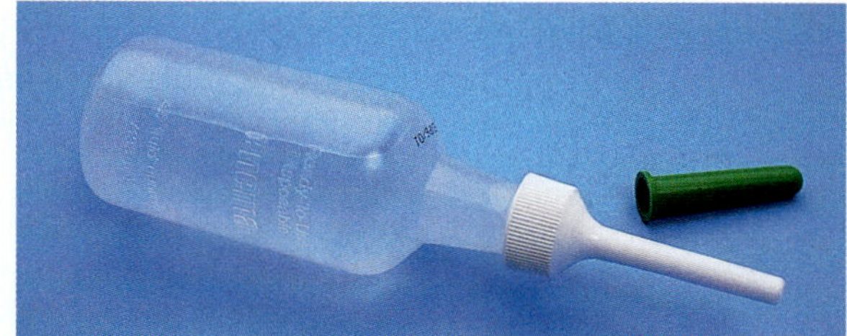

FIG 19-3 Prepackaged enema container with rectal tip and cap.

IMPLEMENTATION *for* ADMINISTERING AN ENEMA

STEPS	RATIONALE
1. **See Standard Protocol (inside front cover).**	
2. If enema is medicated, check accuracy and completeness of each medication administration record (MAR) with health care provider's written medication or procedure order. For all enemas, check patient's name, type of enema, and time for administration. Compare MAR with label of enema solution.	The order sheet is the most reliable source and only legal record of drugs or procedure the patient is to receive. Ensures that patient receives correct medication/enema.
3. With side rail raised on patient's right side and bed raised to appropriate working height, help patient turn onto left side-lying (Sims') position with right knee flexed. Encourage patient to remain in position until procedure is completed. Children are also positioned in dorsal recumbent position.	Allows enema solution to flow downward by gravity along natural curve of sigmoid colon and rectum, improving retention of solution.

> **SAFE PATIENT CARE** Patients with poor sphincter control require placement of a bedpan under the buttocks. Administering enema with patient sitting on toilet is unsafe because curved rectal tubing can abrade rectal wall.

STEPS	RATIONALE
4. Apply clean gloves. Place waterproof pad absorbent side up under hips and buttocks.	Prevents soiling linen.
5. Cover patient with bath blanket, exposing only rectal area and allowing anus to be visualized clearly.	Provides warmth, reduces exposure of body parts, and allows patient to feel more relaxed and comfortable. Provides access to anus.
6. Separate buttocks and examine perianal region for abnormalities, including hemorrhoids, anal fissure, and rectal prolapse.	Findings influence nurse's approach to insertion of enema tip. Rectal prolapse contraindicates an enema. Hemorrhoids can obscure anal opening.
7. Place bedpan or commode in easily accessible position. If patient will be expelling contents into toilet, ensure that toilet is available, and place patient's slippers and bathrobe in easily accessible location.	Bedpan is used if patient unable to get out of bed.
8. Administer enema.	
a. Administer prepackaged disposable enema.	
(1) Remove plastic cap from tip of container. Tip may already be lubricated. Apply more water-soluble lubricant if needed.	Lubrication provides for smooth insertion of tip without rectal irritation or trauma.
(2) Gently separate buttocks and locate anus. Instruct patient to relax by breathing out slowly through mouth.	Breathing out promotes relaxation of external rectal sphincter. Presence of hemorrhoids obscures location of anus.

Continued

(3) Carefully expel any air from enema container.

Air entering colon from the enema container causes further distention and discomfort.

(4) Insert lubricated tip of container gently into anal canal toward umbilicus (see illustration). Insert distance of container tip.

Gentle insertion prevents trauma to rectal mucosa.

> **SAFE PATIENT CARE** If pain occurs or you feel resistance during insertion, stop and discuss with health care provider. Do not force insertion.

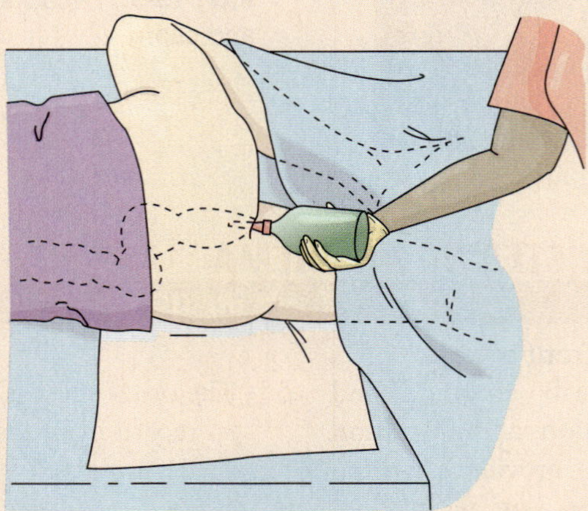

STEP 8a(4) With patient in left lateral Sims' position, insert the tip of the commercial enema into the rectum. (From Sorrentino SA: *Mosby's textbook for nursing assistants,* ed 6, St Louis, 2006, Mosby.)

(5) Roll plastic bottle from bottom to tip until all of solution has entered rectum and colon. Instruct patient to retain solution for 2 to 5 minutes until urge to defecate.

Hypertonic solutions require only small volumes to stimulate defecation. Intermittent squeezing results in return of solution to bottle.

b. Administer enema in standard enema bag.

(1) Add warmed solution to enema bag: Warm tap water as it flows from faucet, place saline container in basin of warm water before adding saline solution to enema bag, and check temperature of solution by pouring small amount of solution over inner wrist.

Hot water can burn intestinal mucosa. Cold water can cause abdominal cramping and is difficult to retain.

(2) If soapsuds enema is ordered, add castile soap after the water.

Prevents suds in enema bag.

(3) Raise container, release clamp, and allow solution to flow long enough to fill tubing.

Removes air from tubing.

(4) Reclamp tubing.

(5) Lubricate 6 to 8 cm (2½ to 3 inches) of tip of tubing with lubricant.

Eases tube insertion through anus.

(6) Gently separate buttocks and locate anus. Instruct patient to relax by breathing out slowly through mouth.

Breathing out promotes relaxation of external anal sphincter.

(7) Insert tip of rectal tube slowly by pointing tip in direction of patient's umbilicus. Length of insertion varies:
Adult: 7.5 to 10 cm (3 to 4 inches)
Adolescent: 7.5 to 10 cm (3 to 4 inches)
Child: 5 to 7.5 cm (2 to 3 inches)
Infant: 2.5 cm (1 inch)

Careful insertion prevents trauma to rectal mucosa from accidental lodging of tube against rectal wall. Forceful insertion beyond recommended length can cause bowel perforation.

> **SAFE PATIENT CARE** If tube does not pass easily, do not force. Consider allowing a small amount of fluid to infuse and trying to reinsert tube slowly. The instillation of fluid may relax the sphincter and provide added lubrication.

STEPS	**RATIONALE**

(8) Hold tubing in rectum constantly until end of fluid instillation.

Bowel contraction can cause expulsion of rectal tube.

(9) Open regulating clamp and allow solution to enter slowly with container at patient's hip level.

Rapid infusion can stimulate evacuation of tubing and cause cramping.

(10) Raise height of enema container slowly to appropriate level above anus: 30 to 45 cm (12 to 18 inches) for high enema; 30 cm (12 inches) for regular enema (see illustration); 7.5 cm (3 inches) for low enema. Instillation time varies with volume of solution administered (e.g., 1 L may take 10 minutes). Hang container on IV pole.

Allows for continuous, slow instillation of solution. Raising container too high causes rapid infusion and possible painful distention of colon. High pressure can cause rupture of bowel in infant.

> **SAFE PATIENT CARE** Temporary cessation of infusion minimizes cramping and promotes ability to retain all of the solution. Lower container or clamp tubing if patient complains of abdominal cramping or if fluid escapes around rectal tube.

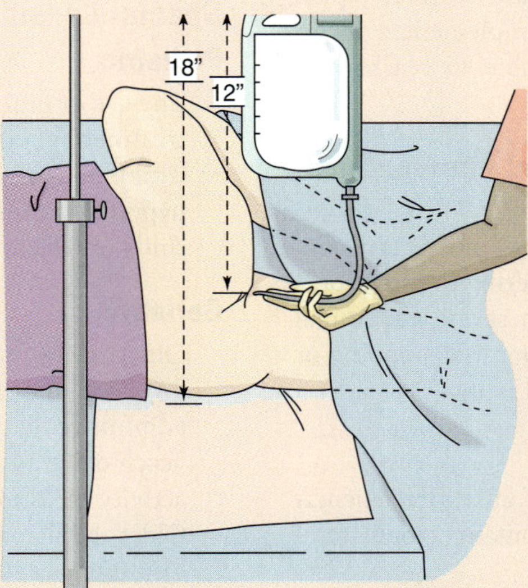

STEP 8b(10) IV pole is positioned so that the enema bag is 30 cm (12 inches) above the anus and approximately 45 cm (18 inches) above the mattress (depending on size of patient). (Adapted from Sorrentino SA: *Mosby's textbook for nursing assistants,* ed 7, St Louis, 2008, Mosby.)

(11) Instill all of solution and clamp the tubing. Tell patient that the procedure is completed and that you will be removing the rectal tube.

Prevents entrance of air into rectum. Patients may misinterpret the sensation of removing the tube as loss of control.

9. Place layers of toilet tissue around tube at anus and gently remove tubing.

Provides for patient's comfort and cleanliness.

10. Explain to patient that feeling of distention is normal. Ask patient to retain solution as long as possible until urge to defecate occurs. This usually takes only a few minutes. Stay at bedside. Have patient lie quietly in bed if possible. (For infant or young child gently hold buttocks together for a few minutes.)

Solution distends bowel. Length of retention varies with type of enema and patient's ability to contract rectal sphincter. Longer retention promotes more effective stimulation of peristalsis and defecation.

11. Assist patient to bathroom or commode if possible. If using the bedpan, assist to as near the normal position for evacuation as possible.

Normal squatting position promotes defecation.

Continued

STEPS	RATIONALE
12. Observe character of stool and solution passed (caution patient against flushing toilet before inspection).	Determines if enema was effective.
13. Assist patient as needed to wash anal area with warm soap and water. Assist patient with hand hygiene.	Fecal contents can irritate skin. Hygiene promotes patient's comfort.
14. **See Completion Protocol (inside front cover).**	

EVALUATION

1. Ask patient if abdominal discomfort was relieved.
2. Inspect color, consistency, and amount of stool; odor; and characteristics of fluid passed.
3. Palpate for abdominal distention.
4. Use *Teach Back:* State to the patient, "I want to be sure I explained what you need to do to develop a regular pattern for moving your bowels. Can you tell me two things you can do to keep your stool soft and moving regularly?" Evaluates what the patient is able to explain or demonstrate. Revise your instruction now or develop plan for revised patient teaching to be implemented at an appropriate time if patient is not able to teach back correctly.

Unexpected Outcomes and Related Interventions

1. Patient is unable to hold enema solution.
   a. If this occurs during instillation, slow rate of infusion.
   b. Position on bedpan while administering the solution.
2. Severe cramping, bleeding, or sudden severe abdominal pain occurs and is unrelieved by temporarily stopping or slowing flow of solution.
   a. Stop enema.
   b. Notify health care provider.
3. With an order for "enemas until clear," after three enemas the water is highly colored or contains solid fecal material.
   a. Notify health care provider.

Recording and Reporting

- Record the time, type, and volume of enema administered; patient's signs and symptoms; response to enema; and results, including color, amount, and appearance of stool.
- Document your evaluation of patient learning.
- Report failure of patient to defecate or any adverse reactions to health care provider.

Sample Documentation

2000 Last bowel movement 5 days ago. Complains of abdominal fullness and rectal pressure. Abdomen distended, firm; 1000-mL soapsuds enema given with "mild" abdominal cramping during administration. Solution returned with large amount of dark brown, soft-formed stool.
2100 States, "I feel better now." Abdomen soft, nondistended. Resting in bed with side rails up × 2 and call light within reach of patient.

Special Considerations
Pediatric

- The use of oral stool softeners is the initial recommended treatment of constipation in children.
- Children and infants usually do not receive prepackaged hypertonic enemas because the solutions cause rapid fluid shifts (Hockenberry and Wilson, 2013).

Geriatric

- Older adults may tire more quickly and are at greater risk for fluid and electrolyte imbalances; use caution when administering enemas "until clear."
- Teach older adults and their family caregivers dietary and activity measures to avoid constipation.
- Older adults may have difficulty in retaining enema solution.

Home Care

- Assess ability and motivation of patient and family caregiver to administer enema in the home and provide instruction as needed.
- Assess patient's ability to manipulate equipment to self-administer enema.
- Instruct patient and family caregiver not to exceed number and volume of enemas.

PROCEDURAL GUIDELINE 19.2
Applying a Fecal Containment Device

A fecal containment device (FCD) is a useful intervention for patients with severe fecal incontinence, such as patients with *Clostridium difficile*–associated diarrhea. Consultation with a health care provider is recommended before applying the device, but a health care provider's order is usually not required (see facility policy). FCDs are an effective way to prevent skin damage resulting from moisture and enzyme action on perianal tissues (Cooper, 2013). There are both indwelling devices (e.g., Flexi-Seal [ConvaTec Inc.], ACTIFLO [Hollister Global]) and topical

PROCEDURAL GUIDELINE 19.2
Applying a Fecal Containment Device—cont'd

containment pouches, which this skill addresses. A risk associated with use of an indwelling device is mucosal pressure ulcer, in this case, inside the rectal wall.

Delegation and Collaboration

The skill of applying a topical (external) FCD cannot be delegated to nursing assistive personnel (NAP). The NAP can assist the nurse by helping with positioning of a patient during device application. The nurse instructs the NAP about:

- Reporting to the nurse any instances of leakage or change in appearance of skin around device noted during routine care.

Equipment

- FCD kit (save the adhesive remover from the kit at the bedside after initial application to aid in removing the device)
- Drainage bag
- Nonsterile gloves
- Protective bed pad
- Bath basin

Procedural Steps

1. **See Standard Protocol (inside front cover).**
2. Identify patient using two identifiers (e.g., name and birthday or name and account number) according to facility policy. *Rationale: Ensures correct patient. Complies with The Joint Commission standards and improves patient safety (TJC, 2014).*
3. *Apply the FCD.*
   a. Observe the anal region for swelling, hemorrhoids, redness, irritation, or drainage. Presence of these findings may contraindicate placement of the FCD or may indicate the need for other interventions to the perianal skin.
   b. Assess frequency and amount of diarrhea. Consider use of extra protective skin cream to perineal area or consult with health care provider about use of antidiarrheal medication.
   c. Assess patient for allergy to latex because many FCDs contain latex.
   d. Apply clean gloves. Fill bath basin with warm water. Position patient in side-lying position with upper leg bent at knee to expose anal area. Place protective bed pad under patient's dependent hip.
   e. Open FCD kit (contents vary by manufacturer). Use the liquid adhesive in thirds: Apply ⅓ of liquid adhesive in kit to the bag area around the small opening. Extend adhesive down all sides of the "cap" or top of the applicator.
   f. Gently separate the patient's buttocks (NAP can assist), exposing the perianal area for the entire procedure.

   g. Cleanse the perianal area with water and the bar soap from the kit and dry thoroughly. Other soaps may leave a film on the skin. Moisture (water, diaphoresis, excoriation, lotions) decreases or prevents adherence by the liquid adhesive.
   h. Spread half the powder onto gloves and apply to the skin around the anus to dry the area where the latex bag will be placed.
   i. Dust off any excess powder. Your gloved hands should slide easily over the area if enough powder has been applied.
   j. Apply the second ⅓ of the clear liquid adhesive. Use the applicator and apply only to the anal area, being certain to encircle the anus completely.
   k. Apply remaining half of the powder to the anal area over the layer of liquid adhesive.
   l. Apply the remaining ⅓ of the clear liquid adhesive to the skin around the anus. Wait 2 full minutes, allowing the solvent to evaporate, ensuring good adhesion.
   m. Grip the handle of the bag-covered applicator and press it firmly onto the external anal area so that the anus is centered with the hole in the bag.
   n. Hold in place, closing the buttocks tightly for 15 seconds to allow the adhesive to set.
   o. Reach into the bag and gently remove the FCD obturator.
   p. Check for patency by placing gloved fingers in the FCD (see illustration) to determine that the bag has been properly centered around the anus and that the anus remains unobstructed.

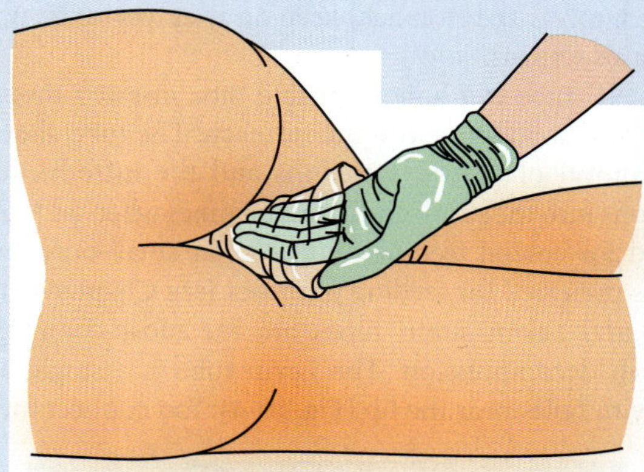

STEP 3p Checking for patency with gloved fingers.

   q. Apply the closure clip. Fold the open end of the FCD collection bag one time without wrinkling it. Clamp it in the closure clip, ensuring that only the metal bars of the clip are compressing the bag.
   r. If a drainage bag is desired (see illustration), place the white plastic "ring" around the "thumb" of the FCD. Cut a small hole in the end of the "thumb," insert the drainage bag tubing into the "thumb," and tighten the ring around the tubing.

Continued

PROCEDURAL GUIDELINE 19.2
Applying a Fecal Containment Device—cont'd

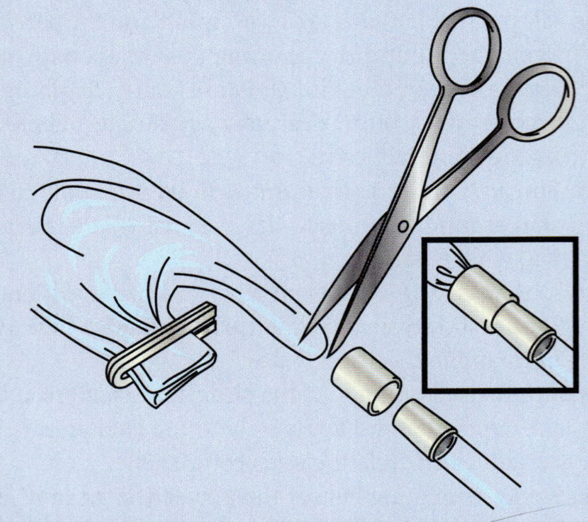

STEP 3r Cut a small hole in the end of the "thumb," insert the drainage bag tubing into the "thumb," and tighten the ring around the tubing.

    s. Leave the adhesive remover at the bedside to aid in later removal of the device.

4. ***Remove FCD collection bag:***
   a. Apply clean gloves. If the patient's bowel control and consistency and frequency of stool return to normal, discontinue the FCD.
   b. Wipe adhesive remover along the adhesive seal.
   c. Gently and slowly peel the FCD from the skin. Place the device in a biohazard container.
   d. Thoroughly cleanse the perianal area making sure to remove all adhesive.
5. **See Completion Protocol (inside front cover).**
6. Monitor patient for diarrhea, and record amounts on I&O record every shift.
7. Record application of device and appearance of skin.
8. Report amount of diarrhea to the health care provider if the volume is greater than 1000 mL/day.

SKILL 19.3 INSERTION, MAINTENANCE, AND REMOVAL OF A NASOGASTRIC TUBE FOR GASTRIC DECOMPRESSION

• **Nursing Skills Online: Enteral Nutrition Module, Lesson 2**

Normal peristalsis is sometimes temporarily altered, either following major surgery or from conditions affecting the GI tract. When peristalsis is slowed or absent, a patient cannot eat or drink fluids without causing abdominal distention. The temporary insertion of an NG tube into the stomach serves to decompress the stomach, keeping it empty until normal peristalsis returns.

An NG tube is a hollow, pliable tube inserted through a patient's nasopharynx into the stomach. The tube allows for the removal of gastric secretions and the introduction of solutions into the stomach. There are times when an NG tube is used for enteral feedings, but a softer small-bore feeding tube is preferred for feeding purposes (see Chapter 12). The Levin and Salem sump tubes are the most common for stomach decompression. The Levin tube is a single-lumen tube with holes near the tip (Fig. 19-4). You connect the tube to a drainage bag or an intermittent suction device to drain stomach secretions. The Salem sump tube is preferable for stomach decompression. The tube has two lumina: one for removal of gastric contents and one to provide an air vent, which prevents suctioning of gastric mucosa into eyelets at the distal tip of the tube. A blue "pigtail" is the air vent that connects with the second lumen (Fig. 19-5). When the main lumen of the sump tube is connected to suction, the air vent permits free, continuous drainage of secretions. ***Never clamp off the air vent, connect to suction, or use for irrigation.*** The health care provider orders the suction setting, which is usually low intermittent.

Insertion of an NG tube requires clean technique. During insertion, patients experience a burning sensation as the tube passes through the sensitive nasal mucosa. One of the greatest nursing care challenges is keeping a patient comfortable during the procedure and after tube placement. When a tube is in place, routinely assess the condition of the naris and

FIG 19-4 Levin tube. (Courtesy Bard Medical, Covington, Georgia.)

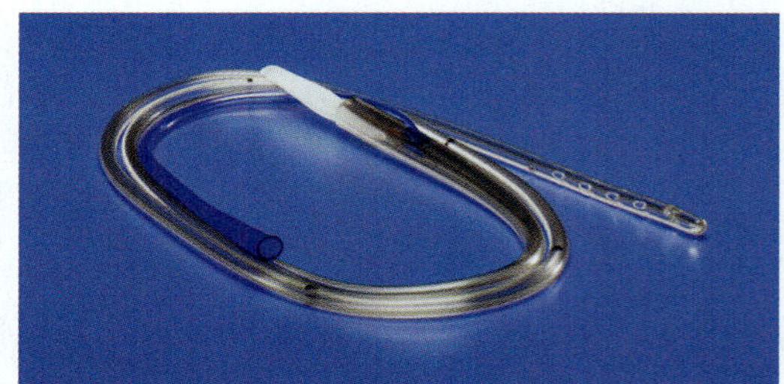

FIG 19-5 Salem sump tube. (Copyright © 2010 Covidien. All rights reserved. Used with permission of Covidien.)

mucosa for inflammation and excoriation. An NG tube often causes a medical device–related pressure ulcer. A pressure ulcer can develop for many reasons: rigidity of device rubbing against mucosa, difficulty in securing or adjusting the device to the body, increased moisture surrounding the tubing, tight securement of the device, and poor positioning or fixation of the device (Norman, 2013). Supportive care includes changing soiled tape or fixation devices, keeping the naris lubricated and clean, and providing frequent mouth care to minimize dehydration from mouth breathing.

ASSESSMENT

1. Identify patient using two identifiers (e.g., name and birthday or name and account number) according to facility policy. *Rationale: Ensures correct patient. Complies with The Joint Commission standards and improves patient safety (TJC, 2014).*
2. Inspect condition of patient's nasal and oral cavity. *Rationale: Determines need for special nursing hygiene measures after tube placement.*
3. Ask if patient has history of nasal surgery or congestion and allergies, and note if deviated nasal septum is present. *Rationale: Alerts nurse of potential obstruction or localized inflammation. Insert tube into uninvolved nasal passage. Procedure may be contraindicated if surgery is recent.*
4. Auscultate for bowel sounds. Palpate patient's abdomen for distention, pain, and rigidity. *Rationale: Provides baseline measure for any abdominal distention, GI ileus, or general GI function.*
5. Assess patient's level of consciousness and ability to follow instructions. *Rationale: Determines patient's ability to assist in procedure.*

> **SAFE PATIENT CARE**   If patient is confused, disoriented, or unable to follow commands, obtain assistance from another staff member to insert the tube.

6. Determine if patient had previous NG tube and which naris was used. *Rationale: Patient's previous experience complements any explanations and prepares patient for NG tube placement.*
7. Verify health care provider order for type of NG tube to be placed and whether tube is to be attached to suction or drainage bag. *Rationale: Requires an order from health care provider. Adequate decompression depends on NG suction.*

PLANNING

Expected Outcomes focus on decompression of the stomach, patient comfort, and prevention of complications related to NG intubation.

1. Abdomen is soft without distention.
2. Patient's level of comfort improves or remains the same.
3. NG tube remains patent.
4. Patient's nasal mucosa is moist and intact.

Delegation and Collaboration

The skill of inserting and maintaining an NG tube cannot be delegated to nursing assistive personnel (NAP). The nurse instructs the NAP about the following:

- When to measure and record the drainage from an NG tube.
- How often to provide oral hygiene.
- Selected comfort measures such as positioning or offering ice chips if allowed.
- How to anchor a tube correctly to the patient's gown during routine care to prevent accidental displacement and pulling on the naris.
- Reporting to the nurse any signs of redness or skin irritation at nares.

Equipment

- 14 Fr or 16 Fr NG tube (smaller lumen catheters are not used for decompression in adults because they must be able to remove thick secretions)
- Water-soluble lubricating jelly
- pH test strips 1.0 to 11.0 (measure gastric aspirate acidity)
- Tongue blade
- Flashlight
- Emesis basin
- Asepto bulb or catheter-tipped syringe
- Commercial fixation device or hypoallergenic tape 1 inch (2.5 cm) wide (option: Bridle nasal tube system)
- Rubber band and plastic clip to attach tube to gown
- Clamp, drainage bag, or suction machine or pressure gauge if wall suction is to be used
- Towel
- Glass of water with straw
- Facial tissues
- Normal saline
- Tincture of benzoin (optional)
- Suction equipment
- Clean gloves

IMPLEMENTATION *for* INSERTION, MAINTENANCE, AND REMOVAL OF A NASOGASTRIC TUBE FOR GASTRIC DECOMPRESSION

STEPS	RATIONALE
1. **See Standard Protocol (inside front cover).**	
2. Place patient in high-Fowler's position. Place pillows behind head and shoulders. Raise bed to horizontal level comfortable for accessing patient.	Promotes patient's ability to swallow during procedure.

Continued

STEPS	RATIONALE

3. Place bath towel over patient's chest; give facial tissues to patient. Place emesis basin within reach. Inform patient that procedure may cause gagging and there will be a burning sensation in nasopharynx as tube is passed.

Prevents soiling patient's gown. Tube insertion through nasal passages may cause tearing and coughing with increased salivation. Increases patient's ability to cooperate and anticipate your actions.

4. Wash bridge of nose with soap and water or alcohol swab.

Removes oils from nose to allow fixation device to adhere.

5. Stand on patient's right side if right-handed or left side if left-handed. Lower side rail.

Allows easiest manipulation of tubing.

6. Instruct patient to relax and breathe normally while occluding one naris. Then have him or her repeat action for other naris. Select nostril with greater airflow.

Tube passes more easily through naris that is more patent.

7. Measure distance to insert tube:
   a. *Traditional method:* Measure distance from tip of nose to earlobe to xiphoid process (see illustration).

Tube extends from naris to stomach; distance varies with each patient.

   b. *Hanson method:* First mark 50-cm (20-inch) point on tube, and then measure traditionally. Tube insertion is a midway point between 50 cm (20 inches) and traditional mark.

8. With a small piece of tape placed around tube or using an indelible marker, mark end of length that you will insert.

Indicates amount of tube to be inserted.

9. Perform hand hygiene and apply clean gloves. Curve 10 to 15 cm (4 to 6 inches) of end of tube tightly around index finger and release.

Aids insertion and decreases stiffness of tube.

10. Lubricate 7.5 to 10 cm (3 to 4 inches) of end of tube with water-soluble lubricating gel.

Minimizes friction against nasal mucosa and aids insertion of tube. Water-soluble lubricant is less toxic than oil-soluble lubricant if aspirated.

11. Alert patient when procedure will begin.

Decreases patient anxiety and increases patient cooperation.

12. Initially instruct patient to extend neck back against pillow; insert tube slowly through naris with curved end pointing downward (see illustration).

Facilitates initial passage of tube through naris and maintains clear airway for open naris.

13. Continue to pass tube along floor of nasal passage, aiming down toward ear. When you feel resistance, apply gentle downward pressure to advance tube (do not force past resistance).

Minimizes discomfort of tube rubbing against upper nasal turbinates. Resistance caused by posterior nasopharynx. Downward pressure helps tube curl around corner of nasopharynx.

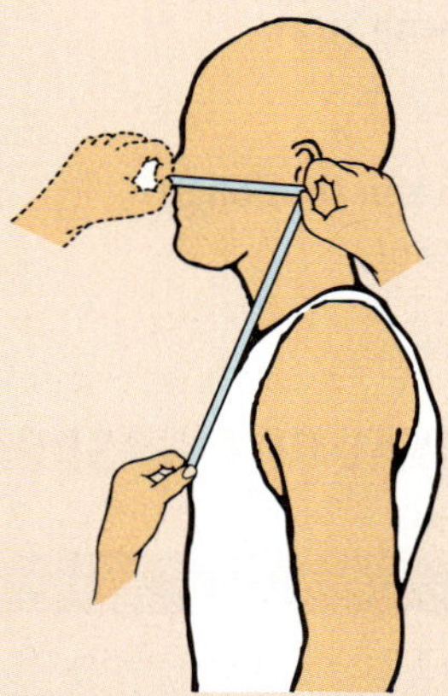

STEP 7a Technique for measuring distance to insert NG tube.

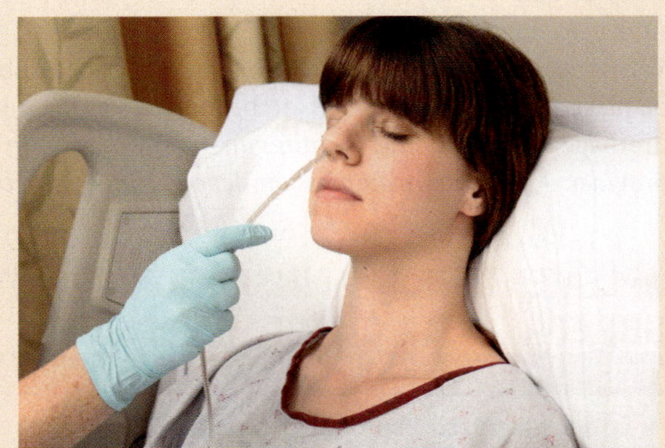

STEP 12 Insert NG tube with curved end pointing downward.

STEPS	RATIONALE

14. If you meet continued resistance, try to rotate tube and see if it advances. If still resistant, withdraw tube, allow patient to rest, lubricate tube again, and insert into other naris.

Forcing against resistance causes trauma to mucosa. Allowing patient to rest helps relieve anxiety.

> **SAFE PATIENT CARE** If unable to insert tube in either naris, stop procedure and notify health care provider.

15. Continue insertion of tube until just past nasopharynx by gently rotating tube toward opposite naris.

   a. Once past nasopharynx, stop tube advancement, allow patient to relax, and provide tissues.

Relieves patient's anxiety; tearing is natural response to mucosal irritation, and excessive salivation may occur because of oral stimulation.

   b. Explain to patient that next step requires that patient swallow. Give patient glass of water unless contraindicated.

Sipping water aids passage of NG tube into esophagus.

16. With tube just above oropharynx, instruct patient to flex head forward, take a small sip of water, and swallow. Advance tube 2.5 to 5 cm (1 to 2 inches) with each swallow of water. If patient is not allowed fluids, instruct to dry swallow or suck air through straw. Advance tube with each swallow.

Flexed position closes off upper airway to trachea and opens esophagus. Swallowing closes epiglottis over trachea and helps move tube into esophagus. Swallowing water reduces gagging or choking. Remove water from stomach by suction after insertion.

17. If patient begins to cough, gag, or choke, withdraw slightly and stop tube advancement. Instruct patient to breathe easily and take sips of water.

Cough reflex is initiated when tube accidentally enters larynx. Withdrawal of the tube reduces risk of laryngeal entry. Small sips of water frequently reduce gagging. Give water cautiously to reduce the risk of aspiration.

> **SAFE PATIENT CARE** If vomiting occurs, assist patient in clearing airway. Perform oral suctioning as needed until airway is clear.

18. If patient continues to cough during insertion, pull tube back slightly.

Tube may enter larynx and obstruct airway.

19. If patient continues to gag and cough or complains that tube feels as though it is coiling behind throat, check back of oropharynx using flashlight and tongue blade. Withdraw tube until tip is back in oropharynx if coiled. Then reinsert with patient swallowing.

Tube may coil around itself in the back of the throat and stimulate gag reflex.

20. After patient relaxes, continue to advance tube with swallowing until you reach tape or mark on tube, which signifies that tube is in the desired distance. Temporarily anchor tube to patient's cheek with piece of tape until tube placement is verified.

Tip of tube needs to be within stomach to decompress properly. Anchoring the tube prevents accidental displacement while tube placement is verified.

21. Verify tube placement: Check facility policy for recommended methods of checking tube placement.

   a. Order bedside x-ray film examination of chest and abdomen.

Radiography is the gold standard for verification of initial placement of the tube (Tho et al., 2011).

   b. While waiting for x-ray, perform the following procedures: Attach Asepto or catheter-tipped syringe to end of tube. Aspirate gently back on syringe to obtain gastric contents, observing color (see illustration).

Observation of gastric contents is useful to determine initial tube placement (Hockenberry and Wilson, 2013). Gastric contents are usually green but are sometimes off-white, tan, bloody, or brown in color. Other common aspirate appearances include yellow or bile-stained (duodenal placement) or possibly saliva-appearing (esophagus) (Hockenberry and Wilson, 2013; Wathen and Peyton, 2014).

Continued

<table>
<tr><td>STEPS</td><td>RATIONALE</td></tr>
</table>

c. A quick check to rule out if tube is in back of throat is to inspect posterior pharynx using tongue blade and pen light.

Tube is pliable and may coil up behind pharynx instead of passing into esophagus.

d. Use gastric (Gastroccult) pH test paper to measure aspirate for pH with color-coded pH paper. Be sure that paper range of pH is at least from 1 to 11 (see illustration).

Evidence supports pH test to be used as indicator for placement (Wathen and Peyton, 2014; Tho et al., 2011) A pH reading of 5.0 or less is a reliable indicator of stomach placement, especially when gastric acid inhibitor is not being used (Wathen and Peyton, 2014). Respiratory secretions are usually 6.0 or greater

e. If tube is not in stomach, advance another 2.5 to 5 cm (1 to 2 inches) and repeat Steps 21a to 21d to check initial tube position; verify with radiography.

Tube must be in stomach to provide decompression.

22. Anchor tube and mark it.

Proper anchoring and marking of tube helps prevent migration of tube and medical device, pressure ulcers, and allows for identification of change in placement of tube.

a. Clamp end of tube or connect tube to drainage bag or suction machine after properly inserted.

Use gravity for drainage bag. Intermittent suction is most effective for decompression. Patient going to operating room often has tube clamped.

b. Secure tube to nose; avoid putting pressure on naris.

Proper placement helps to reduce tissue necrosis.

(1) Apply tube fixation device:

Positions tubing to lessen rubbing against soft palate and naris.

(a) Apply wide end of patch to bridge of nose.
(b) Slip connector around NG tube as it exits nose (see illustration).

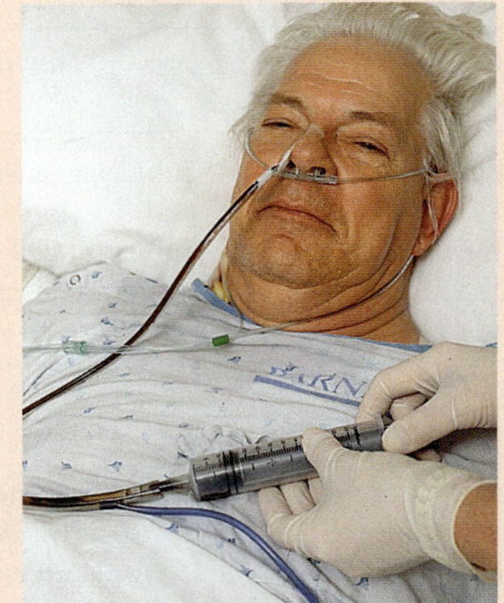

STEP 21b Aspiration of gastric contents.

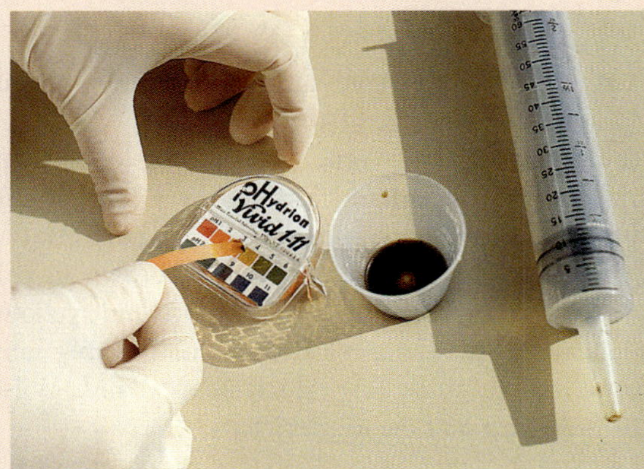

STEP 21d Checking pH of gastric contents.

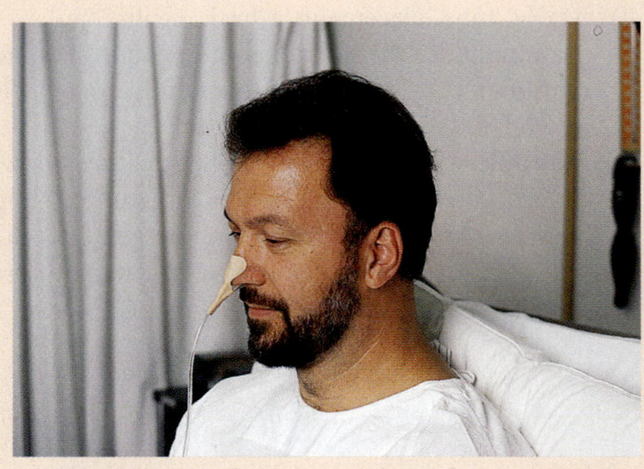

STEP 22b(1)(b) Patient with tube fixation device.

STEPS	RATIONALE

(2) Tape application:
  (a) Cut strip of tape about 10 cm (5 inches) and split down the middle halfway.

Tape anchors tube securely.

  (b) Apply small amount of tincture of benzoin to lower end of nose and allow it to dry (optional). Apply end of prepared tape to nose, leaving split end free. Be sure that top end of tape over nose is secure.
  (c) Carefully wrap two split ends of tape around the tube in opposite directions (see illustrations). Avoid taping tube flush against surface of nasal mucosa if possible.

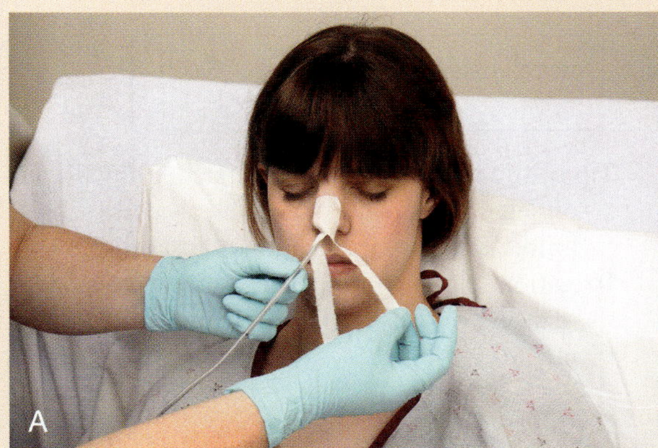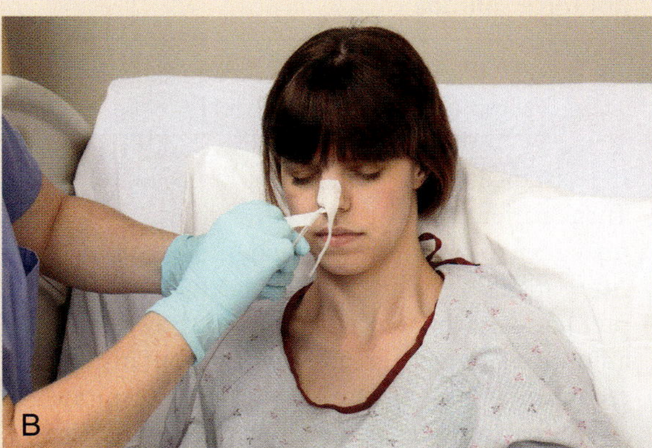

STEP 22b(2)(c) A and **B,** Tape is crossed over and around NG tube.

c. Fasten end of NG tube to patient's gown by looping rubber band around tube in slipknot. Provide some slack so there is no pulling on tube. Clip to gown.

Reduces pressure on naris if tube moves. Provides slack for movement without dislodging NG tube.

d. Keep the pigtail of a Salem sump tube above level of the stomach.

Prevents siphoning action that clogs the tube.

e. Unless health care provider orders otherwise, elevate head of bed 30 degrees.

Helps prevent esophageal reflux and minimizes irritation of tube against posterior pharynx.

23. Explain to patient that sensation of tube decreases with time.

Helps patient to adapt to continued sensory stimulus.

24. Once placement is confirmed:
  a. Place a mark, using either red ink or tape, on tube to indicate where tube exits nose. Alternative: Measure length of tube from naris to connector.

The mark on tube is a guide to indicate if tube remains in correct position.

  b. Document length of tube in patient's record.

Information assists in determining tube placement.

> **SAFE PATIENT CARE** Never reposition an NG tube of a patient who has had gastric surgery because positioning can rupture the suture line.

25. Attach NG tube to suction as ordered.

Suction setting is usually ordered low intermittent, which decreases gastric irritation from NG tube.

> **SAFE PATIENT CARE** If lumen of tube is narrow and secretions are thick, NG tube will not drain as desired. Irrigate tube (see Step 26). Consult with health care provider for higher suction setting if unable to irrigate tube because of thick secretions.

26. *NG tube irrigation:*
  a. Perform hand hygiene and apply clean gloves.

Reduces transmission of microorganisms.

Continued

STEPS	RATIONALE

b. Check for tube placement in stomach by aspirating contents (see Step 21b). Temporarily clamp tube or reconnect to connecting tube and remove syringe.

Prevents accidental entrance of gastric residual into lungs.

c. Empty syringe of aspirant and use it to draw up 30 mL of normal saline.

Use of saline minimizes loss of electrolytes from stomach fluids.

d. Clamp NG tube. Disconnect from connection tubing and lay end of connection tubing on clean towel.

Reduces soiling of patient's gown and bed linen.

e. Insert tip of irrigating syringe into end of NG tube. Remove clamp. Hold syringe with tip pointed at floor and inject saline slowly and evenly. Do not force solution.

Position of syringe prevents introduction of air into vent tubing, which causes gastric distention. Solution introduced under pressure causes gastric trauma.

> **SAFE PATIENT CARE** Do not introduce saline through blue "pigtail" air vent of Salem sump tube.

f. If resistance occurs, check for kinks in tubing. Turn patient onto left side. Report repeated resistance to health care provider.

Tip of tube may lie against stomach lining. Repositioning on left side may dislodge tube away from the stomach lining. Buildup of secretions causes distention.

g. After instilling saline, immediately aspirate or pull back slowly on syringe to withdraw fluid. If amount aspirated is greater than amount instilled, record difference as output. If amount aspirated is less than amount instilled, record difference as intake.

Irrigation clears tubing; the stomach remains empty. Measure and document irrigation inserted in tube as intake.

h. Use an Asepto syringe to place 10 mL of air into blue pigtail of Salem sump tube.

Ensures patency of air vent.

i. Reconnect NG tube to drainage or suction. (Repeat irrigation if solution does not return.)

Reestablishes drainage collection; may repeat irrigation or repositioning of tube until NG tube drains properly.

27. *Removal of NG tube:*

a. Verify order to remove NG tube.

A health care provider's order is required for procedure.

b. Explain procedure to patient, and reassure that removal is less distressing than insertion.

Minimizes anxiety and increases cooperation. Tube passes out smoothly.

c. Perform hand hygiene and apply clean gloves.

Reduces transmission of microorganisms.

d. Stand on patient's right side if right-handed or left side if left-handed.

Allows easiest manipulation of tube.

e. Turn off suction and disconnect NG tube from drainage bag or suction. Take irrigating syringe and insert 20 mL of air into lumen of NG tube. Remove fixation device or tape from bridge of nose and unclip tube from gown.

Have tube free of connections before removal. Clears gastric fluids from tube to prevent aspirating contents or soiling clothing and bedding.

f. Hand patient facial tissue; place clean towel across chest. Instruct patient to take and hold breath.

Some patients wish to blow nose after tube is removed. Towel keeps gown from soiling. Temporary airway obstruction occurs during tube removal.

g. Clamp or kink tubing securely and pull tube out steadily and smoothly into towel held in other hand while patient holds breath.

Clamping prevents tube contents from draining into oropharynx. Reduces trauma to mucosa and minimizes patient's discomfort. Towel covers tube, which is an unpleasant sight. Holding breath helps to prevent aspiration.

h. Inspect intactness of tube.

i. Measure amount of drainage, and note character of content. Dispose of tube and drainage equipment into proper container.

Provides accurate measure of fluid output. Reduces transfer of microorganisms.

STEPS	RATIONALE
j. Clean naris and provide mouth care.	Promotes comfort.
k. Position patient comfortably and explain procedure for drinking fluids if not contraindicated. Instruct patient to notify you if nausea occurs.	Sometimes patients are not allowed anything by mouth (NPO) for 24 hours. When fluids are allowed, orders usually begin with small amount of ice chips each hour, and amounts are increased as patient is able to tolerate more.
28. **See Completion Protocol (inside front cover).**	

EVALUATION

1. Observe amount and character of contents draining from NG tube. Ask if patient feels nauseated.
2. Auscultate for presence of bowel sounds, being sure to turn off suction while doing so. Palpate patient's abdomen periodically. Note any distention, pain, and rigidity.
3. Inspect condition of naris and nose.
4. Observe position of tubing.
5. Ask if patient feels sore throat or irritation in pharynx.
6. Use **Teach Back:** State to the patient, "I want to be sure I explained why you need the NG tube and the importance of letting me know if you are nauseated." Evaluates what the patient is able to explain or demonstrate. Revise your instruction now or develop plan for revised patient teaching to be implemented at an appropriate time if patient is not able to teach back correctly.

Unexpected Outcomes and Related Interventions

1. Patient's abdomen is distended and painful.
   a. Assess patency of NG tube. NG tube may not be in stomach, or it may be kinked and not draining.
   b. Irrigate NG tube. If drainage does not increase or distention unrelieved in 15 to 20 minutes, notify health care provider.
   c. Verify that suction is on as ordered.
2. Patient complains of sore throat from dry, irritated mucous membranes.
   a. Perform oral hygiene more frequently.
   b. Ask health care provider whether patient can suck on ice chips or throat lozenges or if a local anesthetic medication can be used.
3. Patient develops irritation or pressure ulcer of skin around naris.
   a. Provide frequent skin care to area.
   b. Change type of securement device to avoid pressure.
   c. Consider switching tube to other naris.
4. Patient develops signs and symptoms of pulmonary aspiration: fever, shortness of breath, or pulmonary congestion.
   a. Perform complete respiratory assessment.
   b. Notify health care provider.
   c. Obtain chest x-ray film examination as ordered.

5. Tube slips or is pulled out.
   a. Reinsert new tube if decompression is still necessary.
   b. Option: The AMT Bridle device is for patients who attempt to pull at the tube or when taping is difficult because of sores or burns on the nose. A health care provider's order is needed (Parks et al., 2013). The bridle is easily placed by passing magnets within the nasopharynx, which allows umbilical tape to be looped around the vomer bone of the nose and then anchored to the NG tube with a clip.

Recording and Reporting

- Record length, size, type of gastric tube inserted, and naris in which tube was introduced. Also record patient's tolerance of procedure, confirmation of tube placement, character and pH of gastric contents, results of x-ray film, whether the tube is clamped or connected to drainage bag or to suction, and amount of suction supplied.
- Document your evaluation of patient learning.
- Record difference between amount of normal saline instilled and amount of gastric aspirate removed on I&O sheet. Record amount and character of contents draining from NG tube every shift in nurses' notes or flow sheet.
- Record removal of tube "intact," patient's tolerance to procedure, and final amount and character of drainage.
- Report occurrence of abdominal distention, unexpected increase or sudden stoppage in gastric drainage, and patient complaining of gastric distress to health care provider.

Sample Documentation

1000   Inserted 16 Fr NG tube into left naris, advanced to 55-cm (22 inches) mark. Patient assisted with insertion by swallowing and states he is comfortable. 50 mL of light green secretions aspirated, pH 4.0. Tube secured with securement device and attached to low intermittent suction. Tube placement verified by x-ray. Bowel sounds absent. Abdomen is slightly round and nontender.

Special Considerations
Pediatric

- Consider the use of sedation before tube insertion in a child (Hockenberry and Wilson, 2013).

- Consider the child's developmental stage, and prepare child and family before initiating the procedure. Never surprise the child with this procedure (Hockenberry and Wilson, 2013).

Geriatric

- Check for ill-fitting dentures and remove them for patient's safety and comfort during the insertion.

- Oral and nasal mucosal drying is sometimes present. Adequately lubricate the tube for insertion.
- If patient wears a hearing aid, be sure that the aid is in place during preprocedure explanation and insertion of the tube so that patient is able to hear any instructions.

CRITICAL THINKING EXERCISES

Case Study

A 37-year-old man is admitted to the hospital with severe vomiting and abdominal pain. He has a preliminary diagnosis of pancreatitis. The health care provider ordered a series of laboratory tests and abdominal scans. However, before the scan the health care provider wants an NG tube inserted for gastric decompression and placed on low intermittent suction.

1. During the nursing history, the patient tells you that he broke his nose playing college football 9 years ago. Based on this information, what is the next step?
   1. Add extra lubricant to the tube during insertion.
   2. Assess patency of each naris.
   3. Call the health care provider for an order for local anesthetic.
   4. Tell the patient that the prior injury will prevent the tube insertion.
2. Once the tube is inserted and an x-ray has been ordered to verify placement, which of the following aspirates indicates that the tube is properly placed in the stomach?
   1. Clear aspirate with pH 6.7
   2. Yellow-brown aspirate with pH 5.8
   3. Green aspirate with pH 3.2
   4. Mucus-colored aspirate with pH 6.5
3. You are performing measures to ensure NG tube function. The patient asks the reason for injecting air into the blue-colored tube on the Salem sump tube. Your best answer is:
   1. "It will allow me to check the tube's position in your stomach."
   2. "I need to inject air to clear the tube before I remove any fluid."
   3. "By injecting air, this air vent stays clean."
   4. "The air creates a vacuum to make sure the suction is working."

Review Questions

1. While receiving a soapsuds enema, a patient complains of abdominal cramping. Which of the following techniques helps relieve this sensation? Select all that apply.
   1. Ask the patient to hold his or her breath.
   2. Ask the patient to breathe slowly.
   3. Lower the fluid container.
   4. Raise the fluid container.

2. When a patient is suspected to have hardened feces from prolonged constipation, which of the following enemas would the nurse anticipate administering?
   1. Kayexalate
   2. Oil retention
   3. Soapsuds
   4. Tap water
3. A patient comes to the clinic complaining of abdominal discomfort. Which of the following would contribute to functional constipation? Select all that apply.
   1. Regular physical activity
   2. Reduced fluid intake
   3. Maintaining a daily routine
   4. Eating a low-fiber diet
   5. Ignoring the urge to have a bowel movement
4. The nurse sees an order for digital removal of stool in an 83-year-old patient with fecal impaction. The nurse knows there is a risk associated with digital removal of impacted stool secondary to stimulation of the vagus nerve. When this nerve is stimulated, what can occur?
   1. Reflex bradycardia
   2. Reflex tachycardia
   3. Reflex urination
   4. Reflex vomiting
5. When measuring length of insertion for an NG tube, which is the correct measurement technique?
   1. Corner of mouth to earlobe to xiphoid process
   2. Tip of nose to earlobe to xiphoid process
   3. 40 cm (16 inches) from tip of tube
   4. Tip of nose to umbilicus
6. A patient has had an NG tube for 2 days and is complaining about abdominal pain and severe nausea. The NG output has decreased over the past 3 hours, and the nurse is concerned that the tube is not draining properly. What is the nurse's next action?
   1. Irrigate the tube with saline and withdraw the instilled fluid.
   2. Notify the health care provider.
   3. Turn the patient to his left side to promote drainage.
   4. Withdraw the tube 5 to 7.5 cm (2 to 3 inches).

7. A nurse is placing a Salem sump NG tube to low intermittent suction for a 49-year-old female patient who just had three episodes of emesis consisting of bile and partially digested food. The patient reports her last bowel movement was 4 to 5 days ago. Her abdomen is slightly distended, and no active bowel sounds are auscultated. Place the steps of the procedure to place a Salem sump NG tube in proper order.
    1. Place patient in high-Fowler's position
    2. Verify tube placement (check hospital policy)
    3. Measure distance to insert tube (tip of nose to earlobe to xiphoid process)
    4. Assess patient's nares and history of nasal and facial injury
    5. Check for health care provider's order for the procedure
    6. Properly identify the patient

8. On day 2 of hospitalization of the 49-year-old female patient described in the previous question, the Salem sump NG tube is set to low intermittent suction; the patient is assessed to have a distended, firm abdomen and complains of pain in the abdomen. Select appropriate interventions that apply to this situation. Select all that apply.
    1. Pull the tube out 3 cm (1.2 inches) and retape
    2. Increase suction to high intermittent suction
    3. Irrigate the tube with 30 mL normal saline
    4. Ask patient if she is having flatulence
    5. Verify suction is on as ordered

9. A student nurse has been asked by her instructor to describe evidence-based strategies for reducing the risk of a patient developing a mucosal pressure ulcer from an NG tube. Which of the following are appropriate evidence-based strategies? Select all that apply.
    1. Select a 14 Fr or 16 Fr NG tube for insertion
    2. Remove the tape around the tube to assess the skin daily
    3. Avoid placement of NG tube over any scar tissue or abrasion in a naris
    4. Secure NG tube firmly against mucosal surface of naris

10. A patient with Parkinson's disease is admitted; his primary diagnosis is abdominal pain, nausea, and diarrhea. The patient has taken in less than 1000 mL of fluid daily for the last week. The patient reports his last regular bowel movement was 5 days ago. Which of the following is the patient most likely experiencing?
    1. Constipation
    2. Diarrhea
    3. Fecal impaction
    4. Indigestion

REFERENCES

Cooper KL: Evidence-based prevention of pressure ulcers in the intensive care unit, *Crit Care Nurse* 33(6):57, 2013.

Giger J: *Transcultural nursing: assessment and intervention*, ed 6, St Louis, 2013, Mosby.

Hockenberry MJ, Wilson D: *Wong's essentials of pediatric nursing*, ed 9, St Louis, 2013, Mosby.

Hodin R, et al: Nasogastric and nasoenteric tubes, *UpToDate* 2014. http://pmtwww.uptodate.com/contents/nasogastric-and-nasoenteric-tubes.

Mayo Clinic: *Dietary fiber: essential for a healthy diet*, 2012, www.mayoclinic.com/health/fiber/NU00033. Accessed December 25, 2013.

McKay S, Fravel M, Scanlon C: Management of constipation, *J Gerontol Nurs* 38(7):9, 2012.

National Pressure Ulcer Advisory Panel (NPUAP): *Mucosal pressure ulcers: an NPUAP Position Statement*, 2012, http://www.npuap.org/wp-content/uploads/2012/03/Mucosal_Pressure_Ulcer_Position_Statement_final.pdf. Accessed January 25, 2014.

Ness W, Hibberts F: *Management of lower bowel dysfunction, including DRE and DRF: RCN guidance for nurses*, London, 2012, Royal College of Nursing. Available at: https://www.rcn.org.uk/__data/assets/pdf_file/0007/157363/003226.pdf.

Norman J: *MDR pressure ulcers: who thought plastic tubing could be harmful?* 2013, www.Medline.com. Accessed December 28, 2013.

Parks J, et al: Outcomes of nasal bridling to secure enteral tubes in burn patients, *Am J Crit Care* 22(2):136, 2013.

Seidel HM, et al: *Mosby's guide to physical examination*, ed 8, St Louis, 2015, Mosby.

The Joint Commission (TJC): *National Patient Safety Goals*, Oakbrook Terrace, IL, 2014, The Commission. Available at: http://www.jointcommission.org/standards_information/npsgs.aspx.

Tho PC, et al: Implementation of the evidence review on best practice for confirming the correct placement of nasogastric tube in patients in an acute care hospital, *Int J Evid Based Healthc* 9(1):51, 2011.

Wathen B, Peyton C: Pediatric nasogastric tube placement, *Nurs Crit Care* 9(3):14, 2014.

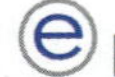

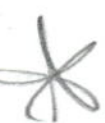

Conditions such as cancer, inflammatory bowel disease, infections such as diverticulitis that lead to perforation of the colon, neurological disease, and trauma alter normal elimination either temporarily or permanently. As a result, surgery becomes necessary to create an opening into the abdominal wall for fecal or urinary elimination. Feces and urine can flow through a segment of the colon or small intestine and out through the opening (called a *stoma*) on the abdomen. The output from the stoma is called the *effluent.*

The opening and stoma created from the ileal portion of the small intestine is called an *ileostomy* (Fig. 20-1); the fecal effluent is watery-to-thick liquid and contains some digestive enzymes. The opening and stoma from the large intestine or colon is called a *colostomy;* the fecal effluent varies in consistency, depending on where the opening in the colon is created. If the opening is in the ascending or transverse colon, the effluent varies from thick liquid to semiformed stool. A colostomy in the descending or sigmoid colon (Fig. 20-2) generally results in a stool similar to that normally passed through the rectum. Fecal ostomies can be temporary or permanent, depending on the underlying condition and the surgical procedure performed.

A urostomy or ileal conduit (Fig. 20-3) is surgically created from a portion of the intestine that is resected from the ileum. One end of the conduit is sutured closed, and the ureters are implanted through the mucosa. The other end is brought out on the abdominal wall, and a stoma is formed for urine to exit the body. This ostomy is permanent. A patient with a colostomy, ileostomy, or ileal conduit has no sensation or control over the time or frequency of the output and wears a pouch to collect the effluent.

Some people with a descending colostomy may be able to regulate their bowel movement with a process called *irrigation* so that most of their bowel movement comes at the same time every day. Irrigation is an enema given through the stoma with an enema bag and a silicone cone specifically designed for persons with colostomies. Warm water instilled into the colon stimulates the bowels to move. The procedure takes about an hour, and because there are so many more reliable ostomy pouches available now, very few people are motivated to learn this procedure today. People who do irrigate may be able to wear a small pouch or a stoma cap over the stoma that would contain gas or small amounts of stool.

PATIENT-CENTERED CARE

Surgery that results in an ostomy can be life-changing. Patient-centered care requires you to consider how an ostomy will affect a patient's lifestyle, self-image, and personal relationships. Listen to patients and learn their values and beliefs that will shape how they will be able to adapt to living with an ostomy. For patients with ostomies, respect what they have learned in self-care. If the patient has an established routine of care that makes him or her feel comfortable, this should be respected, and you should assist the patient as needed.

If possible, a physician or certified ostomy care nurse will meet with a patient before ostomy surgery to mark a stoma site, talk to the patient about the surgery, and answer any

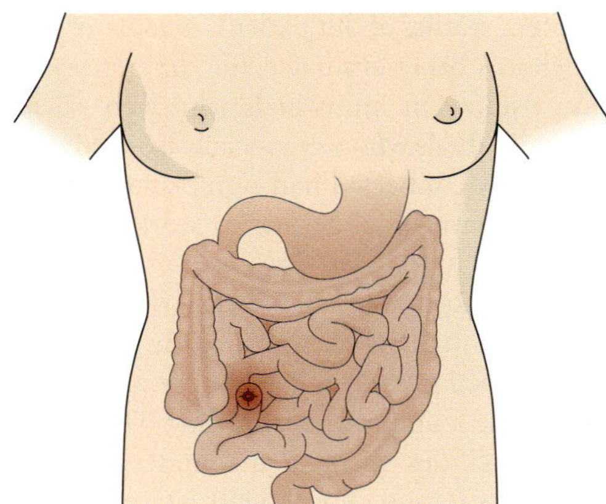

FIG 20-1 Ileostomy.

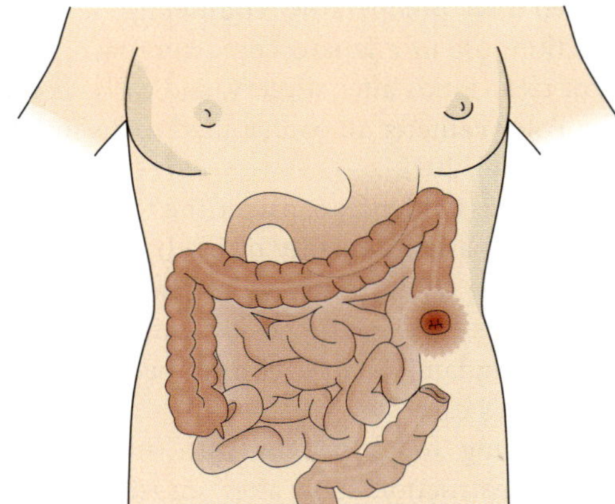

FIG 20-2 Sigmoid colostomy.

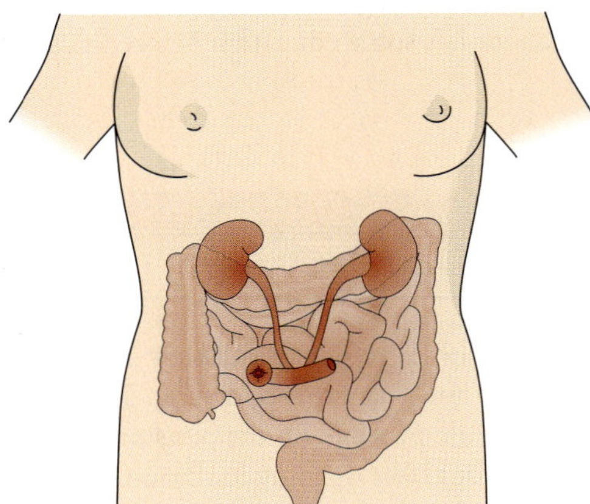

FIG 20-3 Urostomy (ileal conduit).

concerns or questions. Evaluating a patient's abdomen while lying, sitting, and standing allows the health care staff and the patient to find an optimal location and avoid having a stoma that is difficult to pouch (Goldberg et al., 2010). Poor stoma placement causes undue hardship and has a negative impact on a patient's psychological and emotional health (Zimnicki, 2013).

Stoma care has improved because pouching systems are now more effective and adhesive technology is more advanced. With any pouching system, a secure seal to prevent leakage of the effluent and protect the skin around the stoma

(peristomal skin) is vital to helping patients resume normal activities and accept the changes in their bodies as a result of the surgery. In addition to the stress of illness and surgical recovery, patients with ostomies face body image changes, fear of social rejection, and concern about sexual function and intimacy. Often these patients need help with personal care. Do not act offended by the odor or appearance of the effluent in the pouch. A negative reaction from caregivers reinforces the patient's feelings that this alteration in bodily function makes him or her personally and socially unacceptable; however, a supportive nurse can make the initial period of adjustment easier (Erwin-Toth et al., 2012). It is very important to provide an effective pouching system to facilitate the emotional adjustment to the ostomy (Danielsen et al., 2013). Encourage the patient who has cared for an ostomy independently to resume self-care as soon as possible. Respect the patient's routine of care even if it differs from usual care in the health care facility.

A patient's ethnic background can pose unique challenges for ostomy care. New ostomies require monitoring and observation, and this is invasive and embarrassing for some patients. Most cultures consider bowel and urinary secretions unfit for public display. For example, some cultures avoid exposure of the lower torso, which is needed for ostomy care (Black, 2011). Learn whether your patient holds these types of views. If so, it is helpful to assign gender-congruent caregivers if possible and allow the presence of a family member if requested by the patient.

As you communicate with the patient during any care procedure, be sensitive and avoid communicating anything that the patient may interpret as disrespect or disgust. As always, prepare adequately for the procedure; seek necessary assistance; and maintain a calm, professional demeanor.

SAFETY

Safety is a concern when determining proper stoma placement. Proper stoma placement reduces the risk of poor stomal healing, skin irritation, and impaired skin integrity related to drainage. Proper placement also enhances a patient's management of a stoma. When a stoma is properly placed, the patient can visualize the stoma, cleanse the stoma and peristomal site, and easily remove and reapply the new appliance (Zimnicki, 2013).

Skin and stomal care are basic to the safety of a patient with an ostomy. Immediately after surgery, assess a new stoma to determine that the opening on the pouch fits around the stoma but does not allow exposure of the peristomal skin to the fecal or urinary output from the stoma. Effluent is very irritating to the skin. Postoperative edema in the stoma and abdominal distention may require pouch changes to cut the opening in the pouch to fit more appropriately.

It is important to observe the same hygiene measures that you would use for any patient using the bathroom. A patient should be allowed to wash his or her hands before and after participating in ostomy care. Although a new stoma is created surgically, care of the stoma and surrounding skin is not a sterile procedure. Make sure to position patients comfortably to allow them to observe their care and learn from your instruction.

There have been innovations in ostomy care for improving patient safety and comfort. The current trend is to apply a pouch to clean, dry skin without other skin preparations, paste, or adhesives, unless a patient has a specific problem keeping a pouch intact. The adhesives on the skin barriers are pressure-sensitive and heat-sensitive; have the patient apply gentle pressure with the hand over the skin barrier for several minutes to facilitate the adherence of the barrier to the skin. Barriers are available that can be molded with the fingers to make the opening the right size rather than having to cut them to fit. There are new and improved accessory products such as rings or seals for managing abdominal contours that are uneven or peristomal skin that is not intact. Some pouches have effective gas filters that absorb odors and allow for flatus to escape slowly from the pouch through a charcoal filter. The pouch does not allow leakage of liquid effluent through the filter. All ostomy companies now have pouches with integrated closures. An integrated closure is made from a Velcro-like product and eliminates the need for a clip to close the bottom of the pouch. These integrated closures require less manual dexterity to empty the pouch.

EVIDENCE-BASED PRACTICE

Aarts MA et al: Adoption of enhanced recovery after surgery (ERAS) strategies for colorectal surgery at academic teaching hospitals and impact on total length of hospital stay, *Surg Endosc* 26(2):442, 2012.

Nichols T: Social connectivity in those 24 months or less postsurgery, *J Wound Ostomy Continence Nurs* 38(1):63, 2011.

There are recent studies about patients' quality of life with an ostomy. Nichols (2011) evaluated the differences in adjustment to an ostomy in individuals who were socially connected and individuals who were socially isolated. Individuals who were socially connected had significantly better adjustment to the ostomy, faster return to work, and higher life satisfaction scores.

The Enhanced Recovery After Surgery (ERAS) pathway is being explored in many countries as a way to facilitate faster recovery after elective abdominal surgery and decrease cost by shortening the length of hospital stay. The pathway is in use in many facilities for patients undergoing colorectal surgery and more recently for patients having radical cystectomy. Although concrete data about the effectiveness of all aspects of the pathway are not yet available, a more recent study showed that preoperative counseling, intraoperative fluid restriction, use of a laparoscopic approach, immediate initiation of clear fluids after surgery, and early discontinuation of the Foley catheter all contributed to a shorter length of stay (Aarts et al, 2012).

In applying this evidence, consider the following:

- Promote a patient's quality of life by encouraging the patient to be open to help from family members and close friends early in the postoperative period and by encouraging family and friends to become involved in the patient's care.
- When caring for a patient with an ostomy, begin self-care instruction soon after surgery and be aware that the patient may be leaving the hospital in 2 to 5 days.
- When possible, begin teaching preoperatively so that the patient has some education before the surgery.

• Nursing Skills Online: Bowel Elimination/Ostomy Module, Lessons 1, 3, 4

Immediately after a fecal surgical diversion, it is necessary to place a pouch over the newly created stoma to contain effluent when the stoma begins to function. The pouch keeps the patient clean and dry, protects the skin from drainage, and provides a barrier against odor. It is best to use a "cut-to-fit," transparent pouching system that covers the peristomal skin without constricting the stoma and allows for visibility of the stoma. In the immediate postoperative period, the stoma may be edematous, and the abdomen may be distended. These symptoms resolve over a 4- to 6-week period after surgery, but during this time it is necessary to revise the pouching system to adapt to changes in the size of the stoma and the body contours. Consult an ostomy nurse for pouch changing so that teaching may be done at the time of the pouch change.

There are many types of pouching systems. All have a protective layer that adheres to the skin called a *skin barrier* and a pouch. A one-piece pouching system (Fig. 20-4, *A*) has the two parts integrated together. A two-piece system (Fig. 20-4, *B*) has a separate skin barrier and pouch that snaps in

place. The flush or retracted stoma may require a convex wafer (Fig. 20-5) for successful pouching. This type of skin barrier places gentle pressure on the peristomal skin to push the stoma up through the opening in the wafer. You apply the pouch to the skin barrier by attaching it to a flange (a plastic ring) on the barrier. You must use the skin barrier with flange with the corresponding size pouch from the same manufacturer so the pieces fit together properly to avoid leakage between the skin barrier and the pouch.

Some pouching systems have precut openings in the barrier for the stoma, whereas others need to be custom cut to size for the patient's stoma measurement. There is also a new moldable Durahesive skin barrier available with a hydrocolloid flexible collar that replaces the cut-to-fit barriers. Learn how to use the different pouching systems before applying them on patients. The websites for the companies that make ostomy supplies have patient and health care provider instructions that are helpful in understanding how to use the pouching systems.

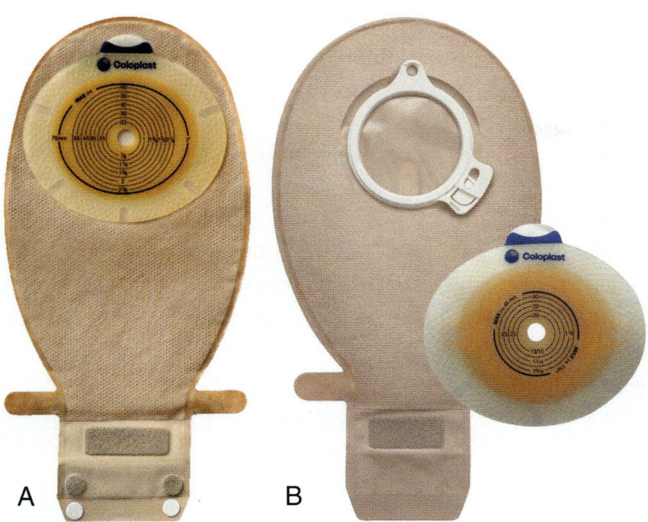

FIG 20-4 **A,** One-piece pouch with Velcro closure. **B,** Two-piece pouching system with separate skin barrier and attachable pouch. (Courtesy Coloplast, Minneapolis, Minnesota.)

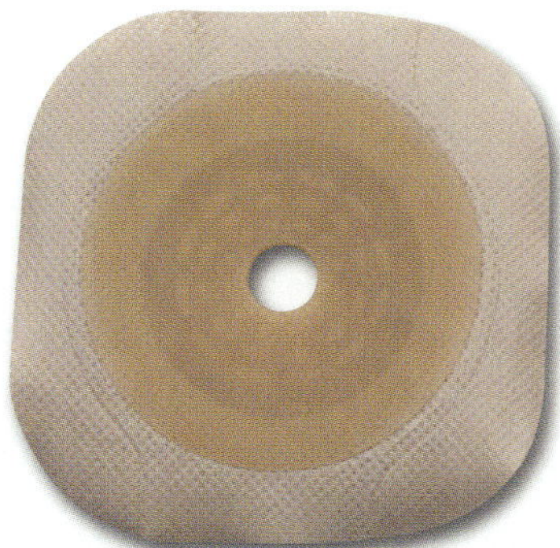

FIG 20-5 Convex skin barrier wafer. (Courtesy Hollister, Inc., Libertyville, Illinois.)

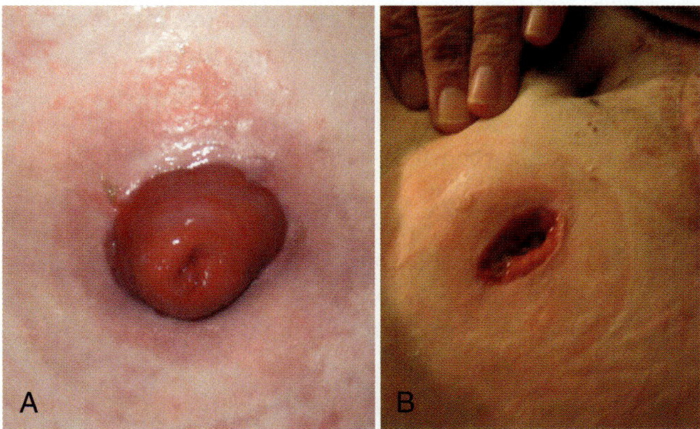

FIG 20-6 **A,** Budded stoma. **B,** Retracted stoma. (Courtesy Jane Fellows.)

ASSESSMENT

1. Identify patient using two identifiers (e.g., name and birthday or name and account number) according to facility policy. *Rationale: Ensures correct patient. Complies with The Joint Commission standards and improves patient safety (TJC, 2014).*
2. Observe existing skin barrier and pouch for leakage, and note the length of time in place. Change the pouch every 3 to 7 days, not daily. *Rationale: Assesses effectiveness of pouching system for determining frequency of change. If an ostomy pouch is leaking, change it. Taping or patching it to contain effluent leaves the skin exposed to chemical or enzymatic irritation (Goldberg et al., 2010).*
3. Apply clean gloves. Observe amount of effluent in the pouch, and empty the pouch if it is more than ⅓ to ½ full by opening the clip or integrated Velcro-like closure and draining it into a container for measurement of the output. *Rationale: Decreases the weight of the pouch and the chance of the pouch loosening or spilling when changing it.*
4. Observe stoma for color, swelling, trauma, and condition of the peristomal skin. If you cannot observe the stoma due to the effluent, apply clean gloves and remove pouch by gently pushing skin away from the adhesive barrier. Properly dispose of soiled pouch and save the clamp if the pouch does not have an integrated closure. Assess type of stoma and whether it is budded (protruding above the skin surface [Fig. 20-6, *A*]), flush with the skin surface, or retracted (below the skin surface [Fig. 20-6, *B*]). Clear pouches permit viewing of a stoma without removal of the pouch. *Rationale: Stoma characteristics aid in determining the appropriate pouching system.*
5. Observe the abdominal contour, and note the presence of scars or incisions. *Rationale: Determines type of pouching system needed. Abdominal contours, scars, or incisions affect the type of system and how the system adheres to the patient's skin.*
6. Assess patient for latex allergy. *Rationale: History of allergy requires use of latex-free pouch.*
7. Observe patient's readiness to learn by willingness to look at stoma and ask questions. If patient is apprehensive about touching or looking at stoma, encourage him or her to observe the pouch change procedure initially. Whenever possible, consult the ostomy care nurse. *Rationale: Determines patient's readiness to learn and facilitates self-care at home.*

PLANNING

Expected Outcomes focus on maintaining integrity of stoma and peristomal skin, promoting normal elimination, and promoting patient's ability to manage ostomy.
1. Stoma is moist and reddish pink. Skin is intact and free of burning or irritation; sutures are intact.
2. Stoma drains moderate amount of liquid or soft stool and flatus in pouch.
3. Patient or family caregiver observes and returns demonstration of pouch change.
4. Patient and family caregiver ask questions about procedure and learn to change pouch.

Delegation and Collaboration
The skill of pouching a new bowel diversion cannot be delegated to nursing assistive personnel (NAP). In some facilities, care of an established ostomy (4 to 6 weeks after surgery) can be delegated. The nurse instructs the NAP about:

- Expected appearance of the stoma and the amount, color, and consistency of drainage from the ostomy.
- Special equipment needed to complete procedure.
- Changes in patient's stoma and surrounding skin integrity that should be reported.

Equipment

- Pouch: clear drainable one-piece or two-piece, cut-to-fit or precut size, or moldable
- Pouch closure device such as a clip if needed
- Measuring guide
- Adhesive remover (optional)
- Clean gloves
- Washcloth
- Towel or disposable waterproof barrier
- Basin with warm tap water
- Scissors
- Waterproof bag for disposal of pouch
- Gown and goggles (if there is a risk of splashing when emptying the pouch)

IMPLEMENTATION *for* POUCHING A BOWEL DIVERSION

STEPS	RATIONALE
1. **See Standard Protocol (inside front cover).**	
2. Position patient semireclining or supine during assessment and pouching. (Note: Some patients with established ostomies prefer to stand.) If possible, provide patient a mirror for observation.	Position ensures there are fewer skin wrinkles, which allows for ease of application of pouching system.
3. Apply clean gloves. Place towel or disposable waterproof barrier under patient and across patient's lower abdomen.	Protects bed linen.
4. If not removed during assessment, remove used pouch and skin barrier gently by pushing skin away from barrier. An adhesive remover may be used to facilitate removal of skin barrier. Dispose of pouch.	Reduces skin trauma. Improper removal of pouch and barrier can cause peristomal skin irritation or breakdown.
5. Cleanse peristomal skin gently with warm tap water using a washcloth; do not scrub skin. Minor bleeding from a stoma is normal during cleansing. Pat the skin dry. Dispose of gloves and perform hand hygiene.	Soap leaves residue on skin, which interferes with pouch adhesion (Goldberg et al., 2010). Pouch does not adhere to wet skin. Reduces transmission of infection.
6. Measure stoma (see illustration). Expect size of stoma to change over first 4 to 6 weeks after surgery.	Allows for proper fit of pouch that will protect peristomal skin.
7. Trace pattern of stoma measurement on adhesive backing of pouch (see illustration).	Prepares for cutting opening in the pouch.
8. Cut opening in pouch (see illustration).	Customizes pouch to provide appropriate fit over stoma.
9. Remove protective backing from adhesive (see illustration).	
10. Apply one-piece pouch (see illustration). Note: Apply clean gloves if stoma is oozing stool.	
a. Press adhesive backing of pouch smoothly against skin, starting from bottom and working up around sides.	Ensures smooth, wrinkle-free seal.

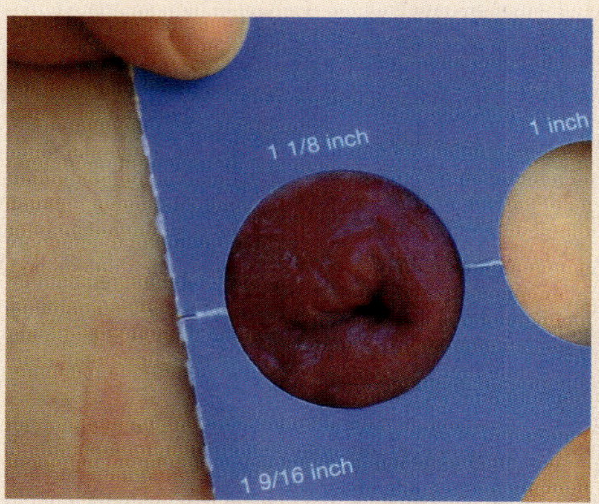

STEP 6 Measure stoma. (Courtesy Coloplast, Minneapolis, Minnesota.)

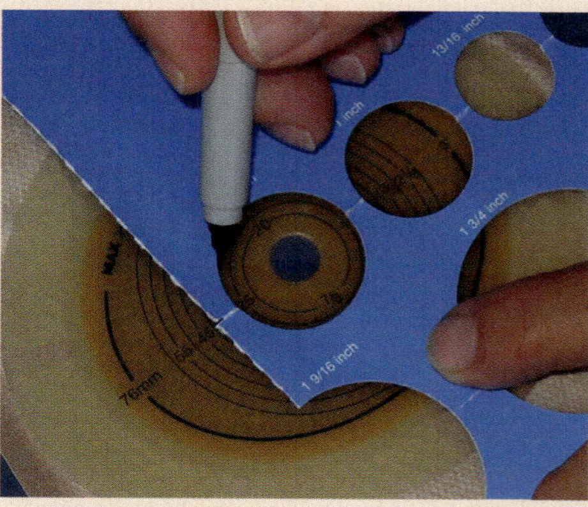

STEP 7 Trace measurement. (Courtesy Coloplast, Minneapolis, Minnesota.)

STEPS	RATIONALE

   b. Hold firmly into place around stoma and outside edges. Bottom of pouch points toward patient's knees when sitting.

   c. Teach patient to hold hand over pouch to apply heat and light pressure to secure seal. Hold for about 1 to 2 minutes.

Pouch adhesives are activated by heat and pressure and hold more securely at body temperature.

11. If using a two-piece barrier wafer and pouch:

   a. Apply clean gloves. Apply the barrier to the skin first (see illustration) and then attach the pouch.

   b. Snap on pouch ensuring it is attached all around the flange.

Ensures pouch is securely fastened.

12. Close end of pouch with clip or integrated closure. Remove and dispose of gloves (if worn)

Closure contains effluent.

13. **See Completion Protocol (inside front cover).**

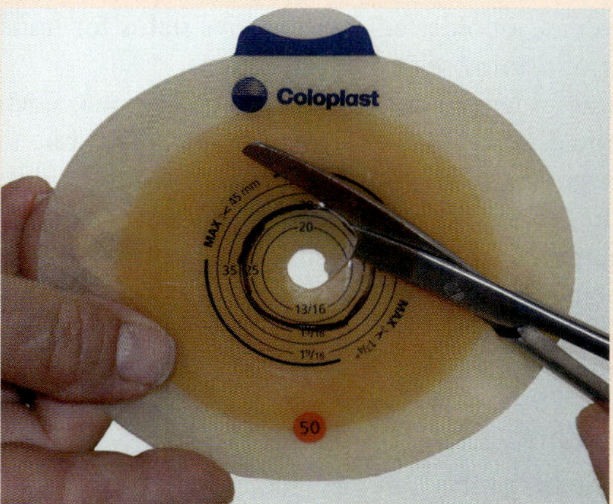

STEP 8 Cut-to-fit, one-piece drainable ostomy pouch. (© 2010 Convatec Inc. Reprinted with permission.)

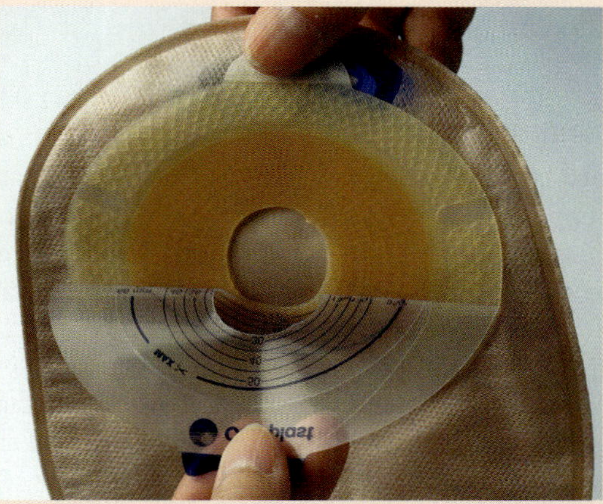

STEP 9 Removing the backing paper for the barrier on a one-piece pouch. (© 2010 Convatec Inc. Reprinted with permission.)

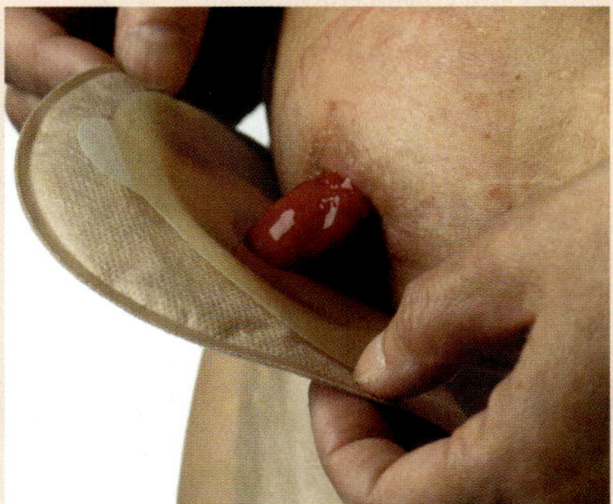

STEP 10 Patient applying a one-piece pouch. (© 2010 Convatec Inc. Reprinted with permission.)

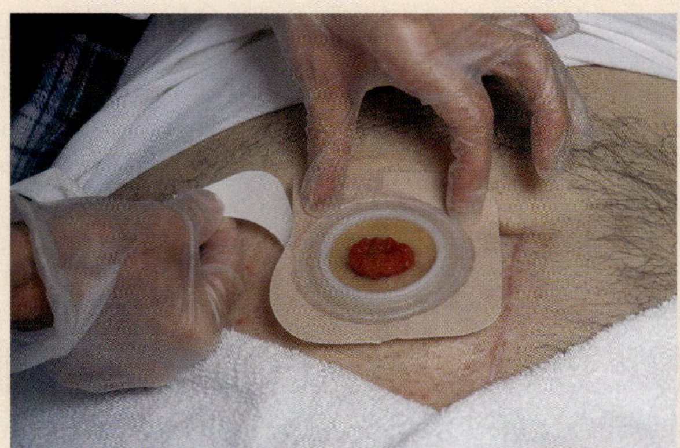

STEP 11a Application of barrier-paste flange for two-piece pouch.

EVALUATION

1. Observe appearance of stoma, peristomal skin, abdominal contours, and suture line during pouch change.
2. Observe willingness of patient and family member or significant other to view stoma and ask questions about the procedure.
3. Use *Teach Back:* State to the patient, "I want to be sure I explained the way to change a pouch correctly to you. Show me how to change your pouch." Evaluates what the patient is able to explain or demonstrate. Revise your instruction now or develop plan for revised patient teaching to be implemented at an appropriate time if patient is not able to teach back correctly.

Unexpected Outcomes and Related Interventions

1. Skin around the stoma is blistered or bleeding, or a rash is noted secondary to hypersensitive reaction to one of the products used, yeast rash, or exposure of the skin to fecal effluent.
   a. Remove pouch carefully.
   b. Consult ostomy nurse.
2. Necrotic stoma is manifested by purple or black color, dry rather than moist texture, failure to bleed when washed gently, or presence of tissue sloughing.
   a. Report to health care provider.
   b. Consult with ostomy nurse.
3. Patient refuses to look at stoma or participate in care.
   a. Explore patient's feelings and enlist family support.
   b. Consult ostomy nurse.
   c. Knowledge and acceptance by staff facilitate understanding and adjustment.

Recording and Reporting

- Record type of pouch and skin barrier applied, amount and appearance of effluent in pouch, size and appearance of stoma, and condition of peristomal skin. Record what patient and family caregivers are able to demonstrate and level of participation.
- Document your evaluation of patient learning.
- Report any of the following to health care provider: abnormal appearance of stoma, suture line, peristomal skin, or volume and character of output.

Sample Documentation

1600   Ileostomy stoma, budded, round, 3.12 cm (1¼ inch) in diameter, appears edematous, red in color. Emptied 200 mL of dark brown liquid from pouch. Two-piece ostomy system intact, without leakage. Ostomy nurse scheduled to begin instruction today. Patient denies itching or burning of peristomal area, declines to view stoma at this time.

Special Considerations

Pediatric

- Ostomy pouches designed especially for neonates, infants, and children are smaller and have a more skin-sensitive adhesive on the barrier.
- Children and adolescents may have ostomy surgery for cancer, inflammatory bowel disease, and trauma.
- Neonates often have multiple stomas on their abdomens that are the result of corrective bowel surgeries. Select a cut-to-fit pouch that allows multiple stoma openings in skin barrier yet still fits on the neonate's small abdomen.
- Peristomal skin of a preterm infant is not fully developed; as a result, you should not use skin sealants and adhesive removers because they damage the epithelium.

Geriatric

- Evaluate an older adult's cognitive status for understanding of ostomy self-care instructions.
- Some older patients have impaired manual dexterity or limited vision; make adaptations for this while teaching. For patients who are unable to custom cut the size of their skin barriers, consider having barriers precut by ostomy equipment supplier or using a precut two-piece system.
- Financial concerns about cost of ostomy supplies and reimbursement are an important issue for patients on fixed income.

Home Care

- Evaluate patient's home toileting facilities and ability to position self to empty pouch directly into the toilet.
- Patient may shower without covering pouch.
- Instruct patient and family caregiver that ostomy care does not require any sterile supplies.
- Family caregivers should wear gloves to avoid contact with stool.
- Patients should avoid placing pouches in extremely hot or cold locations because temperature affects barrier and adhesive materials.

<hr>

SKILL 20.2   POUCHING AN INCONTINENT UROSTOMY

Because urine flows continuously from an incontinent urinary diversion, a urinary pouch is placed over the opening immediately after surgery. Placement of the pouch may be more challenging than with a fecal diversion because urine flow keeps the skin moist. In the immediate postoperative period, urinary stents extend out from the stoma (Fig. 20-7). The surgeon places these stents into the ureters to keep them from becoming stenosed or closed at the site where the ureters are attached to the conduit. The stents are removed during the hospital stay or at the first postoperative visit with the surgeon. The stoma of a urinary diversion is normally red and moist. It is made from a portion of the intestinal tract, usually the ileum. It should protrude above the skin. An ileal conduit is usually located in the right lower abdominal quadrant. While the patient is in bed, the pouch may be connected to a bedside drainage bag to decrease the need for frequent emptying. When the patient goes home, the bedside drainage bag may be used at night to avoid having to get up to empty the pouch. Each type of urostomy pouch (Fig. 20-8) comes with a connector for the bedside drainage bag. Incorrect pouch placement, large volumes of urine in the pouch, or a urinary pouch without an antireflux valve promotes reflux and the risk of infection. You can reduce the risk of reflux by attaching the urinary pouch to straight drainage when high urinary output is expected. A patient must understand the importance of draining the pouch when it is ⅓ to ½ full and using clean technique during stomal and skin care.

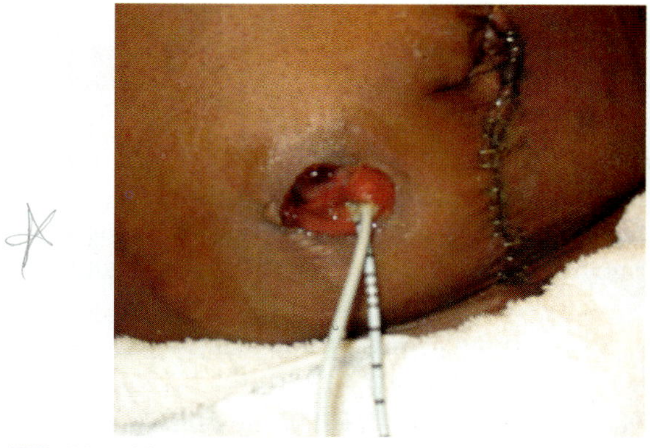

FIG 20-7 Urostomy stoma with stents in place. (Courtesy Jane Fellows.)

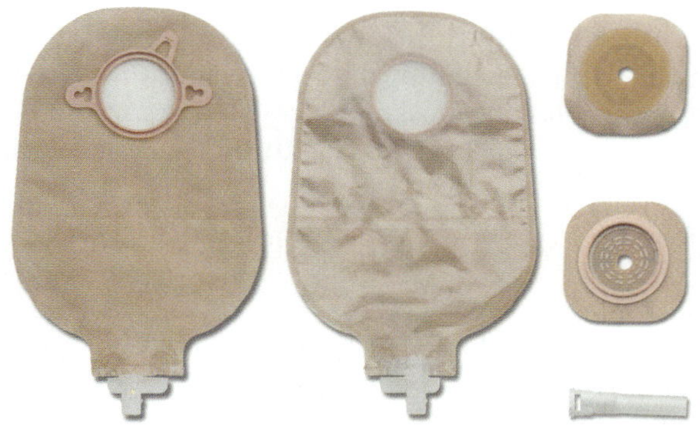

FIG 20-8 Urostomy pouching system with adapter to connect pouch to bedside drainage bag. (Courtesy Hollister, Inc., Libertyville, Illinois.)

ASSESSMENT

1. Identify patient using two identifiers (e.g., name and birthday or name and account number) according to facility policy. *Rationale: Ensures correct patient. Complies with The Joint Commission standards and improves patient safety (TJC, 2014).*

2. Apply clean gloves. Observe existing skin barrier and pouch for leakage of urine and length of time in place. Change the pouch every 3 to 7 days, not daily. *Rationale: Assesses effectiveness of pouching system and determines frequency for changing pouch.*

3. Observe amount of urine in the pouch, and empty it if it is more than $\frac{1}{3}$ to $\frac{1}{2}$ full by opening the tap at the end of the pouch and draining it into a container for measurement. *Rationale: Decreases the weight of the pouch and chance of it loosening or spillage occurring during change. Urine output provides information about renal status.*

4. Observe stoma for color, swelling, trauma, and healing of the peristomal skin. Assess type of stoma. Clear pouches permit viewing of stoma without their removal. If pouch is not clear, remove pouch by gently pushing skin away from the adhesive barrier. Apply clean gloves. Properly dispose of soiled pouch and save any clamps. *Rationale: Stoma characteristics are one of the factors to consider in selecting an appropriate pouching system. Convexity in the skin barrier is often necessary with a flush or retracted stoma.*

5. Assess patient for latex allergy. *Rationale: History of allergy requires use of latex-free pouch.*

6. Observe patient's readiness to learn by willingness to look at stoma and ask questions. If patient is apprehensive about touching or looking at stoma, encourage him or her to observe the pouch change procedure initially. Whenever possible, consult the ostomy care nurse. *Rationale: Assesses patient's reaction to stoma and readiness to begin learning self-care.*

PLANNING

Expected Outcomes focus on maintaining integrity of stoma and peristomal skin, condition of stents, and normal urine output and on promoting patient's ability to manage ostomy.

1. Stoma is moist and reddish pink with stents protruding from it in the postoperative period. Skin is intact and free of irritation; sutures are intact.
2. Urine drains freely from stents or stoma. Urine is yellowish with mucus shreds and is without foul odor. The urine may be pink or contain small blood clots after surgery.
3. Volume of output is within acceptable limits (30 mL/hr).
4. Patient and family caregiver observe and return demonstrate steps of procedure.
5. Patient asks questions about procedure and may attempt to assist with pouch change.

Delegation and Collaboration

The skill of pouching a new incontinent urostomy cannot be delegated to nursing assistive personnel (NAP). In some facilities, care of an established urostomy (≥ 4 to 6 weeks after surgery) can be delegated. The nurse instructs the NAP about:

- Expected appearance of the stoma and amount, color, and consistency of urine from the ostomy.
- Special equipment needed to complete procedure.
- Changes in patient's stoma and surrounding skin integrity that should be reported.

Equipment

- Urinary pouch (with antireflux flap) and skin barrier; clear, drainable one-piece or two-piece, cut-to-fit or precut size with appropriate adapter for connection to bedside drainage bag (see Fig. 20-8)
- Measuring guide
- Bedside urinary drainage bag
- Clean gloves
- Washcloth
- Towel or disposable waterproof barrier
- Basin with warm tap water
- Scissors
- Adhesive remover
- Absorbent wick made from gauze rolled tightly in the shape of a tampon
- Waterproof bag for disposal of pouch
- Gown and goggles (if there is a risk of splashing when emptying the pouch)

IMPLEMENTATION *for* POUCHING AN INCONTINENT UROSTOMY

STEPS	RATIONALE

1. **See Standard Protocol (inside front cover).**

2. Position patient semireclining or supine. If possible provide patient a mirror for observation.

Position ensures there are fewer skin wrinkles, which allows for ease of pouch application.

3. Apply clean gloves. Place towel or disposable waterproof barrier under patient and one across patient's lower abdomen.

Protects bed linen because there will be a continuous flow of urine from the stoma. Maintains patient's dignity.

4. Remove used pouch and skin barrier (if not removed during assessment) by gently pushing skin away from barrier. If stents are present, *do not pull on them.*

Reduces risk of trauma to skin and risk of dislodging stents. Stents are necessary to keep the ureters patent during the immediate postoperative period.

5. Place rolled gauze or wick at stoma opening. Maintain gauze at the stoma opening continuously during pouch measurement and change. If possible, have patient or family caregiver hold this gauze in place.

Rolled gauze absorbs the urine from the stoma site. The gauze forms a wick; using a wick at stoma opening keeps urine from leaking onto the skin and prevents peristomal skin from becoming wet with urine during pouching change procedure. Patient and family participation in care facilitates adjustment to stoma and self-care.

6. While keeping rolled gauze in contact with the stoma, cleanse peristomal skin gently with warm tap water using washcloth; do not scrub skin; avoid using soap. Minor bleeding of the stoma during washing is normal. Pat the skin dry. Remove gloves and perform hand hygiene.

Soap leaves residue on skin, which interferes with pouch adhesion (Goldberg et al., 2010). Pouch does not adhere to wet skin.

7. Measure stoma (see illustration, Skill 20.1, Step 6). Expect size of stoma to change over first 4 to 6 weeks following surgery.

Allows for proper fit of pouch that will protect peristomal skin.

8. Trace pattern on pouch/skin barrier on adhesive of pouch (see illustration, Skill 20.1, Step 7).

Prepares for cutting opening in the pouch.

9. Cut opening in pouch (see illustration, Skill 20.1, Step 8).

Customizes pouch to provide appropriate fit over stoma.

10. Remove protective backing from adhesive surface (see illustration, Skill 20.1, Step 9). Apply clean gloves. Remove wick from stoma.

Prepares pouch for adhesion to the skin. Pouch adhesives are heat-activated and hold more securely at body temperature.

11. Apply pouch (see illustration, Skill 20.1, Step 11a). Press adhesive barrier firmly into place around stoma and outside edges. Have patient hold hand over pouch 1 to 2 minutes to apply heat to secure seal.

Pouch adhesives are heat-activated to create a secure seal on skin.

12. Use adapter provided with pouches to connect pouch to bedside urinary bag. Remove and dispose of gloves.

Provides for collection and measurement of urine. Allows patient to rest without frequent emptying of the pouch.

13. **See Completion Protocol (inside front cover).**

▮ EVALUATION

1. Observe volume and character of urine and appearance of stoma, peristomal skin, abdominal contours, and suture line during pouch change.

2. Observe willingness of patient and family member or significant other to view stoma and ask questions about the procedure.

3. Use **Teach Back:** State to the patient, "Let's go over what we discussed so I know you understand. Tell me why it is important to keep the skin dry. Show me now how to do a pouch change." Evaluates what the patient is able to explain or demonstrate. Revise your instruction now or develop plan for revised patient teaching to be implemented at an appropriate time if patient is not able to teach back correctly.

Unexpected Outcomes and Related Interventions (see Skill 20.1)

1. There is no urinary output for several hours, or output is less than 30 mL/hr. Urine has foul odor.
   a. Notify health care provider.
   b. Determine patency of stents or stoma by observing urine flow.

c. Obtain urine specimen if ordered by health care provider for culture and sensitivity to test for possible infection (see Skill 20.3).

2. Necrotic stoma is manifested by purple or black color, dry rather than moist texture, failure to bleed when washed gently, or presence of tissue sloughing.

   a. Report to health care provider.

   b. Document findings.

Recording and Reporting

* Record type of pouch and skin barrier applied, amount and appearance of urine emptied from pouch, size and appearance of stoma, and condition of peristomal skin.
* Record what patient and family caregivers are able to demonstrate and level of participation.
* Document your evaluation of patient learning.
* Report any of the following to nurse or health care provider: abnormal appearance of stoma, suture line, or peristomal skin or change in volume, color, or odor of urine output.

Sample Documentation

0800 Ileal conduit stoma is red and moist. 250-mL clear yellow urine with white mucus present in pouch. Peristomal skin intact. Suture line dry and approximated. Pouch changed with patient assisting. Patient correctly applied pouch.

Special Considerations
Pediatric

* In neonates, urinary diversions are less common than fecal ostomies.

* Select pediatric pouches designed especially for neonates, infants, and children, which are smaller and have a more skin-sensitive adhesive on the barrier.

Geriatric

* Evaluate an older adult's cognitive status for understanding of ostomy self-care instructions.
* Some older patients have impaired manual dexterity or limited vision; make adaptations for this while teaching. For patients who are unable to custom cut the size of their skin barriers, consider having barriers precut by ostomy equipment supplier or using a precut two-piece system.
* Financial concerns about cost of ostomy supplies and reimbursement are an important issue for patients on fixed income.

Home Care

* Evaluate patient's home toileting facilities and ability to position self to empty pouch directly into the toilet.
* Patient may shower without covering pouch.
* Ostomy care does not require sterile supplies.
* Family caregivers should wear gloves to avoid contact with urine.
* At home, patient can open pouch spout and connect it to straight drainage at night. Make sure that patient understands that adapter will be needed to connect pouch to the bedside drainage bag.

SKILL 20.3 CATHETERIZING A URINARY DIVERSION

Catheterization of a urinary diversion is the only way to obtain an accurate culture and sensitivity specimen when screening for infection. When it is necessary to obtain a urine specimen from a urinary diversion, the best method is to insert a sterile catheter into the stoma (Mahoney et al., 2013). Obtaining a specimen from urine in the pouch does not provide accurate results because of the risk for contamination. With the use of strict sterile asepsis, catheterization is relatively safe and easy. If a patient uses a two-piece pouch, remove the pouch from the skin barrier and replace it after the catheterization. If a patient uses a one-piece pouch, you have to remove the pouch to obtain the specimen and replace with a new pouch afterward. Understand how the stoma and implanted ureters are constructed to prevent trauma of tissues. Reflux of urine into the ureters can cause infection.

ASSESSMENT

1. Identify patient using two identifiers (e.g., name and birthday or name and account number) according to facility policy. *Rationale: Ensures correct patient. Complies with The Joint Commission standards and improves patient safety (TJC, 2014).*

2. Observe signs and symptoms of urinary tract infection, such as elevated temperature, chills, foul-smelling urine, and elevated white blood cell count. *Rationale: Determines need to perform catheterization to obtain a sterile specimen from urinary diversion.*

3. Obtain health care provider's order for catheterization. *Rationale: Procedure and laboratory test requires health care provider's order.*

4. Assess patient's understanding of the need for procedure and how procedure is done. *Rationale: Determines patient's willingness to cooperate and reduces his or her anxiety.*

PLANNING

Expected Outcomes focus on obtaining an uncontaminated urine specimen.

* Urine is obtained correctly.
* Laboratory results are accurate.

Delegation and Collaboration

The skill of catheterizing a urinary diversion cannot be delegated to nursing assistive personnel (NAP). The nurse instructs the NAP to:

- Inform the nurse if patient complains of peristomal or back pain.
- Inform the nurse if there is a change in color, odor, or amount of urine or if there is blood in the urine.

Equipment
- Urinary catheterization supplies (may be contained in prepackaged sterile catheter kit or may need to be gathered separately):
- 14 to 16 Fr sterile catheter
- Water-soluble lubricant
- Antiseptic swabs (e.g., chlorhexidine)
- Sterile gloves
- Sterile specimen container
- Absorbent gauze wick
- Gauze pad
- Towels or disposable waterproof barrier
- Urinary diversion pouch if patient is using one-piece system (if using two-piece system, same pouch can be removed and replaced for procedure as long as skin barrier adhesive remains intact)
- Clean gloves

IMPLEMENTATION *for* CATHETERIZING A URINARY DIVERSION

STEPS	RATIONALE
1. **See Standard Protocol (inside front cover).**	
2. If possible, position patient sitting and drape towel across lower abdomen.	Gravity facilitates flow of urine. Maintains patient's dignity. Towel absorbs urine.
3. Apply clean gloves. Remove pouch. If patient uses two-piece system, remove pouch only and leave barrier attached to skin.	Access to stoma.
4. Remove and discard gloves. Perform hand hygiene. Open sterile catheterization set according to instructions or open needed equipment and place on sterile barrier. If not using catheterization kit, place gauze pad on sterile field and squeeze small amount of lubricant onto gauze.	Avoids contamination.
5. **Apply sterile gloves.**	
6. If needed, have patient hold absorbent wick over stoma while waiting.	Prevents leakage of urine on peristomal skin, linens, and clothing.
7. Cleanse surface of stoma with antiseptic swabs using circular motion from center outward. Using new swab each time; repeat twice. Allow antiseptic to dry.	Removes surface bacteria.
a. If patient has stents in place, use antiseptic swab to cleanse the ends of the stents and place the stents in the sterile cup. Allow urine to drip into the cup until an adequate amount for a specimen has been obtained. Then go directly to Step 13.	Maintains sterility of stent and specimen.
8. Lubricate tip of catheter with water-soluble lubricant.	Lubricant facilitates passage of catheter through stoma.
9. Remove lid from specimen container. Place distal end of catheter into specimen container. Hold catheter in container with nondominant hand.	The conduit is for passage of urine, and only a small volume of urine is obtained.
10. With your dominant hand, gently insert catheter into stoma until urine begins to flow (15 to 30.5 cm [6 to 12 inches]). Do not force catheter; redirect course as needed. Use gentle but firm pressure similar to regular catheterization of urethra. Have patient cough or turn slightly to facilitate flow of urine.	Use care to avoid trauma to conduit.
11. Maintain container below level of stoma. Have patient cough as needed. Urine may flow around and through catheter. This is acceptable, but only urine from catheter is desired. Normally wait 5 minutes; if no urine is in container, pinch catheter and remove; direct any urine "trapped" in catheter into cup.	Facilitates drainage of urine. Culture and sensitivity studies require only 3 to 5 mL of urine.

STEPS	RATIONALE
12. After withdrawing catheter, place absorbent pad over stoma.	Keeps skin dry.
13. Apply lid to specimen container.	Prevents accidental spillage.
14. Reapply new urostomy pouch or reattach pouch if patient uses a two-piece system.	Pouch is necessary to contain urine.
15. Remove gloves; perform hand hygiene. Label and send specimen to laboratory at once.	Avoids transmission of infection. Labeling ensures acceptance of specimen by laboratory and processing. Allowing urine to sit for long periods at room temperature affects laboratory results.
16. See Completion Protocol (inside front cover).	

EVALUATION

1. Refer to laboratory report and compare results of culture and sensitivity with normal expected findings. Remember that mucus is a normal finding in the urine of a patient with an ileal or colon conduit. If specimen is contaminated, a second specimen will be needed.

Unexpected Outcomes and Related Interventions

1. Unable to obtain urine.
   a. Reposition patient.
   b. Encourage fluids and try again later.

Recording and Reporting

- Record time specimen was collected; patient's tolerance of procedure; and appearance of urine, skin, and stoma.

- Report results of laboratory test to nurse in charge or health care provider.

Sample Documentation

0700   Ileal conduit stoma catheterized for urine specimen. 150 mL cloudy urine with a foul odor obtained. Specimen sent to the laboratory.

Special Considerations
Home Care

- Explain common symptoms of urinary tract infection: flank pain, dark or bloody urine, foul-smelling urine, fever ($\geq$38.3°C [101°F]), confusion.
- Encourage patient to notify health care provider if symptoms of infection develop.
- Reinforce importance of fluid intake (2 L/day).

CRITICAL THINKING EXERCISES

Case Study

The nurse is assigned to care for a 28-year-old woman who was admitted to the hospital with abdominal pain. She was diagnosed with Crohn's disease when she was 16 and has had numerous hospital admissions and tried many medications, but now she needs surgery to remove part of her intestine and will have an ileostomy.

1. When the patient returns from surgery, the nurse assesses the stoma. Which of the following normal findings should the nurse expect to see?
   1. Red and moist
   2. Located just below the skin level
   3. Have a stent protruding from it
   4. Pink and dry
2. Which of the following instructions should the nurse teach this patient when discussing changing and emptying her pouch?
   1. Change pouch daily
   2. Empty every 4 to 6 hours
   3. Empty when it is $\frac{1}{3}$ to $\frac{1}{2}$ full
   4. Change every 10 days

3. When it is time to do the first ostomy pouch change, the nurse should:
   1. Delegate this to the NAP to do when she does the rest of the patient's personal care.
   2. Request that the physician do the first pouch change.
   3. Have the patient or her family do the pouch change.
   4. Have an ostomy nurse do the pouch change and begin teaching the patient self-care.

Review Questions

1. A patient with a total colectomy and new ileostomy notices that the bowel movement is always liquid and asks when it will be formed like it was before surgery. How should the nurse respond?
   1. Tell the patient that it will be formed after complete recovery from the surgery.
   2. Tell the patient to eat foods that are constipating until the bowel movement is a firm consistency.
   3. Tell the patient that this is a normal output for an ileostomy.
   4. Tell the patient to reduce fluid intake and it will become more formed.

2. From the following list, select the most important task to be done before surgery to promote patient adjustment to an ostomy.
   1. Give the patient a chance to empty a pouch.
   2. Make sure that the patient has a nutrition consultation.
   3. Schedule stoma site marking with a certified ostomy nurse.
   4. Administer a barium enema.

3. To obtain a urine specimen for culture and sensitivity from a patient with a urostomy, which of the following should be done?
   1. Catheterize the stoma
   2. Take the specimen from a clean pouch
   3. Take a specimen before changing the pouch
   4. Attach the pouch to a bedside drainage bag and take the specimen through the port in the tubing

4. The nurse is changing the pouch on a urostomy. Place the following steps in the correct order.
   1. Prepare the pouch by cutting the opening to the size of the stoma and removing the backing.
   2. Dispose of used pouch
   3. Maintain gentle finger pressure around barrier for 1 to 2 minutes
   4. Cleanse skin around stoma with warm tap water
   5. Wick stoma with a rolled gauze
   6. Press adhesive barrier firmly but gently on the skin

5. A patient has a new colostomy. Which of the following statements is true for this patient? Select all that apply.
   1. The patient will be able to take a shower.
   2. Someone else will always have to change the patient's pouch.
   3. The skin around the stoma will always be red and itchy.
   4. The pouch will be emptied only once a day.
   5. The pouch can be changed only once a week.
   6. The pouches are disposable.
   7. A rash or skin breakdown around the stoma is not normal and requires treatment.

6. An ostomy stoma should be measured with each pouch change because it may change size:
   1. For several months after surgery
   2. For the first few days after surgery
   3. For as long as the patient has a stoma
   4. In the first 4 to 6 weeks after surgery

7. To which factor is an ostomy patient's ability to achieve a good quality of life *most* closely related?
   1. Age
   2. Level of education
   3. Support of spouse, family, and significant others
   4. Manual dexterity

8. A patient with a new ostomy begins crying as the nurse helps her change her pouch for the first time. What should the nurse do?
   1. Tell her that no one will know that she has an ostomy.
   2. Allow her to express her grief over this change in her body.
   3. Request a psychiatric consultation.
   4. Reassure her that it could be worse if the surgeon had not removed all the cancer.

9. A stoma formed from a section of the ileum or small intestine to which the ureters are attached is called:
   1. A nephrostomy
   2. An ascending colostomy
   3. An ileostomy
   4. An ileal conduit

10. A patient with a sigmoid colostomy asks about how to regulate her bowel movement so that she does not have to empty the pouch while she is at work. Which of the following recommendations should the nurse make?
    1. Have the patient wear a larger pouch.
    2. Refer the patient to an ostomy nurse to teach her how to irrigate the colostomy.
    3. Tell the patient to fast for several hours before going to work.
    4. Suggest over-the-counter medications to induce constipation.

REFERENCES

Black P: Understanding religious beliefs of patients needing a stoma, *Gastrointestinal Nursing* 9(10):17, 2011.

Danielsen A, et al: Learning to live with a permanent ostomy, *J Wound Ostomy Continence Nurs* 40(4):407, 2013.

Erwin-Toth P, Thompson SJ, Davis JS: Factors impacting the quality of life of people with an ostomy in North America, *J Wound Ostomy Continence Nurs* 39(4):417, 2012.

Goldberg M, et al: *Management of the patient with a fecal ostomy: best practice guideline for clinicians*, Mt. Laurel, NJ, 2010, Wound Ostomy and Continence Nurses Society (WOCN).

Mahoney M, et al: Procedure for obtaining a urine sample from urostomy, ileal conduit, and colon conduit: best practice guideline for clinician, *J Wound Ostomy Continence Nurs* 40(3):277, 2013.

The Joint Commission (TJC): *National Patient Safety Goals*, Oakbrook Terrace, IL, 2014, The Commission. Available at: http://www.jointcommission.org/standards_information/npsgs.aspx. Accessed August 3, 2014.

Zimnicki K: Preoperative stoma site marking in the general surgery population, *J Wound Ostomy Continence Nurs* 40(5):501, 2013.

Preparation for Safe Medication Administration

Safe and accurate medication administration is a challenging and important nursing responsibility. As a nurse, you are responsible for having a full understanding of medication therapy and the related nursing implications. The nursing process is a useful framework for administering medications. Assessment and planning involve identifying any patient risks for receiving medications, factors that influence the way you administer medications, and how to instruct patients on self-administration. Nursing diagnoses communicate problems related to drug therapy and direct interventions for appropriate nursing care. Implementation includes administering medications correctly and safely and, in many cases, teaching patients how to self-administer medications. Evaluation involves monitoring patients' responses to medications and measuring learning. This chapter includes basic information for safely preparing to administer medications.

PATIENT-CENTERED CARE

Regardless of the health care setting, nurses are responsible for administering medications, evaluating their effects on each patient's health status, and teaching patients about medications and their side effects. You are also responsible for giving patients information to help ensure that they will follow medication regimens and for evaluating their self-administration techniques. Before discharge, be sure that patients or family caregivers are adequately prepared to administer medications in the home. This requires understanding their willingness and ability to adhere to medication therapy and factors within the home that may create barriers.

Culturally, a patient's values and beliefs affect medication response and adherence. Ethnicity, financial resources, education, and previous experiences are additional factors to consider when assisting patients with medication management. A family's influence on a patient's behaviors, such as their attitudes about health care or demands on a patient's daily schedule, can influence medication adherence. Regarding ethnicity, there are cultures in which it is unacceptable to verbalize complaints about stomach problems; it is common for these patients not to report nausea, vomiting, and bowel changes related to medication side effects. For patients whose cultures support the use of herbal and homeopathic remedies, it is important for them to know how these agents alter their responses to medications. In a study involving children, researchers found there was a significant association between decreased adherence and ethnic minorities (Vasbinder et al., 2013). As a nurse, consider each of your patient's backgrounds, including their education, language, and health care beliefs (Vasbinder et al., 2013).

SAFETY

Medication administration safety is a priority goal for safe nursing practice. It begins by having a thorough understanding of the medications you administer and whether patients have any drug allergies. It is then important for you to follow safe preparation and administration standards, which are part of the six rights of medication administration. Box 21-1 summarizes common causes of medication errors. Medication safety also requires you to understand the principles of pharmacokinetics, growth and development, nutrition, and mathematics.

The Joint Commission (2014) has specific national patient safety goals for using medications safely. The 2014 goals include the following:

- Before a procedure, label medicines that are not labeled, such as medicines in syringes, cups, and basins. Do this in the area where medicines and supplies are set up.
- Immediately discard any medication you find that is unlabeled.
- Take extra care with patients who take anticoagulants (e.g., aspirin-containing drugs, warfarin [Coumadin], heparin) because of the risk of bleeding.
- Record and pass along correct information about a patient's medicines to all health care providers. Find out what medicines the patient is taking. Compare those medicines with new medicines given to the patient. Make sure the patient knows which medicines to take when they are at home. Tell the patient it is important to bring their up-to-date list of medicines every time they visit a health care provider.

BOX 21-1 COMMON CAUSES OF MEDICATION ERRORS

- Distraction while preparing medications
- Ambiguous strength designation on labels or in packaging
- Drug product nomenclature (look-alike or sound-alike names, use of lettered or numbered prefixes and suffixes in drug names)
- Equipment failure or malfunction (e.g., infusion pumps)
- Illegible handwriting
- Improper transcription
- Inaccurate dosage calculation
- Inadequately trained personnel
- Inappropriate abbreviations used in prescribing
- Labeling errors
- Excessive workload
- Lapses in individual performance
- Medication unavailable

EVIDENCE-BASED PRACTICE

Agency for Healthcare Research and Quality (AHRQ): *Computerized provider order entry,* 2012, http://www.psnet.ahrq.gov/primer.aspx?primerID=6. Accessed February 2014.

Radley DC et al: Reduction in medication errors in hospitals due to adoption of computerized provider order entry systems, *J Am Med Inform Assoc* 20(3):470, 2013.

Woods AD et al: Clinical decision support for atypical orders: detection and warning of atypical medication orders submitted to a computerized provider order entry system, *J Am Med Inform Assoc* 21:569–573, 2014.

As a part of the American Recovery and Reinvestment Act of 2009, the Healthcare Information Technology for Economic and Clinical Health (HITECH) was developed. One of the requirements of HITECH is the implementation of computerized provider order entry (CPOE). The Institute of Medicine recommends the use of CPOE, which is also known as "e-prescribing." A CPOE system is one in which clinicians directly enter medication orders (and, increasingly, tests and procedures) into a computer system, which transmits the order directly to the pharmacy. These systems have become increasingly common in inpatient settings as a strategy to reduce medication errors. A CPOE system, at a minimum, ensures standardized, legible, and complete orders and has the potential to reduce greatly errors at the ordering and transcribing stages (AHRQ, 2012; Radley et al., 2013). CPOE software allows for automatic drug allergy checks, dosage indications, baseline laboratory result checks, and identification of potential drug interactions.

- Do not overly depend on this technology. Follow the six rights of medication administration.
- Continue to communicate with health care providers directly if you question a medication order.
- Decision support alerts can prevent harmful drug-drug interactions and promote use of evidence-based tests and treatments, but excessive and nonspecific warnings can lead to "alert fatigue." Do not ignore critical warnings (Woods et al., 2014).

PHARMACOKINETICS

When administering medications, know the mechanism of action, the therapeutic and desired effects of the drugs, and the purpose of the medications for each specific patient. It is equally important to be knowledgeable of possible side effects and adverse reactions. Pharmacokinetics is the study of how drugs enter the body (absorption), reach the site of action (distribution), are metabolized, and are excreted from the body. Absorption describes how a drug enters the body and passes into body fluids and tissues. Absorption influences the route of drug administration. Distribution is the way drugs move to the sites of action in the body. Metabolism refers to the chemical reactions by which a medication is broken down (e.g., in the liver) until it becomes chemically inactive. Excretion is the process of drug elimination from the body through the gastrointestinal tract, kidneys, or other body secretions (Skidmore-Roth, 2014).

DRUG ACTIONS

Mechanism of Action

When giving a drug to a patient, you can expect a predictable chemical reaction that changes the physiological activity of the body. This reaction occurs as the medication bonds chemically at a specific site in the body called a *receptor site.* The reactions are possible only when the receptor site and the chemical fit together like a key in a lock. When the chemical fits well, the chemical response is initiated. These drugs are called *agonists* (Lehne, 2013). Some drugs attach at the receptor site but do not produce a new chemical reaction. These drugs are called *antagonists.* Other drugs attach and produce only a small response or prevent other reactions from occurring. These drugs are called *partial agonists.*

Understanding pharmacokinetics enables you to make the decisions necessary to ensure that drugs are given by the appropriate route and to recognize and act based on the nature and extent of drug actions, interactions, and adverse actions. In addition, this knowledge helps in planning drug administration schedules. For example, knowing when the peak action of an analgesic occurs allows you to administer the drug at a time when you anticipate that the patient's pain will increase (e.g., before ambulation or a painful dressing change). Most health care facilities have standard administration schedules.

Medication Dose Responses

Pharmacokinetics affects how much of a drug dose reaches the site of action. Except when administered intravenously, medications take time to enter the bloodstream. The goal in administering a medication is to achieve a constant blood level within a safe therapeutic range. The minimum effective concentration (MEC) is the plasma level of the medication below which the effect of the medication does not occur. The toxic concentration is the level at which toxic effects occur. The safe therapeutic range is between the MEC and the toxic concentration (Fig. 21-1). When a medication is administered repeatedly, its serum level fluctuates between doses. The highest level is called the *peak concentration,* and the lowest level is the *trough concentration.* After peaking, the serum concentration falls progressively. With intravenous (IV) infusions, the peak concentration occurs quickly, but the serum level also begins to decrease immediately. Some medications (e.g., vancomycin or gentamicin [Garamycin]) are based on peak and trough serum levels. You obtain a patient's trough level in a blood sample drawn 30 minutes before administering the drug. You draw a peak level whenever the drug is expected to reach its peak concentration. In the example of vancomycin, a peak is 1.5 to 2.0 hours after completing an IV infusion (Lehne, 2013). Results of peak and trough tests reveal if a drug is reaching its therapeutic level.

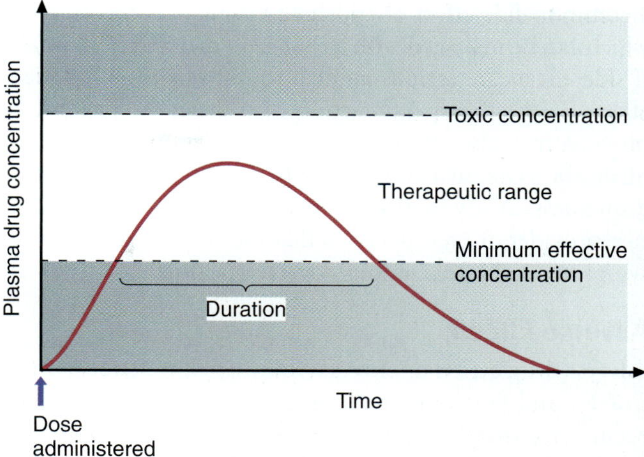

FIG 21-1 The therapeutic range of medication occurs between the minimum effective concentration and the toxic concentration. (From Lehne R: *Pharmacology for nursing care,* ed 8, St Louis, 2013, Saunders.)

All medications have a biological half-life, which is the time it takes for excretion processes to decrease the serum medication concentration by half. To maintain a therapeutic plateau, a patient needs regular fixed doses. The patient and nurse must follow regular dosage schedules and administer prescribed doses at correct intervals. Knowledge of the following time intervals of drug action helps you to anticipate the effect of a drug:

1. *Onset of action:* The time interval between when a drug is given and the first sign of its effect
2. *Peak action:* The time it takes for a drug to reach its highest effective concentration
3. *Duration of action:* The time period from onset of drug action to the time when a response is no longer seen
4. *Plateau:* Blood serum concentration reached and maintained after repeated, fixed doses
5. *Therapeutic range:* The range of plasma concentration that produces the desired drug effect without toxicity (see Fig. 21-1)

TYPES OF MEDICATION ACTION

Therapeutic Effects

A therapeutic effect is the intended or desired physiological response of a medication. A single medication may have many therapeutic effects. For example, aspirin creates analgesia, reduces inflammation and fever, and slows blood clotting. Other drugs have more limited therapeutic effects. For example, an antihypertensive medication lowers blood pressure.

Side Effects

Every medication has potential for harming a patient. Side effects are predictable and often unavoidable secondary effects produced at a usual therapeutic dose. Some side effects may be harmless, whereas others cause injury. For example, a common side effect of codeine phosphate is constipation, which can be managed with a change in diet and fluid intake. If side effects are serious enough to outweigh the beneficial effects of the therapeutic action of a drug, the health care provider may discontinue the drug. Patients often stop taking medications because of side effects such as fatigue, anorexia, drowsiness, or dry mouth. Report any side effects to a health care provider or pharmacist so that they can determine if the symptoms indicate a serious adverse reaction.

Adverse Effects

Adverse drug events or effects (ADEs) are unintended, undesirable, and often unpredictable. Some adverse reactions occur immediately, whereas others take weeks or months to develop. Early clinical recognition of ADEs is the important first step in identification. ADEs range from mild (e.g., rashes or photosensitivity to light) to severe (fatal anaphylaxis). Prompt recognition and reporting of ADEs prevents serious injury to patients. Always assess patients who may be at high risk for an ADE, such as pregnant women and patients with chronic disorders (e.g., hypertension, epilepsy, heart disease, psychoses) (Lehne, 2013). When adverse responses to medications occur, the health care provider discontinues the medication immediately. Health care providers report ADEs to the U.S. Food and Drug Administration (FDA) using the Med-Watch program (FDA, 2014).

Toxic Effects

Toxic medication effects develop after prolonged intake of high doses of medication, after ingestion of drugs intended for external application, or when a drug builds up in the blood because of impaired metabolism or excretion. Toxic effects may be lethal, depending on the action of a drug. For example, morphine, an opioid analgesic, relieves pain by depressing the central nervous system. However, toxic levels of morphine cause severe respiratory depression and death.

Idiosyncratic Reactions

An idiosyncratic reaction is an unpredictable overreaction or underreaction to a drug. Predicting which patients will have an idiosyncratic response is impossible. For example, lorazepam (Ativan), an antianxiety medication, when given to an older adult may worsen anxiety and cause agitation and delirium.

Allergic Reactions

Allergic reactions are also unpredictable responses to medications. Taking a medication the first time may cause an immunological response. When this response occurs, the drug acts as an antigen, causing the production of antibodies. With repeated administration of the medication, the patient develops an allergic response to the drug, its chemical preservatives, or a metabolite of it.

The antibodies create a mild or severe reaction, depending on the patient and the drug. Among the different classes of drugs, antibiotics cause a high incidence of allergic reactions. Table 21-1 summarizes common allergy symptoms. Severe,

TABLE 21-1	COMMON ALLERGIC REACTIONS
SYMPTOM	**DESCRIPTION**
Angioedema	Acute, painless, dermal, subcutaneous, or submucosal swelling involving the face, neck, lips, larynx, hands, feet, or genitalia
Eczema (rash)	Small, raised vesicles that are usually reddened; often distributed over the entire body
Pruritus	Itching of the skin; accompanies most rashes
Rhinitis	Inflammation of mucous membranes lining the nose, causing swelling and clear watery discharge
Urticaria (hives)	Raised, irregularly shaped skin eruptions with varying sizes and shapes; eruptions have reddened margins and pale centers
Wheezing	Constriction of smooth muscles surrounding bronchioles that decreases diameter of airways; occurs primarily on expiration because of severely narrowed airways; development of edema in pharynx and larynx further obstructs airflow

or anaphylactic, reactions are characterized by sudden constriction of bronchiolar muscles, edema of the pharynx and larynx, and severe wheezing and shortness of breath. The patient may become severely hypotensive, necessitating emergency resuscitation measures.

It is common practice for hospitalized patients with known drug allergies to have their allergy information recorded in a clearly identifiable place; this allows all caregivers to be aware of the patient's allergies. In many facilities, this information is recorded on the front of the patient's medical record on a brightly colored sticker. The patient also wears a wristband that contains the name of the medications to which he or she is allergic. Patient allergies must be recorded on the patient's medication administration record (MAR). Patients cared for in other settings (e.g., home) and who have a known history of an allergy to a medication should wear an identification bracelet or medal that alerts all health care providers to the allergy in case the patient is unconscious when receiving medical care.

Medication Interactions

When one medication modifies the action of another, a medication interaction occurs. A medication can enhance or reduce the action of other medications and alter the way in which the body absorbs, metabolizes, or eliminates the drug. When two drugs have a synergistic effect, the effect of the two medications combined is greater than the effect of one drug given separately. For example, alcohol is a central nervous system depressant that has a synergistic effect with antihistamines, antidepressants, and opioid analgesics.

A drug interaction may be desirable. Often a health care provider orders combination drug therapy to create a drug interaction for therapeutic benefit. For example, a patient with moderate hypertension may receive several drugs such as diuretics and vasodilators, which act together to keep blood pressure at a desirable level.

Medication Tolerance and Dependence

Medication tolerance occurs over time. A patient receives the same medication for long periods of time and then requires higher doses to produce the same desired effect. Patients taking various pain medications may develop tolerance over time. It may take a month or longer for tolerance to occur.

Medication tolerance is not the same as medication dependence. Two types of medication dependence exist: psychological (or addiction) and physical. In psychological dependence, the patient desires the medication for a benefit other than the intended effect. Physical dependence implies that a patient will suffer withdrawal effects if the medication is stopped abruptly. When patients receive medications for a short time, such as for postoperative pain, dependence is rare.

Medication Misuse

Misuse of medication includes overuse, underuse, and nonadherence. Patients of all ages misuse medications. Older adults are at greatest risk because of polypharmacy. The incidence of prescription and over-the-counter (OTC) drug misuse and abuse is also increasing. The most commonly abused prescription medications are opioids, stimulants, tranquilizers, and sedatives (Formulary Watch, 2010; Traynor, 2013). You are ethically and legally responsible to understand the problems of persons using medications improperly. When caring for patients with suspected medication abuse or dependence, be aware of your values and attitudes about the willful use of harmful substances. Do not let your personal values interfere with understanding a patient's needs and concerns.

ADMINISTERING MEDICATIONS

Nursing Skills Online: Safe Medication Administration Module, Lesson 1

You are not solely responsible for medication administration. The health care provider and pharmacist also help to ensure that the right medication gets to the right patient. You are accountable for knowing what medications are ordered, understanding their therapeutic effects, recognizing undesired effects, and administering medications correctly.

Medication Orders

A health care provider's order is required for all medications to be administered by a nurse (except in states where Nurse Practice Acts allows advanced practice nurses and nurse practitioners to prescribe). A health care provider's order sheet is in written or electronic form. The health care provider writes the date, time, and medication order, including:

1. The name of the medication, which may be either the trade name (e.g., Percocet) or the generic name (e.g., oxycodone)
2. The dose (e.g., 5 mg)
3. The route (e.g., by mouth [PO])
4. The frequency (e.g., every 4 hours [q4h])
5. Orders for medications to be given prn (as needed) also include the reason they are to be given (e.g., for pain)
6. The signature of the health care provider

Verbal and telephone orders are optional forms of orders when written or electronic communication between a health care provider and nurse is not possible. Student nurses cannot accept verbal or telephone orders. When a nurse receives a verbal or telephone order, he or she enters the order on the health care provider's order sheet. The name of the health care provider and the nurse's signature are included. The health care provider countersigns the order at a later time, usually within 24 hours after making the order (see facility policy). Box 21-2 provides guidelines for safely taking verbal or telephone orders for medications.

There are five common types of medication orders. The type of order is based on the frequency or urgency of medication administration.

You carry out a *standing order* until the health care provider cancels it by another order or until a prescribed number of days elapse. A standing order sometimes indicates a final date or number of doses. Many facilities have a policy for automatically discontinuing standard orders.

A health care provider may order a medication to be given only when a patient requires or requests it. This is a *prn* order. As a nurse, you assess a patient thoroughly to determine whether the patient needs the medication, based on the indication for the drug (e.g., pain or nausea). Sometimes a different type of therapy is more appropriate. A prn order usually has minimum intervals set for the time of administration. This means that you cannot give the drug any more frequently than what is prescribed.

BOX 21-2 GUIDELINES FOR TELEPHONE ORDERS AND VERBAL ORDERS

- Only authorized staff receives and record telephone or verbal orders. Facility identifies in writing the staff that are authorized.
- Clearly identify patient's name, room number, and diagnosis.
- Read back all orders to health care provider (TJC, 2014).
- Use clarification questions to avoid misunderstandings.
- Write "TO" (telephone order) or "VO" (verbal order), including date and time, name of patient, and complete order; sign the name of the health care provider and nurse.
- Follow facility policies; some facilities require documentation of the "read-back" or require two nurses to review and sign telephone or verbal orders.
- Health care provider co-signs the order within the time frame required by the facility (usually 24 hours; verify facility policy).

Single (one-time) orders are common for preoperative medications or medications given before diagnostic examinations. The medication is ordered to be given only once at a specified time. A *stat* order means that you give a single dose of a medication immediately and only once. Stat orders are used for emergencies when a patient's condition changes suddenly. A *now order* is more specific than a one-time order. It is used when a patient needs a medication quickly but not as soon as a stat order. When you receive a now order, you have up to 90 minutes to give the drug (see facility policy).

Although The Joint Commission allows the use of range orders, there continue to be concerns about providing enough guidance to nurses, while still allowing them to address the individual needs of patients. An example of a poorly written range order is "give morphine sulfate 2 to 6 mg IV push every 4h prn for pain." This order is not specific with regard to guidelines needed to give a correct dose. A range order must provide objective measures for nurses to use to determine the correct dose. An example of a good order is "give Lortab 1-2 q 4 hours prn pain. For pain 1-5, 1 tab; for pain 5-10, 2 tabs." A range order should include specific indications (e.g., pain rating score, temperature level) especially for use of a medication indicated for more than one reason (e.g., ibuprofen, which could be indicated for pain or fever) (Rosier, 2012).

Communication and Transcription of Orders

After new medication orders are entered into a computer or written, the drugs must be obtained from the pharmacy. A health care provider's order is transmitted to the pharmacy automatically through the use of the electronic health record, but in the case of a written system, copies of orders are sent. Before updating medication orders, pharmacists assess the medication plan and ensure that orders are valid. The pharmacist is responsible for preparing the correct medications and delivering them to the nursing unit where they are stocked in a medication administration station.

Medication Errors

The Joint Commission (2014) defines a medication error as any preventable event that may cause inappropriate medication use or jeopardize patient safety. Medication errors include inaccurate prescribing; administration of the wrong medication, route, and time interval; and administering extra doses or failing to administer a medication. Hospital medication delivery systems have a system of checks, such as warning notifications, that help prevent medication errors. *Conscientious adherence to the six rights of medication administration is your best way to prevent errors.* See Box 21-3.

Many medication errors occur when nurses become distracted or lose focus during preparation and administration of medications. Errors also occur when nurses do not follow best-practice protocols and procedures related to medication administration. Research reveals that nurses are interrupted 10 times per hour or every six minutes (Speroni et al., 2013). Areas where nurses prepare medications are highly visible locations with high levels of staff traffic. Nurses become interrupted while accessing dispensing systems, depositing

<table>
<tr><td colspan="2" style="background:#2e7d4f;color:white">BOX 21-3   STEPS TO PREVENT MEDICATION ERRORS</td></tr>
<tr><td>
<ul>
<li>Prepare medications for only one patient at a time.</li>
<li>Follow the six rights of medication administration.</li>
<li>Read labels at least 3 times (comparing MAR with label) before administering a medication.</li>
<li>Do not allow anyone or anything to interrupt your administration of medication (e.g., phone call, pager, discussions with staff).</li>
<li>Double-check all calculations and verify with another nurse.</li>
<li>Use at least two patient identifiers every time you administer a medication.</li>
<li>Do not interpret illegible handwriting; clarify with health care provider.</li>
<li>Question unusually large or small doses.</li>
<li>Document all medications as soon as they are given.</li>
<li>When you have made an error, reflect on what went wrong; ask how you could have prevented the error. Complete an occurrence report per facility policy.</li>
<li>Learn as much as you can about each medication you administer. Attend in-service programs that focus on the medications you commonly administer.</li>
<li>Follow facility policies and protocols during medication administration; do not take short cuts.</li>
</ul>
</td></tr>
</table>

medications into delivery containers, and confirming orders on computer screens. Work related interruptions and distractions have been identified as questions from staff or family, equipment alarms, and personal conversations (Speroni et al., 2013; Trbovich et al., 2010). Follow these tips:

- Reduce distractions (e.g., turn off pager) and interruptions around automated medication dispensing machines (Anderson and Townsend, 2010).
- In areas where medications are being prepared, use a brightly colored sign to alert staff to avoid interruptions (e.g., discussions).

When an error occurs, acknowledge it immediately, and then assess the patient. You have an ethical and professional obligation to report an error to the patient's health care provider, the nurse manager, and any other persons indicated by the facility policy regarding errors. Appropriate follow-up may include administering an antidote, withholding a subsequent dose, and monitoring the effects of the medication. A patient's medical record should include a notation that indicates what was given, who was notified, the observed effects of the medication, and follow-up measures taken.

You are also responsible for completing a report describing the incident. Most facilities have a policy or protocol for reporting adverse events. This report provides an objective analysis of what went wrong. It provides information for the risk management team to identify factors contributing to errors and develop ways to avoid similar errors in the future.

DISTRIBUTION SYSTEMS

Systems for storing and distributing medications vary. Facilities providing nursing care have special areas for stocking and dispensing medications. Medication storage areas must be locked when unattended.

Unit-Dose System

The standard for medication distribution is the unit-dose system. The system uses an automatic medication dispensing system (AMDS) or a cart containing a drawer with a 24-hour supply of medications for each patient (Fig. 21-2). Each drawer has a label with the name of the patient in each designated room. The unit dose is the ordered dose of medication that the patient receives at one time. Each medication form is wrapped separately. A cart also contains limited amounts of prn and stock medications for special situations. A medication cart can be pushed from room to room to facilitate administration of medications at routine times. The cart is kept locked when not attended. In some settings, medications are kept in a locked cabinet in patient rooms.

Automated Medication Dispensing Systems

Automated medication dispensing systems (AMDS) within a health care facility are networked with each other and with other computer systems in the facility (e.g., the computerized medical record). AMDS control the dispensing of all medications, including narcotics. Each nurse has a personal security code, allowing access to the system. If your facility uses a system that requires bioidentification, you have to place your finger on a screen to access the computer. Once logged onto the AMDS, you select the patient's name and medication profile. Then you select the medication, dosage, and route from a list on the computer screen. The system opens the medication drawer or dispenses the medication to the nurse, records the event, and charges it to the patient. If the system is connected to the patient's medical record, information about the medication (e.g., name, dose, time) and the name of the nurse who retrieved the medication from the AMDS is recorded in the patient's medical record. Some systems require nurses to scan bar codes before recording this information in the patient's computerized medical record. AMDS and bar code scanning improve accuracy of patient identification, correct medication administration, and medical record

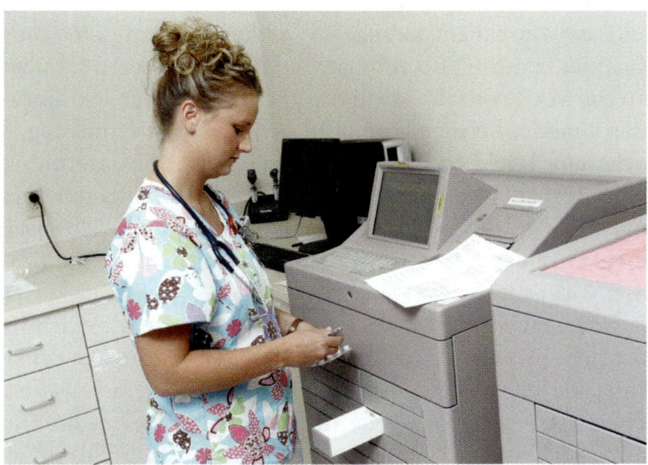

FIG 21-2 Automated medication dispensing system.

keeping, reducing the chance of medication errors (Mandrack et al., 2012; Poon et al., 2010).

MEDICATION ADMINISTRATION RECORD

The medication administration record (MAR) is a form used to verify that the right medications are being administered at the correct times. The process of verification of medications varies among health care facilities. During the transcription process, the nurse and pharmacist check all medication orders for accuracy and thoroughness several times, and the health care provider's complete order is placed on the appropriate MAR. The MAR includes the patient's name, room, and bed number and the names, doses, frequencies, and routes of administration for each medication. Most health care facilities have computers to generate and display electronic MARs. If the MAR is handwritten, a registered nurse (RN) completes or updates the MAR routinely. Nurses record medications administered on the MAR. In many facilities, computer stations in patient rooms allow for easy accessible entry.

Regardless of the type of MAR your facility uses, be sure that you refer to the MAR each time you prepare a medication and have the MAR available at the patient's bedside when administering medications. It is essential that you verify the accuracy of every medication you give to the patient with the patient's orders. If the medication order is incomplete, incorrect, or inappropriate or if there is a discrepancy between the written order and what is on the MAR, consult with the health care provider. Do not give a medication until you are certain that you are able to follow the six rights of medication administration. When you give the wrong medication or an incorrect dose, *you* are legally responsible for the error.

SIX RIGHTS OF MEDICATION ADMINISTRATION

Preparing and administering medications require accuracy and your full attention. To ensure safe medication administration, be aware of the six rights of medication administration.

Right Medication

The Joint Commission includes medication reconciliation as a national patient safety goal for 2014 (TJC, 2014). When a patient enters a hospital setting, a complete list of the patient's current medications must be reviewed and documented with the patient involved. You will compare the medications health care providers order with medications on a patient's list. When the patient is transferred to another service or health care setting, you again must reconcile the patient's current list of medications. The goal of medication reconciliation is to ensure one list of medications and to address or correct any discrepancies before discharge from the health care setting (TJC, 2014).

In 2004, The Joint Commission created its "do not use" list of abbreviations (Table 21-2) as part of the requirements for meeting a National Safety Goal set in 2001. The list of

TABLE 21-2	**PROHIBITED AND ERROR-PRONE ABBREVIATIONS***	
DO NOT USE	**PROBLEM**	**USE INSTEAD**
U (unit) or u	Mistaken for "0" (zero), the number "4" (four), or "cc"	Write "unit"
IU (international unit)	Mistaken for IV (intravenous), the number 10 (ten), or unit	Write "international unit"
q.d. or QD (daily)	Mistaken for qid	Write "daily"
Q.O.D., QOD, q.o.d., qod (every other day)	Mistaken for qd (daily) or qid (4 times daily) if "o" is poorly written	Write "every other day"
Trailing zero (e.g., 1.0 mg)†	Decimal point is missed	Write X mg (e.g., 1 mg)
Lack of leading zero (e.g., .1 mg)	Decimal point is missed	Write 0.X mg (e.g., 0.1 mg)
MS	Can mean morphine sulfate or magnesium sulfate	Write "morphine sulfate" or write "magnesium sulfate"
MSO_4 and $MgSO_4$	Confused for one another	Write "morphine sulfate" or write "magnesium sulfate"

*Applies to all orders and medication-related documentation that is handwritten (including free-text computer entry or on preprinted forms).
†Exception: A "trailing zero" may be used only where required to show precision of a reported value (e.g., laboratory test results), studies that report the size of lesions, or catheter and tube sizes. A "trailing zero" cannot be used in medication orders or medication-related documentation (ISMP, 2013; reprinted with permission).
From The Joint Commission (TJC): Facts about the Official "Do Not Use" List of Abbreviations, 2014, http://www .jointcommission.org/topics/patient_safety.aspx. Accessed February 2014.

unacceptable abbreviations contains abbreviations that have been found to increase the incidence of errors in medication administration. You are responsible for using correct abbreviations and verifying that an order was accurately transcribed. Electronic medical records using CPOE are now incorporating the "do not use" abbreviations. Many facilities have a policy that requires nurses on a specific shift to verify the accuracy of MAR forms printed for each patient each day. Whenever new orders are handwritten on the MAR, the nurse adding the orders must verify that they are added accurately. When verification is complete, you initial and sign the order.

During medication administration, you compare a health care provider's order with the MAR when a medication is ordered initially. Nurses verify information whenever new MARs are written or distributed or when patients transfer from one nursing unit to another or a different health care setting. At the time of medication administration, you compare the label of a medication (Fig. 21-3) with the MAR three times: (1) when removing the medication from the storage bin, (2) before placing the medication in the medicine cup or before taking the medication to the patient's room, and (3) again at the bedside before giving the medication to the patient. If the medication is ordered by trade name and dispensed from the pharmacy by generic name, verify that there is no discrepancy.

If a patient questions a medication, stop and recheck to be certain that there is no mistake. In most cases, the medication order has been changed. Never give a medication until you investigate the patient's concerns and recheck it against the health care provider's order. Attention to a patient's question is how errors are identified and prevented.

Right Dose

The unit-dose system is designed to minimize errors. When a medication is prepared from a larger volume or strength than needed or when the health care provider's orders a system of measurement different from that which the pharmacist supplies, the chance of error increases. After calculating a dose of a high-risk medication such as insulin or warfarin (Coumadin), compare the calculation with one done independently by a second nurse. This verification is especially important if it is an unusual calculation or involves a potentially toxic drug.

After calculating dosages, prepare the medication using standard measurement devices. Use graduated cups, syringes, and scaled droppers. At home, teach patients to use kitchen measuring spoons rather than household teaspoons and tablespoons, which vary in volume. Key principles to observe for preparing medications are reviewed in Chapter 22.

Right Patient

Before administering a medication, identify the patient using two patient identifiers, such as the patient's name or hospital account number. The patient's room number or his or her physical complaint cannot be used as identifiers (TJC, 2014). Check the MAR against the patient's identification bracelet, and ask the patient to state his or her full name. In some facilities, a nurse also compares the medical record number on the MAR with the identification bracelet. If an identification bracelet becomes smudged or illegible or is missing, a new one should be obtained for the patient. In health care settings that are not acute care, The Joint Commission does not require use of armbands for identification. However, there must be a system in place to verify a patient's identification with at least two identifiers.

Some facilities use a wireless bar code scanner to identify the right patient. This system requires you to scan a personal bar code that is commonly placed on your name tag first. Then you scan a bar code on the single-dose medication package. Finally, you scan the patient's armband. This information is stored in a computer for documentation purposes.

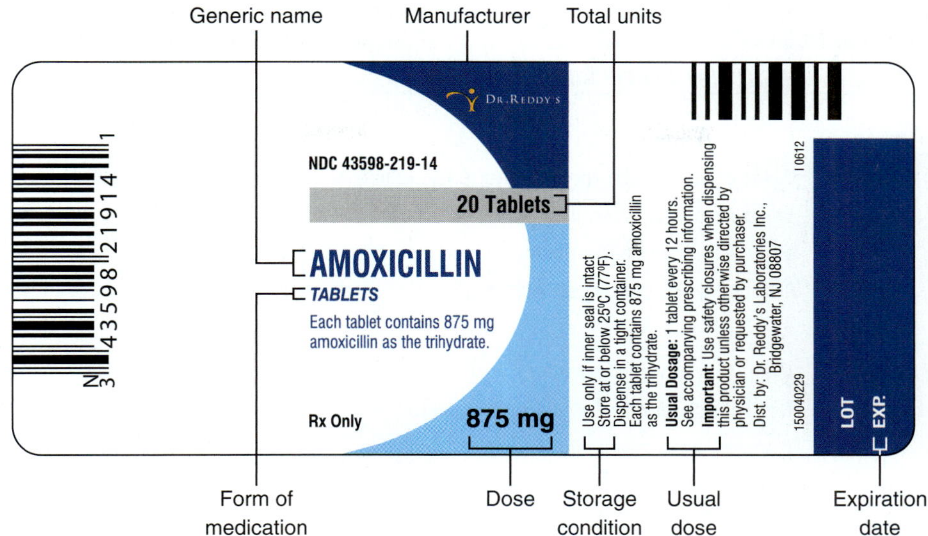

FIG 21-3 Interpreting a medication label. (Courtesy Dr. Reddy's Laboratories, Inc.)

This system helps eliminate medication errors because it provides another step to ensure that the right patient receives the right medication (Glover, 2013).

Right Route

The health care provider's order must designate a route of administration (Table 21-3). If the route of administration is missing or if the specified route is not the recommended route, you must consult the health care provider immediately. Evidence shows that medication errors involving the wrong route are common (Teunissen et al., 2013). When oral medications are prepared in syringes, there is a risk of giving the medication through the parenteral route. When injections are administered, use only preparations intended for parenteral use. Injection of a liquid intended for oral use can produce local complications such as sterile abscess or fatal systemic effects. Medication companies label parenteral medications "for injectable use only."

Right Time

Safe medication administration involves adherence to prescribed doses and dosage schedules. Some facilities set schedules for medication administration. For example, medications to be given three times a day (tid) may be routinely scheduled for 0800, 1400, and 2000 or 0900, 1300, and 1900, depending on facility policy. Nurses are able to alter this schedule based on knowledge about a medication. For example, a medication ordered for once a day might typically be given at 9:00 A.M., but if the medication works best for a patient at bedtime, the nurse can administer it before the patient goes to sleep. Acute care settings use guidelines from the ISMP and Centers for Medicaid and Medicare Services (CMS, 2011; ISMP, 2011) to determine safe, effective, and timely administration of scheduled medications.

According to ISMP (2011) and CMS (2011) guidelines, hospitals need to determine which medications are not eligible for scheduled dosing times and must be given at precise times (e.g., stat doses or first-time loading doses). In addition, hospitals must determine which medications are time-critical scheduled and which are non–time-critical scheduled. With time-critical medications (e.g., antibiotics, insulin, anticoagulants), early or delayed administration of maintenance doses of more than 20 minutes before or after the scheduled dose will most likely cause harm or result in subtherapeutic responses in a patient. Non–time-critical medications (e.g., stool softeners, vitamins) include medications in which the timing of administration most likely will not affect the desired effect of the medication if the drug is given 1 to 2 hours before or after its scheduled time. You administer time-critical scheduled medications at a precise time or within 30 minutes before or after the scheduled time. You administer non–time-critical medications within 1 to 2 hours of their scheduled time.

A medication may be ordered for special circumstances. A preoperative medication may be ordered stat (to be given immediately); now, which means as soon as available, usually within an hour; or on call, which means that the operating or procedure room personnel will notify the nurse when it is the appropriate time. A drug may be ordered before meals (ac) or after meals (pc).

Give priority to medications that must act at certain times. For example, give insulin at a precise interval before a meal. Give antibiotics on time around the clock to maintain therapeutic blood levels.

Right Documentation

To ensure the right documentation, first make sure that the information on your patient's MAR corresponds exactly with the health care provider's order and the label on the medication container. Do not give medications that have incomplete or illegible orders. Verify inaccurate orders before giving medications. It is better to give the correct medication at a later time than to give your patient the wrong medication. Record the administration of each medication on the MAR

TABLE 21-3   FORMS OF MEDICATION BY ROUTE OF ADMINISTRATION

ROUTE	DESCRIPTION OF MEDICATION
Oral	
Solid Forms	
Caplet	Solid dosage form for oral use; shaped like a capsule and coated for ease of swallowing
Capsule	Medication encased in a gelatin shell
Tablet	Powdered medication compressed into hard disk or cylinder
Enteric-coated	Tablet that is coated so that it does not dissolve in stomach; meant for intestinal absorption
Liquid Forms	
Elixir	Clear fluid containing water and alcohol; designed for oral use; usually has sweetener added
Syrup	Medication dissolved in a concentrated sugar solution
Extract	Concentrated medication form made by removing the active portion of medication from its other components
Aqueous solution	Substance dissolved in water and syrups
Other Oral Forms	
Troche (lozenge)	Flat, round dosage form containing medication that dissolves in mouth; not meant for ingestion
Aerosol	Aqueous medication sprayed and absorbed in mouth and upper airway; not meant for ingestion
Topical	
Ointment (salve or cream)	Semisolid, externally applied preparation, usually containing one or more medications
Lotion	Semiliquid suspension often used to cool, protect, or clean skin
Transdermal patch	Medicated disk or patch absorbed through the skin over a designated period of time (e.g., 24 hours)
Parenteral	
Solution	Sterile preparation that contains water with one or more dissolved compounds
Powder	Sterile particles of medication that are dissolved in a sterile solution (e.g., water, normal saline) before administration
Body Cavity	
Intraocular disk	Medicated disk (similar to a contact lens) that is inserted into the patient's eye; medication absorbed over a designated period of time
Suppository	Solid dosage form mixed with gelatin and shaped in the form of a pellet for insertion into a body cavity (rectum or vagina); melts when it reaches body temperature, allowing medication to be absorbed

as soon as you give it. Never document that you have given a medication until you have actually given it. Document the name of the medication, the dose, the time of administration, and the route. Also document the site of any injections you give. Document the patient's response to the medication in the nurses' notes.

MEDICATION PREPARATION

It is legally advisable to administer only the medications that you prepare. Administering a medication prepared by another nurse increases the opportunity for error. The nurse who gives the wrong medication or an incorrect dose is legally responsible for the error. The importance of checking similar patient names and verifying for the correct drug cannot be overemphasized.

Interpreting Medication Labels

Medication labels include several basic pieces of information: the trade name of the drug in large letters, the generic name in smaller letters, the form of the drug, the dosage, the expiration date, the lot number, and the name of the manufacturer. The trade name given by the manufacturer often suggests the action of the drug, and the generic name is the chemical name (see Fig. 21-3).

Dosage Calculations

To administer medications safely, use your mathematics skills to calculate medication dosages and mix solutions. The ability to calculate doses safely is important because you will not always dispense medications in the unit of measure in which they are ordered. Medication companies package and bottle certain standard equivalents. For example, a patient's health care provider orders 250 mg of a medication that is available only in grams. You are responsible for converting available units of volume and weight to the desired doses. Be aware of approximate equivalents in all major measurement systems and use conversion tables. An example follows:

The order reads: vancomycin (Vancocin) 1 g IV.

The pharmacy supplies vancomycin in 500-mg vials.

Because the dose on the medication label is in milligrams, conversion should be from grams to milligrams; 1 g = 1000 mg.

Systems of Measurement

The proper administration of medication depends on your ability to compute drug dosages accurately and measure medications correctly. A careless mistake in placing a decimal point or adding a zero to a dosage can lead to a fatal error. The health care provider and patient depend on you to check the dosage before giving a drug. The metric system is the most common system used in the measurement of medications.

Metric System

As a decimal system, the metric system is the most logically organized of the measurement systems. Each basic unit of measure is organized into units of 10. Multiplying or dividing by 10 forms secondary units. In multiplication, the decimal point moves to the right; in division, the decimal moves to the left. To convert grams to milligrams you multiply by 1000 or move the decimal point three places to the right (0.5 g = 500 mg). Conversely, to convert milligrams to grams, you divide by 1000 or move the decimal point three places to the left (500 mg = 0.5 g).

The basic units of measure in the metric system are the meter (length), liter (volume), and gram (weight). For drug calculations, you will use primarily volume and weight units. In the metric system, small or large letters designate the basic units:

Gram: g or gm

Liter: l or L

Small letters are abbreviations for subdivisions of major units:

Milligram: mg

Milliliter: mL

Household Measurements

Household measures are familiar to most people, but these measures are not recommended for medication administration because of the variability in the size of household utensils. Included in household measures are drops, teaspoons, tablespoons, and cups for volume and ounces and pounds for weight. Before the actual administration of medication, you may need to convert units within a system or between systems and calculate drug dosages (Table 21-4).

Solutions

Solutions are used for injections, irrigations, and infusions. A solution is a given mass of solid substance dissolved in a known volume of fluid or a given volume of liquid dissolved

TABLE 21-4	EQUIVALENTS OF MEASUREMENT	
METRIC	**HOUSEHOLD**
1 mL	15 drops (gtt)
5 mL	1 teaspoon (tsp)
15 mL	1 tablespoon (tbsp)
30 mL	2 tablespoons (tbsp)
240 mL	1 cup (c)
480 mL (approximately 500 mL)	1 pint (pt)
960 mL (approximately 1 L)	1 quart (qt)
3785 mL (approximately 4 L)	1 gallon (gal)

BOX 21-4 FORMULA METHOD

$$\frac{D}{H} \times V = \text{Amount to give}$$

D is the desired dose or the dose ordered by the health care provider for the patient (e.g., 250 mg of penicillin PO 4 times daily).

H is the drug dose on hand or available for use. The dose is on the drug label (e.g., penicillin tablets of 250 mg each).

V is the volume (liquid) or vehicle (number of tablets, capsules) that delivers the available dose (e.g., 1 tablet).

Note: The desired dose **(D)** and the on-hand dose **(H)** must be in the same unit of measurement. If they are in different units, you must perform conversions before completing the formula.

---

in a known volume of another fluid. Solutions are available in units of mass per units of volume (e.g., g/mL, g/L). You can also express a concentration of a solution as a percentage. A 10% solution is 10 g of solid dissolved in 100 mL of solution.

Dosage Calculations

Dosage calculations are necessary when the dose on the medication label differs from the dosage ordered. There are several dosage calculation methods, including formula (Box 21-4) and dimensional analysis (Box 21-5). Dimensional analysis is a method for dosage calculation that involves simple multiplication and division and not algebra.

Example 1

When the dose ordered has the same label as the dose available:

Dose ordered: 0.5 g

Tablets available: 0.25 g per tablet

Step 1. The starting factor is 0.5 g.

The answer label is tablets (i.e., how many tablets should be given).

Step 2. Formulate the conversion equation:

The equivalent needed is 1 tablet = 0.25 g.

$$\frac{0.5\,g}{1} \times \frac{1\,tab}{0.25\,g} = tabs$$

BOX 21-5   DIMENSIONAL ANALYSIS

Follow these steps to solve medication problems using dimensional analysis:

1. Identify the unit of measure that you need to administer. For example, if you are giving a pill, you will usually be giving a tablet or a capsule; for parenteral or oral medications, the unit is milliliters.
2. Estimate the answer in your mind.
3. Place the name or appropriate abbreviation for x on the left side of the equation (e.g., x tab, x mL).
4. Place available information from the problem in a fraction format on the right side of the equation. Place the abbreviation or unit that matches what you are going to administer (determined in Step 1) in the numerator.
5. Look at the medication order and add other factors into the problem. Set up the numerator so that it matches the unit in the previous denominator.
6. Cancel out like units of measurement on the right side of the equation. You should end up with only one unit left in the equation, and it should match the unit on the left side of the equation.
7. Reduce to the lowest terms if possible and solve the problem or solve for x. Label your answer.
8. Compare your estimate from Step 1 with your answer in Step 2.

Cancel labels (g).

    Note: If properly written, all labels except the answer label will cancel.

Step 3. Solve the equation: Reduce the numerical values, and multiply the numerators and denominators.

$$\frac{^{2}\cancel{0.5\,g}}{1} \times \frac{1\ tab}{\cancel{0.25\,g}} = 2\ tabs$$

Example 2

When the dose ordered has a different label than the dose available:

    Dose ordered: 0.5 g

    Tablets available: 250 mg per tablet

Step 1. The starting factor is 0.5 g.

    The answer label is tablets (i.e., how many tablets should be given).

Step 2. Formulate the conversion equation:

    The equivalents needed are 1 g = 1000 mg and 1 tab = 250 mg.

$$\frac{0.5\,g}{1} \times \frac{1000\,mg}{1\,g} \times \frac{1\,tab}{250\,mg} = tabs$$

    Cancel labels (g, mg).

Step 3. Solve the equation:

    Reduce the values and multiply the numerators and denominators.

$$\cancel{0.5\,g} \times \frac{^{4}\cancel{1000\,mg}}{\cancel{1\,g}\ _{2}} \times \frac{1\,tab}{\cancel{250\,mg}} = \frac{4}{2} = 2\ tabs$$

Example 3

When the dose ordered is available in a liquid form:

    Dose ordered: Cephalexin (Keflex) 250 mg PO

    Available: 125 mg per 5 mL

Step 1. The starting factor is 250 mg.

    The answer label is mL.

Step 2. Formulate the conversion equation:

    The equivalent needed is 125 mg = 5 mL.

$$\frac{250\,mg}{1} \times \frac{5\,mL}{125\,mg} = mL$$

    Cancel labels (mg).

Step 3. Solve the equation:

    Reduce and multiply.

$$\frac{^{2}\cancel{250\,mg}}{1} \times \frac{5\,mL}{\cancel{125\,mg}} = 10\ mL$$

NURSING PROCESS

Applying the nursing process to medication administration ensures that you use critical thinking and clinical judgment. As a nurse, your role extends beyond simply giving drugs to a patient. You are responsible for monitoring patients' responses to medications; providing education to the patient and family about the medication regimen; and informing the health care provider when medications are effective, ineffective, or no longer necessary.

Assessment

Begin your assessment by reviewing a patient's medical history and performing a focused physical assessment (for obvious problems); this will yield information about any indications or contraindications for medication therapy. Certain diseases or illnesses place patients at risk for adverse medication effects. For example, if a patient has a gastric ulcer, forms of aspirin increase the chance of bleeding. Long-term health problems require specific medications. This knowledge helps you anticipate the medications that your patient requires.

    Include an assessment of patient allergies. Determine if a patient has actual allergic reactions or drug intolerances, which are uncomfortable side effects. *Never give a patient a medication when there is a known allergy.* Many medications have ingredients found in food sources. For example, if your patient is allergic to shellfish, he or she may be sensitive to products containing iodine such as Betadine or dyes used in radiological testing. In an acute care setting, patients with allergies wear identification bands that list each medication allergy. All allergies and the types of reactions are noted on the patient's admission notes, medication records, and history and physical examination.

    Your assessment also involves identifying all medications that the patient takes every day at home, including prescriptions, over-the-counter (OTC) preparations, and herbal supplements. Determine how long the patient has taken each medication, the current dosage schedule, and whether the patient has had any adverse effects to any of the medications. The patient should know the name, purpose, dosage, route, and side effects of medications and supplements that are being taken. Often patients take many medications and carry a list that includes this information. Patients have different levels of understanding. One patient may describe a diuretic as a "water pill," whereas another may describe it as a drug to minimize swelling and lower blood pressure. Still another may describe it as "the little white pill I take in the morning." By assessing the patient's level of knowledge, you determine the need for teaching. If a patient is unable to understand or remember pertinent information, it may be necessary to involve a family member.

Complete appropriate assessments, which may include, but are not limited to, vital signs, laboratory data, or nature and severity of symptoms. If data contraindicate medication administration, hold the drug and notify the health care provider.

Planning

During planning, organize nursing activities to ensure the safe administration of medications. Current evidence shows that distractions or hurrying during medication preparation administration increases the risk of medication errors (Yoder and Schadewald, 2012). Suggestions to reduce distraction include signage identifying the medication administration area, development of a checklist that includes all the components of medication administration, an educational program for nursing staff, and wearing some identifying clothing (e.g., vest) when preparing medications (Yoder and Schadewald, 2012). The following are general goals of medication administration:
1. Patient achieves therapeutic effect of the prescribed medication.
2. Patient complications related to the prescribed medication are absent.
3. Patient and family caregivers understand medication therapy.
4. Patient and family caregivers administer medication safely (when appropriate).

Implementation

Nursing interventions for safe and effective drug administration include careful medication preparation, accurate and timely administration, and relevant patient education.

Preadministration Activities

1. Identify the medication action, purpose, side effects, and nursing implications for administering and monitoring. Ensure that the medication order has not expired.
2. Minimize distractions (e.g., discussion with staff, phone call, use of pager), close the door of medication room, and post "do not disturb" signage. Do not perform other tasks while preparing medications.
3. Make sure the information on the electronic MAR or printed MAR corresponds exactly with the health care provider's order and with the medication container label. Clarify orders that are unclear or illegible.

4. Calculate medication doses accurately, and use appropriate measuring devices. Verify that the dose prescribed is within a safe dosage range and is appropriate for the patient situation.
5. Take medications to patient at correct time (see six rights of medication administration), including time-critical and non–time-critical medications (see facility policy).
6. Review any preadministration assessments (e.g., vital signs, review laboratory test result).
7. Use thorough hand hygiene technique. Avoid touching tablets and capsules. Wear clean gloves if you are administering oral chemotherapy agents.
8. Use sterile technique for parenteral medications. Wear clean gloves when administering parenteral medications and certain topical medications.
9. Administer only medications that you personally prepare. Do not ask another nurse to administer medications that you prepare. Keep medications secure, and do not administer medications prepared by someone else.
10. When preparing medications, be sure that the label is clear and legible and that the drug is properly mixed; has not changed in color, clarity, or consistency; and has not expired.
11. Keep tablets and capsules in their wrappers and open them at the patient's bedside. This allows you to review each medication with the patient. If a patient refuses medication, there is no question about which one is withheld.

Drug Administration

1. Follow the *six rights* for medication administration.
2. Inform the patient of the name, purpose, action, and common side effects of each medication. Evaluate the patient's knowledge of the medication, and provide appropriate teaching using teach back technique.
3. Stay with the patient until the medication is taken. Provide assistance as necessary. Do not leave medication without a health care provider's order at the bedside. For example, some patients may take their own vitamins or birth control pills while in the hospital.
4. Respect the patient's right to refuse medication. If the medication wrapper is intact, the medication may be returned to the patient's storage bin. When medication is refused, determine the reason for this and take action accordingly. For example, if the patient has unpleasant side effects, it may be possible to eliminate them by giving the pills with food or using a different time schedule.

Postadministration Activities

1. Properly document medications administered (see six rights of medication administration).
2. Document data pertinent to a patient's response; this is especially important when giving drugs ordered prn. Include ability of patient and family caregiver to teach back the education provided.
3. If a medication is refused, document that it was not given, the reason for the refusal, and when the health care provider was notified.

Evaluation

1. Monitor for evidence of therapeutic effects, side effects, and adverse reactions. Monitor physical responses (e.g., heart rhythm, blood pressure, urine output).
2. When a medication is given for relief of symptoms, ask patient to report if symptoms have diminished or been relieved. In the case of pain, has severity lessened?
3. Observe injection sites for bruises, inflammation, localized pain, numbness, or bleeding.
4. Evaluate patient's understanding of medication therapy and ability to self-administer medication.

PATIENT AND FAMILY TEACHING

A well-informed patient is more likely to take medications correctly. However, many patients have limited health literacy, meaning that they have difficulty reading medication labels or calculating doses. Provide an individualized approach to teaching, using visual aids, instructional booklets, or videos. Involve the primary family caregiver when you teach patients about their medications; this may include family members, partners, or home care providers. Specific nursing interventions for educating about self-administration within the home setting are summarized in Box 21-6.

Teaching Patients About Side Effects

You are responsible for teaching a patient and family caregiver about possible side effects associated with each prescribed medication. If you do not inform the patient properly about medications or if your patients have problems with health literacy, it is possible that they will take their medications incorrectly or they will not take their medications at all. Because medications can have many side effects, teaching a patient about all of them can be overwhelming. Remember that patient learning is a continual process. When beginning to teach a patient about a new medication, evaluate each of the side effects. Then teach the patient about the ones that are most likely to occur and occur early after administration. For example, some antibiotics cause hypersensitivity reactions, hepatotoxicity, nephrotoxicity, and platelet dysfunction. Hypersensitivity reactions are likely to occur shortly after taking a few doses of an antibiotic. The other side effects tend to occur after long-term antibiotic administration. Teach patients about side effects in terms of things that they can see, feel, touch, or hear. For example, thrombocytopenia,

---

BOX 21-6   MEDICATION ADMINISTRATION IN HOME CARE

1. Assess all of the patient's prescription and nonprescription medications at each visit. Review information about medications, including desired effect, dose, frequency, adverse effects, and what to do if adverse effects develop.
2. Assess patient's health literacy. Adapt your instructional approach, have patient read a medication label or an instruction pamphlet to determine his or her ability to read and complete simple medication calculations. If health literacy is poor, present information at a level the patient can understand, and arrange for help from family, friends, or home health nurses.
3. Teach the complications and interactions of all food, OTC medications, and herbal medications to patients and family caregivers.
4. Collaborate with social workers to identify community resources for financial assistance with pharmaceutical needs.
5. Monitor and evaluate the effectiveness of the prescribed medications:
   a. Note changes in physical and functional status (e.g., vital signs, sleeping, elimination).
   b. Note changes in mental status (e.g., level of alertness, memory).
   c. Monitor blood levels as needed.
   d. Communicate potential problems to health care provider.
6. Monitor urinary output status of patients because changes in renal excretion may require a decrease or increase in medication dosage.
7. For patients who cannot remember when to take medications, make a chart that lists the times to take each medication or prepare a special container that organizes and stores medications according to days and times when the patient needs to take them.
8. Reduce the chance of medication error by labeling or color-coding medication bottles.
9. Keep an accurate record of a homebound patient's weight, especially an older adult patient, because many medication dosages are calculated by body weight.
10. Teach medication safety in the home environment:
    a. Keep medications in original, labeled containers. Read labels carefully and follow all instructions.
    b. Follow specific disposal instructions on the prescription drug label or patient information that comes with the medicine. *Do not flush* medicines down the sink or toilet unless this information specifically instructs you to do so. Have patients use community drug take-back programs that allow the public to bring unused drugs to a central location for proper disposal. If there are no disposal instructions on a prescription drug label and no take-back program is available, have patient throw the drugs in the household trash following these steps: (1) Remove drugs from their original containers and mix them with an undesirable substance, such as used coffee grounds or kitty litter. (2) Place the mixture in a sealable bag, empty can, or other container to prevent the drug from leaking or breaking out of a garbage bag (FDA, 2013).
11. Never "share" medications with friends or family members.
12. Always finish a prescribed medication; do not save it for a future illness.
13. Instruct patients with arthritis or debilitating illness who have difficulty opening child-proof containers to request non-childproof containers from their health care providers.

Data from Touhy T, Jett K: *Ebersole and Hess's gerontological nursing and healthy aging,* ed 4, St Louis, 2013, Mosby.

a reduction in the number of platelets in the blood, can be a medication side effect. The patient cannot see, feel, touch, or hear thrombocytopenia. However, thrombocytopenia can cause bleeding with petechiae visible on the skin. Teach the patient how to look for petechiae. Be sure to teach the patient what to do about side effects when they are discovered.

Patient's Activities of Daily Living

Evaluate a patient's activities of daily living and the effect they will have on his or her ability to comply with medication schedules. When medications are initiated in the acute care setting, they are often given around the clock. In the home, it may be unreasonable for patients to administer medications according to this schedule. In collaboration with the health care provider or the pharmacist, teach the patient and family caregiver how to adjust medication schedules to be compatible with the patient's lifestyle. Include what to do for missed doses.

Evaluating Teaching Effectiveness

Evaluating the effectiveness of teaching tells you if a patient understands the information needed to self-administer medications safely and correctly. One method of evaluating patient understanding is to create medication cards with the generic and trade names of the medication on the front of the card and all pertinent medication information on the back of the card. You can flash the card in front of the patient and ask him or her to read the names of the medication. Another method is to have patients read labels on prepared medications. Medication bottles often have fine print and are difficult to read for patients with impaired vision. If the patient correctly identifies the name of the medication, ask him or her the following questions:

- Why are you taking this medicine?
- How often do you take this medicine?
- What side effects can occur with this medicine?
- If this side effect occurs, what are you going to do about it?

Also, be sure to assess a patient's sensory, motor, and cognitive functions. Impairments may affect the patient's ability to self-administer medications safely (e.g., open pill containers, prepare a syringe). A family caregiver or home health aides may need to assist with medication administration. Many self-help devices are also available for purchase (e.g., pill boxes with times displayed and electronic dispensers).

SPECIAL HANDLING OF CONTROLLED SUBSTANCES

As a nurse, you are responsible for following legal regulations when administering controlled substances (medications with potential for abuse). Controlled substances must be properly stored to prevent diversion. Violations of the Controlled Substances Act may result in fines, imprisonment, and loss of license. Health care facilities have policies for the proper storage and distribution of controlled substances, including opioids (Box 21-7). Most facilities use computerized systems for medication access and distribution.

BOX 21-7   STORAGE AND ACCOUNTABILITY FOR CONTROLLED SUBSTANCES

- All controlled substances are stored in a securely locked, substantially constructed cabinet (i.e., automated medication dispensing system [AMDS] or safe) or a locked room.
- Authorized nurses carry a computer entry code for an AMDS or a set of keys.
- An inventory record is kept to record all controlled substances used, including patient's name, date, name of medication, and time of medication administration.
- Before any medication is removed from the cabinet, the number actually available is compared with the number indicated on the controlled substance record. If a discrepancy exists, it must be rectified before proceeding.
- If any part of a dose of a controlled substance is discarded, a second nurse witnesses disposal of the unused portion, and the record is signed by both nurses.
- At change of shift, one nurse going off duty counts all controlled substances with a nurse coming on duty. Both nurses sign the record to indicate that the count is correct. (Computerized storage has eliminated this process.)
- Discrepancies in controlled substance counts are reported immediately.

Handling Chemotherapy Medications

A common treatment for cancer is chemotherapy, antineoplastic drugs that act by killing cells that divide rapidly, one of the main properties of most cancer cells. Chemotherapy is administered in both IV and oral forms. Nurses must undergo certification to administer IV chemotherapy. However, oral chemotherapy is becoming more common and can be administered by any RN.

Oral chemotherapy has the same exposure risks to health care providers, patients, and their family caregivers as IV forms (Goodin et al., 2011). Physically touching a chemotherapy tablet is dangerous. Chemotherapy is highly toxic not only to cancer cells but also to normal cells. Chemotherapy drugs cause DNA damage leading to cell death or cell growth arrest. The damage to others may not be known for months or years because the injuries could include cancer, birth defects, or immune dysfunction. It is critical for health care providers, patients, and family caregivers to use proper protective techniques to avoid exposure to oral chemotherapy tablets.

A patient excretes chemotherapy chemicals through urine, stool, vomit, sweat, and saliva (ACS, 2013; Pharma Cycle, 2013). When patients self-administer chemotherapy at home, families should be warned of the dangers of exposure. For example, patients' toilets should be double-flushed after use, during and 48 hours after discontinuing chemotherapy (ACS, 2013). Toilets are a hazard for children and pets.

Accidental exposure to oral chemotherapeutic agents can occur during handling (i.e., unpacking, storage, handling, administration, and disposal) (Goodin et al., 2011). Guidelines for health care providers, patients, and family caregivers to handle these drugs safely and appropriately are essential:

- In health care facilities, cytotoxic agents should be stored in a designated area per the manufacturer's instructions and separate from noncytotoxic agents
- Use disposable gloves when preparing and handling chemotherapy medications and after handling any body secretions.
- Perform thorough hand hygiene before and after glove application.
- Do not crush, cut, or split chemotherapy drugs.
- Use separate equipment to prepare chemotherapy and regular medicines.
- All disposable protective clothing as well as any disposable materials used while handling oral chemotherapeutic agents should be disposed of as cytotoxic waste according to the local waste disposal regulatory guidelines.
- Patients and their family members should avoid deep kissing and sharing food or drinks because chemotherapy can be in saliva. Clean flatware and dishes thoroughly with soap and warm water and rinse well before washing a second time with other dishes.
- Any clothes or sheets that have body fluids on them should be washed in a washing machine—not by hand. Wash them twice in hot water with regular laundry detergent. Do not wash them with other clothes. If they cannot be washed right away, seal them in a plastic bag. (Guidelines are adapted from ACS, 2013; Goodin et al., 2011.)

SPECIAL CONSIDERATIONS

Pediatric

Children vary in age; weight; and ability to absorb, metabolize, and excrete medications. Children's doses are lower than doses for adults, and caution is needed in preparing medications. Medication may or may not be prepared and packaged in doses appropriate for children. Preparing appropriate doses often requires calculation based on body weight (Hockenberry and Wilson, 2013). A child's parents may be helpful in determining the best way to give a child medication.

Geriatric

Individuals older than age 65 are the largest users of prescription and OTC medication (Touhy and Jett, 2013). Because of the physiological changes associated with aging, nursing interventions are needed to promote safe and effective medication administration, including spacing medication times to not interfere with meals, substituting liquid preparation for solid form if the older adult has difficulty swallowing, or providing memory aids in large print. Always observe an older adult opening and preparing his or her medication safely. Be aware of the following patterns related to medication use:

- *Polypharmacy.* Polypharmacy involves taking two or more medications to treat the same illness, taking two or more medications from the same chemical class, or taking two or more medications with the same or similar actions to treat different illnesses (Touhy and Jett, 2013). Polypharmacy also occurs when a patient mixes nutritional supplements or herbal products with medications. To decrease the risks associated with polypharmacy, work with your patient's health care provider's to ensure that the patient's medication regimen is as simple as possible.
- *Self-prescribing.* Older adults often attempt to seek relief from a variety of problems with OTC preparations, folk medicines, and herbs.
- *Misuse of drugs.* Misuse by older adults includes overuse, underuse, erratic use, and contraindicated use.
- *Nonadherence.* Deliberate misuse of medication is considered to be nonadherence. Older adults alter doses because of ineffectiveness, unpleasant side effects, and lack of financial resources.

CRITICAL THINKING EXERCISES

Case Study

A 70-year-old patient was just admitted to the hospital with a medical diagnosis of heart failure. The patient is complaining of recently needing three pillows to sleep at night (orthopnea) and ankle swelling (peripheral edema). While reviewing his home medications, the nurse notes the patient takes five different medicines. One of his medication prescriptions, a diuretic (furosemide), is full, whereas his other medications are not. When the nurse probes further about the patient's medications, she discovers that the patient discontinued his diuretic about 2 weeks ago because it made him "get up all night to use the bathroom."

1. The patient says to the nurse, "I do not know what is wrong. I have been taking my medicines." What should the nurse address with the patient?

2. Which of the following factors should the nurse consider that might also affect the patient's adherence to taking the diuretic? Select all that apply.
    1. The patient's belief that the diuretic does not help him breathe
    2. Insurance coverage for his medications
    3. The patient's age
    4. Patient's ability to remember medication schedule

Review Questions

1. A nurse enters a medication room to prepare a patient's 10 A.M. ordered medications. The patient has three medicines ordered for 10 A.M. Which of the following increase the nurse's risk for making a medication error? Select all that apply.
   1. A nurse colleague entering the medication room asking about a health care provider order.
   2. One of the medications missing from the automatic dispensing cabinet.
   3. The nurse hoping to return to another patient who requires a new IV solution to be started.
   4. The use of a computer code to access the automatic dispensing cabinet.

2. The nurse uses a current drug index to look up a pain medication and finds that the onset of action of the drug is 30 minutes, it peaks in 60 minutes, and the duration of action is 3 hours. The patient asks the nurse to administer this medication so it will be most effective when the patient participates in a strenuous hour-long physical therapy session later in the day. When should the nurse give this medication to the patient?
   1. Stat
   2. 15 minutes before the physical therapy session
   3. 1 hour before the physical therapy session
   4. Just before the patient begins the physical therapy session

3. The nurse finds the following new medication order written in a patient's hospital chart: "3/17/09 0800 furosemide 40 mg twice a day." What should the nurse do first?
   1. Enter the order in the hospital computer
   2. Administer the medication
   3. Contact the health care provider
   4. Review the order with a pharmacist

4. A patient returns from an x-ray procedure at 10:30 A.M. and was due to receive a stool softener at 10 A.M. When should the nurse administer this drug?
   1. Immediately
   2. Within the next 90 minutes
   3. At 10 A.M. the next day
   4. The medication should be held and the health care provider contacted

5. A health care provider's order for a medication states: "Percocet (oxycodone/acetaminophen) 1 or 2 tabs BID and prn." The health care provider is very busy, does not like to be bothered, and is known for being difficult to work with. What should the nurse do?
   1. Consult a pharmacist to interpret the order.
   2. Call the health care provider and have the order verified.
   3. Administer the medication twice a day and as the patient needs.
   4. Talk to the unit secretary on the floor who is good at reading the health care provider's handwriting.

6. A patient has an order for 1 tbsp of Robitussin for a cough. Converting this to the metric system, what dose would the nurse give to the patient?
   1. 5 mL
   2. 10 mL
   3. 30 mL
   4. 15 mL

7. A patient is to receive Keflex (cephalexin), 500 mg PO. The drawer of the automated medication dispensing system opens. There are five tablets, each labeled 250 mg cephalexin in the drawer. What should the nurse give to the patient?
   1. ½ tablet
   2. 1 tablet
   3. 1½ tablets
   4. 2 tablets

8. A nurse has to give the following medications to her patients. To which patient should she give medications first? A patient who:
   1. Is to receive 325 mg of aspirin who has a history of coronary artery disease
   2. Needs 2 tablets of acetaminophen/hydrocodone (Vicodin) who is rating his incisional pain 8 on a pain scale of 0 to 10
   3. Is to get captopril (Capoten) 25 mg for a history of hypertension whose current blood pressure is 125/72 mm Hg
   4. Is receiving trimethoprim/sulfamethoxazole (Bactrim DS) for a urinary tract infection

9. The safe administration of a chemotherapy tablet requires a nurse to do which of the following? Select all that apply.
   1. Wear disposable gloves when preparing a tablet
   2. Perform thorough hand hygiene
   3. Crush a tablet and mix food to reduce difficulty swallowing the drug
   4. Dispose of any used medication cups or gloves in cytotoxic waste container

10. An older adult states that she cannot see her medication bottles clearly to determine when to take her prescription. What should the nurse do? Select all that apply.
    1. Provide a dispensing container for each day of the week.
    2. Provide larger, easier-to-read labels.
    3. Tell the patient what is in each container.
    4. Have a family caregiver administer the medication.

REFERENCES

American Cancer Society (ACS): *Chemotherapy principles: an in-depth discussion of the techniques and its role in cancer treatment*, 2013, http://www.cancer.org/acs/groups/cid/documents/webcontent/002995-pdf.pdf. Accessed February 2014.

Anderson P, Townsend T: Medication errors: don't let them happen to you, *Am Nurse Today* 5(3):23, 2010.

Centers for Medicare and Medicaid (CMS): *Medication administration guidance update*, 2011, https://www.cms.gov/Surveycertificationgeninfo/downloads/SCLetter12_05.pdf. Accessed February 2014.

Formulary Watch: *FDA's safe use initiative to address preventable harm due to medication misuse errors and other related problems*, 2010, http://formularyjournal.modernmedicine.com/formulary-journal/news/clinical/clinical-pharmacology/fdas-safe-use-initiative-address-preventable-h. Accessed December 2013.

Glover N: Challenges implementing bar-coded medication administration in the emergency room in comparison to medical-surgical units, *Comput Inform Nursing* 31(3):133, 2013.

Goodin S, et al: Safe handling of oral chemotherapeutic agents in clinical practice: recommendations from an international pharmacy panel, *J Oncol Pract* 7(1):7, 2011.

Hockenberry MJ, Wilson D: *Wong's essentials of pediatric nursing*, ed 9, St Louis, 2013, Mosby.

Institute of Safe Medication Practices (ISMP): *Never use parenteral syringes for oral medications*, 2010, http://www.accessdata.fda.gov/psn/transcript.cfm?show=94#9. Accessed February 2014.

Institute of Safe Medication Practices (ISMP): *Acute care guidelines for timely administration of scheduled medications*, 2011, http://www.ismp.org/tools/guidelines/acutecare/tasm.pdf. Accessed February 2014.

Institute of Safe Medication Practices (ISMP): *List of error prone abbreviations, symbols, and dose designations*, 2013, http://www.ismp.org/tools/errorproneabbreviations.pdf. Accessed February 9, 2014.

Lehne RA: *Pharmacology for nursing care*, ed 8, St Louis, 2013, Saunders.

Mandrack M, et al: Nursing best practices using automated dispensing cabinets: nurses' key role in improving medication safety, *Medsurg Nurs* 21(3):134, 2012.

Pharma Cycle: *Extreme danger for family members if bodily fluids from chemotherapy patients are not controlled*, 2013, http://www.pharma-cycle.com/familydangers.html. Accessed February 2014.

Poon EG, et al: Effect of bar-code technology on the safety of medication administration, *N Engl J Med* 362(18):1698, 2010.

Rosier PK: Facing up to the challenge of range orders, *Nursing* 42(12):64, 2012.

Skidmore-Roth L: *Mosby's 2014 nursing drug reference*, ed 27, St Louis, 2014, Mosby.

Speroni K, et al: What causes near-misses and how are they mitigated, *Nursing* 43(4):353–2013, 2013.

Teunissen R, et al: Clinical relevance of and risk factors associated with medication administration time errors, *Am J Health Syst Pharm* 70(12):1052, 2013.

The Joint Commission (TJC): *National Patient Safety Goals*, Oakbrook Terrace, IL, 2014, The Commission. Available at: http://www.jointcommission.org/standards_information/npsgs.aspx.

Touhy T, Jett K: *Ebersole and Hess's gerontological nursing and healthy aging*, ed 4, St Louis, 2013, Mosby.

Traynor K: IMS report calls medication misuse a $200 billion problem, *Am J Health Syst Pharm* 70(15):1268, 2013.

Trbovich P, et al: Interruptions during the delivery of high-risk medications, *J Nurs Adm* 40(5):211–218, 2010.

U.S. Food and Drug Administration (FDA): *How to dispose of unused medicines*, 2013, http://www.fda.gov/forconsumers/consumerupdates/ucm101653.htm. Accessed December, 2013.

U.S. Food and Drug Administration (FDA): *Med Watch, the FDA safety information and adverse event reporting program*, 2014, http://www.fda.gov/Safety/MedWatch/. Accessed February 2014.

Vasbinder E, et al: The association of ethnicity with electronically measured adherence to inhaled corticosteroids in children, *Eur J Clin Pharmacol* 69(3):683, 2013.

Woods AD, et al: Clinical decision support for atypical orders: detection and warning of atypical medication orders submitted to a computerized provider order entry system, *J Am Med Inform Assoc* 21:569–573, 2014.

Yoder M, Schadewald D: The effect of a safe zone on nurse distractions, interruptions, and medication administration errors, *West J Nurs Res* 34(8):1068, 2012.

Administration of Nonparenteral Medications

Nonparenteral medications include medications that are not given by injection, such as oral medications, skin preparations, eyedrops, and eardrops. The route chosen depends on the properties and desired effects of the medication and the physical and mental condition of the patient. The oral route (by mouth) is the easiest and most desirable way to administer medications. Each route has advantages and disadvantages (Table 22-1). There are many reasons why you may find it necessary to recommend a change from one route to another. When the need to recommend a change occurs, you are responsible for consulting with the health care provider for an order or conferring with a pharmacist to meet the patient's needs safely.

Topical administration of medications involves applying drugs directly to skin, mucous membranes, or tissue membranes. You apply medications to the skin by painting, spraying, or spreading medication over a localized area. Transdermal patches (adhesive-backed medicated disks) applied to the skin continuously release medication over several hours or days. The topical administration route avoids puncturing the skin and lessens tissue injury and risk of infection that may occur with injections. When applying a transdermal patch, it is essential to rotate the application site to reduce the incidence of a localized skin reaction.

Medications applied to membranes such as the cornea of the eye or rectal mucosa are absorbed quickly because of the vascularity of the membrane. When drug concentrations are high, systemic effects can occur. For example, bradycardia and hypotension may occur after instillation of ophthalmic beta blockers such as timolol (Timoptic). Mucous and tissue membranes differ in their sensitivity to medications. For example, the cornea of the eye is extremely sensitive to chemicals. Patients commonly experience burning sensations during administration of eyedrops and nose drops. Medications applied to the vaginal or rectal mucosa are generally less irritating.

PATIENT-CENTERED CARE

An excellent time to provide patient education is during medication administration. Most patients discharged from hospitals are placed on new medications, and they often continue previously ordered medications. The goal of patient education is to improve patient adherence to medication regimens. This requires a patient-centered approach because patients have different reasons for failure to adhere to their medication regimens include patient, medication, and health care provider issues (Berben et al., 2011). Patient issues

TABLE 22-1   NONPARENTERAL ROUTES OF ADMINISTRATION

ROUTE	ADVANTAGES	DISADVANTAGES
Inhalation	Directly acts on lung tissues and provides rapid relief of respiratory distress	It is difficult for some patients to hold or manipulate inhaler canisters correctly. Patients must be taught how to use equipment.
Mucous membranes: eyes, ears, nose; vaginal, rectal	Local application to involved site; limited side effects; rectal route is an alternative when oral route unavailable	Insertion of vaginal or rectal products may cause embarrassment. Rectal suppositories are contraindicated in patients with rectal surgery or active rectal bleeding.
Oral (swallowed)	Easy, comfortable, economical; may produce local or systemic effects	Some drugs are destroyed by gastric secretions. Cannot be given if patient is NPO, is unable to swallow, is nauseated, has gastric suction, or is unconscious or confused and unwilling to cooperate. Drugs may irritate lining of GI tract, discolor teeth, or have unpleasant taste.
Skin: topical application or transdermal patches	Provides primarily local effect; painless; limited side effects; transdermal application provides systemic effects and bypasses the liver and its first-pass effects	Extensive topical applications may be bulky or cause difficulty in maneuvering. They may leave oily or pasty substance on skin and may soil clothing. Systemic absorption can be unreliable. Allergies to adhesive in transdermal patches may develop.

GI, Gastrointestinal; *NPO*, nothing by mouth.
Modified from Lehne RA: *Pharmacology for nursing care*, ed 8, St Louis, 2011, Mosby.

include cognitive impairment, depression, health care literacy, physical limitation, social and financial issues, and lack of knowledge. Medication issues include multiple medications, medication discrepancies, and side effects. Health care provider issues include inappropriate prescriptions, poor instruction, and lack of health care provider knowledge about adherence. Simply explaining medications and offering printed information are not enough. You must adapt your instructional approach to the patient's values, beliefs, readiness and willingness to learn, and resources available. For example, repetition of information is important, especially when caring for older adults and patients with cognition problems (e.g., changes in consciousness, inability to attend because of symptoms).

Involve family caregivers in education sessions because they may be the ones administering medications. Using a "teach back" approach, which is shown in the evaluation step of the skills, is a way to evaluate what the patient or family caregiver is able to explain or demonstrate. The information obtained during the teach back session determines what, if any, patient education must be modified.

Health and cultural beliefs are different for each patient and influence how patients manage and adhere to medication therapy. For example, herbal remedies and alternative therapies may be common practice, and health care providers need to include questions in a patient's medication history to obtain information regarding the use of herbs and alternative practices. In addition, some herbal medications interfere with prescribed medications. If a patient is not responding to drug therapy as expected, it is important to consider cultural influences on drug response, metabolism, and side effects (Qureshi, 2010).

SAFETY

The physical environment where you prepare medications contributes to medication errors. Often the most critical drug calculations, judgments, and medication preparations are made in noisy, dimly lit, and chaotic areas of a nursing unit (Sulosaari et al., 2011; Tzeng et al., 2013). Be aware of the conditions in the area where you prepare medications. Because we rely on visual stimulation to make critical decisions, both artificial light and natural light are important to patient safety. Always have sufficient lighting when locating equipment, reading labels, calculating doses, and preparing medications. Increased noise and disruptions increase your cognitive workload, making it difficult to perform safely (Tzeng et al., 2013). Construction noise, foot traffic, monitoring machines, telephones, and hallway conversations are some of the factors that decrease your ability to concentrate and attend properly to medication administration. In some facilities, policies have been established that do not allow anyone to approach or interrupt a nurse who is in the process of preparing medications.

EVIDENCE-BASED PRACTICE

Bonkowski J et al: Effect of barcode-assisted medication administration on emergency department medication errors, *Acad Emerg Med* 20(8):801, 2013.

Kim J, Bates DW: Medication administration errors by nurses: adherence to guidelines, *J Clin Nurs* 22(3-4):590, 2013.

Mandrack M et al: Nursing best practices using automated dispensing cabinets: nurses' key role in improving medication safety, *Medsurg Nurs* 21(3):134, 2012.

Sulosaari V et al: An integrative review of the literature on registered nurses' medication competence, *J Clin Nurs* 20(3-4):464, 2011.

Teunissen R et al: Clinical relevance of and risk factors associated with medication administration time errors, *Am J Health Syst Pharm* 70(12):1052, 2013.

Tzeng HM et al: Medication error-related issues in nursing practice, *Medsurg Nurs* 22(1):13, 2013.

Wulff K et al: Medication administration technologies and patient safety: a mixed method systematic review, *J Adv Nurs* 67(10):2080, 2011.

Medication administration is an essential role of the nurse. Nurses must be competent in all aspects of administering medications, evaluating the effectiveness of medications, and observing for adverse effects. Medication administration technologies are designed to assist nurses in administering medications safely. However, these technologies are not without risk (Bonkowski et al., 2013; Mandrack et al., 2012). Knowledge of the technology and nurse competencies is essential in increasing patient safety and promotion of best

medication administration practices (Kim and Bates, 2013; Sulosaari et al., 2011).

- Be vigilant when implementing new medication administration technologies. Ensure that all nurses are properly educated and knowledgeable about the system (Bonkowski et al., 2013; Wulff et al., 2011).
- Ensure that the medication nurse is free of distractions. Inform all members of the health care team not to interrupt the nurse during medication administration (Tzeng et al., 2013).
- Use best practices when calculating medications, double-check calculations, and do not give medication if the dosage appears incorrect (Kim and Bates, 2013; Sulosaari et al., 2011).
- Critically evaluate why a patient is receiving a specific medication and what outcome is expected during or after the medication regimen.
- Best-practice guidelines for safe medication administration include clinical decision-making, and theoretical and clinical practice competencies (Teunissen et al., 2013).
- Follow facility policy for a "no interruption zone," an area in which only those nurses preparing medications can stand (Mandrack et al., 2012)

SKILL 22.1   ADMINISTERING ORAL MEDICATIONS

• Nursing Skills Online: Nonparenteral Medication Administration, Lesson 1

Patients usually are able to ingest or self-administer oral medications with few problems. However, situations may arise that contraindicate patients receiving medications by mouth, including the presence of gastrointestinal (GI) alterations, the inability of a patient to swallow food or fluids, and the use of gastric suction. An important precaution to take when administering any oral preparation is to protect patients from aspiration (see Chapter 12, Skill 12-4).

Absorption of an oral medication after it is ingested depends largely on its form or preparation. Solutions and suspensions that are already in a liquid state (Fig. 22-1) are absorbed more readily than tablets or capsules. Oral medications are absorbed more easily when administered between meals and when the stomach is not filled with food, which slows absorption. When effective absorption in the stomach is required, give drugs at least 1 hour before or 2 hours after meals or antacids.

Some drugs are not absorbed until reaching the small intestine. Enteric coatings on some tablets resist being dissolved by gastric juices and prevent digestion in the upper GI tract. The coating protects the stomach lining from irritation by the medication. The drug is eventually absorbed in the intestine. Do *not* crush or dissolve enteric-coated medications before administration. Crushing enteric-coated medication causes the medication to be released

too early; the medication may become inactive in the stomach or fail to reach the intended site of action (Paparella, 2010). The website of the Institute for Safe Medication Practices, http://www.ismp.org/Tools/doNotCrush.pdf, contains a complete list of medications that cannot be crushed (ISMP, 2013).

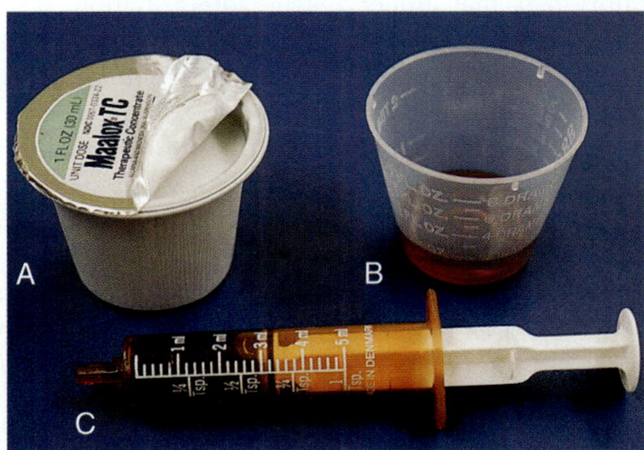

FIG 22-1 A, Liquid medication in a single-dose package. **B,** Liquid measured in a medicine cup. **C,** Oral medicine in syringe.

ASSESSMENT

1. Check accuracy and completeness of each medication administration record (MAR) with health care provider's medication order. Check patient's name, drug name and dosage, route of administration, and time for administration. Clarify incomplete or unclear orders with health care provider before administration. Recopy or reprint any portion of a printed MAR that is difficult to read. *Rationale: The health care provider's order is the most reliable source and only legal record of drugs the patient is to receive. Ensures that patient receives the right medications (Mandrack et al., 2012; Sulosaari et al., 2011). Handwritten MARs are a source of medication errors (Alassaad et al., 2013).*

2. Review pertinent information related to medication, including action, purpose, normal dose and route, common side effects, time of onset and peak action, and nursing implications. *Rationale: Allows you to anticipate effects of drug and observe patient's response.*

3. Assess for any contraindications to oral medication, including being on NPO (nothing by mouth) status, inability to swallow, nausea or vomiting, bowel inflammation, reduced peristalsis, recent GI surgery, gastric suction, and decreased level of consciousness (LOC). Notify the health care provider if any contraindications are discovered. *Rationale: Alterations in GI function can interfere with drug absorption, distribution, and excretion. Patients with impaired swallowing or decreased LOC are at increased risk for aspiration of oral medications.*

4. Assess risk for aspiration using a dysphagia screening tool if available (see Skill 12.2 in Chapter 12) (Box 22-1). *Rationale: Patients with dysphagia are at risk for aspirating oral medication.*

5. Assess patient's medical history, history of allergies, medication history, and diet history. List any drug allergies on each page of the MAR. When allergies are present, patient should wear an allergy bracelet. *Rationale: These factors influence how drugs act, and information reveals any previous problems with medication administration.*

6. Gather and review physical assessment findings and laboratory data that influence drug administration, such as vital signs and results of renal and liver function tests. *Rationale: Data may lead to holding a medication or reveal that a certain drug is contraindicated.*

7. Assess patient's knowledge about health and medication use. *Rationale: Determines patient's need for medication education and guidance needed to achieve appropriate drug adherence.*

8. Assess patient's preferences for fluids and determine if medications can be given with these fluids. Maintain fluid restrictions as prescribed. *Rationale: Some fluids interfere with medication absorption. Offering fluids during drug administration is an excellent way to increase patient's fluid intake. Fluids ease swallowing and facilitate absorption from the GI tract. However, fluid restrictions must be maintained.*

BOX 22-1	PROTECTING A PATIENT FROM ASPIRATION

- Assess patient's ability to swallow and cough, and check for presence of gag reflex.
- Prepare oral medication in form that is easiest to swallow.
- Allow patient to self-administer medications if possible.
- If patient has unilateral (one-sided) weakness, place medication in stronger side of mouth.
- Administer pills one at a time, ensuring that each medication is properly swallowed before next one is introduced.
- Thicken regular liquids or offer fruit nectars if patient cannot tolerate thin liquids.
- Avoid straws because they decrease control patient has over volume intake, which increases risk of aspiration.
- Have patient hold and drink from a cup if possible.
- Time medications to coincide with mealtimes or when patient is well rested and awake if possible.
- Administer medications using another route if risk of aspiration is severe.

PLANNING

Expected Outcomes focus on safe, accurate, and effective drug therapy.

1. Patient responds appropriately with the desired medication effect.
2. Patient denies any GI discomfort or symptoms of alterations.
3. Patient correctly explains purpose of medication and drug dosage schedule.

Delegation and Collaboration

The skill of administering oral medications cannot be delegated to nursing assistive personnel (NAP). In some long-term care settings, trained and certified nursing assistants administer certain nonopioid, nonparenteral medications to stable patients. The nurse instructs the NAP about:

- Potential side effects of medications and reporting their occurrence.
- Informing the nurse if patient's condition changes or worsens after medication administration.

Equipment

- Automated, computer-controlled drug dispensing system or medication cart
- Disposable medication cups
- Glass of water, juice, or preferred liquid and drinking straw
- Pill-crushing device (optional)
- Paper towels
- Medication administration record (MAR)
- Clean gloves (if handling an oral medication)

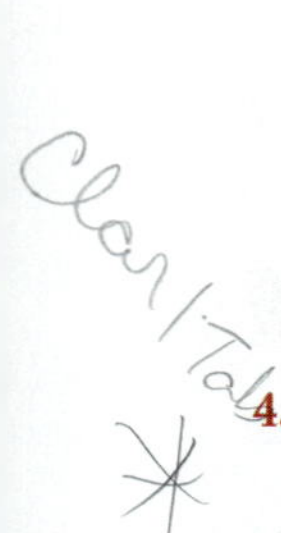

IMPLEMENTATION *for* ADMINISTERING ORAL MEDICATIONS

STEPS	RATIONALE

1. **See Standard Protocol (inside front cover).**
2. Prepare medications.

   a. Plan preparation to avoid interruptions, keep door to medication room closed, do not take phone calls; follow facility policy for a "No Interruption Zone."

   Interruptions and distractions contribute to medication administration errors (Mandrack et al., 2012; Popescu et al., 2011).

   b. Arrange medication tray and cups in medication preparation area or move medication cart to position outside patient's room.

   Organization of equipment saves time and reduces error.

   c. Access automated dispensing system (ADS) or unlock medicine drawer or cart.

   Unauthorized access to medications is prevented when dispensing systems are locked.

   d. Prepare medications for *one patient at a time.* Follow the six rights of medication administration. Keep all pages of MARs or computer printouts for one patient together or look at one patient's medication computer screen at a time.

   Prevents preparation errors (Kim and Bates, 2013).

   e. Select correct drug from ADS, stock supply, or unit-dose drawer. Compare name of medication on the label with MAR or computer printout (see illustration).

   Reading label and comparing it against transcribed order reduce errors. *This is the first check for accuracy.*

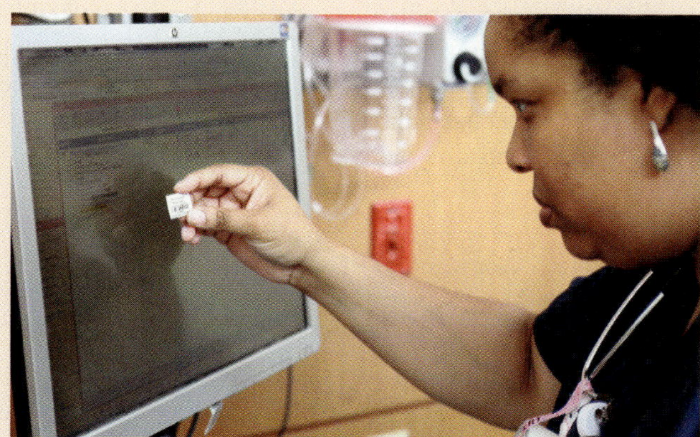

STEP 2e The nurse compares MAR with medication label.

   f. Check expiration date on each medication one at a time. Log off ADS after removing medication. Return all outdated drugs to pharmacy.

   Medications used past expiration date may be inactive or harmful to patient. Logging off the ADS ensures that no one else can remove medications using your identity.

   g. Check or calculate drug dose as needed. Double-check any calculation. Ask another nurse to check calculation if needed.

   Double-checking pharmacy calculations reduces risk of error. Some facilities require nurses to check calculations of certain medications (e.g., insulin) with another nurse (Kim and Bates, 2013).

> **SAFE PATIENT CARE** If preparing a controlled substance, check record for previous medication count and compare current count with supply available. Note: Controlled drugs may be stored in computerized locked cart (see Chapter 21).

   h. *Prepare solid forms of oral medications.*

   (1) To prepare tablets or capsules from a floor stock bottle, pour required number into bottle cap and transfer medication to medication cup. Do not touch medication with fingers. Return extra tablets or capsules to bottle.

   Maintains clean technique required of medication administration.

Continued

STEPS	RATIONALE

(2) To prepare unit-dose tablets or capsules, place packaged tablet or capsule directly into medicine cup without removing wrapper. Administer medications only from containers with labels that are clearly marked and legible.

Wrapper identifies drug name and dose, which can facilitate teaching.

(3) When using a blister pack, "pop" medications through foil or paper backing into a medication cup (see illustration).

Blister packs provide about a 1-month supply. Each "blister" usually contains a single dose.

(4) If it is necessary to give half a tablet or pill for a proper dose, the pharmacy should split the tablet, repackage, and send to the unit. If you must split the tablet, use a clean, gloved hand to break the tablet or cut with a clean pill-cutting device (check facility policy). Break only tablets prescored by the manufacturer (line transverses the center of the tablet).

For inpatient settings, the Institute for Safe Medication Practices (2006) recommends that if a pill *must* be split, the pharmacist should split the pill, repackage and label it, and send it to the nurse for administration. Nurses *should not* split pills (ISMP, 2006, 2008). Tablets that are not prescored cannot be broken into equal halves, resulting in an inaccurate dose.

(5) Place all tablets or capsules that patient will receive at one time in one medicine cup. Exception: Use separate cup for each medication requiring preadministration assessments (e.g., pulse rate, blood pressure).

Serves as a reminder to complete appropriate assessment and facilitates withholding drugs (if necessary).

(6) If patient has difficulty swallowing and liquid medications are not an option, use a pill-crushing device to grind pills (see illustration). Crush each medication separately. Clean device before and after use. Mix ground tablet in small amount (teaspoon) of soft food (custard or applesauce).

Large tablets are often difficult to swallow. A ground tablet mixed with palatable soft food is usually easier to swallow. Mixing with larger amount of food may result in a dose error if patient refuses to eat all food.

> **SAFE PATIENT CARE** Not all drugs can be crushed (e.g., capsules, enteric-coated drugs). Consult pharmacist or "Do Not Crush List" when in doubt (ISMP, 2013).

i. *Prepare liquids.*

(1) Gently shake the container before administering. **NOTE:** If drug is in a unit-dose container with the correct volume, shaking is not needed. Administer directly from single dose cup. Do not pour into a medicine cup.

Mixing liquid suspensions just before pouring ensures that the correct amount of medication, and not just the solvent, is measured for the dose.

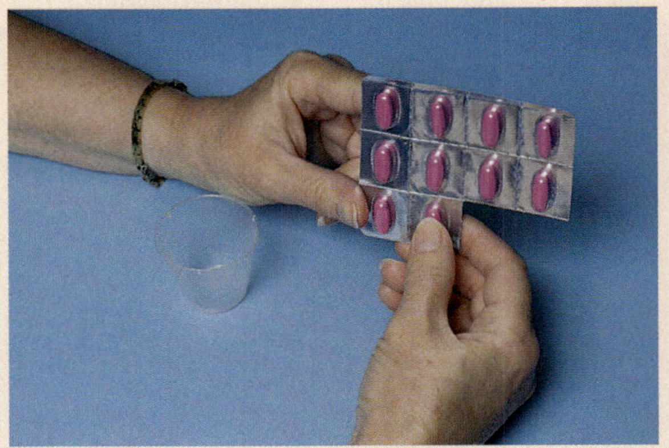

STEP 2h(3) Place tablet into medicine cup without removing wrapper.

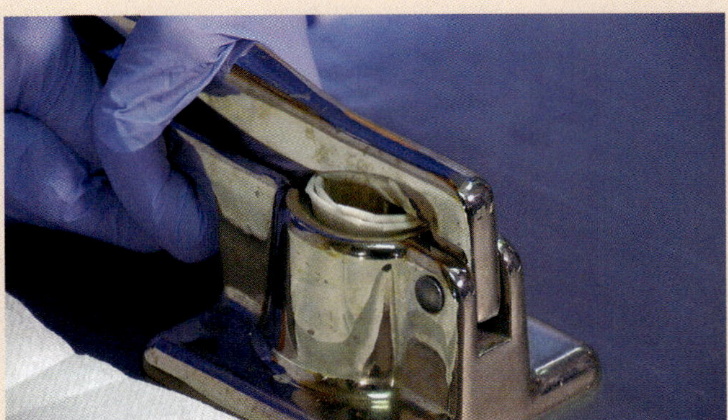

STEP 2h(6) Crushing a tablet with pill-crushing device.

(2) If drug is in a multidose bottle, remove cap from container and place it upside down on the work surface. Check and discard medications that are cloudy or have changed color.

Prevents contamination of inside of cap.

(a) Hold bottle with label against palm of hand while pouring.

Prevents spilled liquid from dripping and obscuring label.

(b) Place medication cup on countertop at eye level or, when necessary, in hand, and fill to desired level on scale. Scale should be even with fluid level at its surface or base of meniscus, not edges (see illustration). For small doses of liquid medications, draw liquid into a calibrated 10-mL syringe designed for enteral administration (see Fig. 22-1, *C*).

Ensures accuracy of measurement. Use of special syringe for oral medications is more accurate for measuring small doses of liquid medications and prevents accidental parenteral administration (ISMP, 2010).

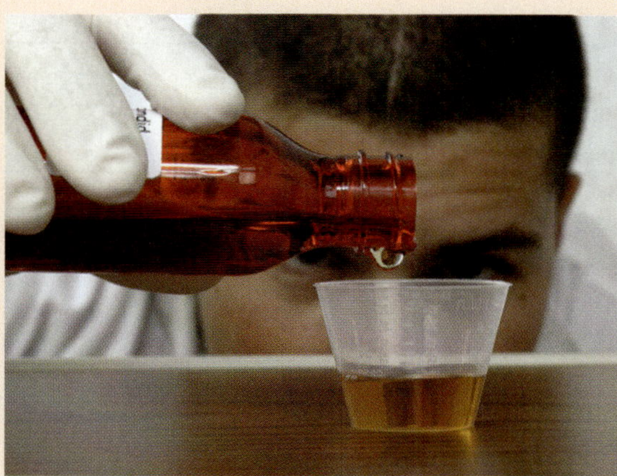

STEP 2i(2)(b) Measuring liquid medication. Look at meniscus at eye level.

(c) Discard any excess liquid into sink or designated area. Wipe lip of bottle with paper towel. Recap the bottle.

Prevents contamination of contents of bottle and prevents bottle cap from sticking.

j. Return stock containers or unused unit-dose medications to shelf or drawer. Label medication cups and poured medications with patient's name before leaving medication preparation room. Do not leave drugs unattended.

Ensures that correct medications are prepared for correct patient.

k. Before going to patient's room, compare MAR with labels on prepared drugs for drug name and patient name.

Reading labels a second time reduces errors. *This is the second check for accuracy.*

3. Administer medications.

a. Take medications to patient at correct time (see facility policy). Medications that require exact timing include STAT, first-time or loading, and one-time doses. Give time-critical scheduled medications (e.g., antibiotics, anticoagulants, insulin, anticonvulsants, immunosuppressive agents) at exact time ordered (no later than 30 minutes before or after scheduled dose). Give non–time-critical scheduled medications within a range of either 1 or 2 hours of scheduled dose (ISMP, 2011). During administration, apply the six rights of medication administration.

Hospitals must adopt medication administration policy and procedure for timing of medication administration that considers nature of the prescribed medication, specific clinical application, and patient needs (DHHS, 2011; ISMP, 2011). Time-critical scheduled medications are medications where early or delayed administration of maintenance doses of greater than 30 minutes before or after the scheduled dose may cause harm or result in substantial suboptimal therapy or pharmacological effect. Non–time-critical medications *are medications where early or delayed administration within a specified range of either 1 or 2 hours* should not cause harm or result in substantial suboptimal therapy or pharmacological effect (DHHS, 2011; ISMP, 2011).

Continued

STEPS	RATIONALE
b. At the patient's bedside, identify patient using two identifiers (e.g., name and birthday or name and account number) according to facility policy. Compare identifiers with information on the patient's MAR or medical record. Then compare MAR or computer printout with the names of medications on the medication labels and patient name.	Ensures the correct patient. Complies with The Joint Commission standards and improves patient safety (TJC, 2014). *This is the third check for accuracy* and ensures that the patient receives the correct medication.
c. Explain the purpose of each medication, action, and most common possible adverse effects. Allow patient to ask any questions about drugs.	Patient has the right to be informed, and patient's understanding of each medication improves adherence with drug therapy.
d. Perform necessary preadministration assessment (e.g., blood pressure, pulse) for specific medications. Ask patient if he or she has allergies.	Determines whether specific medications should be withheld at that time. Confirms patient's allergy history.

> **SAFE PATIENT CARE** If patient or family caregiver expresses any concern regarding the accuracy of a medication, do not give the medication. Explore the patient's concern, and verify health care provider's order.

STEPS	RATIONALE
e. Assist patient to sitting or Fowler's position. Use side-lying position if patient is unable to sit. Have patient stay in position for 30 minutes.	Position decreases risk of aspiration during swallowing.

> **SAFE PATIENT CARE** If in doubt about a patient's ability to swallow, check swallow, cough, and gag reflexes (see Skill 12.2). If these reflexes are impaired or if the patient is unable to swallow pills without choking, withhold the medication, keep the patient NPO, and notify the health care provider.

STEPS	RATIONALE
f. Administer medication.	
(1) For tablets: Patient may wish to hold solid medications in hand or cup before placing in mouth. Offer water or juice to help patient swallow medications. Give a full glass of water if not contraindicated.	Patient becomes familiar with medications by seeing each drug. Choice of fluid can improve fluid intake.
(2) For orally disintegrating formulations (tablets or strips): Remove medication from blister packet just before use. Do not push the tablet through the foil. Place medication on top of patient's tongue and caution against chewing the medicine.	Orally disintegrating formulations begin to dissolve when placed on the tongue. Water is not needed. Careful removal from packaging is needed because the tablets and strips are thin and fragile.
(3) For sublingual medications: Have patient place medication under tongue and allow it to dissolve completely (see illustration). Caution patient against swallowing tablet or saliva.	Drug is absorbed through blood vessels of undersurface of tongue. If swallowed, drug is destroyed by gastric juices or rapidly detoxified by liver, preventing therapeutic blood level.
(4) For buccal medications: Have patient place medication in mouth between mucous membranes of cheek and gums until it dissolves (see illustration).	Buccally administered drugs act locally or systemically as they are swallowed in saliva.
(5) For powdered medications: Mix with liquids at bedside and give to patient to drink.	When prepared in advance, powdered drugs thicken, and some even harden, making swallowing difficult.
(6) For crushed medications mixed in food: Give each medication separately in teaspoon of food.	Ensures that patient swallows all of the medicine.

STEPS	RATIONALE

(7) For effervescent medications: Add tablet or powder to glass of liquid. Give immediately after dissolving.

Effervescence improves unpleasant taste and often relieves GI problems.

(8) For lozenges: Caution patient against chewing or swallowing lozenges.

Lozenges act through slow absorption through oral mucosa, not gastric mucosa.

g. If patient is unable to hold medications, place medication cup to the lips and gently introduce each drug into the mouth, one at a time. A spoon can also be used to place the pill in the patient's mouth. Do not rush or force medications.

Administering a single tablet or capsule eases swallowing and decreases risk for aspiration.

> **SAFE PATIENT CARE** If a tablet or capsule falls to the floor, discard it and repeat preparation. Drug is contaminated.

h. Stay until patient completely swallows each medication or takes it by prescribed route. Ask patient to open mouth if you are uncertain whether medication was swallowed.

Nurse is responsible for ensuring that patient receives ordered dose. If left unattended, patient may not take dose or may save drugs, causing health risk.

i. For highly acidic medications (e.g., aspirin), offer patient a nonfat snack (e.g., crackers) if not contraindicated by patient's condition.

Reduces gastric irritation. The fat content of foods may delay drug absorption.

j. Replenish stock such as cups and straws, return cart to medicine room if used, and clean work area.

Clean working space helps other staff complete duties efficiently.

4. See Completion Protocol (inside front cover).

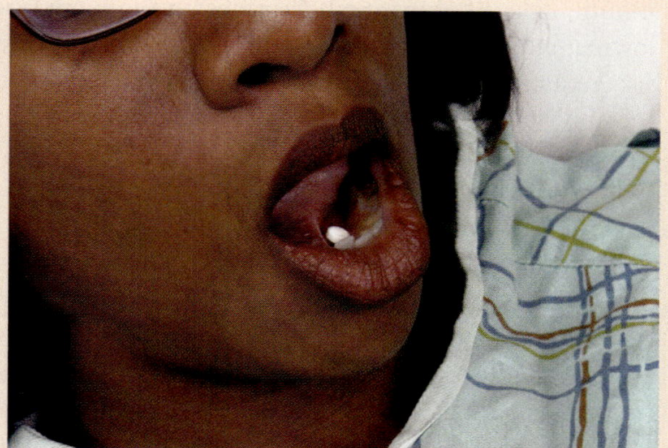

STEP 3f(3) Proper placement of sublingual tablet in sublingual pocket.

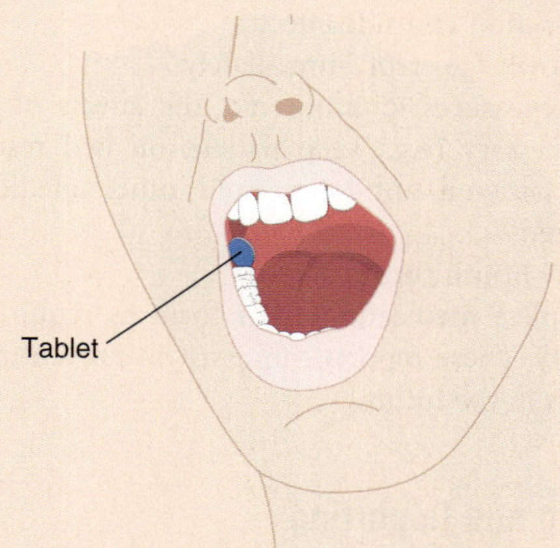

STEP 3f(4) Buccal administration of tablet.

EVALUATION

1. Return within appropriate time to determine patient's response to medications, including therapeutic effects, side effects or allergy, and adverse reactions. Sublingual and buccal medications act in 15 minutes; most oral medications act in 30 to 60 minutes.

2. Ask patient or family member to identify drug name and explain purpose, action, dosage schedule, and potential side effects of drug.

3. Use *Teach Back:* State to the patient, "I want to be sure you understand what I explained about how to use your sublingual nitroglycerin medication. Can you show me how you would take a dose?" Evaluates what the patient is able to explain or demonstrate. Revise your instruction now or develop plan for revised patient teaching to be implemented at an appropriate time if patient is not able to teach back correctly.

Unexpected Outcomes and Related Interventions

1. Patient exhibits adverse effects (e.g., side effect, toxic effect, allergic reaction).
   a. Withhold further doses and assess vital signs.
   b. Notify health care provider and pharmacy.
   c. Symptoms such as urticaria, pruritus, rhinitis, and wheezing may indicate emergency medications for allergic reaction.
2. Patient is unable to explain drug information.
   a. Further assess knowledge of the patient and/or family caregiver of medications and guidelines for drug safety.
   b. Provide further instruction as necessary; offer alternative instructional option.
3. Patient refuses medication.
   a. Assess why patient is refusing medication (e.g., health beliefs, values, symptoms such as nausea, disagreement with treatment plan, side effects).
   b. Educate patient about the purpose of the medication and the potential effects of not taking the drug.
   c. Notify health care provider.
   d. Record information taught, refusal of medication, and patient's stated reason.
4. Administration error occurs (wrong drug, dose, patient, route, or time).
   a. Evaluate patient for untoward effects according to the drug action and side effects.
   b. Acknowledge error immediately.
   c. Take measures to counteract the effects of the error if necessary (e.g., keep patient on bed rest, administer ordered antidotes, hold other medications if ordered).
   d. Notify health care provider.
   e. Complete medication error form as required by the facility. These reports can assist in preventing similar errors in the future.

Recording and Reporting

- Record drug, dose, route, and time administered on MAR immediately *after* administration, not before. Include initials or signature.
- Document your evaluation of patient learning.
- If drug is withheld, record reason in nurses' notes. Follow facility policy for marking held medications on the MAR. Most facilities require that you circle the time the drug normally would have been given on the MAR or computer printout.
- Report adverse effects or patient response and withheld drugs to nurse in charge or health care provider.

Sample Documentation

Note: Documentation of medications is usually done on the MAR. Other documentation occurs only if a problem is noted.

0900   Apical pulse 50 beats/min and regular; c/o nausea; skin cool and moist to touch. Digoxin held, health care provider notified. Patient able to demonstrate correct method for taking nitroglycerin tablet.

Special Considerations

Pediatric

- Liquid medications are safer to swallow to avoid aspiration of small pills.
- Pediatric doses are usually calculated based on body weight.
- Children will refuse bitter or distasteful oral medicines. Mix the drug with a small amount (about 1 teaspoon) of a sweet-tasting substance such as jam, applesauce, sherbet, or fruit puree. Do not use honey in infants because of the risk of botulism. Offer the child juice or an ice pop after medication administration. Do not place medication in an essential food item such as milk or formula; the child may refuse the food at a later time.
- Measure small amounts of liquid medications using a plastic calibrated spoon or syringe. Amounts less than 1 teaspoon are more accurately measured with a calibrated oral syringe (Beckett et al., 2012).

Geriatric

- Physiological changes of aging influence distribution, absorbtion, and excretion. Common changes include dry mouth; delayed esophageal clearance and impaired swallowing; reduction in gastric acidity and stomach peristalsis; reduced liver function, resulting in altered drug metabolism; and reduced renal function and colon motility, slowing drug excretion (Lehne, 2013).
- Give with a full glass of water (unless restricted) to aid passage of the drug. Give patient time to swallow.
- Patients may have several health problems or chronic conditions that require the use of multiple drugs, often prescribed by different health care providers. Polypharmacy creates a high risk for drug interactions and adverse reactions. Assess for potential drug interactions.
- When instructing patients about their medication regimen, include the patient's spouse or another family caregiver.
- If possible, provide a written medication schedule for the patient to follow at home. Use large print in written materials if vision is impaired.

Home Care

- Instruct patient/family caregiver about specific drug regimen (purpose, action, dose, dosage intervals, side effects, food to avoid or take with drugs).
- Help patients/family caregivers to set up medication reminders at home (e.g., pill boxes arranged by day of week)
- When measuring liquid medications at home, provide patients and family members with calibrated spoons and oral syringes (Beckett et al., 2012).

SKILL 22.2 ADMINISTERING MEDICATIONS THROUGH A FEEDING TUBE

• *Nursing Skills Online: Enteral Nutrition Module, Lesson 5*

Patients who have enteral feeding tubes are unable to receive food or medication by mouth. Chapter 12 describes the clinical indications and nursing care implications for enteral feeding tubes. Medications administered by enteral tubes preferably should be in liquid form. If a medication is unavailable in a liquid, you need to prepare an oral medication tablet or capsule by crushing or dissolving it. However, you cannot crush sublingual, slow-release, chewable, long-acting, or enteric-coated medications. Check with a pharmacist about whether you can crush or dissolve a medication (ISMP, 2013). Always verify the position of an enteral tube before administering any medication (see Skill 12.4).

If a medication is to be administered through an NG tube inserted for decompression, consult the health care provider because the tube must be clamped for 30 minutes to 1 hour after instillation of the medication. In most cases, do not give medications into NG or nasointestinal tubes that are inserted for decompression of the stomach.

ASSESSMENT

1. Check accuracy and completeness of each MAR with health care provider's medication order. Check patient's name, drug name and dosage, route of administration, and time for administration. Clarify incomplete or unclear orders with health care provider before administration. *Rationale: The health care provider's order is the most reliable source and only legal record of drugs a patient is to receive. Ensures that patient receives the right medications (Mandrack et al., 2012; Sulosaari et al., 2011). Handwritten MARs are a source of medication errors (Alassaad et al., 2013).*

2. Review pertinent information related to medication, including action, purpose, normal dose and route, common side effects, time of onset and peak action, and nursing implications. If medication is in a solid dose form, determine if it can be crushed. *Rationale: Allows you to anticipate effects of drug and observe patient's response. Enteric-coated or sustained-release medications cannot be crushed.*

3. Assess for any contraindications to patient receiving medication enterally, including presence of bowel inflammation or reduced peristalsis, recent GI surgery, or presence of gastric suction that cannot be temporarily turned off. *Rationale: Alterations in GI function interfere with drug distribution, absorption, and excretion. Patients with GI suction do not benefit from the medication because it may be suctioned from GI tract before it can be absorbed.*

4. Assess patient's medical history, including history of allergies, medication history, and diet history. If you identify contraindications for a medication, withhold and inform health care provider. *Rationale: History may reveal past problems with medication tolerance and response. Historical data allow you to anticipate how certain drugs might act.*

5. Gather and review physical assessment data (e.g., bowel sounds, abdominal distention) and laboratory data (e.g., renal and liver function) that may influence drug administration. *Rationale: Physical examination findings or laboratory data may contraindicate drug administration.*

6. Assess for potential drug-food interactions. *Rationale: Some drugs, such as phenytoin (Dilantin), warfarin (Coumadin), and fluoroquinolone antimicrobials, may require that tube feeding be stopped for 1 hour before and 2 hours after the dose (Lehne, 2013).*

7. Assess patient's knowledge about medication. *Rationale: Determines level of instruction needed.*

8. Avoid complicated medication schedules that frequently interrupt enteral feedings. Investigate and use alternative routes of medication administration if possible (e.g., intravenous, rectal)

9. Check with the pharmacy for availability of liquid preparations for patient's medications. An order from the health care provider may be needed to change the dosage form.

PLANNING

Expected Outcomes focus on administration of appropriate medication; avoidance of tube clogging; and safe, accurate, and effective drug therapy.

1. Patient experiences desired medication effect within period of onset of medication.
2. Patient's feeding tube remains patent after medication administration.
3. Patient does not aspirate during or after medication administration.

Delegation and Collaboration

The skill of administering medications by enteral feeding tubes cannot be delegated to nursing assistive personnel (NAP). The nurse instructs the NAP to:
• Keep the head of the bed elevated for a minimum of 30 degrees (preferably 45 degrees for 1 hour after medication administration; follow facility policy).
• Report immediately to the nurse coughing, choking, gagging, or drooling of liquid.

Equipment
• MAR
• 60-mL syringe, catheter tip for large-bore tubes, Luer-Lok tip for small-bore tubes
• Gastric pH test strip (scale of 1 to 11.0)
• Graduated container

- Medication to be administered
- Pill crusher if medication in tablet form
- Water or sterile water for immunocompromised patients
- Tongue blade or straw to stir dissolved medication
- Clean gloves
- Stethoscope (for evaluation)

IMPLEMENTATION *for* ADMINISTERING MEDICATIONS THROUGH A FEEDING TUBE

STEPS	RATIONALE
1. Determine if medication interacts with enteral feeding. If interaction occurs, stop the feeding 30 minutes before medication administration.	Facilitates absorption of medication (Phillips and Endacott, 2011).
2. Perform hand hygiene. Prepare medications for instillation into feeding tube (see Skill 22-1). Check label of medication against MAR two times. Fill graduated container with 50 to 100 mL of tepid water (sterile water for immunocompromised patients [Bankhead et al., 2009]).	*This includes the first and second checks for accuracy.* Preparation process ensures that right patient receives right medication. Tepid water prevents abdominal cramping, which can occur with cold water.

> **SAFE PATIENT CARE** Whenever possible, use liquid medications instead of crushed tablets. If you have to crush tablets, flush the tubing before and after medication administration to prevent the drug from adhering to the inside of the tube. Never add crushed medications directly to a tube feeding (Wilson and Best, 2011; Phillips and Endacott, 2011).

STEPS	RATIONALE
a. Liquid medication: prepare according to Skill 22-1.	
b. Tablets: Crush each tablet into a fine powder, using a pill-crushing device. If a pill-crushing device is unavailable, place tablet between two medication cups and grind with a blunt instrument. Dissolve each tablet in separate cup of 30 mL of warm water.	Fine powder dissolves more readily, reducing chance of occluding feeding tube.
c. Capsules: Ensure that contents of capsule (granules or gelatin) can be expressed from the covering (check with pharmacist). Open capsule or pierce gel cap with sterile needle and empty contents into 30 mL of warm water (or solution designated by drug company). Gel caps dissolve in warm water, but this may take 15 to 20 minutes.	Dissolved medication does not occlude feeding tube.
3. **Never add a medicaton directly to tube-feeding formula. Sometimes the feeding needs to be held before and/or after medication administration. Verify this and the amount of time that you hold a feeding with facility policy, pharmacist, or medication reference manual.**	Maximizes therapeutic effect of medication.
4. Take medications to patient at correct time (see facility policy). Give STAT, first-time or loading, and one-time doses at time ordered. Give time-critical scheduled medications (e.g., antibiotics, anticoagulants, anticonvulsants, immunosuppressive agents) no later than 30 minutes before or after scheduled dose. Give non–time-critical scheduled medications within a range of either 1 or 2 hours of scheduled dose (ISMP, 2011). During administration, apply the six rights of medication administration.	Hospitals must adopt medication administration policy and procedure for timing of medication administration that considers nature of the prescribed medication, specific clinical application, and patient needs (DHHS, 2011; ISMP, 2011). Time-critical scheduled medications are medications where early or delayed administration of maintenance doses of greater than 30 minutes before or after the scheduled dose may cause harm or result in substantial suboptimal therapy or pharmacological effect. Non–time-critical medications *are medications where early or delayed administration within a specified range of either 1 or 2 hours* should not cause harm or result in substantial suboptimal therapy or pharmacological effect (DHHS, 2011; ISMP, 2011).

STEPS	RATIONALE

5. See Standard Protocol (inside front cover).

6. At patient's bedside, identify patient using two identifiers (e.g., name and birthday or name and account number) according to facility policy. Compare identifiers with information on the patient's MAR or medical record. Then again compare MAR or computer printout with the names of medications on medication labels. Ask patient if he or she has allergies.

Ensures correct patient. Complies with The Joint Commission standards and improves patient safety (TJC, 2014). *This is the third check for accuracy* and ensures that the patient receives correct medication. Confirms patient's allergy history.

7. Discuss the purpose of each medication, action, and possible adverse effects. Allow patient to ask any questions about drugs.

Patient has the right to be informed, and patient's understanding of each medication improves adherence with drug therapy.

8. Elevate head of bed to 45 degrees (unless contraindicated) or sit the patient up in a chair (Bankhead, 2009). Position in reverse Trendelenburg's position if spinal injury is present.

Reduces risk of aspiration, keeping head above stomach.

9. Apply clean gloves. If continuous enteral tube feeding is infusing, adjust infusion pump to hold tube feeding. Check placement of feeding tube (see Skill 12.4) by observing gastric contents and checking pH of aspirated contents. A properly obtained pH value of 0 to 4.0 is a good indication of gastric placement.

Ensuring tube placement reduces the risk of introducing fluids into the respiratory tract (Phillips and Endacott, 2011; Williams, 2012).

10. Check for gastric residual volume (GRV). Draw up 30 mL of air into 60-mL syringe and connect to feeding tube. Flush tube with air, then pull back slowly to aspirate gastric contents (see illustration) (see Chapter 12). Determine GRV using either the scale on the syringe or the graduated container. Return aspirated contents to stomach unless volume exceeds 250 mL (check facility policy) (Metheney et al, 2010). When GRV is excessive, hold medication and contact health care provider for orders.

GRV categories have been identified as significant in studies when patients have two or more GRV values of at least 250 mL or one or more GRV values exceeding 500 mL (Bankhead, 2009). Large residuals indicate delayed gastric emptying and put patient at increased risk for aspiration (Metheney et al., 2010). In addition, GRV has the potential to interfere with enteral medications (Zhu and Zhou, 2013).

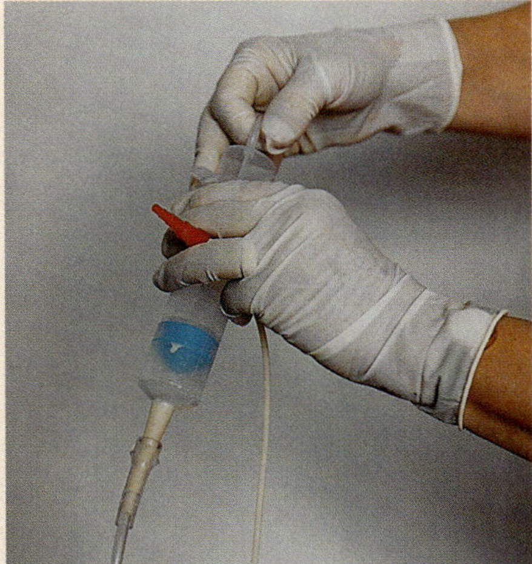

STEP 10 Aspirate stomach contents for residual volume.

11. Irrigate the tubing.
   a. Pinch or clamp enteral tube and remove syringe. Draw up 30 mL of water into syringe. Reinsert tip of syringe into tube, release clamp, and flush tubing. Clamp tube again and remove syringe.

Pinching the tubing or using a valve prevents leakage or spillage of stomach contents. Flushing ensures that tube is patent.

Continued

STEPS	RATIONALE

b. Some enteral tubes are connected to continuous feeding tubing with a stopcock apparatus such as a Lopez valve that contains a medication port (see illustration). Attach the tip of a syringe to medication port on stopcock; turn the "off" setting of stopcock away from the patient and toward the infusion tubing. Flush the feeding tube and set stopcock "off" again toward medication port. Remove syringe.

12. Remove bulb or plunger from syringe and reinsert syringe into tip of feeding tube.

Removal of bulb or plunger prepares syringe for delivery of medication.

13. Administer first liquid or dissolved medication by pouring into syringe (see illustration). Do not mix medications together. Allow to flow by gravity.

> **SAFE PATIENT CARE** If medication does not flow freely, raise the height of the syringe to increase the rate of flow or try having the patient change position slightly because the end of the feeding tube may be against gastric or intestinal mucosa. If still not flowing, try a gentle push with bulb or plunger of the syringe.

a. If giving only one dose of medication, flush with 30 mL of water after administration.

Rinsing is necessary to wash out any active material from the tubing, and it maintains patency of enteral tube and ensures that medication passes through tube to stomach (Zhu and Zhou, 2013).

b. To administer more than one medication, give each separately and flush between medications with 15 to 30 mL of water.

Allows for accurate identification of medication if a dose is spilled. In addition, some medications may be incompatible (Klang et al., 2013).

c. Follow last medication with 30 to 60 mL of water.

Avoids tube clogging with medication and ensures that medication enters stomach (Klang et al., 2013).

14. Clamp proximal end of feeding tube if a tube feeding is not being administered, and cap end of tube.

Prevents air from entering stomach between medication doses.

15. Restart tube feeding if appropriate or hold feeding for 30 minutes or longer if needed to avoid changes in bioavailablity of drugs (Bankhead et al., 2009).

Allows for adequate absorption of medication and avoids potential drug-food interaction between medication and enteral feeding.

16. Assist patient to comfortable position and keep head of bed elevated for at least 1 hour (per facility policy).

Promotes adequate passage of medication through stomach and reduces risk of aspiration.

17. **See Completion Protocol (inside front cover).**

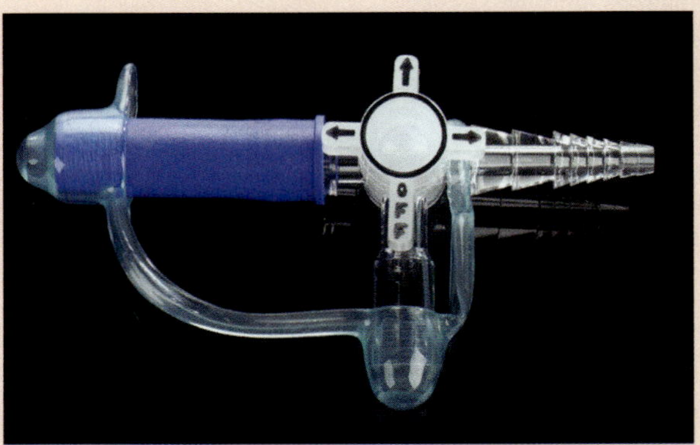

STEP 11b Lopez valve with medication port. (Courtesy ICU Medical Inc, San Clemente, California.)

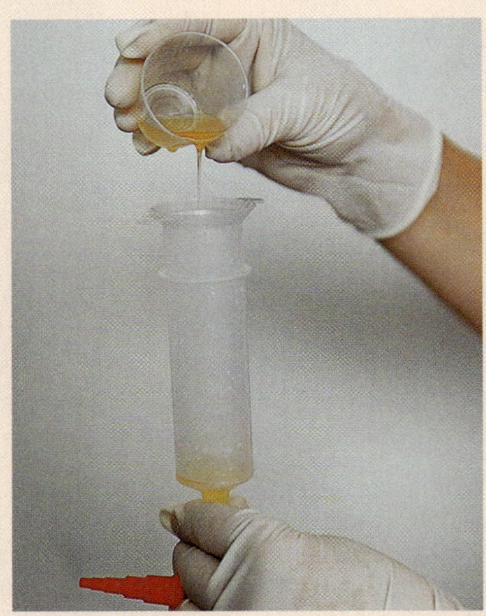

STEP 13 Pour liquid medication into syringe.

EVALUATION

1. Return within 30 minutes to evaluate patient's response to medications.
2. Observe tube patency after medication administration.
3. Monitor patient for signs of aspiration, such as dyspnea, choking, gurgling speech, or congested breath sounds, during and after medication administration.

Unexpected Outcomes and Related Interventions

1. Patient is unable to receive medication because of blocked enteral tube.
   a. For newly inserted tube, notify health care provider and obtain x-ray film confirmation of positioning.
   b. Attempt to flush tube gently with large-bore syringe and warm water to clear clog. (Avoid using a small-bore syringe because this exerts large amounts of pressure and may rupture tube.)
   c. If irrigation is ineffective, obtain an order for a declogging stylus (see facility policy).
   d. Tube may have to be removed and a new one inserted.
2. Patient shows signs of aspiration, such as respiratory distress, changes in vital signs, and decreased oxygen saturation.
   a. Stop the administration of all fluids and medications through feeding tube.
   b. Elevate the head of the bed and stay with the patient. Have another staff member notify the patient's health care provider.
   c. Assess vital signs, oxygen saturation, and breath sounds.

Recording and Reporting

- Record in nurses' notes method used to check for tube placement, GRV, and pH of aspirate. Record drug, dose, route, and time administered on MAR immediately *after* administration, not before. Include initials or signature. Record patient teaching and validation of understanding in nurses' notes. Record total amount of water used for medication administration on proper intake and output (I&O) form.

- Report adverse effects or patient response and withheld drugs to nurse in charge or health care provider.

Sample Documentation

Note: Documentation for medications via feeding tube is usually done on the MAR. Fluids given without medications must be recorded as intake on I&O form. Other documentation occurs only if a problem is noted.

1300   Unable to administer medication because of clogged feeding tube despite attempts to irrigate with 60 mL tap water. Health care provider notified; medications and tube feeding held pending placement of new tube.

Special Considerations
Geriatric

- Assess patient for use of medications that may affect the pH of gastric secretions such as H_2 receptor antagonists or antacids. H_2 receptor antagonists reduce volume of gastric acid secretion and acid content of secretions, causing the pH value to be higher or more basic (Klang et al., 2013).

Home Care

- Teach patient or family caregiver:
  - How to store medications and tube feeding supplements.
  - How to check placement of tube before administering any medication.
  - How to administer medication through feeding tube.
  - Importance of giving medication and to notify health care provider if there is any doubt concerning the placement of the tube.
  - About importance of consistent irrigation of feeding tube before, during, and after medications are given.
- Provide patient or primary caregiver with resources to determine which medications can be crushed, which medications should not be crushed, and how to obtain liquid formulations of medications.

• **Nursing Skills Online: Nonparenteral Medication Administration, Lesson 2**

Topical administration of medications involves applying drugs directly to skin, mucous membranes, or tissues. Topical drugs such as lotions, patches, pastes, and ointments primarily produce local effects, but they can also create systemic effects if absorbed through the skin (Lawton, 2013). Systemic effects are more likely to occur if the skin is thin, drug concentration is high, contact with the skin is prolonged, or the drug is applied to broken skin. To protect from accidental exposure, apply topical drugs using gloves and applicators. Skin encrustations and dead tissue harbor microorganisms and block contact of medications with the affected tissue or membrane. Applying new medications over previously applied drugs does little to prevent infection or provide a therapeutic benefit. Always cleanse the skin or a wound thoroughly before applying a dose of a topical drug. Apply each type of medication—ointment, lotion, or patch—in the proper way to ensure penetration and absorption.

ASSESSMENT

1. Check accuracy and completeness of each MAR with health care provider's medication order. Check patient's

name, drug name and dosage, route of administration, and time for administration. Clarify incomplete or unclear orders with health care provider before administration. *Rationale: The health care provider's order is the most reliable source and only legal record of drugs the patient is to receive. Ensures that patient receives the right medications (Mandrack et al., 2012; Sulosaari et al., 2011). Handwritten MARs are a source of medication errors (Alassaad et al., 2013).*

2. Review pertinent information related to medication, including action, purpose, normal dose and route, time of onset and peak action, common side effects, and nursing implications. *Rationale: Allows you to anticipate effects of drug and observe patient's response.*

3. Assess condition of skin or membrane where medication is to be applied (see Chapter 7). You can assess skin or membrane just before applying the medication. If there is an open wound, apply clean gloves. First wash site thoroughly with mild, nondrying soap and warm water; rinse; and dry. Remove any previously applied medication or debris. Also remove any blood, secretions, excretions, or other body fluids. Assess for symptoms of skin irritation such as pruritus or burning. Remove gloves. *Rationale: Cleansing thoroughly promotes correct skin assessment. Assessment provides baseline to determine change in condition of skin after therapy. Topical agents can lessen or aggravate these symptoms. Topical medications applied to damaged skin can cause harmful effects, such as burns, blistering, and increased systemic absorption (Cohen, 2013).*

4. Assess patient's medical history, history of allergies (including latex or topical agent), and medication history. Ask if patient has had a reaction to a cream or lotion applied to the skin. *Rationale: Allergic contact dermatitis is common and can worsen existing dermatological condition. Latex allergy requires use of latex-free gloves.*

5. Determine amount of topical agent required for application by assessing skin site, reviewing health care provider's order, and reading application directions carefully (a thin, even layer is usually adequate). *Rationale: An excessive amount of topical agent can chemically irritate the skin, negate the effectiveness of the drug, or cause adverse systemic effects such as decreased white blood cell counts.*

6. Determine if patient or family caregiver is physically able to apply medication by assessing grasp, hand strength, reach, and coordination. *Rationale: This is necessary if patient is to self-administer drug in the home.*

7. Assess patient's knowledge of action and purpose of medication being given and willingness to adhere to drug regimen. *Rationale: Determines if patient or caregiver can administer drug in the home.*

PLANNING

Expected Outcomes focus on safe, accurate, and effective drug therapy.

1. With repeated application, patient's condition improves (e.g., relief of pain, inflammation, or drainage).
2. Patient or caregiver explains purpose of medication, dosage schedule, and most common possible side effects.
3. Patient or family caregiver administers topical medication or patch correctly.

Delegation and Collaboration

The skill of administering most topical preparations, including patches, cannot be delegated to nursing assistive personnel (NAP). However, some facilities (e.g., long-term care) may allow NAP to apply some forms of topical agents to irritated skin or for the protection of the perineum during morning or perineal care. Check facility policies. The nurse instructs the NAP to:

- Report any skin irritation, burning, blistering, or increased itching immediately to nurse.
- Not apply any dressing over the agent unless instructed to do so.

Equipment

- Clean gloves (for intact skin) or sterile gloves (for nonintact skin)
- Cotton-tipped applicators, tongue blades (optional), or gauze pad/dressing
- Ordered medication (powder, cream, lotion, ointment, spray, patch)
- Basin of warm water, washcloth, towel, nondrying soap
- Sterile dressing, tape (if needed)
- Felt-tip pen
- MAR

IMPLEMENTATION *for* APPLYING TOPICAL MEDICATIONS TO THE SKIN

STEPS	RATIONALE
1. Perform hand hygiene. Prepare medications for application. Check label of medication against MAR two times (see Skill 22-1). Preparation usually involves taking bottle or tube of lotion, cream, or ointment or patch out of storage and then to patient's room. Check expiration date on containers.	*This includes the first and second checks for accuracy.* Process for preparation ensures that right patient receives right medication.

STEPS	RATIONALE

2. Take medications to patient at correct time (see facility policy). Medications that require exact timing include STAT, first-time or loading, and one-time doses. Give time-critical scheduled medications (e.g., antibiotics) no later than 30 minutes before or after scheduled dose. Give non–time-critical scheduled medications within a range of either 1 or 2 hours of scheduled dose (ISMP, 2011). During administration, apply the six rights of medication administration.

Hospitals must adopt medication administration policy and procedure for timing of medication administration that considers nature of the prescribed medication, specific clinical application, and patient needs (DHHS, 2011; ISMP, 2011). Time-critical scheduled medications are medications where early or delayed administration of maintenance doses of greater than 30 minutes before or after the scheduled dose may cause harm or result in substantial suboptimal therapy or pharmacological effect. Non–time-critical medications *are medications where early or delayed administration within a specified range of either 1 or 2 hours* should not cause harm or result in substantial suboptimal therapy or pharmacological effect (DHHS, 2011; ISMP, 2011).

3. See Standard Protocol (inside front cover).

4. At the patient's bedside, identify patient using two identifiers (e.g., name and birthday or name and account number) according to facility policy. Compare identifiers with information on the patient's MAR or medical record. Then compare MAR or computer printout with the names of medications on the medication labels and patient name.

Ensures the correct patient. Complies with the Joint Commission Standards and improves patient safety (TJC, 2014). *This is the third check for accuracy* and ensures that the patient receives the correct medication.

5. Discuss the purpose of each medication, action, and possible adverse effects. Allow patient to ask any questions.

Patient has the right to be informed, and patient's understanding of each medication improves adherence with drug therapy.

6. If skin is broken, **apply sterile gloves.** Otherwise, apply clean gloves.

SAFE PATIENT CARE Do not administer topical medications to the skin or membranes if integrity is altered unless indicated by health care provider (Cohen, 2013).

---

7. *Apply topical creams, ointments, and oil-based lotions.*

 a. Expose affected area while keeping unaffected areas covered.

Adequate visualization is necessary for application. Protects patient privacy.

 b. Wash, rinse, and dry affected area before applying medication (see Assessment, Step 3).

Cleansing removes microorganisms resident in remaining debris and allows for visualization of the patient's skin (Lawton, 2013).

 c. If skin is excessively dry and flaking, apply topical agent while skin is still damp.

Retains moisture within skin layers.

 d. Remove gloves and apply new clean or sterile gloves.

Changing gloves prevents cross-contamination of infected or contagious lesions. Applying gloves protects you from absorption of medication and drug effects (Cohen, 2013). Use sterile gloves when applying agents to open, noninfectious skin lesions.

 e. Place required amount of medication in palm of gloved hand and soften by rubbing briskly between hands.

Softening of topical agent makes it easier to apply to skin.

 f. Tell patient that skin will feel soothed by application, but initially it might feel cold. Once softened, spread it evenly over skin surface, using long, even strokes that follow direction of hair growth. Do not rub skin vigorously. Apply thickness as directed by manufacturer's instructions.

Ensures even distribution of medication. Technique prevents irritation of hair follicles.

Continued

STEPS	RATIONALE

g. Explain to patient that skin may feel greasy after application.

Ointments often contain oil.

8. *Apply antianginal (nitroglycerin) ointment.*

a. Remove previous dose paper. Fold used paper containing any residual medication with used sides together and dispose in biohazard trash container. Wipe off residual medication with a tissue, then discard.

Prevents overdose that can occur with multiple-dose papers left in place. Proper disposal protects others from accidental exposure to medication.

b. Write date, time, and nurse's initials on new application paper.

Label provides reference to prevent missing doses.

c. Antianginal (nitroglycerin) ointments are usually ordered in inches and can be measured on small sheets of paper marked off in 1.25-cm [½ inch]) markings. Apply desired number of inches of ointment to paper measuring guide (see illustration).

Ensures correct dose of medication.

> **SAFE PATIENT CARE** Unit-dose packages are available. (Warning: One package equals 2.5 cm [1 inch]; smaller amount should not be measured from this package.)

d. Select application site: Apply nitroglycerin to chest area, back, abdomen, or anterior thigh (Lehne, 2013). Do not apply on hairy surfaces or over scar tissue.

Application on hairy surfaces or scar tissue may interfere with absorption.

e. Rotate application sites.

Minimizes skin irritation.

f. Apply ointment to skin surface by holding edge or back of paper measuring guide and placing ointment and paper directly on skin (see illustration).

Minimizes chance of ointment covering gloves and later touching nurse's hands (Lawton, 2013).

g. Do not rub or massage ointment into skin.

Medication is designed to absorb slowly over several hours; massaging may increase absorption.

h. Secure ointment and paper with transparent dressing or strip of tape; plastic wrap is an option. Apply dressing or plastic wrap only when instructed by pharmacy (Lawton, 2013).

Prevents staining of clothes or accidental removal of medication. Covering some topical medications with dressing or plastic wrap increases heat and thus drug absorption (Cohen, 2013).

9. *Apply transdermal patches (e.g., analgesic, nicotine, nitroglycerin, estrogen).*

a. If an old patch is present, remove it, and cleanse the area. Be sure to check between skin folds for a patch.

Failure to remove old patches may result in overdose. Many patches are small, clear, or flesh-colored and can easily be hidden beneath skin folds. Cleansing removes traces of previous dose.

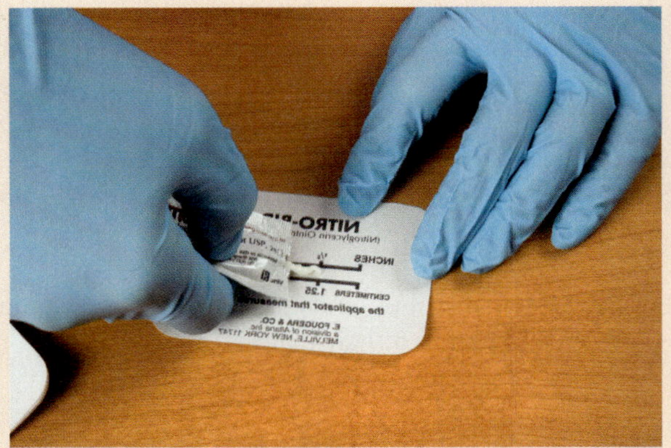

STEP 8c Ointment spread in inches over measuring guide.

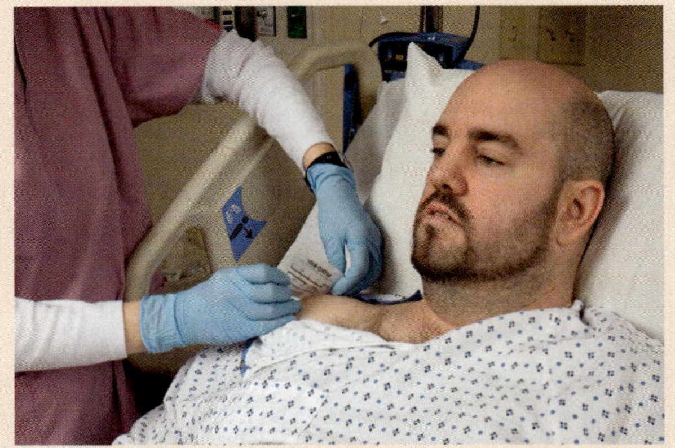

STEP 8f Nurse applies measuring guide with medication on patient's skin.

STEPS	RATIONALE
b. Dispose of old patch by folding in half with sticky sides together. Some facilities require the patch to be cut before disposal (see facility policy). Dispose in biohazard trash bag.	Proper disposal prevents accidental exposure to medication.
c. Date and initial the outer side of the new patch before applying it, and note time of administration. Use a soft-tip or felt-tip pen.	Visual reminder prevents missing or extra doses. A ballpoint pen damages the patch and alters medication delivery.
d. Choose a new site that is clean, dry, and free of hair. Some patches have specific instructions for placement locations (e.g., Testoderm patches are placed on scrotum; a scopolamine patch is placed on back of the ear; never apply an estrogen patch to the breast tissue or waistline (Cohen, 2013). Do not apply a patch on skin that is oily, burned, cut, or irritated in any way.	Ensures complete medication absorption. Hormone patches should never be placed on the breasts, on the genitals, or over the reproductive organs. Because of the systemic absorption of hormones, there is an increased risk for breast, testicular, or ovarian cancers (Cohen, 2013).

> **SAFE PATIENT CARE** Never apply heat such as with a heating pad over a transdermal patch because this results in an increased rate of absorption with potentially serious adverse effects (Cohen, 2013).

STEPS	RATIONALE
e. Carefully remove the patch from its protective covering by pulling off the liner. Hold the patch by the edge without touching the adhesive.	Touching only the edges ensures that the patch will adhere and that the medication dose has not been changed. Removing the protective covering allows the medication to be absorbed through the skin.
f. Apply the patch, pressing firmly with the palm of one hand for 10 seconds. Make sure that it sticks well, especially around the edges. Apply overlay if provided with patch.	Adequate adhesion prevents loss of the patch, which results in decreased dose and effectiveness.
g. Do not apply patch to previously used site for at least 1 week.	Rotation of site reduces skin irritation from medication and adhesive (Lawton, 2013).
h. Instruct patient never to cut transdermal patches in half; a change in dose would require a prescription for a new strength of transdermal medication.	Cutting a transdermal patch in half would alter the intended medication delivery of the transdermal system, resulting in inadequate or altered drug levels.

> **SAFE PATIENT CARE** It is recommended to have a daily "patch-free" interval of 10 to 12 hours because tolerance develops if patches are used 24 hours a day every day (Lehne, 2013). Apply a new patch each morning, leave in place for 12 to 14 hours, and remove in the evening. Consult the health care provider.

STEPS	RATIONALE
i. Instruct patient always to remove old patch before applying new one. Patients should not use alternative forms of medications when using patches. For example, patients should not smoke while using a nicotine patch. Patients should not apply nitroglycerin ointment in addition to the patch unless specifically ordered to do so by health care provider.	Use of patch with an additional/alternative drug preparation can result in toxicity and other side effects (Cohen, 2013).
10. *Administer aerosol sprays (e.g., local anesthetic sprays).*	
a. Shake container vigorously. Read container label for distance recommended to hold spray away from area, usually 15 to 30 cm (6 to 12 inches).	Mixing ensures delivery of a fine, even spray. Proper distance ensures that fine spray hits skin surface. Holding container too close results in thin, watery distribution.

Continued

STEPS	RATIONALE
b. Ask patient to turn face away from spray or cover face briefly with towel when spraying neck or chest.	Prevents inhalation of spray.
c. Spray medication evenly over affected site (spray is timed for period of seconds in some cases).	Entire affected area of skin should be covered with thin spray.
11. *Apply suspension-based lotion.*	
a. Follow Steps 7a to 7d to cleanse skin. Shake container vigorously.	Mixes powder throughout liquid to form well-mixed suspension.
b. Apply small amount of lotion to small gauze dressing or pad and apply to skin by stroking evenly in direction of hair growth.	Method of application leaves protective film of powder on skin after water base of suspension dries. Technique prevents irritation of hair follicles.
c. Explain to patient that area will feel cool and dry.	Water evaporates to leave thin layer of powder.
12. *Apply a powder.*	
a. Be sure that skin surface is thoroughly dry. With your nondominant hand, fully spread apart any skin folds such as between toes or under axilla and dry with a towel.	Minimizes caking and crusting of powder. Fully exposes skin surface for application.
b. If area of application is near the face, ask patient to turn face away from powder or briefly cover face with towel.	Prevents inhalation of powder.
c. Dust skin site lightly with dispenser so that area is covered with fine, thin layer. Option: Cover skin area with dressing if ordered by health care provider.	Thin layer of powder has slight lubricating properties to reduce friction and promote drying (Lilley et al., 2011).
13. **See Completion Protocol (inside front cover).**	

EVALUATION

1. Inspect condition of skin between applications.
2. Observe patient or family caregiver apply topical medication.
3. Ask patient or family caregiver to name the medication and its purpose, dosage, schedule, and common side effects.
4. Use **Teach Back:** State to the patient, "I want to be sure you understand what I explained about how to apply your nitroglycerin paste. It is time for your dose; can you show me now how to apply the medication?" Evaluates what the patient is able to explain or demonstrate. Revise your instruction now or develop plan for revised patient teaching to be implemented at an appropriate time if patient is not able to teach back correctly.

Unexpected Outcomes and Related Interventions

1. Skin site appears inflamed and edematous with blistering and oozing of fluid from lesions, or patient continues to complain of pruritus and tenderness. These signs can indicate subacute inflammation, eczema, or an adverse reaction to the topical agent (Cohen, 2013).
   a. Stop using the product and notify health care provider; additional or alternative therapies may be needed.
2. Patient is unable to explain information about topical application or does not administer as prescribed.

   a. Identify possible reasons for nonadherence and explore alternative approaches (e.g., family caregiver) or options.

Recording and Reporting

- Record drug, dose or strength, site of application, and time administered on MAR immediately after administration, not before. Include initials or signature.
- Document your evaluation of patient learning.
- Describe condition of skin before each application in nurses' notes. Do not chart medication administration until after administration.
- Report adverse effects or changes in appearance and condition of skin lesions to health care provider.

Sample Documentation

0930   Skin on chest dry and intact. Patient correctly cleaned patch site and applied nitroglycerin paste.

Special Considerations
Geriatric

- Changes in the skin of an older adult include increased wrinkling, dryness, flaking, and tendency to bruise. Handle fragile skin gently when applying topical medications.

Home Care

- Instruct patient on safe disposal techniques at home. Fold used patches with medication sides together and wrapped in newspaper before discarding. Used applicators or patches are placed into cardboard or plastic disposable containers. Children and pets may become ill if they ingest or handle used patches; careful disposal is necessary to ensure safety in the home.
- Instruct patient never to apply a heating pad or apply plastic wrap (unless instructed to do so). Both of these actions can cause burning, blistering, and in some cases increased absorption of the medications (Cohen, 2013).

SKILL 22.4 INSTILLING EYE AND EAR MEDICATIONS

• Nursing Skills Online: Nonparenteral Medication Administration, Lessons 3 and 4

Common eye (ophthalmic) medications are in the form of drops and ointments, including over-the-counter (OTC) preparations such as artificial tears and vasoconstrictors (e.g., Visine, Murine). However, many patients receive prescribed ophthalmic drugs for eye conditions such as glaucoma and eye infections and after cataract extraction. In addition, a third type of delivery system is the intraocular disk. Medications delivered by disk resemble a contact lens, but the disk is placed in the conjunctival sac, not on the cornea, and it remains in place for up to 1 week.

The eye is the most sensitive organ to which you apply medications. The cornea is richly supplied with sensitive nerve fibers. Care must be taken to prevent instilling medication directly onto the cornea. The conjunctival sac is much less sensitive and a more appropriate site for medication instillation.

Any patient receiving topical eye medications should learn correct self-administration of the medication, especially patients with glaucoma, who must often undergo lifelong medication administration for control of the disease. You can easily instruct patients and family caregivers while administering medications. Family caregivers often administer eye medications when patients are unable to manipulate applicators and immediately after eye surgery, when a patient's vision is blurred, making it difficult to assemble needed supplies and read medication labels.

When administering ear medications, be aware of certain safety precautions. Internal ear structures are sensitive to temperature extremes; administer eardrops at room temperature. Administering cold eardrops can cause severe dizziness (vertigo) or nausea, either of these conditions can debilitate a patient for several minutes. Although structures of the outer ear are not sterile, use sterile drops and solutions in case the eardrum is ruptured. A final safety precaution is to avoid forcing any solution into the ear. Do not occlude the ear canal with a medicine dropper because this can cause pressure within the canal during instillation and subsequent injury to the eardrum. Follow these precautions to administer eardrops safely and effectively.

ASSESSMENT

1. Check accuracy and completeness of each MAR with health care provider's medication order. Check patient's name, drug name and dosage, route of administration, and time for administration. Clarify incomplete or unclear orders with health care provider before administration. *Rationale: The health care provider's order is the most reliable source and only legal record of drugs the patient is to receive. Ensures that patient receives the right medications (Mandrack et al., 2012; Sulosaari et al., 2011). Handwritten MARs are a source of medication errors (Alassaad et al., 2013).*

2. Review pertinent information related to medication, including action, purpose, normal dose and route, common side effects, time of onset and peak action, and nursing implications. *Rationale: Allows you to anticipate effects of drug and observe patient's response.*

3. Assess condition of external eye or ear structures (see Chapter 7). If drainage is present, apply clean gloves. *Rationale: This assessment may be done just before drug instillation. Provides a baseline to determine later if local response to medications occurs. This also indicates the need to clean the area before drug application.*

4. Determine whether patient has symptoms of eye or ear discomfort or visual or hearing impairment. *Rationale: Certain eye medications can act either to lessen or to increase symptoms. Occlusion of external ear canal by swelling, drainage, or cerumen can impair hearing acuity and is painful.*

5. Assess patient's medical history, history of allergies (including latex), and medication history. *Rationale: Factors influence how certain drugs act. Reveals patient's need for medication.*

6. Assess patient's LOC and ability to follow instructions. *Rationale: Patient must lie still during drug administration. Sudden movements can cause injury from dropper.*

7. Assess patient's knowledge regarding drug therapy and desire to self-administer medication. *Rationale: Findings indicate need for health teaching and involvement of family caregiver. Motivation influences teaching approach. Reflects patient's ability to learn to self-administer medication.*

8. Assess patient's ability to manipulate and hold eye or ear medication dropper or ocular disks. *Rationale: Reflects patient's ability to self-administer drug.*

PLANNING

Expected Outcomes focus on relief of symptoms without unpleasant adverse reactions and on safe, accurate, and effective drug therapy.

1. Patient experiences desired effect of medication and states that symptoms (e.g., irritation, dryness) are relieved.

2. Patient denies discomfort or unpleasant side effects or adverse reactions.

3. Patient describes medication effects and technique of application.
4. Patient correctly demonstrates self-instillation of eyedrops or eardrops.

Delegation and Collaboration

The skills of administering eyedrops or eardrops cannot be delegated to nursing assistive personnel (NAP). The nurse instructs the NAP about:

- Potential side effects of medications, including hearing changes or vision impairment, and how to report their occurrence.

Equipment

- Appropriate medication (eyedrops with sterile dropper, ointment tube, medicated intraocular disk, or eardrops)
- Clean gloves (for eyedrops and if ear has drainage)
- MAR

Eyedrops or Ointment

- Cotton balls or facial tissue
- Warm water and washcloth
- Eye patch and tape (optional)

Eardrops

- Cotton-tipped applicator, cotton balls

IMPLEMENTATION *for* INSTILLING EYE AND EAR MEDICATIONS

STEPS	RATIONALE
1. *Perform hand hygiene.* Prepare medications for application. Check label of medication against MAR two times (see Skill 22-1).	*This includes the first and second checks for accuracy.* Ensures that right patient receives right medication.
a. Check expiration date on medication.	Medications used past expiration date may be inactive or harmful to patient.
b. Check drug dose (number of drops) and concentration. If the dose or concentration printed on package differs from what is ordered, consult with pharmacy. Drugs are typically given in drops. Double-check the eye or ear to receive medication.	Double-checking pharmacy calculations and ordered route reduces risk of error.
2. Take medications to patient at correct time (see facility policy). Medications that require exact timing include STAT, first-time or loading, and one-time doses. Give time-critical scheduled medications (e.g., antibiotics) no later than 30 minutes before or after scheduled dose. Give non–time-critical scheduled medications within a range of either 1 or 2 hours of scheduled dose (ISMP, 2011). During administration, apply the six rights of medication administration.	Hospitals must adopt medication administration policy and procedure for timing of medication administration that considers nature of the prescribed medication, specific clinical application, and patient needs (DHHS, 2011; ISMP, 2011). Time-critical scheduled medications are medications where early or delayed administration of maintenance doses of greater than 30 minutes before or after the scheduled dose may cause harm or result in substantial suboptimal therapy or pharmacological effect. Non–time-critical medications *are medications where early or delayed administration within a specified range of either 1 or 2 hours* should not cause harm or result in substantial suboptimal therapy or pharmacological effect (DHHS, 2011; ISMP, 2011).
3. **See Standard Protocol (inside front cover).**	
4. At the patient's bedside, identify patient using two identifiers (e.g., name and birthday or name and account number) according to facility policy. Compare identifiers with information on the patient's MAR or medical record. Then compare MAR or computer printout with the names of medications on the medication labels and patient name.	Ensures the correct patient. Complies with the Joint Commission Standards and improves patient safety (TJC, 2014). *This is the third check for accuracy* and ensures that the patient receives the correct medication.
5. Discuss the purpose of each medication, action, and possible adverse effects. Allow patient to ask any questions. Explain procedure. Patients who self-instill medications may be allowed to give drops under nurse's supervision (check facility policy). Tell patients receiving eyedrops (e.g., mydriatics) that vision will be temporarily blurred and sensitivity to light may occur.	Patient has the right to be informed, and patient's understanding of each medication improves adherence with drug therapy. Patients often become anxious about medication being instilled into eye because of potential discomfort.

> **SAFE PATIENT CARE** Reinforce that patient should not drive or attempt to perform any activity that requires acute vision or sensitivity to light until vision returns to normal.

6. *Instill eye medications.*

a. Perform hand hygiene. Apply clean gloves. Ask patient to lie supine or sit back in chair with neck slightly hyperextended.

Position provides easy access to eye or ear for medication instillation and minimizes drainage of eye medication into tear duct.

> **SAFE PATIENT CARE** Do not hyperextend the neck of a patient with a cervical neck injury.

b. If crusting or drainage is present along eyelid margins or inner canthus, gently wash away. Soak any dried crusts with a warm, damp washcloth or cotton ball over eye for several minutes. Always wipe clean from inner to outer canthus (see illustration). Remove gloves. Perform hand hygiene and apply new pair of clean gloves.

Cleansing eye from inner to outer canthus avoids introducing microorganisms into lacrimal ducts (Lilley et al., 2011). Soaking allows easy removal of crusts without applying pressure to eye.

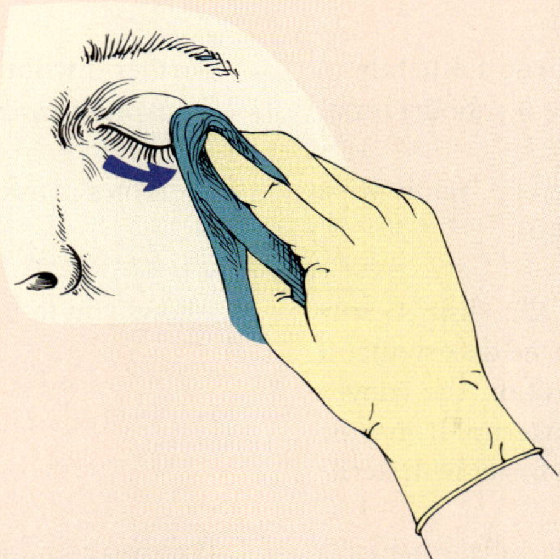

STEP 6b Cleanse eye, washing from inner to outer canthus, before administering drops or ointment.

c. Explain that there might be a temporary burning sensation from eyedrops.

Cornea is highly sensitive.

d. *Instill eyedrops.*

(1) Gently rotate drop container between hands.

Ensures medication is mixed before administration.

(2) Hold a cotton ball or clean tissue in nondominant hand on patient's cheekbone just below lower eyelid.

Tissue absorbs medication that escapes eye.

(3) With tissue resting below lower lid, gently press downward with thumb or forefinger against bony orbit, exposing conjunctival sac. Never press directly against patient's eyeball.

Prevents pressure and trauma to eyeball, and prevents fingers from touching eye.

(4) Ask patient to look at ceiling.

Action moves sensitive cornea up and away from conjunctival sac into which you instill medication. Reduces stimulation of blink reflex.

(5) Rest dominant hand gently on patient's forehead and hold filled medication eyedropper approximately 1 to 2 cm (½ to ¾ inch) above conjunctival sac.

Prevents accidental contact of eyedropper with eye and reduces risk of injury and transfer of microorganisms to dropper. Contact of eyedropper with eye contaminates the container (ophthalmic medications are sterile).

Continued

STEPS	**RATIONALE**
(6) Drop prescribed number of drops into conjunctival sac (see illustration).	Conjunctival sac normally holds 1 or 2 drops. Provides even distribution of medication across eye.
(7) If patient blinks or closes eye, causing drops to land on outer lid margins, repeat procedure.	Therapeutic effect of drug is obtained only when drops enter conjunctival sac.
(8) When giving drops that may cause systemic effects, apply gentle pressure to patient's nasolacrimal duct with a clean tissue for 30 to 60 seconds over each eye, one at a time. Avoid pressure directly against patient's eyeball.	Prevents overflow of medication into nasal and pharyngeal passages. Minimizes absorption into systemic circulation.
(9) After instilling drops, ask patient to close eyes gently.	Helps to distribute medication. Squinting or squeezing eyelids forces medication from conjunctival sac.
e. Instill eye ointment.	
(1) Ask patient to look up.	Moves sensitive cornea up and away from conjunctival sac and reduces stimulation of the blink reflex during ointment application.
(2) Holding applicator above lower lid margin, apply thin ribbon of ointment evenly along inner edge of lower eyelid on conjunctiva (see illustration) from inner canthus to outer canthus.	Distributes medication evenly across eye and lid margin.
(3) Have patient close eye and rub lid lightly in circular motion with a tissue if rubbing is not contraindicated.	Further distributes medication without traumatizing eye. Avoid pressure directly against patient's eyeball.
(4) If excess medication is on eyelid, gently wipe it from inner to outer canthus.	Promotes comfort and prevents trauma to eye.
f. Apply intraocular disk.	
(1) Open package containing the disk. Gently press your fingertip against the disk so that it adheres to your finger. Position the convex side of the disk on your fingertip. It may be necessary to moisten gloved finger with sterile saline.	Allows you to inspect disk for damage or deformity.
(2) With your other hand, gently pull the patient's lower eyelid away from the eye. Ask patient to look up.	Prepares conjunctival sac for receiving medicated disk and moves sensitive cornea away.
(3) Place the disk in the conjunctival sac so that it floats on the sclera between the iris and lower eyelid (see illustration).	Ensures delivery of medication.
(4) Pull patient's lower eyelid out and over the disk. You should not be able to see the disk at this time. Repeat if you can see the disk (see illustration).	Ensures accurate medication delivery.

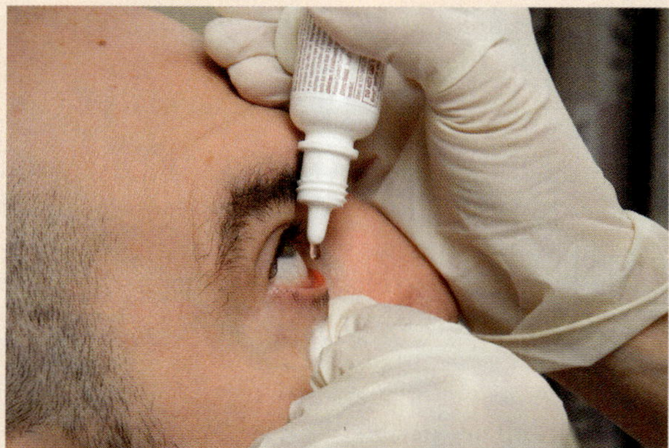

STEP 6d(6) Hold eyedropper over lower conjunctival sac.

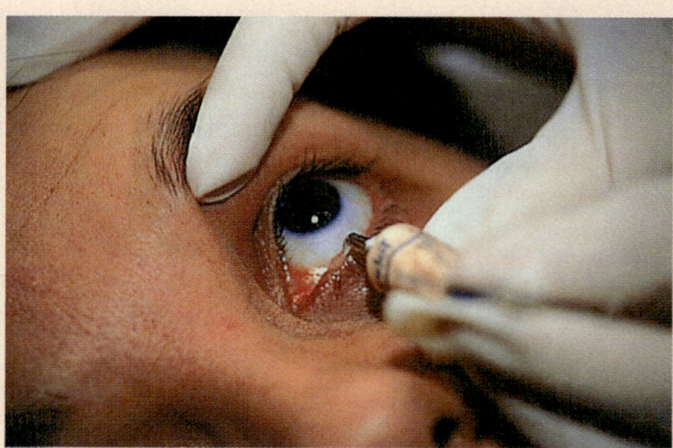

STEP 6e(2) Apply eye ointment along inside edge of lower eyelid on conjunctiva from inner to outer canthus.

STEPS	RATIONALE

7. *Remove intraocular disk.*

  a. Perform hand hygiene and apply clean gloves. Gently pull downward on lower eyelid using the nondominant hand.

Exposes disk.

  b. Using the forefinger and thumb of your dominant hand, pinch the disk and lift it out of patient's eye (see illustration).

8. If excess eye medication is on eyelid, gently wipe it from inner to outer canthus.

Promotes comfort and prevents trauma to eye.

9. After administering eye medications, remove and dispose of gloves and soiled supplies. Perform hand hygiene.

Reduces spread of microorganisms.

10. If patient had eye patch, apply clean one by placing it over affected eye so that entire eye is covered. Tape securely without applying pressure to eye.

Clean eye patch reduces chance of infection.

11. *Instill eardrops.*

  a. Perform hand hygiene and apply clean gloves (only when drainage is present).

Reduces spread of microorganisms.

  b. Warm medication to room temperature by running warm water over bottle (making sure not to damage the label or allow water to enter the bottle).

Ear structures are very sensitive to temperature extremes. Cold may cause vertigo and nausea.

  c. Position patient on side (if not contraindicated) with ear to be treated facing up, or patient may sit in a chair or at the bedside. Stabilize patient's head with his or her hand.

Facilitates distribution of medication into ear.

  d. Straighten ear canal by pulling pinna upward and outward (adult or child >3 years of age) or down and back (child ≤3 years of age).

Straightening of ear canal provides direct access to deeper external ear structures. Anatomical differences in younger children and infants require different methods of positioning canal (Hockenberry and Wilson, 2013).

  e. If cerumen or drainage occludes outermost portion of ear canal, wipe out cerumen that you can see by gently using a cotton-tipped applicator. Take care not to force wax into canal (see illustration).

Cerumen and drainage harbor microorganisms and can block distribution of medication into canal. Occlusion blocks sound transmission.

  f. Instill prescribed drops, holding dropper 1 cm (½ inch) above ear canal.

Avoiding contact prevents contamination of dropper, which could contaminate the medication in container.

  g. Ask patient to remain in side-lying position for a few minutes. Apply gentle massage or pressure to tragus of ear with finger (see illustration).

Allows complete distribution of medication. Pressure and massage move medication inward.

  h. If ordered, gently insert a portion of cotton ball into outermost part of canal. Do not press cotton into canal.

Prevents escape of medication when patient sits or stands.

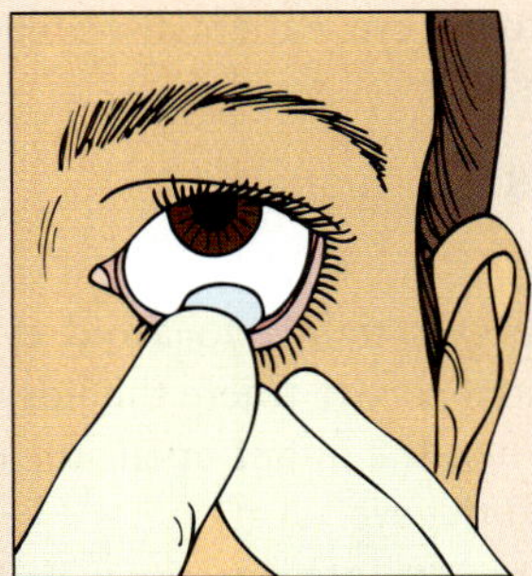

STEP 6f(3) Place disk in conjunctival sac between iris and lower eyelid.

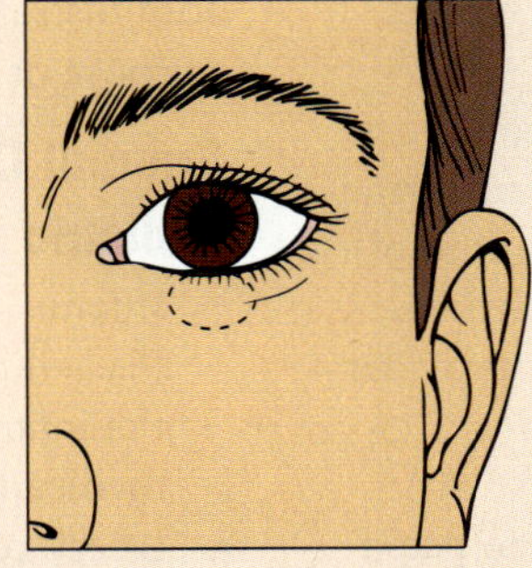

STEP 6f(4) Gently pull lower eyelid over disk.

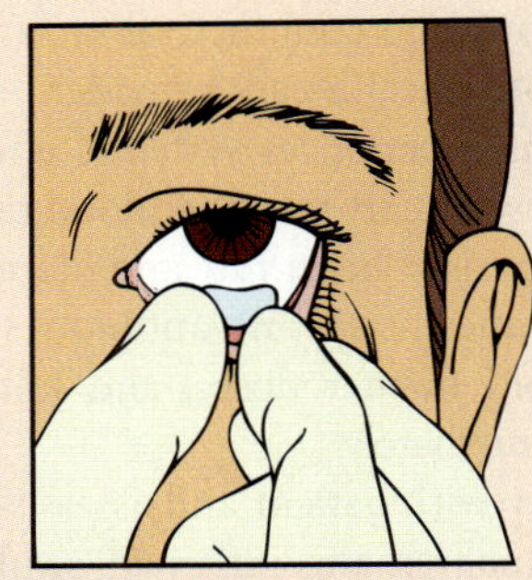

STEP 7b Carefully pinch disk to remove it from patient's eye.

Continued

STEPS	RATIONALE

   i. Remove cotton after 15 minutes. Assist patient to comfortable position after drops are absorbed.   Allows time for drug distribution and absorption.

12. See Completion Protocol (inside front cover).

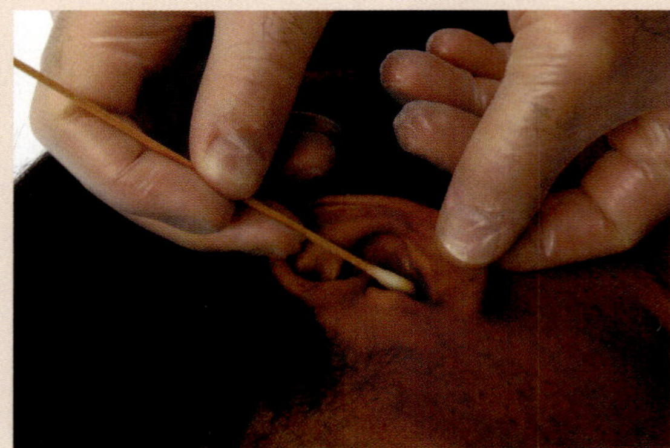

STEP 11e Always cleanse outer canal only. Do not push secretions into ear.

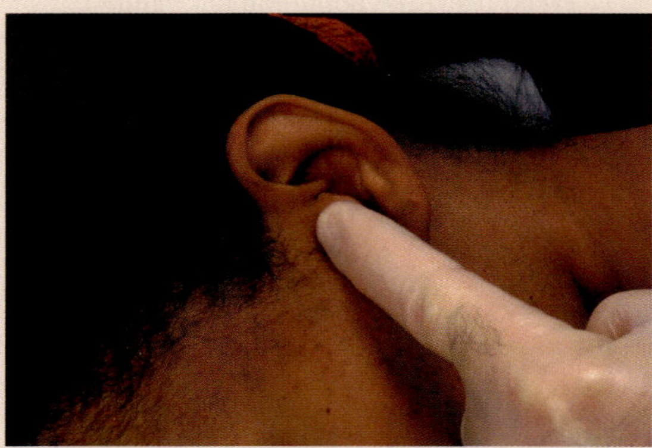

STEP 11g Nurse applies gentle pressure to tragus of ear after instilling drops.

EVALUATION

1. Evaluate for desired effects of medication by questioning patient and inspecting the eyes/ears (e.g., level of eye irritation or inflammation, ear pain and drainage).
2. Note patient's response to instillation, observe for side effects, and ask if any discomfort was felt.
3. Use **Teach Back:** State to the patient, "I want to be sure you understand what I explained about your eye medication and how to administer eyedrops. Can you explain why you apply the drops only to your left eye? Can you show me now how to place the drops in your left eye?" Evaluates what the patient is able to explain or demonstrate. Revise your instruction now or develop plan for revised patient teaching to be implemented at an appropriate time if patient is not able to teach back correctly.

Unexpected Outcomes and Related Interventions

1. Patient complains of burning or pain or experiences local side effects (e.g., headaches, bloodshot eyes) after administration of eyedrops.
   a. Evaluate condition of eyes.
   b. Use greater caution during next instillation to instill drops into conjunctival sac and not onto the cornea.
   c. Notify health care provider.
2. Patient experiences systemic effects from eyedrops (e.g., increased heart rate and blood pressure from epinephrine or decreased heart rate and blood pressure from timolol). Local anesthetics and antibiotics can cause anaphylaxis.
   a. Hold further doses, and notify health care provider immediately.
   b. Stay with patient and assess vital signs.
3. Ear canal remains inflamed, swollen, and tender to palpation. Drainage is present.
   a. Notify health care provider.

4. Patient's hearing acuity continues to be reduced.
   a. Wax may be impacted. Ear irrigation can remove cerumen (see Chapter 11).
   b. Notify health care provider.

Recording and Reporting

- Record drug, dose or strength, site of application (e.g., right eye, left eye, both), and time administered on MAR immediately after administration, not before. Include initials or signature.
- Document your evaluation of patient learning.
- Record objective data related to condition of tissues involved (e.g., redness, drainage, irritation), any subjective data (e.g., pain, itching, altered vision or hearing), and patient's response to medications. Note evidence of any side effects experienced in nurses' notes.
- Report any side effects or continued complaints of visual or hearing deficits to nurse in charge or health care provider.

Sample Documentation

1300   Complaining of dry and irritated eye; some yellowish drainage in lacrimal sac. Patient able to demonstrate correct administration of eyedrop to left eye. Patient also able to state purpose of medication correctly.

Special Considerations
Pediatric

- Infants often clench the eyes tightly to avoid eyedrops. Place the drops in the nasal corner where the lids meet as the infant lies supine. When the infant opens the eye, the medication will flow into the eye.
- Insert cotton pledgets loosely into ear canal to prevent medication from flowing out of the external ear canal. To prevent cotton from absorbing medication in ear,

premoisten cotton with a few drops of medication (Hockenberry and Wilson, 2013).

- Ensure that parents and other caregivers are aware of the proper method of administration (e.g., for children <3 years old, gently pull the pinna of the ear downward and straight back).
- Restrain infants or young children in supine position with head turned to expose affected ear. Hold child in this position until drug has time to be absorbed (Hockenberry and Wilson, 2013).
- Teach the signs of hearing loss and the need for frequent follow-ups to parents with children who have chronic otitis media.

Geriatric

- Many older adults accumulate cerumen in the ear. This should be removed by irrigation before administration of medication (see Chapter 11).

Home Care

- Have patients with chronic health problems consult their health care provider before using OTC eye medications. When using OTC medications, encourage patient to follow manufacturer's directions closely.
- Patients should not share eyedrops with other family members. Risk of infection transmission is high.

SKILL 22.5   USING METERED-DOSE INHALERS

• Nursing Skills Online: Nonparenteral Medication Administration, Lesson 5

Medications administered with handheld inhalers are dispersed through an aerosol spray, mist, or powder that penetrates the airways. Pressurized metered-dose inhalers (MDIs), breath-actuated MDIs, and dry powder inhalers (DPIs) deliver medications that produce local effects such as bronchodilation. Some of these medications are absorbed rapidly through the pulmonary circulation and create systemic side effects; for example, albuterol (Proventil) may cause palpitations, tremors, or tachycardia. Patients who receive drugs by inhalation frequently have chronic respiratory disease. Because they depend on these medications for disease control, they must learn about them and how to administer them safely. Inhalers and small-volume nebulizers (see Skill 22-6) are devices that deliver inhaled medications.

MDIs are small, handheld devices that disperse medication into the airways through an aerosol spray or mist by activation of a propellant. Dosing is usually achieved with 1 or 2 puffs. DPIs deliver inhaled medication in a fine powder formulation to the respiratory tract, and as a result more medication is delivered to the lungs and less to the oropharynx. Fig. 22-2 shows examples of MDIs and DPIs. The deeper passages of the respiratory tract provide a large surface area for drug absorption, and the alveolar-capillary network absorbs medication rapidly.

An MDI delivers a measured dose of a drug with each push of a canister. Approximately 5 to 10 pounds of pressure is needed to activate the aerosol; this is difficult for some older adults because hand strength diminishes with age. Use of an MDI requires coordination during the breathing cycle, and consequently many patients spray only the back of their throats and fail to receive a full dose. The inhaler must be depressed to expel medication just as the patient inhales; this ensures that the medication reaches the lower airways. The problem of poor coordination can be solved by the use of spacer devices (e.g., AeroChamber, Inspirease) or a breath-activated MDI (e.g., Maxair Autohaler). A spacer device

decreases the amount of medication deposited into the oropharyngeal mucosa. Some spacers have a one-way valve that activates on inhalation, removing the need for good hand-breath coordination (Lehne, 2013). Box 22-2 summarizes common problems that occur when using an inhaler.

ASSESSMENT

1. Check accuracy and completeness of each MAR with health care provider's medication order. Check patient's name, drug name and dosage (number of inhalations), route of administration, and time for administration. Clarify incomplete or unclear orders with health care provider before administration. *Rationale: The health care provider's order is the most reliable source and only legal record of drugs the patient is to receive. Ensures that patient receives the right medications (Mandrack et al., 2012;*

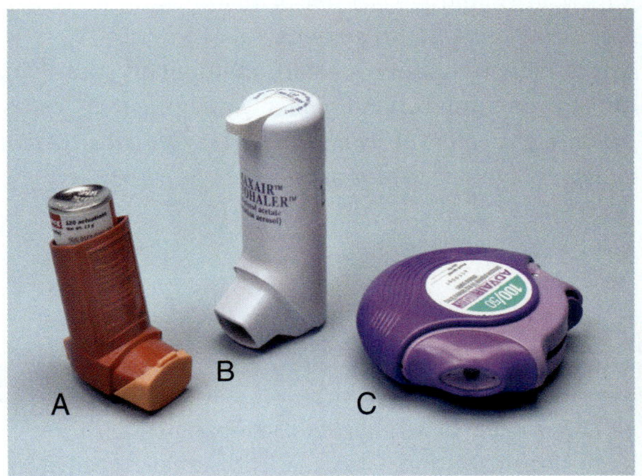

FIG 22-2 Types of inhalers. **A,** Metered-dose inhaler (MDI). **B,** Breath-activated inhaler. **C,** Dry powder inhaler (DPI). (From Lilley LL et al: *Pharmacology and the nursing process,* ed 6, St Louis, 2011, Mosby.)

> **BOX 22-2**   **COMMON PROBLEMS WHEN USING AN INHALER**
>
> - *Not taking medication as prescribed:* Either too much or too little is taken.
> - *Incorrect activation:* This usually occurs through pressing the canister before taking a breath. These actions should be done simultaneously so the drug can be carried down to the lungs with the breath.
> - *Forgetting to shake the inhaler:* The drug is in a suspension, and particles may settle. If the inhaler is not shaken, it may not deliver the correct dose of the drug.
> - *Not waiting long enough between puffs:* The whole process should be repeated when taking the second puff; otherwise, an incorrect dose may be delivered, or the drug may not penetrate into the lungs.
> - *Failure to clean the valve:* Particles may jam the valve in the mouthpiece unless it is cleaned occasionally. This is a frequent cause of failure to get 200 puffs from one inhaler.
> - Failure to observe whether the inhaler is actually releasing a spray: If it is not, this should be checked with the pharmacist.
> - *Failure to recognize when the canister is empty.* This occurs when the MDI has no built-in dose counter or instructions in dose counting.

Sulosaari et al., 2011). Handwritten MARs are a source of medication errors (Alassaad et al., 2013).

2. Review pertinent information related to medication, including action, purpose, normal dose and route, common side effects, time of onset and peak action, and nursing implications. *Rationale: Allows you to anticipate effects of drug and observe patient's response.*

3. Assess patient's medical history, history of allergies, and medication history. *Rationale: Factors influence how certain drugs act. Reveals patient's need for medication.*

4. Assess respiratory pattern and auscultate breath sounds. *Rationale: Establishes baseline of airway status for comparison during and after treatment.*

5. Assess patient's ability to hold, manipulate, and depress canister and inhaler. *Rationale: Impairment of grasp or presence of tremors of hands interferes with patient's ability to depress canister within inhaler.*

6. Assess patient's readiness to learn: Patient asks questions about medication, requests education in use of inhaler, is mentally alert, and participates in own care.

7. Assess patient's ability to learn: Patient should not be fatigued, in pain, or in respiratory distress; assess level of understanding of medical terms.

8. Assess patient's knowledge and understanding of disease and purpose and action of prescribed medications. *Rationale: May assist in assessing patient's potential for compliance with self-administration.*

PLANNING

Expected Outcomes focus on relief of symptoms; promoting knowledge for self-administration of inhalers; and safe, accurate, and effective drug therapy.

1. Patient correctly self-administers metered dose.

2. Patient describes proper time during respiratory cycle to inhale spray and number of inhalations for each administration.

3. Patient's breathing pattern improves, and airways become less restrictive with adequate gas exchange.

4. Patient lists common side effects of medications and criteria for calling health care professional if dyspnea develops.

Delegation and Collaboration

The skill of administering MDIs cannot be delegated to nursing assistive personnel (NAP). The nurse instructs the NAP about:

- Potential side effects of medications and reporting their occurrence.
- Signs of breathing difficulties (e.g., paroxysmal coughing, audible wheezing).

Equipment

- Inhaler device with medication canister (MDI or DPI) (see Fig. 22-2)
- Spacer device such as AeroChamber or Inspirease (optional)
- Facial tissues (optional)
- MAR
- Stethoscope
- Pulse oximeter (optional)

IMPLEMENTATION *for* USING METERED-DOSE INHALERS

STEPS	RATIONALE
1. Perform hand hygiene. Prepare medications for administration. Check label of inhaler against MAR two times (see Skill 22-1). Preparation involves taking inhaler device out of storage and into patient room. Check expiration date on container.	*This includes the first and second checks for accuracy.* Ensures that right patient receives right medication. Medications used past expiration date may be inactive or harmful to patient.

2. Take medications to patient at correct time (see facility policy). Medications that require exact timing include STAT, first-time or loading, and one-time doses. Give time-critical scheduled medications (e.g., antibiotics, bronchodilators, steroids) no later than 30 minutes before or after scheduled dose. Give non–time-critical scheduled medications within a range of either 1 or 2 hours of scheduled dose (ISMP, 2011). During administration, apply the six rights of medication administration.

Hospitals must adopt medication administration policy and procedure for timing of medication administration that considers nature of the prescribed medication, specific clinical application, and patient needs (DHHS, 2011; ISMP, 2011). Time-critical scheduled medications are medications where early or delayed administration of maintenance doses of greater than 30 minutes before or after the scheduled dose may cause harm or result in substantial suboptimal therapy or pharmacological effect. Non–time-critical medications *are medications where early or delayed administration within a specified range of either 1 or 2 hours* should not cause harm or result in substantial suboptimal therapy or pharmacological effect (DHHS, 2011; ISMP, 2011).

3. **See Standard Protocol (inside front cover).**

4. At the patient's bedside, identify patient using two identifiers (e.g., name and birthday or name and account number) according to facility policy. Compare identifiers with information on the patient's MAR or medical record. Then compare MAR or computer printout with the names of medications on the medication labels and patient name.

Ensures the correct patient. Complies with the Joint Commission Standards and improves patient safety (TJC, 2014). *This is the third check for accuracy* and ensures that the patient receives the correct medication.

> **SAFE PATIENT CARE** When the patient is scheduled to receive inhaled bronchodilators and inhaled corticosteroids at the same time, the bronchodilators should be given first to promote opening of the airways. After 5 minutes, administer the second drug (Lehne, 2013).

5. Discuss the purpose of each medication, action, and possible adverse effects. Allow patient to ask any questions. Explain what a metered dose is and how to administer. Warn about overuse of inhaler, including side effects.

Patient has the right to be informed, and patient's understanding of each medication improves adherence with drug therapy. Makes patient a participant and reduces anxiety in learning new skill.

6. Allow adequate time for patient to manipulate inhaler, canister, and spacer device (if provided). Explain and demonstrate how canister fits into inhaler.

Patient must be familiar with how to assemble and use equipment.

> **SAFE PATIENT CARE** If using an MDI that is new or has not been used for several days, push a "test spray" into the air to prime the device before using. This ensures that the MDI is patent. You do not need to do this for a DPI.

7. *Explain steps for administering MDI, without spacer* (demonstrate when possible).

Simple step-by-step explanation allows patient to ask questions at any point during procedure.

  a. Remove mouthpiece cover from inhaler after inserting MDI canister into holder.

  b. Shake inhaler well for 2 to 5 seconds (five or six shakes).

Ensures mixing of medication in canister.

  c. Hold inhaler upright in dominant hand.

  d. Instruct patient to position inhaler in one of two ways:

  (1) Place mouthpiece in mouth with opening toward back of throat, closing lips tightly around it (see illustration).

Directs aerosol toward airways.

  (2) Position mouthpiece 2 to 4 cm (1 to 2 inches) in front of widely opened mouth (see illustration), with opening of inhaler aimed toward back of throat. Lips do not touch inhaler.

Directs aerosol spray toward airway. This is the best way to deliver the medication without a spacer.

Continued

STEPS	RATIONALE
e. Have patient take a deep breath and exhale completely.	Prepares airway to receive medication.
f. With inhaler positioned, have patient hold inhaler with thumb at the mouthpiece and index and middle fingers at the top. This is a three-point or bilateral hand position.	Hand position ensures proper activation of MDI (Lehne, 2013).
g. Instruct patient to tilt head back slightly and inhale slowly and deeply through the mouth for 3 to 5 seconds while depressing the canister fully.	Medication is distributed to airways during inhalation.
h. Have patient hold breath for about 5 to 10 seconds (Roy et al., 2011).	Allows the tiny drops of aerosol spray to reach deeper branches of airways (Mayo Clinic, 2011a).
i. Remove MDI from mouth and hold breath another 5 to 10 seconds before exhaling (Roy et al., 2011). Exhale slowly through nose or pursed lips.	Keeps small airways open during exhalation.

8. *Explain steps to administer MDI using a spacer device* (demonstrate when possible).

STEPS	RATIONALE
a. Remove mouthpiece cover from MDI and mouthpiece of spacer device. Inspect the spacer for foreign objects.	Inhaler fits into end of spacer device.
b. Shake inhaler well for 2 to 5 seconds (five or six shakes).	Mixes medication in canister.
c. Insert MDI into end of spacer device.	Spacer device traps medication released from MDI; patient then inhales the drug from the device. Spacers break up and slow down the particles increasing absorption of the medication into the airway (Mayo Clinic, 2011b).
d. Instruct patient to place spacer device mouthpiece into mouth and close lips. Do not insert beyond raised lip on mouthpiece. Avoid covering small exhalation slots with the lips.	Medication should not escape through mouth.
e. Have patient breathe normally through spacer device mouthpiece (see illustration).	Allows patient to relax before delivering medication.

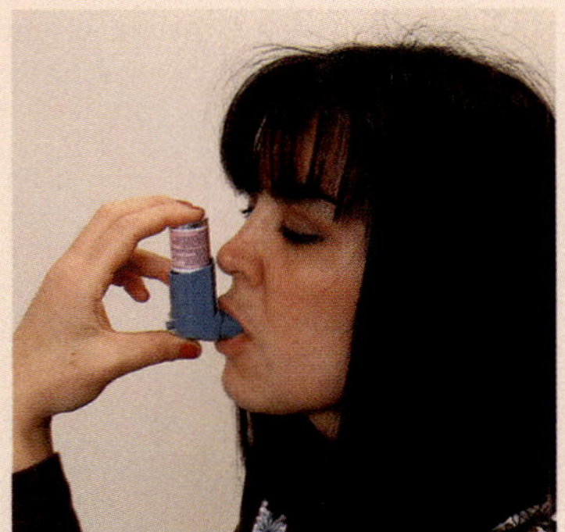

STEP 7d(1) Using MDI.

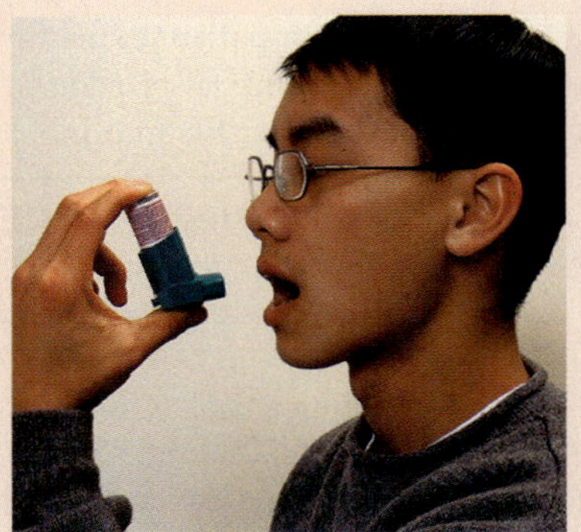

STEP 7d(2) Alternative technique for using MDI.

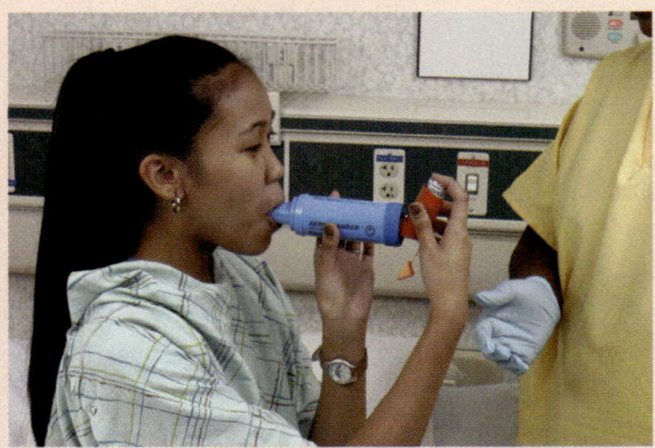

STEP 8e Using spacer device with MDI. (From Lilley LL et al: *Pharmacology and the nursing process*, ed 6, St Louis, 2011, Mosby.)

STEPS	RATIONALE

    f. Instruct patient to depress medication canister, spraying 1 puff into spacer device.

Device contains fine spray and allows patient to inhale more medicine.

    g. Instruct patient to breath in slowly and deeply through mouth for 3 to 5 seconds.

Particles of medication are able to distribute to deeper airways.

    h. Instruct patient to hold breath for 10 seconds.

Ensures full drug distribution.

  9. *Explain steps to administer DPI or breath-activated MDI (demonstrate when possible).*

Use of simple step-by-step explanations allows patient to ask questions at any point during the procedure.

    a. Remove mouthpiece cover. *Do not shake* inhaler.

    b. Prepare medication as directed by manufacturer (e.g., hold inhaler upright and turn wheel to the right and then to the left until a click is heard; load medication pellet).

Primes inhaler, ensuring that medication is delivered to patient (Mayo Clinic, 2011b).

    c. Exhale away from inhaler.

Prevents loss of powder.

    d. Position mouthpiece between lips.

Keeps medication from escaping through mouth.

    e. Inhale deeply and forcefully through mouth.

Creates aerosol.

    f. Hold full breath for 5 to 10 seconds.

Allows distribution of medication.

 10. Instruct patient to wait 20 to 30 seconds between inhalations (if same medication) or 2 to 5 minutes between inhalations (if different medication).

Drugs must be inhaled sequentially. Always administer bronchodilators before steroids so that dilators can open airway passages (Lehne, 2013).

 11. Instruct patient not to repeat inhalations before next scheduled dose.

Drugs are prescribed at intervals during the day to provide a constant drug level and minimize side effects. Beta-adrenergic bronchodilator MDIs are used either on an "as needed" basis or regularly every 4 to 6 hours.

 12. Explain that patient might feel a gagging sensation in throat caused by droplets of medication on pharynx or tongue.

This occurs if medication is sprayed or inhaled incorrectly.

 13. After use of the MDI, instruct patient to rinse mouth out with warm water and spit the water out about 2 minutes after last dose.

Inhaled bronchodilators may cause dry mouth and taste alterations. Steroids may alter the normal flora of the oral mucosa and lead to development of fungal infection (Lehne, 2013).

 14. Have patient refer to manufacturer's instructions for cleaning. Most recommend weekly. Instruct patient to remove MDI medication canister, rinse the inhaler and cap with warm running water. Shake off excess water and allow to dry completely. Do not get the valve mechanism of the canister wet. Do not wash a DPI. Instead, clean the mouthpiece with a dry cloth.

Removes residual medication and decreases transfer of microorganisms. Do not place inhalers holding cromolyn, nedocromil, or hydrofluoroalkane in water.

 15. Ask if patient has any questions.

 16. **See Completion Protocol (inside front cover).**

EVALUATION

1. Ask patient to explain drug schedule and dose of medication.
2. After medication instillation, assess patient's respirations, breath sounds, and peak flow measures if ordered.
3. Observe patient self-administer an inhaled dose of medication.
4. Ask patient to describe side effects and criteria for calling health care provider.
5. Use **Teach Back:** State to the patient, "I want to be sure you understand how to use and clean your inhaler the right way. Can you show me now how to clean the device?" Evaluates what the patient is able to explain or demonstrate. Revise your instruction now or develop plan for revised patient teaching to be implemented at an appropriate time if patient is not able to teach back correctly.

Unexpected Outcomes and Related Interventions

1. Patient's breathing pattern is ineffective; respirations are rapid and shallow.
     a. Obtain vital signs and respiratory status.
     b. Evaluate type of medication or patient's administration technique.
     c. Notify health care provider.

2. Patient experiences paroxysms of coughing.
  a. Observe and evaluate patient's administration technique.
  b. Notify health care provider.
3. Patient has cardiac dysrhythmias (light-headedness, syncope).
  a. Evaluate cardiac and pulmonary status (see Chapter 7).
  b. Withhold all further doses of medication.
  c. Notify health care provider.
4. Patient is unable to self-administer medication correctly.
  a. Explore alternative delivery routes.
  b. Assess potential benefits of a spacer device.
  c. Revise your instruction now or develop plan for revised patient teaching to be implemented at an appropriate time if patient is not able to teach back correctly.

Recording and Reporting

- Record drug, dose or strength, number of inhalations, and time administered on MAR immediately after administration, not before. Include initials or signature.
- Document your evaluation of patient learning.
- Record in nurses' notes patient's response to MDI (e.g., respiratory rate and pattern, breath sounds), evidence of side effects (e.g., arrhythmia, patient's feelings of anxiety), and patient's ability to use MDI.
- Report any side effects of medication to health care provider.

Sample Documentation

0900 Coughing violently and reports difficulty breathing. Wheezing noted throughout all lung fields. R 32, P 98 and regular. Self-administered albuterol per MDI (2 puffs) correctly with no verbal coaching. Needed reminder to clean inhaler after use. Reported relief from shortness of breath within 1 minute.

0915 Reports breathing more at ease, R 24, P 94 and regular. Wheezing remains in left upper lobe, right lung fields are clear.

Special Considerations
Pediatric

- A spacer is beneficial to young children because they have difficulty coordinating the activation of the inhaler and inhaling (Hockenberry and Wilson, 2013).
- Educate child and parent about the need to use inhaler during school hours. Help family find resources within the school or day care facility. Many school systems do not permit self-administration of MDIs. Follow school policy. A health care provider's order is required.

Geriatric

- An older adult may be unable to depress the medication canister because of weakened grasp. If there is difficulty with coordinating activation of the inhaler and inhalation, the use of a spacer device may be helpful.

Home Care

- The patient's health care provider often will order use of a small, handheld peak flowmeter to regularly monitor if lung disease is under control and to monitor response to therapy (Barrons et al., 2011). The patient blows into the device and it gives a score, or peak flow number. The score shows how well the patient's lungs are working at the time of the test.
- Teach patients how to count doses in MDI and how to plan for renewal of medication. Failure to do so might result in a patient using an empty inhaler during an acute episode of a respiratory problem. To track doses:
  - Note first day of use on a calendar.
  - Note number of inhalations in the canister (e.g., 200 inhalations per MDI).
  - Note number of inhalations used per day (e.g., 2 inhalations a day, 3 times a day, equals 6 inhalations a day).
  - Divide the total number of inhalations in canister by the number of inhalations needed per day to determine number of days inhaler should last (e.g., 200/6 = 33 days of 3 times-a-day dosing).
  - Mark on calendar the date inhaler will be empty; obtain a refill a few days before.

SKILL 22.6 USING SMALL-VOLUME NEBULIZERS

Nebulization is a process of adding medications or moisture to inspired air by mixing particles of various sizes with air. Adding moisture to the respiratory system through nebulization improves clearance of pulmonary secretions (Tai et al., 2011). Medications such as bronchodilators, mucolytics, and corticosteroids are often administered by nebulization. Small-volume nebulizers are machines that convert a drug solution into a mist that a patient then inhales into the tracheobronchial tree. The droplets in the mist are much finer than the droplets created by MDIs or DPIs. Inhalation of the nebulized mist is delivered via face mask or a mouthpiece held between the teeth. A nebulized medication is designed to create a local effect, but it can be absorbed into the bloodstream through the alveoli. As a result, systemic effects from the medications may occur.

ASSESSMENT

1. Check accuracy and completeness of each MAR with health care provider's medication order. Check patient's name, drug name and dosage, route of administration, and time for administration. Clarify incomplete or unclear orders with health care provider before administration. *Rationale: The health care provider's order is the most reliable source and only legal record of drugs the patient is to receive. Ensures that patient receives the right medications*

(Mandrack et al., 2012; Sulosaari et al., 2011). Handwritten MARs are a source of medication errors (Alassaad et al., 2013).

2. Review pertinent information related to medication, including action, purpose, normal dose and route, time of onset and peak action, common side effects, and nursing implications. *Rationale: Allows you to anticipate effects of drug and observe patient's response.*

3. Assess patient's medical history (e.g., history of cardiac disease), history of allergies, and medication and diet history. *Rationale: Factors influence how certain drugs act. Reveals patient's need for medication and risk for side effects.*

4. Assess patient's grasp and ability to assemble, hold, and manipulate the nebulizer equipment. Option: Assess family caregiver's ability to assemble equipment for patient. *Rationale: Patient can still use a nebulizer if caregiver sets up equipment. However, any impairment of grasp or hand tremors interfere with ability to use nebulizer.*

5. Assess pulse, respirations, breath sounds, pulse oximetry, and peak flow measurement (if ordered). *Rationale: Provides baseline to determine effect of medication.*

6. Assess patient's knowledge of medication and readiness to learn (e.g., patient is alert, asks questions about medication, and requests education in use of nebulizer).

| PLANNING

Expected Outcomes focus on safe, accurate, and effective drug therapy; relief of symptoms; and patient's ability to self-administer small-volume nebulizer.

1. Patient's breathing pattern is effective.
2. Patient's oxygen saturation level is adequate.
3. Patient is able to demonstrate self-administration of nebulized dose of medication correctly.
4. Patient is able to describe common side effects of medication and criteria for calling health care provider.

Delegation and Collaboration

In many facilities, a respiratory therapist performs the skill of administering medications by nebulizer. The nurse must be aware of the type and actions of the inhaled medication that the patient is receiving. The skill of administering medications by nebulizer cannot be delegated to nursing assistive personnel (NAP). The nurse instructs the NAP about:

- Potential side effects of medications and to report their occurrence to the nurse.
- Reporting paroxysmal coughing, ineffective breathing patterns, and other respiratory difficulties.

Equipment

- Medication ordered and diluent (if needed)
- Medicine dropper or syringe
- Nebulizer bottle and tubing assembly
- Small-volume nebulizer machine (often called *handheld nebulizer* or simply *nebulizer*)
- Pulse oximeter and peak flow device
- Stethoscope
- MAR

IMPLEMENTATION *for* USING SMALL-VOLUME NEBULIZERS

STEP	RATIONALE
1. Prepare medications for administration. Check label of nebulized medication against MAR two times (see Skill 22-1). Preparation may involve taking medication vial out of storage. Check expiration date on container.	*This includes the first and second checks for accuracy.* Ensures that right patient receives right medication.
2. Take medications to patient at correct time (see facility policy). Medications that require exact timing include STAT, first-time or loading, and one-time doses. Give time-critical scheduled medications (e.g., corticosteroids) no later than 30 minutes before or after scheduled dose. Give non–time-critical scheduled medications within a range of either 1 or 2 hours of scheduled dose (ISMP, 2011). During administration, apply the six rights of medication administration.	Hospitals must adopt medication administration policy and procedure for timing of medication administration that considers nature of the prescribed medication, specific clinical application, and patient needs (DHHS, 2011; ISMP, 2011). Time-critical scheduled medications are medications where early or delayed administration of maintenance doses of greater than 30 minutes before or after the scheduled dose may cause harm or result in substantial suboptimal therapy or pharmacological effect. Non–time-critical medications *are medications where early or delayed administration within a specified range of either 1 or 2 hours* should not cause harm or result in substantial suboptimal therapy or pharmacological effect (DHHS, 2011; ISMP, 2011).

Continued

STEP	RATIONALE

3. See Standard Protocol (inside front cover).

4. At the patient's bedside, identify patient using two identifiers (e.g., name and birthday or name and account number) according to facility policy. Compare identifiers with information on the patient's MAR or medical record. Then compare MAR or computer printout with the names of medications on the medication labels and patient name.

Ensures the correct patient. Complies with the Joint Commission Standards and improves patient safety (TJC, 2014). *This is the third check for accuracy* and ensures that the patient receives the correct medication.

5. Discuss the purpose of each medication, action, and possible side effects. Allow patient to ask any questions. Explain to patient how to assemble nebulizer.

Patient has the right to be informed, and patient's understanding of each medication improves adherence with drug therapy. Makes patient a participant in care and minimizes anxiety. Enables patient to self-administer drug if physically able and motivated.

6. Explain use of nebulizer.

Makes patient more knowledgeable about how treatment affects respirations.

7. Assemble nebulizer equipment per manufacturer's directions.

Assembly may vary slightly with different manufacturers. Proper assembly ensures safe delivery of medication.

8. Add prescribed medication using medicine dropper or syringe and diluent (if needed) to nebulizer cup.

Ensures proper dose and delivery of ordered medication.

9. Attach the cap of the nebulizer cup. Connect the tubing connector and mouthpiece or face mask to the cup.

10. Connect the tubing to both the aerosol compressor and the nebulizer cup.

11. Have patient hold mouthpiece between lips with gentle pressure (see illustration).

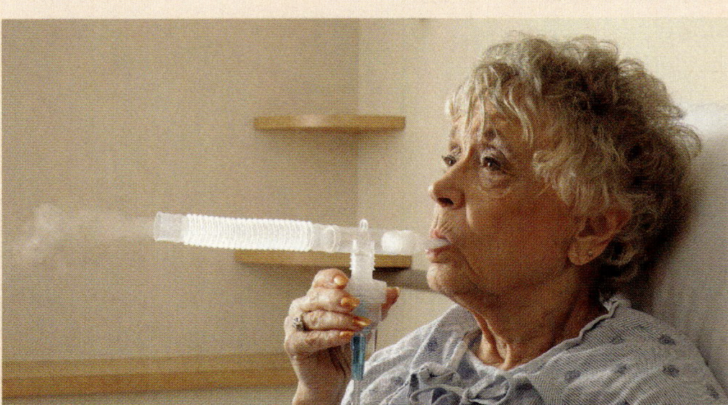

STEP 11 Nebulizer mouthpiece placed between patient's lips during treatment.

a. If patient is an infant, child, or fatigued adult or unable to follow instructions, use a face mask.

Use of a face mask does not require patient to remember to hold mouthpiece correctly. Correct delivery ensures sufficient deposition of medication.

b. Use special adapters for patients with a tracheostomy.

Promotes greater deposition of medication in the airways.

12. Turn on the small-volume nebulizer machine and ensure that a sufficient mist is formed.

Verifies that equipment is working properly during delivery of medication.

13. Instruct patient to take a deep breath, slowly, to a volume slightly greater than normal. Encourage a brief, end-inspiratory pause; then have patient exhale passively.

Improves effectiveness of medication.

a. If patient is dyspneic, encourage him or her to hold every fourth or fifth breath for 5 to 10 seconds.

Maximizes effectiveness of medication.

STEP	RATIONALE
b. Remind patient to repeat the breathing pattern until the drug is completely nebulized. This usually takes about 10 minutes.	Maximizes effectiveness of medication.
(1) Some health care providers set a time limit for the length of the treatment rather than waiting for the medication to nebulize completely.	
c. Tap the nebulizer cup occasionally during treatment and toward the end of treatment.	Releases droplets that are clinging to the side of the cup, allowing for renebulization of the solution.
d. Monitor patient's pulse during procedure, especially if beta-adrenergic bronchodilators are used.	Enables nurse to observe for potential side effects of medications.

> **SAFE PATIENT CARE** Some respiratory medications can cause systemic effects such as restlessness, nervousness, and palpitations. Administer these medications with caution to patients with cardiac disease because of the possibility of hypertension, dysrhythmias, or coronary insufficiency. If severe bronchospasm occurs during treatment, discontinue drug immediately, and notify health care provider.

STEP	RATIONALE
14. When medication is completely nebulized, turn off machine. Rinse the nebulizer cup per facility guidelines. Dry completely. Store tubing assembly per facility policy. Also check facility policy for daily cleansing.	Proper cleaning and storage reduces transfer of microorganisms. A soak-then-rinse method after each medication administration is frequently adequate (Tai et al., 2013).
15. If steroids are nebulized, instruct patient to rinse mouth and gargle with warm water after nebulizer treatment.	Removes medication residue from oral cavity and helps to prevent oral candidiasis, an adverse effect of inhaled steroid therapy.
16. After nebulization, have patient take several deep breaths and cough to expectorate mucus.	A nebulized medication is often ordered to open airways and promote expectoration of mucus.
17. See Completion Protocol (inside front cover).	

EVALUATION

1. Assess patient's respirations, breath sounds, cough effort, sputum production, and pulse oximetry; assess peak flow measures if ordered.
2. Ask patient to explain drug schedule.
3. Ask patient to describe side effects of medication and criteria for calling health care provider.
4. Use *Teach Back:* State to the patient, "I want to be sure you understand what I explained about how to use a small-volume nebulizer the right way. Can you show me now how to prepare the nebulizer and take a dose?" Evaluates what the patient is able to explain or demonstrate. Revise your instruction now or develop plan for revised patient teaching to be implemented at an appropriate time if patient is not able to teach back correctly.

Unexpected Outcomes and Related Interventions

1. Patient's breathing pattern is ineffective; respirations are rapid and shallow; breath sounds indicate wheezing.
   a. Reassess type of medication or delivery method.
   b. Notify health care provider.
2. Patient experiences paroxysms of coughing. Aerosolized particles can irritate posterior pharynx.
   a. Reassess type of medication or delivery method.
   b. Notify health care provider.
3. Patient experiences cardiac dysrhythmias (syncope, lightheadedness), especially if receiving beta-adrenergic bronchodilators.
   a. Withhold all further doses of medication. Assess vital signs.
   b. Notify health care provider for reassessment of type of medication and delivery method.
4. Patient is unable to self-administer medication properly. Revise your instruction now or develop plan for revised patient teaching to be implemented at an appropriate time if patient is not able to teach back correctly.

Recording and Reporting

- Record drug, dose or strength, length of treatment, route, and time administered on MAR immediately after administration, not before. Include initials or signature.
- Document your evaluation of patient learning.
- Document patient's response to treatment.

- Report adverse effects or patient response and withheld drugs to nurse in charge or health care provider.

Sample Documentation

0900 Reports that he "has trouble catching my breath" after walking down hallway. Observed patient correctly prepare nebulizer with budesonide 500 mcg. Patient successfully administered nebulizer over 20 minutes.

0930 Postnebulizer R 26, P 100; wheezes decreased. States he is "breathing easier now."

Special Considerations

Pediatric

- Use a nebulizer mask if child is too young to hold mouthpiece correctly for the duration of the treatment (Hockenberry and Wilson, 2013).
- Educate child and parent about the use of a nebulizer during school or day care hours. Help family find resources within the school or day care facility. Follow school policy regarding having the nebulizer and medication available

for use during school hours. A health care provider's order may be necessary.

Geriatric

- Patients may have weakened grasp, hand tremors, or coordination problems that make it difficult to hold nebulizer. A family caregiver might be able to assist.

Home Care

- Rinse the nebulizer and allow to air dry after each use. For daily cleansing, soak the nebulizer for 10 minutes in soapy tap water, change the water, then rinse for 30 seconds and allow to air dry (Tai et al., 2011).
- Follow manufacturer's recommendations for maintenance of small-volume nebulizer machine, including changing the filters when they become discolored (grayish).
- Advise patients taking long-acting beta agonists, which are used for long-term control of symptoms, about possible adverse effects, such as nervousness, restlessness, tremor, headache, nausea, rapid or pounding heart rate, and dizziness. Emphasize that the drug should be taken only as ordered to avoid developing a tolerance.

PROCEDURAL GUIDELINE 22.1
Administering Vaginal Medications

- **Nursing Skills Online: Nonparenteral Medication Administration Module, Lesson 6**

Patients who develop vaginal infections often require topical application of antiinfective agents. Vaginal medications are available in foam, jelly, cream, or suppository form. Medicated irrigations or douches can also be given. However, excessive use of irrigations or douches can lead to vaginal irritation.

Vaginal suppositories are oval-shaped and come individually packaged in foil wrappers. They are larger and more oval than rectal suppositories (Fig. 22-3). Storage in a refrigerator prevents the solid suppositories from melting. You insert a suppository into the vagina either with an applicator or a gloved hand. After insertion, body temperature causes the suppository to melt, and the medication is distributed. Foam, jellies, and creams are administered with an inserter or applicator. Patients often prefer administering their own vaginal medications, and you should give them privacy to do so. After instillation of the drug, a patient may wish to wear a perineal pad to collect excess drainage. Because vaginal medications are frequently given to treat infection, any discharge is often foul-smelling. Follow good aseptic technique, and offer the patient frequent opportunities for perineal hygiene (see Chapter 10).

Delegation and Collaboration

The skill of administering vaginal instillations cannot be delegated to nursing assistive personnel (NAP). The nurse instructs the NAP about:

- Potential side effects of medications and to report their occurrence to the nurse.
- Reporting a change in comfort level or new or increased vaginal discharge or bleeding to the nurse.

Equipment

- Vaginal cream, foam, jelly, tablet, suppository, or irrigating solution
- Applicators (Fig. 22-4) (if needed)
- Clean gloves
- Tissues
- Towels and washcloths
- Perineal pad; drape or sheet
- Water-soluble lubricants
- Bedpan
- Irrigation or douche container (if needed)
- MAR

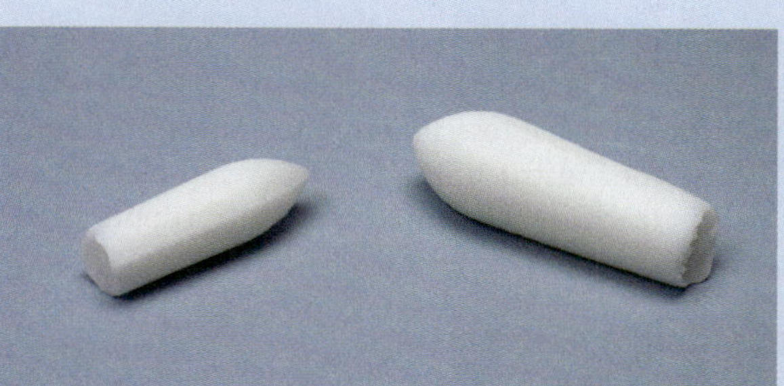

FIG 22-3 Vaginal suppositories *(right)* are larger and more oval than rectal suppositories *(left)*. (From Lilley LL et al: *Pharmacology and the nursing process,* ed 4, St Louis, 2004, Mosby.)

PROCEDURAL GUIDELINE 22.1
Administering Vaginal Medications—cont'd

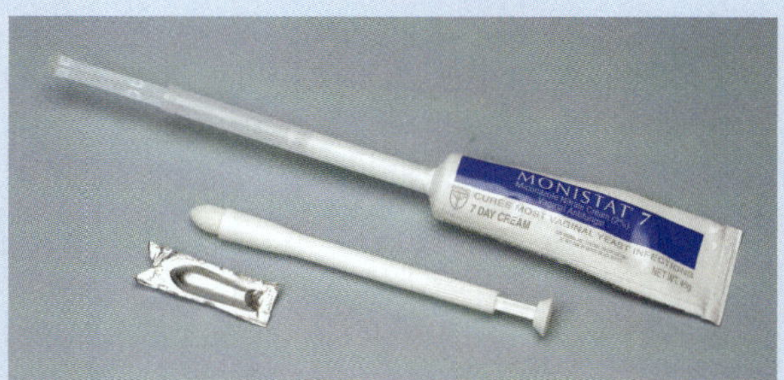

FIG 22-4 *From top:* Vaginal cream with applicator, applicator, and vaginal suppository. (From Lilley LL et al: *Pharmacology and the nursing process,* ed 6, St Louis, 2011, Mosby.)

Procedural Steps

1. Check accuracy and completeness of each MAR with health care provider's medication order. Check patient's name, drug name and dosage, route of administration, and time for administration. Clarify incomplete or unclear orders with health care provider before administration.
2. Review pertinent information related to medication, including action, purpose, normal dose and route, common side effects, time of onset and peak action, and nursing implications.
3. Assess patient's medical history, history of allergies, and medication history.
4. Ask if patient is experiencing any symptoms of pruritus, burning, discharge, or discomfort.
5. Assess patient's knowledge of medication and readiness to learn (e.g., patient asks questions about medication, requests education in use of suppository).
6. Assess patient's ability to insert suppository (cognitive level and hand coordination).
7. Prepare suppository for administration. Check label of medication against MAR two times (see Skill 22-1). Preparation usually involves removing suppository from refrigerator and taking to patient room. Verify expiration date on container. *These are the first and second checks for accuracy.*
8. Take medications to patient at correct time (see facility policy). Medications that require exact timing include STAT, first-time or loading, and one-time doses. Give time-critical scheduled medications (e.g., antibiotics) no later than 30 minutes before or after scheduled dose. Give non–time-critical scheduled medications within a range of either 1 or 2 hours of scheduled dose (ISMP, 2011). During administration, apply the six rights of medication administration.
9. **See Standard Protocol (inside front cover).**
10. At patient's bedside, again compare MAR or computer printout with the names of medications on the medication labels. *This is the third check for accuracy.* Also, ask patient if he or she has allergies.
11. Discuss the purpose of each medication, action, and possible adverse effects. Allow patient to ask questions. Explain procedure to patient and be specific if patient plans to self-administer medication.
12. Have patient void to prevent accidental passing of urine during insertion.
13. Assist patient with lying in dorsal recumbent position. Patients with restricted mobility in knees or hips may lie supine with legs abducted. Keep abdomen and lower extremities draped.
14. Be sure that vaginal orifice is well illuminated by room light, or position a portable gooseneck lamp if needed.
15. Perform hand hygiene, and apply clean gloves. Inspect condition of external genitalia and vaginal canal; note if drainage is present (see Chapter 7).
16. Insert vaginal suppository.
    a. Remove suppository from foil wrapper, and apply liberal amount of water-soluble lubricant to smooth or rounded end. Be sure that suppository is at room temperature. Lubricate gloved index finger of dominant hand.
    b. With nondominant gloved hand, gently separate labial folds in the front-to-back direction.
    c. With dominant gloved hand, insert rounded end of suppository along posterior wall of vaginal canal entire length of finger (7.5 to 10 cm [3 to 4 inches]) (see illustration).

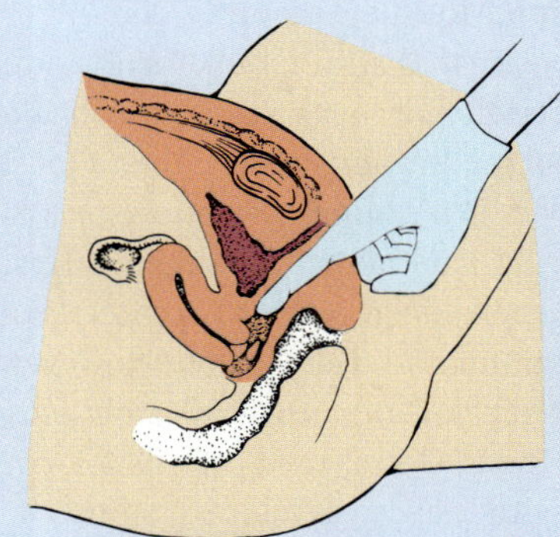

STEP 16c Vaginal suppository insertion.

    d. Withdraw finger, and wipe away remaining lubricant from around orifice and labia with a tissue or cloth.
17. Insert cream or foam.
    a. Fill cream or foam applicator following package directions.
    b. With nondominant gloved hand, gently separate labial folds. Insert applicator approximately 5 to 7.5 cm (2 to 3 inches). Push applicator plunger to deposit medication into vagina (see illustration).

Continued

PROCEDURAL GUIDELINE 22.1
Administering Vaginal Medications—cont'd

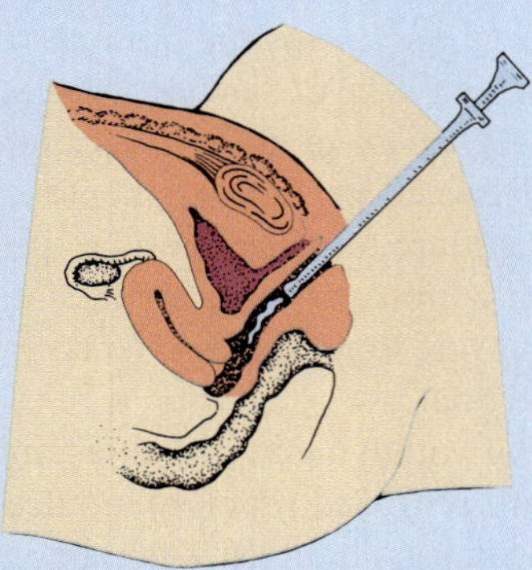

STEP 17b Applicator with cream inserted into vaginal canal.

   c. Withdraw applicator, and place on paper towel. Wipe off residual cream from labia or vaginal orifice with a tissue or cloth.

18. Instruct patient who received suppository or cream to remain on her back for at least 10 minutes.
19. If using an applicator, wash with soap and warm water, rinse, and store for future use.
20. Offer perineal pad when patient resumes ambulation.
21. **See Completion Protocol (inside front cover).**
22. Apply clean gloves. Between applications, inspect condition of vaginal canal and external genitalia 30 minutes after administration. Assess character of vaginal discharge if present. Remove gloves, and perform hand hygiene.
23. Question patient regarding continued pruritus, burning, discomfort, or discharge.
24. Use ***Teach Back:*** State to the patient, "I want to be sure you understand what I explained about the medication. Can you tell me the purpose, action, and side effects of the medication and show me how to use the applicator?" Evaluates what the patient is able to explain or demonstrate. Revise your instruction now or develop plan for revised patient teaching to be implemented at an appropriate time if patient is not able to teach back correctly.
25. Record drug, dose or strength, length of treatment, route, and time administered on MAR immediately after administration, not before. Include initials or signature. Record patient teaching and validation of understanding and ability to self-administer medication in nurses' notes.
26. Report to health care provider if patient states that symptoms do not disappear or that symptoms get worse.
27. Report adverse effects or patient response and withheld drugs to nurse in charge or health care provider.

PROCEDURAL GUIDELINE 22.2
Administering Rectal Suppositories

- **Nursing Skills Online: Nonparenteral Medication Administration Module, Lesson 6**

A rectal suppository is a thin, bullet-shaped form of medication that acts when it melts and is absorbed into the rectal mucosa. Rectal medications exert either a local effect on GI mucosa, such as promoting defecation, or systemic effects, such as relieving nausea or providing analgesia. The rectal route is not as reliable as oral or parenteral routes in terms of drug absorption and distribution. However, the medications are relatively safe because they rarely cause local irritation or side effects. Rectal medications are contraindicated in patients with newly developed stomach pain (cause unknown); recent surgery on the rectum, bowel, or prostate gland; rectal bleeding or prolapse; and very low platelet counts (Lehne, 2013). In addition, patients with acute coronary conditions should not receive rectal suppositories because of the risk of vagal stimulation during insertion.

Rectal suppositories are thinner and more bullet-shaped than vaginal suppositories (see Fig. 22-3). The rounded end prevents anal trauma during insertion. When administering a rectal suppository, place it past the internal anal sphincter and against the rectal mucosa. Improper placement can result in expulsion of the suppository before the medication dissolves and is absorbed into the mucosa. If a patient prefers to self-administer a suppository, give specific instructions so the medication is deposited correctly. Do not cut the suppository into sections to divide the dosage; the active drug may not be distributed evenly within the suppository, and the result may be an inaccurate dose (Lehne, 2013).

Delegation and Collaboration

The skill of rectal medication administration cannot be delegated to nursing assistive personnel (NAP). The nurse instructs the NAP about:

- Reporting expected fecal discharge or bowel movement to the nurse.
- Reporting occurrence of specific potential side effects of medications to the nurse.
- Informing the nurse of any rectal discharge, pain, or bleeding.

Equipment

- Rectal suppository
- Water-soluble lubricating jelly
- Clean gloves
- Tissue
- Drape
- MAR

PROCEDURAL GUIDELINE 22.2
Administering Rectal Suppositories—cont'd

Procedural Steps

1. Check accuracy and completeness of each MAR with health care provider's medication order. Check patient's name, drug name and dosage, route of administration, and time for administration. Clarify incomplete or unclear orders with health care provider before administration.
2. Review pertinent information related to medication, including action, purpose, normal dose and route, common side effects, time of onset and peak action, and nursing implications.
3. Assess patient's medical history for rectal surgery or bleeding, cardiac problems, history of allergies, and medication history.
4. Ask patient if he or she has symptoms of rectal irritation, pain, or bleeding.
5. Review any presenting signs and symptoms of GI alterations (e.g., constipation or diarrhea).
6. Assess patient's ability to hold suppository and position self to insert medication.
7. Review patient's knowledge of purpose of drug therapy and interest in self-administering suppository.
8. Prepare suppository for administration. Check label on medication against MAR two times (see Skill 22-1). *These are the first and second checks for accuracy.*
9. Take medications to patient at correct time (see facility policy). Medications that require exact timing include STAT, first-time or loading, and one-time doses. Give time-critical scheduled medications no later than 30 minutes before or after scheduled dose. Give non–time critical scheduled medications within a range of either 1 or 2 hours of scheduled dose (ISMP, 2011). During administration, apply the six rights of medication administration.
10. **See Standard Protocol (inside front cover).**
11. At patient's bedside, again compare the MAR or computer printout with the names of medications on the medication labels. Ask patient if he or she has allergies. *This is the third check for accuracy.*
12. Discuss the purpose of each medication, action, and possible adverse effects. Allow patient to ask any questions. Explain procedure to patient. Be specific if patient plans on self-administering medication.
13. Apply clean gloves. Assist patient in assuming a left side-lying Sims' position with upper leg flexed upward. Position exposes anus and relaxes anal sphincter.
14. If patient has mobility impairment, assist him or her to a left lateral position. Obtain assistance from another health care provider to help patient turn, and use pillows under patient's upper arm and leg for support and comfort.
15. Keep patient draped with only anal area exposed.

16. Examine condition of anus externally and palpate rectal walls as needed (e.g., if impaction is suspected) (see Chapter 7). Dispose of gloves if they become soiled. Turn them inside out and dispose in trash receptacle.

> **SAFE PATIENT CARE** Do not palpate patient's rectum if patient has had rectal surgery (Lehne, 2013).

17. Apply clean gloves if previous gloves were soiled and discarded.
18. Remove suppository from foil wrapper, and lubricate rounded end with water-soluble lubricant (see illustration). Lubricate gloved index finger of dominant hand. If patient has hemorrhoids, use a liberal amount of lubricant and handle area gently.

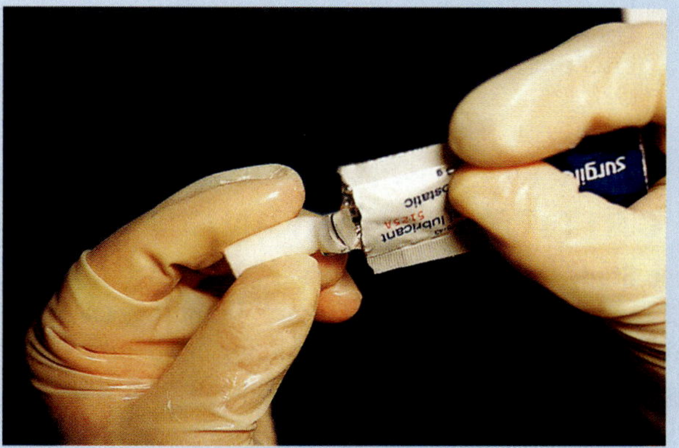

STEP 18 Lubricate tip of suppository.

19. Ask patient to take slow, deep breaths through mouth and relax anal sphincter.
20. Retract patient's buttocks with nondominant hand. With gloved index finger of dominant hand, insert suppository gently through anus, past internal sphincter, and against rectal wall, 10 cm (4 inches) in adults (see illustration) or 5 cm (2 inches) in infants and children.

> **SAFE PATIENT CARE** Do not insert suppository into a mass of fecal material; this reduces effectiveness of medication.

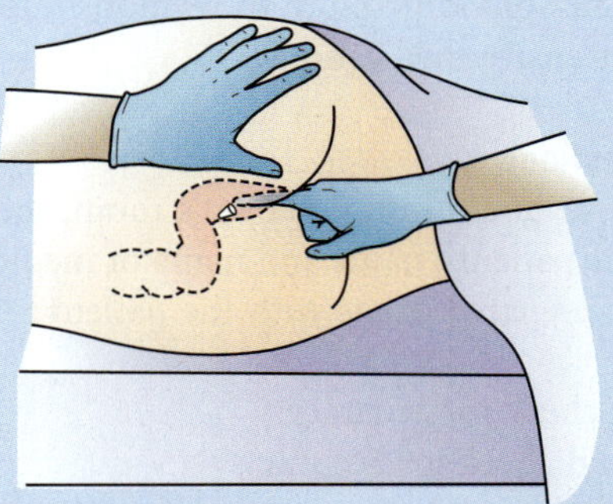

STEP 20 Inserting rectal suppository.

Continued

PROCEDURAL GUIDELINE 22.2
Administering Rectal Suppositories—cont'd

21. Withdraw finger, and wipe patient's anal area.
22. Option: A suppository may be given through a colostomy (not ileostomy) if ordered. Patient should lie supine. Use a small amount of water-soluble lubricant for insertion.
23. Ask patient to remain flat or on side for 5 minutes to prevent expulsion of suppository.
24. If suppository contains laxative or fecal softener, place call light within reach so that patient can obtain assistance to reach bedpan or toilet.
25. If suppository was given for constipation, remind patient *not* to flush the commode after the bowel movement.
26. **See Completion Protocol (inside front cover).**
27. Return to bedside within 5 minutes to determine if suppository was expelled.
28. Ask if patient is experiencing any localized anal or rectal discomfort.
29. Evaluate patient for relief of symptoms for which medication was prescribed.
30. Use *Teach Back:* State to the patient, "I want to be sure you understand what I explained about how to take a rectal suppository. At your next dose will you show me how to insert a rectal suppository?" Evaluates what the patient is able to explain or demonstrate. Revise your instruction now or develop plan for revised patient teaching to be implemented at an appropriate time if patient is not able to teach back correctly.
31. Record drug, dose or strength, length of treatment, route, and time administered on MAR immediately after administration, not before. Include initials or signature. Record patient teaching and validation of understanding and ability to self-administer medication in nurses' notes.
32. Report adverse effects or patient response and withheld drugs to nurse in charge or health care provider.

CRITICAL THINKING EXERCISES

Case Study

A 55-year-old woman with contact dermatitis on her right forearm is visiting a medicine clinic for her regular checkup. She is also hypertensive and takes a diuretic and a beta-adrenergic blocker for her blood pressure.

1. The nurse in the clinic provides instruction to the patient on how to apply a topical cream for her dermatitis. Which of the following statements, if made by the patient, would indicate that she needs further instruction?
   1. "I should wash, rinse, and dry my arm before applying the cream."
   2. "If the skin seems dry, it helps to apply the cream when the skin is still damp."
   3. "I should soften the cream in the palm of my hand before applying to the skin."
   4. "I will spread the cream on the skin and rub it in vigorously so that it will absorb."
2. The nurse practitioner taught the patient how to measure her own blood pressure at home. When should she measure her blood pressure in relationship to taking her antihypertensive medications?

Review Questions

1. Just before going into a patient's room, the nurse compares the patient's name and name of medication on the label of prepared drugs with the patient's MAR. This is the:
   1. First check for accuracy
   2. Second check for accuracy
   3. Third check for accuracy
   4. None of the above
2. A toddler is to receive 2.5 mL of an antipyretic by mouth. Which equipment is the most appropriate for medication administration for this child?
   1. A medication cup
   2. A teaspoon
   3. A 5-mL syringe
   4. An oral-dosing syringe
3. A patient has difficulty swallowing tablets and wants to chew his medications or have them crushed. One of the medications is an extended-release preparation. Which of the following actions is appropriate?
   1. Cut medication into halves or quarters to facilitate swallowing
   2. Crush medication and mix with applesauce or pudding
   3. Contact pharmacy for possible alternatives
   4. Encourage patient to swallow this one preparation
4. A patient has a prescored medication that must be split in half to ensure accurate dosage. What is the recommended approach to splitting the medication?
   1. Use a pill-cutting device to ensure an even split of the medication
   2. Request that the pharmacy split the medication and repackage
   3. Place the medication on a hard surface and cut with a sterile blade
   4. Use your fingers to break apart the medication

5. The nurse is instructing a patient on the proper method for using an MDI with spacer. The patient is to receive a bronchodilator and a corticosteroid, 2 puffs each three times a day. The two medications are prescribed for the same time each day. The patient takes the bronchodilator first. Which of the following steps for self-administering the MDI are correct in this patient's situation? Select all that apply.
   1. Shake inhaler well for 2 to 5 seconds (five or six shakes) and insert MDI into end of spacer.
   2. Place spacer device mouthpiece into mouth and close lips. Pass mouthpiece into the back of the pharynx. Avoid covering small exhalation slots with the lips.
   3. Breathe normally through spacer device mouthpiece.
   4. Depress medication canister, spraying 1 puff into spacer device.
   5. Breathe in slowly and fully (for 5 seconds) and then hold breath for 10 seconds.
   6. Wait 30 seconds after the second puff of bronchodilator and then take the steroid.
6. A nurse is administering ophthalmic ointment to a patient. Place the following steps in correct order for the administration of the ointment.
   1. Clean eye, washing from inner to outer canthus.
   2. Assess patient's level of consciousness and ability to follow instructions.
   3. Apply thin ribbon of ointment evenly along inner edge of lower eyelid on conjunctiva.
   4. Have patient close eye and rub lightly in a circular motion with a cotton ball.
   5. Ask patient to look at ceiling and explain the steps to patient.
7. The nurse should include which instruction when teaching a patient about using transdermal patches for management of chronic pain?
   1. Apply the patch to the same spot each day for consistent dosing.
   2. If the patient experiences severe sedation, cut the patch in half for the next dose.
   3. If pain is not relieved, apply a second patch without removing the first one.
   4. Remove the old patch and cleanse the area before applying a new patch.
8. The nurse is caring for a patient who has an order for an acetaminophen (Tylenol) rectal suppository. Which of the following findings in the nurse's assessment would contraindicate administration?
   1. Rectal hemorrhoids
   2. Presence of a fever
   3. Rectal bleeding
   4. Diarrhea
9. A patient comes to the clinic and is told that he is receiving a new medication that switches him from an MDI to a DPI for delivery of an inhalant. Which of the following steps used in administering an MDI are part of DPI administration? Select all that apply.
   1. Do not repeat an inhalation until next scheduled dose.
   2. Always count remaining doses.
   3. Hold your breath for 10 seconds after an inhalation.
   4. Be sure to coordinate a puff with inhalation.
10. When administering eardrops to a 5-year-old child, how should the nurse hold the child's ear?
    1. Pull the pinna down and back before administering the eardrops
    2. Pull the pinna up and outward before administering the eardrops
    3. Retract the tragus out from ear canal
    4. Have the child sit up and pull the pinna forward

REFERENCES

Alassaad A, et al: Prescription and transcription errors in multidose-dispensed medication on discharge from hospital: an observational and interventional study, *J Eval Clin Pract* 19(1):185, 2013.

Bankhead R: Enteral nutrition administration: ASPEN enteral nutrition practice recommendations, *J Parenter Enteral Nutr* 33(2):149, 2009.

Barrons R, et al: Inhaler device selection: special considerations in elderly patients with chronic obstructive pulmonary disease, *Am J Health Syst Pharm* 68(13):1221, 2011.

Beckett VL, et al: Accurately administering oral medication to children isn't child's play, *Arch Dis Child* 97(9):838, 2012.

Berben L, et al: Which interventions are used by health care professionals to enhance medication adherence in cardiovascular patients? A survey of current clinical practice, *Eur J Cardiovasc Nurs* 10(1):14, 2011.

Cohen H: Prevent adverse drug events from topical medications, *Nursing* 43(7):68, 2013.

Department of Health and Human Services (DHHS): *Updated guidance on medication administration, Hospital Appendix A of the State Operations Manual (SOM)*, Baltimore, MD, 2011, Centers for Medicare & Medicaid Services. Available at: http://www.compass-clinical.com/hospital-accreditation/ wp-content/uploads/2011/11/SCLetter12-pdfMedication -administration-guidance-Update-11182.pdf. Accessed December 18, 2013.

Hockenberry M, Wilson D: *Wong's essentials of pediatric nursing*, ed 9, St Louis, 2013, Mosby.

Institute for Safe Medication Practices (ISMP): Tablet splitting: do it only if you "half" to, and then do it safely, *ISMP Medication Safety Alert* 11(10):2006. http://www.ismp.org/Newsletters. Accessed December 18, 2013.

Institute for Safe Medication Practices (ISMP): *Splitting tablets challenges you and your patients*, 2008, http://www.ismp.org/ newsletters/nursing/Issues/NurseAdviseERR200806.pdf. Accessed December 18, 2013.

Institute for Safe Medication Practices (ISMP): *Never use parenteral syringes for oral medications,* 2010, http://www.accessdata.fda.gov/psn/transcript.cfm?show=94#9. Accessed December 18, 2013.

Institute for Safe Medication Practices (ISMP): *Acute care guidelines for timely administration of scheduled medications,* 2011, http://www.ismp.org/Tools/guidelines/acutecare/tasm.pdf. Accessed December 18, 2013.

Institution for Safe Medication Practices (ISMP): *Oral forms that should not be crushed,* 2013, http://www.ismp.org/tools/donotcrush.pdf. Accessed December 18, 2013.

Kim J, Bates DW: Medication administration errors by nurses: adherence to guidelines, *J Clin Nurs* 22(3–4):590, 2013.

Klang M, et al: Osmolality, pH, and compatibility of selected oral liquid medications with an enteral nutrition product, *J Parenter Enteral Nutr* 37(5):689, 2013.

Lawton S: Safe and effective application of topical treatments to the skin, *Nurs Stand* 27(42):49, 2013.

Lehne RA: *Pharmacology for nursing care,* ed 8, Philadelphia, 2013, Saunders.

Lilley LL, et al: *Pharmacology and the nursing process,* ed 6, St Louis, 2011, Mosby.

Mandrack M, et al: Nursing best practices using automated dispensing cabinets: nurses' key role in improving medication safety, *Medsurg Nurs* 21(3):134, 2012.

Mayo Clinic: *Asthma inhalers: which one's right for you?* 2011a, http://www.mayoclinic.com/health/asthma-inhalers/HQ01081. Accessed December 18, 2013.

Mayo Clinic: *Using a metered dose asthma inhaler and spacer,* 2011b, http://www.mayoclinic.com/health/asthma/MM00608. Accessed December 18, 2013.

Metheney A, et al: Effectiveness of an aspiration risk-reduction protocol, *Nurs Res* 59(1):18, 2010.

Paparella S: Identified safety risks with splitting and crushing oral medications, *J Emerg Nurs* 36(2):158, 2010.

Phillips NM, Endacott R: Medication administration via enteral tubes: a survey of nurse's practices, *J Advanced Nurs* 67(12):2586, 2011.

Popescu A, et al: Multifactorial influences on and deviations from medication administration safety and quality in the acute medical/surgical context, *Worldviews Evid Based Nurs* 8(1):15, 2011.

Qureshi B: Cultural, religious, and ethnic issues in prescribing, *Practice Nurse* 39(5):35, 2010.

Roy A, et al: Inhaler device, administration technique, and adherence to inhaled corticosteroids in patient with asthma, *Prim Care Respir J* 20(2):148, 2011.

Sulosaari V, et al: An integrative review of the literature on registered nurses' medication competence, *J Clin Nurs* 20(3–4):464, 2011.

Tai CH, et al: Cleaning small-volume nebulizers: the efficacy of different reagents and application methods, *J Nurs Res* 19(1):61, 2011.

The Joint Commission (TJC): *National Patient Safety Goals,* Oakbrook Terrace, IL, 2014, The Commission. Available at: http://www.jointcommission.org/standards_information/npsgs.aspx.

Tzeng HM, et al: Medication error-related issues in nursing practice, *Medsurg Nurs* 22(1):13, 2013.

Williams T: Administering enteral tube medications—room for improvement, *Evid Based Nurs* 15(4):126, 2012.

Wilson N, Best C: Administration of medicines via an enteral feed tube, *Nurs Times* 107(41):18, 2011.

Zhu L, Zhou Q: Therapeutic concerns with oral medication are administered nasogastrically, *J Clin Pharm Ther* 38(4):272, 2013.

Administration of Parenteral Medications

The route of medication administration is the path by which a drug comes in contact with the body. Medications administered by the *parenteral* route enter body tissues and the circulatory system by injection. Injected medications are more quickly absorbed than oral medications; parenteral routes are used when patients are vomiting, cannot swallow, or are restricted from taking oral fluids. There are four routes for parenteral administration:

1. *Subcutaneous injection:* Injection into tissues just under the dermis of the skin
2. *Intramuscular (IM) injection:* Injection into the body of a muscle
3. *Intradermal (ID) injection:* Injection into the dermis just under the epidermis
4. *Intravenous (IV) injection or infusion:* Injection into a vein

PATIENT-CENTERED CARE

Injections are invasive and involve some discomfort. Because risk of tissue or nerve damage exists, selection of the site of injection is an important nursing concern. Prepare patients by explaining the procedure, and use good communication techniques to distract them in a way to minimize discomfort. Additional ways to minimize a patient's discomfort when giving an injection include the following:

- Use sharp, beveled needles in the shortest length and smallest gauge possible.
- Change the needle if liquid medication coats its shaft or is irritating to the tissues.
- Position and flex a patient's limbs to reduce muscular tension.
- Apply a vapocoolant spray (e.g., Fluori-Methane spray or ethyl chloride) or topical anesthetic (e.g., EMLA cream) to the injection site when possible or place wrapped ice on the site for a minute before injection.
- Insert the needle at the proper angle, smoothly and quickly. Do not hesitate, and slowly push the needle into tissue.
- Inject the medication slowly but smoothly.
- Hold the syringe steady once the needle is in the tissue to prevent tissue damage.
- Withdraw the needle smoothly at the same angle used for insertion.
- Gently apply an antiseptic pad (e.g., alcohol) or dry, sterile gauze pad to the site.
- Apply gentle pressure at the injection site.
- Rotate subsequent injection sites to prevent the formation of indurations and abscesses.

Research demonstrates that ethnicity, genetics, and culture influence drug response, pharmacokinetics, pharmacodynamics, and patient adherence and education (Giger, 2013;

Lehne, 2013). Knowledge about variations in therapeutic dose and adverse effects is essential in administering medications to different ethnic groups. For example, some patients experience a therapeutic response at a lower dose than recommended and require careful monitoring (Ng et al., 2013; Silva, 2013). You need skill in communicating with and educating diverse patient populations. For example, if a patient values patience and modesty, make your questions specific, and take time when assessing their knowledge of drug effects. Cultural assessment also yields information about dietary preferences and use of tobacco, alcohol, and herbal remedies that affect drug action and response. Cultural context is essential in planning education for patients and families (Lehne, 2013).

SAFETY

Patient safety in administering medication involves following the six rights of medication administration (see Chapter 21). When managing a patient's medications, communicate clearly with members of the interdisciplinary team, assess and incorporate the patient's priorities of care and preferences, and use the best evidence when making decisions about patient care. Follow these guidelines to ensure safe medication administration:

- Be vigilant during medication administration. Avoid distractions while preparing a parenteral medication.
- Be sure that your patients receive the appropriate medications. Know why your patient is receiving each medication; know what you need to do before, during, and after medication administration; and evaluate the effectiveness of medications and any adverse effects after your patient takes medications.
- Verify that medications have not expired by checking labels.
- Use at least two identifiers before administering medications and check against the medication administration record (MAR). Follow facility policy for patient identification.
- Clarify unclear medication orders, and ask for help whenever you are uncertain about an order or calculation. Consult with your peers, pharmacists, and other health care providers, and be sure that you have resolved all concerns related to medication administration before preparing and giving medications.
- Use the technology (e.g., bar scanning, electronic MARs) available in your facility when preparing and giving medications. Follow all policies related to use of the technology, and do not use "workarounds." A *workaround* bypasses a procedure, policy, or problem in a system. Nurses who use "workarounds" fail to follow facility protocols, policies, or procedures during medication administration in an attempt to get medications administered to patients in a more timely fashion.
- Use strict aseptic technique during parenteral medication preparation and administration.
- Educate patients about each medication they take while you are administering medications. It is important for a patient to know each medication with respect to purpose, daily dose and when to take the medications, most common side effects, and the problems to report to the health care provider. Make sure that you answer all of their questions before administering medications. Educate family caregivers if appropriate.
- Most of the time you cannot delegate medication administration. Ensure that you follow standards set by the Nurse Practice Act in your state and guidelines established by your health care facility. Licensed practical nurses or licensed vocational nurses usually can administer medications via the oral (po), subcutaneous, IM, and ID routes. Sometimes they can give medications intravenously if they have had special training and if the medications are not high-alert medications. Some states also allow certified medical assistants to administer some types of medications (e.g., oral medications) in long-term care facilities.
- No-interruption zones (NIZs) have been recommended by the Institute for Safe Medication Practices (2012). NIZs are created by placing signs, red tape, or tile borders on the floor around medication carts or areas. Nurses standing in these zones are not to be interrupted (Freeman et al., 2013).

NEEDLESTICK PREVENTION

The most frequent route of exposure to bloodborne disease is from needlestick injuries (Hadaway, 2012). These injuries occur when health care workers recap needles, mishandle IV lines and needles, or leave needles at a patient's bedside. The use of safer needle devices and implementation of education about needle safety can prevent injuries (ANA, 2013). The Needlestick Safety and Prevention Act is a federal law that mandates health care facilities to use safe needle devices to reduce the frequency of needlestick injury. Employers must update their exposure control plans, maintain a sharps injury log, and seek employees' input when evaluating and selecting safer medical devices (OSHA, 2012).

A sharp with engineered sharps injury protection (SESIP) is a device effective in preventing needlesticks. One type of SESIP is a blunt-end cannula; another is a safety syringe equipped with a plastic guard or sheath that slips over the needle as it is withdrawn from the skin (Fig. 23-1). The guard immediately covers the needle, eliminating the chance for a needlestick injury. A variety of other SESIP devices are found in needleless IV line connection systems (see Chapter 27). Box 23-1 lists recommendations for health care workers to reduce their risk of needlestick injuries.

Special puncture-proof and leak-proof containers are available in health care facilities for the disposal of sharps. Containers are made so that only one hand needs to be used when disposing of uncapped needles. In addition, containers must stand upright, not be allowed to overfill, and be colored red or labeled with a biohazard symbol (Fig. 23-2).

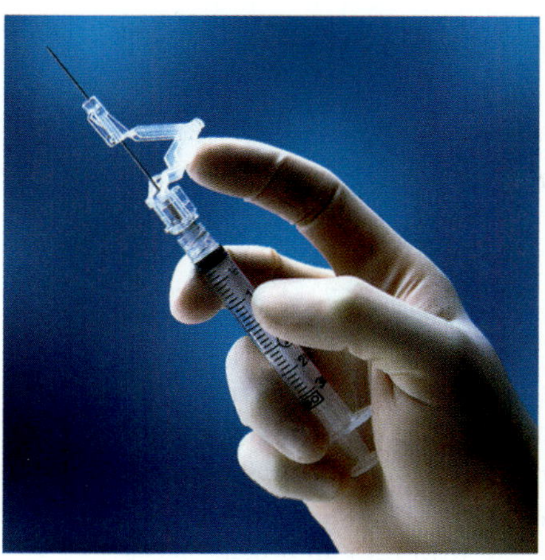

FIG 23-1 Needleless system. Safety syringe with guard.

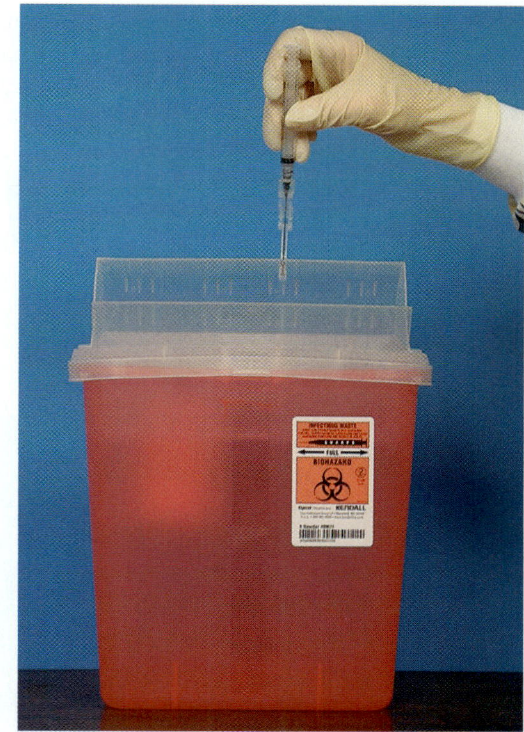

FIG 23-2 Sharps disposal using only one hand.

<table>
<tr><td>

BOX 23-1 **RECOMMENDATIONS FOR PREVENTION OF NEEDLESTICK INJURIES**

1. Avoid using needles when effective needleless systems or SESIP devices are available.
2. Do not recap needles after medication administration.
3. Plan safe handling and disposal of needles before beginning a procedure that requires the use of a needle.
4. Immediately dispose of used needles, needleless systems, and SESIP into puncture- and leak-proof sharps disposal containers.
5. Maintain a sharps injury log (see facility policy).
6. Attend educational offerings regarding bloodborne pathogens and follow recommendations for infection prevention, including receiving the hepatitis B vaccine.
7. Report all needlestick and sharps-related injuries immediately, according to facility policies.
8. Participate in the selection and evaluation of SESIP devices with safety features within your facility whenever possible.

</td></tr>
</table>

Data from Occupational Safety and Health Administration (OSHA): *Bloodborne pathogens and needlestick injuries, 77 FR 19934,* 2012, https://www.osha.gov/FedReg_osha_pdf/FED20120403.pdf. Accessed July 2013.

EVIDENCE-BASED PRACTICE

Crawford C, Johnson J: To aspirate or not: an integrative review of the evidence, *Nursing* 42(3):20, 2012.

The practice of aspirating for blood before an injection has been a standard of nursing practice for decades. The goal of aspiration was to ensure that an artery or vein had not been penetrated to prevent medication from being injected directly into the circulatory system. Both literature reviews and integrative reviews demonstrate that aspiration before injection of medication into tissues is not based on current scientific evidence (Crawford and Johnson, 2012). The Academy of Pediatrics, the Advisory Committee on Immunization Practices, and the World Health Organization have stated that aspiration is unnecessary. Recommendations from the integrative review of aspiration practices suggest:

- Use of a rapid injection without aspiration is less painful for routine IM immunizations.
- Aspiration is not indicated for subcutaneous injections of immunizations, insulin, and heparin.
- Aspiration may be indicated for specific medications such as penicillin.
- Until a standard of practice is established, injection technique must be individualized and based on best practices to reduce injection complications.

• **Nursing Skills Online: Injections Module, Lessons 1 and 2**

SYRINGES

Syringes are single use, disposable, and with tips that are either Luer-Lok or non–Luer-Lok. They are packaged separately, in paper wrappers or rigid plastic containers. Syringes come with or without a sterile needle or with a needleless SESIP device. The parts of a syringe are shown in (Fig. 23-3). Non–Luer-Lok syringes use needles or needleless

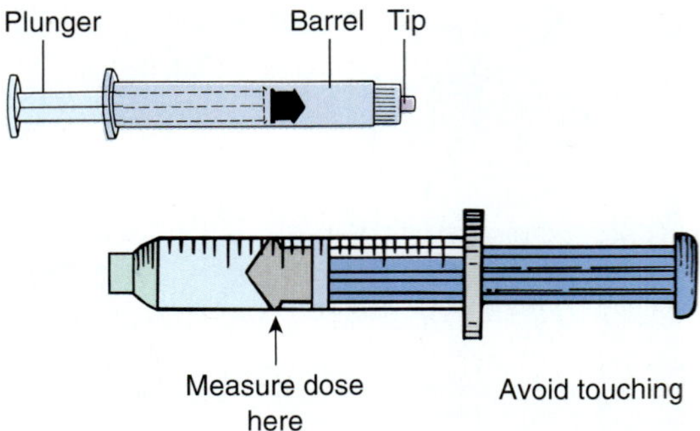

FIG 23-3 Parts of a syringe.

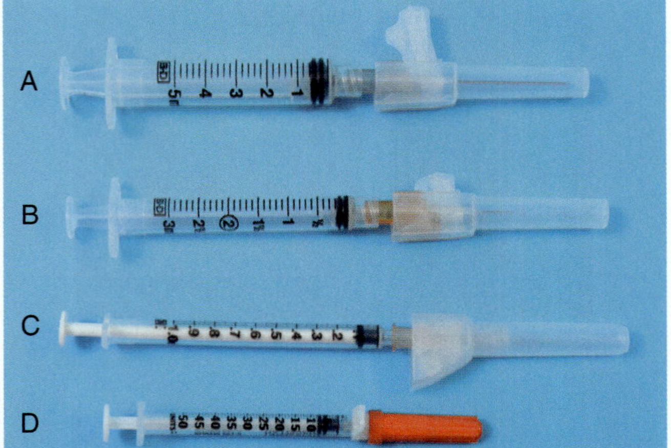

FIG 23-4 Types of syringes. **A,** 5-mL syringe. **B,** 3-mL syringe. **C,** Tuberculin syringe marked in 0.01 (hundredths) for doses less than 1 mL. **D,** Insulin syringe marked in units (50).

devices that slip onto the tip. Luer-Lok syringes (Fig. 23-4, *A*) use standard needles or needleless devices that twist onto the syringe tip and lock in place to prevent the accidental removal of the needle from the syringe.

Syringes come in various sizes, ranging in capacity from 0.5 to 60 mL (see Fig. 23-4). Always select the smallest syringe size possible to improve accuracy of medication preparation. In addition, avoid injecting a large volume of fluid into tissues. It is unusual to use a syringe larger than 5 mL for IM injections. Larger volumes create discomfort for a patient. Syringes are most commonly marked in a scale by tenths of a milliliter (see Fig. 23-4, *A, B*). You use tuberculin syringes to prepare small amounts of medications. You also use them for ID and subcutaneous injections (see Fig. 23-4, *C*). Insulin syringes (see Fig. 23-4, *D*) hold 0.3 to 1 mL, come with preattached needles, and are calibrated in units. Most insulin syringes are U-100s, designed for use with U-100 strength insulin. Each milliliter of solution contains 100 units of insulin.

NEEDLES

Some needles come attached to syringes. Others come packaged individually to allow flexibility in selecting the right needle for a patient. Needles are disposable, and most are made of stainless steel. A needle has three parts: the hub,

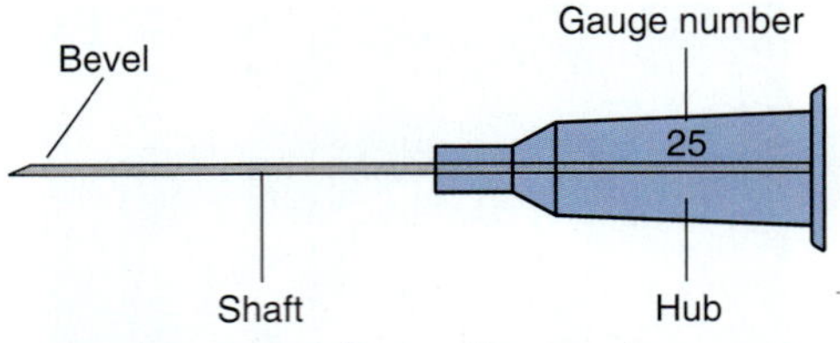

FIG 23-5 Parts of a needle.

which fits onto the tip of the syringe; the shaft, which connects to the hub; and the bevel, or slanted tip (Fig. 23-5). The needle hub, shaft, and bevel must remain sterile at all times. To prevent contamination, use gentle force to place the needle onto a syringe with the cap intact.

The tip of a needle, or the bevel, is always slanted. The bevel creates a narrow slit when injected into tissue that quickly closes as the needle is removed to prevent leakage of medication, blood, or serum. Longer beveled tips are sharper and narrower, which minimizes discomfort from a subcutaneous or IM injection.

Most needles vary in length from ⅜ to 3 inches. Use longer needles (1 to 1½ inches) for IM injections and shorter needles (⅜ to ⅝ inch) for subcutaneous injections. Choose the needle length according to a patient's size and weight, type of tissue to be injected, and route of administration. Children and very small, thin adults generally require a shorter needle. The smaller the needle gauge, the larger the needle diameter. Needle caps and hubs are color coded for ease of selection. The selection of a gauge depends on the viscosity of fluid to be injected. For example, use a larger 22-gauge, 1½-inch needle for IM injections. Use a smaller 25-gauge, ⅝-inch needle for subcutaneous injections.

DISPOSABLE INJECTION UNITS

Single-dose, prefilled, disposable syringes are available for some medications. You do not need to prepare medication doses except perhaps to expel unneeded portions of medication or air. However, it is important to check the medication and concentration carefully because prefilled syringes appear very similar. Prefilled unit-dose systems such as Tubex and Carpuject include reusable plastic syringe holders and disposable, prefilled, sterile, glass cartridge units (Fig. 23-6). To assemble a prefilled system, place the cartridge barrel first, into the plastic syringe holder. Following manufacturer's instructions, turn the plunger rod to the left (counterclockwise) and the lock to the right (clockwise) until it "clicks." Finally, remove the needle guard and advance the plunger to expel air and excess medication, as with a regular syringe. The cartridge may be used with SESIP needles. After administering a medication, dispose of the glass cartridge safely in a puncture-proof and leak-proof container.

AMPULES AND VIALS

Ampules contain single doses of injectable medication in a liquid form and are available in sizes ranging from 1 to 10 mL

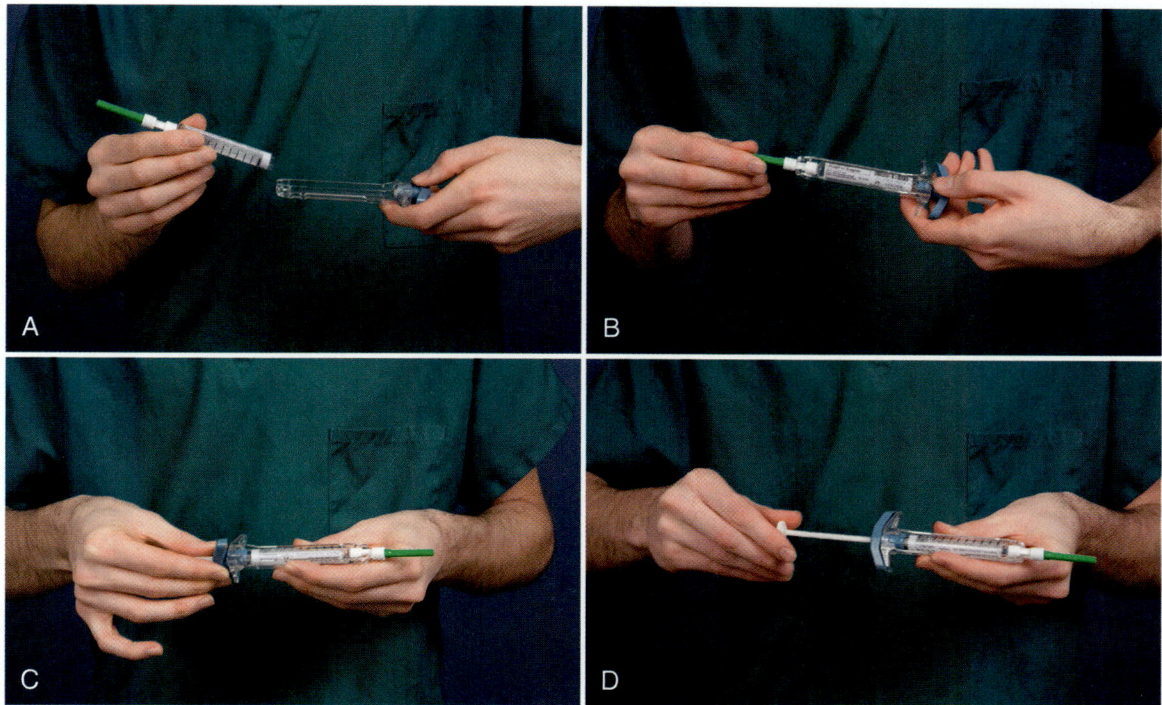

FIG 23-6 **A-D,** Carpuject syringe holder and needleless, prefilled, sterile cartridge.

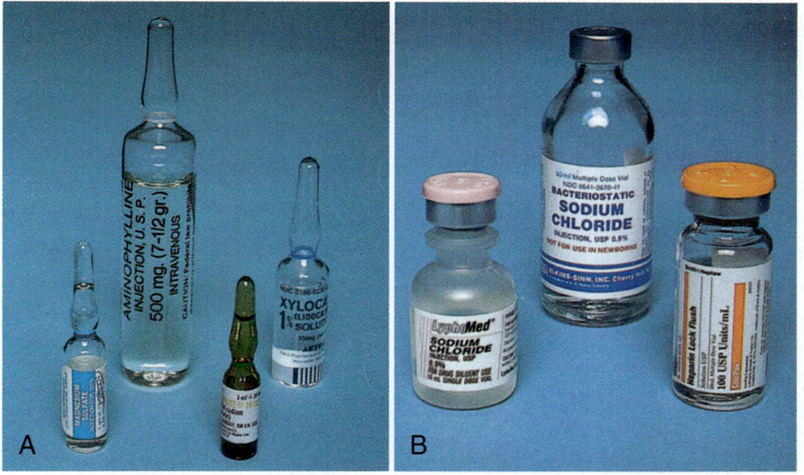

FIG 23-7 **A,** Medication in ampules. **B,** Medication in vials.

or more. An ampule is made of glass with a constricted, pre-scored neck that is snapped off to allow access to the medication (Fig. 23-7, *A*). A colored ring around the neck indicates where the ampule is prescored to be broken easily. Medication is easily withdrawn from an ampule by aspirating the fluid with a filter needle and syringe. Filter needles must be used when preparing medication from a glass ampule to prevent glass particles from being drawn into the syringe (Alexander et al., 2014). *Do not* use a filter needle to administer a medication. Place an appropriate-size needle on the syringe after withdrawing the medication.

A vial is a single-dose or multi-dose plastic or glass container with a rubber seal at the top (see Fig. 23-7, *B*). After you open a single-dose vial, discard it, regardless of the amount of medication used (Alexander et al., 2014). A multi-dose vial contains several doses of medication and can be entered several times, although only for a single patient (Alexander et al., 2014). When using a multi-dose vial, write the date that the vial is opened on the vial label. Verify with the facility how long an opened multi-dose vial may be used. Vials that exceed the time allowed by facility policy must be properly discarded.

A metal or plastic cap protects a rubber seal of the vial. Remove the cap when you first prepare the vial for use. Vials may contain liquid or dry forms of medications; medications that are unstable in solution are packaged in dry form. The vial label specifies the solvent or diluents used to dissolve the dry medication and the amount needed to prepare a desired medication concentration. Normal saline and distilled water are the most common diluents.

Some vials have two chambers separated by a rubber stopper. One chamber contains a diluent, and the other chamber contains a dry medication. Before preparing a medication, push on the upper chamber to dislodge the rubber stopper and allow the powder and the diluent to mix. In contrast to an ampule, a vial is a closed system. You must inject air into the vial to permit easy withdrawal of the solution. Some medications, even when in a vial, may need to be drawn up with a filter needle because of the nature of the medication. Facility policies and package inserts from the manufacturer indicate drugs that should be prepared with a filter needle.

A health care provider may order an injectable medication that requires reconstitution because it comes in a powdered form. Time-sensitive injectable medications, which must be administered within a specific time period to guarantee full drug effectiveness, are frequently ordered in this way.

ASSESSMENT

1. Check accuracy and completeness of each MAR or computer printout with health care provider's written medication order. Check patient's name, drug name and dosage, route of administration, and time for administration. Recopy or reprint any portion of the MAR that is difficult to read. *Rationale: The health care provider's order is the most reliable source and only legal record of patient's medications. Ensures that patient receives the right medications. Handwritten MARs are a source of medication errors (ISMP, 2011a; Tzeng et al., 2013).*

2. Assess patient's medical and medication history and history of allergies. *Rationale: Determines need for medication or possible contraindications for medication administration.*

3. Review medication reference information for action, purpose, side effects, and nursing implications. *Rationale: Allows you to administer drug properly and monitor patient's response. This is particularly important if you are unfamiliar with the drug.*

4. Assess patient's body build, muscle size, and weight if giving subcutaneous or IM medication. *Rationale: Determines type and size of syringe and needle for injection.*

PLANNING

Expected Outcomes focus on safe preparation of medication from ampules and vials.

1. Proper dose is prepared. No air bubbles are in syringe barrel.

Delegation and Collaboration
The skill of preparing injections from ampules and vials cannot be delegated to nursing assistive personnel (NAP).

Equipment
Medication in an Ampule
- Syringe, needle, and filter needle
- Small sterile gauze pad or alcohol swab

Medication in a Vial
- Syringe and two needles
- Needles:
  - Needleless blunt-tip vial-access cannula or needle for drawing up medication (if needed)
  - Filter needle if indicated
- Small sterile gauze pad or alcohol swab
- Diluent (e.g., 0.9% sodium chloride or sterile water if indicated)

Both
- Sharps with SESIP safety needle for injection
- MAR or computer printout
- Medication in vial or ampule
- Puncture-proof container for disposal of syringes, needles, and glass

IMPLEMENTATION for PREPARING INJECTIONS: VIALS AND AMPULES

STEP	RATIONALE
1. **See Standard Protocol (inside front cover).**	
2. Prepare medications:	
a. If using a medication cart, move it outside patient's room.	Organization of equipment saves time and reduces error.
b. Unlock medicine drawer or cart, or log onto computerized medication dispensing system.	Medications are safeguarded when locked in a medication dispensing system.
c. Follow facility NIZ policy. Prepare medications for one patient at a time. Keep all pages of MARs or computer printouts for one patient together or look at only one patient's electronic MAR at a time.	Preventing distractions reduces medication preparation errors (Freeman et al., 2013).
d. Select correct drug from stock supply or unit-dose drawer. Compare label of medication with MAR computer printout or computer screen.	Reading label and comparing it with transcribed order reduce errors. *This is the first check for accuracy.*
e. Check expiration date on each medication, one at a time.	Medications used past their expiration date are sometimes inactive, less effective, or harmful to patients.

  f. Calculate drug dose as necessary. Double-check calculation. Ask another nurse to check calculations if needed.

Double-checking reduces risk of error. Refer to facility policy regarding medications that must be double checked.

  g. If preparing a controlled substance, check record for previous drug count, and compare with supply available.

Controlled substance laws require careful monitoring of dispensed narcotics.

  h. Do not leave drugs unattended.

Nurse is responsible for safekeeping of drugs.

3. *Prepare ampule:*

  a. Tap top of ampule lightly and quickly with finger until fluid moves from neck of ampule (see illustration).

Dislodges any fluid that collects above neck of ampule. All solution moves into lower chamber.

  b. Place small gauze pad or unopened alcohol swab around neck of ampule (see illustration).

Protects fingers from trauma as glass tip is broken off. *Do not use opened alcohol swab to wrap around top of ampule because alcohol may leak into ampule.*

  c. Snap neck of ampule quickly and firmly away from hands (see illustration).

Protects your fingers and face from shattering glass.

  d. Draw up medication quickly, using a filter needle long enough to reach bottom of ampule to access medication.

System is open to airborne contaminants. Filter needles filter out any fragments of glass (Alexander et al., 2014).

  e. Hold ampule upside down or set it on a flat surface. Insert filter needle into center of ampule opening. Do not allow needle tip or shaft to touch rim of ampule.

Broken rim of ampule is considered contaminated. When ampule is inverted, solution dribbles out if needle tip or shaft touches rim of ampule.

  f. Aspirate medication into syringe by gently pulling back on plunger (see illustration).

Withdrawal of plunger creates negative pressure within syringe barrel, which pulls fluid into syringe.

  g. Keep needle tip under surface of liquid. Tip ampule to bring all fluid within reach of needle.

Prevents aspiration of air bubbles.

  h. If you aspirate air bubbles, do not expel air into ampule.

Air pressure forces fluid out of ampule, and medication is lost.

  i. To expel excess air bubbles, remove needle from ampule. Hold syringe with needle pointing up. Tap side of syringe to cause bubbles to rise toward needle. Draw back slightly on plunger and push plunger upward to eject air. Do not eject fluid.

Withdrawing plunger too far removes it from barrel. Holding syringe vertically allows fluid to settle in bottom of barrel. Pulling back on plunger allows fluid within needle to enter barrel. You then expel air at top of barrel and within needle.

  j. If syringe contains excess fluid, use sink for disposal. Hold syringe vertically with needle tip up and slanted slightly toward sink. Slowly eject excess fluid into sink. Recheck fluid level in syringe by holding it vertically.

Safely disperses medication into sink. Position of needle allows you to expel medication without it flowing down needle shaft. Rechecking fluid level ensures proper dose.

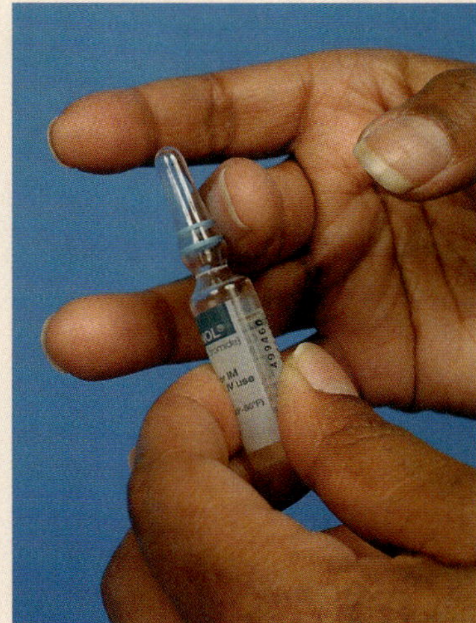

STEP 3a Tapping ampule moves fluid down neck.

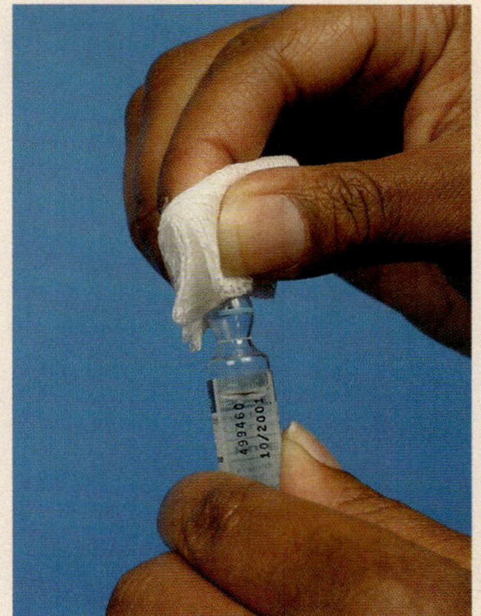

STEP 3b Gauze pad placed around neck of ampule.

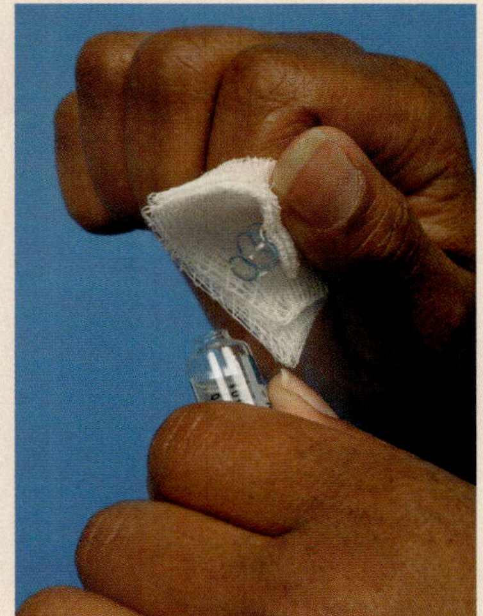

STEP 3c Neck snapped away from hands.

Continued

STEP	RATIONALE

k. Cover needle with its safety sheath or cap. Replace filter needle with regular SESIP needle.

Minimizes needlesticks. Filter needles cannot be used for injection.

4. *Prepare vial containing a solution:*

a. Remove cap covering top of unused vial to expose sterile rubber seal. If a multi-dose vial has been used before, cap is already removed. Firmly and briskly wipe surface of rubber seal with alcohol swab and allow it to dry.

Vial comes packaged with cap that cannot be replaced after seal removal. *Not all drug manufacturers guarantee that caps of unused vials are sterile.* Swabbing reduces transmission of microorganisms. Allowing alcohol to dry prevents it from coating needle and mixing with medication.

b. Pick up syringe and remove needle cap or cap covering needleless access device (see illustration). Pull back on plunger to draw amount of air into syringe equivalent to volume of medication to be aspirated from vial.

Injecting air into vial prevents buildup of negative pressure in vial when aspirating medication.

> **SAFE PATIENT CARE** Some medications and some facilities require use of filter needle when preparing medications from vials. Check facility policy or medication reference. If you use a filter needle to aspirate medication, you need to change it to a regular SESIP needle of the appropriate size to administer the medication (Alexander et al., 2014).

c. With vial on flat surface, insert tip of needleless device or needle through center of rubber seal (see illustration). Apply pressure to tip of needle during insertion.

Center of seal is thinner and easier to penetrate. Using firm pressure prevents dislodging rubber particles that could enter vial or needle.

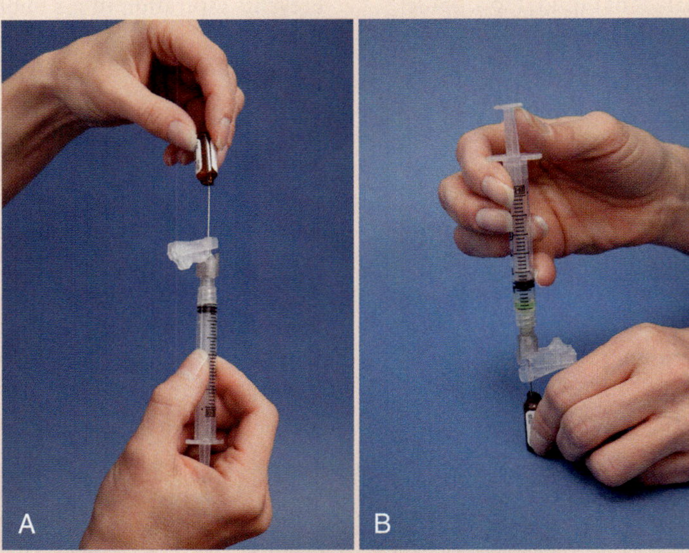

STEP 3f A, Medication aspirated with ampule inverted. **B,** Medication aspirated with ampule on flat surface.

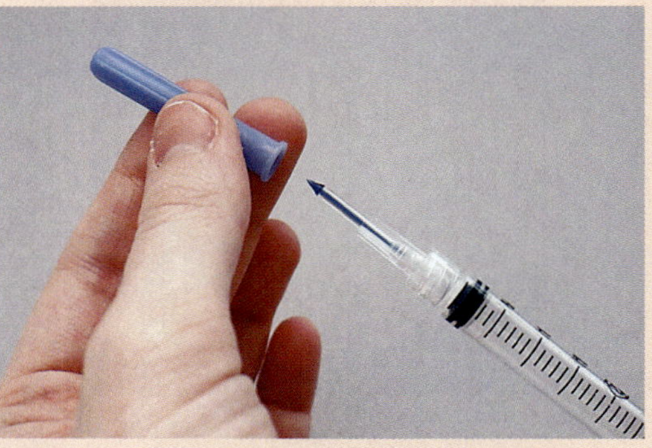

STEP 4b Syringe with needleless access device.

STEP	RATIONALE

d. Inject air into the air space of vial, holding on to plunger. Hold plunger with firm pressure; plunger sometimes is forced backward by air pressure within the vial.

Injection of air creates vacuum needed to get medication to flow into syringe. Injecting into air space of vial prevents formation of bubbles and inaccurate dose.

e. Invert vial while keeping firm hold on syringe and plunger. Hold vial between thumb and index finger of nondominant hand. Grasp end of syringe barrel and plunger with thumb and forefinger of dominant hand to counteract pressure in vial.

Inverting vial allows fluid to settle in lower half of container. Position of hands prevents forceful movement of plunger and permits easy manipulation of syringe.

f. Keep tip of needle or needleless access device below fluid level.

Prevents aspiration of air.

g. Allow air pressure from vial to fill syringe gradually with medication (see illustration). If necessary, pull back slightly on plunger to obtain correct amount of solution.

Positive pressure within vial forces fluid into syringe.

h. When desired volume is obtained, position needle into air space of vial; tap side of syringe barrel carefully to dislodge any air bubbles. Eject any air remaining at top of syringe into vial.

Forcefully striking barrel while needle is inserted in vial may bend needle. Accumulation of air displaces medication and causes dose errors.

i. Remove needle or needleless access device from vial by pulling back on barrel of syringe.

Pulling plunger rather than barrel would cause plunger to separate from barrel, resulting in loss of medication.

j. Hold syringe at eye level at 90-degree angle to ensure correct volume and absence of air bubbles. Remove any remaining air by tapping barrel to dislodge any air bubbles. Draw back slightly on plunger and push plunger upward to eject air. Do not eject fluid. Recheck volume of medication.

Holding syringe vertically allows fluid to settle in bottom of barrel. Pulling back on plunger allows fluid within needle to enter barrel so that you do not expel fluid. You then expel air at top of barrel and within needle.

k. If you need to inject medication into patient's tissue, change needle to appropriate gauge and length according to route of medication administration. An IV medication will be injected with the needleless adapter.

Inserting needle through a rubber stopper dulls beveled tip. New needle is sharper, and because no fluid is along shaft, it does not track medication through tissues.

l. For multi-dose vial, make label that includes date of opening vial concentration of drug per milliliter and your initials.

Ensures that other nurses will prepare future doses correctly. You discard some drugs within a certain time frame after mixing or opening a vial.

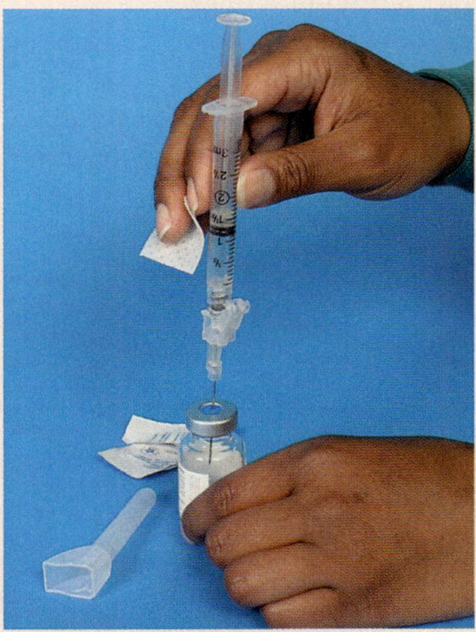

STEP 4c Insert safety needle through center of vial diaphragm (with vial flat on surface).

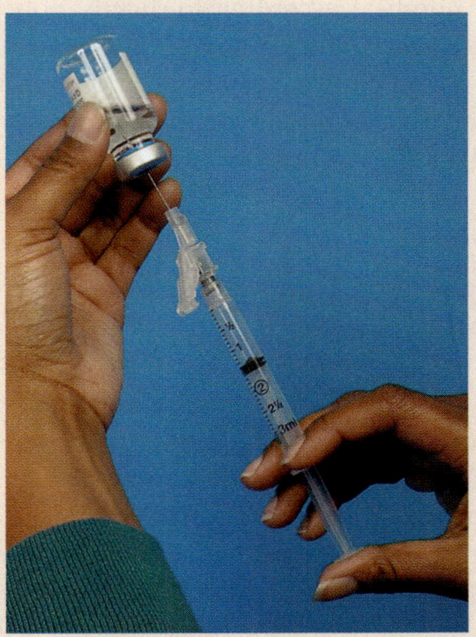

STEP 4g Withdraw fluid with vial inverted.

Continued

STEP	RATIONALE

5. Prepare vial containing a powder (reconstituting medications):

a. Remove cap covering vial of powdered medication and cap covering vial of proper diluent. Firmly swab both rubber seals with alcohol swab and allow to dry. — Allowing alcohol to dry prevents it from coating needle and mixing with medication.

b. Draw up volume of desired diluent into syringe following Steps 4b through 4j. — Prepares diluents for injection into vial containing powdered medication.

c. Insert tip of needleless access device or needle through center of rubber seal of vial of powdered medication. Inject diluents into vial. Remove needle. — Diluent begins to dissolve and reconstitute medication.

d. Mix medication thoroughly. Roll in palms. Do not shake. — Ensures proper dispersal of medication throughout solution and prevents formation of air bubbles.

e. Reconstituted medication in vial is ready to be drawn into new syringe. Read label carefully to determine dose after reconstitution. — Once you add diluent, concentration of medication (milligrams/milliliters) determines dose you give. Reading medication label carefully decreases administration errors.

f. Draw up reconstituted medication in syringe. Insert needleless access device or needle into vial. Do not add additional air. Follow Steps 4e to 4k. — Prepares medication for administration.

> **SAFE PATIENT CARE** Some facilities require that you verify dose of certain medications (e.g., insulin and heparin) for accuracy with another nurse. Check facility guidelines before administering medication.

6. Compare label of medication with MAR, computer screen, or computer printout. — *This is the second check for accuracy.*

7. See Completion Protocol (inside front cover).

EVALUATION

1. Just before administering drug to patient, identify patient using two identifiers (e.g., name and birthday or name and account number) according to facility policy. Compare identifiers with information on the patient's MAR or medical record. *Rationale: Ensures correct patient. Complies with The Joint Commission standards and improves patient safety (TJC, 2014).* Compare MAR with label of prepared drug, and compare dose in syringe with desired dose. *This is the third check for accuracy and occurs at patient's bedside.*

Unexpected Outcomes and Related Interventions

1. Air bubbles remain in syringe.
   a. Expel air from syringe, and add medication to syringe until you prepare the correct dose.
2. Incorrect dose of medication is prepared.
   a. Discard prepared dose and prepare new corrected dose.

PROCEDURAL GUIDELINE 23.1
Mixing Parenteral Medications in One Syringe

Some medications need to be mixed from two vials or from a vial and an ampule. Mixing compatible medications avoids the need to give a patient more than one injection. Most nursing units have medication compatibility charts, which are in drug reference guides, posted within patient care areas or available electronically. If you are uncertain about medication compatibilities, consult a pharmacist. When mixing medications, you must correctly aspirate fluid from each type of container. When using multi-dose vials, do not contaminate the contents of the vial with medication from another vial or ampule.

When you mix medications from a vial and an ampule, you prepare medications from the vial first. Then you withdraw medication from the ampule using the same syringe and a filter needle. When mixing medications from two vials, do not contaminate one medication with another, ensure that the final dose is accurate, and maintain aseptic technique.

PROCEDURAL GUIDELINE 23.1
Mixing Parenteral Medications in One Syringe—cont'd

Give special consideration to the proper preparation of insulin, which comes in vials. Insulin is the hormone used to treat diabetes mellitus. Insulin is classified by rate of action, including short or rapid duration, intermediate duration, and long duration. Often patients with diabetes mellitus receive a combination of different types of insulin to control their blood glucose levels. Before preparing insulin, gently roll cloudy insulin preparation (Humulin N) between the palms of the hands to resuspend the insulin (Lehne, 2013).

If more than one type of insulin is required to manage a patient's diabetes, you can mix them in one syringe if they are compatible. Always prepare the short- or rapid-acting insulin first to prevent it from becoming contaminated with the longer acting insulin (Lehne, 2013). In some settings, insulin is not mixed.

Delegation and Collaboration

The skill of mixing medications in one syringe cannot be delegated to nursing assistive personnel (NAP). The nurse instructs the NAP about:
- Potential side effects of medications and the need to report their occurrence to the nurse.

Equipment

- Single-dose or multi-dose vials and ampules containing medication
- Syringe and two needles
- Needles:
  - Needleless blunt-tip vial-access cannula or needle for drawing up medication
  - Filter needle if indicated
  - SESIP needle for injection
- Alcohol swab
- Puncture-proof container for disposing of syringes, needles, and glass
- MAR or computer printout
- Medication in vial or ampule

Procedural Steps

1. **See Standard Protocol (inside front cover).**
2. Check accuracy and completeness of MAR or computer printout with health care provider's written medication order. Check patient's name, medication name and dosage, route of administration, and time of administration. Recopy or reprint any portion of MAR that is difficult to read.
3. Review pertinent information related to medication including action, purpose, side effects, and nursing implications.
4. Assess patient's body build, muscle size and weight if giving subcutaneous or IM injections.
5. Consider compatibility of medications to be mixed and type of injection.

6. Check medication's expiration date printed on vial or ampule.
7. Perform hand hygiene.
8. Prepare medication for one patient at a time following the six rights of medication administration (see Chapter 21). Select an ampule or a vial from the unit-dose drawer or automated dispensing system. Compare the label of the medication with MAR or computer printout. *This is the first check for accuracy.*
9. *Mixing medications from two vials:*
   a. Take syringe with needleless access device or filter needle and aspirate volume of air equivalent to first medication dose (vial A).
   b. Inject air into vial A, making sure that needleless access device or needle does not touch solution (see illustration).

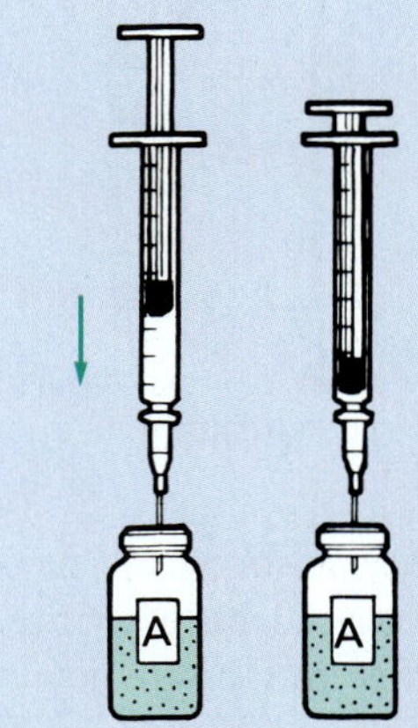

STEP 9b Injecting air into vial A.

   c. Holding on to plunger, withdraw needleless access device or needle and syringe from vial A. Aspirate air equivalent to second medication dose (vial B) into syringe.
   d. Insert needleless access device or needle into vial B, inject volume of air into vial B, and withdraw medication from vial B into syringe (see illustration).

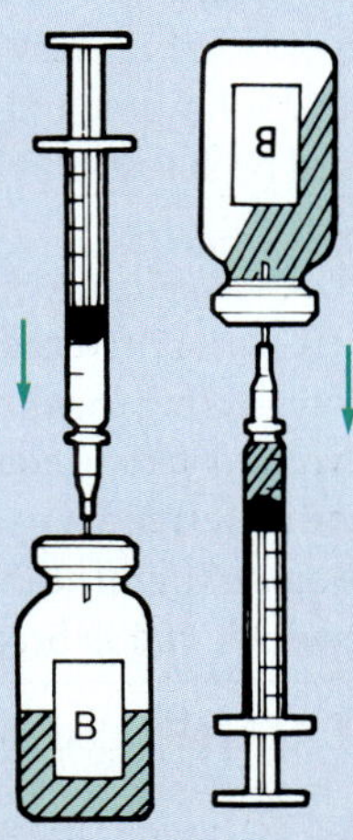

STEP 9d Injecting air into vial B and withdrawing dose.

Continued

PROCEDURAL GUIDELINE 23.1
Mixing Parenteral Medications in One Syringe—cont'd

e. Withdraw needleless access device or needle and syringe from vial B. Ensure that proper volume has been obtained.

f. Determine on syringe scale what the combined volume of medications should measure.

g. Insert needleless access device or needle into vial A, being careful not to push plunger and expel medication within syringe into vial. Invert vial and carefully withdraw the desired amount of medication from vial A into syringe (see illustration).

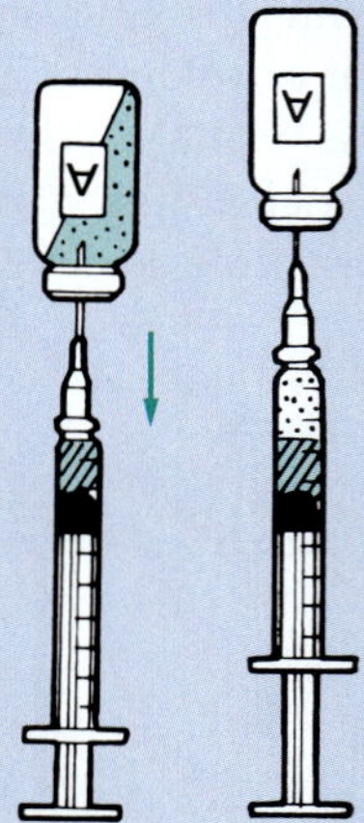

STEP 9g Withdrawing medication from vial A; medications are now mixed.

h. Withdraw needleless access device or needle and expel any excess air from syringe. Check fluid level in syringe. Medications are now mixed.

SAFE PATIENT CARE If too much medication is withdrawn from second vial, discard syringe and start over. Do not push medication back into either vial.

i. Change needleless access device or needle for appropriate-size needle if medication is being injected. Keep new needleless device or needle capped until administration time.

10. *Mixing insulin:*
   a. If patient takes insulin that is cloudy (Humulin N), roll the bottle of insulin gently between the hands to resuspend the insulin preparation.
   b. Wipe off tops of both insulin vials with alcohol swab and allow to dry.
   c. Verify insulin dose against MAR.
   d. If mixing rapid- or short-acting insulin with intermediate- or long-acting insulin, take insulin syringe and aspirate volume of air equivalent to dose to be withdrawn from intermediate- or long-acting insulin first. If two long-acting insulins are mixed, it makes no difference which vial is prepared first.

SAFE PATIENT CARE If long-acting insulin glargine (Lantus) is ordered, note this is a clear insulin that should not be mixed with other insulin preparations.

e. Insert needle and inject air into vial of intermediate- or long-acting insulin. Do not let the tip of the needle touch solution.

f. Remove syringe from vial of insulin without aspirating medication.

g. With the same syringe, inject air equal to the dose of rapid- or short-acting insulin into the vial and withdraw the correct dose into the syringe.

h. Remove the syringe from the rapid- or short-acting insulin, and remove any air bubbles to ensure accurate dose.

SAFE PATIENT CARE Some facilities require the dose of clear insulin verified before proceeding with mixing of insulin. After the medications are mixed, have dose verified a second time.

i. *Verify* insulin doses with MAR, and show insulin prepared in syringe to another nurse to verify that correct dose of insulin was prepared. Determine which point on syringe scale the combined units of insulin should measure by adding the number of units of both insulins together (e.g., 4 units regular + 10 units NPH = 14 units total). Verify combined dosage.

j. Place the needle of the syringe back into the vial of intermediate- or long-acting insulin. Be careful not to push plunger and inject insulin in syringe into the vial.

k. Invert the vial and carefully withdraw the desired amount of insulin into syringe.

l. Withdraw needle and check fluid level in syringe. Keep needle of prepared syringe sheathed or capped until ready to administer medication.

11. *Mixing medications from a vial and an ampule:*
   a. Prepare medication from vial first, following Skill 23.1, Step 4.
   b. Determine on syringe scale what the combined volume of medications should measure.

SAFE PATIENT CARE If needleless access device is used in preparing medication from vial, change needleless system to filter needle.

c. Using same syringe, prepare medication from ampule following Step 3 in Skill 23.1.

d. Withdraw filter needle from ampule, and verify fluid level in syringe. Change filter needle to appropriate SESIP needle. Keep needleless access device or needle sheathed or capped until administering medication.

e. Check syringe carefully for total combined dose of medications.

12. Compare MAR, computer printout, or computer screen with prepared medication and labels on vials and ampules. *This is the second check for accuracy.*
13. **See Completion Protocol (inside front cover).**
14. Just before administering drug to patient, identify patient using two identifiers (e.g., name and birthday or name and account number) according to facility policy. Compare identifiers with information on the patient's MAR or medical record. Compare MAR with label of prepared drug, and compare dose in syringe with desired dose. *This is the third check for accuracy and occurs at patient's bedside.*

SKILL 23.2   ADMINISTERING SUBCUTANEOUS INJECTIONS

• **Nursing Skills Online: Injections Module, Lesson 3**

Subcutaneous injections involve depositing medication into the loose connective tissue underlying the dermis. Because subcutaneous tissue does not contain as many blood vessels as muscles, medications are absorbed more slowly than with IM injections. Physical exercise or application of hot or cold compresses influences the rate of drug absorption by altering local blood flow to tissues. Any condition that impairs blood flow is a contraindication for subcutaneous injections.

You give subcutaneous medications in small doses of less than 2 mL that are isotonic, nonirritating, nonviscous, and water-soluble. Limited research indicates that volumes up to 2 mL may be given without tissue damage (Dychter et al., 2012; Walker et al., 2010). In infants and children, the recommendation is to administer amounts up to 0.5 mL in one site (Hockenberry and Wilson, 2013). Examples of subcutaneous medications include epinephrine, insulin, allergy medications, opioids, and heparin. Because subcutaneous tissue contains pain receptors, the patient often experiences some discomfort.

The best subcutaneous injection sites include the outer aspect of the upper arms, the abdomen from below the costal margins to the iliac crests, and the anterior aspects of the thighs (Fig. 23-8). These areas are easily accessible and are large enough to rotate multiple injections within each anatomical location.

Choose an injection site that is free of skin lesions, bony prominences, and large underlying muscles or nerves. Site rotation prevents the formation of lipohypertrophy or lipoatrophy in the skin. A patient's body weight and amount of adipose tissue indicate the depth of the subcutaneous layer. Base the needle length and angle of needle insertion on the patient's weight and an estimate of subcutaneous tissue. Generally, a 25-gauge, ⅝-inch needle inserted at a 45-degree angle or a ½-inch needle inserted at a 90-degree angle deposits medications into the subcutaneous tissue of a normal-size patient (Fig. 23-9). A child usually requires a 26- to 30-gauge needle inserted at a 90-degree angle (Hockenberry and Wilson, 2013). If the patient is obese, grasp the tissue and use a needle long enough to insert through the fatty tissue at the base of the skin fold. Thin patients sometimes have insufficient tissue for subcutaneous injections. The upper abdomen is the best injection site for patients with little peripheral subcutaneous tissue. Aspiration after a subcutaneous injection, including heparin and insulin, is not necessary because piercing a blood vessel and causing hematoma formation are rare (Crawford and Johnson, 2012).

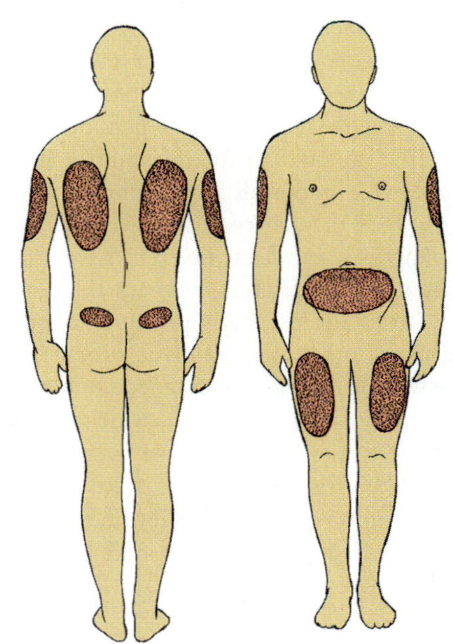

FIG 23-8 Common sites for subcutaneous injections.

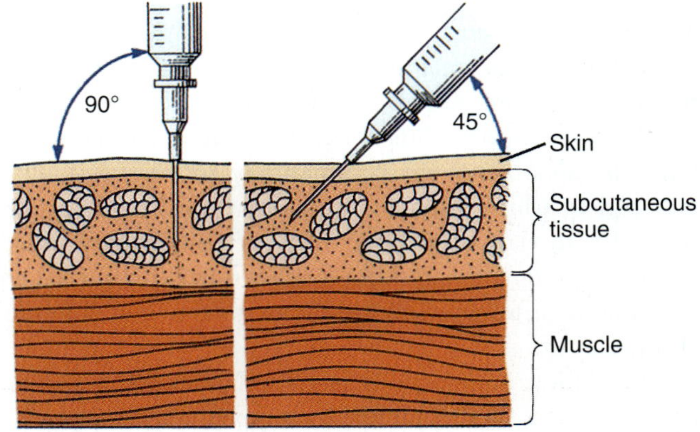

FIG 23-9 Subcutaneous injection. Angle and needle length depend on thickness of skin fold.

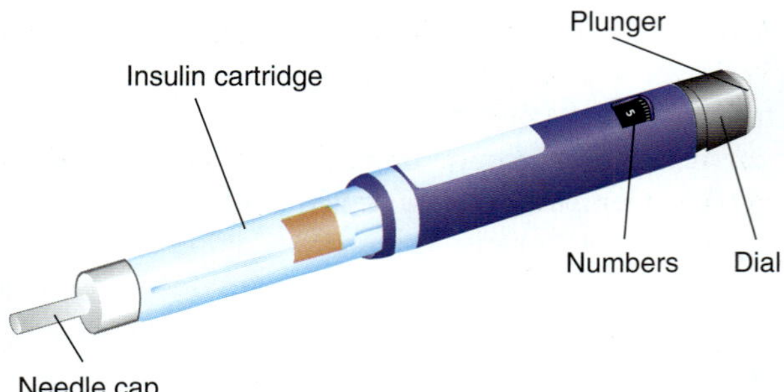

FIG 23-10 Insulin injection pen.

Several technologies are available for administration of subcutaneous injections. *Injection pens* are a technology that patients can use to self-administer medications (e.g., epinephrine, insulin, or interferon) subcutaneously (Fig. 23-10). Injection pens offer a convenient delivery method using prefilled, disposable cartridges. The patient grasps the skin, inserts the needle, releases the skin, and injects a predetermined medication dose. Teaching is essential to ensure that patients use the correct injection technique and deliver the correct dose of medication. Instruct patients that it is important to purge the pen before a dose is given. The disadvantages to this technology include users' lack of knowledge and skill in administration technique and how to store the device (Mitchell et al., 2012). One new technology is a *needleless injection system* that administers subcutaneous medications without the use of needles. Needle-free injections use high pressure to penetrate the skin and disperse medication into the subcutaneous tissue. Another new advance in subcutaneous injection is the *subcutaneous device* (e.g., Insuflon), which is inserted into the subcutaneous tissue; the needle is removed, leaving the cannula in the tissue to provide an avenue for administering medications for 3 days without having to puncture the skin with each injection (Riley and Raup, 2010).

SPECIAL CONSIDERATIONS FOR ADMINISTRATION OF INSULIN

Most patients manage type 1 diabetes mellitus with injections. Rotation of anatomical injection sites is no longer necessary because newer human insulins carry a lower risk for hypertrophy. Patients choose one anatomical area (e.g., the abdomen) and systematically rotate sites within that region, which maintains consistent insulin absorption from day to day. Absorption rates of insulin vary based on the injection site. Insulin is most quickly absorbed in the abdomen, followed by the arms, thighs, and buttocks (Lehne, 2013).

The timing of injections is critical for correct insulin administration. Health care providers plan insulin injection times based on blood glucose levels and when the patient will eat. When developing an effective diabetes management plan,

it is essential to know the peak action and duration of the insulin. Box 23-2 provides general guidelines for insulin administration.

SPECIAL CONSIDERATIONS FOR ADMINISTRATION OF HEPARIN

Heparin therapy provides therapeutic anticoagulation to reduce the risk of thrombus formation by suppressing clot formation. Patients receiving heparin are at risk for bleeding, including bleeding gums, hematemesis, hematuria, or melena. Results from coagulation blood tests (e.g., activated partial thromboplastin time, partial thromboplastin time) allow you to monitor the desired therapeutic range for heparin therapy.

Before administering heparin, know the preexisting conditions that contraindicate its use, including cerebral or aortic aneurysm, cerebrovascular hemorrhage, severe hypertension, and blood dyscrasias. In addition, assess for conditions in which increased risk of hemorrhage is present, such as recent childbirth; severe diabetes and renal disease; liver disease; severe trauma; and active ulcers or lesions of the gastrointestinal, genitourinary, or respiratory tract. Assess the patient's current medication regimen, including use of over-the-counter and herbal medications (e.g., garlic, ginger, ginkgo, horse chestnut, or feverfew), for possible interaction with heparin. Other medications that interact with heparin include aspirin, nonsteroidal antiinflammatory drugs, cephalosporins, antithyroid agents, probenecid, and thrombolytics.

Heparin is administered subcutaneously or intravenously. In some patients, low-molecular-weight heparins (LMWHs) (e.g., enoxaparin [Lovenox]) are more effective than heparin. The anticoagulant effects are more predictable (Lehne, 2013). LMWHs have a longer half-life and require less laboratory monitoring, but they are expensive. To minimize the pain and bruising associated with LMWH, it is given subcutaneously on the right or left side of the abdomen at least 5 cm (2 inches) away from the umbilicus. Administer LMWH in its prefilled syringe with the attached needle; do not expel the air bubble in the syringe before administration.

ASSESSMENT

1. Check accuracy and completeness of each MAR with health care provider's original medication order. Check patient's name, drug name and dosage, route of administration, and time for administration. Recopy or reprint any portion of printed MAR that is difficult to read. *Rationale: The health care provider's order is the most reliable source and only legal record of the patient's medications. Ensures that patient receives the right medications. Handwritten MARs are a source of medication errors (ISMP, 2011a; Tzeng et al., 2013).*

2. Assess patient's medical and medication history. *Rationale: Identifies need for medication or possible contraindications for medication administration.*

3. Review medication reference information for medication action, purpose, side effects, normal dose, rate of administration, time of peak onset, and nursing implications. *Rationale: This knowledge allows you to give medication safely and monitor patient's response to therapy. This is especially important if you are unfamiliar with the medication.*

4. Assess patient's history of allergies; known type of allergens, and normal allergic reaction. *Rationale: Certain substances have similar compositions; it may harm patients to give a medication if there is a known allergy.*

5. Observe patient's previous verbal and nonverbal responses to injection. *Rationale: Anticipating patient's anxiety allows you to use distraction to reduce pain awareness.*

6. Assess for contraindications to subcutaneous injections, such as circulatory shock or reduced local tissue perfusion. *Rationale: Reduced tissue perfusion interferes with drug absorption and distribution.*

7. Assess patient's symptoms before initiating medication therapy. *Rationale: Provides information to evaluate desired effect of the medication.*

8. Assess amount and condition of patient's adipose tissue. *Rationale: The amount of adipose tissue influences methods for administering injections.*

9. Assess patient's knowledge of medication. *Rationale: Reveals needs for patient education.*

PLANNING

Expected Outcomes focus on safe administration of subcutaneous injections.

1. Patient experiences no pain or mild burning at injection site.
2. Patient achieves desired effect of medication with no signs of allergies or undesired effects.
3. Patient explains purpose, dosage, and effects of medication.

Delegation and Collaboration

The skill of administering subcutaneous injections cannot be delegated to nursing assistive personnel (NAP). The nurse instructs the NAP about:

- Potential medication side effects and reporting their occurrence to the nurse.

Equipment

- Proper-size syringe and SESIP needle:
  - Subcutaneous: syringe (1- to 3-mL) and needle (25- to 27-gauge, $\frac{3}{8}$- to $\frac{5}{8}$-inch)
  - Subcutaneous U-100 insulin: insulin syringe (1 mL) with preattached needle (28- to 31-gauge, $\frac{5}{16}$- to $\frac{1}{2}$-inch)
  - Subcutaneous U-500 insulin: 1 mL tuberculin syringe with needle (25- to 27-gauge, $\frac{1}{2}$- to $\frac{5}{8}$-inch)
- Small gauze pad (optional)
- Alcohol swab
- Medication vial or ampule
- Clean gloves
- MAR or computer printout
- Puncture-proof container

IMPLEMENTATION *for* ADMINISTERING SUBCUTANEOUS INJECTIONS

STEP	RATIONALE
1. Perform hand hygiene and prepare medication for one patient at a time using aseptic technique (see Skill 23.1). Keep all pages of MARs or computer printouts for one patient together or look at only one patient's electronic MAR at a time. Check label of medication carefully with MAR or computer printout two times while preparing medication.	Ensures that medication is sterile. Preventing distractions reduces medication errors (Freeman et al., 2013). *These are the first and second checks for accuracy* and ensure that the correct medication is administered.

Continued

STEP	RATIONALE

2. Take medications to patient at correct time (see facility policy). Medications that require exact timing include STAT, first-time or loading doses, and one-time doses. Give time-critical scheduled medications (e.g., antibiotics, anticoagulants, insulin, anticonvulsants, immunosuppressive agents) at exact time ordered (no later than 30 minutes before or after scheduled dose). Give non–time-critical medications within a range of 1 or 2 hours of scheduled dose (ISMP, 2011b). During administration, apply six rights of medication administration.

Hospitals must adopt medication administration policy and procedure for timing of medication administration that considers the nature of the prescribed medication, specific clinical application, and patient needs (DHHS, 2011; ISMP, 2011b). Time-critical scheduled medications are medications for which early or delayed administration of maintenance doses of greater than 30 minutes before or after the scheduled dose may cause harm or result in substantial suboptimal therapy or pharmacological effect. Non–time-critical medications are medications for which early or delayed administration within a specific range of either 1 or 2 hours should not cause harm or result in substantial suboptimal therapy or pharmacological effect (DHHS, 2011; ISMP, 2011b).

3. See Standard Protocol (inside front cover).

4. At the patient's bedside, identify patient using two identifiers (e.g., name and birthday or name and account number) according to facility policy. Compare identifiers with information on the patient's MAR or medical record. Then compare the MAR or computer printout with the names of medications on the medication labels and patient name one more time. Ask patient if he or she has allergies.

Ensures correct patient. Complies with The Joint Commission standards and improves patient safety (TJC, 2014). *This is the third check for accuracy* and ensures that patient receives correct medication. Confirms patient's allergy history.

5. Discuss the purpose of each medication, action, and most common possible adverse effects. Allow patient to ask any questions. Tell patient that injection will cause a slight burning or sting.

Patient has the right to be informed, and patient's understanding of each medication improves adherence with drug therapy. Helps minimize patient's anxiety.

6. Apply clean gloves. Keep sheet or gown draped over body parts not requiring exposure.

Reduces transmission of microorganisms. Respects dignity of patient while exposing injection area.

7. Select appropriate injection site. Inspect skin surface over sites for bruises, inflammation, or edema. Do not use an area that is bruised or has signs associated with infection.

Injection sites are free of abnormalities that interfere with drug absorption. Sites used repeatedly become hardened from lipohypertrophy (increased growth in fatty tissue).

8. Palpate sites, and avoid sites with masses or tenderness. Ensure that needle is correct size by grasping skin fold at site with thumb and forefinger. Measure fold from top to bottom. Make sure that needle is one-half length of fold.

You can mistakenly give subcutaneous injections in the muscle, especially in the abdomen and thigh sites. Appropriate size of needle ensures that you inject the medication in the subcutaneous tissue (Black, 2013; Gibney et al., 2010).

a. When administering insulin or heparin, make the abdominal injection site your first choice, followed by thigh injection site.

Risk for bruising and pain is affected by site (Pourghaznein et al., 2014).

b. When administering LMWH subcutaneously, choose a site on the right or left side of the abdomen at least 5 cm (2 inches) away from the umbilicus.

Injecting LMWH on the side of the abdomen helps decrease pain and bruising at the injection site (Pourghaznein et al., 2014).

9. Assist patient into comfortable position. Have patient relax arm, leg, or abdomen, depending on site selection.

Relaxation of site minimizes discomfort.

10. Relocate site using anatomical landmarks.

Injection into correct anatomical site prevents injury to nerves, bone, and blood vessels.

11. Cleanse site with antiseptic swab. Apply swab at center of site and rotate outward in circular direction for about 5 cm (2 inches) (see illustration).

Mechanical action of swab removes secretions containing microorganisms.

STEP	**RATIONALE**
12. Hold swab or gauze between third and fourth fingers of nondominant hand.	Remains readily available for use when withdrawing needle after injection.
13. Remove needle cap or protective sheath by pulling it straight off.	Preventing needle from touching sides of cap prevents contamination.
14. Hold syringe between thumb and forefinger of dominant hand; hold as a dart (see illustration).	Quick, smooth injection requires proper manipulation of syringe parts.
15. Administer injection:	
a. For average-size patient, hold skin across injection site or grasp skin with nondominant hand.	Needle penetrates tight skin more easily than loose skin. Pinching skin elevates subcutaneous tissue and desensitizes area.
b. Inject needle quickly and firmly at 45- to 90-degree angle. Release skin if pinched. Option: When using injection pen, continue to grasp skin while injecting medication.	Quick, firm insertion minimizes discomfort. (Injecting medication into compressed tissue irritates nerve fibers.) Correct angle prevents accidental injection into muscle.
c. For obese patient, grasp skin at site and inject needle at 90-degree angle below tissue fold.	Obese patients have fatty layer of tissue above subcutaneous layer.
d. After needle enters site, grasp lower end of syringe barrel with nondominant hand to stabilize it. Move dominant hand to end of plunger, and slowly inject medication over several seconds. Avoid moving syringe.	Movement of syringe may displace needle and cause discomfort. Slow injection of medication minimizes discomfort.
e. Release stabilizing fingers while withdrawing needle quickly and place antiseptic swab or gauze gently over site.	Supporting tissues around injection site reduces discomfort. Dry gauze may minimize patient discomfort associated with alcohol on nonintact skin.
16. Apply gentle pressure to site. Do not massage site. (If heparin is given, hold alcohol swab or gauze to site for 30 to 60 seconds.)	Aids absorption. Massage can damage underlying tissue. Time interval prevents bleeding at site.
17. Discard uncapped needle or needle enclosed in safety shield (see Fig. 23-1) and attached syringe into a puncture-proof and leak-proof receptacle.	Prevents injury to patients and health care personnel. Recapping needle increases risk for a needlestick injury (OSHA, 2012).
18. **See Completion Protocol (inside front cover).**	
19. Stay with patient for several minutes and observe for any allergic reactions.	Dyspnea, wheezing, and circulatory collapse are signs of severe anaphylactic reaction.

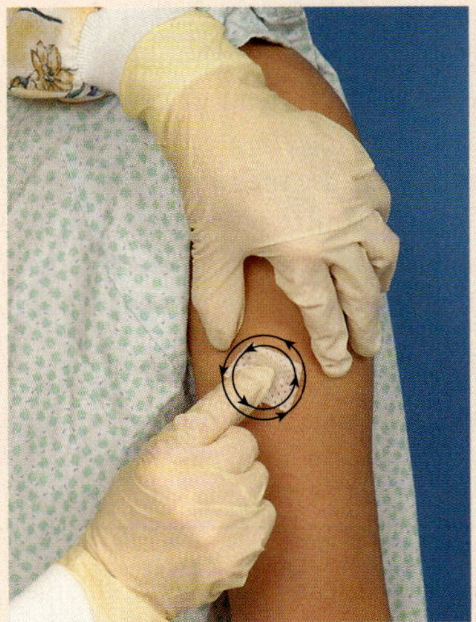

STEP 11 Cleansing site with circular motion.

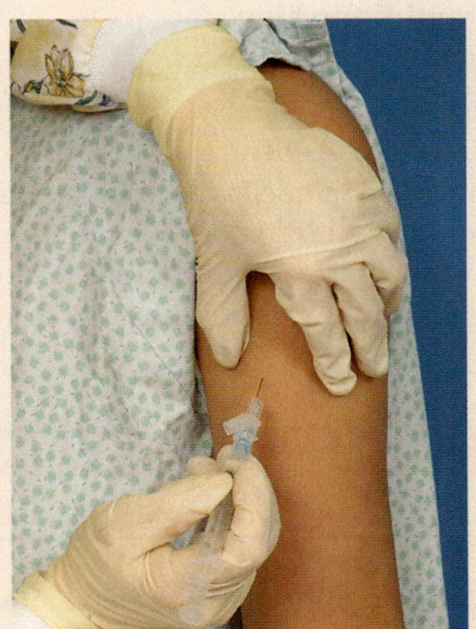

STEP 14 Holding syringe as if grasping a dart.

EVALUATION

1. Return to room in 15 to 30 minutes and ask if patient feels any acute pain, burning, numbness, or tingling at injection site.
2. Inspect site, noting bruising or induration.
3. Observe patient's response to medication at times that correlate with onset, peak, and duration of medication.
4. Use *Teach Back:* State to the patient, "I want to be sure I clearly explained the purpose and effects of this medication. Can you tell me some of the reasons you received this medication?" Evaluates what the patient is able to explain or demonstrate. Revise your instruction now or develop plan for revised patient teaching to be implemented at an appropriate time if patient is not able to teach back correctly.

Unexpected Outcomes and Related Interventions

1. Patient complains of localized pain, numbness, tingling, or burning at injection site.
   a. Assess injection site; may indicate potential injury to nerve or tissues.
   b. Notify patient's health care provider.
   c. Do not reuse site.
2. Patient displays adverse reaction with signs of urticaria, eczema, pruritus, wheezing, and dyspnea.
   a. Monitor patient's heart rate, respirations, blood pressure, and temperature.
   b. Follow facility policy for appropriate response to allergic reactions (e.g., administration of antihistamine or epinephrine), and notify patient's health care provider immediately.
   c. Add allergy information to patient's record.
3. Hypertrophy of skin develops from repeated subcutaneous injection.
   a. Do not use site for future injections.
   b. Instruct patient not to use site for 6 months.

Recording and Reporting

- Immediately after administration, record medication, dose, route, site, time, and date given on MAR. Sign MAR according to facility policy.
- Record patient's response to medication in nurses' notes.
- Document your evaluation of patient learning.
- Report any undesirable effects from medication to patient's health care provider, and document adverse effects in record.

Sample Documentation

0730   Blood glucose 320 mg/dL; 8 units Humalog insulin administered subcutaneously in RLQ of abdomen. Patient able to teach back why he was receiving insulin.

0800   Patient complaining of dizziness and sweating; health care provider notified.

Special Considerations
Pediatric

- Children can be anxious or afraid of needles. Assistance with properly positioning and holding the child is sometimes necessary. Distraction such as blowing bubbles and pressure at the injection site before giving the injection helps reduce the child's anxiety.

Geriatric

- Aging patients have less elastic skin and reduced subcutaneous skin fold thickness. The upper abdominal site is the best site to use when a patient has little subcutaneous tissue.

Home Care

- Improper disposal of used needles and sharps in the home setting poses a health risk to the public and waste workers. Several options for safe sharps disposal at home exist, including allowing patients to transport their own sharps containers from home to collection sites (e.g., doctor's office, a hospital, or a pharmacy); mailing their used syringes to a collection site (mail-back programs); syringe exchange programs; or special devices that destroy the needle on the syringe, rendering it safe for disposal. If the patient cannot implement any of these options, have patient dispose of needles and other sharps in a hard plastic or metal container with a tightly sealed lid (e.g., empty detergent bottle, soda bottle, or coffee can).
- Most insulin preparations have bacteriostatic properties that inhibit bacterial growth on the skin. Patients with diabetes may reuse their syringes at home if they can safely recap their needles. Syringes should be discarded when the needles become dull or bent or contact any surface other than the skin. Wiping the needle off with alcohol is not recommended because the silicon coating on the needle is removed, making injections more painful. Patients with poor personal hygiene, acute illness, or open hand wounds or immunocompromised patients should not reuse syringes (ADA, 2014).

- **Nursing Skills Online: Injections Module, Lesson 5**

The IM injection route deposits medication into deep muscle tissue, which has a rich blood supply, allowing medication to absorb more quickly than the subcutaneous route. However, there is an increased risk of injecting drugs directly into blood vessels. Any factor that interferes with local tissue blood flow affects the rate and extent of drug absorption.

An IM injection requires a longer and larger gauge needle to penetrate deep muscle tissue. The viscosity of a medication, injection site, patient's weight, and amount of adipose tissue influence selection of needle size. Determine needle gauge by the medication to be administered. Note that the most common intramuscular injections are immunizations.

You administer adult immunizations and parenteral medications that are in aqueous solutions with a 20- to 25-gauge needle. Give viscous or oil-based solutions with an 18- to 21-gauge needle. Use a small-gauge needle (22- to 25-gauge) for children. The U.S. Centers for Disease Control and Prevention (2012a) current recommendations for needle length are based on patient weight. An adult patient who is thin (less than 59 kg [130 pounds]) requires a needle length of $\frac{5}{8}$ to 1 inch, whereas an average-weight patient (59 to 80 kg [130 to 200 pounds] [female]; 59 to 118 kg [130 to 260 pounds] [male]) requires a 1- to $1\frac{1}{2}$-inch needle; patients weighing more than 80 kg (200 pounds [female]) or 118 kg (260 pounds [male]) require a $1\frac{1}{2}$-inch needle. Recommendations for needle length in children include use of a needle sufficient to deposit the medication in the body of the muscle (Hockenberry and Wilson, 2013). The Centers for Disease Control and Prevention (2012a) guidelines for immunizations recommend a 1-inch needle for infants (1 to 12 months old) in the anterolateral thigh and a 1- to $1\frac{1}{4}$-inch needle for toddlers (1 to 2 years) and children and adolescents (3 to 18 years) in the anterolateral thigh or a $\frac{5}{8}$- to 1-inch needle in the deltoid. A $\frac{5}{8}$-inch needle can be used for toddlers and older children weighing less than 59 kg (130 pounds). Length varies by injection site. The CDC (2012a) recommends the anterolateral thigh (vastus lateralis) as the preferred IM injection site for immunizations of newborns, infants, children, and teens. The deltoid is recommended for immunizations in adults and is an option for toddlers, children, and teens (CDC, 2012a).

Muscle is less sensitive to irritating and viscous medications. A normal, well-developed adult can safely tolerate 2 to 5 mL of medication in larger muscles such as the ventrogluteal (Dychter et al., 2012). However, clinically it is unusual to administer greater than 3 mL of medication in a single injection because the body does not absorb it well. Older adults and thin patients often tolerate only 2 mL in a single injection. The muscles of older infants and small children can tolerate 1 mL of medication in a single site. Children with larger muscles are often able to tolerate a maximum volume of 2 mL of medication (Hockenberry and Wilson, 2013).

Administer IM injections so that the needle is perpendicular to the patient's body and as close to a 90-degree angle as possible (Davidson and Rourke, 2013). Rotate IM injection sites to decrease the risk for hypertrophy. Emaciated or atrophied muscles absorb medication poorly; avoid their use when possible. The Z-track method, a technique for pulling the skin during an injection, is recommended for IM injections (Zimmermann, 2010). This technique prevents leakage of medication into subcutaneous tissue, seals medication in the muscle, and minimizes irritation. The zigzag path seals the needle track wherever tissue planes slide across each other (Fig. 23-11). The medication is sealed in the muscle tissue.

INJECTION SITES

When selecting an IM site, determine that the site is free of pain, infection, necrosis, bruising, and abrasions. Also consider the location of underlying bones, nerves, and blood

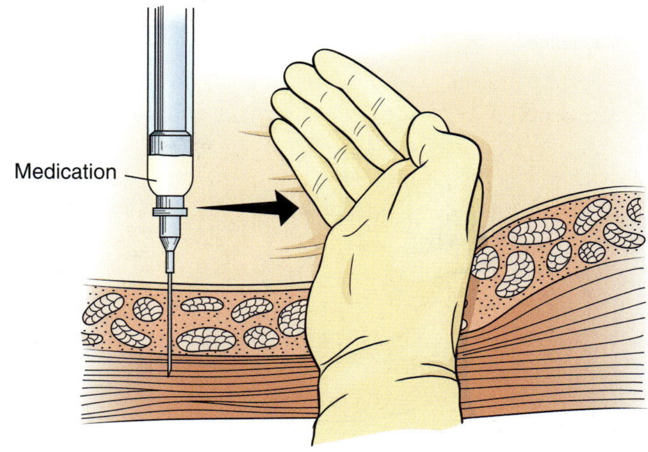

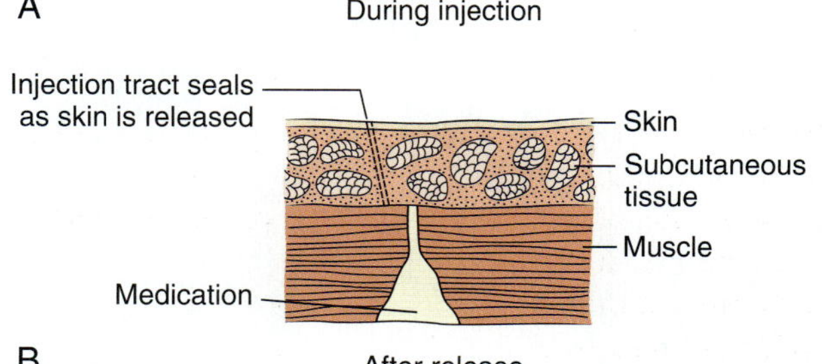

FIG 23-11 A, Pulling on overlying skin with dorsum of hand during IM injection moves tissue to prevent later tracking. **B,** The Z-track left after injection prevents the deposit of medication through sensitive tissue.

vessels and the volume of medication you will administer. Because of the sciatic nerve location, the dorsogluteal muscle is not recommended as an injection site, except in the case of immunizations (CDC, 2012a). If a needle hits the sciatic nerve, the patient may experience partial or permanent paralysis of the leg (Walters and Furyk, 2012; Zimmermann, 2010).

Ventrogluteal Muscle

The ventrogluteal muscle involves the gluteus medius and minimus and is a safe injection site for adults and children of all ages (Hockenberry and Wilson, 2013; Zimmermann, 2010). Research has shown that pain and nerve and tissue injury and pain are associated with inappropriate site selection (Dychter et al., 2012; Walters and Furyk, 2012; Zimmerman, 2010).

To locate the ventrogluteal muscle, have a patient lie in either supine or lateral position; place the heel of your hand over the greater trochanter of the patient's hip with the wrist almost perpendicular to the femur. Use your right hand for the left hip and left hand for the right hip. Point the thumb toward the patient's groin, point the index finger to the anterior superior iliac spine, and extend the middle finger back along the iliac crest toward the buttock. The index finger, the middle finger, and the iliac crest form a V-shaped triangle. The injection site is the center of the triangle (Fig. 23-12). To relax this muscle, patients lie on their side or back, flexing the knee and hip.

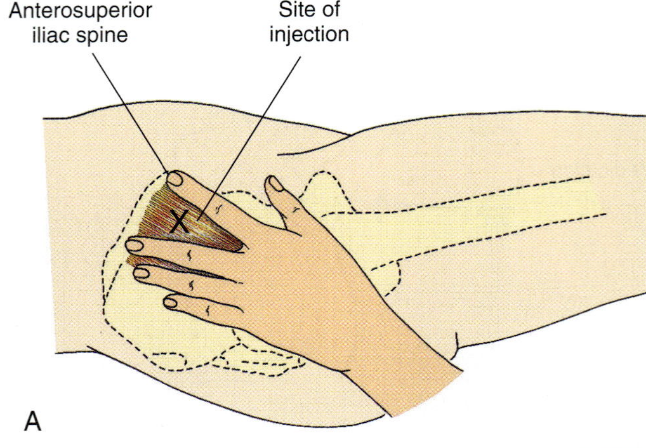

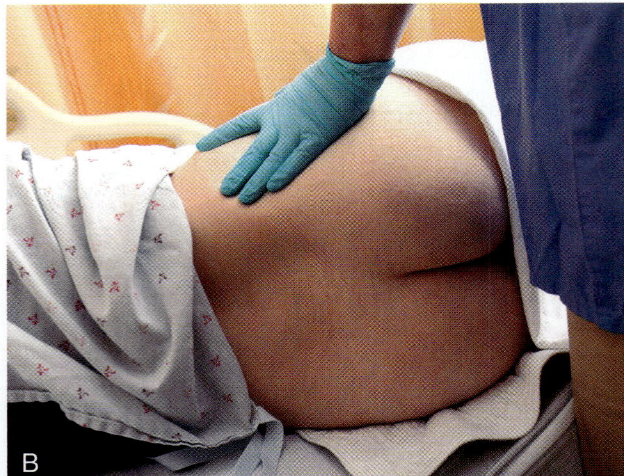

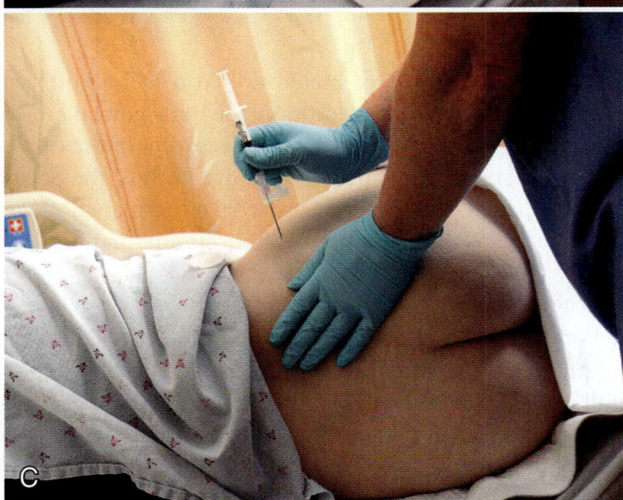

FIG 23-12 A, Landmarks for ventrogluteal site. **B,** Locating ventrogluteal site in patient. **C,** Giving intramuscular injection in ventrogluteal muscle using Z-track method.

Vastus Lateralis Muscle

The vastus lateralis muscle is another injection site used in adults and is the preferred site for administration of biologicals (e.g., immunizations) to infants, toddlers, and children (CDC, 2012; Hockenberry and Wilson, 2013). The muscle is thick and well developed; it is located on the anterolateral aspect of the thigh. It extends in an adult from a hand breadth above the knee to a hand breadth below the greater trochanter of the femur (Fig. 23-13). Use the middle third of the muscle for injection. The width of the muscle usually extends from the midline of the thigh to the midline of the outer side of the thigh. With young children or cachectic patients, it helps to grasp the body of the muscle during injection to ensure that the medication is deposited in muscle tissue. To help relax the muscle, ask the patient to lie flat with the knee slightly flexed and foot externally rotated or assume a sitting position.

Deltoid Muscle

Although the deltoid site is easily accessible, the muscle is not well developed in many adults. There is potential for injury because the axillary, radial, brachial, and ulnar nerves and the brachial artery lie within the upper arm under the triceps and along the humerus (Fig. 23-14). *Carefully assess the condition of the deltoid muscle, consult medication references for suitability of medication, and carefully locate the injection site using anatomical landmarks.* Use this site for small medication volumes (less than 2 mL); administration of routine immunizations in toddlers, older children, and adults; or when other sites are inaccessible because of dressings or casts (CDC, 2012).

Locate the deltoid muscle by fully exposing the patient's upper arm and shoulder and asking him or her to relax the arm at the side or by supporting the patient's arm and flexing the elbow. Do not roll up any tight-fitting sleeve. Allow the patient to sit or lie down. Palpate the lower edge of the acromion process, which forms the base of a triangle in line with the midpoint of the lateral aspect of the upper arm. The injection site is in the center of the triangle, about 3 to 5 cm (1 to 2 inches) below the acromion process (see Fig. 23-14, *B*). You locate the apex of the triangle by placing four fingers across the deltoid muscle, with the top finger along the acromion process. The injection site is three finger widths below the acromion process.

ASSESSMENT

1. Check accuracy and completeness of each MAR with health care provider's original medication order. Check patient's name, drug name and dosage, route of administration, and time for administration. Recopy or reprint any portion of printed MAR that is difficult to read. *Rationale: The health care provider's order is the most reliable source and only legal record of patient's medications. Ensures that patient receives the right medications. Handwritten MARs are a source of medication errors (ISMP, 2011a; Tzeng et al., 2013).*
2. Assess patient's medical and medication history. *Rationale: Identifies need for medication or possible contraindications for medication administration.*
3. Review medication reference information for action, purpose, common side effects, normal dose, rate of administration, time of peak onset, and nursing implications. *Rationale: Knowledge of medication allows you to give medication safely and monitor patient's response to therapy.*

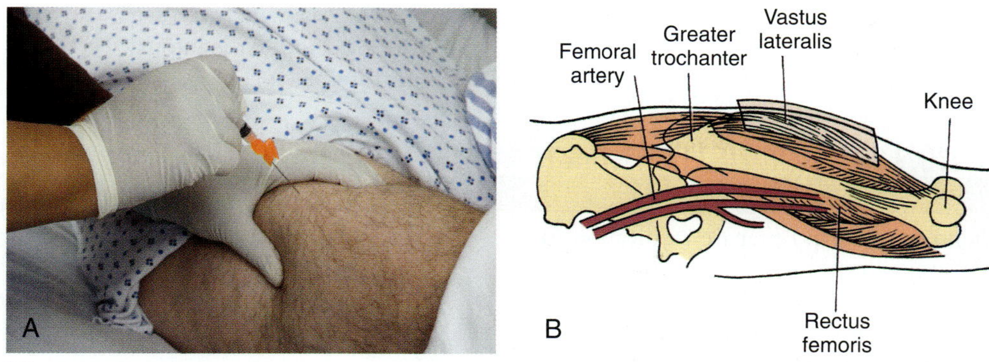

FIG 23-13 A, Injection into the vastus lateralis muscle. **B,** Landmarks for vastus lateralis site.

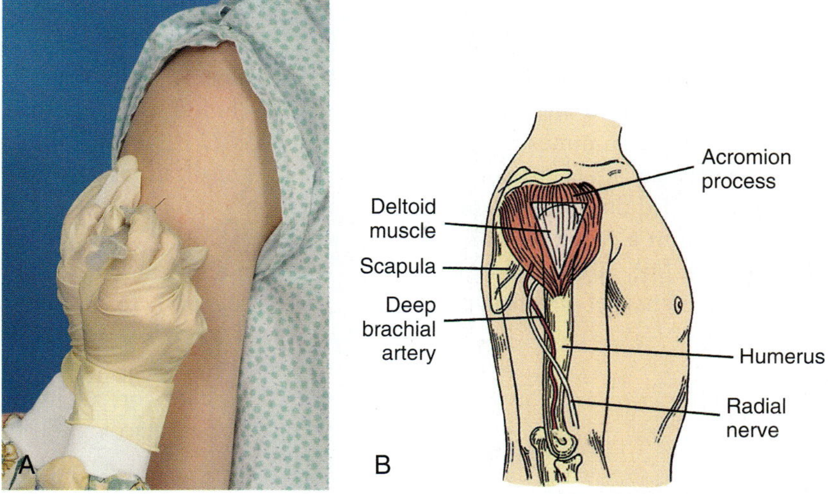

FIG 23-14 A, Administering IM injection in deltoid site. **B,** Anatomical view of the deltoid muscle.

4. Assess patient's history of allergies, known type of allergens, and normal allergic reaction. *Rationale: Certain substances have similar compositions; it may harm patients to give a medication if there is a known allergy.*

5. Observe patient's previous verbal and nonverbal responses toward injection. *Rationale: Injections are sometimes painful. Anticipating patient's anxiety allows you to use distraction to reduce pain awareness.*

6. Assess for contraindication to IM injections, such as muscle atrophy, reduced blood flow, or circulatory shock. *Rationale: Atrophied muscle absorbs medication poorly. Factors interfering with blood flow to muscles impair drug absorption.*

7. Assess patient's symptoms before initiating medication therapy. *Rationale: Provides information to evaluate desired effect of medication.*

8. Assess patient's knowledge regarding medication. *Rationale: Reveals need for patient instruction.*

▌PLANNING

Expected Outcomes focus on safe administration of IM injection.

1. Patient experiences no pain or mild burning at injection site.

2. Patient achieves desired effect of medication with no signs of allergies or undesired effects.

3. Patient explains purpose, dosage, and effects of medication.

Delegation and Collaboration

The skill of administering IM injections cannot be delegated to nursing assistive personnel (NAP). The nurse instructs the NAP about:

- Potential medication side effects and to report their occurrence to the nurse.
- Reporting any change in the patient's condition to the nurse.

Equipment

- Proper size syringe and SESIP needle:
  - 2 to 3 mL for adult
  - 0.5 to 1 mL for infants and small children
- Needle: length corresponds to site of injection and age and size of patient
- Needle gauge depends on length of needle; administer most biologicals and medications in aqueous solutions with 20- to 25-gauge needle; give viscous or oil-based solutions with an 18- to 21-gauge needle in adults. Use a 22- to 25-gauge needle in children.

- Alcohol swab
- Small gauze pad
- Vial or ampule of medication
- Clean gloves
- MAR or computer printout
- Puncture-proof container

IMPLEMENTATION *for* ADMINISTERING INTRAMUSCULAR INJECTIONS

STEP	RATIONALE
1. Perform hand hygiene and prepare medication for one patient at a time using aseptic technique (see Skill 23.1). Keep all pages of MARs or computer printouts for one patient together or look at only one patient's electronic MAR at a time. Check label of medication carefully with MAR or computer printout two times while preparing medication.	Ensures that medication is sterile. Preventing distractions reduces medication errors (Freeman et al., 2013). *These are the first and second checks for accuracy* and ensure that the correct medication is administered.
2. Take medications to patient at correct time (see facility policy). Medications that require exact timing include STAT, first-time or loading doses, and one-time does. Give time-critical scheduled medications (e.g., antibiotics, anticonvulsants, immunosuppressive agents) at exact time ordered (no later than 30 minutes before or after scheduled dose). Give non–time-critical medications within a range of 1 or 2 hours of scheduled dose (ISMP, 2011b). During administration, apply six rights of medication administration.	Hospitals must adopt medication administration policy and procedure for timing of medication administration that considers the nature of the prescribed medication, specific clinical application, and patient needs (DHHS, 2011; ISMP, 2011b). Time-critical scheduled medications are medications for which early or delayed administration of maintenance doses of greater than 30 minutes before or after the scheduled dose may cause harm or result in substantial suboptimal therapy or pharmacological effect. Non–time-critical medications are medications for which early or delayed administration within a specific range of either 1 or 2 hours should not cause harm or result in substantial suboptimal therapy or pharmacological effect (DHHS, 2011; ISMP, 2011b).
3. **See Standard Protocol (inside front cover).**	
4. At the bedside, identify patient using two identifiers (e.g., name and birthday or name and account number) according to facility policy. Compare identifiers with information on the patient's MAR or medical record. Again compare MAR or computer printout with the names of medications on the medication labels and patient name. Ask patient if he or she has allergies.	Ensures correct patient. Complies with The Joint Commission standards and improves patient safety (TJC, 2014). *This is the third check for accuracy* and ensures that patient receives correct medication. Confirms patient's allergy history.
5. Discuss the purpose of each medication, action, and common possible adverse effects. Allow patient to ask any questions. Tell patient that injection will cause a slight burning or sting.	Patient has the right to be informed, and patient's understanding of each medication improves adherence with drug therapy. Helps minimize patient's anxiety.
6. Apply clean gloves. Keep sheet or gown draped over body parts not requiring exposure.	Reduces transmission of microorganisms. Respects dignity of patient while exposing injection area.
7. Select appropriate site. Note integrity and size of muscle. Palpate for tenderness or hardness and avoid these areas. If patient receives frequent injections, rotate sites.	Ventrogluteal site preferred for all ages (Hockenberry and Wilson, 2013; Zimmerman, 2010). Exception: use vastus lateralis for immunizations in children and deltoid in adults (CDC, 2012). Condition of tissue and muscle determines site selection.
8. Assist patient to comfortable position. Position patient depending on chosen site (e.g., sit, lie flat, on side, or prone).	Reduces strain on muscle and minimizes injection discomfort.

SAFE PATIENT CARE Ensure that medical condition (e.g., circulatory shock) does not contraindicate patient's position for injection.

STEP	RATIONALE
9. Relocate site using anatomical landmarks.	Injection into correct anatomical site prevents injury to nerves, bone, and blood vessels.
a. Option: Apply EMLA cream to injection site for at least 1 hour before IM injection or use a vapocoolant spray (e.g., ethyl chloride) just before injection.	Decreases pain at injection site.
10. Cleanse site with antiseptic swab. Apply swab at center of site and rotate outward in circular direction for about 5 cm (2 inches).	Mechanical action of swab removes secretions containing microorganisms.
11. Hold swab or gauze between third and fourth fingers of nondominant hand.	Swab or gauze remains readily accessible for use when withdrawing needle after injection.
12. Remove needle cap or sheath by pulling it straight off.	Preventing needle from touching sides of cap prevents contamination.
13. Hold syringe between thumb and forefinger of dominant hand; hold as a dart, palm down.	Quick, smooth injection requires proper manipulation of syringe parts.
14. Administer injection:	
a. Position ulnar side of nondominant hand just below site and pull skin laterally approximately 2.5 to 3.5 cm (1 to 1½ inches). Hold position until medication is injected. With dominant hand, inject needle quickly at 90-degree angle into muscle (see Fig. 23-11, *A*).	Z-track creates zigzag path through tissues that seals the needle track to avoid tracking medication. A quick, dart-like injection reduces discomfort (Davidson and Rourke, 2013).
b. Option: If patient's muscle mass is small, grasp body of muscle between thumb and forefingers.	Ensures that medication reaches the muscle mass (CDC, 2012a; Hockenberry and Wilson, 2013).
c. After needle pierces skin, while still pulling on skin with nondominant hand, grasp lower end of syringe barrel with fingers of nondominant hand to stabilize it. Move dominant hand to end of plunger. Avoid moving syringe.	Smooth manipulation of syringe reduces discomfort from needle movement. Skin remains pulled until after medication is injected to ensure Z-track administration.
d. NOTE: For immunizations, Do Not Aspirate. For other medications (e.g., Interferon), pull back on plunger quickly for 2 to 5 seconds. If no blood appears, proceed with injection. Inject medication slowly at a rate of 10 sec/mL (Zimmermann, 2010).	Use of a rapid injection without aspiration is less painful for routine IM immunizations (Crawford and Johnson, 2012). The CDC no longer recommends aspiration after administering a vaccine (2012a). Aspiration of blood into syringe indicates possible placement into a vein. Slow injection reduces pain and tissue trauma.

> **SAFE PATIENT CARE** If blood appears in syringe, remove needle, dispose of medication and syringe properly, and prepare another dose of medication for injection.

STEP	RATIONALE
e. Wait 10 seconds, and smoothly and steadily withdraw needle, release skin, and apply alcohol swab or gauze gently over site.	Allows time for medication to absorb into muscle before syringe is removed and skin is released. Dry gauze minimizes discomfort associated with alcohol on nonintact skin.
15. Apply gentle pressure to site. Do not massage site. Apply bandage if needed.	Massage damages underlying tissue.
16. Discard uncapped needle or needle enclosed in safety shield and attached syringe into a puncture-proof and leak-proof receptacle.	Prevents injury to patients and health care personnel. Recapping needle increases risk for a needlestick injury (OSHA, 2012).
17. **See Completion Protocol (inside front cover).**	
18. Stay with patient for several minutes and observe for any allergic reactions.	

EVALUATION

1. Return to room in 15 to 30 minutes and ask if patient feels any acute pain, burning, numbness, or tingling at injection site.
2. Inspect site; note any bruising or induration.
3. Observe patient's response to medication at times that correlate with the onset, peak, and duration of medication.
4. Use *Teach Back:* State to the patient, "I want to be sure I explained why you were receiving this injection in your muscle and what to expect during and after the injection. Can you tell me what to expect after the injection?" Evaluates what the patient is able to explain or demonstrate. Revise your instruction now or develop plan for revised patient teaching to be implemented at an appropriate time if patient is not able to teach back correctly.

Unexpected Outcomes and Related Interventions

1. Patient complains of localized pain or continued burning at injection site, indicating potential injury to nerve or vessels.
   a. Assess injection site.
   b. Notify patient's health care provider.
2. Blood is aspirated during injection.
   a. Immediately stop injection and remove needle.
   b. Prepare new syringe of medication for administration.
3. Patient displays adverse reaction with signs of urticaria, eczema, pruritus, wheezing, and dyspnea.
   a. Follow facility policy for appropriate response to adverse drug reactions (e.g., administration of antihistamine such as diphenhydramine [Benadryl] or epinephrine).
   b. Notify patient's health care provider immediately.
   c. Add allergy information to patient's record.

Recording and Reporting

- Record medication, dose, route, site, time, and date given on MAR immediately after administration, not before. Correctly sign MAR according to facility policy.
- Record patient's response to medication in nurses' notes.
- Document your evaluation of patient learning.
- Report any undesirable effects from medication to patient's health care provider, and document adverse effects in record.

Sample Documentation

0800   Administered 100 mcg cyanocobalamin for vitamin B_{12} deficiency IM in right ventrogluteal muscle. Patient reports some burning during and after administration. Patient able to discuss what to expect after the injection and to report any excess pain at injection site to nurse.

Special Considerations
Pediatric

- Children can be anxious or fearful of needles. Assistance with proper positioning and holding the child is sometimes necessary. Distraction such as blowing bubbles and pressure at the injection site before giving the injection can help alleviate the child's anxiety (Hockenberry and Wilson, 2013).

Geriatric

- Older patients may have decreased muscle mass, which reduces drug absorption from IM injections. In addition, older adults may have loss of muscle tone and strength that impairs mobility, placing them at high risk for falls from guarding an injection site.

Home Care

- Self-administration of an IM injection is difficult, especially in the ventrogluteal. Teach primary family caregiver to identify and administer injections in this site or to use vastus lateralis.
- Instruct adult patients who require frequent injections to apply EMLA cream to the injection site 1 hour before administration.
- Patients need instruction about safe disposal of syringes and needles (see Skill 23.2, Special Considerations, Home Care).
- See Chapter 31 for information about modifying safety risks in the home.

SKILL 23.4   ADMINISTERING INTRADERMAL INJECTIONS

• Nursing Skills Online: Injections, Lesson 4

ID injections are typically administered for skin testing (e.g., tuberculosis [TB] screening and allergy tests). Because such medications are potent, you inject them into the dermis, where blood supply is reduced and drug absorption occurs slowly. A patient may have an anaphylactic reaction if a medication enters the circulation too rapidly. The health care provider may perform skin testing in patients with a history of numerous allergies. Skin testing often requires you to inspect the test site visually; you need to ensure that ID sites are free of lesions and injuries and are relatively hairless. The inner forearm and upper back are ideal locations.

To administer an ID injection, use a tuberculin or small syringe with a short ($\frac{3}{8}$ to $\frac{5}{8}$ inch), fine-gauge (25- to 27-gauge) needle. The angle of insertion for an ID injection is 5 to 15 degrees (Fig. 23-15). Inject only small amounts of medication (0.01 to 0.1 mL) intradermally. If a bleb does not appear or if the site bleeds after needle withdrawal, the

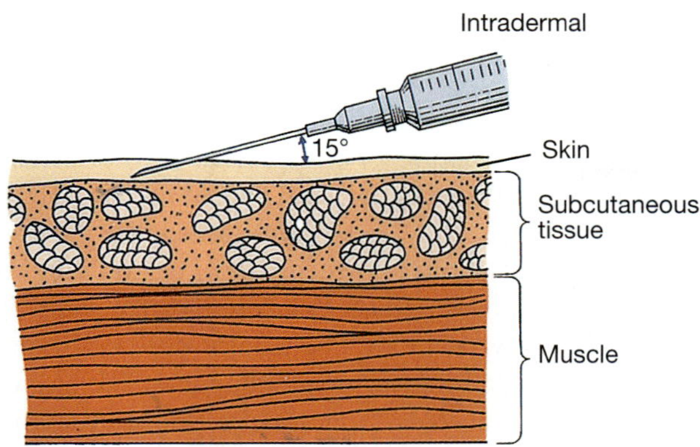

FIG 23-15 Intradermal needle tip inserted into dermis.

medication may have entered subcutaneous tissues. In this situation, skin test results will not be valid.

ASSESSMENT

1. Check accuracy and completeness of each MAR with health care provider's original medication order. Check patient's name, drug name and dosage, route of administration, and time for administration. Recopy or reprint any portion of printed MAR that is difficult to read. *Rationale: The health care provider's order is the most reliable source and only legal record of patient's medications. Ensures that patient receives the right medications. Handwritten MARs are a source of medication errors (ISMP, 2011a; Tzeng et al., 2013).*

2. Assess patient's medical and medication history. *Rationale: Identifies need for medication and possible contraindication for medication.*

3. Review medication reference information for action, purpose, side effects, normal dose, rate of administration, time of peak onset, and nursing implications. *Rationale: Type of reaction depends on patient's ability to mount a cell-mediated response. Knowledge of expected and adverse reactions to skin testing helps you determine which symptoms to monitor, how frequently, and when to reassess patient.*

4. Assess patient's history of allergies, known type of allergens, and normal allergic reaction. *Rationale: Certain substances have similar compositions; it may harm patients to give a medication if there is a known allergy.*

5. Observe patient's previous verbal and nonverbal responses to injection. *Rationale: Injections are sometimes painful. Anticipating patient's anxiety allows you to use distraction to reduce pain awareness.*

6. Assess for contraindication to ID injections, such as reduced local tissue perfusion. Assess for history of severe adverse reactions or necrosis that occurred after previous ID injection. *Rationale: Medications are potent and can cause severe anaphylaxis.*

7. Assess patient's knowledge of purpose and response to skin testing. *Rationale: Patients need to know when to come back for follow-up reading of skin test and when and how to report any reaction.*

PLANNING

Expected Outcomes focus on safe ID injection.

1. Patient experiences very mild burning sensation during injection but no discomfort after injection.
2. Small, light-colored bleb approximately 6 mm (¼ inch) in diameter forms at site and gradually disappears. Minimal bruising is present.
3. Patient is able to identify signs of skin reaction and their significance.

Delegation and Collaboration

The skill of administering ID injections cannot be delegated to nursing assistive personnel (NAP). The nurse instructs the NAP about:

- Potential medication side effects and reporting their occurrence to the nurse.
- Reporting any change in the patient's condition to the nurse.

Equipment

- Syringe: 1-mL tuberculin syringe with preattached 25- to 27-gauge, ⅜- to ⅝-inch needle
- Alcohol swab
- Small gauze pad
- Vial or ampule of medication
- Clean gloves
- MAR or computer printout
- Puncture-proof container

IMPLEMENTATION *for* ADMINISTERING INTRADERMAL INJECTIONS

STEP	RATIONALE
1. Perform hand hygiene, and prepare medication for one patient at a time using aseptic technique (see Skill 23.1). Keep all pages of MARs or computer printouts for one patient together or look at only one patient's electronic MAR at a time. Check label of medication carefully with MAR or computer printout two times while preparing medication.	Ensures that medication is sterile. Preventing distractions reduces medication errors (Freeman et al., 2013). *These are the first and second checks for accuracy and ensure that the correct medication is administered.*

Continued

STEP	RATIONALE
2. Take medications to patient at correct time (see facility policy). Medications that require exact timing include STAT, first-time or loading doses, and one-time doses. Give time-critical scheduled medications at exact time ordered (no later than 30 minutes before or after scheduled dose). Give non–time-critical medications within a range of 1 or 2 hours of scheduled dose (ISMP, 2011b). During administration, apply six rights of medication administration.	Hospitals must adopt medication administration policy and procedure for timing of medication administration that considers nature of the prescribed medication, specific clinical application, and patient needs (DHHS, 2011; ISMP, 2011b). Time-critical scheduled medications are medications for which early or delayed administration of maintenance doses of greater than 30 minutes before or after the scheduled dose may cause harm or result in substantial suboptimal therapy or pharmacological effect. Non–time-critical medications are medications for which early or delayed administration within a specific range of either 1 or 2 hours should not cause harm or result in substantial suboptimal therapy or pharmacological effect (DHHS, 2011; ISMP, 2011b).
3. See Standard Protocol (inside front cover).	
4. At the bedside, identify patient using two identifiers (e.g., name and birthday or name and account number) according to facility policy. Compare identifiers with information on the patient's MAR or medical record. Again compare MAR or computer printout with the names of medications on the medication labels. Ask patient if he or she has allergies.	Ensures correct patient. Complies with The Joint Commission standards and improves patient safety (TJC, 2014). *This is the third check for accuracy* and ensures that patient receives correct medication. Confirms patient's allergy history.
5. Discuss the purpose of each medication, action, and common possible adverse effects. Allow patient to ask any questions. Tell patient that injection will cause a very mild burning.	Patient has the right to be informed, and patient's understanding of each medication improves adherence with drug therapy. Helps minimize patient's anxiety.
6. Apply clean gloves. Keep sheet or gown draped over body parts not requiring exposure.	Reduces transmission of microorganisms. Respects dignity of patient while exposing injection area.
7. Select appropriate site. Note lesions or discolorations of skin. If possible, select site three to four finger widths below antecubital space and one hand width above wrist. If you cannot use the forearm, inspect the upper back. If necessary, use sites appropriate for subcutaneous injections.	An ID injection site is free of discolorations or hair so you can see the results of skin test and interpret them correctly (CDC, 2012b).
8. Assist patient to comfortable position. Have patient extend elbow and support it and forearm on flat surface.	Stabilizes injection site for easiest accessibility.
9. Cleanse site with antiseptic swab. Apply swab at center of site and rotate outward in circular direction for about 5 cm (2 inches).	Mechanical action of swab removes secretions containing microorganisms.
a. Option: Use a vapocoolant spray (e.g., ethyl chloride) just before injection.	Decreases pain at injection site.
10. Hold swab or gauze between third and fourth fingers of nondominant hand.	Swab or gauze remains readily accessible when withdrawing needle.
11. Remove needle cap from needle by pulling it straight off.	Preventing needle from touching sides of cap prevents contamination.
12. Hold syringe between thumb and forefinger of dominant hand. Hold bevel of needle pointing up.	With bevel up, you are less likely to deposit medication into tissues below dermis.
13. Administer injection:	
a. With nondominant hand, stretch skin over site with forefinger or thumb.	Needle pierces tight skin more easily.

STEP	RATIONALE

b. With needle almost against patient's skin, insert it slowly at a 5- to 15-degree angle until resistance is felt. Advance needle through epidermis to approximately 3 mm (⅛ inch) below skin surface. You will see bulge of needle tip through skin.

Ensures that needle tip is in dermis. You will obtain inaccurate results if you do not inject needle at correct angle and depth (CDC, 2012b).

c. Inject medication slowly. Normally you feel resistance. If not, needle is too deep; remove and begin again.

Slow injection minimizes discomfort at site. Dermal layer is tight and does not expand easily when you inject solution.

d. While injecting medication, note that small bleb (approximately 6 mm [¼ inch]) resembling mosquito bite appears on skin surface (see illustration).

Bleb indicates that you deposited medication in dermis.

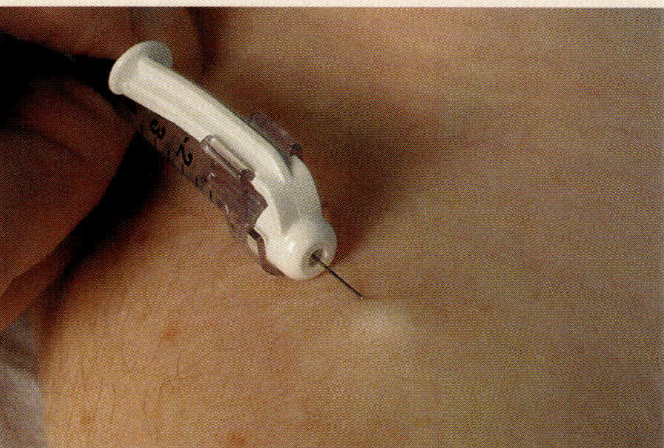

STEP 13d Injection creates a small bleb.

e. After withdrawing needle, apply alcohol swab or gauze over site. Do not massage site. Apply bandage if needed.

14. Discard uncapped needle or needle enclosed in safety shield and attached syringe into a puncture-proof and leak-proof receptacle.

Prevents injury to patients and health care personnel. Recapping needle increases risk for a needlestick injury (OSHA, 2012).

15. See Completion Protocol (inside front cover).

16. Stay with patient for several minutes and observe for any allergic reactions.

Dyspnea, wheezing, and circulatory collapse are signs of severe anaphylactic reaction.

▌EVALUATION

1. Return to room in 15 to 30 minutes and ask if patient feels any acute pain, burning, numbness, or tingling at injection site.
2. Use *Teach Back:* State to the patient, "I want to be sure I explained the purpose of TB skin testing and what you might see after the test. Can you explain to me what the injection site might look like in 2 to 3 days?" Evaluates what the patient is able to explain or demonstrate. Revise your instruction now or develop plan for revised patient teaching to be implemented at an appropriate time if patient is not able to teach back correctly.
3. Inspect bleb. Option: Use skin pencil and draw circle around perimeter of injection site. Read TB test at 48 to 72 hours; look for induration (hard, dense, raised area) of skin around injection site of:
   - 15 mm or more in patients with no known risk factors for TB.
   - 10 mm or more in patients who are recent immigrants; injection drug users; residents and employees of high-risk settings; patients with certain chronic illnesses; children younger than 4 years of age; and infants, children, and adolescents exposed to high-risk adults.
   - 5 mm or more in patients who are positive for human immunodeficiency virus (HIV), have fibrotic changes on chest x-ray film consistent with previous TB infection, have had organ transplants, or are immunosuppressed (CDC, 2012b).

Unexpected Outcomes and Related Interventions

1. Patient complains of localized pain or continued burning at injection site, indicating potential injury to nerve or vessels.
   a. Assess injection site.
   b. Notify patient's health care provider.

2. Raised, reddened, or hard zone (induration) forms around ID test site.
   a. Notify health care provider.
   b. Document sensitivity to injected allergen or positive test if TB skin testing was completed.
3. Patient has adverse reaction with signs of urticaria, eczema, pruritus, wheezing, and dyspnea.
   a. Follow facility policy for appropriate response to adverse drug reactions (e.g., administration of antihistamine or epinephrine).
   b. Notify patient's health care provider immediately.
   c. Add allergy information to patient's record.

Recording and Reporting

- Immediately after administration, record drug, dose, route, site, time, and date administered. Correctly sign MAR according to facility policy.
- Record patient's response to medication.
- Document your evaluation of patient learning.
- Report any undesirable effects from medication to patient's health care provider, and document adverse effects in record.

Sample Documentation

0900 Patient's ID site, right forearm noted 10-mm raised, reddened zone. Health care provider notified, and patient sent for chest radiograph at 1000. Patient unable to explain why there was a need for TB testing. Provided a pamphlet on testing and will allow patient time to read.

Special Considerations

Pediatric

- Children who are exposed to persons with confirmed or suspected infectious TB should be tested for TB immediately after exposure (Hockenberry and Wilson, 2013).
- Children who are exposed to high-risk individuals (e.g., HIV-infected, homeless, incarcerated) should be tested for TB every 2 to 3 years (Hockenberry and Wilson, 2013).

Geriatric

- The skin of older adults is less elastic and must be held taut to ensure that ID injection is administered correctly.

SKILL 23.5 ADMINISTERING MEDICATIONS BY INTRAVENOUS BOLUS

• Nursing Skills Online: Intravenous Medication Administration, Lessons 1 and 3

In the past, nurses often mixed medications into large volumes of IV fluids (500 to 1000 mL). However, today's safety standards and evidence-based practice no longer support this practice on a routine basis (Alexander et al., 2014; INS, 2011; ISMP, 2011a; TJC, 2014). Best practices for administration of IV solutions and medications include using standardized concentrations and dosages of medications, administering solutions and medications prepared and dispensed from the pharmacy as commercially prepared, using standardized infusion concentrations of "high-alert" medications (e.g., heparin, potassium, dopamine), and using standardized label practices (INS, 2011; ISMP, 2010; Manrique-Rodriguez et al., 2012).

An IV bolus is one method of medication administration currently practiced on patient care units. It introduces a concentrated dose of a medication directly into a vein via an existing IV access (see Chapter 27). An IV bolus or "push" usually requires a small volume of fluid, which is an advantage for patients at risk for fluid overload. Administering medications by IV bolus is common in emergencies when you need to deliver a fast-acting medication quickly. Because these medications act quickly, it is essential that you monitor patients closely for adverse reactions. Facilities have policies and procedures that identify the medications that nurses are allowed to administer by IV push and other IV routes. These policies are based on the medication, capability and availability of staff, and type of monitoring equipment available.

The IV bolus is a dangerous method to administer medications because it allows no time to correct errors. Administering an IV push medication too quickly can cause death. Be very careful in calculating the correct amount of the medication to give. In addition, a bolus may cause direct irritation to the lining of blood vessels; always confirm placement of an IV catheter or needle. Never give an IV bolus if the insertion site appears edematous or reddened or if the IV fluids do not flow at the ordered rate. Accidental injection of some medications into tissues surrounding a vein can cause pain, sloughing of tissues, and abscesses.

Verify the rate of administration of IV push medication using facility guidelines or a medication reference manual. The Institute for Safe Medication Practices (2014) has identified practices to reduce harm from IV push medications, including improving access to information about the medications, reducing access to "high-alert" medications, using labels, using computerized alerts, standardizing ordering and administration, and using technology and double checks of doses by nurses. Review the amount of medication the patient will receive each minute, the recommended concentration, and the rate of administration. For example, if a patient is to receive 6 mL of a medication over 3 minutes, give 2 mL of the IV bolus medication every minute. Understand the purpose of the medication and any potential adverse reactions related to the rate and route of administration. Some IV medications can be pushed safely only when the patient is continuously monitored for dysrhythmias, blood pressure changes, or other adverse effects. You can push some medications only in specific areas within a health care facility (e.g., critical care unit). Confirm facility guidelines about requirements for special monitoring.

IV push medications are given through either an existing continuous IV infusion or an intermittent venous access (commonly called a *saline lock*). A saline lock is an IV catheter with a small "well" or chamber covered by a rubber cap. An IV catheter can be converted into a lock by inserting a special rubber-seal injection cap into the end of the catheter (see Chapter 27). Use of a lock saves time by eliminating constant monitoring of an IV line. It also offers better mobility, safety, and comfort for patients by eliminating the need for a continuous IV line. After you administer an IV bolus through an intermittent venous access, flush with a normal saline solution to keep it patent.

ASSESSMENT

1. Check accuracy and completeness of each MAR with health care provider's original medication order. Check patient's name, drug name and dosage, route of administration, and time for administration. Recopy or reprint any portion of printed MAR that is difficult to read. *Rationale: The health care provider's order is the most reliable source and only legal record of patient's medications. Ensures that patient receives the right medications. Handwritten MARs are a source of medication errors (ISMP, 2011a; Tzeng et al., 2013).*
2. Assess patient's medical and medication history. *Rationale: Identifies need for medication or contraindication for medication.*
3. Review medication reference information for medication action, purpose, common side effects, normal dose, time of peak onset, how slowly to give the medication, and nursing implications such as the need to dilute the medication or administer it through a filter. *Rationale: Knowledge of medication allows you to give it safely and monitor patient's response to therapy.*
4. If you give medication through an existing IV line, determine compatibility of medication with IV fluids and any additives within IV solution. *Rationale: IV medication is sometimes incompatible with IV solution or additives or both; a new site may need to be initiated.*
5. Perform hand hygiene. Assess condition of IV needle insertion site for signs of infiltration or phlebitis. *Rationale: Do not administer medication if site is edematous or inflamed.*
6. Assess patency of patient's existing IV infusion line or saline lock (see Chapter 27). *Rationale: For medication to reach the venous circulation effectively, IV line must be patent, and fluids must infuse easily.*

7. Assess patient's history of medication allergies, known type of allergens, and normal allergic reaction. *Rationale: IV medications may cause rapid response. Allergic response is immediate.*
8. Assess patient's symptoms before administering medication. *Rationale: Provides information to evaluate desired effect of medication.*
9. Assess patient's understanding of purpose of IV medication therapy. *Rationale: Reveals need for patient instruction.*

PLANNING

Expected Outcomes focus on safe administration of an IV bolus medication.
1. Desired effect of medication achieved with no signs of adverse reactions.
2. IV site remains intact without signs of swelling or inflammation or symptoms of tenderness at site.
3. Patient explains purpose and side effects of medication.

Delegation and Collaboration
The skill of administering medications by IV bolus cannot be delegated to nursing assistive personnel (NAP). The nurse instructs the NAP about:
- Potential medication actions and side effects of the medications and to report their occurrence to the nurse.
- Obtaining any required vital signs and reporting them to the nurse.
- Reporting any patient complaints of moisture or discomfort around IV insertion site.

Equipment
- Watch with secondhand
- Clean gloves
- Antiseptic swab
- Medication in vial or ampule
- Proper size syringes for medication and saline flush with needleless device or SESIP needle (21- to 25-gauge)
- Intravenous lock: Vial of normal saline flush solution (saline recommended [Alexander et al., 2014]; if facility continues to use heparin flush, the most common concentration is 10 units/mL; check facility policy)
- MAR or computer printout
- Puncture-proof container

IMPLEMENTATION *for* ADMINISTERING MEDICATIONS BY INTRAVENOUS BOLUS

STEP	RATIONALE
1. Perform hand hygiene and prepare medication for one patient at a time using aseptic technique (see Skill 23.1). Keep all pages of MARs or computer printouts for one patient together or look at only one patient's electronic MAR at a time. Check label of medication carefully with MAR or computer printout two times while preparing medication.	Ensures that medication is sterile. Preventing distractions reduces medication errors (Freeman et al., 2013). *These are the first and second checks for accuracy* and ensure that the correct medication is administered.

Continued

STEP	RATIONALE

> **SAFE PATIENT CARE** Some IV medications require dilution before administration. Verify with facility policy or pharmacist. If a small amount of medication is given (e.g., less than 1 mL), dilute medication in small amount (e.g., 5 mL) of normal saline or sterile water so that the medication does not collect in the "dead spaces" (e.g., Y-site injection port, IV cap) of the IV delivery system.

2. Take medications to patient at correct time (see facility policy). Medications that require exact timing include STAT, first-time or loading doses, and one-time doses. Give time-critical scheduled medications (e.g., scheduled opioids, antibiotics, anticonvulsants, insulin, and immunosuppressive agents) at exact time ordered (no later than 30 minutes before or after scheduled dose). Give non–time-critical medications within a range of 1 or 2 hours of scheduled dose (ISMP, 2011b). During administration, apply six rights of medication administration.

   Hospitals must adopt medication administration policy and procedure for timing of medication administration that considers the nature of the prescribed medication, specific clinical application, and patient needs (DHHS, 2011; ISMP, 2011b). Time-critical scheduled medications are medications for which early or delayed administration of maintenance doses of greater than 30 minutes before or after the scheduled dose may cause harm or result in substantial suboptimal therapy or pharmacological effect. Non–time-critical medications are medications for which early or delayed administration within a specific range of either 1 or 2 hours should not cause harm or result in substantial suboptimal therapy or pharmacological effect (DHHS, 2011; ISMP, 2011b).

3. **See Standard Protocol (inside front cover).**

4. At the patient's bedside, identify patient using two identifiers (e.g., name and birthday or name and account number) according to facility policy. Compare identifiers with information on the patient's MAR or medical record. Again compare the names of medications on the medication label with the MAR or computer printout one more time at patient's bedside. Ask patient if he or she has any allergies.

   Ensures correct patient. Complies with The Joint Commission standards and improves patient safety (TJC, 2014). *The third check for accuracy* ensures that the correct medication is administered. Confirms patient's allergy history.

5. Discuss the purpose of each medication, action, and possible adverse effects with patient. Allow patient to ask any questions about drugs. Explain procedure to patient. Encourage patient to report symptoms of discomfort at IV site.

   Patient has the right to be informed, and patient's understanding of each medication improves adherence with drug therapy. Helps identify possible IV infiltration early.

6. *IV push (existing IV line):*

   a. Apply clean gloves. Select injection port of IV tubing closest to patient. Use needleless injection port.

      Reduces transmission of microorganisms. Follows provisions of the Needle Safety and Prevention Act of 2001 (OSHA, 2012).

> **SAFE PATIENT CARE** Never administer IV medications through tubing that is infusing blood, blood products, or parenteral nutrition solutions.

   b. Clean injection port with antiseptic swab. Allow to dry.

      Prevents transfer of microorganisms during blunt cannula insertion.

   c. *Connect syringe to IV line:* Insert needleless tip of syringe through center of port (see illustration).

      Prevents introduction of microorganisms. Prevents damage to port diaphragm and possible leakage from site.

   d. Occlude IV line by pinching tubing just above injection port (see illustration). Pull back gently on plunger of syringe to aspirate for blood return.

      Aspiration ensures that medication is delivered into bloodstream.

> **SAFE PATIENT CARE** In the case of smaller gauge IV needles, blood return sometimes is not aspirated, even if IV line is patent. If IV site shows no signs of infiltration and IV fluid is infusing without difficulty, give IV push.

STEP	RATIONALE

e. Release tubing and inject medication within amount of time recommended by facility policy, pharmacist, or medication reference manual. Use a watch to time administrations. You can pinch the IV line while pushing medication and release it when not pushing medication. Allow IV fluids to infuse when not pushing medication.

Ensures safe medication infusion. Rapid injection of IV drug can be fatal. Allowing IV fluids to infuse while pushing IV drug enables medication to be delivered to patient at prescribed rate.

f. After injecting medication, withdraw syringe and recheck fluid infusion rate.

Injection of bolus often alters rate of fluid infusion. Rapid fluid infusion causes circulatory fluid overload.

g. If IV medication is incompatible with IV fluids, stop IV fluids, clamp IV line, and flush with 10 mL of normal saline or sterile water (see facility policy). Give IV bolus over the appropriate amount of time and flush with another 10 mL of normal saline or sterile water at the same rate as medication was administered.

Allows IV bolus to be administered without risks associated with IV incompatibilities. Ensure that facility guidelines permit flushing lines with incompatible medications. A new site may need to be initiated.

7. *IV push (IV lock):*

a. Apply clean gloves. Prepare flush solution according to facility policy.

   (1) *Saline flush method (preferred):* Prepare two syringes filled with 2 to 3 mL of normal saline (0.9%). Many facilities do not provide prefilled normal saline syringes for flushing IV lines.

Normal saline is effective in keeping IV locks patent and is compatible with a wide range of medications.

   (2) *Heparin flush method (not recommended; refer to facility policy)*

b. Administer medication:

   (1) Clean injection port with antiseptic swab and allow to dry.

Prevents transfer of microorganisms during needle insertion.

   (2) Insert needleless tip of syringe with normal saline (0.9%) flush through injection port of IV lock.

   (3) Pull back gently on syringe plunger and check for blood return.

Indicates if needle or catheter is in vein.

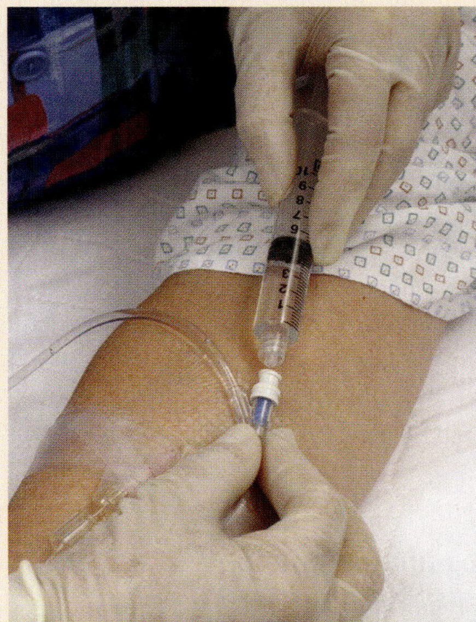

STEP 6c Connecting syringe to IV line with needleless blunt cannula tip.

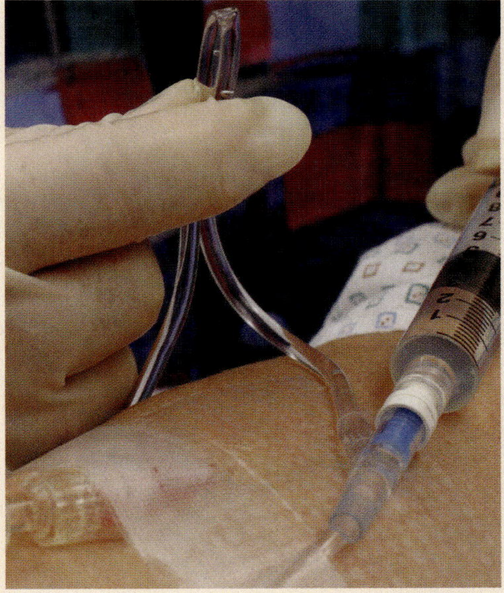

STEP 6d Occluding IV tubing above injection port.

Continued

STEP	RATIONALE
(4) Flush IV site with normal saline by pushing slowly on plunger.	Clears needle and reservoir of blood. Flushing without difficulty indicates patent IV line.
(a) Carefully observe the area of skin above the IV catheter. Note any puffiness or swelling as you flush the IV line.	Swelling indicates infiltration into the vein and requires removal of catheter.
(5) Remove saline-filled syringe.	
(6) Clean injection port of lock with antiseptic swab and allow to dry.	Prevents transmission of microorganisms.
(7) Insert needleless tip of syringe containing prepared medication through injection port of IV lock.	Allows administration of medication.
(8) Inject medication within amount of time recommended by facility policy, pharmacist, or medication reference manual. Use a watch to time administration.	Many medication errors are associated with IV pushes being administered too quickly. Following guidelines for IV push rates promotes patient safety.
(9) After administering bolus, withdraw syringe.	
(10) Clean injection site of lock with antiseptic swab and allow to dry.	Prevents transmission of microorganisms.
(11) Flush injection port. Attach second syringe with normal saline and inject flush at the same rate the medication was delivered.	Flushing IV line with saline prevents occlusion of IV access device and ensures that all medication is delivered. Flushing IV site at same rate as medication ensures that any medication remaining within IV needle is delivered at the correct rate.
8. Dispose of SESIP covered needles and syringes in puncture-proof and leak-proof container.	Prevents accidental needlestick injuries and follows CDC guidelines for disposal of sharps (OSHA, 2012).
9. **See Completion Protocol (inside front cover).**	
10. Stay with patient for several minutes and observe for any allergic reactions.	Dyspnea, wheezing, and circulatory collapse are signs of severe anaphylactic reaction.

EVALUATION

1. Observe patient closely for adverse reactions during administration and for several minutes thereafter.
2. Observe IV site during injection for sudden swelling and for 48 hours after IV push.
3. Assess patient's status after giving medication to evaluate the effectiveness of the medication.
4. Use *Teach Back:* State to the patient, "I want to be sure I explained why you were receiving an IV push medication and what to expect from this medication. Could you tell me why you received this medication?" Evaluates what the patient is able to explain or demonstrate. Revise your instruction now or develop plan for revised patient teaching to be implemented at an appropriate time if patient is not able to teach back correctly.

Unexpected Outcomes and Related Interventions

1. Patient develops adverse reaction to medication.
   a. Stop delivering medication immediately and follow facility policy for appropriate response (e.g., administration of antihistamine or epinephrine) and reporting of adverse drug reactions.
   b. Notify patient's health care provider of adverse effects immediately.
   c. Add allergy information to patient's medical record per facility policy.
2. IV site shows symptoms of infiltration or phlebitis (see Chapter 27).
   a. Stop IV infusion immediately. If administration is still necessary, discontinue access device and restart in another site.
   b. Determine how much damage the IV medication can produce in subcutaneous tissue.
   c. Provide IV extravasation care (e.g., injecting phentolamine [Regitine] around IV infiltration site) as indicated by facility policy; use a medication reference or consult pharmacist to determine appropriate follow-up care.

Recording and Reporting

- Record medication administration, including dose, route, time administered, and date, on MAR immediately after administration, not before. Correctly sign MAR according to facility policy.

- Record condition of IV site and patient teaching about medication in nurses' notes.
- Record patient's response to medication in nurses' notes.
- Document your evaluation of patient learning.
- Report any adverse reactions to patient's health care provider. Patient's response may indicate need for additional medical therapy.

Sample Documentation

1400   Furosemide (Lasix) 20 mg IVP administered over 2 minutes via IV in right forearm. Site free from redness and edema. Patient denies any pain at IV insertion site. Patient able to teach back that medication was given to remove excess fluids from the body.

Special Considerations
Pediatric

- The therapeutic dose of IV push medications for infants and children is often small and difficult to prepare accurately even with a tuberculin syringe. Infuse these medications slowly and in small volumes because of the risk for fluid volume overload (Hockenberry and Wilson, 2013). To maintain pediatric safety, carefully follow facility guidelines when administering IV bolus medication.

Geriatric

- The renal and metabolic systems do not function as efficiently in older patients because of the aging process. To reduce the risk of adverse effects of IV push medications, administer them over longer periods of time.

Home Care

- IV push medications are frequently given in the home. Nurses, pharmacists, and health care providers need to collaborate closely in the care of these patients. Patients and families who are independently responsible for managing IV medications need to understand all aspects of administration safety. Adequate eyesight and manual dexterity are necessary to manipulate a syringe. Patients and family caregivers need to understand the venous access device, rate to give medications, and how to flush the access device. Patients need to store medications safely, dispose of IV supplies appropriately, and know whom to contact in case of an emergency.

SKILL 23.6   ADMINISTERING INTRAVENOUS MEDICATIONS BY PIGGYBACK AND SYRINGE PUMPS

• **Nursing Skills Online: Intravenous Medication Administration Module, Lesson 4**

One method of administering IV medications uses small volumes (25 to 250 mL) of compatible IV fluids infused over a desired period of time. This method reduces the risk of rapid dose infusion and provides independence for patients. Patients must have an established IV line that is kept patent by either a continuous infusion or intermittent flushes of normal saline.

PIGGYBACK

A piggyback is a small (25 to 250 mL) IV bag connected to a short tubing line that connects to the *upper* Y-port of a primary infusion line or to an intermittent venous access such as a saline lock. The IV container that holds the medication is labeled following the IV piggyback medication format of the Institute for Safe Medication Practices (2010). The piggyback tubing is a microdrip or macrodrip system. The set is called a piggyback because the small bag is set higher than the primary infusion bag when administered by gravity. The port of the primary IV line contains a back-check valve that automatically stops the flow of the primary infusion when the piggyback infusion flows, preventing the primary infusion from flowing. After the piggyback solution infuses and the solution within the tubing falls below the level of the primary infusion drip chamber, the back-check valve opens, and the primary infusion begins to flow again.

SYRINGE PUMP

The syringe pump is battery operated and delivers medications in very small amounts of fluid (5 to 60 mL) within controlled infusion times using standard syringes (Fig. 23-16).

ASSESSMENT

1. Check accuracy and completeness of each MAR with health care provider's original medication order. Check patient's name, drug name and dosage, route of administration, and time for administration. Recopy or reprint any portion of printed MAR that is difficult to read. *Rationale: The health care provider's order is the most reliable source and only legal record of the patient's medications. Ensures that patient receives the right medications. Handwritten MARs are a source of medication errors (ISMP, 2011a; Tzeng et al., 2013).*
2. Assess patient's medical and medication history. *Rationale: Identifies need for medication or contraindications for medication.*
3. Review medication reference information for medication action, purpose, common side effects, normal dose, time of peak onset, how slowly to give the medication, and nursing implications (e.g., need to dilute the medication

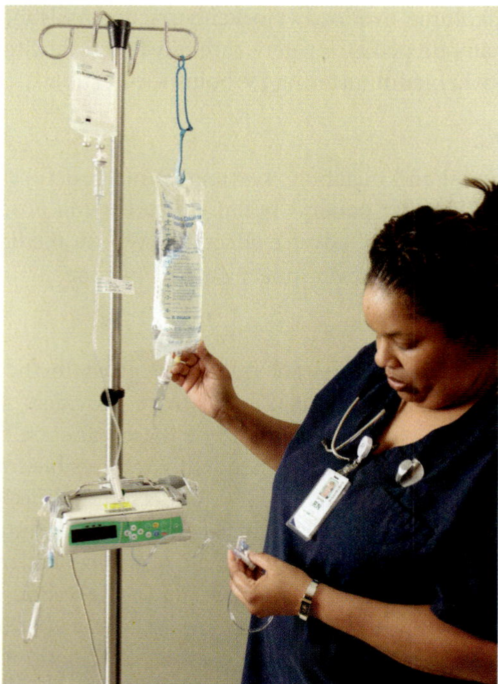

FIG 23-16 Syringe pump.

or administer it through a filter). *Rationale: Knowledge of medication allows you to give medication safely and monitor patient's response to therapy.*

4. If you give medication through existing IV line, determine compatibility of medication with IV fluids and any additives within IV solution. *Rationale: IV medication is sometimes incompatible with IV solution or additives or both.*

> **SAFE PATIENT CARE** Never administer IV medications through tubing that is infusing blood, blood products, or parenteral nutrition solutions.

5. Assess patency and placement of patient's existing IV infusion line (see Chapter 27). *Rationale: Do not administer medication if site is edematous or inflamed.*
6. Assess patient's history of medication allergies, known type of allergens, and normal allergic reaction. *Rationale: IV administration of medications may cause rapid response. Allergic response is immediate.*

7. Assess patient's symptoms before initiating medication therapy. *Rationale: Provides information to evaluate desired effect of medication.*
8. Assess patient's knowledge of medication. *Rationale: Reveals need for instruction.*

PLANNING

Expected Outcomes focus on safe administration of a piggyback or syringe pump IV medication.

1. Medication is administered safely with desired therapeutic effect achieved.
2. Medication infuses within desired time frame.
3. IV site remains intact without signs of swelling, inflammation, or symptoms of tenderness at site.
4. Patient explains the purpose and the side effects of medication.

Delegation and Collaboration

The skill of administering IV medications by piggyback and syringe pumps cannot be delegated to nursing assistive personnel (NAP). The nurse instructs the NAP about:

- Potential medication actions and side effects and to report their occurrence to the nurse.
- Reporting any change in the patient's condition or vital signs to the nurse.
- Reporting any patient complaints of moisture or discomfort around IV insertion site.

Equipment

- Adhesive tape (optional)
- Antiseptic swab
- Clean gloves
- IV pole
- MAR or computer printout
- Puncture-proof container

Piggyback or Syringe Pump

- Medication prepared in 5- to 250-mL labeled infusion bag or syringe
- Prefilled syringe containing normal saline flush solution (for saline lock only)
- Short microdrip, macrodrip, or syringe IV tubing set, with blunt-end needleless cannula attachment
- Needleless device
- Syringe pump if indicated

IMPLEMENTATION *for* ADMINISTERING INTRAVENOUS MEDICATIONS BY PIGGYBACK AND SYRINGE PUMPS

STEP	RATIONALE
1. Perform hand hygiene and prepare medication for one patient at a time using aseptic technique (see Skill 23.1). Keep all pages of MARs or computer printouts for one patient together or look at only one patient's electronic MAR at a time. Check label of medication carefully with MAR or computer printout two times while preparing medication.	Ensures that medication is sterile. Preventing distractions reduces medication errors (Freeman et al., 2013). *These are the first and second checks for accuracy* and ensure that the correct medication is administered.

2. Take medications to patient at correct time (see facility policy). Medications that require exact timing include STAT, first-time or loading doses, and one-time doses. Give time-critical scheduled medications (e.g., antibiotics, anticoagulants, scheduled opioids, insulin, anticonvulsants, immunosuppressive agents) at exact time ordered (no later than 30 minutes before or after scheduled dose). Give non–time-critical medications within a range of 1 or 2 hours of scheduled dose (ISMP, 2011b). During administration, apply six rights of medication administration.

Hospitals must adopt medication administration policy and procedure for timing of medication administration that considers the nature of the prescribed medication, specific clinical application, and patient needs (DHHS, 2011; ISMP, 2011b). Time-critical scheduled medications are medications for which early or delayed administration of maintenance doses of greater than 30 minutes before or after the scheduled dose may cause harm or result in substantial suboptimal therapy or pharmacological effect. Non–time-critical medications are medications for which early or delayed administration within a specific range of either 1 or 2 hours should not cause harm or result in substantial suboptimal therapy or pharmacological effect (DHHS, 2011; ISMP, 2011b).

3. **See Standard Protocol (inside front cover).**

4. At the bedside, identify patient using two identifiers (e.g., name and birthday or name and account number) according to facility policy. Compare identifiers with information on the patient's MAR or medical record. Again compare MAR or computer printout with the names of medications on the medication labels and patient name. Ask patient if he or she has allergies.

Ensures correct patient. Complies with The Joint Commission standards and improves patient safety (TJC, 2014). *This is the third check for accuracy* and ensures that patient receives correct medication. Confirms patient's allergy history.

5. Discuss the purpose of each medication, action, and possible common adverse effects. Allow patient to ask any questions. Explain that you will give medication through existing IV line. Encourage patient to report symptoms of discomfort at site.

Keeps patient informed of planned therapies, minimizing anxiety. Patients who verbalize pain at the IV site help detect IV infiltrations early, lessening damage to surrounding tissues.

6. Administer infusion:

  a. *Piggyback infusion:*

    (1) Connect infusion tubing to medication bag (see Chapter 27). Fill tubing by opening regulator flow clamp. When tubing is full, close clamp and cap end of tubing.

Filling infusion tubing with solution and freeing air bubbles prevent air embolus.

    (2) Hang piggyback medication bag above level of primary fluid bag (see illustration). (Use hook to lower main bag.)

Height of fluid bag affects rate of flow to patient.

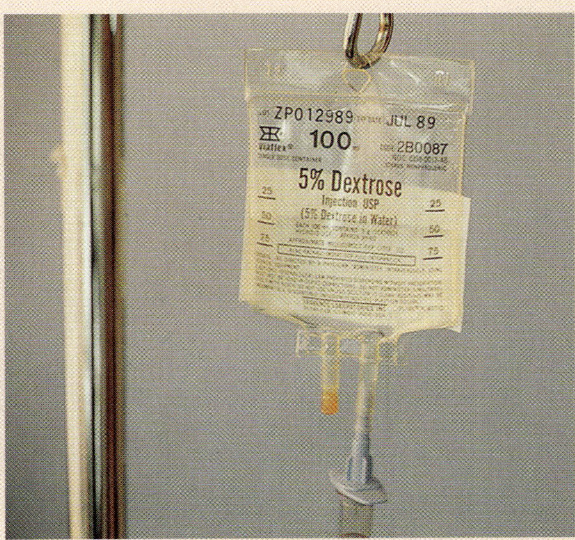

STEP 6a(2) Small-volume mini-bag for piggyback infusion.

Continued

STEP	RATIONALE

(3) Connect tubing of piggyback infusion to appropriate connector on upper Y-port of primary infusion line:

Connection allows IV medication to enter main IV line.

    (a) *Needleless system:* Wipe off needleless port of main IV with alcohol swab, allow to dry. Remove cap and insert cannula tip of piggyback infusion tubing (see illustrations).

Use needleless connections to prevent accidental needlestick injuries (OSHA, 2012).

(4) Connect tubing of piggyback infusion to a saline lock:

Flushing of lock ensures patency.

    (a) Follow Steps 7a(1) through 7b(5) in Skill 23.5 to flush and prepare lock.

    (b) Wipe off port of lock with alcohol swab, let dry. Remove cap and insert tip of piggyback infusion tubing via needleless access to port of saline lock.

(5) Regulate flow rate of medication solution by adjusting regulator clamp or IV pump infusion rate (see Chapter 27). Infusion times vary. Refer to medication reference or facility policy for safe flow rate.

Provides slow, safe infusion of medication and maintains therapeutic blood levels.

(6) Once medication has infused:

    (a) *Continuous infusion:* Check flow rate on primary infusion. The primary infusion automatically begins to flow after the piggyback solution is empty.

Back-check valve on piggyback stops flow of the primary infusion until medication infuses. Checking flow rate ensures proper administration of IV fluids.

    (b) *Saline lock:* Disconnect tubing and apply cap. Cleanse port with alcohol, and flush IV line with 2 to 3 mL of sterile 0.9% sodium chloride. Maintain sterility of IV tubing between intermittent infusions.

Ensures lock remains patent.

(7) Regulate continuous main infusion line to ordered rate.

Infusion of piggyback sometimes interferes with main line infusion rate.

(8) Leave IV piggyback bag and tubing in place for future drug administration (see facility policy) or discard in puncture-proof and leak-proof containers.

Establishment of secondary line produces route for microorganisms to enter main line. Repeated changes in tubing increase risk of infection transmission.

b. *Syringe pump administration:*

    (1) Connect prefilled syringe to syringe pump tubing; remove end cap of tubing.

Special tubing designed to fit syringe delivers medication to main IV line.

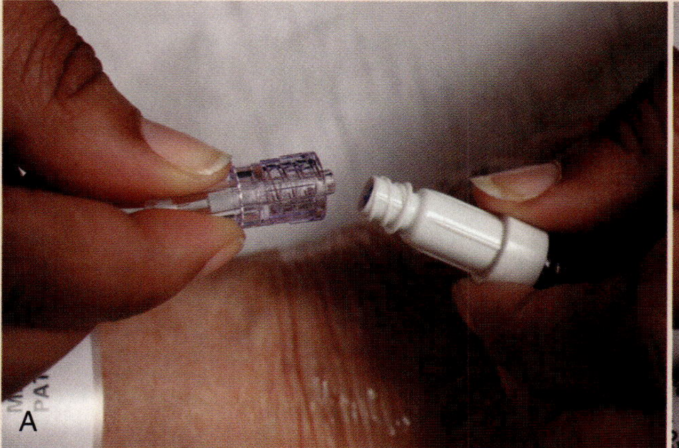
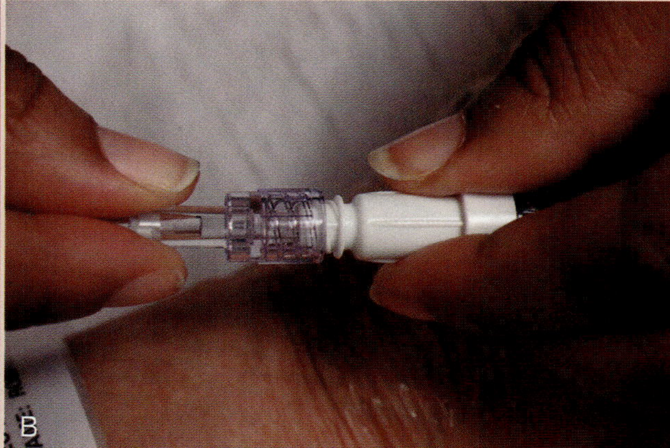

STEP 6a(3)(a) A, Needleless lock cannula system. **B,** Blunt-end cannula inserts into port and locks.

STEP	RATIONALE

(2) Carefully apply pressure to syringe plunger, allowing tubing to fill with medication. Reapply cap.

Ensures that tubing is free of air bubbles to prevent air embolus.

(3) Place syringe into syringe pump (follow product directions) and hang on IV pole. Ensure that syringe is secured (see illustration).

Correct placement is necessary for proper infusion.

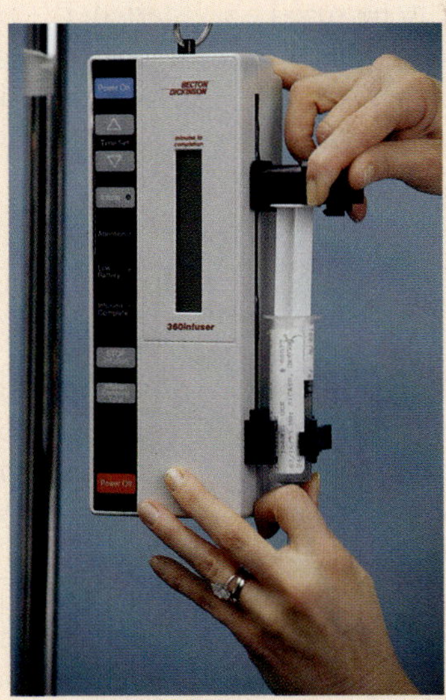

STEP 6b(3) Ensure that syringe is secure after placing it into syringe pump.

(4) Remove cap and connect end of syringe pump tubing to main IV line or saline lock.

   (a) *Existing IV line:* Wipe off needleless port on main IV line with alcohol swab, let dry, and insert tip of the syringe pump tubing through center of port.

Needleless connections reduce risk of needlestick injuries (OSHA, 2012).

   (b) *Saline lock:* Follow Steps 7a(1) through 7b(5) in Skill 23.5 to flush and prepare lock. Wipe off port with alcohol swab, allow to dry, and insert tip of syringe pump tubing.

(5) Set pump to deliver medication within time recommended by facility policy, pharmacist, or medication reference manual. Press button on pump to begin infusion.

Pump automatically delivers medication at safe, constant rate based on volume in syringe.

(6) Once medication has infused:

Maintains patency of primary IV line.

   (a) *Main IV infusion:* Check flow rate. Infusion automatically begins to flow when the pump stops. Regulate infusion to desired rate as needed.

   (b) *Saline lock:* Disconnect tubing and apply cap, cleanse port with alcohol, and flush IV line with 2 to 3 mL of sterile 0.9% sodium chloride.

(7) Dispose of supplies in puncture-proof and leak-proof container.

Prevents accidental needlesticks (OSHA, 2012).

7. See Completion Protocol (inside front cover).

8. Stay with patient for several minutes and observe for any allergic reactions.

Dyspnea, wheezing, and circulatory collapse are signs of severe anaphylactic reaction.

EVALUATION

1. Observe patient closely for adverse reactions during administration and for several minutes thereafter.
2. During infusion, periodically check infusion rate and condition of IV site.
3. Assess patient's status after giving medication to evaluate the effectiveness of the medication.
4. Use **Teach Back:** State to the patient, "I want to be sure I explained the reasons for this medication and what to expect. Can you tell me one of the reasons you are receiving this medication?" Evaluates what the patient is able to explain or demonstrate. Revise your instruction now or develop plan for revised patient teaching to be implemented at an appropriate time if patient is not able to teach back correctly.

Unexpected Outcomes and Related Interventions

1. Patient develops adverse or allergic reaction to medication.
   a. Stop medication infusion immediately.
   b. Follow facility policy for appropriate response and reporting of allergic or adverse medication reactions.
   c. Notify patient's health care provider of adverse effects immediately.
   d. Add allergy information to patient's medical record.
2. Medication does not infuse over established time frame.
   a. Determine reason (e.g., improper calculation of flow rate, poor positioning of IV needle at insertion site, infiltration) (see Chapter 27).
   b. Take corrective action as indicated.
3. IV site shows symptoms of infiltration or phlebitis (see Chapter 27).
   a. Stop infusion immediately and discontinue access device.
   b. Treat IV site as indicated by facility policy.
   c. For infiltration, determine how harmful the IV medication is to subcutaneous tissue. Provide IV extravasation care (e.g., injecting phentolamine [Regitine] around IV infiltration site) as indicated by facility policy, or consult pharmacist to determine appropriate follow-up care.

Recording and Reporting

- Immediately record medication, dose, route, infusion rate, and date and time administered on MAR or computer printout. Correctly sign name according to facility policy.
- Record volume of fluid in medication bag or syringe pump as fluid intake.
- Report any adverse reactions to patient's health care provider.
- Document your evaluation of patient learning.

Sample Documentation

1600 Furosemide (Lasix) 10 mg IV via syringe pump started. IV insertion site left forearm free from redness, pain, or edema. Primary IV D_5 ½ normal saline infusing at 100 mL/hr without difficulty. Patient able to teach back reasons why he is receiving this medication and what to expect after infusion.

Special Considerations
Pediatric

- Infants and young children are more vulnerable to alterations in fluid balance and do not adjust quickly to changes in fluid balance. Monitor intake and output carefully when infusing IV medications (Hockenberry and Wilson, 2013).

Geriatric

- Altered pharmacokinetics of medications and the effects of polypharmacy place older adults at risk for medication toxicity. Carefully monitor the response of older adults to IV medication therapy (Touhy and Jett, 2014).
- Older adults are at risk for developing fluid volume overload and require careful assessment for signs of overload and heart failure.

Home Care

- Patients or family caregivers who administer IV medications at home require education about the steps of medication administration. The patient or family caregiver needs to perform several return demonstrations of IV medication administration before performing this skill independently. In addition, patients and family caregivers need to know signs of IV medication administration complications such as phlebitis and infiltration and what to do for any problems.

SKILL 23.7   **ADMINISTERING MEDICATIONS BY CONTINUOUS SUBCUTANEOUS INFUSION**

The continuous subcutaneous infusion (CSQI or CSCI) route of medication administration is used for selected medications (e.g., opioids, insulin). The route is also effective with medications to stop preterm labor (e.g., terbutaline [Brethine]) and to treat pulmonary hypertension (e.g., treprostinil sodium [Remodulin]). One factor that determines the infusion rate of CSQI is the rate of medication absorption. Most patients can absorb 3 to 5 mL/hr of medication, but the rate of absorption is more dependent on osmotic pressure than the rate of administration (Alexander et al., 2014; INS, 2011; Kuensting, 2011).

With CSQI, patients are able to manage their illness or pain without the risks and expenses involved with IV medication administration. This route is relatively easy for patients and families to learn and understand in the home setting. CSQI improves oncologic and postoperative pain control in

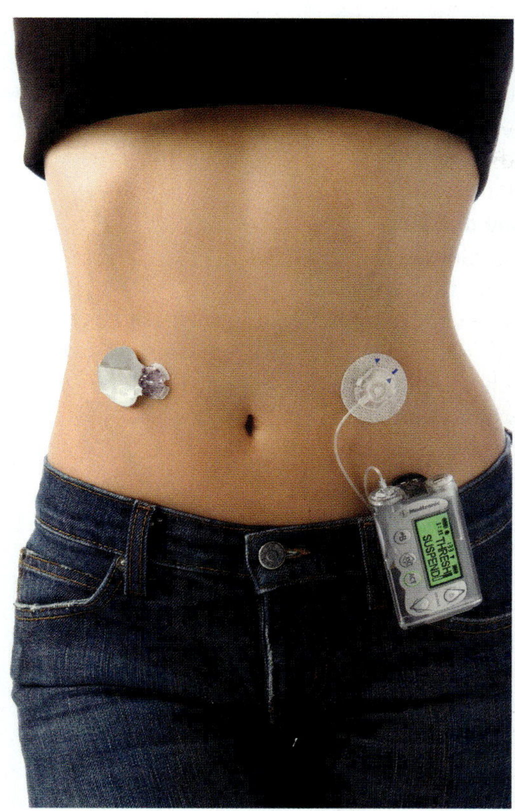

FIG 23-17 Minimed Paradigm REAL-Time Insulin CSQI Pump and Continuous Glucose Monitoring System. (Courtesy Medtronic MiniMed, Northridge, California.)

different patients, including infants, children, and adults (Oldenmenger et al., 2012).

Patients with diabetes mellitus using CSQI for management of blood glucose levels receive intense diabetes self-management education from qualified diabetic educators and insulin pump trainers. The newest system integrates an insulin pump with real-time continuous glucose monitoring (Fig. 23-17) (Medtronic MiniMed, 2013). Patients with diabetes mellitus using insulin pumps generally require less insulin because insulin is absorbed and used more efficiently (Buchko et al., 2012).

The procedure to initiate and discontinue CSQI therapy is similar, regardless of the type of medication being delivered. However, nursing assessment and interventions vary, depending on the type of medication administered. For example, if the medication is for diabetes glucose management, you evaluate the patient's blood glucose levels and episodes of hypoglycemia or hyperglycemia (Carchidi et al., 2011).

Use a small-gauge (25- to 27-gauge) winged butterfly IV needle or special commercially prepared polytetrafluoroethylene (Teflon) cannula to deliver medications. Although Teflon cannulas are generally more expensive, they tend to be more comfortable and have lower rates of complications than winged IV needles. The cannulas are associated with fewer needlestick injuries. Base the choice of needle type on facility guidelines or patient preference. Use the needle with the shortest length and the smallest gauge needed to start and maintain the infusion.

Use the same anatomical sites as for subcutaneous injections and the upper chest (see Skill 23.2). Site selection depends on a patient's activity level and the type of medication. For example, pain medications given to ambulatory patients are best delivered in the upper chest, which allows patients to move freely. Insulin is absorbed most consistently in the abdomen; choose a site in the abdomen away from the waistline. Always avoid sites where the tubing of the pump could be disturbed. Rotate sites at least every 24 to 48 hours or after 1.5 to 2.0 L of fluid has infused or every 2 to 7 days for medication infusions (Alexander et al., 2014; INS, 2011).

The CSQI route requires a computerized pump with safety features, including lockout intervals and warning alarms. Ideally, medication pumps are individualized based on the medication being delivered and the patient's needs. You also need to consider the availability and cost of the pump and its supplies. When possible, have patients select the pump that fits their individual and home needs and is easiest to use.

ASSESSMENT

1. Check accuracy and completeness of each MAR with health care provider's original medication order. Check patient's name, drug name and dosage, route of administration, and time for administration. Recopy or reprint any portion of printed MAR that is difficult to read. *Rationale: The health care provider's order is the most reliable source and only legal record of the patient's medication. Ensures that patient receives the right medications. Handwritten MARs are a source of medication errors (ISMP, 2011a; Tzeng et al., 2013).*

2. Assess patient's medical and medication history. *Rationale: Identifies need for medication or contraindication for medication.*

3. Review medication reference to administer drug safely, including action, purpose, side effects, normal dose, time of peak onset, rate to give the medication, and nursing implications. *Rationale: Knowledge of medication allows you to give medication safely and monitor patient's response to therapy.*

4. Assess for contraindications to CSQI (e.g., thrombocytopenia or reduced local tissue perfusion). *Rationale: Reduced tissue perfusion interferes with medication absorption and distribution.*

5. Assess adequacy of patient's adipose tissue to determine appropriate site. *Rationale: Physiological changes of aging or effect of illness on subcutaneous tissue affects choice of catheter insertion site.*

6. Assess patient's history of medication allergies, known type of allergens, and normal allergic reaction. *Rationale: CSQI administration of medications may cause rapid response. Allergic response is immediate.*

7. Assess patient's symptoms before initiating medication therapy. Determine severity of pain (if using analgesia) or

measure blood glucose level (if using insulin). *Rationale: Provides information to evaluate desired effect of medication.*

8. Assess patient's knowledge of medication and medication delivered by CSQI. *Rationale: Provides information about patient's understanding of medication and need for instruction.*

PLANNING

Expected Outcomes focus on safe administration of CSQI.
1. Needle insertion site remains free from infection.
2. Patient achieves desired effect of medication with no signs of adverse reactions.
3. Patient explains purpose, dosage, and effects of medication and verbalizes understanding of CSQI therapy.

Delegation and Collaboration

The skill of administering CSQI medications cannot be delegated to nursing assistive personnel (NAP). The nurse instructs the NAP about:
- Potential medication side effects or reactions and to report their occurrence to the nurse.
- Reporting complications (e.g., leaking, redness, discomfort) at the CSQI needle insertion site to the nurse.
- Obtaining any required vital signs and reporting them to the nurse.

Equipment
Initiation of CSQI
- Clean gloves
- Alcohol swab
- Antibacterial skin preparation such as chlorhexidine
- Small-gauge (25- to 27-gauge) winged IV catheter with attached tubing or CSQI-designed catheter (e.g., Sof-Set)
- Infusion pump
- Occlusive, transparent dressing
- Tape
- Medication in appropriate syringe or container
- MAR or computer printout

Discontinuing CSQI
- Clean gloves
- Small, sterile gauze dressing
- Tape or adhesive bandage
- Alcohol swab and chlorhexidine (optional)
- Puncture-proof container

IMPLEMENTATION *for* ADMINISTERING MEDICATIONS BY CONTINUOUS SUBCUTANEOUS INFUSION

STEP	RATIONALE
1. Review manufacturer's directions for pump.	Ensures proper use of equipment.
2. Perform hand hygiene and prepare medication for one patient at a time using aseptic technique (see Skill 23.1). Keep all pages of MARs or computer printouts for one patient together or look at only one patient's electronic MAR at a time. Check label of medication carefully with MAR or computer printout two times while preparing medication.	Ensures that medication is sterile. Preventing distractions reduces medication errors (Freeman et al., 2013). *These are the first and second checks for accuracy* and ensure that the correct medication is administered.
3. Obtain and program medication administration pump. Place syringe in pump.	Ensures that medication dose administered is accurate.
4. Take medications to patient at correct time (see facility policy). Medications that require exact timing include STAT, first-time or loading doses, and one-time doses. Give time-critical scheduled medications (e.g., anticoagulants, insulin) at exact time ordered (no later than 30 minutes before or after scheduled dose). Give non–time-critical medications within a range of 1 or 2 hours of scheduled dose (ISMP, 2011b). During administration, apply six rights of medication administration.	Hospitals must adopt medication administration policy and procedure for timing of medication administration that considers the nature of the prescribed medication, specific clinical application, and patient needs (DHHS, 2011; ISMP, 2011b). Time-critical scheduled medications are medications for which early or delayed administration of maintenance doses of greater than 30 minutes before or after the scheduled dose may cause harm or result in substantial suboptimal therapy or pharmacological effect. Non–time-critical medications are medications for which early or delayed administration within a specific range of either 1 or 2 hours should not cause harm or result in substantial suboptimal therapy or pharmacological effect (DHHS, 2011; ISMP, 2011b).
5. **See Standard Protocol (inside front cover).**	

STEP	RATIONALE

6. At the bedside, identify patient using two identifiers (e.g., name and birthday or name and account number) according to facility policy. Compare identifiers with information on the patient's MAR or medical record. Again compare the MAR or computer printout with the names of medications on the syringe medication label. Ask patient if he or she has allergies.

Ensures correct patient. Complies with The Joint Commission standards and improves patient safety (TJC, 2014). *This is the third check for accuracy* and ensures that patient receives correct medication. Confirms patient's allergy history.

7. Discuss the purpose of each medication, action, and possible adverse effects. Allow patient to ask any questions. Tell patient that needle insertion will cause slight burning or stinging.

Patient has the right to be informed, and patient's understanding of each medication improves adherence with drug therapy.

8. Initiate CSQI:

  a. Assist patient to comfortable lying or sitting position.

  Eases pain associated with insertion of needle.

  b. Select appropriate insertion site free of irritation and away from bony prominences and waistline. Most common sites are subclavicular and abdomen.

  Ensures proper medication absorption.

  c. Apply clean gloves. Cleanse injection site with alcohol using a circular motion, followed by antiseptic, using straight cleansing strokes. Allow both agents to dry.

  Reduces risk of infection at insertion site.

  d. Hold needle in dominant hand and remove needle guard.

  Prepares needle for insertion.

  e. Gently grasp or lift up skin with nondominant hand.

  Ensures that needle will enter subcutaneous tissue.

  f. Gently and firmly insert needle at a 45- to 90-degree angle (see illustration). Some shorter prepackaged needles (e.g., Sof-Set, Subcutaneous Set) are inserted at a 90-degree angle. Refer to manufacturer's directions.

  Decreases pain related to insertion of needle.

  g. Release skinfold and apply tape over "wings" of needle.

  Secures needle.

> **SAFE PATIENT CARE** Some cannulas have a sharp needle covered with a plastic catheter. In this case, remove the needle and leave the plastic catheter in the skin.

  h. Place occlusive, transparent dressing over insertion site (see illustration).

  Protects site from infection and allows you to assess site during medication infusion.

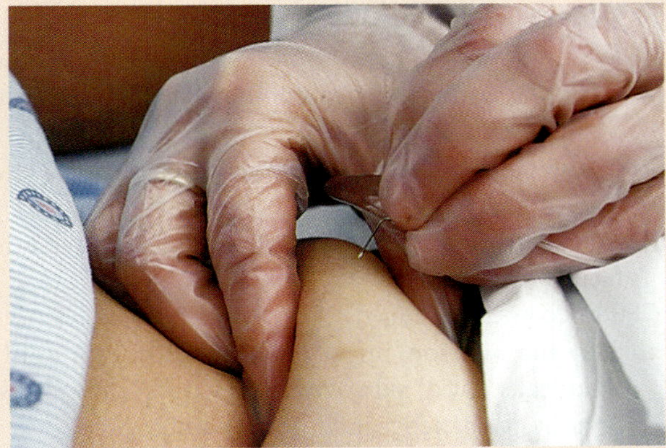

STEP 8f Insertion of needle into subcutaneous tissue of abdomen.

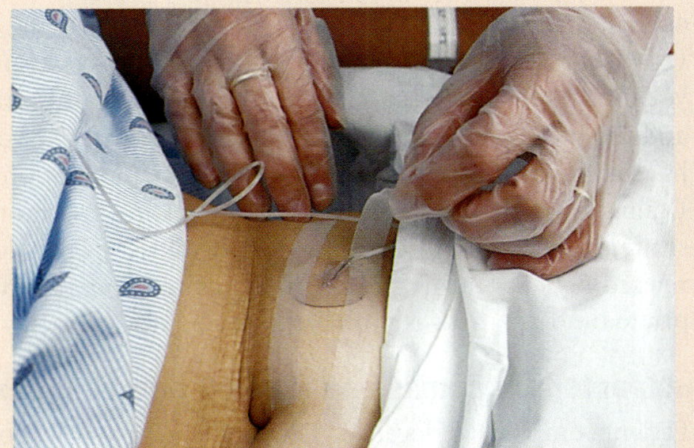

STEP 8h Placement of transparent dressing over insertion site.

Continued

STEP	RATIONALE
i. Attach tubing from needle to tubing from infusion pump and turn on pump.	Allows you to administer medication.
j. Dispose of any sharps in appropriate leak-proof and puncture-proof container.	Prevents accidental needlestick injuries and follows CDC guidelines for disposal of sharps (OSHA, 2012).
k. Inspect site before leaving patient and instruct patient to inform you if site becomes red or begins to leak.	Initiate a new site with a new needle whenever erythema or leaking occurs. If the site is free from complications, rotate the needle used for fluids every 1 to 2 days and for medication every 2 to 7 days (Alexander et al., 2014; INS, 2011).
9. Stay with patient for several minutes and observe for any allergic reactions.	Dyspnea, wheezing, and circulatory collapse are signs of severe anaphylactic reaction.
10. Discontinue CSQI:	
a. Verify order and establish alternative method for medication administration if applicable.	If medication will be required after discontinuing CSQI, a different medication or route is often necessary to continue to manage patient's illness or pain.
b. Stop infusion pump.	Prevents medication from spilling.
c. Perform hand hygiene and apply clean gloves.	Follows CDC recommendations to prevent accidental exposure to blood and body fluids (OSHA, 2012).
d. Remove dressing without dislodging or removing the needle.	Exposes needle.

> **SAFE PATIENT CARE** If site is infected or if included in facility guidelines, cleanse site with alcohol and antiseptic. Apply triple antibiotic cream to site if it is excoriated (abraded).

STEP	RATIONALE
e. Remove tape from the wings of needle and pull needle out at the same angle it was inserted.	Minimizes patient discomfort.
f. Apply gentle pressure at site until no fluid leaks out of skin.	Dressing adheres to site if skin remains dry.
g. Apply small sterile gauze dressing or adhesive bandage to site.	Prevents bacterial entry into puncture site.
11. Dispose of uncapped needles and syringe in puncture-proof and leak-proof container.	Prevents accidental needlestick injuries and follows CDC guidelines for disposal of sharps (OSHA, 2012).
12. See Completion Protocol (inside front cover).	

▌EVALUATION

1. Evaluate patient's response to medication.
2. Assess site at least every 4 hours for redness, pain, drainage, or swelling.
3. Use *Teach Back:* State to the patient, "I want to be sure you understand your continuous infusion into the skin and the medication you receive. Can you tell me why you have a continuous infusion to receive your medication?" Evaluates what the patient is able to explain or demonstrate. Revise your instruction now or develop plan for revised patient teaching to be implemented at an appropriate time if patient is not able to teach back correctly.

Unexpected Outcomes and Related Interventions

1. Patient complains of localized pain or burning at insertion site of needle or site appears red or swollen or is leaking, indicating potential infection or needle dislodgment.
   a. Remove needle and place new needle in a different site.
   b. Continue to monitor original site for signs of infection and notify health care provider if you suspect infection.
2. Patient displays signs of allergic reaction to medication.
   a. Stop delivering medication immediately and follow facility policy for appropriate response (e.g., administration of antihistamine or epinephrine) and reporting of adverse drug reactions.
   b. Notify patient's health care provider of adverse effects immediately.
   c. Add allergy information to patient's medical record per facility policy.
3. CSQI becomes dislodged.
   a. Stop the infusion, apply pressure at the site until no fluid leaks out of skin, cover site with a gauze dressing or adhesive bandage, and initiate a new site.
   b. Assess patient to determine effects of not receiving medication (e.g., assess patient's pain level using age-appropriate pain scale, obtain blood glucose level).

Recording and Reporting

- After initiating CSQI, immediately chart medication, dose, infusion rate, route, site, time, date, and type of medication pump in patient's MAR and in nurse's notes. Correctly sign name following facility guidelines.
- If medication is an opioid, follow facility policy to document waste.
- Record patient's response to medication and appearance of site every 4 hours or according to facility policy in nurses' notes.
- Document your evaluation of patient learning.
- Report any adverse effects from medication or infection at insertion site to patient's health care provider and document according to facility policy. Patient's condition often indicates need for additional medical therapy.

Sample Documentation

1400   CSQI initiated with 25-gauge Teflon catheter in RLQ of abdomen. Infusing morphine sulfate at 0.05 mg/hr. Site free from redness and edema. Patient able to teach back why he is receiving medication via the CSQI route.

Special Considerations

Pediatric

- Insulin pumps offer flexibility for adolescents, placing the responsibility of diabetes management on the child.

Extensive child and family education is needed in using CSQI (Hockenberry and Wilson, 2013).
- Clean and rotate sites in children every 48 to 72 hours or at the first sign of inflammation (Hockenberry and Wilson, 2013).

Geriatric

- Hypodermoclysis is an easy-to-use, safe, and cost-effective alternative to IV hydration for older adults (Scales, 2011).

Home Care

- Patients in the home using CSQI need a responsible family caregiver if available. Educate the patient or family caregiver about the desired effect of the medication, side effects and adverse effects of the medication, operation of the pump, how to evaluate the effectiveness of the medication, when and how to assess and rotate insertion sites, and when to call a health care provider for problems. Patients need to know where and how to obtain and dispose of all required supplies.
- Patients managing CSQI at home may use an antibacterial soap (e.g., Hibiclens, pHisoHex) instead of alcohol and chlorhexidine to cleanse insertion site.

CRITICAL THINKING EXERCISES

Case Study

The nurse is developing a plan of care for a patient with thrombophlebitis of the left leg who is scheduled to receive heparin 5000 units subcutaneously on admission to the unit and every 8 hours thereafter. The heparin comes prepared from the pharmacy in a single-dose vial.

1. What information does the nurse need to know about the medication and the vial before administration?
2. What information does the nurse need to know about the patient before administration of the heparin?
3. What is the preferred site for this patient's heparin injection, and what is the primary difference between a vial and ampule when preparing a dose?

Review Questions

1. The nurse is to administer morphine sulfate 1 mg IV push every 8 hours as needed for pain. What does the nurse need to assess before administering the morphine? Select all that apply.
   1. The compatibility of the morphine with what is running in the existing line
   2. The IV rate per hour of administration
   3. The level of the patient's pain
   4. The condition of the IV site

2. The nurse is mixing two medications in one syringe, one from a vial and one from an ampule. What is the first step to prepare the medication?
   1. Check the volume of medication in syringe.
   2. Draw up medication from the ampule first.
   3. Shake the medication in the vial to ensure that there is no cloudiness.
   4. Draw up the medication from the vial first.

3. Which assessment finding indicates a positive tuberculin reaction in a patient with no known risk factors for TB?
   1. A large area of redness and swelling at the injection site
   2. An induration of 18 mm
   3. Frequent, productive cough accompanied by fever
   4. Sudden onset of shortness of breath and wheezing

4. Which symptoms may indicate that a patient has sustained an injury to a nerve after an IM injection?
   1. Pain, numbness, and tingling at the injection site 2 hours after the injection
   2. Pain experienced during the injection
   3. Urticaria, eczema, wheezing, and dyspnea
   4. Nausea, vomiting, and diarrhea

5. Match the needle size to use when administering an injection in each situation listed.
   1. 25-gauge, 1-inch _______
   2. 22-gauge, 1½ inch _______
   3. 27-gauge, ⅝ inch _______

   a. Intradermal Mantoux test
   b. Child older than 1 year receiving IM immunization
   c. Average-size woman receiving IM injection

6. A patient is to receive a subcutaneous injection of heparin. The patient is 5 feet, 2 inches tall and weighs 61 kg (135 pounds). The nurse plans to administer the injection in the abdomen. The most appropriate needle size to use for this injection is:
   1. 18 gauge, 1¼ inch
   2. 20 gauge, 1 inch
   3. 22 gauge, 1½ inch
   4. 25 gauge, ⅝ inch

7. The nurse needs to reconstitute a medication for a subcutaneous injection. Which action would indicate the procedure is completed correctly?
   1. The nurse shakes the vial after the fluid is injected into the vial to mix it completely.
   2. The nurse determines the amount of prepared medication and concentration before adding the appropriate diluent.
   3. The powder is injected into the vial of diluent.
   4. The nurse evaluates the concentration after the diluent and powder are mixed.

8. When assessing a patient's IV site before giving an IV push medication, the nurse notes that the site is cool, pale, and swollen. What should the nurse do?
   1. Stop the IV infusion and change it to another site.
   2. Slow the rate of the IV infusion.
   3. Flush the IV line with a normal saline flush.
   4. Take off the IV dressing and place a new one on that is not as tight.

9. What is the most important action for the nurse to implement before giving a medication via IV push?
   1. Assess the IV insertion site.
   2. Stop the primary (maintenance) fluid infusion.
   3. Dilute the medication to minimize vein irritation.
   4. Ensure that the correct filter needle is used to withdraw the medication from the vial.

10. Place the steps for administering an ID injection in the correct order.
    1. With the needle almost against patient's skin, insert it slowly at a 5- to 15-degree angle.
    2. Withdraw needle and apply gauze gently over site.
    3. Hold syringe between thumb and forefinger of dominant hand with bevel up.
    4. Inject medication slowly.
    5. Note a small bleb resembling a mosquito bite.
    6. Advance needle through epidermis to approximately 3 mm (⅛ inch) below skin surface.
    7. With nondominant hand, stretch skin over site with forefinger and thumb.

REFERENCES

Alexander M, et al: *Core curriculum for infusion nursing*, ed 4, Philadelphia, 2014, Lippincott Williams & Wilkins.

American Diabetes Association (ADA): *Insulin storage and syringe safety*, 2014. http://www.diabetes.org/living-with-diabetes/treatment-and-care/medication/insulin/insulin-storage-and-syringe-safety.html. Accessed August 14, 2014.

American Nurses Association (ANA): *Sharps safety: recommendations for progress*, Washington, DC, 2013, ANA. Available at: http://nursingworld.org/MainMenuCategories/WorkplaceSafety/Healthy-Work-Environment/SafeNeedles/SharpsSafety.

Black L: Ditch the pinch: bilateral exposure injuries during subcutaneous injection, *Am J Infect Control* 41(9):815, 2013.

Buchko B, et al: Improving care of patients with insulin pumps during hospitalization: translating the evidence, *J Nurs Care Qual* 27(4):333, 2012.

Carchidi C, et al: Clinical effectiveness and cost-effectiveness of continuous subcutaneous insulin infusion for diabetes: systematic review and economic evaluation, *Am J Matern Child Nurs* 36(1):32, 2011.

Centers for Disease Control and Prevention (CDC): *Administering vaccines: dose, route, site, and needle size*, 2012a. http://www.immunize.org/catg.d/p3085.pdf. Accessed August 20, 2014.

Centers for Disease Control and Prevention (CDC): *Diagnosis of tuberculosis disease*, 2012b. http://www.cdc.gov/tb/publications/factsheets/testing/diagnosis.htm. Accessed July 21, 2013.

Crawford C, Johnson J: To aspirate or not: an integrative review of the evidence, *Nursing* 42(3):20, 2012.

Davidson KM, Rourke L: Teaching best-evidence: deltoid intramuscular injection technique, *J Nurs Educ Pract* 3(7):121, 2013.

Department of Health and Human Services, Centers for Medicare & Medicaid Services (DHHS): *Updated guidance on medication administration, Hospital Appendix A of State Operations Manual*, Baltimore, 2011, Department of Health and Human Services.

Dychter S, Gold D, Haller M: Subcutaneous drug delivery, *J Infus Nurs* 35(3):155, 2012.

Freeman R, Lee-Lehner B, Pesenecker J: Reducing interruptions to improve medication safety, *J Nurs Care Qual* 28(2):176, 2013.

Gibney M, et al: Skin and subcutaneous adipose layer thickness in adults with diabetes at sites used for insulin injections: implications for needle length recommendation, *Curr Med Res Opin* 26(6):1520, 2010.

Giger J: *Transcultural nursing: assessment and intervention*, ed 6, St Louis, 2013, Mosby.

Hadaway L: Needlestick injuries, short peripheral catheters, and health care worker risks, *J Infus Nurs* 35(3):165, 2012.

Hockenberry MJ, Wilson D: *Wong's essentials of pediatric nursing*, ed 9, St Louis, 2013, Mosby.

Infusion Nurses Society (INS): Infusion nursing standards of practice, *J Infus Nurs* 34(1 Suppl):S1, 2011.

Institute for Safe Medication Practices (ISMP): *Principles of designing a medication label for injectable syringes for patient specific, inpatient use*, 2010. http://www.ismp.org/Tools/guidelines/labelFormats/Injectable.asp. Accessed August 14, 2014.

Institute for Safe Medication Practices (ISMP): *Root causes: a roadmap to actions*, 2011a. http://www.psqh.com/marchapril-2011/798-ismp.html. Accessed July 20, 2013.

Institute for Safe Medication Practices (ISMP): *Acute care guidelines for timely administration of scheduled medications*, 2011b. http://www.ismp.org/tools/guidelines/acutecare/tasm.pdf. Accessed July 20, 2013.

Institute for Safe Medication Practices (ISMP): *ISMP list of high-alert medications in acute care settings*, 2014. http://www.ismp.org/Tools/institutionalhighAlert.asp. Accessed August 14, 2014.

Institute for Safe Medication Practices (ISMP): *Side tracks on the safety express. Interruptions lead to errors and unfinished … Wait, what was I doing?* 2012. https://www.ismp.org/Newsletters/acutecare/showarticle.aspx?id=37. Accessed August 17, 2014.

Kuensting L: Subcutaneous infusion of fluid in children, *J Emerg Nurs* 37:346, 2011.

Lehne R: *Pharmacology for nursing*, ed 8, St Louis, 2013, Elsevier.

Manrique-Rodriguez S, et al: Development of a compatibility chart for intravenous Y-site drug administration in a pediatric intensive care unit, *J Infus Nurs* 35(2):109, 2012.

Medtronic MiniMed: *MiniMed Paradigm REAL-Time Insulin Pump and Continuous Glucose Monitoring System*, 2013. http://www.medtronicdiabetes.com/products/paradigmrevelpump. Accessed July 22, 2013.

Mitchell V, Porter K, Beatty S: Administration technique and storage of disposable insulin pens reported by patients with diabetes, *Diabetes Educ* 38(5):651, 2012.

Ng C, et al: *Ethno-psychopharmacology: advances in current practice*, New York, 2013, Cambridge University Press.

Occupational Safety and Health Administration (OSHA): *Bloodborne pathogens and needlestick injuries, 77 FR 19934*, 2012. https://www.osha.gov/FedReg_osha_pdf/FED20120403.pdf. Accessed July 2013.

Oldenmenger W, et al: Efficacy of opioid rotation to continuous parenteral hydromorphone in advanced cancer patients failing on other opioids, *Support Care Cancer* 20(8):1639, 2012.

Pourghaznein T, Azimi A, Jafarabadi M: The effect of injection duration and injection site on pain and bruising of subcutaneous injection of heparin, *J Clin Nurs* 23(7–8):1105, 2014.

Riley D, Ramp G: Impact of subcutaneous injection device on improving patient care, *Nurs Manage* 41(6):49, 2010.

Scales K: Use of hypodermoclysis to manage dehydration, *Nurs Older People* 23(5):16, 2011.

Silva H: Ethnopsychopharmacology and pharmacogenomics, *Adv Psychosom Med* 33:88, 2013.

The Joint Commission (TJC): *National Patient Safety Goals*, Oakbrook Terrace, IL, 2014, The Commission. Available at: http://www.jointcommission.org/standards_information/npsgs.aspx.

Touhy TA, Jett KF: *Ebersole and Hess' gerontological nursing & healthy aging*, ed 4, St Louis, 2014, Mosby.

Tzeng H, Yin C, Schneider T: Medication error-related issues in nursing practice, *Medsurg Nurs* 22(1):14, 2013.

Walker J, et al: Evidence-based practice guidelines: a survey of subcutaneous dexamethasone administration, *Int J Palliat Nurs* 16(10):494, 2010.

Walters M, Furyk J: Paediatric intramuscular injections for developing world settings: a review of the literature for best practices, *J Transcult Nurs* 23(4):406, 2012.

Zimmermann PG: Revisiting IM injections, *Am J Nurs* 110(2):60, 2010.

CHAPTER 24

Wound Care and Irrigation

Proper wound care promotes wound healing that results in an intact skin layer (Fig. 24-1). Nurses play a vital role in wound care management. Wound healing is extremely complex, involving a series of physiological processes among cells and tissues. The location, severity, and extent of an injury and the tissue layers involved all affect the wound healing process (Doughty and Sparks-Defriese, 2012). Like-wise, the rate of healing depends on numerous internal and external factors (Box 24-1). Effective wound management requires you to understand the processes of wound healing, the factors that interfere with healing, and how to perform a comprehensive wound assessment. Assessment of a wound provides you with information needed to recognize changes in a wound so that you can institute appropriate wound care measures. The wound assessment is the foundation for the wound plan of care and helps to determine wound healing progress or deterioration.

A partial-thickness wound (loss of the epidermis and superficial dermal layers) heals by regeneration. However, a full-thickness wound (total loss of epidermis and dermis and in some cases as deep as the muscle layer or bone) heals by scar formation. In a full-thickness wound, healing occurs in four phases (Box 24-2). Collagen deposition begins during inflammation and peaks during proliferation. It is important for nurses to assess for the presence of this new tissue, called the "healing ridge" (Fig. 24-2). This "healing ridge" is composed of newly formed collagen, and you can usually feel it

along the edges of an intact suture line by days 5 to 9 (Doughty and Sparks-Defriese, 2012). Types of healing are primary, secondary, and tertiary intention (Fig. 24-3). Healing by primary intention occurs when the wound edges of a clean surgical incision remain close together. Wounds left open and allowed to heal by scar formation are classified as healing by secondary intention. Healing by tertiary intention is often called delayed primary intention. It occurs when surgical wounds are not closed immediately but left open for 3 to 5 days to allow edema or infection to diminish. The wound edges are then stapled or sutured closed. The type of wound and the manner in which it heals dictate the types of treatment and wound support required.

PATIENT-CENTERED CARE

Wound assessment is the first essential step in planning care for a patient with a wound. Discuss with the patient and family the importance of a thorough and periodic wound assessment so that they understand the need for this procedure. It is important for them to understand that wounds heal in an organized fashion and that the ongoing assessments aid in determining wound progress and treatments. Determine what effect the wound may have from the patient's cultural perspective; for example, some cultures believe that the use of herbs or other folk remedies help to support wound healing. It is important to be culturally sensitive to the

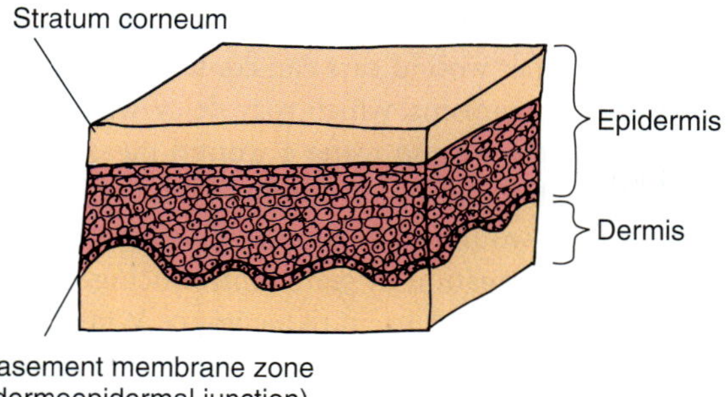

FIG 24-1 Diagram of layers of the skin and subcutaneous tissue.

BOX 24-1 FACTORS THAT INFLUENCE WOUND HEALING

- With increasing age, there is a reduction in collagen deposition, which is thought to contribute to the development of dermal atrophy and poor wound healing (Baranoski et al., 2012a).
- Inadequate nutrition, including proteins, carbohydrates, lipids, vitamins, and minerals, impairs wound healing resulting in severe alterations in healing such as dehiscence (Stotts, 2012).
- Obesity results in a higher risk for incidence of wound complications such as surgical site infection and wound dehiscence. Fat tissue has less vascularization, which decreases transport of nutrients and cellular elements required for healing (Gallagher Camden, 2012).
- A hematocrit value less than 20% and a hemoglobin value less than 10 g/100 mL negatively influence tissue repair because of decreased oxygen delivery. Oxygen release to tissue is reduced in smokers and in patients with peripheral vascular diseases.
- Diabetes causes impaired wound healing from reduced collagen synthesis and deposition, decreased wound strength, and impaired leukocyte (white blood cell) function.
- Wound infection prolongs the inflammatory response, and the microorganisms use nutrients and oxygen that are intended for repair.
- Long-term steroid therapy and chemotherapy or the use of immunosuppressive medications may diminish the inflammatory response and reduce the healing potential.
- An open wound must be maintained in a moist environment, and a closed wound must be protected from microorganisms and stress.

BOX 24-2 PHASES OF WOUND HEALING (FULL-THICKNESS WOUNDS)

Hemostasis

Blood vessels constrict; clotting factors activate coagulation to stop bleeding. Clot formation seals disrupted vessels so that blood loss is controlled and acts as a temporary bacterial barrier. Growth factors are released, which attract cells needed to begin tissue repair.

Inflammatory Phase

Vasodilation occurs, allowing plasma and blood cells to leak into the wound, noted as edema, erythema, and exudate. Leukocytes (white blood cells) arrive in the wound to begin cleanup. Macrophages appear and regulate the wound repair. The purpose of inflammation is to ensure a clean wound bed in a noncomplicated wound.

Proliferative/Rebuilding Phase

New capillaries are created, restoring the delivery of oxygen and nutrients to the wound bed. At the same time, new granulation tissue forms. Collagen is synthesized and begins to provide strength and structural integrity to a wound. Contraction reduces the size of the wound. Epithelial resurfacing (construction of new epidermis) begins to cover the wound.

Maturation/Remodeling Phase

Collagen is remodeled to become stronger and provide tensile strength to the wound. Outer appearance in an uncomplicated wound is that of a well-healed scar.

Data from Doughty DB, Sparks-Defriese B: Wound healing physiology. In Bryant RA, Nix DP, editors: *Acute and chronic wounds: current management concepts,* ed 4, St Louis, 2012, Mosby.

---

patient's and family's beliefs; for example, some skin substitutes (used in severe wounds) are pork based and may be unacceptable in some cultures.

As in all clinical situations, approach wound assessment through the "patient's eyes," especially in the case of chronic wounds. Patients with chronic wounds have often seen multiple care providers and have used various therapies to manage their wounds. Become familiar with what they have used in the past, determine whether the therapies that they use are safe, and if the therapies are not safe, explain why.

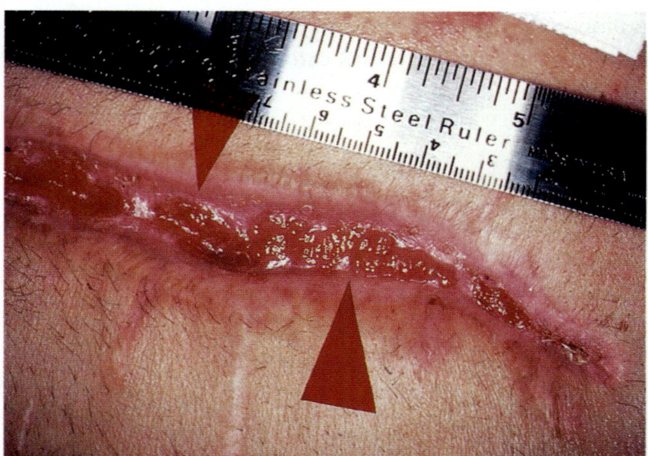

FIG 24-2 Surgical wound with epithelialization occurring, epithelial healing ridge apparent. (From Bryant RA, Nix DP: editors: *Acute and chronic wounds current management concepts,* ed 3, St Louis, 2007, Mosby.)

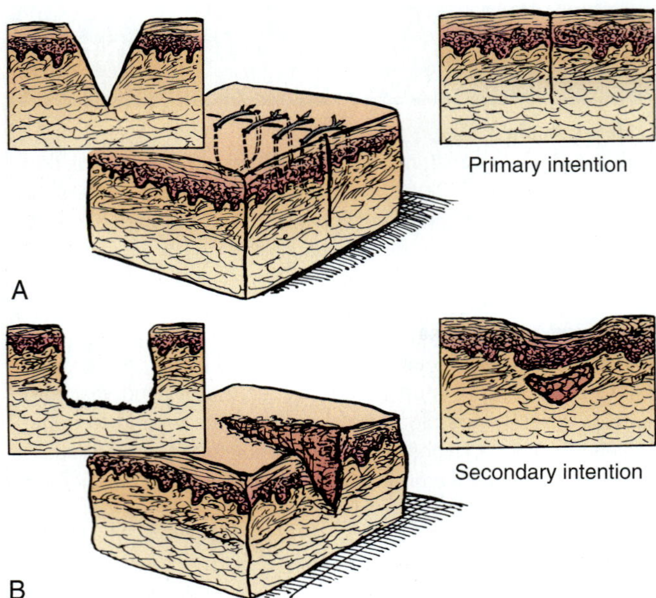

FIG 24-3 A, Wound healing by primary intention, such as with a surgical incision. Wound healing edges are pulled together and approximated with sutures, staples, or adhesive, and healing occurs by connective tissue deposition. **B,** Wound healing by secondary intention. Wound edges are not approximated, and healing occurs by granulation tissue formation and contraction of the wound edges. (Used with permission from Bryant RA, editor: *Acute and chronic wounds: nursing management,* ed 2, St Louis, 2000, Mosby.)

Always value and apply any expertise patients may have in managing their wound.

SAFETY

When you perform a wound assessment, wound irrigation, emptying of a wound collection device, or removal of staples or stitches, safety is a priority. One risk to a patient's safety is the risk for infection. When a wound is present, the patient no longer has the protection of intact skin. When you assess a wound or provide wound care, remember to use proper infection control practices to reduce the risk for a wound infection. Improper wound care can contaminate the wound bed with microorganisms, which may delay wound healing. When measuring a wound using a wound measuring guide or cotton-tipped applicator, gently insert the guide over the perimeter of the wound so as not to cause any tissue injury. Perform wound irrigation by gently introducing the ordered fluid into the wound to prevent tissue injury. When removing staples or stitches, use the correct instruments to prevent trauma to the newly healed incision.

EVIDENCE-BASED PRACTICE

Institute for Healthcare Improvement: *How to prevent surgical site infection,* 2012, http://www.ihi.org/resources/Pages/Tools/HowtoGuidePreventSurgicalSiteInfection.aspx. Accessed August 25, 2014.

Institute for Healthcare Improvement (IHI): *Surgical site infection,* 2014, http://www.ihi.org/topics/ssi/pages/default.aspx. Accessed August 25, 2014.

It has been found that the use of razors before surgery increases the incidence of wound infection compared with clipping, depilatory use, or no hair removal at all (IHI, 2012). Razors have been shown to cause small skin cuts that may not be visible to the human eye. These small cuts serve as a portal for skin bacteria to enter the skin and contribute to a surgical site infection. Hair removal has been a carryover technique with little evidence to support the procedure and may be unnecessary for many procedures. When hair must be removed to perform the procedure safely, use of a razor should be avoided. It is preferable to use clippers rather than shaving with a razor because this results in fewer surgical site infections (IHI, 2014).

Evidence-based interventions for hair removal before surgery or when providing wound care include:

- Discontinue the use of razors in the operating room and in the entire facility.
- Use clippers for hair removal and train staff members in proper use.
- Educate patients not to shave preoperatively or when doing wound care.

- **Nursing Skills Online: Wound Care Module, Lesson 1**

Wound assessment is the collection of data that characterizes the status of a wound and the periwound skin to determine the phase of healing (Nix, 2012). This information is used to continue the plan of care or alter the type of intervention (e.g., type and frequency of dressing; use of adjunct wound therapies, such as appropriate nutrition and antibiotics; or interventions such as débridement, a pressure redistribution device, or a surgical referral). The frequency of wound assessment depends on the condition of the wound as well as the standards of practice within the patient's health care setting.

Acute care settings generally require assessment daily or with each dressing change. Long-term care facilities may require an initial admission assessment and a weekly assessment for a chronic wound. Home care assessments depend on the frequency of visits. The type of wound assessment tool used by staff members depends on the facility. Regardless of the setting, determine the frequency of wound assessment by the wound characteristics observed at the previous

PROCEDURAL GUIDELINE 24.1
Performing a Wound Assessment—cont'd

dressing change, facility protocols, and the health care provider's orders. The effectiveness of interventions cannot be determined unless baseline assessment data are compared with follow-up data (Baranoski et al., 2012b).

Delegation and Collaboration

The skill of wound assessment cannot be delegated to nursing assistive personnel (NAP). The nurse instructs the NAP to:

- Report any drainage outside of the wound dressing to the nurse for further assessment.
- Report any dressing that is no longer adherent.
- Report the presence of odor in the area of the wound.

Equipment

- Protective equipment: clean gloves, gown, and goggles if splash or spray risk exists
- Facility tool to document assessment: measuring guide
- Cotton-tipped applicator
- Dressing supplies (as ordered)
- Disposable biohazard bag

Procedural Steps

1. **See Standard Protocol (inside front cover).**
2. Identify patient using two identifiers (e.g., name and birthday or name and account number) according to facility policy.
3. Examine the medical record for the last wound assessment to use as a comparison for this wound assessment. Also, review the record to determine the etiology of the wound.
4. Assess comfort level or pain on a scale of 0 to 10.
5. Apply clean gloves. Remove soiled dressings, examine dressings for quality of drainage (color, consistency), presence of odor, and quantity of drainage (note if dressings were saturated, slightly moist, or had no drainage). Discard dressings in waterproof biohazard bag; remove and discard gloves. Perform hand hygiene.
6. Apply clean gloves. Inspect the wound, and determine the type of wound healing (e.g., primary or secondary intention).
7. Use the facility-approved assessment tool and assess the following:
   a. Wound healing by primary intention (surgical wound):
      (1) Assess the anatomical location of the wound on the body.
      (2) Note if the incisional wound margins are approximated (closed together). The wound edges should be together with no gaps.
      (3) Observe for the presence of drainage. A closed incision should not have any drainage.

(4) Look for evidence of infection (presence of erythema, odor, or wound drainage).

(5) Lightly palpate along the incision to feel a healing ridge (see Fig. 24-2). The ridge is newly formed connective tissue beneath the skin, extending to about 1 cm (½ inch) on each side of the wound 5 to 9 days after the onset of the wound. This is an expected positive sign (Doughty and Sparks-Defriese, 2012).

   b. Wound healing by secondary intention (e.g., pressure ulcer or contaminated surgical or traumatic wound):
      (1) Assess the anatomical location of the wound.
      (2) Assess wound dimensions. Measure the size of the wound, including length, width, and depth, using a centimeter measuring guide. Measure length by placing the measurement tool over the wound at the point of greatest length (or head to toe). Measure width at the point of greatest width (or side to side) (see illustration) (Nix, 2012). Measure depth by inserting a cotton-tipped applicator in the area of greatest depth and placing a mark on the applicator at skin level. Discard the measuring guide and the cotton-tipped applicator in a trash bag.

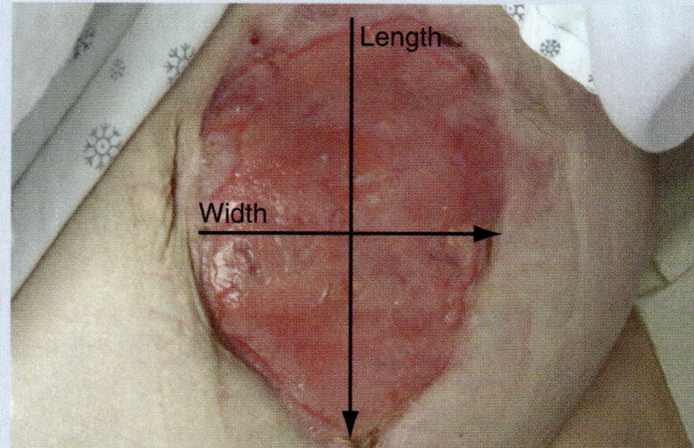

STEP 7b(2) Measuring wound length and width.

      (3) Assess for undermining. Use a cotton-tipped applicator to probe the wound edges gently. Measure the depth, and note the location using the face of the clock as a guide. The 12 o'clock position (top of the wound) would be the head of the patient, and the 6 o'clock position would be the bottom of the wound toward the patient's feet. Document the number of centimeters the area of damage extends from the wound edge (e.g., underneath intact skin).
      (4) Assess the extent of tissue loss. If the wound is a pressure ulcer, determine the deepest viable

Continued

PROCEDURAL GUIDELINE 24.1
Performing a Wound Assessment—cont'd

tissue layer in the wound bed and determine the stage. If necrotic tissue does not allow visualization of the base of the wound, the stage cannot be determined. If the wound is not a pressure ulcer determine if there is partial-thickness loss (epidermis and part of the dermis) or full-thickness loss (loss of both the epidermis and the dermis). If it is a pressure ulcer, use the staging system of the European Pressure Ulcer Advisory Panel (EPUAP) and the National Pressure Ulcer Advisory Panel (NPUAP) (EPUAP and NPUAP, 2009).

(5) Note the tissue type including the percentage of granulation, slough, and necrotic tissue present in the wound.

(6) Note the presence of exudate—amount, color, consistency, and odor. Indicate amount of exudate by using part of dressing saturated or in terms of quantity (e.g., scant, moderate, or copious).

(7) Note if wound edges are rounded toward the wound bed; this may be an indication of delayed wound healing. Describe the presence of epithelialization at wound edges (if present) because this indicates healing.

(8) Inspect the periwound skin, including color, texture, and temperature, and describe skin integrity (e.g., open macerated areas). Periwound assessment provides clues about the effectiveness of wound treatment and possible wound extension (Nix, 2012).

8. Reapply dressing per order. Place time, date, and initials on the new dressing. Discard gloves and perform hand hygiene.

9. Reassess level of comfort or pain using a scale of 0 to 10 after dressing is reapplied.

10. **See Completion Protocol (inside front cover).**

11. Record wound assessment findings, and compare assessment with previous wound assessments to monitor wound healing.

SKILL 24.1   PERFORMING A WOUND IRRIGATION

Wound irrigation cleanses and irrigates surgical wounds or chronic wounds such as pressure ulcers by removing debris from a wound surface, decreasing bacterial counts, and loosening and removing necrotic tissue (Smith et al., 2013; Ramundo, 2012). The cleansing solution is introduced directly into the wound with a syringe, a syringe and catheter, or a pulsed lavage device. If a patient has a deep wound with a narrow opening, attach a soft catheter (a rubber catheter that is flexible and can easily be introduced into the wound without causing trauma) to the syringe to permit the fluid to enter the wound. Irrigation should not cause tissue injury or discomfort. Avoid fluid retention in the wound by positioning a patient on the side to encourage the flow of the irrigant away from the wound. Use a 35-mL syringe with a 19-gauge angiocatheter to facilitate optimal pressure for cleansing with minimal risk for tissue injury (Ramundo, 2012). Pulsatile high-pressure lavage is an alternative to using the 35-mL syringe and the 19-gauge angiocatheter. A pulsatile lavage machine combines intermittent high-pressure lavage with suction to loosen necrotic tissue and facilitate its removal by other methods of débridement (Ramundo, 2012).

Solutions used for irrigations include normal saline, warm water, and commercially available wound cleansers. Typically, you use sterile technique for cleansing and irrigating surgical wounds and clean technique for certain chronic wounds,

such as a pressure ulcer that has not shown evidence of healing over a 2-week period.

▌ASSESSMENT

1. Identify patient using two identifiers (e.g., name and birthday or name and account number) according to facility policy. *Rationale: Ensures correct patient. Complies with The Joint Commission standards and improves patient safety (TJC, 2014).*

2. Review health care provider's order for wound irrigation, noting the type and amount of fluid and irrigation device. *Rationale: Open wound irrigation requires medical order, including the type of solution to use.*

3. Assess patient's level of comfort on a scale of 0 to 10. If patient is uncomfortable, offer an analgesic at least 30 minutes before removal. *Rationale: Provides baseline to determine tolerance to procedure.*

4. Examine recent documented assessment of patient's wound. *Rationale: Provides basis for comparing assessment findings with baseline to determine progress toward healing.*

5. Apply clean gloves. Perform wound assessment (see Procedural Guideline 24.1). Keep wound uncovered or apply a single layer of gauze over wound.

6. Assess patient for history of allergies to antiseptics, medications, tapes, or dressing materials. *Rationale: Known*

allergies suggest application of a sample of prescribed wound treatment as skin test before flushing wound with large volume of solution.

PLANNING

Expected Outcomes focus on promoting wound healing.
1. Patient states acceptable level of comfort on pain scale of 0 to 10 during and after wound irrigation.
2. Wound is free of excessive drainage, exudate, and inflammation.
3. Skin integrity is maintained; no redness, edema, or inflammation is noted in surrounding tissue.

Delegation and Collaboration
The skill of sterile wound irrigation cannot be delegated to nursing assistive personnel (NAP). However, the cleansing of chronic wounds using clean technique can be delegated. It is the nurse's responsibility to assess and document wound characteristics. The nurse instructs the NAP to:

- Report observations when a wound is cleansed (e.g., wound color, presence of bleeding, drainage).
- Report patient pain.

Equipment
- Irrigation/cleansing solution per order (volume 1.5 to 2 times the estimated wound volume)
- Irrigation delivery system (per order), depending on amount of desired pressure: sterile irrigation 35-mL syringe with sterile soft angiocatheter or 19-gauge needle (WOCN, 2010) or handheld shower.
- Protective equipment: sterile gloves, gown, and goggles if splash or spray risk exists
- Waterproof underpad if needed
- Dressing supplies
- Disposable waterproof biohazard bag
- Wound assessment supplies (see Procedural Guideline 24.1)

IMPLEMENTATION *for* PERFORMING A WOUND IRRIGATION

STEPS	RATIONALE
1. **See Standard Protocol (inside front cover).**	
2. Explain procedure to patient and family.	Decreases patient anxiety and teaches the patient and family the correct procedure.
3. Position patient comfortably with wound vertical to collection basin to permit gravitational flow of irrigating solution over wound and into collection receptacle. Remove layer of gauze (if present).	Directing solution from top to bottom of wound and from clean to contaminated area prevents further infection.
4. Place underpad under area where irrigation will take place. Then remove clean gloves.	Prevents bed linen from becoming wet.
5. Perform hand hygiene. Apply gown and goggles. **Apply sterile gloves** for Steps 6 and 7, and use sterile precautions.	Reduces transmission of microorganisms. Protects from splashes or sprays of body fluids.

6. Irrigate wound with wide opening:
  a. Fill 35-mL syringe with irrigation solution.
  b. Attach 19-gauge angiocatheter.
	Wound irrigation facilitates wound healing.
	
	Catheter lumen delivers ideal pressure for cleansing and removal of debris (Ramundo, 2012).

c. Hold angiocatheter tip 2.5 cm (1 inch) above upper end of wound and over area to be cleansed.	Prevents syringe contamination. Careful placement of syringe prevents unsafe pressure of flowing solution.
d. Using continuous pressure, flush wound; repeat Steps 6a to 6c until prescribed solution is used.	Flushing wound helps to remove debris; clear solution indicates removal of all debris.
7. Irrigate deep wound with a very small opening: a. Attach soft catheter, such as a rubber straight catheter, to filled irrigation syringe.	Catheter permits direct flow of irrigant into wound. Expect wound to take longer to empty when opening is small.
b. Gently insert tip of catheter into opening of wound, about 1.3 cm (0.5 inch).	Prevents tip from touching fragile inner wall of wound.

SAFE PATIENT CARE Do not force catheter into the wound because this causes tissue damage.

Continued

STEPS	RATIONALE

c. Using slow, continuous pressure, flush wound.

Use of slow mechanical force of a stream of solution loosens particulate matter on the wound surface and promotes healing (Ramundo, 2012).

> **SAFE PATIENT CARE** Pulsatile high-pressure lavage is often the irrigation of choice for necrotic wounds. Pressure settings should be set per provider order, usually between 4 and 15 psi, and should not be used on skin grafts, exposed blood vessels, muscle, tendon, or bone. Use with caution if patient has coagulation disorder or is taking anticoagulants (Ramundo, 2012).

d. Remove and refill syringe. Reconnect to catheter, and repeat until prescribed solution is used.

8. Cleanse wound with a handheld shower:

a. Apply clean gloves. With patient seated comfortably in shower chair, adjust spray to gentle flow; make sure that water is warm.

Helps patients shower with assistance or independently. May be accomplished at home.

b. Shower for 5 to 10 minutes with shower head 30 cm (12 inches) away from wound.

Ensure that wound is cleansed thoroughly.

9. When indicated, obtain wound cultures after cleansing with nonbacteriostatic solution (see Skill 8.5).

Documents presence or absence of pathogens in the wound.

10. Dry wound edges with gauze; dry patient after shower.

Prevents maceration of surrounding tissue from excess moisture.

11. Apply dressing per health care provider's order, and label with date, time, and nurse's initials.

Maintains protective barrier and healing environment for wound. Indicates time of most recent dressing change.

12. Assist patient to comfortable position.

13. **See Completion Protocol (inside front cover).**

EVALUATION

1. Have patient rate level of comfort on a scale of 0 to 10.
2. Monitor type of tissue in wound bed and presence of drainage and inflammation. This assessment can identify where the wound is in the wound healing trajectory and helps determine the best dressing.
3. Use *Teach Back:* State to the patient, "I want to be sure I clearly explained how to use a handheld shower to clean your wound. Can you describe for me now how to do wound cleaning?" Evaluates what the patient is able to explain or demonstrate. Revise your instruction now or develop plan for revised patient teaching to be implemented at an appropriate time if patient is not able to teach back correctly.

Unexpected Outcomes and Related Interventions

1. Bleeding or serosanguineous drainage appears.
   a. Flush wound during next irrigation using less pressure.
   b. Notify health care provider of bleeding.
2. Patient reports increased pain or discomfort during irrigation.
   a. Decrease force of pressure during wound irrigation.
   b. Assess patient for need for additional analgesia before wound care.

Recording and Reporting

- Record wound assessment before and after irrigation, amount and type of solution used, irrigation device used, patient tolerance of the procedure, and type of dressing applied after irrigation.
- Document your evaluation of patient learning.
- Immediately report to attending health care provider any evidence of fresh bleeding, sharp increase in pain, retention of irrigant, or signs of shock.

Sample Documentation

0900   Patient rates abdominal wound pain as 3 on a scale of 0 to 10. Abdominal wound 5 cm (2 inches) × 15.2 cm (6 inches) with 1.2 cm (0.5 inches) of depth, wound base completely covered with granulation tissue, minimal serous drainage. Wound irrigated with 150 mL of NS, using irrigating syringe. Irrigant clear at end of procedure. Wound lightly packed with moist sterile gauze and covered with one abdominal dressing. Patient had no complaints; rates abdominal wound pain as 3 postprocedure.

Special Considerations
Pediatric

- Some children may become frightened and may either verbally or physically attempt to prevent the wound irrigation. Describing the wound irrigation using a doll may help to alleviate the fear. When possible, include parents in procedure.

- Neonatal skin is immature and easily damaged from pressure irrigation. Check that products are approved for this patient population.

Geriatric

- Wound irrigation can be frightening for older adults with cognitive impairment and in some cases painful. Assess patient's cooperation before irrigating the wound.
- A 20% loss in dermal thickness occurs with aging. The skin is less resilient, and wound irrigation can easily result in skin tears and other trauma (Baranoski et al., 2012a).

Home Care

- Assess patient's home environment to determine adequacy of facilities for performing wound care; check especially for adequate lighting, running water, and storage of supplies.
- Provide support for patient and caregiver during the wound-healing process. Chronic wounds do not heal properly and do not close in a timely manner (Doughty and Sparks-Defriese, 2012).

SKILL 24.2 MANAGING WOUND DRAINAGE EVACUATION

When wound drainage accumulates in a wound bed, it interferes with wound healing. Wound drainage is facilitated when the surgeon inserts a drain directly through the suture line into the wound or through a small stab wound near the surgical site. Jackson-Pratt and Hemovac drains are portable drainage self-contained suction devices that are connected to a drainage tube within the wound and provide constant low-pressure suction to remove and collect drainage. A Jackson-Pratt drain (Fig. 24-4) is used for small amounts of drainage (100 to 200 mL per 24 hours). A Hemovac or ConstaVac drainage system is used for larger amounts of drainage (500 mL per 24 hours). When a drainage device is more than half full, it should be emptied, and the volume of the exudate measured. After measurement reset the suction on the drainage device and verify that the drainage tubes exiting the wound are patent. If the patient has more than one drain, number each to report drainage amount accurately.

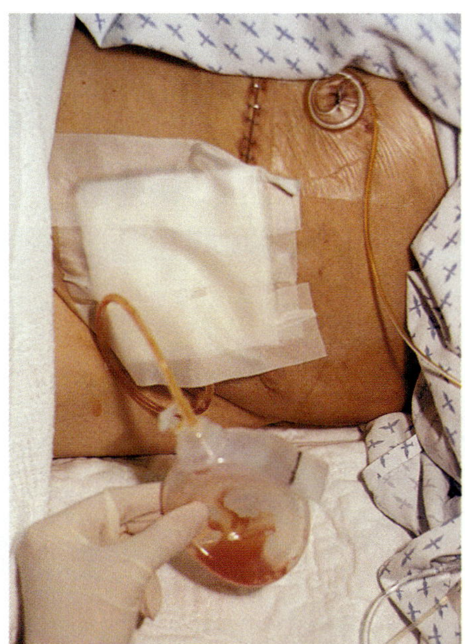

FIG 24-4 Jackson-Pratt drainage tube and reservoir.

▌ASSESSMENT

1. Identify patient using two identifiers (e.g., name and birthday or name and account number) according to facility policy. *Rationale: Ensures correct patient. Complies with The Joint Commission standards and improves patient safety (TJC, 2014).*
2. Identify the number and type of drainage systems present when patient returns from surgery or from interventional radiology. *Rationale: Awareness of drain placement is needed to plan and identify type and quantity of dressing supplies required.*
3. Perform wound assessment, wearing clean gloves (see Procedural Guideline 24.1). *Rationale: Provides baseline to determine progress of wound healing.*
4. Inspect drainage system to verify proper functioning. Observe drainage tube for patency by observing drainage movement through tubing in direction of the reservoir, patency of drainage tubing, airtight connection sites, and the presence of any leaks or kinks in the system. Ensure that there is no pulling on the tubing. Confirm that the tube is secure. Remove gloves and perform hand hygiene. *Rationale: Properly functioning system maintains suction until reservoir is filled or drainage is no longer being produced or accumulated. Tension on drainage tubing causes injury to underlying tissue or skin.*

▌PLANNING

Expected Outcomes focus on promoting wound healing and comfort and preventing infection.

1. Quantity and appearance of wound drainage remain within expected guidelines based on type of surgery or involved area.
2. Vacuum is reestablished.
3. Patient reports less pain than initially assessed (scale of 0 to 10).

Delegation and Collaboration

Assessment of wound drains and drainage systems cannot be delegated to nursing assistive personnel (NAP). However, the skill of emptying a closed drainage container, measuring the amount of drainage, and reporting the amount on the patient's intake and output (I&O) record may be delegated. The nurse instructs the NAP to:

- Report to the nurse the appearance of drain contents and amount, odor of drainage, and patient's report of discomfort at drain site.
- Increase the frequency of emptying the drain other than once a shift.

Equipment

- Graduated measuring cylinder
- Alcohol wipes
- Split gauze sponges (for drain site)
- Dressing materials (for surgical incision)
- Nonallergenic tape
- Clean gloves
- Safety pin(s)
- Protective equipment: goggles, mask, and gown if risk of spray from drain is present
- Disposable drape or barrier
- *Option:* Normal saline for cleansing tube insertion site

IMPLEMENTATION *for* MANAGING WOUND DRAINAGE EVACUATION

STEPS	RATIONALE
1. **See Standard Protocol (inside front cover).**	
2. Apply clean gloves. Place measuring container on bed between you and patient.	Reduces transmission of microorganisms.
3. *Empty Hemovac or ConstaVac:*	
a. Maintain asepsis while opening plug on port indicated for emptying drainage reservoir. Tilt evacuator in direction of plug. Slowly squeeze the two flat surfaces together, tilting container toward measuring container.	Vacuum is broken, and reservoir pulls air in until chamber is fully expanded. Squeezing empties reservoir of drainage.
b. Drain contents into measuring container (see illustration).	Contents counted as fluid output.
c. Place evacuator on a flat surface and press downward until bottom and top are in contact (see illustration).	Compression of surface of Hemovac recreates vacuum.
d. Holding surfaces together with one hand, use other hand to cleanse port; immediately replace plug.	Cleansing plug reduces transmission of microorganisms.

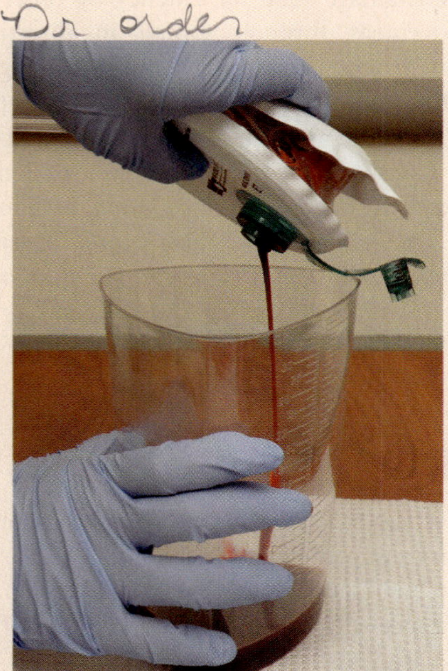

STEP 3b Emptying Hemovac contents into measuring container.

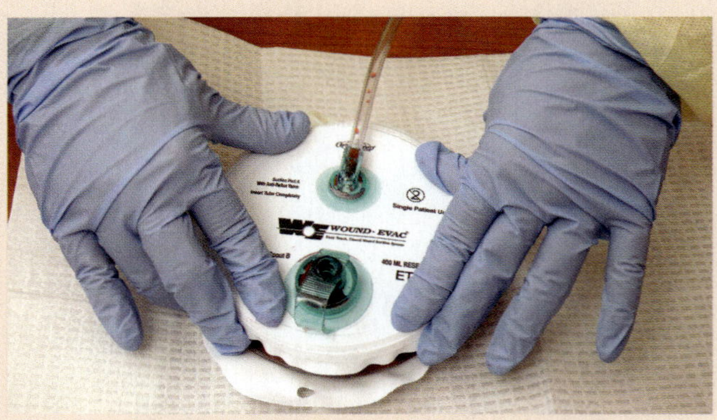

STEP 3c Hemovac suction.

STEPS	**RATIONALE**

   e. Check suction device for reestablishment of vacuum, patency of drainage tubing, and absence of tension on tubing.

Facilitates wound drainage and prevents pressure and trauma to tissues.

4. *Empty Hemovac with wall suction:*

   a. Turn off suction.

   b. Disconnect suction tubing from Hemovac port.

   c. Empty Hemovac as described in Step 3.

   d. Cleanse port opening and end of suction tubing with alcohol wipe; reconnect suction tubing to open port of Hemovac.

Empties drainage and reestablishes suction to wound bed. Cleansing plug reduces transmission of microorganisms.

   e. Set suction level as prescribed or on low if health care provider does not specify suction level.

5. *Empty Jackson-Pratt drain:*

   a. Open port on the end of bulb-shaped reservoir (see illustration).

Breaks vacuum.

   b. Tilt bulb toward direction of port and drain toward opening to empty drainage into measuring container (see illustration). Gently squeeze bulb to empty completely. Cleanse end of emptying port and plug with alcohol wipe.

Reduces transmission of microorganisms into drainage evacuator.

   c. Compress bulb over drainage container. While compressing bulb, replace plug immediately.

Establishes vacuum.

6. Place and secure drainage system below exit site with safety pin to patient's gown.

Pinning system to patient's gown prevents tension or pulling on tubing and insertion site.

> **SAFE PATIENT CARE** Ensure that there is slack in the tubing from the reservoir to the wound, allowing patient movement and no tension at the insertion site.

7. Inspect condition of skin at drain insertion site. (*Option:* Cleanse with gauze and saline [as needed]). Apply new clean split gauze around tube. Secure with tape. Apply new dressing to surgical wound (see Chapter 28).

Drainage is irritating to skin and increases risk of skin breakdown.

8. Note characteristics of drainage; measure volume and discard by flushing in commode. Rinse or discard measuring container.

Contents counted as fluid output.

9. Remind patient to keep drain lower than insertion site when ambulating, sitting, and lying.

Facilitates drainage.

10. **See Completion Protocol (inside front cover).**

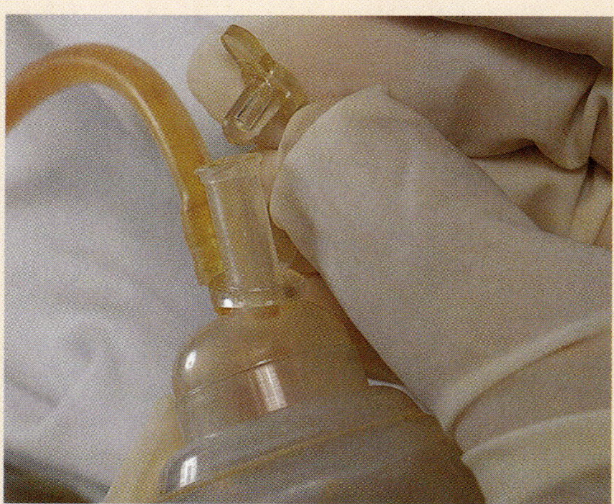

STEP 5a Opening port of Jackson-Pratt drain.

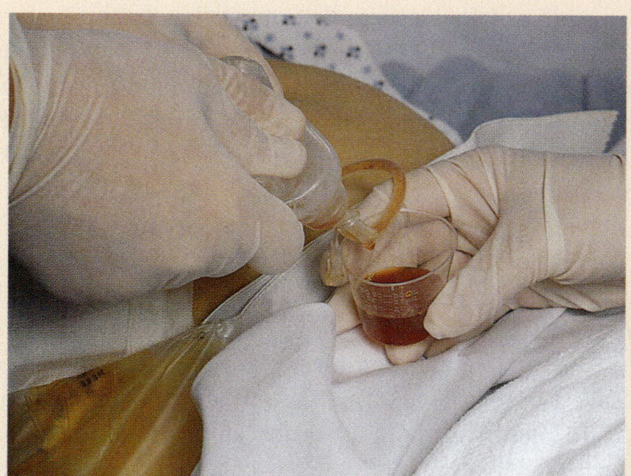

STEP 5b Emptying contents from Jackson-Pratt drainage device.

Continued

EVALUATION

1. Compare amount and characteristics of drainage with what is expected to determine patency of tubing and functioning of drainage evacuator.
2. Inspect for drainage around tubing, which may indicate lack of vacuum or obstruction of drainage system.
3. Ask patient to describe level of comfort using a scale of 0 to 10 in relation to drain site.
4. Use **Teach Back:** State to the patient, "I want to be sure I explained clearly how to empty the drainage system. Can you tell me how to reestablish the suction after you empty the system?" Evaluates what the patient is able to explain or demonstrate. Revise your instruction now or develop plan for revised patient teaching to be implemented at an appropriate time if patient is not able to teach back correctly.

Unexpected Outcomes and Related Interventions

1. Drainage is not accumulating in drainage system.
   a. Position tubing to enhance gravity flow and eliminate kinks or pressure on tubing.
   b. Check for loss of suction.
2. Excessive amount of bright bloody drainage accumulates over a short time (e.g., 4 hours). Drainage that is bright red in large amounts may indicate hemorrhage.
   a. Report excessive bright red drainage to surgeon.
   b. Confirm with surgeon and keep patient on nothing-by-mouth (NPO) status because it may be necessary for patient to return to surgery for suturing of a bleeding vessel.

Recording and Reporting

- Record results from emptying wound drainage system and dressing change in progress notes and I&O record. Note characteristics of insertion site and drainage. Record patient's level of comfort.
- Report presence of functioning drainage system and emptying frequency at end-of-shift report to oncoming nurse.
- Document your evaluation of patient learning.

Sample Documentation

1800 Skin around tube site is pink. Drain is secure with one suture. 200 mL of dark red drainage emptied from Hemovac. 4 × 4 drain dressing applied around drainage site. No reports of pain or discomfort with procedure.

Special Considerations
Pediatric

- Advise family members to keep drainage container less than one-third full to prevent tugging of drainage collector.
- Because children are very active, be sure to secure drainage device to avoid accidental removal.

Geriatric

- Patients with large amounts of drainage need additional fluid intake to prevent dehydration.
- Measures may need to be taken to prevent a confused patient from pulling out drain.

Home Care

- Instruct how to change dressings around drainage tube. Ask patient or caregiver to record the amount of drainage, and bring the record to the health care provider at the next outpatient visit.

SKILL 24.3 REMOVING SUTURES AND STAPLES

Sutures are used to close a surgical incision both within tissue layers in deep wounds and for the outer skin layer. A patient's history of wound healing, site of incision, tissues involved, and purpose of the sutures determine the closure material selected (Whitney, 2012). Deep sutures are a material that is absorbed or an inert wire that remains indefinitely. Nonabsorbable sutures (sutures that require removal) are available in silk, cotton, Prolene, wire, nylon, and Dacron. Removable skin sutures are interrupted or continuous. Interrupted sutures are separate stitches, each with its own knot (Fig. 24-5, *A*). A continuous suture is one long "thread" that spirals along the entire suture line at evenly spaced intervals. The surface appearance is very similar to a line of interrupted sutures except that each section crossing the incision line does not have a knot (see Fig. 24-5, *B*). Another type of continuous stitch is a blanket continuous suture. This suture spirals along the incision with each turn pulled over to one side. The suture is looped around the thread of the previous stitch before making the next turn in spiral (see Fig. 24-5, *C*). When appearance and minimal scarring are important, very fine Dacron or subcutaneous sutures beneath the skin are used. An obese patient with abdominal surgery may have retention sutures covered with rubber tubing to provide greater strength (see Fig. 24-5, *D*).

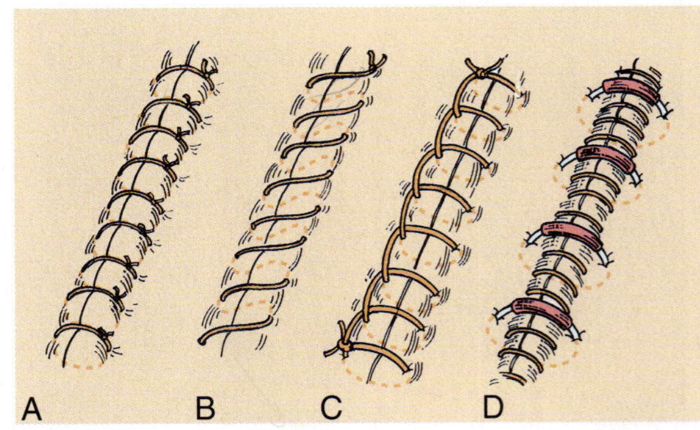

FIG 24-5 Sutures. **A,** Interrupted. **B,** Continuous. **C,** Blanket continuous. **D,** Retention.

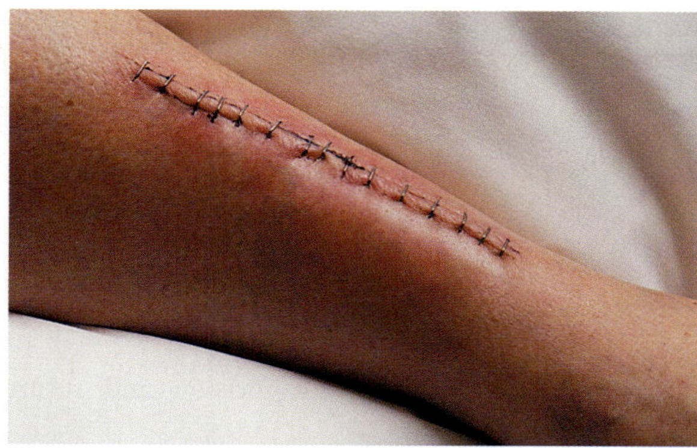

FIG 24-6 Suture line secured with staples.

Staples are made of stainless steel, are quick to use, and provide ample strength. They are used for skin closure of abdominal incisions and orthopedic surgery when appearance of the incision is not critical (Fig. 24-6). The time of removal is based on the stage of incisional healing and extent of surgery.

Facility policy determines which health care providers may remove sutures and staples. Sutures and staples generally are removed within 7 to 10 days after surgery if healing is adequate. Retention sutures are left in place longer (≥14 days). Timing the removal of sutures and staples is important. They must remain in place long enough to ensure initial wound closure. If any sign of suture line separation is evident during the removal process, the remaining sutures are left in place, and a description is documented and reported to the health care provider. In some cases these sutures are removed several days to 1 week later. After sutures are removed, the nurse applies Steri-Strips over the incision to provide support. The strips loosen over time (5 to 7 days) and can be removed when half of the strip is no longer attached to the skin.

ASSESSMENT

1. Identify patient using two identifiers (e.g., name and birthday or name and account number) according to facility policy. *Rationale: Ensures correct patient. Complies with The Joint Commission standards and improves patient safety (TJC, 2014).*

2. Review health care provider's order for specific directions related to suture or staple removal, including which sutures are to be removed (e.g., every other). *Rationale: Order is required because of the risk of premature or improper suture removal leading to wound damage.*
3. Assess patient for history of allergies. *Rationale: Determines if patient is sensitive to antiseptic or latex.*
4. Assess patient's level of comfort on a scale of 0 to 10. If patient is uncomfortable, offer an analgesic at least 30 minutes before removal. *Rationale: Provides baseline to determine tolerance to procedure.*
5. Inspect surgical incision for healing ridge (see Fig. 24-2) and skin integrity of suture line for uniform closure of wound edges, normal color, and absence of drainage and inflammation. *Rationale: Adequate healing needs to occur before sutures or staples are removed.*

PLANNING

Expected Outcomes focus on maintaining skin integrity, preventing infection, and promoting comfort.
1. Patient's incision is intact with edges well approximated after suture or staple removal.
2. Patient states an acceptable level of comfort on a scale of 0 to 10 after removal of sutures or staples.
3. Patient is able to perform incisional self-care by discharge.

Delegation and Collaboration

The skill of staple or suture removal cannot be delegated to nursing assistive personnel (NAP). The nurse instructs the NAP about:
- Specific wound hygiene measures.
- Reporting any patient complaints of discomfort, pressure, or wound drainage at the site.

Equipment
- Disposable waterproof biohazard bag
- Sterile suture removal set (forceps and scissors) or sterile staple remover
- Sterile antiseptic applicators or swabs
- Gauze pads
- Steri-Strips
- Clean gloves

IMPLEMENTATION *for* REMOVING SUTURES AND STAPLES

STEPS	RATIONALE
1. **See Standard Protocol (inside front cover).**	
2. Ensure there is direct lighting on suture line.	Aids visibility.
3. Apply clean gloves. Remove dressing (if present) and discard; remove gloves and dispose of them directly into waterproof bag. Perform hand hygiene.	Reduces transmission of microorganisms.

Continued

STEPS	RATIONALE

4. Prepare materials for suture/staple removal:
   a. Open sterile suture removal kit or staple extractor kit.
   b. Open sterile antiseptic swabs and place on inside surface of kit.
   c. Open gloves (sterile if facility policy indicates).
5. Apply clean gloves.

Reduces transmission of infection.

6. Cleanse sutures/staples and healed incision with antiseptic swabs. Wipe across sutures using a clean swab for each swipe.

Removes surface bacteria from incision and sutures/staples.

7. *Remove staples:*
   a. Place lower tip of staple extractor under first staple. As you close handles, upper tip of extractor depresses center of staple, causing both ends of staple to be bent upward and exit their insertion sites in the dermal layer simultaneously (see illustration).

Avoids excess pressure to suture line and secures smooth removal of each staple.

   b. Carefully control staple extractor.
   c. As soon as both ends of staple are visible, move it away from skin surface (see illustration).
   d. Release handles of staple remover over disposable waterproof bag, allowing staple to drop into bag.
   e. Repeat Steps 7a to 7d for removal of remaining staples as ordered.

Avoids suture line pressure and pain.
Prevents scratching tender skin surface with sharp pointed ends of staple for comfort and infection control.
Avoids contamination of sterile field with used staples.

Minimizes risk of separation of wound edges.

8. *Remove interrupted sutures:*
   a. Place gauze a few inches from suture line. Hold scissors in dominant hand and forceps (clamp) in nondominant hand.

Gauze serves as a receptacle for removed sutures. Placement of scissors and forceps allows for efficient suture removal.

   b. Grasp knot of suture with forceps and gently pull up knot while slipping tip of scissors under suture near skin (see illustration).
   c. Snip suture as close to skin as possible at end distal to knot. With knot grasped with forceps, use one continuous smooth action to pull suture through from the other side. Place removed suture on gauze.

Smoothly removes suture without additional tension to suture line.

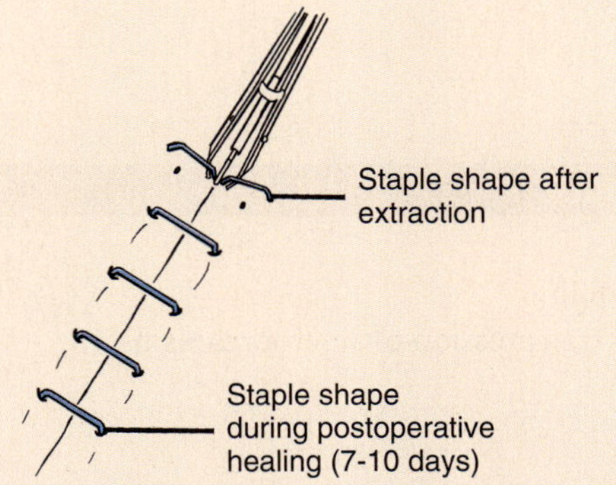

STEP 7a Staple extractor placed under staple.

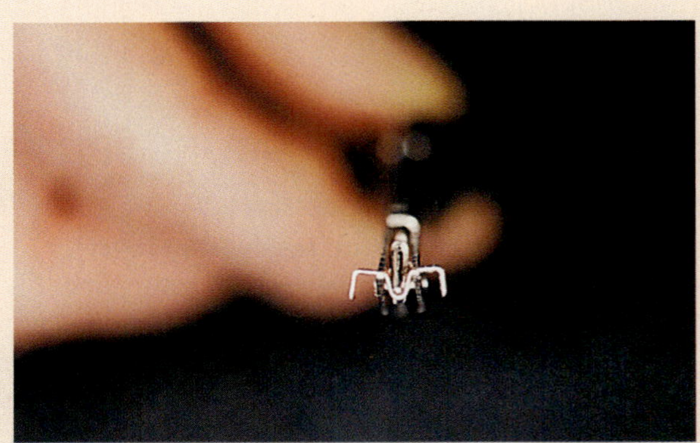

STEP 7c Staple removed by extractor.

STEPS	RATIONALE

> **SAFE PATIENT CARE** Never snip both ends of a suture because there will be no way to remove the part of the suture situated below the skin surface. Never pull exposed surface of any suture into tissue below dermis. The exposed surface of any suture is considered contaminated.

d. Repeat Steps 8a to 8c until every other suture has been removed.

9. *Remove continuous and blanket stitch sutures:*

a. Place sterile gauze a few inches from suture line. Grasp scissors in dominant hand and forceps in nondominant hand.

Gauze serves as a receptacle for removed sutures. Placement of scissors and forceps allows for efficient suture removal.

b. Snip first suture close to skin surface at end distal to knot.

Releases suture. Prevents pulling contaminated portion of suture through skin.

c. Snip second "suture" on same side.

d. Grasp knotted end and gently pull with continuous smooth action, removing suture from beneath the skin. Place suture on gauze.

Smoothly removes sutures without additional tension to suture line.

e. Repeat Steps 9a to 9d until entire line is removed.

10. Inspect incision site to ensure that all sutures are removed and identify any trouble areas. Gently wipe suture line with antiseptic swabs to remove debris and cleanse wound. Cleanse in a direction out and away from incision.

Reduces risk of incision separation. Prevents contamination of incision.

11. Apply Steri-Strips according to facility policy or surgeon's preference.

Supports wound by distributing tension across wound.

a. Cut Steri-Strips to allow strips to extend 4 to 5 cm ($1\frac{1}{2}$ to 2 inches) on each side of the incision.

b. Remove backing and apply across incision (see illustration).

c. Inform patient to take showers rather than soak in the bathtub according to surgeon's preference.

Steri-Strips are not removed and are allowed to fall off gradually.

12. Apply light dressing if drainage is apparent or if clothing may rub and irritate suture line.

13. Instruct patient about local and systemic signs of infection, and tell patient to notify health care provider if these occur after discharge.

Provides information to patient for reporting wound infection to health care provider.

14. **See Completion Protocol (inside front cover).**

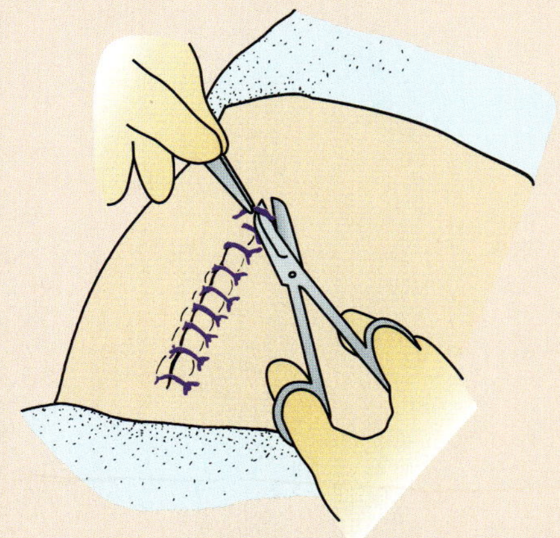

STEP 8b Removal of interrupted suture. Nurse cuts suture as close to skin as possible, away from the knot.

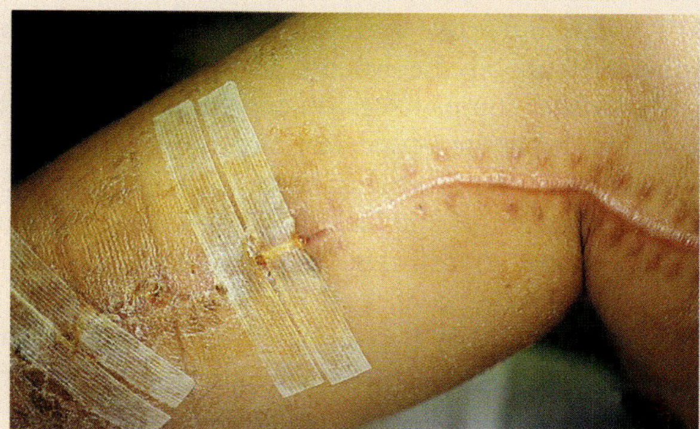

STEP 11b Steri-Strips over incision.

EVALUATION

1. Inspect incision for approximation of wound edges.
2. Ask patient to rate pain using a scale of 0 to 10.
3. Use *Teach Back:* State to the patient, "I want to be sure that I have adequately explained the signs of a wound or incision infection before you are discharged. Can you tell me the signs of infection and what you need to tell your health care provider if this happens?" Evaluates what the patient is able to explain or demonstrate. Document your evaluation of patient learning. Revise your instruction now or develop plan for revised patient teaching to be implemented at an appropriate time if patient is not able to teach back correctly.

Unexpected Outcomes and Related Interventions

1. Patient exhibits wound separation or dehiscence (surgical wound breaks, separates, and opens to the fascial level) and reports something "gave way."
   a. Notify surgeon.
   b. Keep any remaining sutures or staples in place.
2. Evisceration develops, involving protrusion of visceral organs through wound opening. This is a serious emergency because blood supply to tissues may be compromised when organs protrude.
   a. Keep organs moist by applying sterile towels that have been saturated in warm sterile saline solution.
   b. Immediately notify surgeon so that surgical intervention can be arranged.

Recording and Reporting

- Record condition of wound, number of sutures removed, and patient's response in patient's progress note.

- Notify health care provider immediately of any of the following findings: suture line separation, evisceration, bleeding, or new purulent drainage.
- Document your evaluation of patient learning.

Sample Documentation

1300   Wound edges well approximated. Healing ridge palpated on either side of abdominal incision. No redness, swelling, or wound drainage. All sutures removed. Steri-Strips applied. Patient instructed to shower (avoid baths), avoid tension on incision, and avoid heavy lifting. Patient instructed to return to health care provider in 1 week, and appointment slip given to wife.

Special Considerations
Pediatric

- Young children need reassurance before suture removal. Involve parent; demonstrate removal technique before actual removal.
- Talk to patient while removing sutures; reassure patient to remain inactive and calm.

Geriatric

- Older adults may need reassurance about the suture removal procedure. Assess mental status for comprehension of the procedure.
- There may be a higher risk for dehiscence after sutures are removed because of delayed healing of aging skin.
- Skin tears related to use of adhesives may occur in older patients.

SKILL 24.4 NEGATIVE-PRESSURE WOUND THERAPY

Negative-pressure wound therapy (NPWT) expedites wound healing through the use of controlled subatmospheric pressure using the body's own defense mechanisms to enhance moist wound healing (Figs. 24-7 and 24-8) (Netsch, 2012). NPWT assists and accelerates wound healing by generating negative pressure at the wound surface, which removes wound exudate, stimulates granulation tissue, reduces the bacterial burden in the wound, contracts the wound bed, and provides a moist wound environment. NPWT is available in several different forms and includes a wound filler dressing, suction catheter, transparent adhesive dressing, suction source, and collection container (Fig. 24-9).

Wounds managed by NPWT include acute (surgical) and traumatic wounds, surgical dehiscence, pressure ulcers, surgical flaps, and compromised flaps. When NPWT is selected for wound treatment, it is applied and changed every 48 hours for most wounds. The dressing is applied to the wound; the clear adhesive drape is placed over the dressing and secured to the periwound skin. Depending on the type of device used,

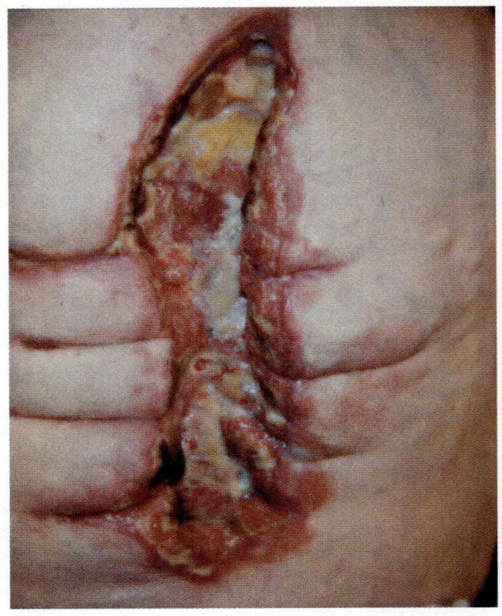

FIG 24-7 Dehisced wound before NPWT.

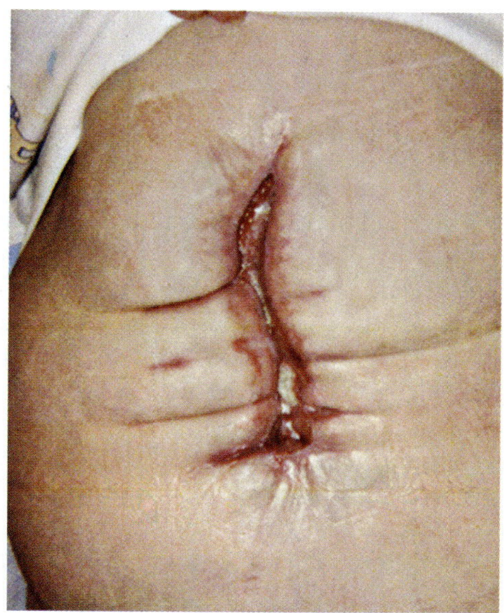

FIG 24-8 Dehisced wound after NPWT.

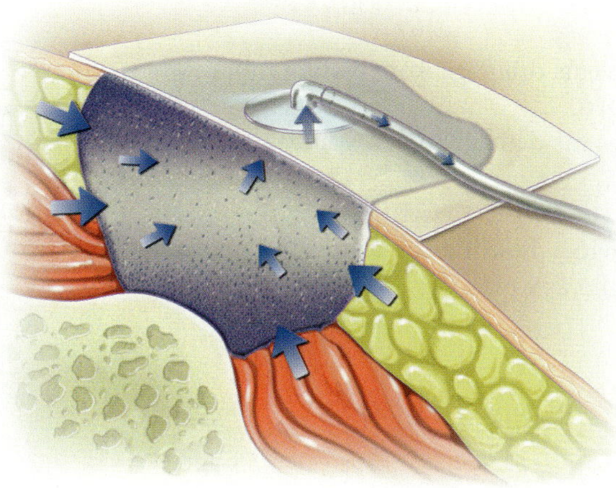

FIG 24-9 Wound NPWT in place. This is a wound vacuum-assisted closure (V.A.C.) system using negative pressure to remove fluid from the area surrounding the wound reducing edema and improving circulation to the area. (Courtesy KCI, San Antonio, Texas.)

evacuation tubing is placed over or into the dressing and attached to a suction source. The amount of suction or negative pressure varies from −75 mm Hg to −125 mm Hg, depending on the device and the characteristics of the wound. An airtight seal is necessary to maintain a negative-pressure environment. A snug and tight application of the dressing must be applied to ensure a good seal.

ASSESSMENT

1. Identify patient using two identifiers (e.g., name and birthday or name and account number) according to facility policy. *Rationale: Ensures correct patient. Complies with The Joint Commission standards and improves patient safety (TJC, 2014).*

2. Review health care provider's order for NPWT, including the amount of suction to be used, the type of wound filler dressing, and scheduled changes. *Rationale: Determines frequency of dressing change, negative pressure setting, and special instructions. Health care provider's order is also necessary for reimbursement.*

3. Assess patient's and caregiver's knowledge of purpose of dressing change. *Rationale: Determines level of support and explanation required.*

4. Assess patient's level of comfort on a scale of 0 to 10. If patient is uncomfortable, offer an analgesic at least 30 minutes before removal. *Rationale: Provides baseline to determine tolerance to procedure.*

5. Assess location, appearance, and size of wound (see Procedural Guideline 24.1). *Rationale: Provides information regarding status of wound healing, presence of complications, and the proper type of supplies and assistance needed.*

PLANNING

Expected Outcomes focus on promoting comfort, wound healing, and preventing infection.

1. Patient's wound begins to close with smaller measurements, presence of granulation tissue, and there is less drainage or edema.

2. Dressing remains intact with airtight seal and prescribed negative pressure.

3. Patient states an acceptable level of comfort on a scale of 0 to 10 during and after dressing change.

Delegation and Collaboration

The skill of removal and application of NPWT cannot be delegated to nursing assistive personnel (NAP). The nurse instructs the NAP to:

- Use caution in positioning and turning patient to avoid tubing displacement.
- Report any change in the dressing shape or if the dressing is not flat to the wound.
- Report any wound fluid leakage around the edges of the adhesive drape.

Equipment

- NPWT unit (requires health care provider's order)
- NPWT dressing (gauze or foam, depending on manufacturer's recommendations; transparent dressing, adhesive drape)
- NPWT suction device
- Tubing for connection between NPWT unit and NPWT dressing
- 3 pairs gloves, clean and sterile
- Sterile scissors
- Skin preparation/skin barrier protectant/hydrocolloid dressing/skin barrier
- Protective equipment: gown, mask, and goggles if splashing is a risk
- Waterproof, disposable trash biohazard bag

IMPLEMENTATION *for* NEGATIVE-PRESSURE WOUND THERAPY

STEPS	RATIONALE

1. **See Standard Protocol (inside front cover).**
2. Discuss procedure with patient. — Decreases patient anxiety.
3. Verify that patient received analgesia at least 20 to 30 minutes before dressing change. — Pain has been reported with NPWT removal and application; pain medication given before dressing change can reduce procedural pain (Upton and Andrews, 2013).
4. Position patient comfortably, and drape to expose only wound site. Instruct patient not to touch wound or sterile supplies. Place a disposable waterproof bag within reach of work area. — Maintaining patient comfort assists in completing skill smoothly. Draping provides access to wound while minimizing unnecessary exposure.
5. Apply clean gloves. If risk for spray exists, apply protective gown, goggles, and mask or face shield. — Reduces transmission of microorganisms.
6. Follow manufacturer's directions for removal and replacement because each unit varies slightly with regard to removal and application. *Turn off NPWT unit by pushing therapy on/off button:* — Deactivates therapy and allows for proper drainage of fluid in drainage tube.
   a. Raise tubing above unit and clamp, and engage clamp on dressing tubing. — Prevents backflow of any drainage in tubing.
   b. Engage clamp on dressing tubing.
   c. Allow drainage to flow from tubing into drainage collector. — Prevents drainage from exiting tubing when removed.
   d. Gently stretch drape horizontally, and remove slowly from dressing and skin. — Prevents damage to periwound skin.
   e. Remove old dressing and discard.
7. Perform wound assessment (see Procedural Guideline 24.1). Remove gloves and discard in proper receptacle. — Provides baseline for change or maintenance of wound therapy plan.
8. Perform hand hygiene and apply clean gloves.
9. Cleanse wound per facility policy. Gently blot periwound dry with gauze.
   a. Apply clean or sterile gloves depending on facility policy and wound status.
   b. If ordered, irrigate wound with normal saline or other solution as ordered by health care provider. Gently blot periwound with gauze and dry thoroughly. — Irrigation removes wound debris and cleans wound bed. Cleaning periwound area helps to maintain a tight seal.
10. Apply a skin protectant product to periwound surface. — Protects periwound from moisture associated skin damage. Contact dermatitis may result if suction is applied directly to skin (Netsch, 2012).
11. Application of NPWT (there are several manufacturers of NPWT; follow manufacturers' directions):
    a. Prepare NPWT filler dressing. — The filler dressing depends on the NPWT used and can include foam or gauze dressings with or without antimicrobials such as silver. The type of dressing may be adjusted based on undermining, tunneling, or sinus tracts present (Netsch, 2012). Consult with wound care expert for appropriate type.
       (1) Measure wound, and select appropriate size of dressing. — Establishes baseline for wound dimensions and dressing choice.
       (2) Using sterile scissors, cut filler dressing to wound size. — The wound should be completely covered with filler dressing.

> **SAFE PATIENT CARE** In some instances an antimicrobial product, such as sliver impregnated gauze or topical antibiotic is order. These products help reduce the bioburden of the wound.

b. Place filler dressing in wound following manufacturer's instructions. Count the number of filler dressings and document in chart.

Dressing edges should be in direct contact with wound tissue. A dressing count provides the nurse who removes the dressing with the number that should be removed.

c. Place suction device per manufacturer's recommendations. Some devices use the suction device over the dressing, and others use the suction device after the transparent dressing is applied.

d. Apply NPWT transparent dressing over the wound dressing (and suction drain). Trim dressing to cover wound dressing, and extend onto periwound skin approximately 2.5 to 5 cm (1 to 2 inches) (see illustration).

Ensure that wound is properly covered and a negative pressure seal is achieved (Box 24-3).

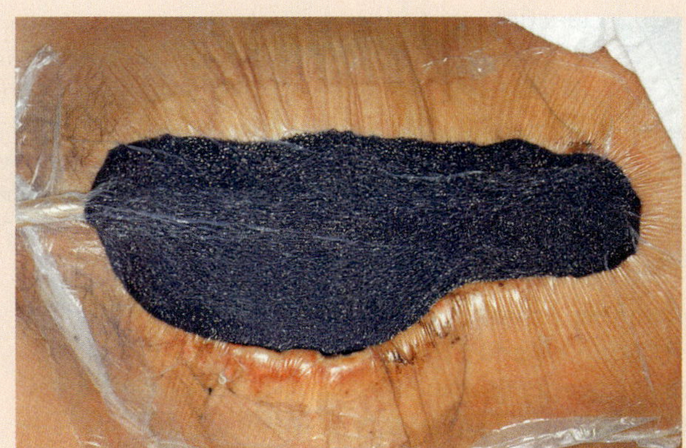

STEP 11d Foam wound filler, transparent dressing over existing wound.

(1) If using NPWT that has drain tubing that is applied after transparent dressing, cut hole in dressing large enough to accommodate tubing. Place into dressing, and seal with adhesive drape.

Dressing should be airtight with no tunnels or gaps; this ensures a good seal when the suction is activated.

12. After the wound is completely covered, connect tubing from the dressing to the tubing from the NPWT unit and set at ordered suction level. Examine the system to be sure that the seal is intact and the therapy is working; this is different for each type of NPWT unit. For example, on some units the display screen shows "Therapy On." Check facility policy and procedure for specific information.

Optimal negative pressure levels should be between −75 and −125 mm Hg (WOCN, 2010).

13. Record initials and date on new dressing.

14. **See Completion Protocol (inside front cover).**

EVALUATION

1. Perform wound inspection; compare appearance of wound with previous assessment.
2. Ask patient to rate pain using a scale of 0 to 10.
3. Verify airtight dressing seal and proper negative pressure.

Unexpected Outcomes and Related Interventions

1. Wound appears inflamed and tender, drainage has increased, and odor is present.
   a. Notify health care provider.
   b. Obtain wound culture per order.
2. Patient reports increase in pain.
   a. Patient may need more analgesic support.
   b. Negative pressure may need to be reduced; confer with health care provider.
3. Negative pressure seal has broken.
   a. Take preventive measures (see Box 24-3).
   b. Consider filling uneven skin surfaces with a skin barrier product to enhance the seal.

Recording and Reporting

- Record appearance of wound (characteristics of and amount of drainage), placement of NPWT, negative pressure setting, and patient's response.
- Report brisk, bright bleeding; evidence of poor wound healing; and possible wound infection to health care provider.

Sample Documentation

1100   Home visit. Wound on lower abdomen is pink, moist, and without edema in periwound region. Wound size is improving, currently 2 × 2.2 cm with 1.5 cm depth. Patient reports decrease in frequency and intensity of pain in wound area. Currently 4 on scale of 0 to 10. Medicated with 600 mg ibuprofen 30 minutes before dressing change. Dressing changed every 48 hours. Observed wife correctly change dressing and activated NPWT to −125 mm Hg. Family has sufficient NPWT supplies for the next week. Reviewed dressing care plan with wife and patient; dressing changes continue every 48 hours.

Special Considerations
Pediatric

- This wound application is not appropriate for fragile neonatal skin.

<table>
<tr><td colspan="2">BOX 24-3   MAINTAINING AN AIRTIGHT SEAL WITH NEGATIVE-PRESSURE WOUND THERAPY</td></tr>
</table>

To avoid loss of suction (negative pressure), the wound and dressing must stay sealed after therapy is initiated. Problem seal areas include wounds around joints; near skin creases and folds; and near moisture such as diaphoresis, wound drainage, and urine or stool. The following points may assist in maintaining an airtight seal:

- Clip hair on skin around wound (check facility policy).
- Fill uneven skin surfaces with a skin barrier product such as paste or strips.
- Make sure that skin surface is dry.
- Cut transparent film to extend 2.5 to 5 cm (1 to 2 inches) beyond wound perimeter.
- Frame periwound area with skin sealant, skin barrier, hydrocolloid, or transparent film dressing.
- Fill uneven skin surfaces with a skin barrier product such as paste or strips.
- Cut or mold transparent dressing to fit wound.
- Avoid wrinkles when applying transparent film.
- Identify any air leaks with a stethoscope, and repair leaks with a sealant dressing (e.g., transparent dressing). Use only one or two additional layers for large leaks. Multiple layers reduces moisture vapor transmission and causes maceration of wound.
- Avoid adhesive remover because it leaves a residue that hinders film adherence.

Geriatric

- Use skin care practices to protect periwound skin. The adhesive film may be irritating to fragile skin. Skin protectant is one method to reduce the risk of tissue injury.
- Visual impairment may prevent self-care, and home care services may be required.

Home Care

- When NPWT is used in the home, the patient and family caregiver may benefit from initial visits with a home care nurse to monitor initial treatments.
- Provide information to family and family caregiver regarding proper disposal of contaminated product.

CRITICAL THINKING EXERCISES

Case Study

A patient underwent an emergency colon resection for a perforated diverticulum 3 days ago. His abdominal wound was closed with staples at the time of surgery. After 24 hours, the postoperative dressing was removed, and the midline abdominal incision was left open to air. The incision and surrounding area was assessed every 8 hours. Today when the wound was assessed and the sides of the incision were palpated for the presence of the healing ridge, serous drainage was expressed in the middle section of the incision, and the area on either side of the incision from top to bottom was warm and red. No healing ridge was palpated.

1. The nurse is assessing the incision and the wound drainage. What should be included in the assessment? Select all that apply.
   1. Color, amount, and odor of drainage
   2. Integrity of the staples, if they are approximating the incision edges
   3. Results of the most recent hemoglobin and hematocrit
   4. Patient's pain when the area is palpated
2. The nurse has consulted with the surgeon about the finding of drainage from the stapled incision. The surgeon has removed the staples in the area of the incision where the drainage and redness were found. There is now an open area in the incision, and the order is to irrigate the open wound. What would be appropriate interventions when irrigating the wound? Select all that apply.
   1. Leave gauze dressing in place and irrigate into the gauze.
   2. Use a 19-gauge angiocatheter and a 35-mL syringe.
   3. Poor warm saline over the wound.
   4. Direct the solution through catheter to the area.
   5. Pour the solution into the wound directly from the container.
3. The portion of the patient's wound that is open is now healing by what method?
   1. Primary intention
   2. Secondary intention
   3. Tertiary intention

Review Questions

1. What would be the appropriate assessments of a wound that is healing by secondary intention? Select all that apply.
   1. Depth
   2. Color and percentage of tissue in the wound
   3. Estimated amount of time the wound will take to heal
   4. Presence of undermining
   5. Condition of the periwound skin
2. When the nurse attempts to empty the Jackson-Pratt bulb drainage collector from a patient with an intraabdominal abscess, she notes no drainage in the collector. Based on the report she received from the outgoing nurse at the beginning of her shift, she knows that he had 100 mL in the drainage collector 8 hours ago. What should her immediate actions be? Select all that apply.
   1. Call the surgeon to report these findings.
   2. Assess the dressing around the tube for drainage.
   3. Observe the tube and the area for 8 hours.
   4. Gently irrigate the tube with 50 mL of normal saline.

3. Which of the following care measures should be provided to a patient with a Jackson-Pratt drain?
   1. Empty the bulb only when it is filled to the top of the container.
   2. When the patient is ambulating, place a knot in the tubing to prevent excess drainage.
   3. Pin the bulb below the insertion site to facilitate drainage.
   4. Lubricate the insertion site to prevent crusting.
4. What is the correct sequence for staple removal from a healing surgical incision?
   a. Using staple remover, gently place under staple and press the extractor down.
   b. Put on clean gloves.
   c. Place Steri-Strips horizontally over incision.
   d. Palpate and verify the presence of the healing ridge.
   e. Explain procedure to patient.
   1. c, d, e, b, a
   2. e, b, d, a, c
   3. e, c, b, a, d
   4. e, d, b, a, c
5. What is the recommended amount of pressure to be used in NPWT?
   1. −100 to −350 mm Hg
   2. −75 to −125 mm Hg
   3. 0 to −55 mm Hg
   4. −350 to −500 mm Hg
6. Which of the following interventions fix or prevent a break in the seal on an NPWT adhesive drape? Select all that apply.
   1. Use pieces of the adhesive drape over the areas where air is leaking.
   2. Stuff small pieces of gauze into the areas that appear to have the leak.
   3. Clip hair on skin surface before application.
   4. Do not use adhesive remover on the skin.
   5. Soap the skin around the wound and allow to air dry.
7. What is the purpose of using Steri-Strips across an incision after staple or suture removal?
   1. To keep the incision dry in the areas where the staples or stitches were removed
   2. To support the wound by distributing tension across it
   3. To keep a 2-cm (about 1 inch) separation together to facilitate healing
   4. To conceal the incision from the patient, reducing anxiety

8. What is the appropriate way to measure the depth of a wound healing by secondary intention?
 1. Lightly pack the wound with dry gauze dressings to determine the volume and record the number of dressings used.
 2. Use a cotton tip applicator at the deepest area, record the depth, and record the location of the deepest part of the wound.
 3. Use a cotton tip applicator in three of the deepest parts of the wound and find the average of the three measurements.
 4. Measure the depth and length of the wound, and multiply together for the depth.

9. What is the correct order of wound healing phases?
 1. Inflammatory, hemostasis, proliferative, maturation
 2. Hemostasis, inflammatory, proliferative, maturation
 3. Proliferative, inflammatory, hemostasis, maturation
 4. Hemostasis, inflammatory, proliferative, maturation

10. Which self-contained wound evacuator drain is used to remove a small amount of fluid?
 1. Hemovac drain
 2. Jackson-Pratt drain
 3. ConstaVac drain
 4. McDonald drain

REFERENCES

Baranoski S, et al: Skin: an essential organ. In Baranoski S, Ayello EA, editors: *Wound care essentials: practice principles*, ed 3, Philadelphia, 2012a, Lippincott Williams & Wilkins.

Baranoski S, et al: Wound assessment. In Baranoski S, Ayello EA, editors: *Wound care essentials: practice principles*, ed 3, Philadelphia, 2012b, Lippincott Williams & Wilkins.

Doughty DB, Sparks-Defriese B: Wound healing physiology. In Bryant RA, Nix DP, editors: *Acute and chronic wounds: current management concepts*, ed 4, St Louis, 2012, Mosby.

European Pressure Ulcer Advisory Panel (EPUAP) and National Pressure Ulcer Advisory Panel (NPUAP): *Treatment of pressure ulcers: quick reference guide*, Washington, DC, 2009, NPUAP. http://www.epuap.org/guidelines/Final_Quick_Treatment.pdf. Accessed August 25, 2014.

Gallagher Camden S: Skin care needs of the obese patient. In Bryant RA, Nix DP, editors: *Acute and chronic wounds: current management concepts*, ed 4, St Louis, 2012, Mosby.

Netsch DS: Negative pressure wound therapy. In Bryant RA, Nix DP, editors: *Acute and chronic wounds: current management concepts*, ed 4, St Louis, 2012, Mosby.

Nix DP: Skin and wound inspection and assessment. In Bryant RA, Nix DP, editors: *Acute and chronic wounds: current management concepts*, ed 4, St Louis, 2012, Mosby.

Ramundo J: Wound debridement. In Bryant RA, Nix DP, editors: *Acute and chronic wounds: current management concepts*, ed 4, St Louis, 2012, Mosby.

Smith MEB, et al: Pressure ulcer treatment strategies: a systematic comparative effectiveness review, *Ann Intern Med* 159(1):39, 2013.

Stotts NA: Nutritional assessment and support. In Bryant RA, Nix DP, editors: *Acute and chronic wounds: current management concepts*, ed 4, St Louis, 2012, Mosby.

The Joint Commission (TJC): *National Patient Safety Goals*, Oakbrook Terrace, IL, 2014, The Commission. Available at: http://www.jointcommission.org/standards_information/npsgs.aspx.

Upton D, Andrews A: Pain and trauma in negative pressure wound therapy: a review, *Int Wound J* 2013. doi: 10.1111/iwj.12059. [Epub ahead of print].

Whitney JD: Acute surgical and traumatic wounds. In Bryant RA, Nix DP, editors: *Acute and chronic wounds: current management concepts*, ed 4, St Louis, 2012, Mosby.

Wound, Ostomy and Continence Nurses Society (WOCN): *Guideline for prevention and management of pressure ulcers, WOCN Clinical Practice Guidelines Series*, Mount Laurel, NJ, 2010, Wound, Ostomy and Continence Nurses Society (WOCN).

Pressure Ulcers

Pressure ulcers are localized areas of tissue destruction caused by the compression of soft tissue over a bony prominence and an external surface for a prolonged time (WOCN, 2010). The term *bedsore* is inaccurate because such ulcers result from positions other than lying. Pressure ulcers can occur when patients are sitting or when an external source such as a cast edge applies unrelieved pressure to the skin. Fig. 25-1 shows pressure points over bony prominences where pressure ulcers can develop in sitting and lying positions. Common sites for the development of pressure ulcers include the sacrum, heels, elbows, lateral malleoli, trochanters, and ischial tuberosities (Ayello et al., 2012). Three pressure-related forces lead to the development of a pressure ulcer: (1) intensity of pressure (how much pressure is applied); (2) duration of pressure (how long pressure is applied); and (3) tissue tolerance (the ability of skin and its supporting structures to endure pressure without adverse effects). The intensity of the pressure must exceed capillary closure pressure, compressing the blood flow to the skin. Both low pressure over a prolonged period and high pressure over a short period can create a pressure ulcer. The greater the pressure and the longer pressure is applied, the greater the likelihood that a pressure ulcer will develop. Special mattresses and support surfaces help reduce or redistribute this pressure (see Procedural Guideline 25.1). The third factor, tissue tolerance, refers to the ability of the tissue to react to the pressure.

Three external factors (i.e., shear, friction, and moisture) make the tissues less tolerant to pressure (Pieper, 2012). Shear is a parallel force that stretches tissue and blood vessels, such as when a patient is in a semi-Fowler's position and slides toward the foot of the bed (Fig. 25-2). The skin over the sacrum sticks to the bed sheets, but the bony structure slides down, occluding the blood vessels, causing deep tissue injury. Friction, the rubbing of the tissue against a surface, abrades the top layer of skin (epidermis), which makes tissue susceptible to pressure injury. Skin moisture (most often from fecal and urinary incontinence) softens skin, creating the risk for skin breakdown. Other factors related to pressure ulcer development include poor nutrition; advanced age; medical conditions causing poor tissue perfusion (e.g., low blood pressure, smoking, elevated temperature, anemia); and psychosocial status, in particular, stress-induced cortisol secretion (Pieper, 2012; WOCN, 2010).

WOUND HEALING

Skin, the largest organ in the body, protects the body from chemical and mechanical insults and bacterial and viral entry and regulates fluid loss and electrolytes. When wounded, the skin and supporting tissue go through a complex repair process. You have an important role in wound healing, supporting patients by providing the appropriate wound-healing

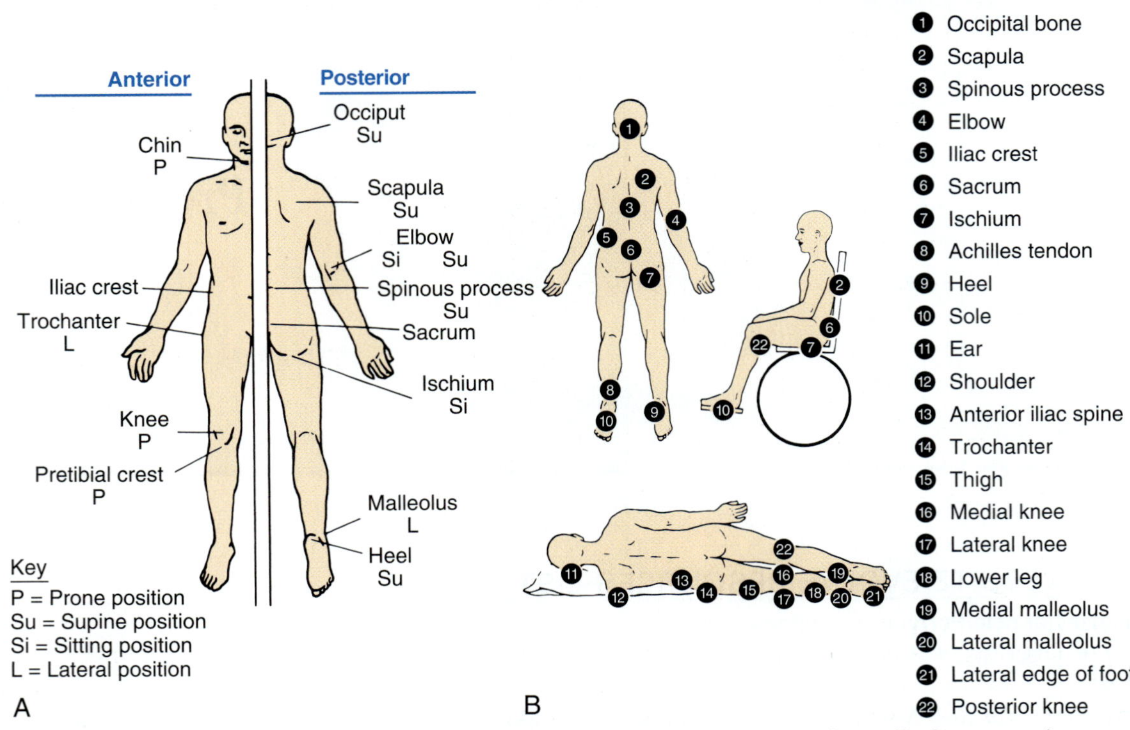

FIG 25-1 A, Bony prominences most frequently underlying pressure ulcers. **B,** Pressure ulcer sites. (Courtesy San Diego Veterans Administration Medical Agency.)

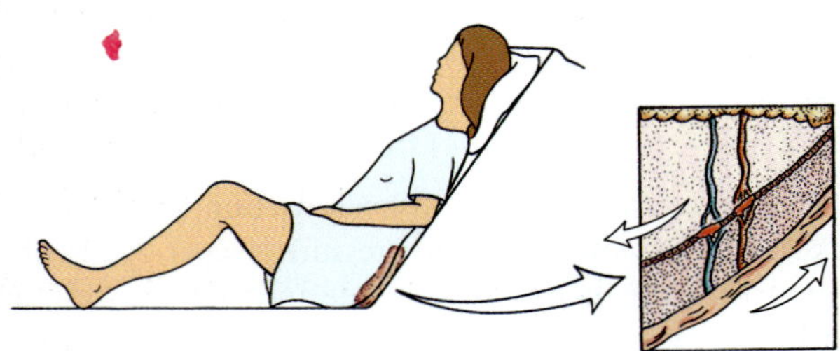

FIG 25-2 Shear exerted in the sacral area.

environment. A comprehensive wound assessment provides information needed for planning wound care for a patient. To provide appropriate wound care, you must understand the process of wound healing. The physiology of wound healing occurs via two mechanisms: (1) regeneration (i.e., replacement of damaged or lost tissue with more of the same as occurs in partial-thickness wounds) or (2) connective tissue repair in wounds with tissue loss where scar formation replaces lost tissue, such as in full-thickness wounds (Doughty and Sparks-Defriese, 2012). See Chapter 24 for a full discussion of wound healing.

Many factors influence wound healing and patient care. Wound healing is a process that requires specific nutrients to fuel healing (Stotts, 2012). Infection prolongs the inflammatory phase, which prevents epithelialization. Medications such as steroids slow the inflammatory process, making wounds more prone to infection and delayed healing (Table 25-1). High levels of stress increase cortisol levels, which reduce the number of lymphocytes and decrease the inflammatory response.

PATIENT-CENTERED CARE

When assessing a patient for pressure ulcer risk, describe to the patient and family members the importance of determining possible risk factors. Informing them of the need to identify risk factors educates them on the increased risk for pressure ulcer development. Describe to patients and family members what interventions will be instituted for prevention and treatment. Be mindful that patients with dark skin may need a close examination for color changes. Also, let patients and family members help identify skin color changes (as appropriate). A patient is familiar with bodily changes and is an important resource in your assessment. In some instances, the change in tissue may be noted only by touching the skin to note temperature changes.

When providing care for a patient with a pressure ulcer, a patient-centered approach attends to the patient's comfort and emotional support. Describe what you are doing when you gently palpate areas of the skin or apply treatments to wounds. Gather all supplies at the bedside just before a procedure so that patients are not left alone with their wounds uncovered.

SAFETY

Preventing skin breakdown and pressure ulcers is essential for safe patient care. Preventing injuries to a patient's skin and underlying muscle tissue not only saves health care resources but also protects the patient's overall level of health, independence, and optimal functioning. When performing a skin

TABLE 25-1	FACTORS THAT DELAY WOUND HEALING
FACTOR	**RATIONALE**
Advanced age	Aging affects all phases of wound healing. The most significant change includes a diminished inflammatory response.
Obesity	Fatty subcutaneous tissue is less vascular.
Diabetes mellitus	Vascular changes reduce blood flow to peripheral tissues; leukocyte malfunction results from hyperglycemia, resulting in high risk for infection.
Inadequate blood supply	Vascular changes decrease delivery of oxygen and nutrients.
Nutritional deficiencies	Inadequate nutrition slows healing because of lack of nutrients (vitamin C, protein, zinc) needed for wound healing (Stotts, 2012).
Corticosteroid drugs	Immunosuppression decreases the inflammatory response and collagen synthesis.
Chemotherapy	Chemotherapy interferes with leukocyte (white blood cell count) production and immune response.
Infection	Infection increases inflammatory response and tissue destruction.
Smoking	Smoking impedes blood flow from vasoconstriction.
Poor general health	When health is poor, factors need for wound healing are absent.

assessment, provide privacy for patients and assist them as necessary in position changes, while keeping areas not under examination covered. Position the patient in bed to assess the skin adequately; when turning the patient onto the side, be sure that the side rail is up on the side of the bed to which the patient is turned to prevent falls. Specific evidence-based measures can be used to reduce pressure ulcer risk (Chou et al, 2013; Sullivan and Schoelles, 2013). The use of an intervention bundle guides identification for patients at risk and identifies early interventions.

EVIDENCE-BASED PRACTICE

Fletcher J: Device related pressure ulcers made easy, *Wounds UK* 8(2):1, 2012.

McNichol L et al: Medical adhesives and patient safety: state of the science: consensus statements for the assessment, prevention, and treatment of adhesive-related skin injuries, *Journal of Wound Ostomy Continence Nurs* 40:365, 2013.

Siddiqui A et al: A continuous bedside pressure mapping system for prevention of pressure ulcer development in the ICU, *Wounds* 25(12):333, 2013.

Although there is an increased awareness of pressure ulcers occurring over bony prominences, very little of the literature focuses on the problem of device-related pressure ulcers, ulcers occurring around and under medical devices as well as under medical adhesives. Medical devices known to contribute to pressure ulcers include nasogastric (NG) tubes; endotracheal (ET) tubes; Foley catheters; and other plastic, rubber, or silicone tubes. It is thought that a device-related pressure ulcer may occur because of poor fixation or positioning of the equipment and from edema in the area of the device. The skin breakdown mimics the shape of the device. To avoid pressure ulcers from occurring, it is important to include inspection of all devices and tubes in all body locations. Care should be taken in placement and securement of the devices (Fletcher, 2012). Work by a consensus group examined skin damage from medical adhesives (McNichol et al., 2013). This group recommended an examination of the type of tape used and the technique for application and removal. The prevalence of adhesive-related injuries is difficult to determine, but there are several reports of tape stripping and skin tears related to the use of tape. Both device-related and adhesive-related skin injuries should be considered when assessing skin for potential areas of skin breakdown.

- Frequently perform skin assessment around and under devices and tubes.
- Frequently assess for edema in the skin underlying a tube or other medical device (Fletcher, 2012).
- Remove adhesive tape and assess underlying skin to determine if another type of tape is needed (McNichol et al., 2013).
- Rotate tubes to different positions to decrease pressure in the area where the tube is in contact with the skin (Fletcher, 2012). For example, ET tubes can be moved from one side of the mouth to the other.
- Double-check and determine that tube or device is properly positioned and has proper fixation to decrease unnecessary tube movement and skin damage.
- Implement care bundle for pressure ulcer prevention (Siddiqui et al., 2013):
  - Comprehensive skin assessment
  - Standardized pressure ulcer risk assessment
  - Implementation plan based on findings of assessments
  - Post and use a turn schedule
  - Choose and use a pressure-redistribution surface
  - Elevate heels
  - Assess nutrition
  - Manage incontinence

SKILL 25.1 PRESSURE ULCER RISK ASSESSMENT AND PREVENTION STRATEGIES

• Nursing Skills Online: Wound Care Module, Lesson 4

A comprehensive program to prevent pressure ulcers includes the use of a risk assessment tool to identify factors that place the patient at risk for skin breakdown. Risk assessment allows you to plan appropriate interventions to reduce or prevent skin breakdown. In addition to the risk assessment tool, a daily skin inspection, including an examination of pressure points, is essential. The Braden Scale for Predicting Pressure Sore Risk (Table 25-2) has six subscales that measure degrees of sensory perception, moisture, activity, mobility, nutrition, friction, and shear (Braden and Bergstrom, 1989). Each sub-scale is given a score, resulting in a total score indicative of the patient's risk for developing a pressure ulcer. The scale is used on admission to a health care facility and at periodic intervals.

Systematically inspect the skin of all patients at risk at least once a day, paying particular attention to bony prominences. Inspect a patient's skin during routine care, and always document your findings.

ASSESSMENT

1. Assess patient's risk for pressure ulcer formation, using facility pressure ulcer risk assessment tool. Determine the risk assessment score, and compare patient's score with established score ranges that indicate high risk for skin breakdown. *Rationale: A validated risk assessment tool is recommended by the Wound, Ostomy and Continence Nurses Society (2010). Identifies patients at risk early so that risk factors can be reduced through interventions (Chou et al, 2013).*

2. Assess patient for presence of potential pressure areas other than bony prominences, such as risks for ulcer development from medical devices, including nares (NG tubes, oxygen cannula), tongue, and lips (oral airway, ET tube) and skin next to drainage tubes or beneath orthopedic devices (braces, casts) (Fletcher, 2012). *Rationale: Pressure from a medical device or how a medical device is secured*

TABLE 25-2 BRADEN SCALE FOR PREDICTING PRESSURE SORE RISK

SENSORY PERCEPTION	1. COMPLETELY LIMITED	2. VERY LIMITED	3. SLIGHTLY LIMITED	4. NO IMPAIRMENT
Ability to respond meaningfully to pressure-related discomfort	Unresponsive (does not moan, flinch, or grasp) to painful stimuli because of diminished level of consciousness or sedation *Or* Limited ability to feel pain over most of body surface	Responds only to painful stimuli; cannot communicate discomfort except by moaning or restlessness *Or* Has a sensory impairment that limits the ability to feel pain or discomfort over ½ of body	Responds to verbal commands but cannot always communicate discomfort or need to be turned *Or* Has some sensory impairment that limits ability to feel pain or discomfort in one or two extremities	Responds to verbal commands; has no sensory deficit that would limit ability to feel or voice pain or discomfort
MOISTURE	**1. CONSTANTLY MOIST**	**2. VERY MOIST**	**3. OCCASIONALLY MOIST**	**4. RARELY MOIST**
Degree to which skin is exposed to moisture	Skin kept moist almost constantly by perspiration, urine; dampness detected every time patient is moved or turned	Skin often but not always moist; must change linens at least once a shift	Skin occasionally moist, requiring an extra linen change approximately once a day	Skin usually dry; must change linens only at routine intervals
ACTIVITY	**1. BEDFAST**	**2. CHAIRFAST**	**3. WALKS OCCASIONALLY**	**4. WALKS FREQUENTLY**
Degree of physical activity	Confined to bed	Ability to walk severely limited or nonexistent; cannot bear own weight and/or must be assisted into chair or wheelchair	Walks occasionally during day but for very short distances, with or without assistance; spends majority of each shift in bed or chair	Walks outside room at least twice a day and inside room at least once every 2 hours during waking hours

TABLE 25-2   BRADEN SCALE FOR PREDICTING PRESSURE SORE RISK—cont'd

MOBILITY	1. COMPLETELY IMMOBILE	2. VERY LIMITED	3. SLIGHTLY LIMITED	4. NO LIMITATION
Ability to change and control body position	Does not make even slight changes in body or extremity position without assistance	Makes occasional slight changes in body or extremity position but unable to make frequent or significant changes independently	Makes frequent although slight changes in body or extremity position independently	Makes major and frequent changes in position without assistance

NUTRITION	1. VERY POOR	2. PROBABLY INADEQUATE	3. ADEQUATE	4. EXCELLENT
Usual food intake pattern	Never eats a complete meal; rarely eats more than ⅓ of any food offered; eats 2 servings or less of protein (meat or dairy products) per day; takes fluids poorly; does not take a liquid dietary supplement *Or* Is NPO and/or maintained on clear liquids or IV fluids for more than 5 days	Rarely eats a complete meal and generally eats only about ½ of any food offered; protein intake includes only 3 servings of meat or dairy products per day; occasionally takes a dietary supplement *Or* Receives less than optimum amount of liquid diet or tube feeding	Eats over half of most meals; eats a total of 4 servings of protein (meat, dairy products) each day; occasionally refuses a meal but usually takes a supplement if offered *Or* Is on a tube feeding or TPN regimen that probably meets most nutritional needs	Eats most of every meal; never refuses a meal; usually eats a total of 4 or more servings of meat and dairy products; occasionally eats between meals; does not require supplementation

FRICTION AND SHEAR	1. PROBLEM	2. POTENTIAL PROBLEM	3. NO APPARENT PROBLEM	
	Requires moderate-to-maximum assistance in moving; complete lifting without sliding against sheets impossible; frequently slides down in bed or chair, requiring frequent repositioning with maximum assistance; spasticity, contractures, or agitation leads to almost constant friction	Moves feebly or requires minimum assistance; during a move skin probably slides to some extent against sheets, chair, restraints, or other devices; maintains relatively good position in chair or bed most of the time but occasionally slides down	Moves in bed and chair independently and has sufficient muscle strength to lift up completely during move; maintains good position in bed or chair	
			Total Score	

Scoring: Very high risk, <9; high risk, 10-12; moderate risk, 13-14; mild risk, 15-18; not at risk, >18 (Ayello and Braden, 2002).
IV, Intravenous; *TPN,* total parenteral nutrition.
© 1988 Barbara Braden and Nancy Bergstrom. Used with permission.

increases the risk for tissue injury under and around the device (McNichol et al., 2013). Frequent assessment of these areas results in timely identification of the potential for or actual early skin injury (Fletcher, 2012).

3. Observe patient for preferred positions when in bed or chair. *Rationale: Weight of body is placed on certain bony prominences, and patient may resist repositioning of these areas.*

4. Observe patient's ability to initiate and assist with position changes. *Rationale: Prolonged lying or sitting in one position can cause capillary compression and tissue loss.*

5. Assess patient's and support person's understanding of risks for the development of pressure ulcers and knowledge of preventive measures. *Rationale: Patient and family are integral to prevention and management of pressure ulcers (WOCN, 2010).*

PLANNING

Expected Outcomes focus on identifying patient's risk for skin breakdown and preventing it.

1. Risk factors are identified.
2. Patient experiences no change from baseline skin assessment.
3. Patient experiences no new areas of erythema or signs of skin loss.
4. Patient has an acceptable comfort level (4 or less on a pain scale of 0 to 10) in pressure-redistribution positions.

Delegation and Collaboration

The skill of pressure ulcer risk assessment may not be delegated to nursing assistive personnel (NAP). The nurse instructs the NAP about the following:

- Explaining frequency of position changes and specific positions individualized for the patient.
- Reviewing need to report to you any redness or break in patient's skin or any abrasion from adhesives, tubes, assistive devices, or other medical devices.

Equipment

- Risk assessment tool
- Positioning aids
- Clean gloves

IMPLEMENTATION *for* PRESSURE ULCER RISK ASSESSMENT AND PREVENTION STRATEGIES

STEPS	RATIONALE
1. **See Standard Protocol (inside front cover).**	
2. Explain procedure to patient and family members.	Helps patient and family understand the importance of risk assessment.
3. Gloves are needed when open draining wounds are present.	Reduces transmission of microorganisms.
4. Inspect skin at least once a day:	
a. Observe patient's skin; pay particular attention to bony prominences. If you find a reddened area, gently press the area with a gloved finger to check for blanching. If the area does not blanch, suspect tissue injury, and recheck in 1 hour. Any discoloration may vary from pink to a deep red.	Routine skin inspection is fundamental to risk assessment and in designing interventions to reduce risk (Berlowitz, 2014a; WOCN, 2010). Persistent redness in lightly pigmented skin when pressed can indicate tissue injury (Baranoski et al., 2012). If an area of redness blanches (lightens in color), this indicates that skin is not at risk for breakdown.
b. If patient has darkly pigmented skin, look for color changes that differ from patient's normal skin color, such as red, blue, or purple tones.	Darkly pigmented skin may not have blanching. Although the skin may not show direct changes in color, the color may differ from the surrounding area (Lewis et al, 2014) (Box 25-1).
5. Check all treatment and assistive devices (catheters, feeding tubes, casts, braces) for potential pressure points. Remove and dispose of gloves.	Pressure from these devices increases risk to all areas of a patient's skin, not just to bony prominences (Fletcher, 2012; Mulgrew et al., 2011).
6. Review patient's pressure ulcer risk score.	Risk score aids in identifying interventions needed to lessen or eliminate the present risk factors.

> **SAFE PATIENT CARE** Do not massage reddened areas because this may cause additional tissue trauma. Reddened areas indicate blood vessel damage; massaging can damage the vessels further.

STEPS	RATIONALE
7. If immobility, inactivity, or poor sensory perception is a risk factor for patient, consider one of the following interventions:	Immobility and inactivity reduce a patient's ability or desire to change position independently. Poor sensory perception decreases the patient's ability to feel the sensation of pressure or discomfort.
a. Reposition patient at least every 2 hours as his or her condition allows; use a written schedule (Berlowitz, 2014a).	Reduces the duration and intensity of pressure. Some patients may require repositioning more often.
b. When patient is in the side-lying position in bed, use the 30-degree lateral position (see illustration).	Reduces direct contact of trochanter with the support surface.
c. When needed, use pillow bridging (see illustration).	Use of pillows prevents direct contact between bony prominences.
d. Place patient (when lying in bed) on pressure-redistribution surface (see Procedural Guideline 25.1).	Reduces amount of pressure exerted against tissues.

STEPS	RATIONALE

e. Place patient (when in a chair) on a pressure-redistribution device, and shift the points under pressure at least every hour.

Reduces amount of pressure on sacral and ischial areas.

8. If friction and shear are identified as risk factors, consider the following interventions:

Friction and shear damage underlying skin.

a. Use two nurses and a pull sheet to lift and reposition patient. Use a slide board (see Chapter 15) to transfer patient from bed to stretcher.

Proper repositioning of patient prevents dragging along the sheets. A slide board provides slippery surface to reduce friction.

b. Ensure that heels are free from the surface of the bed by using a pillow under the calves to elevate the heels.

"Floating" the heels from the bed surface eliminates shear and friction.

c. Maintain head of the bed at 30 degrees.

Lower head levels decrease the potential for patient to slide toward foot of bed and incur a shear injury.

9. If patient receives a low score on a moisture subscale, consider one or more of the following interventions:

Continual exposure of body fluids to the patient's skin increases risk for skin breakdown and pressure ulcer development.

a. Apply a moisture barrier ointment to perineum and surrounding skin after each incontinent episode.

Protects intact skin from fecal or urinary incontinence.

b. If skin is denuded, use a protective barrier paste after each incontinent episode.

Provides a barrier between skin and stool or urine, allowing for healing.

c. If incontinence is ongoing, consider a collection device, such as fecal incontinence collector, bowel management system, or indwelling urinary catheter.

Collection of the irritating substance may be appropriate if cause of incontinence cannot be controlled.

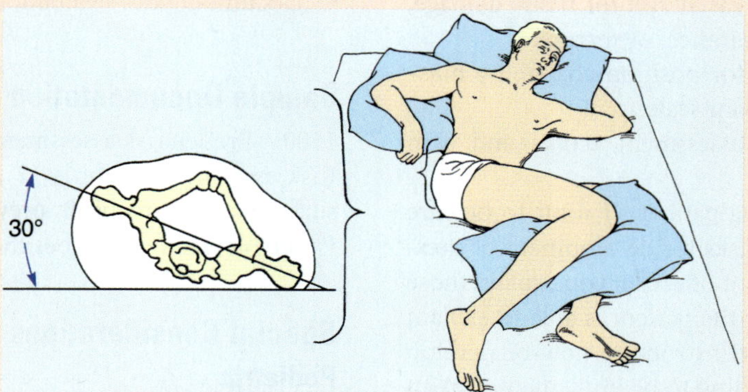

STEP 7b The 30-degree lateral position with pillow placement.

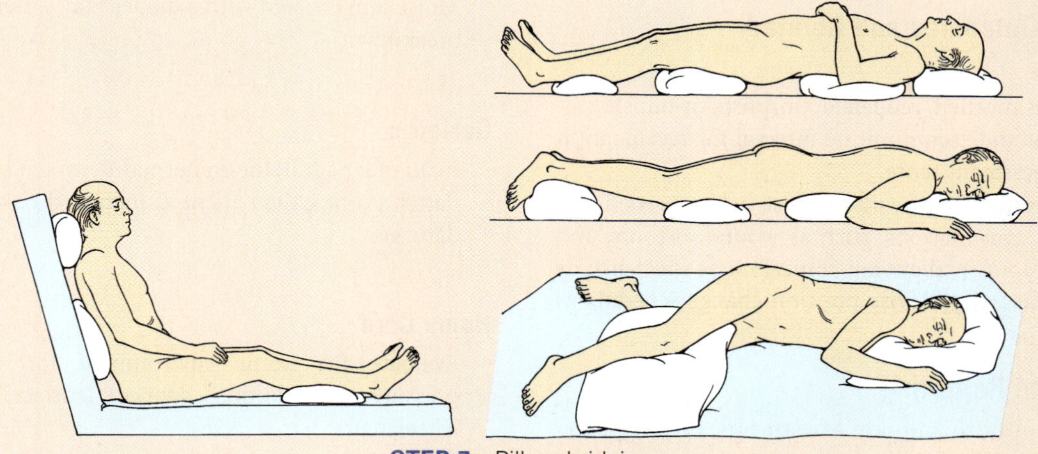

STEP 7c Pillow bridging.

Continued

STEPS	RATIONALE

d. If source of moisture is from wound drainage, consider frequent dressing changes, skin protection with protective barriers, or collection devices.

Removes frequent exposure of skin to wound drainage.

10. If patient scores low on nutrition subscale of the risk assessment, consider the following interventions:

There is a strong relationship between nutrition and pressure ulcer development.

a. Assess patient's nutritional status, including fluid intake. Determine if patient has been receiving nothing by mouth (NPO) recently.

Dehydration can affect albumin levels and tissue integrity.

b. Perform nutritional screening on patients identified to be at risk on nutrition subscale. Consider referral to a registered dietitian per facility policy.

Malnutrition is a risk factor for pressure ulcer development.

c. Offer support with eating (see Chapter 12).

Encourages intake.

d. Institute oral supplements (tube feedings, dietary supplements) per health care provider's order if patient is undernourished.

Oral supplements increase patient's protein intake and calorie count and supply essential vitamins and minerals. Various options are available depending on whether patients have other conditions such as diabetes.

11. Educate patient and family caregiver regarding pressure ulcer risk and prevention.

Assists in adhering to interventions to reduce pressure ulcer risk (Baharestani, 2012; Berlowitz, 2014a).

12. See Completion Protocol (inside front cover).

▌EVALUATION

1. Observe patient's skin for areas at risk for tissue damage, noting change in color, appearance, or texture.
2. Observe patient's tolerance for position change by measuring level of comfort on pain scale.
3. Compare subsequent risk assessment scores and skin assessments.
4. Use **Teach Back:** State to the patient, "I want to be sure that I explained to you the risks for development of pressure ulcers and how to prevent one. Can you explain those to me now?" Evaluates what the patient is able to explain or demonstrate. Revise your instruction now or develop plan for revised patient teaching to be implemented at an appropriate time if patient is not able to teach back correctly.

Unexpected Outcomes and Related Interventions

1. Skin becomes mottled, reddened, purplish, or bluish.
   a. Document and communicate interval for reevaluation of risk assessment score.
   b. Obtain health care provider's order (when needed) for identified consultations, such as wound, ostomy, and continence nurse; dietitian; clinical nurse specialist; or physical therapist. Revise position change schedule as needed.

Recording and Reporting

- Record patient's risk and skin assessments, turning intervals, pressure-redistribution support surface, and moisture protection interventions.
- Report need for additional consultations (if indicated) for high-risk patient.
- Document your evaluation of patient learning.

Sample Documentation

1500   Braden risk assessment scale completed on admission. Risk assessment score is 12 (high risk). Skin intact over all surfaces; pressure ulcer prevention protocol implemented. Patient correctly describes the turn schedule.

Special Considerations
Pediatric

- Immature skin in a pediatric patient is susceptible to skin tears.
- Moist skin covered with a diaper may soften, causing skin breakdown.

Geriatric

- In an older adult, the epidermal-dermal junction becomes flatter, putting the patient at increased risk for epidermal damage.

Home Care

- Evaluate the home environment for the use of a pressure-redistribution support surface (including a wheelchair).
- Evaluate the seating surface for an appropriate pressure-redistribution support surface.

BOX 25-1   SKIN ASSESSMENT FOR PATIENTS WITH DARK SKIN

Patients with darkly pigmented skin cannot be assessed for pressure ulcer risk by examining skin color only. Follow these recommended guidelines:

1. Assess localized skin color changes. Any of the following may appear:
   - Skin color changes are different from usual skin tone.
   - Darkly pigmented skin may not have visible blanching; color may differ from the surrounding area.
   - Color is darker than surrounding skin (purplish, bluish, eggplant).
2. Lighting is important for skin assessment:
   - Use natural or halogen light.
   - Avoid fluorescent lamps, which can give skin a bluish tone.
   - Avoid wearing tinted lenses when assessing skin color.
3. Assess tissue consistency:
   - Skin is taut, shiny, or indurated; edema occurs with induration of more than 15 mm in diameter.
   - Assess for edema, swelling.
   - Assess for firm or boggy feel.
4. Assess sensation:
   - Assess for pain or changes in skin sensation such as burning or itching.
5. Skin temperature:
   - Initially, skin in the area of pressure may feel warmer than surrounding skin.
   - Subsequently, skin may feel cooler than surrounding skin.
   - Feel areas of skin that are not involved in or around a pressure point to serve as a point of temperature reference.

Modified from Lewis S et al: *Medical-surgical nursing: assessment and management of clinical problems*, ed 9, St Louis, 2014, Elsevier; National Pressure Ulcer Advisory Panel (NPUAP): *Pressure ulcer stages revised by NPUAP*, 2007, http://www.npuap.org/pr2.htm. Accessed March 31, 2014.

PROCEDURAL GUIDELINE 25.1
Selection of a Pressure-Redistribution Support Surface

Pressure ulcers can occur in any health care setting. Patients in the operating room are also at risk for injury to the skin and underlying tissue. This injury occurs from a combination of factors, such as surgical positioning and the effects of anesthetic agents. Because the damage resulting from intraoperative pressure is thought to develop in the muscle and subcutaneous tissues and progresses outward, damage is sometimes not visible for several days. Use support surfaces in the operating room for patients at high risk for pressure ulcer development (NPUAP/EPUAP, 2009; Sutton et al, 2013). The use of intraoperative pressure-redistribution devices is associated with a decreased incidence of postoperative pressure ulcers (Pham et al., 2011). When you care for postoperative patients, observe the skin for signs of injury or breakdown, even when a patient is ambulatory in the postoperative setting. In addition, instruct patients having surgery in ambulatory care settings how to observe for signs of skin breakdown when they return home.

In patient care areas, specialized support surfaces are foam, air, or gel mattresses, beds, and cushions (Table 25-3). Pressure-redistribution surfaces are classified as nonpowered or powered support surfaces. Nonpowered support surfaces include mattresses or mattress overlays filled with air, water, gel, foam, or a combination of any of these. Powered support surfaces change the pressure beneath a patient, reducing the duration of any applied pressure (Nix and Mackey, 2012). Mattresses or beds with a slick surface help decrease friction and shear. Surfaces with porous covers allow airflow, which reduces moisture, resulting in decreased risk for skin maceration. Support surfaces are designed to prevent pressure ulcers and through pressure redistribution provide an environment more conducive to pressure ulcer healing (Nix and Mackey, 2012).

Delegation and Collaboration

The selection of a pressure-redistribution support device cannot be delegated to nursing assistive personnel (NAP).

Equipment

- Facility pressure ulcer risk assessment tool (see Skill 25.1)
- Body chart, tape measure, or camera to document existing areas of impaired skin integrity
- Documentation record
- Skin care products

Procedural Steps

1. Assess patient's risk for skin breakdown using a risk assessment tool (e.g., Braden Scale).
2. Assess patient's existing pressure ulcers, including areas of blistering, abnormal reactive hyperemia, and abrasion.
3. Assess patient's level of comfort using a pain scale of 0 to 10.
4. Identify patient using two identifiers (e.g., name and birthday or name and account number) according to facility policy. Ensures correct patient. Complies with The Joint Commission standards and improves patient safety (TJC, 2014).
5. Place "at-risk" patients on a pressure-redistribution surface (Nix and Mackey, 2012; NPUAP/EPUAP, 2009).
6. Identify patient factors when selecting an appropriate surface.
   a. Does the patient need pressure redistribution (e.g., you cannot reposition the patient or there is an existing pressure ulcer)?
   b. Is the surface needed for short-term or long-term care? A short-term surface is usually needed for

Continued

PROCEDURAL GUIDELINE 25.1
Selection of a Pressure-Redistribution Support Surface—cont'd

patients with acute illness and hospitalization. A long-term surface is usually needed for patients receiving extended or home care.

  c. What is the potential comfort level achieved by the surface? If the patient is sensitive to noise, a device with a loud motor would increase his or her discomfort.

  d. Are the patient and family caregiver adherent to repositioning? In addition, are they aware that a support surface should never replace repositioning? In a home setting, a support surface is often necessary when the patient or family caregiver is unable to reposition independently or assist with repositioning.

  e. Does the support surface have a potential to interfere with the patient's independent functioning? The height of the overlay and its soft edge may affect a patient's ability to transfer, and a high-air-loss bed is inappropriate for a patient who needs to get in and out of bed frequently.

  f. What are the patient's financial limitations?

  g. If the patient is using the device in the home, what are the environmental limitations? Will the home and existing electrical service accommodate the surface selected? Can the family caregivers in the home manage the surface?

  h. What is the durability of the product? Is the surface easily subjected to puncture? What is the ease of cleaning the surface?

7. Determine the specific redistribution device (see Table 25-3).

  a. Pressure-redistribution devices redistribute pressure over bony prominences. Surfaces providing pressure redistribution include therapeutic mattress replacements, nonpowered and powered (i.e., moving) surfaces, low-air-loss beds and mattresses, and air-fluidized beds (Nix and Mackey, 2012). Pressure-redistribution surfaces are also used in the operating room for patients who are at high risk or undergoing lengthy procedures.

  b. Use a nonpowered support surface if the patient can assume a variety of positions without bearing weight on a pressure ulcer and without bottoming out. Bottoming out makes the support surface ineffective. To assess for bottoming out, place a hand (palm up) under the mattress or cushion below the area of risk for pressure areas (e.g., patient's pressure points when lying or sitting on surface). If less than 2.5 cm (1 inch) of support material is felt, patient has bottomed out (WOCN, 2010).

  c. Select a powered support surface when patient cannot assume a variety of positions without bearing weight on a pressure ulcer, if patient fully compresses the static support surface, or if the pressure ulcer does not show evidence of healing. Alternating or powered mattresses are associated with a lower incidence of pressure ulcers than standard mattresses (Nix and Mackey, 2012).

  d. Patients with stage III or IV pressure ulcers on multiple turning surfaces may benefit from an air-fluidized bed (Nix and Mackey, 2012; WOCN, 2010).

  e. There is limited evidence that low-air-loss beds reduce the incidence of pressure ulcers in intensive care (WOCN, 2010).

  f. When excess moisture is a potential risk, a support surface that provides airflow is important in drying the skin and reducing the incidence of pressure ulcers (NPUAP/EPUAP, 2009).

8. Check facility policy regarding implementing support surface.

  a. Obtain a health care provider's order; this is usually required for a patient to obtain third-party reimbursement.

  b. Consult with facility case manager or social worker to assist with patient's financial eligibility and terms and length of third-party reimbursement for the surface.

  c. Consult with facility home care or discharge planning if the device is anticipated for long-term use. Specific procedures and evaluations are needed for continuity of surface when patient is transferred to extended care or discharged home.

9. Inspect condition of skin regularly according to facility policy to evaluate changes in skin and effectiveness of therapy.

10. Observe existing pressure ulcers for evidence of healing.

11. Observe for side effects associated with specific pressure-reducing surface (e.g., changes in fluid and electrolyte status).

12. Document pressure ulcer risk assessment and skin assessment in the patient's record.

13. Document the support surface selected and patient response to the surface (see specific skills for recording and reporting details).

CATEGORY AND MECHANISM OF ACTION	INDICATIONS FOR USE	ADVANTAGES	DISADVANTAGES
Support Surfaces and Overlays			
Foam Overlays (Available as Overlay, Full Mattress, or as Chair Cushion)			
Redistributes pressure; the cover (top) reduces friction and shear; base height of 7.5-10 cm (3-4 inches); see manufacturer's guidelines regarding amount of body weight supported.	Use for moderate- to high-risk patients	One-time charge No setup fee Cannot be punctured Available in various sizes (e.g., bed, chair, operating room table) Little maintenance, low cost Does not need electricity	Elevated patient body temperature May trap moisture Limited life span Plastic protective sheet needed for incontinent patients or patients with draining wounds
Fluid Fill Overlays (Available as Overlay or in Full Mattress)			
Chambers filled with water or viscous fluid (gel, silicon elastomer, or polyvinyl). Permit a high degree of immersion allowing the body to sink into the surface, increasing the surface pressure distribution area and lowering the interface pressure.	Use for high-risk patients	Readily available Easy to clean	Easily punctured Heavy Fluid motion (in the water mattress) may make procedures (e.g., dressing changes, CPR) difficult Maintenance needed to prevent microorganism growth (water mattress) Patient transfers out of bed are difficult
Nonpowered Air-Filled Overlays			
Reduce pressure by lowering mean interface pressure between patient's tissues and mattress.	Use for moderate- to high-risk patients Use for patients who can reposition themselves	Easy to clean; multiple-patient use Low maintenance Potential repair of some air-filled products Durable	Damaged by punctures from needles and sharps Require routine monitoring to determine adequate inflation pressure Patient transfers out of bed difficult
Low-Air-Loss Overlays (Available in Full Bed or Overlay)			
Maintain constant and slight air movement against skin to prevent buildup of moisture and skin maceration.	Use for moderate- to high-risk patients	Easy to clean Maintain constant inflation Deflate to facilitate transfer and CPR Control moisture Air permeable, bacteria impermeable, and waterproof fabric covering overlay Reduce shear and friction Setup provided by manufacturer	Damaged by needles and sharps Noisy Require electricity
Specialty Beds			
Air-Fluidized Beds			
Bedframe contains silicone-coated beads and incorporates both air and fluid support. The silicone-coated beads become fluidized when air is pumped through the beads. Air-fluidized beds permit the highest degree of immersion among support surfaces.	Use for high-risk patients Use for patients with stage III or IV pressure ulcers or burns	Quickly become firm for CPR or other treatments when device is turned off Reduce shear, friction, and edema to site May facilitate management of copious wound drainage or incontinence Setup provided by manufacturer	Patient risk for dehydration, especially in patients with severe burns, possibly increased by continuous circulation of warm, dry air Possible increase in room temperature Possible patient disorientation Patient transfer difficult Heavy Expensive May not be wide enough for use for obese patients or patients with contractures

Continued

TABLE 25-3	SUPPORT SURFACES—cont'd		
CATEGORY AND MECHANISM OF ACTION	**INDICATIONS FOR USE**	**ADVANTAGES**	**DISADVANTAGES**
Low-Air-Loss Beds Bedframe with a series of connected air-filled pillows; amount of pressure in each pillow controlled and can be calibrated to patient need. Patient's weight is distributed more evenly for pressure redistribution (Nix and Mackey, 2012).	Use is indicated in patients who cannot be repositioned frequently or patients who have skin breakdown on more than one surface Contraindicated in patients with unstable spinal column	Can raise and lower head and foot of bed Easy transfer in and out of bed Less frequent turning schedule Can transfer pillows to stretcher with patient Setup provided by manufacturer	Requires portable motor that is noisy Bed surface material slippery; patients can easily slide down mattress or out of bed when being transferred
Continuous Lateral Rotation Provides continuous rotation to promote mobilization of pulmonary secretions and provides low air loss, which provides pressure redistribution.	Thought to be useful for pulmonary therapy by positioning patient in such a way that one lung is higher than the other to prevent pneumonia	May reduce pulmonary complications associated with restricted mobility	Does not reduce shear or moisture, and the risk for shear injury exists (NPUAP/EPUAP, 2009)

CPR, Cardiopulmonary resuscitation.
Data from Bryant RA, Nix DP: *Acute and chronic wounds: nursing management,* ed 4, St Louis, 2012, Mosby; and Baranoski S, Ayello EA: *Wound care essentials,* ed 3, Philadelphia, 2012 Lippincott Williams & Wilkins.

SKILL 25.2 TREATMENT OF PRESSURE ULCERS AND WOUND MANAGEMENT

• **Nursing Skills Online: Wound Care Module, Lesson 4**

Treatment of a patient with a pressure ulcer includes systematic support of the patient, reduction or elimination of the cause of the skin breakdown, and wound management that provides an environment conducive to healing. Wound healing does not occur or occurs slowly in a malnourished patient or a patient with poor cardiovascular status; measures are needed to support the patient systemically. Other factors that impede wound healing include immunosuppressive therapy and uncontrolled diabetes mellitus.

The cause of a wound must be assessed before wound therapy is instituted. If the contributing causes of a pressure ulcer (pressure, shear, friction, moisture) are not addressed, the tissue damage continues, and healing does not occur. A wound environment conducive to healing is achieved by using topical wound therapy with the following objectives: control or eliminate causative factors, provide systemic support to reduce existing and potential cofactors, prevent and manage infection, cleanse the wound, remove nonviable tissue, maintain appropriate level of moisture, eliminate dead space, control odor, eliminate or minimize pain, and protect the periwound skin (Berlowitz, 2014b; Rolstad et al., 2012). The choice of topical treatment (dressings and solutions) is dictated by these objectives. Ongoing monitoring evaluates the effectiveness of wound care.

ASSESSMENT

1. Assess patient's level of comfort on a pain scale of 0 to 10. If patient is in pain, determine if a prn medication has been ordered and administer along with appropriate non-pharmacological strategies (see Chapter 13). Ibuprofen-releasing foam dressings are now available for use in conjunction with other routes of pain relief (Berlowitz, 2014b). *Rationale: Maintains patient comfort during the dressing change.*

2. Determine if patient is allergic to topical agents. *Rationale: Topical agents contain elements that may cause localized skin reactions.*

3. Identify reasons for pressure ulcer. *Rationale: Failure to address causative factors results in a nonhealing wound (Rolstad et al., 2012).*
4. Review medical order for topical agents or dressings. *Rationale: Ensures that right patient receives proper medication and treatment.*
5. Identify patient using two identifiers (e.g., name and birthday or name and account number) according to facility policy. *Rationale: Ensures correct patient. Complies with The Joint Commission standards and improves patient safety (TJC, 2014).*
6. ![hand hygiene icon] Perform hand hygiene and apply clean gloves. Assess patient's wounds using the following wound parameters, and continue ongoing wound assessment per facility protocol. Note: This may be done during procedure after dressing removal. *Rationale: Determines effectiveness of wound care and drives the treatment plan of care (Berlowitz, 2014a; WOCN, 2010).*
   a. *Wound location:* Describe the body site where the wound is located.
   b. *Stage of wound:* Describe the extent of tissue destruction (Table 25-4). Staging is not done if the wound etiology is something other than pressure.
   c. *Wound size:* Length, width, and depth of the wound are measured per facility protocol. Use a disposable measuring guide for length and width. Use a cotton-tipped applicator to assess depth (Fig. 25-3).
   d. *Presence of undermining, sinus tracts, or tunnels:* Use a sterile cotton-tipped applicator to measure depth and, if needed, a gloved finger to examine the wound edges.
   e. *Condition of the wound bed:* Describe the type and percentage of tissue in the wound bed.
   f. *Volume of exudate:* Describe the amount, characteristics, odor, and color.
   g. *Condition of periwound skin:* Examine the skin for breaks; dryness; and the presence of a rash, swelling, redness, or warmth.
   h. *Wound edges:* Gives information regarding epithelialization, chronicity, and etiology (Berlowitz, 2014a; Berlowitz, 2014b; Rolstad, 2012).
   i. *Presence of pain:* Note pain at or around the wounded area; have patient rate pain on scale of 0 to 10.
7. Observe for factors affecting wound healing, including poor perfusion, immunosuppression, or preexisting infection.
8. Assess for significant weight loss (>5% change in 30 days or >10% in 180 days) (NPUAP/EPUAP, 2009). *Rationale: Patients with pressure ulcers who are underweight or losing weight need enhanced caloric and protein supplements (Berlowitz, 2014b; WOCN, 2010).*
9. Assess patient's and family caregiver's understanding of pressure ulcer characteristics and purpose of treatment. *Rationale: Explanations relieve anxiety and promote cooperation during procedure.*

PLANNING

Expected Outcomes focus on healing ulcer and preventing further skin breakdown.
1. Ulcer drainage decreases.
2. Granulation tissue is present in wound base.
3. Nutritional intake reaches ordered 24-hour calorie and nutrient level.
4. Patient's skin is protected from further breakdown.

Delegation and Collaboration
The skill of treatment of pressure ulcers and wound management may not be delegated to nursing assistive personnel (NAP). The nurse instructs the NAP about the following:
- Any patient-specific position changes.
- Observing and reporting back to you any redness, break in patient's skin, irritation from adhesive or medical devices, or areas of changing tissue consistency.

Equipment
- Clean gloves
- Sterile gloves (optional)
- Goggles and cover gown (if splash is a risk)
- Plastic bag for dressing disposal
- Wound-measuring device
- Cotton-tipped applicators
- Normal saline or cleansing agent (as ordered)
- Topical agent or solution (as ordered)
- Dressings
- Hypoallergenic tape if needed

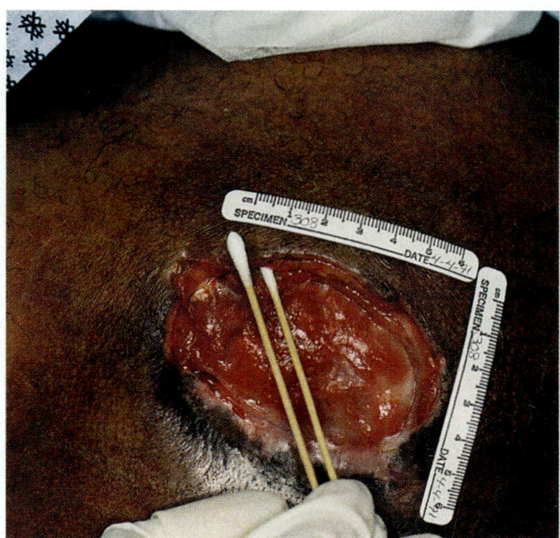

FIG 25-3 Measuring depth of a pressure ulcer.

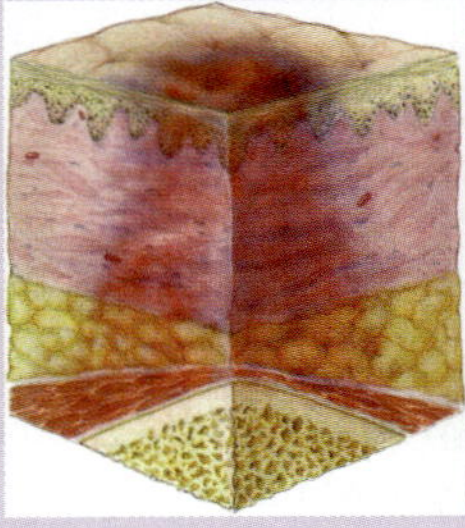 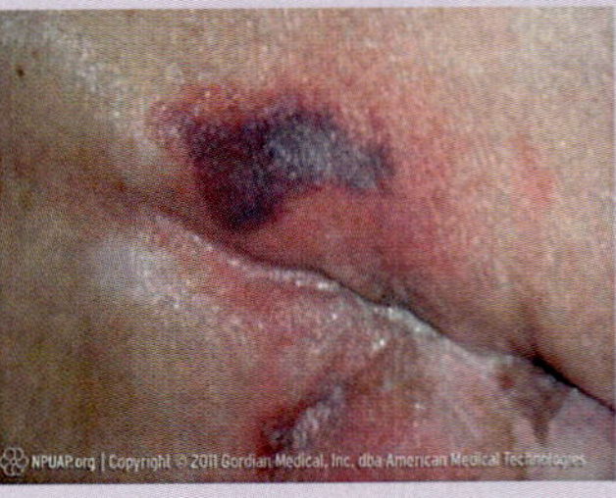

Suspected Deep Tissue Injury

Purple or maroon localized area of discolored intact skin or blood-filled blister resulting from damage of underlying soft tissue from pressure and/or shear. The area may be preceded by tissue that is painful, firm, mushy, boggy, warmer, or cooler compared with adjacent tissue. Deep tissue injury may be difficult to detect in patients with dark skin tones. Evolution may include a thin blister over a dark wound bed. The wound may further evolve and become covered by thin eschar. Evolution may be rapid, exposing additional layers of tissue even with optimal treatment.

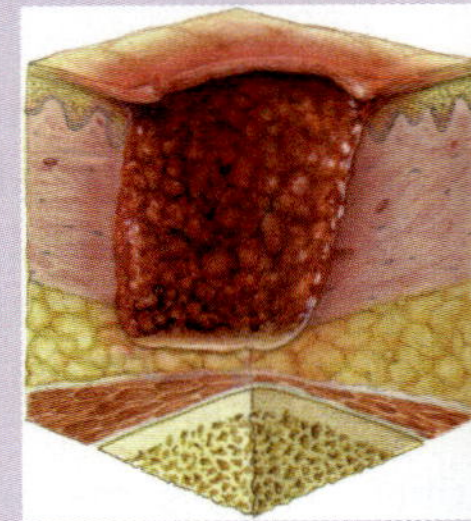 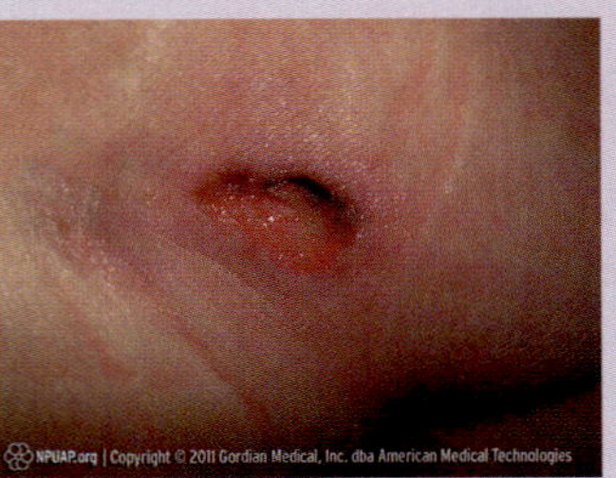

Stage III

Full-thickness tissue loss. Subcutaneous fat may be visible, but bone, tendon, or muscle is *not* exposed. Slough may be present but does not obscure depth of tissue loss. *May* include undermining and tunneling. The depth of a stage III pressure ulcer varies by anatomical location. The bridge of the nose, ear, occiput, and malleolus do not have (adipose) subcutaneous tissue, and stage III ulcers can be shallow. In contrast, areas of significant adiposity can develop extremely deep stage III pressure ulcers. Bone or tendon is not visible or directly palpable.

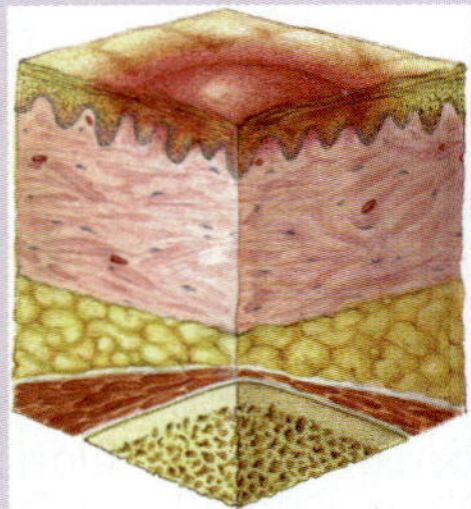 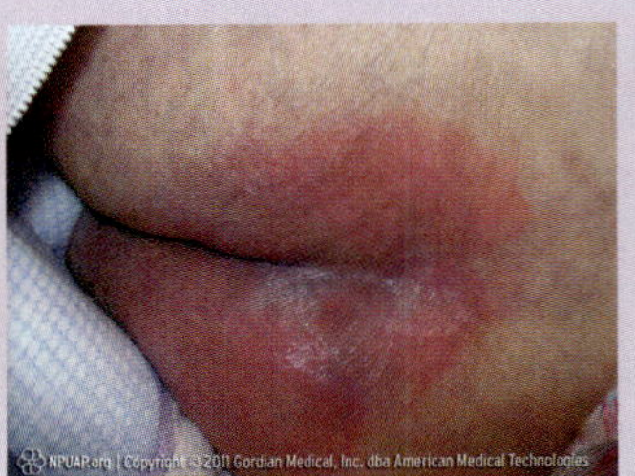

Stage I

Intact skin with nonblanchable redness of a localized area usually over a bony prominence. Darkly pigmented skin may not have visible blanching; color may differ from the surrounding area. The area may be painful, firm, soft, warmer, or cooler compared with adjacent tissue. Stage I may be difficult to detect in patients with dark skin tones. May indicate "at risk" patients.

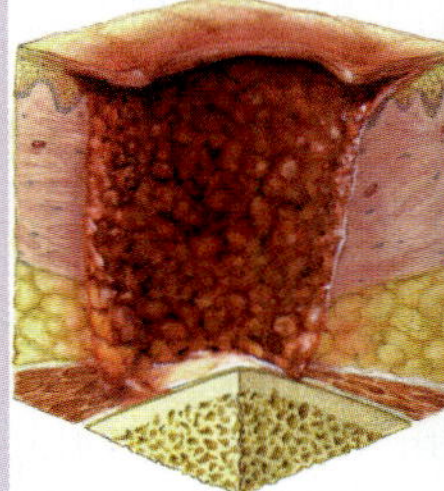 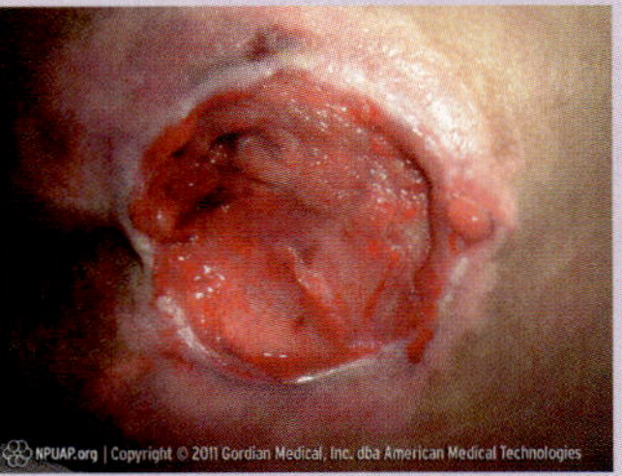

Stage IV

Full-thickness tissue loss with exposed bone, tendon, or muscle. Slough or eschar may be present. Often includes undermining and tunneling. The depth of a stage IV pressure ulcer varies by anatomical location. The bridge of the nose, ear, occiput, and malleolus do not have (adipose) subcutaneous tissue, and these ulcers can be shallow. Stage IV ulcers can extend into muscle or supporting structures (e.g., fascia, tendon, or joint capsule) making osteomyelitis or osteitis likely to occur. Exposed bone or muscle is visible or directly palpable.

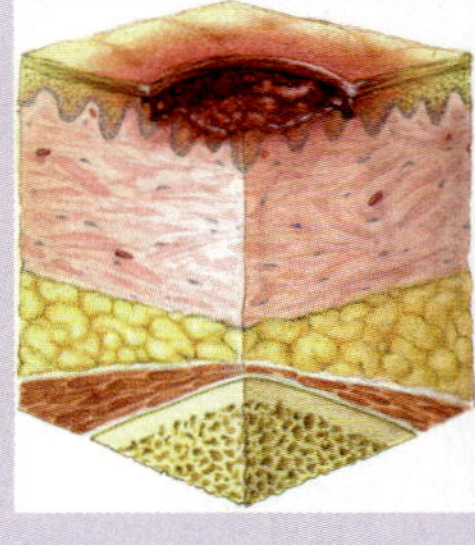 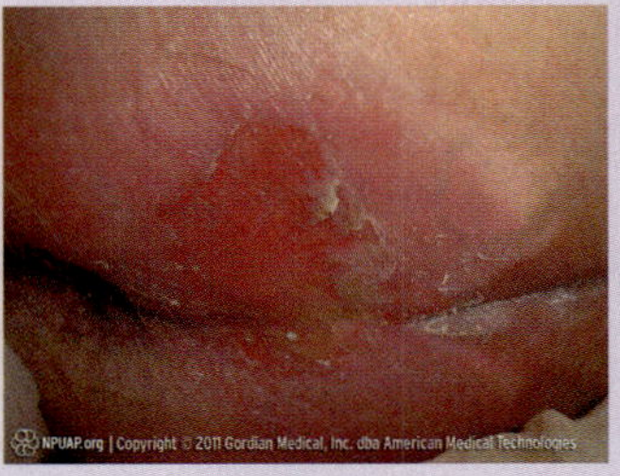

Stage II

Partial-thickness loss of dermis manifesting as a shallow open ulcer with a red-pink wound bed, without slough. May also manifest as an intact or open or ruptured serum-filled or serosanguineous fluid–filled blister. Manifests as a shiny or dry, shallow ulcer without slough or bruising.* This category should not be used to describe skin tears, tape burns, incontinence-associated dermatitis, maceration, or excoriation.

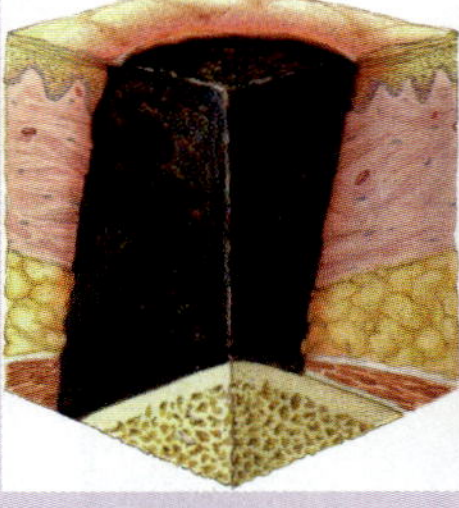 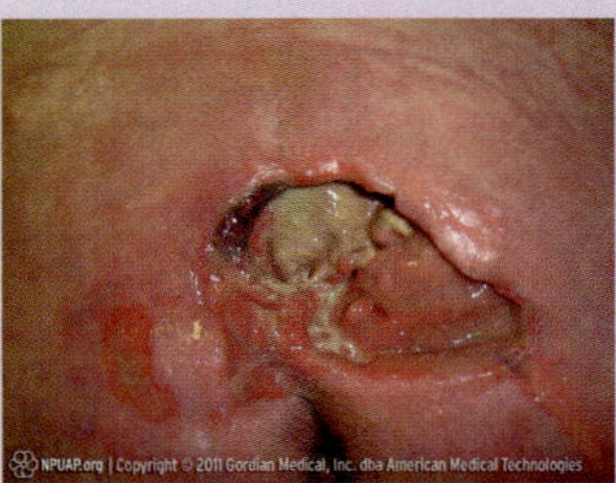

Unstageable

Full-thickness tissue loss in which actual depth of the ulcer is completely obscured by slough (yellow, tan, gray, green, or brown) or eschar (tan, brown, or black) or both in the wound bed. Until enough slough or eschar or both are removed to expose the base of the wound, the true depth cannot be determined, but it will be either a stage III or IV. Stable (dry, adherent, intact without erythema or fluctuance) eschar on the heels serves as "the body's natural (biological) cover" and should not be removed.

*Bruising indicates deep tissue injury.
Data from National Pressure Ulcer Advisory Panel (NPUAP): *Pressure ulcer stages revised by NPUAP,* 2007, http://www.npuap.org/pr2.htm. Accessed March 31, 2014. Photos courtesy Laurel Wiersma, RN, MSN, CNS, Barnes-Jewish Hospital, St Louis, Missouri.

IMPLEMENTATION *for* TREATMENT OF PRESSURE ULCERS AND WOUND MANAGEMENT

STEPS	RATIONALE

1. See Standard Protocol (inside front cover).

2. Select pressure ulcer management based on patient's condition and reason for pressure ulcer care:

a. Prevent and manage infection. — Infected wounds do not heal.

b. Cleanse wound. — Removes surface bacteria.

c. Remove nonviable tissue that promotes infection. — Many dressings support softening and eventual loosening of nonviable tissue.

d. Maintain appropriate level of moisture. — A moist environment supports wound healing.

e. Eliminate dead space. — Prevents exudate buildup.

f. Control odor.

g. Eliminate or minimize pain.

h. Protect periwound skin.

i. Manage incontinence. — Moisture from urine and liquid stool macerates skin and carries microorganisms.

3. Consult with health care provider or wound care specialist in selecting appropriate dressing (Table 25-5) based on pressure ulcer assessment, principles of wound management, and patient care setting. Dressing options include: — The dressing provides an appropriate wound-healing environment (Berlowitz, 2014b; WOCN, 2010).

a. Gauze pads. — Used for wicking, maintaining a moist environment, packing, and delivering solutions to a wound.

b. Transparent film dressings. — Used on shallow partial-thickness wounds with minimal wound exudate.

c. Hydrogel (available in a sheet or in a tube). — Maintains moist environment to facilitate wound healing.

d. Hydrocolloid. — Maintains moist environment to facilitate wound healing while protecting wound base.

e. Alginate dressings. — Highly absorbent of wound exudate in heavily draining wounds.

f. Foam dressings. — Protective and prevent wound dehydration; absorbs drainage. Maintain moist environment.

g. Silver-impregnated dressings and gels. — Control bacterial burden in wound.

h. Enzymatic débriding agents. — Promote removal of devitalized tissue.

i. Wound fillers. — Fill shallow wounds, hydrate, and absorb.

j. Antimicrobials. — Control or decrease bioburden. Include antibacterials and antiseptics.

4. Open packages and topical solution containers. — Prepares supplies for easy application so that you can use supplies without contaminating them.

5. Position patient to expose ulcer, keeping rest of body covered with bed linen. — Prevents unnecessary exposure of body parts.

6. Apply clean gloves. Remove old dressings and discard in plastic bag. Discard gloves; perform hand hygiene. This is a time when you can assess the wound.

7. Apply clean gloves. Cleanse wound with prescribed solution, cleansing from least contaminated to most contaminated area. Rinse with solution; gently wipe wound base and surrounding skin with moistened gauze. Use fresh piece of moistened gauze to clean skin surface; dry with fresh dry gauze. — Reduces surface bacteria; removes wound exudate or dressing residue.

8. Apply topical agents to wound using cotton-tipped applicators or gauze as ordered:

a. *Antibacterials:* Examples include bacitracin, metronidazole, and silver sulfadiazine. — Destroy or stop bacterial growth.

Continued

STEPS	RATIONALE
b. *Antiseptics:* Examples include acetic acid and hypochlorite (Dakin's solution).	Reduce bacteria on the wound surface. Use is limited because of cell toxicity.
c. *Enzyme débriding agents:* Cover wound with débriding agent and apply a moist gauze dressing over wound.	Remove dead tissue. Moisture must be present for enzyme preparation to work.
9. Apply prescribed wound dressing:	
a. *Moist dressing* (see Chapter 26):	
(1) Apply saline to gauze; wring out excess.	Dampens gauze, allowing gauze to "wick" drainage.
(2) Unfold gauze and, if wound has depth, loosely pack it with the dressing; if shallow, lay gauze over wound.	Unfolded gauze allows for wicking of drainage.
(3) Cover with secondary dry dressing; tape dressing over wound.	
b. *Transparent film dressings* (see Chapter 26).	Applied over superficial wounds only.
c. *Hydrogel:*	Hydrogel maintains moist environment to facilitate wound healing.
(1) Cover wound base with a thick layer of amorphous hydrogel or cut a sheet to fit wound base.	
(2) Cover with secondary dressing; tape.	
(3) If using impregnated gauze, pack loosely into wound; cover with secondary gauze dressing, and tape.	Loosely packed dressing delivers gel to the wound base and allows any wound debris to be trapped in the gauze.
d. *Hydrocolloid* (see Chapter 26):	
(1) Choose a hydrocolloid that extends beyond the wound base by 1 inch. The release paper is removed and applied over the cleaned wound (periwound edges must be dry for adherence).	Hydrocolloid forms a gel over the wounded area; the outer edge creates the seal.
e. *Alginate:*	
(1) Cut to size of wound and loosely pack into wound.	Dressing swells and increases in size; tight packing can compromise blood flow to tissues.
(2) Cover with a secondary gauze dressing; apply tape.	
f. *Foam dressings* **(see Chapter 26).**	Protective; prevents wound dehydration; absorbs small-to-moderate amount of drainage.
10. Reposition patient comfortably off wound.	
11. **See Completion Protocol (inside front cover).**	

TABLE 25-5	DRESSING SELECTION BASED ON WOUND ASSESSMENT		
WOUND DESCRIPTION	**REQUIREMENTS**	**RATIONALE**	**DRESSING OPTIONS**
Necrotic tissue	Débridement	Removal of dead tissue decreases risk of bacterial overgrowth and facilitates healing (healing will not take place in the presence of devitalized tissue).	Consider a dressing that traps the moisture from the wound (e.g., hydrogel, impregnated gauze, hydrocolloid) over the necrotic tissue, allowing the tissue to soften and be removed (autolysis). *Or* Consider use of enzyme preparations for chemical débridement.
Granulation tissue	Protection	Support granulation tissue with a moist environment to facilitate healing.	Consider the use of hydrocolloid, hydrogel, or foam dressing to maintain moisture.

TABLE 25-5	**DRESSING SELECTION BASED ON WOUND ASSESSMENT—cont'd**		
WOUND DESCRIPTION	**REQUIREMENTS**	**RATIONALE**	**DRESSING OPTIONS**
Dry wound base	Hydration	A moist wound base facilitates healing by providing a surface for new cells to migrate.	Consider use of a hydrogel to bring moisture to the wound. *Or* Consider use of gauze with saline to provide moisture to the wound.
Moderate-to-heavy exudate	Absorption	Excess wound drainage overhydrates cells, delaying healing and macerating the periwound skin.	Consider the use of a hydrocolloid, foam, alginate, or hydrofiber dressing, all of which absorb various amounts of drainage.
Significant depth	Packing	Packing prevents wound drainage from accumulating in the dead space of the deep wound.	Consider the use of gauze, alginate, or wound filler; pack lightly into the defect to fill the wound.
Erythema, warmth, edema, tenderness	Infection management	Wound infection prolongs the inflammatory response, delaying wound healing.	Antimicrobial dressings or solutions decrease bacterial overload.
Periwound skin maceration	Protection	Maceration can cause further skin breakdown and discomfort.	Skin sealant or barrier ointment provides protection.

EVALUATION

1. Observe skin surrounding wound for inflammation, edema, and tenderness.
2. Inspect dressings and exposed wounds; observe for drainage, foul odor, and tissue necrosis. Monitor patient for signs and symptoms of infection, including fever and elevated white blood cell count.
3. Compare subsequent wound measurements with each dressing change.
4. Ask patient to rate pain on a scale of 0 to 10 during and after pressure ulcer care.
5. Use *Teach Back:* State to the patient, "I want to be sure that I provided you with a clear description of how pressure ulcers develop and why we are cleansing the wound with normal saline and applying a hydrocolloid dressing. Can you and your sister describe the dressing change process to me?" Evaluates what the patient or family caregiver is able to explain or demonstrate. Revise your instruction now or develop plan for revised patient teaching to be implemented at an appropriate time if patient is not able to teach back correctly.

Unexpected Outcomes and Related Interventions

1. Skin surrounding ulcer becomes macerated.
   a. Reduce exposure of surrounding skin to topical agents and moisture.
   b. Consider use of a liquid skin barrier on periwound skin.
2. Ulcer becomes deeper with increased drainage or development of necrotic tissue.

   a. Notify health care provider for possible change in pressure ulcer status.
   b. Additional consultations (e.g., wound care nurse specialist) may be indicated.
   c. Obtain necessary wound cultures.

Recording and Reporting

- Record appearance and condition of ulcer, type of topical agent or dressing used, and patient's response in medical record.
- Report any deterioration in ulcer appearance.
- Document your evaluation of patient learning.

Sample Documentation

0900   Sacral pressure ulcer, stage II, 2 × 3 cm irregular shape. Base of wound covered 100% by granulation tissue; no drainage or odor present. Surrounding skin intact. Wound cleansed with NS and hydrocolloid dressing applied. On a low-air-loss overlay, repositioned q 2 hr as condition allowed. Nutritional supplements taken as offered. Patient and sister instructed in care and prevention of skin breakdown and correctly described wound cleansing and dressing change.

Special Considerations

Pediatric

- Reinforce wound dressings in the diaper zone with a water-resistant tape. Carefully remove this tape to avoid skin stripping.

Geriatric

- Skin in older adults has a slower and less intense inflammatory reaction; closely monitor older patients.

Home Care

- The bed at home should have the appropriate type of support surface.
- Ensure that patient and family caregiver know how to use the wound products chosen.
- Choose a dressing that does not require multiple dressing changes in a 24-hour period. This decreases the amount of time that the family will need to pay to the wound management program, increases compliance, and makes good use of home care resources.

CRITICAL THINKING EXERCISES

Case Study

A man is admitted to a surgical unit after a small bowel resection. He is currently NPO and has had frequent loose stools and several incontinence episodes. He is alert and oriented but notes that he has abdominal discomfort when he moves. He has been wheelchair bound for several months following complications from hip surgery. His wife also has health issues and has been unable to provide direct care to her husband at home.

1. The nurse is assessing the patient for pressure ulcer risk using the Braden Scale. Under the moisture subscale, she has determined that the patient's skin moisture is related to fecal incontinence. What are two interventions that the nurse can consider as the plan of care to reduce the effects of skin moisture?
   1. Application of talcum powder in areas where stool is in contact with the skin
   2. Use of a moisture barrier ointment after each bowel movement
   3. A fecal incontinence collector
   4. Placing several towels under patient's buttocks
2. During the patient's skin assessment, the nurse notes redness with partial-thickness skin loss around the anus and onto the buttocks. The nurse is unsure if this is a pressure ulcer and wonders if the wound needs staging. Which of the following statements is the correct assessment of the patient's skin issues?
   1. This is a nonstageable wound, and the area should be left open to air and assessed at a regularly scheduled interval.
   2. Taking into account the patient's frequent stools, it is likely that the skin breakdown is from incontinence (and not a pressure ulcer), and this type of skin breakdown would not be staged.
3. Consider the stage of this as a partial-thickness pressure ulcer, which would be stage II, III. The nurse assigned to this patient is working with a nursing assistive personnel (NAP). Which of the following activities can be delegated? Select all that apply.
   1. Perianal skin assessment following perineal hygiene
   2. Positioning to 30-degree lateral position
   3. Transfer from bed to chair.
   4. Identification of patient discomfort.

Review Questions

1. Which of the following patients have factors that can impair wound healing? Select all that apply.
   1. A patient whose surgical wound is producing yellowish drainage and whose white blood cell count is elevated
   2. A patient with cancer receiving the antiinflammatory drug cortisol
   3. An older-adult patient who has been advised to add more sources of vitamin C to her diet
   4. A trauma patient who has an open wound that is being treated with a moist dressing
2. A 71-year-old patient has been in the intensive care unit for 48 hours. She has an ET tube inserted through the mouth to maintain ventilation. She has an intravenous (IV) line infusing at 125 mL/hr. Her abdominal incision over the right lower quadrant is dry and intact. The nurses have placed pillows under both calves to suspend the ankles. Turning the patient is difficult because she weighs 145.45 kg (320 pounds). She is most likely to be at risk for pressure ulcers in which of the following locations? Select all that apply.
   1. Heels
   2. Posterior bony prominences
   3. Nose
   4. Mouth
   5. IV site
3. When using gauze moistened in normal saline for a wound dressing, why is the gauze pad wrung out before application?
   1. To prevent excessive delivery of the solution to the wound
   2. To keep the healing wound moist and wick any excessive drainage
   3. To prevent moistening the secondary dressing and causing maceration
   4. To allow the wound to become slightly dry to facilitate healing
4. What is the primary mechanism of action of a hydrocolloid dressing?
   1. It covers the wound, preventing staff members or the patient from viewing the affected area.
   2. It forms a gel over the wound to facilitate moist wound healing.
   3. It forms a temporary membrane over the wound, allowing oxygen transport directly to the wound.
   4. It delivers epithelial growth factors to the wound base.

5. The dressing ordered for a patient's sacral pressure ulcer is a hydrocolloid dressing. Place the following steps in appropriate order for the dressing application:
   a. Cleanse wound with ordered solution.
   b. Remove paper backing from dressing.
   c. Explain to patient the purpose of the dressing change.
   d. Position patient to gain access to the pressure ulcer.
   e. Select hydrocolloid dressing that extends 1 inch beyond wound base.
   f. Place dressing over wound; apply light pressure for 30 to 60 seconds.
   1. a, c, e, f, b, d
   2. c, d, a, e, b, f
   3. c, d, a, e, b, f
   4. e, a, c, d, b, f

6. Which of the following patients is most at risk for developing a pressure ulcer?
   1. An 80-year-old adult with Alzheimer's disease who has poor oral intake
   2. A 45-year-old man who is confined to a wheelchair as a result of paraplegia
   3. A 50-year-old man with type 1 diabetes who underwent major heart surgery 24 hours ago and has diaphoresis
   4. A 60-year-old woman who underwent bladder surgery and now has urinary incontinence

7. A patient is admitted to the intensive care unit with pneumonia and renal failure. He is receiving IV fluids of D_5 ½ NS and is NPO. He has been diaphoretic and febrile and requires linen changes each shift. He is able to turn in bed but requires reminding. He is confined to bed. He is able to respond verbally and describe sources of discomfort. Which category on the Braden Scale is not included in this assessment?
   1. Nutrition
   2. Activity
   3. Frictional shear
   4. Moisture

8. When taking care of a patient on an air fluidized bed, which of the following complications should be considered?
   1. Back pain because of the lack of firm support
   2. Dehydration because of the amount of warm circulating air
   3. Problems moving the patient out of the bed because of the body submersion
   4. Lack of healing of the pressure ulcer because of the high skin/bed pressures
   5. Difficulty moving this bed to another location because of the weight

9. Choose four factors that impede wound healing:
   1. Shear/friction
   2. High calcium levels
   3. Poor nutrition
   4. Hypothyroidism
   5. Lack of family support

10. Which of the following explains why an obese patient is at risk for poor wound healing?
    1. Loose tissue cannot regenerate.
    2. Fat is poorly perfused and cannot heal quickly.
    3. An obese patient stretches the healing tissue when moving.
    4. Dehydration is a problem for an obese patient.

REFERENCES

Ayello EA, et al: Pressure ulcers. In Baranoski S, Ayello EA, editors: *Wound care essentials: practice principles*, ed 3, Philadelphia, 2012, Lippincott Williams & Wilkins.

Ayello EA, Braden B: How and why to do pressure ulcer risk assessment, *Adv Skin Wound Care* 15(3):125, 2002.

Baharestani MM: Quality of life and ethical issues. In Baranoski S, Ayello EA, editors: *Wound care essentials: practice principles*, ed 3, Philadelphia, 2012, Lippincott Williams & Wilkins.

Baranoski S, et al: Wound assessment. In Baranoski S, Ayello EA, editors: *Wound care essentials: practice principles*, ed 3, Philadelphia, 2012, Lippincott Williams & Wilkins.

Berlowitz D: Prevention of pressure ulcers, *UpToDate* 2014a. http://www.uptodate.com/contents/prevention-of-pressure-ulcers.

Berlowitz D: Treatment of pressure ulcers, *UpToDate* 2014b. http://www.uptodate.com/contents/treatment-of-pressure-ulcers.

Braden BJ, Bergstrom N: Clinical utility of the Braden Scale for predicting pressure sore risk, *Decubitus* 2(3):441, 1989.

Chou R, et al: Pressure ulcer risk assessment and prevention, *Ann Intern Med* 159(1):28, 2013.

Doughty D, Sparks-Defriese B: Wound-healing physiology. In Bryant RA, Nix DP, editors: *Acute and chronic wounds: current management concepts*, ed 4, St Louis, 2012, Mosby.

Fletcher J: Device related pressure ulcers made easy, *Wounds UK* 8(2):1, 2012.

Lewis S, et al: *Medical-surgical nursing: assessment and management of clinical problems*, ed 9, St Louis, 2014, Elsevier.

McNichol L, et al: Medical adhesives and patient safety: state of the science: consensus statements for the assessment, prevention, and treatment of adhesive-related skin injuries, *J Wound Ostomy Continence Nurs* 40(4):365, 2013.

Mulgrew S, et al: Pressure necrosis secondary to negative pressure dressing, *Ann R Coll Surg Engl* 93(5):e27, 2011.

National Pressure Ulcer Advisory Panel (NPUAP)/European Pressure Ulcer Advisory Panel (EPUAP): *Prevention and treatment of pressure ulcers: clinical practice guideline*, Washington, DC, 2009, National Pressure Ulcer Advisory Panel.

Nix D, Mackey DM: Support surfaces. In Bryant RA, Nix DP, editors: *Acute and chronic wounds: current management concepts*, ed 4, St Louis, 2012, Mosby.

Pham B, et al: Support surfaces for intraoperative prevention of pressure ulcers in patients undergoing surgery: a cost-effectiveness analysis, *Surgery* 150(1):122, 2011.

Pieper B: Pressure ulcers: impact, etiology and classification. In Bryant RA, Nix DP, editors: *Acute and chronic wounds: current management concepts*, ed 4, St Louis, 2012, Mosby.

Rolstad BS, et al: Topical management. In Bryant RA, Nix DP, editors: *Acute and chronic wounds: current management concepts*, ed 4, St Louis, 2012, Mosby.

Siddiqui A, et al: A continuous bedside pressure mapping system for prevention of pressure ulcer development in the ICU, *Wounds* 25(12):333, 2013.

Stotts NA: Nutritional assessment and support. In Bryant RA, Nix DP, editors: *Acute and chronic wounds: current management concepts*, ed 4, St Louis, 2012, Mosby.

Sullivan N, Schoelles KM: Preventing in facility pressure ulcers as a patient safety strategy: a systematic review, *Ann Intern Med* 158(5 Pt 2):410, 2013.

Sutton S, et al: A quality improvement project for safe and effective patient positioning during robot-assisted surgery, *AORN* 97(4):448, 2013.

The Joint Commission (TJC): *National Patient Safety Goals*, Oakbrook Terrace, IL, 2014, The Commission. Available at: http://www.jointcommission.org/standards_information/npsgs.aspx.

Wound, Ostomy and Continence Nurses Society (WOCN): *Guideline for prevention and management of pressure ulcers*, *WOCN Clinical Practice Guidelines Series*, Mount Laurel, NJ, 2010, Wound, Ostomy and Continence Nurses Society (WOCN).

Dressings, Bandages, and Binders

Wound healing is complex physiologically. Dressings are an important part of this process because of their ability to control moisture, débride dead tissue, and protect a wound. Numerous dressings and products are available for managing acute and chronic wounds (Table 26-1). A primary dressing is a protective cover that comes in direct contact with a wound bed. Secondary dressings cover or secure a primary dressing in place (Rolstad et al., 2011). It is important to match the wound characteristics, goals of wound management, and properties of an "ideal" dressing (Box 26-1).

The type and condition of the wound bed, surrounding periwound, and type and amount of drainage determine the type of dressing to use. For example, alginates are highly absorbent, whereas hydrogels are excellent for wound débridement (Meaume et al., 2011). This chapter reviews principles of wound care, compares wound care products, and reviews the proper techniques for the application of dressings.

The removal of necrotic tissue or slough is a component of wound healing because it allows for growth of new tissue. Certain dressings have débriding properties. The traditional tissue débriding method is the moist-to-dry dressing. Although effective, this type of dressing can be harmful to healthy granulating tissue or the periwound area. This method can be labor-intensive and more costly because of the required frequency of dressing changes (The Wound Healing and Management Node Group, 2011). Advances in wound care therapies have led to the development of many débriding products for use as well as moist gauze for débriding necrotic wounds. Autolytic débriding products contain enzymes that break down dead tissue. Enzymatic products are used in combination with moist-to-dry gauze but may also come as packaged dressings that do not require additional gauze packing.

Dressings protect wounds and guard against contamination, heat loss, further tissue injury, and spread of microorganisms. Some dressings are impregnated with antimicrobial elements such as silver to prevent or treat a wound infection (Meaume et al., 2011). Dressings also control bleeding and drainage. They promote hemostasis by direct pressure and absorption of drainage. They may also serve to support or immobilize a body part.

PATIENT-CENTERED CARE

Acute and chronic wounds present numerous challenges to the health care team and to patients and their families. Wounds frequently are the cause of great distress. As a nurse, identify patients' specific cultural or spiritual practices as they relate to the management of wounds. Ask a patient if

TABLE 26-1   COMPARISON OF WOUND CARE PRODUCTS

PRODUCT CATEGORY	INDICATIONS FOR USE	CONTRAINDICATIONS	ADVANTAGES	DISADVANTAGES	FREQUENCY OF CHANGE (PER MANUFACTURER'S RECOMMENDATIONS)
Gauze Dressings					
Cotton or synthetic material; woven or nonwoven construction	Protection of surgical incisions Mechanical débridement (moist to dry) Secondary dressing for other wound products Packing wounds	Over granulating wounds as primary treatment	Available in many sizes and forms Sterile and nonsterile	May adhere to healthy tissue, causing injury when removed Lint fibers may be left on wound May interfere with wound healing if gauze dries out in moist-to-dry dressing	2-3 times per day as needed
Transparent Films					
Adhesive membrane dressings; waterproof, impermeable to fluids and bacteria; allow oxygen and moisture vapor exchange	Shallow wounds Dry to minimal exudate Promote autolytic débridement Stage I-II pressure ulcers	Infected wounds Wounds that tunnel, undermine, or are full thickness Wounds with moderate-to-heavy exudate Third-degree burns	Easy to apply and remove without damage to underlying tissue Permit viewing of wound Create second skin Protect from friction Waterproof Create a moist environment that softens thin slough and eschar Protective shield to external fluids and bacteria	May cause skin maceration May not adhere to moist areas May cause skin stripping if improperly removed	Change every 3-4 days or as needed. If using to facilitate autolytic débridement, change every 24 hours
Hydrocolloids					
Adhesive dressings that contain gel-forming agents; mold to body contours; considered semi-occlusive dressing	Partial- or full-thickness wound Shallow minimal to moderate exudating wounds Clean stage II and noninfected shallow stage II-IV pressure ulcers Can be used in combination with absorbent powder or alginate	Third-degree burns Acutely infected wounds Arterial or diabetic ulcers (use with caution) Wounds with dry eschar	Reduces pain Available in many sizes Promotes autolytic débridement Impermeable to fluids/bacteria Thermal insulator Easy to apply and remove	Potential for periwound maceration if dressing left in place too long Drainage (gelatinous mass) under dressing often mistaken for pus/infection Adhesive possibly too aggressive for fragile skin	Every 3-5 days

TABLE 26-1   COMPARISON OF WOUND CARE PRODUCTS—cont'd

PRODUCT CATEGORY	INDICATIONS FOR USE	CONTRAINDICATIONS	ADVANTAGES	DISADVANTAGES	FREQUENCY OF CHANGE (PER MANUFACTURER'S RECOMMENDATIONS)
Hydrogel Glycerin- or water-based dressings designed to maintain clean, moist wound; may also absorb small amount of exudate	Partial- or full-thickness wound Shallow or deep wounds Dry to minimally invasive wound with or without clean granular wound base Wounds with undermining Necrotic wounds	Third-degree burns Wounds with heavy exudate	Nonadherent Cool and soothing Decrease pain Facilitate autolysis Conform to wound High water content aids in débridement along with ability to absorb water	Potential for maceration or candidiasis of periwound area	Change daily if adhesive sheets or wound fillers are not used. Change adhesive covers up to 3 times per week
Alginates Highly absorbent nonwoven material that forms a gel when exposed to wound drainage; fibrous product derived from brown seaweed	Moderate to heavily exudating wounds Shallow or deep Partial- and full-thickness wounds Leg ulcers, donor sites, traumatic wounds	Third-degree burns Nondraining wounds Dry, necrotic wounds	Nonadhering Nonocclusive Hemostatic properties May be packed into tunneled areas Promote autolytic débridement in exudating wounds Highly absorbent and biodegradable properties	More expensive than gauze or gauze packing strips Not practical for large wounds Gelled material possibly mistaken for purulence	Change daily or as often as needed, usually every 24 to 48 hours
Foam Dressings Absorbent, nonadherent polyurethane pad used to protect wounds and maintain moist healing environment	Moderate or heavily exudating wounds Partial- and full-thickness wounds Stage II-IV pressure ulcers	Ischemic wound with dry eschar Third-degree burns Wounds that tunnel, with sinus tracts Nondraining wounds	Highly absorbent while maintaining moist wound environment Often used as secondary dressing with films and absorbers Many foams nonadherent to wound bed	Nonadhesive foams require secondary dressing Maceration of periwound if dressing left on too long	Change every 24 hours or as needed

Modified from Collins R et al: Wound care literature review 2011, *J Wound Ostomy Continence Nurs* 39:S4, 2012; Rolstad BS, Bryant RA, Nix DP: Topical management. In Bryant RA, Nix DP (Eds): *Acute and chronic wounds: nursing management*, ed 4, St Louis, 2012, Mosby; Newton H: An introduction to wound healing and dressings, *Br J Healthc Manage* 19(6):270, 2013.

BOX 26-1 CHARACTERISTICS AND OUTCOMES OF AN IDEAL DRESSING

Characteristics
- Able to absorb exudate yet keeps wound bed moist and surrounding periwound dry and intact
- Appropriate for infected wounds
- Can be removed without trauma, pain, or dressing fragments left in wound
- Conforms to the body to allow ease of movement
- Maintains physiologic wound environment
- Keeps surrounding (periwound) skin dry
- Easy to apply and remove with easy-to-follow patient/family caregiver instructions for independence with dressing changes
- Cost-effective

Outcomes
- Reduces volume of exudate and amount of necrotic tissue
- Resolves or prevents periwound erythema
- Reduces wound dimensions or depth
- Reduces pain intensity during dressing changes

Bryant RA, Nix DP: *Acute and chronic wounds: nursing management*, ed 4, St Louis, 2012, Mosby; Benbow M: Addressing pain in wound care and dressing removal, *Nursing & Residential Care* 13(10):474, 2011.

---

there are any special considerations to be aware of before proceeding. This question opens up the discussion and allows you to include the patient in decision making and to focus on individualizing care.

Patients and their families often learn how to become the primary caretakers of wounds. Family members' presence during dressing changes allows them an opportunity to see that their loved one is being cared for and provides the patient a sense of comfort and needed emotional support (Bishop et al., 2013). Use this time to teach the patient and family caregiver about wound care, how to perform a dressing change, and how to evaluate if the dressing change is performed correctly.

Pain management is a part of patient-centered care. Your role is to minimize a patient's discomfort during a dressing change by understanding his or her values and beliefs about pain management (see Evidence-Based Practice).

SAFETY

Many wounds are colonized or contaminated with low levels of bacteria. A biofilm is a fungal or bacteria-embedded slimy matrix of proteins and sugars that adheres to the surface of a wound bed (and other surfaces such as urinary catheters and endotracheal tubes). These biofilms are known to contribute to infections, especially in chronic wounds. Biofilms contribute to inflammation and an increased production of exudates and slough (Jones, 2013; Phillips et al., 2010).

For safe and effective wound care management, follow these guidelines:

1. Know the cause and type of wound to ensure the proper treatment plan is in place and healing outcomes are achieved (see Box 26-1).
2. Know the expected amount and type of wound exudate (see Table 26-2).
3. Be aware of the presence of drainage tubes before removing a dressing to prevent accidental removal.
4. Wear personal protective equipment (PPE, such as gloves, mask, gown, and goggles, as indicated and if risk of splashing exists. Follow isolation protocols to prevent the spread of infection.
5. Dispose of contaminated dressings and supplies properly (see facility policy).

EVIDENCE-BASED PRACTICE

Faucher N et al: Superabsorbent dressings for copiously exudating wounds, *Br J Nurs* 21(12):S22, 2012.

Ljubic A: Cleansing chronic wounds with tap water or saline: a review, *J Community Nurs* 27(1):19, 2013.

Solowiej K, Upton D: Painful dressing changes for chronic wounds: assessment and management, *Br J Nurs* 21(20): S20, 2012.

Pain management is necessary for proper wound care. Research has shown there is a relationship between psychological distress and wound healing. One way to relieve psychological distress is pain control. Controlling pain during dressing changes can reduce the negative impact and stress of subsequent dressing changes. When assessing a patient's level of pain with dressing changes, observe nonverbal and behavior indicators such as the inability to keep still, bracing, moaning, and gasping. Individualize the plan of care for dressing changes because each patient responds differently to pain and discomfort. Wound pain can severely affect a patient's quality of life (Solowiej and Upton, 2012).

- Select a wound care product that minimizes pain while decreasing the risk of infection and controlling exudate.
- Assess a patient's need for an analgesic before dressing changes, and administer 30 to 60 minutes before the dressing change.
- A moist environment promotes wound healing; a wound left open to air is likely to become dry and painful (Solowiej and Upton, 2012).
- Wound cleaning removes debris from a wound bed, especially the periwound. The solution should be at body temperature (37° C) to provide comfort and maintain the temperature in the wound bed during dressing changes (Ljubic, 2013).
- Avoid inflammation, maceration, and excoriation to the periwound, which contains susceptible nerve endings (Faucher et al., 2012).
- Avoid overpacking of a wound bed to minimize pressure.

SKILL 26.1 APPLYING A GAUZE DRESSING (DRY AND MOIST-TO-DRY)

Dry dressings (Fig. 26-1) are for wounds healing by primary intention with little drainage. A dry gauze protects a wound from injury, prevents the introduction and spread of bacteria, reduces discomfort, and speeds healing. Dry woven gauze dressings do not interact with wound tissues and cause little wound irritation. They are commonly used for abrasions and nondraining postoperative incisions. Telfa gauze dressings contain a shiny, nonadherent surface on one side that does not stick to wounds. Drainage passes through the nonadherent surface to the outer gauze dressing (Table 26-2). Dry dressings are not appropriate for débriding wounds. In the presence of drainage, a dry dressing may adhere to the wound bed and surrounding tissue causing pain and trauma on removal (Benbow, 2011). To minimize pain and injury, moisten the dressing with sterile normal saline or sterile water before removing the gauze.

Moist-to-dry dressings include a combination of dry gauze and a gauze layer moistened with an appropriate solution. The use of this method is less common as new wound care products continue to be developed. The primary purpose is to débride wounds mechanically, specifically full-thickness wounds healing by secondary intention and wounds with necrotic tissue. A moist-to-dry dressing has a lightly moistened contact dressing layer that touches the wound surface. The moistened gauze increases the absorptive ability of the dressing to collect exudate and wound debris. This layer dries and adheres to dead cells, débriding the wound when removed. Isotonic solutions such as normal saline or lactated Ringer's solution are best to use to moisten the gauze. The outer absorbent layer of a moist-to-dry dressing is a dry dressing that protects the wound from invasive microorganisms. There is some question as to whether moist-to-dry dressings provide moist wound healing (Wodash, 2012).

You normally secure dressings with tape, which may be paper, plastic, woven, or elastic material with adhesive. Damage to skin may occur with repeated application and removal of adherent products; this is known as skin stripping (Denyer, 2011). Several other techniques are available to reduce tape-related injury. Montgomery straps are wide strips of tape with holes and laces that secure dressings when placed on opposite wound edges and tied. Strips of a Stomahesive or hydrocolloid dressing can be used to create a window around a wound. Then you apply tape over the Stomahesive strips, reducing direct contact with the periwound skin. Pulling tape off of the skin can result in skin tears.

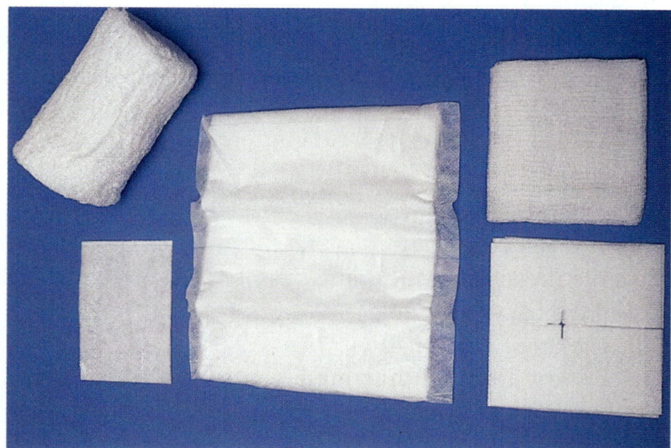

FIG 26-1 Types of gauze dressings: 4 × 4, split, roll, and ABD.

TABLE 26-2	TYPES OF WOUND DRAINAGE

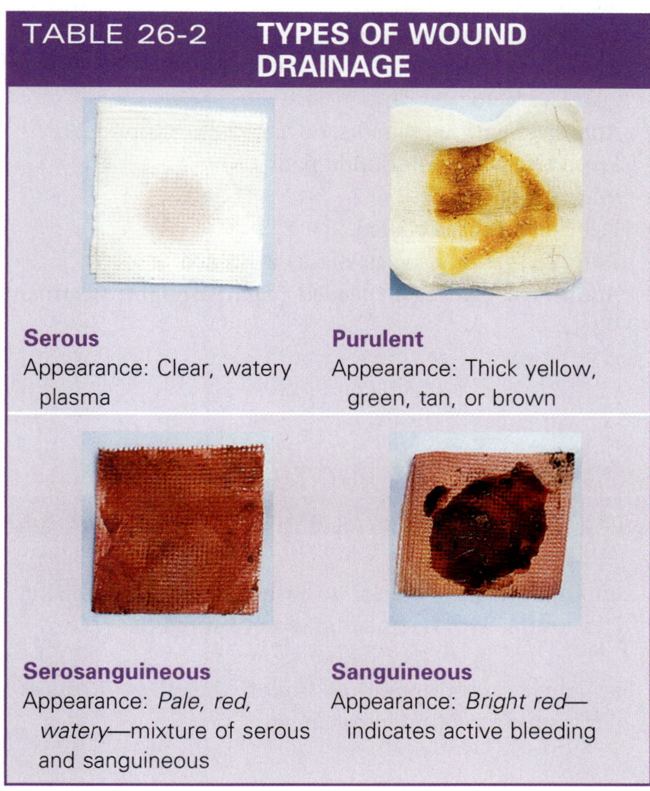

Serous
Appearance: Clear, watery plasma

Purulent
Appearance: Thick yellow, green, tan, or brown

Serosanguineous
Appearance: *Pale, red, watery*—mixture of serous and sanguineous

Sanguineous
Appearance: *Bright red*—indicates active bleeding

▌ASSESSMENT

1. Identify patient using two identifiers (e.g., name and birthday or name and account number) according to facility policy. *Rationale: Ensures correct patient. Complies with The Joint Commission standards and improves patient safety (TJC, 2014).*
2. Ask patient to rate wound pain using a scale of 0 to 10. Administer prescribed analgesic as needed 30 minutes before the dressing change. *Rationale: Giving pain medication before dressing change achieves peak effect of drug during procedure. Superficial wounds with multiple exposed nerves may be intensely painful, whereas deeper wounds with destruction of nerves should be less painful (Krazner, 2011).*
3. Assess knowledge of patient and family caregiver of purpose of dressing change. *Rationale: Determines level of support and explanation required.*

4 Determine the need, readiness, and willingness for patient or family caregiver to participate in dressing wound. *Rationale: Prepares patient or family caregiver if dressing will be changed at home.*

5. Review medical orders for type of dressing. *Rationale: Indicates type of dressing supplies needed.*

6. Review previous nursing notes and electronic medical record (EMR). *Rationale: Data allow you to obtain appropriate supplies and review baseline condition of wound.*

7. Assess patient for presence of allergies to antiseptics, tape, or latex. *Rationale: Prevents localized or systemic reaction to wound care supplies.*

8. Identify risk factors for wound healing, including older age, prematurity (infant), obesity, diabetes mellitus, circulation disorders, nutritional deficit, immunosuppression, radiation therapy, high stress levels, and use of steroids. *Rationale: Physiologic changes and effects of disease and treatment conditions can affect wound healing (Doughty and Sparks-DeFriese, 2011).*

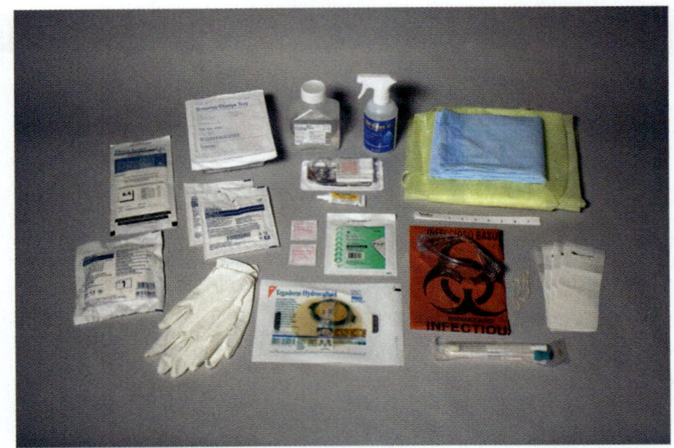

FIG 26-2 Dressing set with PPE and wound cleansers.

- Reporting to the nurse any pain, fever, bleeding, or wound drainage.

PLANNING

Expected Outcomes focus on preventing infection, promoting healing, controlling pain, and patient and family caregiver learning.

1. Patient's wound shows evidence of healing by decrease in size and less drainage, redness, or swelling.
2. Patient reports pain less than previous assessment after dressing change.
3. Dressing remains clean, dry, and intact.
4. Patient or family caregiver explains purpose of dressing and method of dressing application.

Delegation and Collaboration

The skill of applying dry and moist-to-dry dressings may sometimes be delegated to nursing assistive personnel (NAP) if the wound is chronic (see facility policy and Nurse Practice Act). All wound assessments, care of acute new wounds, and wound care requiring sterile technique cannot be delegated. The nurse instructs the NAP about:

- How to adapt the skill for a specific patient, such as need for special tape or technique to secure the dressing.

Equipment

- Clean and sterile gloves
- Centimeter ruler
- Sterile dressing set including scissors and forceps (check facility policy) (Fig. 26-2)
- Sterile drape (optional)
- Necessary dressings: fine-mesh gauze, 4 × 4–inch gauze, abdominal pads (ABDs)
- Sterile basin (optional)
- Antiseptic ointment (as prescribed)
- Wound cleanser (as prescribed)
- Sterile normal saline (or prescribed solution)
- Tape (include nonallergenic tape as necessary), Montgomery ties, or bandages as needed
- Measuring device: cotton-tipped applicator, measuring guide, camera
- Adhesive remover, scissors, or hair clipper (optional)
- Protective waterproof underpad
- Waterproof bag
- Débriding gel as ordered
- PPE (i.e., gown, goggles, mask) if needed
- Additional lighting if needed (e.g., flashlight, treatment light)

IMPLEMENTATION *for* APPLYING A GAUZE DRESSING (DRY AND MOIST-TO-DRY)

STEPS	RATIONALE
1. **See Standard Protocol (inside front cover).**	
2. Position patient comfortably, and drape to expose only wound site. Instruct patient not to touch wound or sterile supplies.	Draping provides access to wound while minimizing exposure. Avoids contamination of supplies.
3. Apply clean gloves. Place disposable waterproof bag within reach of work area. Fold top of bag to make a cuff. Perform hand hygiene. Apply additional PPE if needed.	Facilitates safe disposal of soiled dressings. Reduces transmission of microorganisms.

STEPS	RATIONALE

4. Gently remove tape, bandages, or ties by using your nondominant hand to support the dressing. With your dominant hand, pull tape parallel to the skin and toward the dressing. If dressing is over hairy areas, remove in the direction of hair growth. Get patient's permission to clip or shave area (check facility policy). Remove any adhesive from skin with adhesive remover.

Pulling tape toward dressing reduces stress on suture line or wound edges and reduces irritation and discomfort.

5. With a gloved hand or forceps, remove dressing one layer at a time, observing appearance and drainage on dressing. Use caution to avoid tension on any drains that are present.

Determines dressings needed for replacement. Avoids accidental removal of an underlying drain, which may or may not be sutured in place.

a. If bottom layer of moist-to-dry dressing sticks, alert patient of discomfort and gently free dressing.

Moist-to-dry dressing should débride a wound (The Wound Healing and Management Node Group, 2011).

b. If a dry dressing adheres to a wound that is not to be débrided, moisten with normal saline first and then remove.

Prevents injury to wound edges.

6. Fold dressings with drainage contained inside and remove gloves inside out. With small dressings, remove gloves inside out over dressing (see illustrations). Cover wound lightly with a sterile gauze pad. Dispose of gloves and soiled dressings. Perform hand hygiene.

Contains soiled dressings, prevents contact with drainage; reduces cross-contamination.

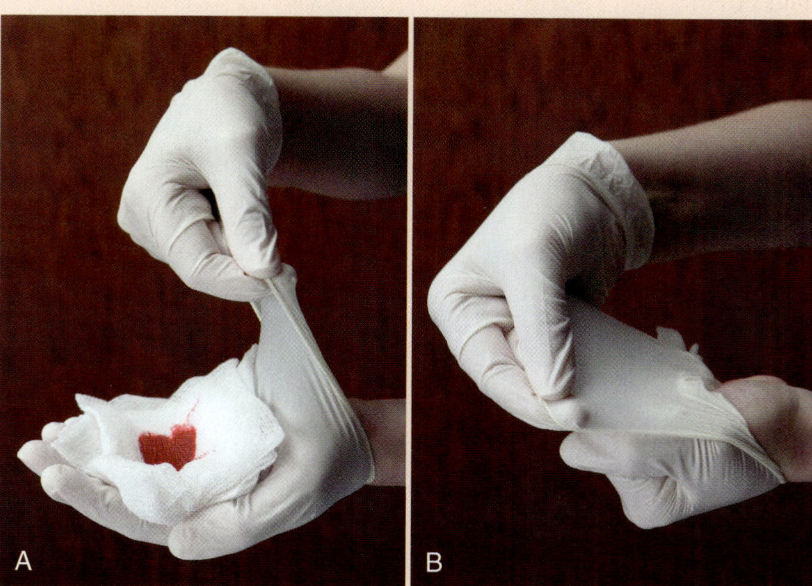

STEP 6 A and **B,** Dispose of soiled dressing and gloves.

7. Create a sterile field with a sterile dressing tray or individually wrapped sterile supplies on over-bed table (see Chapter 5). Pour prescribed solution into sterile basin.

Creates sterile work area.

8. Apply clean gloves. Remove gauze cover over wound, and then cleanse wound.

a. Use gauze or cotton ball moistened in saline or antiseptic swab (per health care provide order) for each cleansing stroke or spray wound surface with wound cleanser.

Prevents transfer of organisms from previously cleaned area.

Continued

STEPS	RATIONALE
b. Clean from least contaminated to most contaminated area (see illustration).	Cleaning in this direction prevents introduction of organisms into wound.
c. Cleanse around drain (if present), using circular strokes starting near the drain and moving outward away from insertion site (see illustration).	Correct aseptic technique in cleaning prevents contamination.
9. Use sterile dry gauze to blot wound dry in same manner as in Step 8.	Drying reduces excess moisture, which eventually harbors microorganisms.
10. Inspect wound and periwound for appearance, color, size (length, width, and depth), drainage, edema, presence and condition of drains, approximation (wound edges are together), granulation tissue, or odor. Use measuring guide or ruler to measure wound size. Gently palpate wound edges for bogginess or patient report of increased pain.	Condition of wound indicates status of healing.
11. Apply antiseptic ointment (if ordered) with sterile cotton-tipped applicator or gauze, using same technique to apply as for cleaning. Dispose of gloves. Perform hand hygiene.	Helps reduce growth of microorganisms.
12. Apply dressing (see facility policy).	
a. Dry sterile dressing:	
(1) Apply clean gloves. Option: **Apply sterile gloves** (if recommended by facility policy).	Some facilities or condition of wounds may require sterile gloves.
(2) Apply loose 4 × 4–inch gauze square as contact layer (see illustration).	Promotes proper absorption of drainage.
(3) If drain is present, apply precut, split 4 × 4–inch gauze around drain.	Secures drain and promotes drainage absorption at site.
(4) Apply additional layers of gauze as needed.	Ensures proper coverage and optimal absorption.
(5) Apply thicker woven pad (e.g., ABD, Surgipad) (see illustration).	This type of cover dressing is used on postoperative wounds when there is excessive drainage.

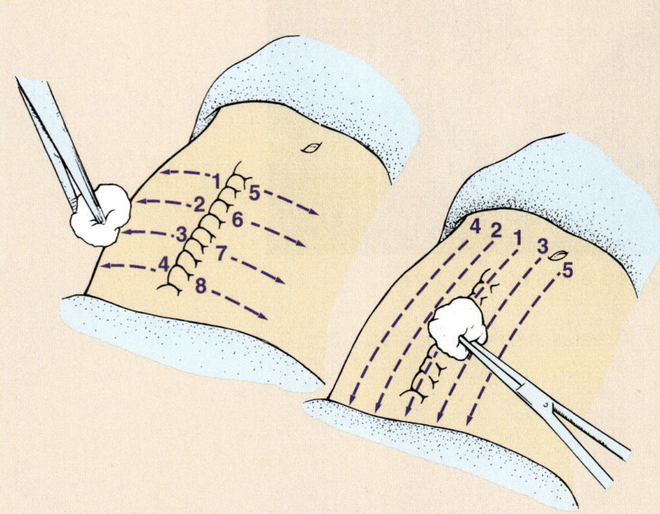

STEP 8b Method for cleansing a wound.

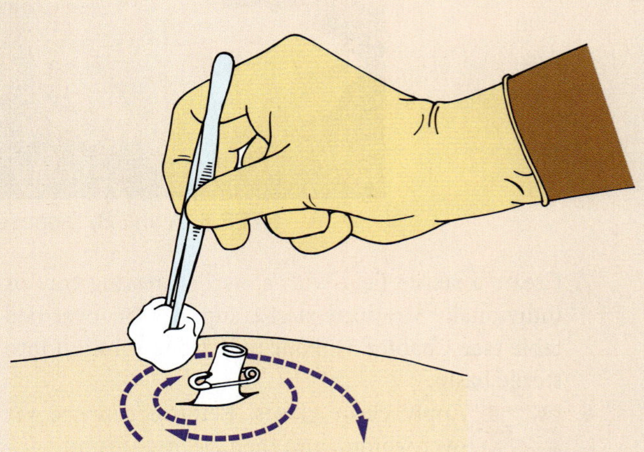

STEP 8c Cleansing a drain site.

STEPS	RATIONALE

b. Moist-to-dry dressing:

(1) **Apply sterile gloves** (see facility policy).

Reduces transmission of infection.

(2) Place fine-mesh or loose 4 × 4–inch gauze in container of prescribed sterile solution. Wring out solution as much as possible. Option: If using packing strips, use sterile scissors to cut the amount of dressing needed to pack wound. Do not let packing strip touch the outside of the bottle. Pour prescribed solution over the packing gauze to moisten and wring out excess solution.

Moist gauze absorbs drainage and when allowed to dry traps debris.

(3) Apply damp fine-mesh or open-weave gauze as a single layer directly onto wound surface. If wound is deep, gently pack gauze into wound with gloved hands or forceps until all wound surfaces are in contact with damp gauze, including dead spaces from sinus tracts, tunneling, and undermining. Be sure that gauze does not touch periwound skin (see illustrations).

Inner gauze should be just moist, not dripping wet, to absorb drainage and adhere to debris. Moisture that escapes the dressing can macerate the periwound skin.

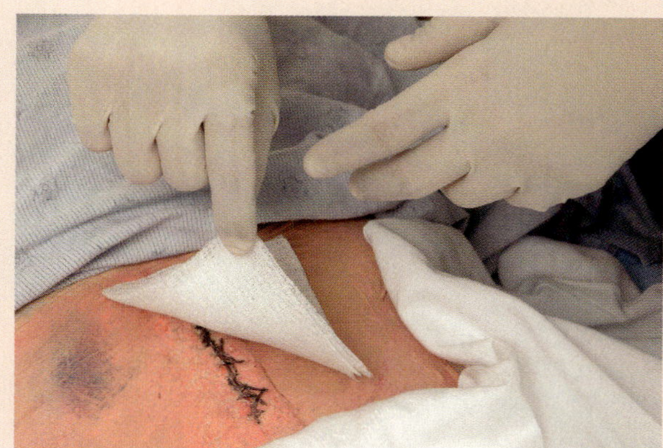

STEP 12a(2) Placing dry gauze dressing over simple wound.

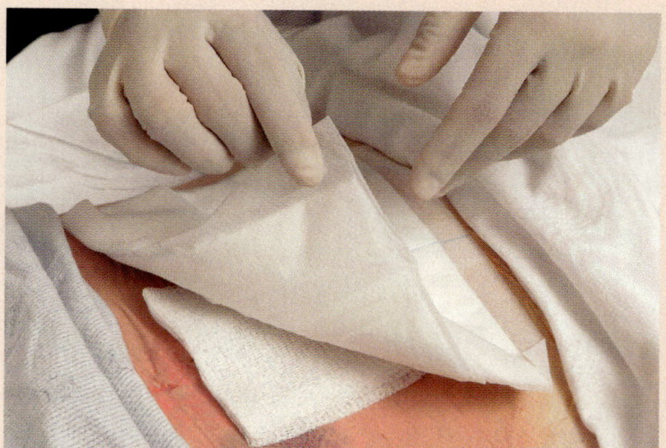

STEP 12a(5) Placing ABD pad over gauze dressing.

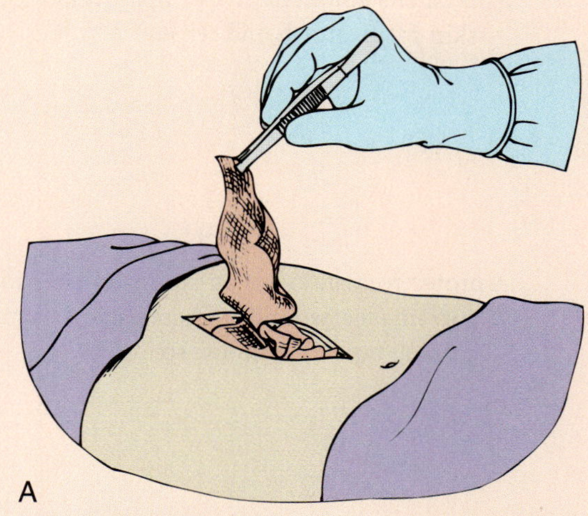

A

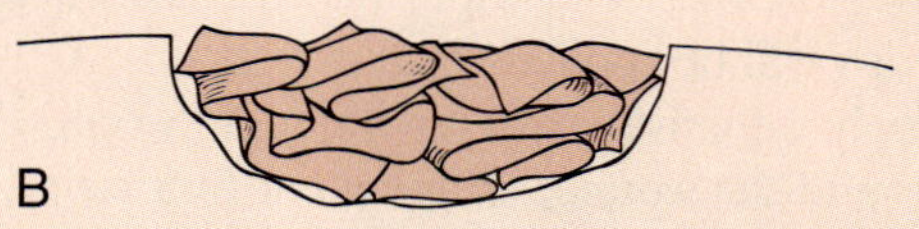

B

STEP 12b(3) A, Packing a wound with fine-mesh gauze. **B,** Cross section of wound packed loosely.

Continued

STEPS	RATIONALE

> **SAFE PATIENT CARE** When packing a wound, gauze should conform to base and side of wound (Rolstad et al., 2011). Wound is loosely packed to facilitate wicking of drainage into absorbent outer layer of dressing. Overpacking the wound can lead to increased pressure within the wound bed, causing tissue damage and delayed healing.

(4) Apply dry, sterile 4 × 4–inch gauze over damp gauze.

Dry layers pull moisture from wound.

(5) Cover with ABD, Surgipad, or gauze.

Protects wound from entrance of microorganisms.

13. Secure dressing.

   a. *Tape:* Apply tape 1 to 2 inches (2.5 to 5 cm) beyond dressing. Use nonallergenic tape when necessary.

Supports wound, ensures placement and stability of dressing.

   b. *Montgomery ties (see illustrations):*

Ties allow for repeated dressing changes without removal of tape.

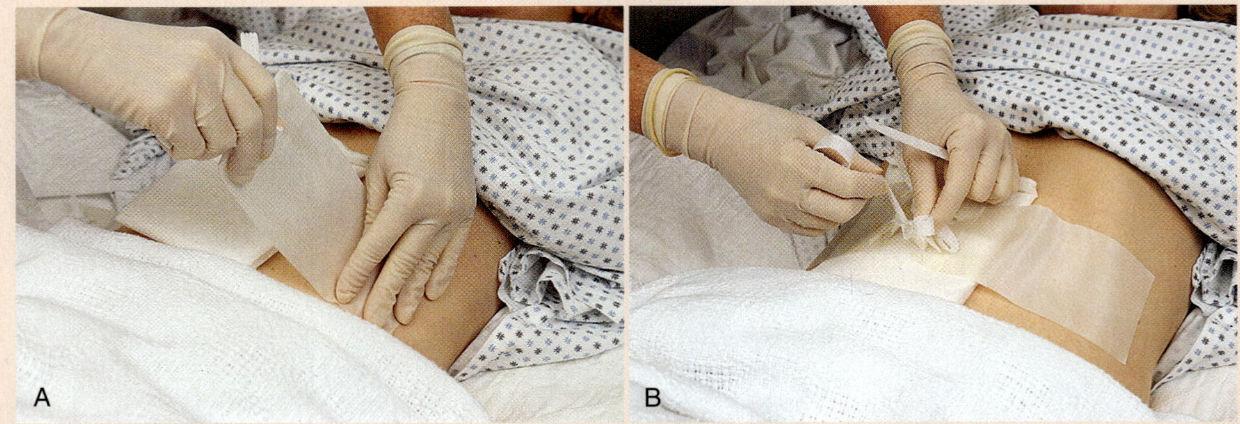

STEP 13b Montgomery ties. **A,** Each tie is placed at side of dressing. **B,** Securing ties encloses dressing.

   (1) Be sure that skin is clean. Application of a skin barrier is recommended.

Skin barrier (Stomahesive or hydrocolloid) protects intact skin from stretch and tension of adhesive tape.

   (2) Expose adhesive surface of tape ends.

   (3) Place ties on opposite sides of dressing over skin or skin barrier.

   (4) Secure dressing by lacing ties across dressing snugly enough to hold dressing secure but without pressure on the skin.

   c. *For protective window:*

A protective window is an alternative to Montgomery ties for smaller wounds. There is less skin irritation by placing tape on window strips.

   (1) Cut strips of the Stomahesive or hydrocolloid pad into 1-cm (½-inch) strips.

   (2) Use skin barrier to wipe areas of skin where strips will be applied.

   (3) Apply adhesive strips to frame a "window" around the wound, using two or four strips.

   (4) Apply the dressing, then secure tape ends to the adhesive strips.

STEPS	RATIONALE

d. *For dressing on an extremity:* Secure with roller gauze (see illustration) or elastic net.

Roller gauze conforms to contour of foot or hand.

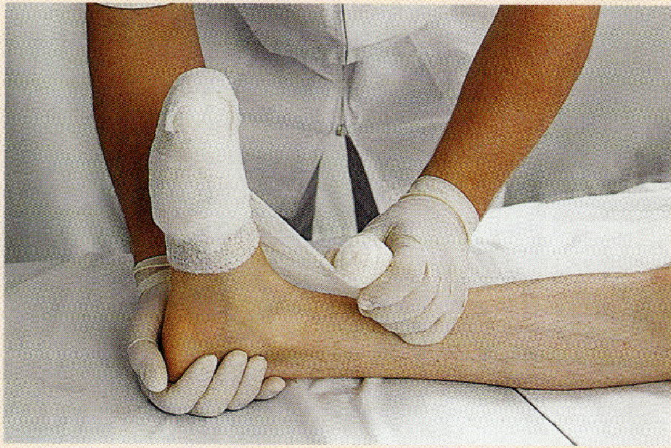

STEP 13d Wrap roller gauze around extremity.

14. Label dressing with your initials and date dressing changed.

Provides timeline for when next dressing change is to be scheduled.

15. See Completion Protocol (inside front cover).

EVALUATION

1. Observe appearance of wound with each dressing change for healing: measure size of wound, and observe amount, color, and type of drainage and periwound erythema or swelling.
2. Ask patient to rate pain using a scale of 0 to 10.
3. Inspect condition of dressing at least every shift or as ordered.
4. Use *Teach Back:* State to the patient, "We covered a lot today with the dressing change, and I want to make sure that I explained things clearly. So let's review what we discussed. What are the steps involved in changing your dressing?" Evaluates what the patient is able to explain or demonstrate. Revise your instruction now or develop plan for revised patient teaching to be implemented at an appropriate time if patient is not able to teach back correctly.

Unexpected Outcomes and Related Interventions

1. Wound appears inflamed and tender, drainage is evident, or an odor is present.
   a. Monitor patient for signs of infection (e.g., fever, increased white blood cell count).
   b. Notify health care provider.
   c. Obtain wound cultures as ordered.
   d. If there is yellow, tan, or brown necrotic tissue, refer to health care provider to determine need for débridement.
2. Wound bleeds during dressing change.
   a. Observe color and amount of drainage. If excessive, may need to apply direct pressure.
   b. Inspect area along dressing and directly underneath to determine the amount of bleeding.

   c. Obtain vital signs as needed and notify health care provider.
3. Patient reports a sensation that "something has given way under the dressing."
   a. Observe wound for increased drainage or dehiscence (partial or total separation of wound layers) or evisceration (total separation of wound layers and protrusion of viscera through the wound opening).
   b. Protect wound by covering with sterile moist dressing.
   c. Instruct patient to lie still.
   d. Stay with patient to monitor vital signs.
   e. Have health care provider notified.

Recording and Reporting

- Record size and appearance of wound, characteristics of drainage, presence of necrotic tissue, type of dressings applied, response to dressing change, and level of comfort in nurses' notes.
- Document your evaluation of patient learning.
- Report any unexpected appearance of wound drainage, bright red bleeding, dehiscence, or evisceration to health care provider.

Sample Documentation

1000   Midline abdominal wound dressing changed. Wound measures 6 cm × 2 cm with 1-cm depth. Wound bed with 90% pink granulation tissue and 10% yellow slough. Minimal amount of serosanguineous drainage, no odor. Periwound skin intact. Wound bed cleansed with wound cleanser spray. Saline-moistened gauze lightly packed into wound. Covered with 4 × 4–inch gauze and ABD. Skin protectant wipe applied to periwound skin. Dressing secured with hypoallergenic cotton tape. Reported 0 pain on scale of 0 to 10 pre and post dressing change, 3/10 during change.

Special Considerations
Pediatric
- Children may be fearful of dressing changes, especially if a child had a bad experience with a wound treatment or dressing change in the past. To avoid long-term fear and distress over dressing changes, look for ways to help a child cope. Allow the child to pick a distraction to use during the dressing change (e.g., playing a video game, listening to music) (Nilsson et al., 2011).

Geriatric
- Consider risk factors in older-adult patients for impaired skin integrity, such as sensory impairment, dry and dehydrated skin, or impaired nutritional status, that will affect wound healing (Jones, 2011).

- Adhesive tape may be too irritating to older adults' skin and cause skin tears. Use paper tape, nonallergenic tape, or wraps or mesh to avoid tape contacting a patient's skin.

Home Care
- Some wounds may be cleansed in the shower. Have patient verify this practice with health care provider before discharge.
- Clean, instead of sterile, dressings may be used in the home.
- Dispose of contaminated dressings consistent with local regulations. Most regulations require placing dressings in sealed plastic bags.

SKILL 26.2   APPLYING A PRESSURE BANDAGE

A pressure bandage is a temporary treatment to control excessive, sudden, unanticipated bleeding. Hemorrhage may occur during or after diagnostic interventions (e.g., cardiac catheterization, arterial puncture, organ biopsy), surgery, or a life-threatening occurrence related to trauma (stabbing, gunshot). Pressure dressings are essential for stopping the flow of blood and promoting clotting at the site (hemostasis) until definitive action can be taken. Given the emergent nature of an acute bleeding episode, the aseptic techniques considered essential in most dressing applications are secondary to the goal of halting the bleeding. A pressure dressing applied in an emergency is usually temporary; the wound can be cleansed and the dressing changed after the bleeding has been controlled. In addition, hemostatic dressings are available to use to assist in controlling bleeding.

ASSESSMENT

1. Anticipate risk factors for unexpected bleeding, including traumatic injury, arterial puncture, donor graft site, postsurgical wound débridement, and surgical patient with history of bleeding disorder. *Rationale: Familiarity with conditions associated with unexpected bleeding allows you to anticipate and respond as needed.*
2. Assess the location and condition of the area where hemorrhage may develop. *Rationale: Allows for early identification. Helps identify proper type and amount of supplies needed.*
3. Assess patient for presence of allergies to antiseptics, tape, or latex. *Rationale: Prevents localized or systemic reaction to dressing supplies.*

> **SAFE PATIENT CARE** If patient is nonresponsive and no history is available, use nonlatex or nonallergenic supplies.

4. Assess patient's anxiety level and knowledge of the clinical situation. *Rationale: Determines need for education and positive reinforcement during procedure.*

5. Assess patient's baseline vital signs as part of monitoring condition or procedure. *Rationale: If data available, baseline vital signs indicate status of circulatory function.*

PLANNING

Expected Outcomes   focus on minimizing blood loss, preventing hemodynamic instability and infection, and promoting patient and family caregiver education.
1. Patient shows complete cessation of bleeding at site of hemorrhage.
2. There is no hematoma formation at site of pressure application.
3. Patient maintains stable blood pressure and heart rate.
4. Distal circulation is maintained, with intact pulse (distal to site of injury).
5. Patient or family caregiver is able to explain risk of rebleeding and how to apply pressure dressing.

Delegation and Collaboration
The skill of applying a pressure bandage cannot be delegated to nursing assistive personnel (NAP). The nurse directs the NAP to:
- Assist the nurse as directed. Observe the pressure dressing during care activities to make sure that it remains in place and there is no visible bleeding from the site, including underneath the patient.
- Report to the nurse any pain, fever, bleeding, or wound drainage.

Equipment
- Clean gloves
- Necessary dressings: fine-mesh gauze, roller gauze, hemostatic dressing (per facility policy), ABD
- Adhesive tape, hypoallergenic if necessary
- Adhesive remover (optional)
- PPE (e.g., gown, goggles) as needed
- Equipment for vital signs

IMPLEMENTATION *for* APPLYING A PRESSURE BANDAGE

STEPS	RATIONALE
1. **See Standard Protocol (inside front cover).**	Maintaining asepsis and privacy are considered only if time and severity of blood loss permit.

Phase I: Immediate Action—First Nurse

STEPS	RATIONALE
2. Identify external bleeding site. Look underneath patient if he or she has large abdominal dressing. Note: Wound to groin area can result in large amounts of blood loss, which is not always visible.	Quick identification increases response time to stop bleeding.
3. Apply immediate manual pressure to the site of bleeding.	Hemostasis maintained as supplies are prepared.
4. Seek assistance.	Bandage must be secured quickly.

Phase II: Applying Pressure Bandage—Second Nurse

STEPS	RATIONALE
5. Quickly identify source of bleeding.	Determines method of application and supplies to use.
a. Arterial bleeding is bright red and gushes forth in waves, related to heart rate; if vessel is very deep, flow will be steady.	
b. Venous bleeding is dark red and flows smoothly.	
c. Capillary bleeding is oozing of dark red blood; self-sealing controls bleeding.	
6. Elevate the affected body part (e.g., extremity) if possible.	Helps slow rate of hemorrhage.
7. First nurse continues to apply direct pressure as second nurse unwraps roller bandage and places within easy reach. Second nurse quickly cuts three to five lengths of adhesive tape and places them within reach. Do not cleanse wound.	Pressure dressing controls bleeding temporarily. Preparation allows nurses to secure pressure bandage quickly.
8. In simultaneous coordinated actions:	
a. Rapidly cover bleeding area with multiple thicknesses of gauze compresses. First nurse slips fingers out as second nurse exerts adequate pressure over gauze to continue controlling bleeding (see illustrations).	Gauze is absorbent. Layers provide bulk against which local pressure can be applied to bleeding site.

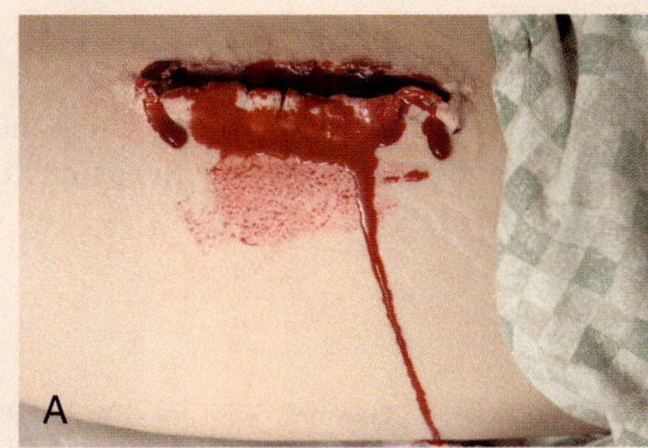 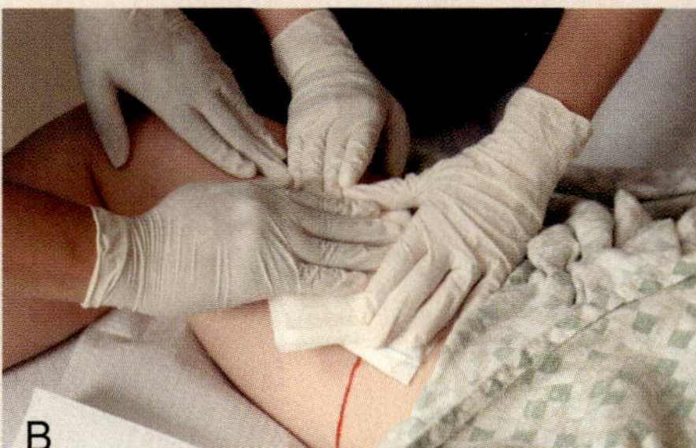 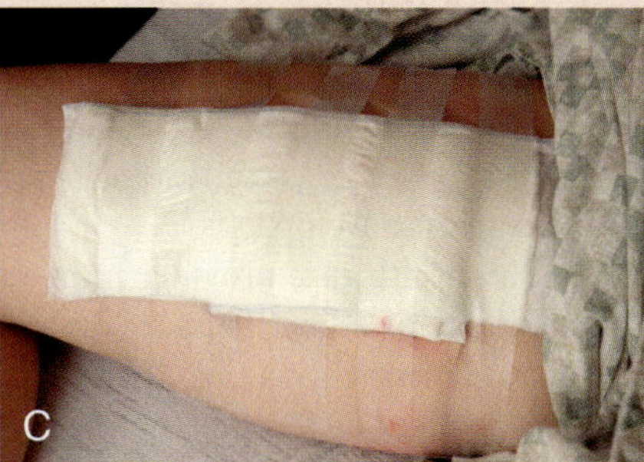

STEP 8a A, Bleeding wound. **B,** Nurses applying pressure dressing. **C,** Dressing applied.

STEPS	RATIONALE
b. First nurse places adhesive strips 7 to 10 cm (3 to 4 inches) beyond width of dressing with even pressure on both sides of fingers as close as possible to central bleeding. Secure tape on distal end, pull tape across dressing. Keep firm pressure as the proximate end of tape is secured.	Tape exerts downward pressure, promoting hemostasis. To ensure blood flow to distal tissues and prevent tourniquet effect, adhesive tape must not be continued around entire extremity.
c. Second nurse removes fingers temporarily. First nurse quickly covers center of area with a third strip of tape.	Provides pressure to source of bleeding.

Continued

STEPS	RATIONALE
d. Continue reinforcing area with tape as each successive strip is overlapped on alternating sides of center strip. Keep applying pressure.	Prevents tape from loosening.
e. When bandage is on extremity, apply roller gauze; apply two circular turns tautly on both sides of nurse's fingers that are pressing the gauze. Compress over bleeding site. Simultaneously remove finger pressure and apply roller gauze over center. Continue with figure-eight turns. Secure end with two circular turns and strip of adhesive (see Procedural Guideline 26.2).	Roller gauze acts as pressure bandage, exerting more even pressure over extremity.
9. See Completion Protocol (inside front cover).	

EVALUATION

1. Observe dressing for control of bleeding.
2. Evaluate adequacy of circulation (distal pulse, skin characteristics).
3. Estimate volume of blood loss (e.g., count number of dressings used, weigh saturated dressing).
4. Measure vital signs.
5. Use **Teach Back:** State to the patient, "I want to be sure that I correctly explained the risks of rebleeding. Can you tell me the things you are going to do to prevent the wound from bleeding again?" Evaluates what the patient is able to explain or demonstrate. Revise your instruction now or develop plan for revised patient teaching to be implemented at an appropriate time if patient is not able to teach back correctly.

Unexpected Outcomes and Related Interventions

1. There is continued bleeding. Fluid and electrolyte imbalance, tissue hypoxia, confusion, hypovolemic shock and cardiac arrest develop.
   a. Notify health care provider immediately.
   b. Reinforce or adjust pressure dressing.
   c. Initiate intravenous (IV) therapy per order.
   d. Place patient in Trendelenburg position; provide covers for warmth, and instruct patient to remain still.
   e. Monitor apical pulse, distal pulses, and blood pressure every 5 to 15 minutes.
2. Pressure dressing is too tight and occludes circulation.
   a. Inspect areas distal to pressure dressing to ensure that circulation has not been occluded.
   b. Adjust dressing as needed.
   c. Notify health care provider.

Recording and Reporting

- Report immediately to health care provider present status of patient's bleeding control, time bleeding was discovered, estimated blood loss, nursing interventions including effectiveness of applied pressure dressing, vital signs, mental status, signs of restlessness, and the need for health care provider to attend to patient immediately.
- Record interventions and patient's response in progress notes and vital sign flow sheet.
- Document your evaluation of patient teaching.

Sample Documentation

2230   Patient noted to have excessive bleeding from left mastectomy site 2 hours postoperatively. Dressing saturated with frank red blood. Two ABDs applied over saturated dressing and held in place with pressure. Dressing then bound tightly with 5-cm (2-inch) surgical tape. No further blood noted on reinforced dressing applied at 2200. Health care provider notified. Vital signs are stable.

Special Considerations
Pediatric

- Maintaining a calm environment will allow the child and parents to remain calm and assists in getting the cooperation needed to control bleeding.

Geriatric

- An older adult has an increased risk for vascular and tissue changes distal to the pressure dressing because of the normal changes of aging. Evaluate skin and pulse distal to the pressure bandage frequently.

Home Care

If patient is at risk for hemorrhage, instruct on the following:
- How patient or family caregiver should apply pressure with clean towel or linens.
- Immediate activation of the emergency (9-1-1) system.
- How to position patient by elevating affected body part (if extremity).

PROCEDURAL GUIDELINE 26.1
Applying a Transparent Dressing

A transparent film dressing is a clear, adherent, nonabsorptive, polyurethane sheet. When it is applied, a moist exudate forms over a wound surface, which prevents tissue dehydration. Rapid effective healing occurs by speeding epithelial cell growth. The dressing adhesive is inactivated by moisture and does not adhere to a wound; it has no absorptive capacity and is impermeable to fluids and bacteria (Rolstad et al., 2011). A transparent dressing is appropriate for preventing skin tears on high-risk intact skin (e.g., high friction areas) and for treating superficial wounds with minimal or no exudate. A transparent film is also used as a dressing over an IV site. The synthetic permeable membrane acts as a temporary second skin, adheres to undamaged skin to contain exudate, minimizes wound contamination, and allows a wound surface to "breathe." It is common to use transparent dressings as secondary dressings to wound products such as alginates and foam.

If a patient's skin is thin and fragile, use a skin barrier on the skin around a wound before application. Because transparent dressings are clear, you can observe a wound without removing the dressing. For best results, apply the dressing over clean, débrided wounds that are not actively bleeding. The accumulation of fluid with a white, opaque appearance and erythema of the surrounding tissue usually indicates an infection. In this case, remove the dressing and obtain a wound culture if ordered by the health care provider.

Delegation and Collaboration

The skill of applying transparent dressings for select wounds can be delegated to nursing assistive personnel (NAP) (refer to facility policy). The assessment of a wound cannot be delegated. The nurse instructs the NAP to:

- Note how to adapt the skill for a specific patient (e.g., size of dressing).
- Report any signs of bleeding, drainage, infection, or poor wound healing immediately to the nurse.

Equipment

- Clean gloves
- Sterile gloves (optional)
- Dressing set (optional)
- Sterile saline or other cleansing agent (as ordered)
- Cotton swabs
- Spray wound cleanser
- Waterproof bag for disposal
- Transparent dressing (size as needed)
- Sterile 4 × 4–inch gauze pads
- Skin barrier and skin preparation materials (optional)
- PPE as needed

Procedural Steps

1. Identify patient using two identifiers (e.g., name and birthday or name and account number) according to facility policy.

2. Review health care provider's orders for frequency and type of dressing change to determine size of transparent dressing and supplies needed.
3. Assess current dressing for condition and size.
4. Assess for allergies, especially antiseptics, tape, or latex.
5. Ask patient to rate level of pain using pain scale of 0 to 10. Administer prescribed pain medication as needed 30 minutes before dressing change.
6. Assess patient's knowledge of purpose of dressing change.
7. Determine need for patient or family caregiver to participate in dressing wound.
8. Assess patient's risk for impaired wound healing (e.g., aging, poor nutrition).
9. **See Standard Protocol (inside front cover).**
10. Position patient comfortably to allow access to dressing site.
11. Move clothing or linen to expose wound site, minimizing exposure. Instruct patient not to touch wound or sterile supplies.
12. Cuff top of disposable waterproof bag and place within reach of work area.
13. Apply clean gloves. Remove old dressing by stretching film in direction parallel to wound rather than pulling. For a skin tear with skin still attached, remove film in direction of the open edge of the wound (Stephen-Hayes et al., 2011).
14. Dispose soiled dressings in waterproof bag, and remove gloves by pulling them inside out and placing in waterproof bag. Perform hand hygiene.
15. Prepare dressing supplies.
16. Pour saline or prescribed cleansing solution over sterile 4 × 4–inch gauze pads.
17. Apply clean gloves. Option: **Apply sterile gloves** (check facility policy).
18. Cleanse wound and periwound area gently with 4 × 4–inch sterile gauze pad moistened with sterile saline or spray wound cleanser. Clean from least contaminated to most contaminated area (see Skill 26.1).
19. Pat skin around wound thoroughly using dry 4 × 4–inch sterile gauze.
20. Inspect wound for tissue type, color, odor, and drainage; measure size if indicated (see Chapter 24). If drainage has increased, consider a different type of dressing.
21. Remove gloves and perform hand hygiene.
22. Apply transparent dressing according to manufacturer's directions. Allow for a 2.5-cm (1-inch) perimeter onto intact skin surrounding the wound (Rolstad et al., 2011).
    a. Apply clean gloves.
    b. Remove paper backing, taking care not to allow adhesive areas to touch each other (see illustration).

Continued

PROCEDURAL GUIDELINE 26.1
Applying a Transparent Dressing—cont'd

   c. Place film smoothly over wound without stretching (see illustration). Avoid wrinkles.

   d. Use your fingers to smooth and adhere the dressing.

   e. Label with date, initials, and time of dressing change on outer label of dressing. For skin tears with flaps, draw arrow to indicate direction to remove dressing (see illustration).

23. **See Completion Protocol (inside front cover).**
24. Record appearance of wound, presence and characteristics of drainage, presence of odor, and dressing applied. Note patient's comfort level and response to dressing change and ability of patient or family caregiver to change dressing.

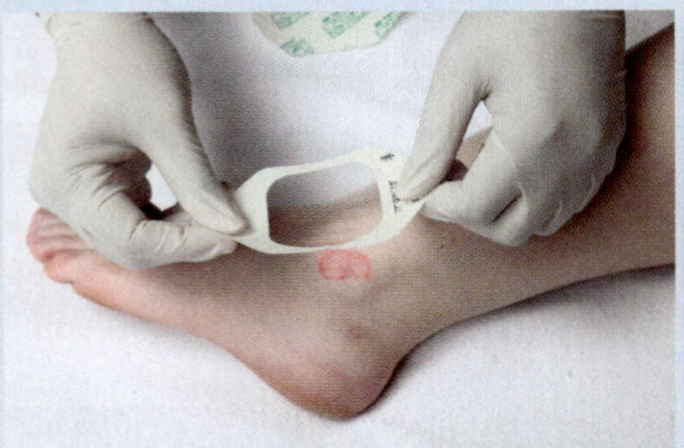

STEP 22b Transparent dressing placed over small wound on ankle.

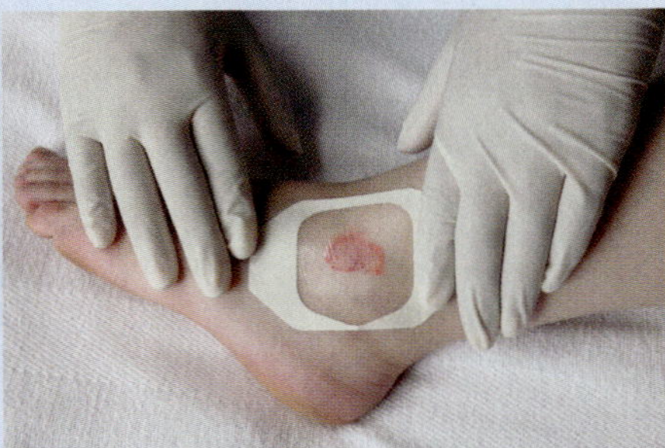

STEP 22c Place film smoothly without stretching.

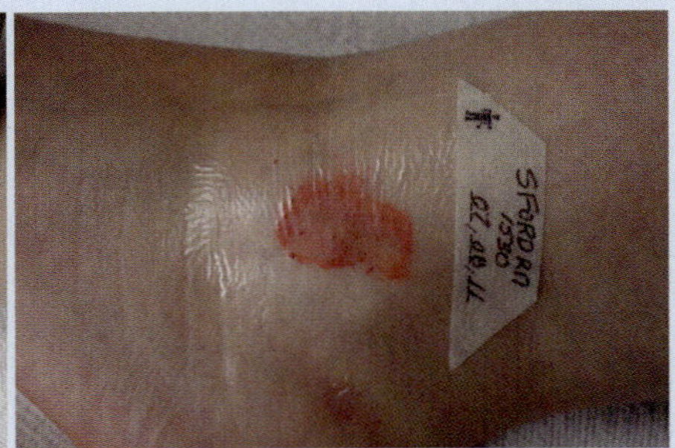

STEP 22e Transparent dressing correctly labeled.

SKILL 26.3   APPLYING HYDROCOLLOID, HYDROGEL, FOAM, OR ALGINATE DRESSINGS

There are numerous classes of dressings to use for wounds with different characteristics. The aim of wound care is to match the properties of a dressing with the characteristics of a wound to enhance healing. Dressings can be divided into two classes: absorbent and hydrating.

A hydrocolloid dressing is a formulation of elastomeric adhesive, and gelling agents. It promotes significantly better wound healing outcomes compared with conventional gauze (Baranoski and Ayello, 2012; Rolstad et al., 2011). Hydrocolloid dressings absorb drainage and hydrate and débride wounds. When in contact with wound drainage, the hydrocolloid forms a gel that promotes a moist environment and facilitates autolytic and enzymatic débridement. The cushioning effect of a hydrocolloid adhesive dressing diminishes pain and protects the wound and periwound skin. This type of dressing conforms well to different body contours and protects the periwound from blister formation when a dressing over a joint (e.g., knee or hip) is flexed with movement (Siddique et al., 2011). Hydrocolloid dressings come in the form of granules, paste, or wafers. Wound exudate is absorbed into the dressing, forming a jelly-like substance next to the wound surface. The dressing maintains a moist, insulated environment for rapid, effective healing.

Hydrogel dressings are glycerin-based or water-based dressings that hydrate wounds, promoting moist wound healing and autolysis (Rolstad et al., 2011). They have some absorptive properties. These dressings are similar to hydrocolloids and come in the form of sheets, amorphous gels, and impregnated gauze. The gel dressings are nonadherent and less painful to remove and must be covered with a secondary dressing to hold them in place.

Examples of absorbent dressings are foam, hydrofiber (alginate), and multilayer. A foam dressing absorbs moderate-to-heavy exudates in superficial or deep wounds, protects friable periwound skin, provides autolytic débridement, and pads high trauma areas. Foam dressings are used with infected wounds after appropriate intervention and close monitoring of wound healing. However, the dressing is not appropriate when there is tunneling of a wound. Some foam dressings are designed to fit around tubes such as a tracheostomy.

Alginate dressings are manufactured from natural substances (seaweed) and are known for their absorptive properties, forming a gel over the wound surface to contain exudate. This dressing may come as a sheet or rope that can be packed into a wound that has moderate-to-heavy drainage. An alginate dressing creates a moist environment and promotes autolysis, granulation, and epithelialization of the wound bed (Rolstad, et al., 2011). A secondary dressing is required.

ASSESSMENT

1. Identify patient using two identifiers (e.g., name and birthday or name and account number) according to facility policy. *Rationale: Ensures correct patient. Complies with The Joint Commission standards and improves patient safety (TJC, 2014).*

2. Ask patient to rate wound pain using a scale of 0 to 10. Administer prescribed analgesic as needed 30 minutes before dressing change. *Rationale: Giving pain medication before dressing change achieves peak effect of drug during procedure. Superficial wounds with multiple exposed nerves may be intensely painful, whereas deeper wounds with destruction of nerves should be less painful (Krazner, 2011).*

3. Assess patient's knowledge of purpose of dressing change and determine need to include family caregiver. *Rationale: Determines level of support and explanation required if a dressing will be changed at home.*

4. Review health care provider's orders for type of dressing. *Rationale: Indicates type of dressing or application to use.*

5. Review previous nursing notes and EMR. *Rationale: Data allow you to obtain appropriate supplies and to review baseline condition of wound.*

6. Assess patient for presence of allergies to antiseptics, tape, or latex. *Rationale: Prevents localized or systemic reaction.*

PLANNING

Expected Outcomes focus on preventing infection, promoting healing, controlling pain, and patient and family caregiver learning wound care.

1. Patient's wound shows evidence of healing by a decrease in size and less drainage, redness, or swelling.

2. Patient reports less pain during and after dressing change.

3. Dressing remains clean, dry, and intact.

4. Patient or family caregiver explains purpose of dressing and method of dressing application.

Delegation and Collaboration

The skill of applying a hydrocolloid, hydrogel, foam, or alginate dressing cannot be delegated to nursing assistive personnel (NAP). The nurse directs the NAP to:

- Assist in positioning patient during dressing change.
- Report to the nurse any pain, fever, bleeding, or wound drainage.

Equipment

- Clean gloves
- Sterile gloves (optional)
- Dressing set (optional)
- Sterile scissors
- Sterile drape (optional)
- Necessary primary dressings: gauze, hydrocolloid, hydrogel, foam, or alginate
- Secondary dressing of choice
- Sterile saline or other cleansing solution (as ordered)
- Skin barrier wipe
- Tape (nonallergenic paper or adhesive), ties as needed
- Measuring guide (tape measure, tracing paper, camera as needed)
- Adhesive remover
- Waterproof bag
- Débriding gel (as ordered)
- Sterile 4 × 4–inch gauze pads or cotton balls
- PPE if needed (when splashing is a risk)

IMPLEMENTATION *for* APPLYING HYDROCOLLOID, HYDROGEL, FOAM, OR ALGINATE DRESSINGS

STEPS	RATIONALE
1. **See Standard Protocol (inside front cover).**	
2. Expose wound site and drape patient. Place disposable waterproof bag within reach of work area. Fold top of bag to make a cuff.	Facilitates safe disposal of soiled dressings.
3. Apply clean gloves. Apply moisture-proof gown, mask, and goggles if there is risk of splashing.	Reduces transmission of microorganisms.
4. Using nondominant hand, gently remove tape, bandages, or ties of existing dressing. Pull tape parallel to the skin and toward the dressing. If dressing is over hairy areas, remove tape in the direction of hair growth and get patient's permission to clip or shave area before applying new dressing (check facility policy). Remove any adhesive from skin.	Pulling tape toward dressing reduces stress on wound edges, irritation, and discomfort.

> **SAFE PATIENT CARE** Check removal directions for specific brand of dressings listed here. Some brands need to have old dressing soaked or moistened before removal. Others require use of adhesive remover, which should not come in direct contact with a wound.

Continued

STEPS	RATIONALE
5. With a gloved hand or forceps, remove dressing one layer at a time. Note amount and character of drainage. Use caution to avoid tension on any drains.	Reduces irritation and possible injury to tissue.
6. Fold dressings with drainage contained inside and remove gloves inside out. With small dressings, remove gloves inside out to enclose dressing (see Skill 26.1). Dispose of gloves and soiled dressing according to facility policy. Cover wound lightly with a sterile 4×4–inch gauze pad. Perform hand hygiene.	Contains soiled dressings; prevents contact of nurse's hands with drainage; reduces cross-contamination.

> **SAFE PATIENT CARE** Hydrocolloid dressings interact with wound fluids and form a soft whitish yellow gel, which is sometimes hard to remove and may have a faint odor. A residual gel substance occurs in wound beds with some absorption dressings; this is normal. Do not confuse these findings with pus or purulent exudates, wound infection, or wound deterioration.

STEPS	RATIONALE
7. Create a sterile field with a sterile dressing tray or individually wrapped sterile supplies on over-bed table (see Chapter 5). Pour prescribed solution into sterile basin.	Creates sterile work area.
8. Remove gauze cover over wound.	
9. Cleanse wound.	
a. Apply clean gloves. Sterile gloves are optional (see facility policy). Use 4×4–inch gauze or cotton ball moistened in saline or use an antiseptic swab (per health care provider order) for each cleansing stroke. Option: Spray wound surface with wound cleanser (see Chapter 24).	Reduces introduction of organisms into wound. Cleaning and irrigating removes residual product without injuring tissue.
b. Clean from least contaminated to most contaminated area.	Cleaning in this direction prevents introduction of organisms.
c. Cleanse around drain (if present), using circular strokes starting near the drain and moving outward away from insertion site.	Correct aseptic technique in cleaning prevents contamination.
10. Use sterile dry gauze to blot dry wound and periwound, using techniques in Step 9.	Drying reduces excess moisture, which can contain microorganisms.
11. Dispose of gloves. Perform hand hygiene.	
12. Inspect appearance and condition of wound and periwound. Measure wound size and depth (see Chapter 24).	Appearance and measurement indicate state of wound healing.
13. Apply dressing.	
a. *Hydrocolloid dressing:*	
(1) Select proper size wafer (see illustration) so that the dressing extends to cover intact periwound skin at least 2.5 cm (1 inch) beyond wound edges. Do not stretch dressing; avoid wrinkles and tenting.	Hydrocolloid dressing prevents shear and friction from loosening edges and circumvents need for tape along dressing borders (Rolstad et al., 2011). Allows molding of wafer to body part.
(2) In the case of a deep wound, apply hydrocolloid granules, impregnated gauze, or paste before applying wafer.	Functions as filler material to ensure contact with all wound surfaces.
(3) Remove paper backing from adhesive side and place over wound. Do not stretch, and avoid wrinkles or tenting. Hold the dressing in place for 30 to 60 seconds after application.	Molds dressing at body temperature (Rolstad et al., 2011).

STEPS	RATIONALE

(4) If cut from a large piece, tape edges with nonallergenic tape to avoid rolling or sticking to clothing. Apply a secondary dressing as needed.

b. *Hydrogel:*

(1) Apply skin barrier wipe to surrounding skin that will come in contact with adhesive or gel.

Protects periwound skin because hydrogel has high water content and can macerate periwound skin (Rolstad et al., 2011).

(2) Apply gel or impregnated gauze directly into the wound, spreading evenly over the wound bed (see illustration). Fill wound cavity with gel about ½ to ⅔ full, or pack the gauze loosely, including undermined or tunneled areas. Cover with a moisture-retentive dressing or hydrocolloid wafer. Option: Hydrogel sheets composed of water should be cut to size of wound only.

Hydrogels hydrate and facilitate autolytic débridement of wounds. Filling wound partially full allows for expansion with exudate (Rolstad et al., 2011).

(3) Cut hydrogel sheet containing glycerin so that it extends 2.5 cm (1 inch) onto intact periwound skin. Cover with a moisture-retentive secondary dressing if needed.

Protects skin around wound from maceration.

(4) Secure dressing with nonallergenic tape if secondary dressing is not self-adhering.

c. *Foam:*

Know removal and application characteristics of specific foam brand.

(1) Apply skin barrier wipe to surrounding skin that will come in contact with thin foam dressing adhesive.

Protects periwound skin from maceration or irritation from adhesive.

(2) Cut foam sheet to extend 2.5 cm (1 inch) onto intact periwound skin. Verify which side of foam dressing should be placed toward wound bed and which side should be facing away.

Ensures proper absorption and keeps wound exudates away from wound bed (Rolstad et al., 2011).

(3) Cut foam to fit around a drain or tube, if present.

(4) Cover with secondary dressing as needed.

Some foam brands need to be covered with a secondary dressing (Rolstad et al., 2011).

STEP 13a(1) Example of hydrocolloid dressings.

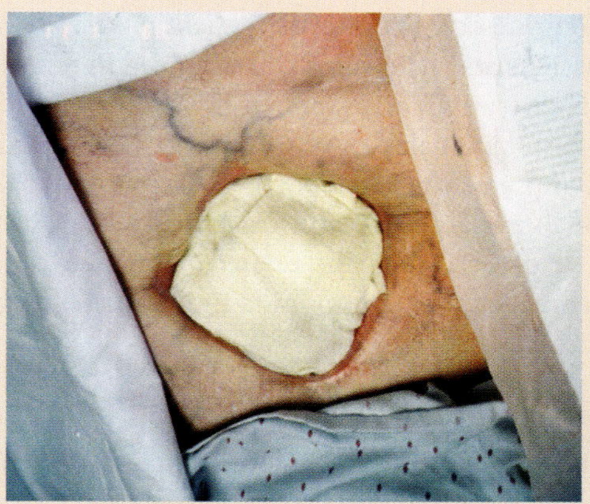

STEP 13b(2) Hydrogel-impregnated gauze packed in open wound.

Continued

STEPS	RATIONALE

   d. Alginate:

     (1) Cut sheet or rope to fit size of wound or loosely pack into wound space (see illustration), filling ½ to ⅔ full.

Expands with absorption of fluid or exudate (Rolstad et al., 2011).

     (2) Apply secondary dressing such as transparent film (see illustration), foam, or hydrocolloid.

Secondary dressing prohibits drainage on bed linens and clothing.

14. Label dressing with your initials and date dressing changed.

Provides timeline for when next dressing change is to be scheduled.

15. See Completion Protocol (inside front cover).

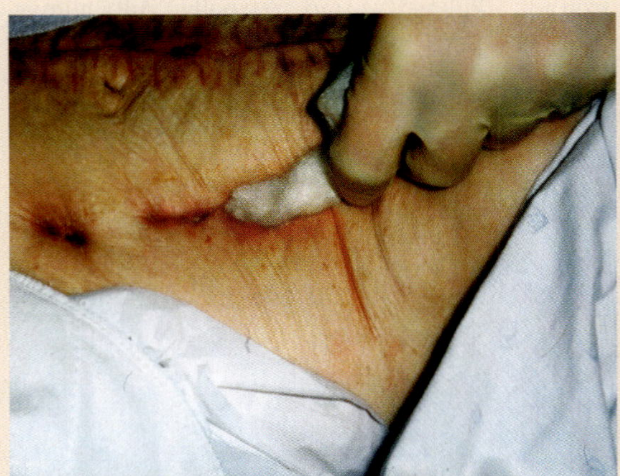

STEP 13d(1) Alginate dressing applied to fill dead space and absorb exudate in full-thickness abdominal wound. (From Bryant R, Nix D: *Acute and chronic wounds: current management and concepts*, ed 4, St Louis, 2012, Mosby.)

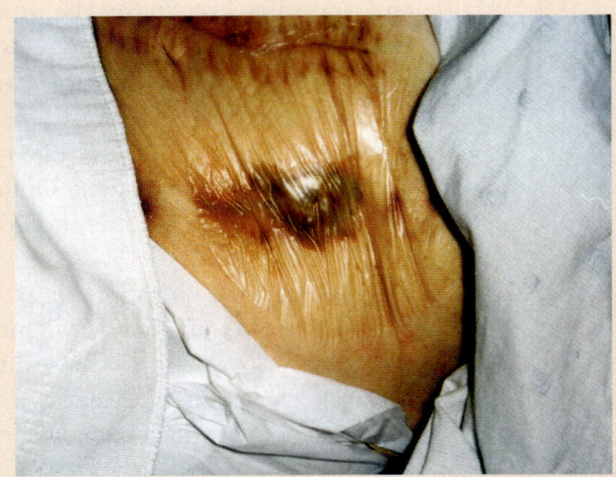

STEP 13d(2) Alginate dressing secured with transparent dressing. (From Bryant R, Nix D: *Acute and chronic wounds: current management and concepts*, ed 4, St Louis, 2012, Mosby.)

EVALUATION

1. Inspect appearance of wound; measure size of wound; observe amount, color, and type of drainage; observe presence of periwound erythema or swelling. Palpate around wound for tenderness.
2. Ask patient to rate pain using a scale of 0 to 10.
3. Inspect condition of dressing at least every shift or as ordered.
4. Use *Teach Back:* State to the patient, "We have reviewed many signs and symptoms you will need to report to your health care provider. I want to be sure that I did a good job of explaining those to you. Can you tell me which signs and symptoms you will report?" Evaluates what the patient is able to explain or demonstrate. Revise your instruction now or develop plan for revised patient teaching to be implemented at an appropriate time if patient is not able to teach back correctly.

Unexpected Outcomes and Related Interventions

1. Wound is inflamed, and patient complains of tenderness. There is yellow, tan, or brown necrotic tissue. Wound size has increased. Drainage is present with or without odor.
   a. Monitor patient for signs of infection (e.g., fever, increased white blood cell count).
   b. In rare cases, some wounds do not tolerate hypoxia induced by hydrocolloid dressings; discontinue use in these cases. Notify health care provider.
   c. Evaluate for other factors impairing wound healing.
2. Dressing does not stay in place.
   a. Evaluate size of dressing used for adequate margin (2.5 to 3.75 cm [1 to 1½ inches]) or dry skin more thoroughly before reapplication.
   b. Consider custom shapes for difficult body parts.
   c. Secure dressing with roll gauze, tape, transparent dressing, or dressing sheet.
3. Periwound skin is macerated.
   a. Assess moisture-control property of dressing or application technique. A new type of dressing may be needed.

Recording and Reporting

- Record size and appearance of wound, characteristics of drainage, presence of necrotic tissue, type of dressings applied, patient's response to dressing change, and level of comfort in nurses' notes.
- Document your evaluation of patient learning.
- Report any unexpected appearance of wound drainage, bright red bleeding, or evidence of wound dehiscence or evisceration.

Sample Documentation

0930   Ulcer on R medial malleolus measuring 4 cm × 2 cm, 0.5 cm in depth. Wound bed with 50% pink granulation tissue and 50% yellow slough tissue. Minimal serous drainage noted. No odor. Surrounding skin intact. Wound cleansed with saline. Hydrogel applied to wound bed. Skin protectant applied to periwound skin. Covered with a 4 × 4–inch hydrocolloid dressing. Patient reported 4/10 pain with removal of old dressing. 0/10 pain at present.

Special Considerations

Pediatric

- See Skill 26.1.

Geriatric

- Avoid early and frequent removal of a hydrocolloid dressing to reduce injury to surrounding intact skin.
- See Skill 26.1.

Home Care

- See Skill 26.1.

PROCEDURAL GUIDELINE 26.2
Applying Gauze and Elastic Bandages

Gauze and elastic bandages secure or wrap hard-to-cover areas of the body, such as dressings on extremities, amputation stumps, and the hands. Bandages are a secondary dressing, providing protection, pressure, immobilization, and anchoring of underlying dressings or splints. There are numerous types of and applications for bandages. Bandages are available in rolls of various widths and materials, including gauze, elastic webbing, elasticized knit, and muslin. Gauze bandages are lightweight and inexpensive, mold easily around body contours, and permit air circulation to prevent skin maceration. Elastic bandages apply compression to a body part. Elastic compression to a lower extremity prevents edema by promoting the return of blood from the peripheral to the central circulation. Muslin bandages are thicker than gauze and stronger for supporting or applying pressure.

When applying a bandage, select a type of bandage turn (Table 26-3) and width depending on the size and shape of the body part to be bandaged. For example, bandages 7.5 cm (3 inches) wide are most commonly used for the adult leg. A smaller 5-cm (2-inch) bandage is normally used for the wrist. When applying an elastic bandage onto an extremity, start at the site farthest from the heart (distal) and proceed toward the heart (proximal).

Delegation and Collaboration

The skill of applying an elastic bandage for compression cannot be delegated to nursing assistive personnel (NAP). The skill of applying bandages to secure nonsterile dressings can be delegated. The nurse instructs the NAP by:

- Explaining how to modify the bandage for a specific patient.
- Reviewing what to observe and report back to the nurse (e.g., patient's complaint of pain, numbness, or tingling after application or changes in patient's skin color or temperature).

Equipment

- Clean gloves (if wound drainage present)
- Correct width and number of gauze or elastic bandages
- Clips or adhesive tape
- Optional: Pillow

Procedural Steps

1. **See Standard Protocol (inside front cover).**
2. Review patient's medical record for specific orders related to application of gauze or elastic bandage. Note area to be covered, type of bandage required, and frequency of change.
3. Identify patient using two identifiers (e.g., name and birthday or name and account number) according to facility policy.
4. Ask patient to rate level of pain using pain scale of 0 to 10. Administer prescribed pain medication as needed 30 minutes before dressing change.
5. Assess patient's knowledge of purpose of bandage and whether there is a need for patient or family caregiver to participate in bandage application.
6. Position patient comfortably in bed or chair.
7. Assess adequacy of circulation by palpating temperature of skin and pulses (distal to area to be bandaged). Inspect for skin color, presence of edema, sensation, and movement.
8. Apply clean gloves (if drainage is present).
9. Inspect condition of primary dressing. Note presence of drainage.
10. *Apply gauze or elastic bandage to secure dressing:*
    a. Elevate dependent extremity for 15 minutes before applying elastic bandage to promote venous return.
    b. Make sure that primary dressing is in place.
    c. Hold roll of bandage in dominant hand and use other hand to hold lightly beginning layer of bandage at most distal body part (see illustration).

Continued

d. Begin with two circular turns to anchor bandage. Continue transferring roll to dominant hand as you wrap the bandage (see illustration).

e. Alternate ascending and descending turns (figure-eight pattern) when wrapping a joint.

f. Ensure that bandage is snug but not tight and that the primary dressing or splint is positioned correctly.

g. While unrolling elastic bandage, stretch bandage slightly. Explain to patient that smooth, even pressure will be applied to improve circulation, reduce swelling, and immobilize body part.

h. Secure end of gauze or elastic bandage to outside layer of bandage, not skin, with tape or clips (see illustration).

> **SAFE PATIENT ALERT** Keep toes and fingers unwrapped and visible for circulatory assessment unless digits are being treated with dressings.

11. *Apply elastic bandage over stump:*
    a. Elevate stump by using a pillow or supporting with the assistance of another person.
    b. Secure bandage by wrapping it twice around proximal end of stump or person's waist (depending on size of stump) (see illustrations).
    c. Make a half turn with bandage perpendicular to its edge.

d. Bring body of bandage over distal end of stump.

e. Continue to fold bandage over stump, wrapping from distal to proximal points.

f. Secure with metal clips, Velcro if provided, or tape.

12. Assess degree of tightness of bandage, wrinkles, looseness, and presence of drainage.

13. **See Completion Protocol (inside front cover).**

14. Evaluate distal circulation when bandage application is complete, at least twice during the next 8 hours, then at least every shift.
    a. Observe skin color for pallor or cyanosis.
    b. Palpate skin for warmth.
    c. Palpate distal pulses and compare bilaterally.
    d. Ask patient to rate pain on scale of 0 to 10 and to describe any numbness, tingling, or other discomfort.
    e. Check bandage for wrinkles, looseness, and presence of drainage.

15. Have patient or family caregiver demonstrate bandage application.

16. Record patient's level of comfort, circulation status, type of bandage applied, presence of swelling, and range of motion at baseline and after bandage application and record type of bandage applied.

17. Report condition of any changes in neurological or circulatory status to health care provider.

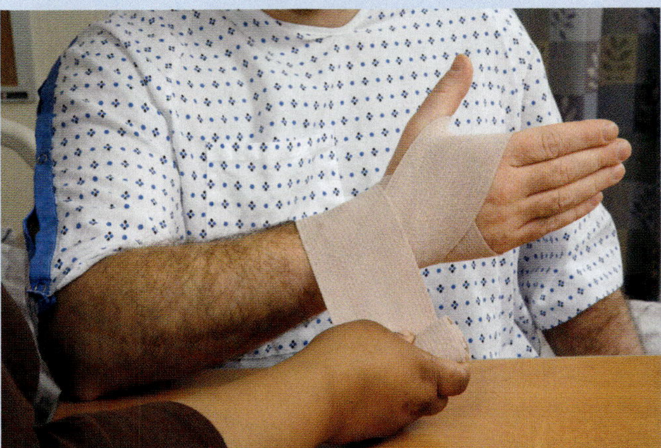

STEP 10c Hold bandage in dominant hand and apply using circular turns.

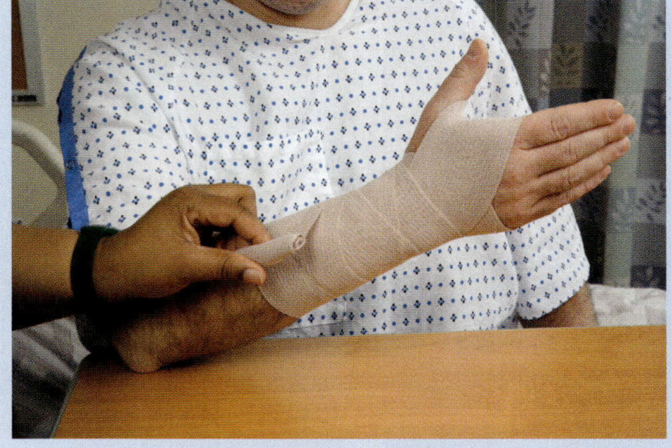

STEP 10d Apply bandage from distal to proximal.

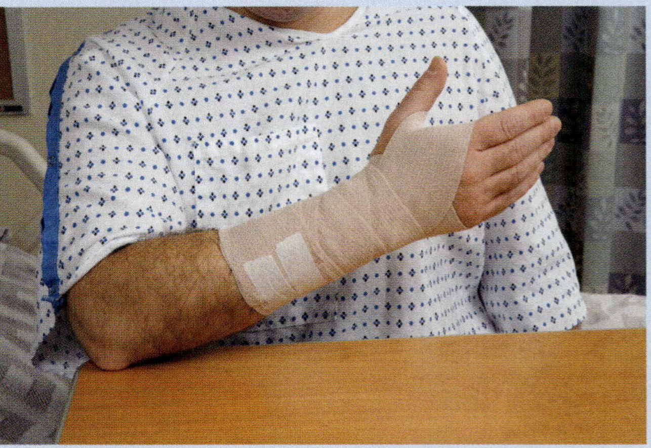

STEP 10h Secure with tape or closure device.

PROCEDURAL GUIDELINE 26.2
Applying Gauze and Elastic Bandages—cont'd

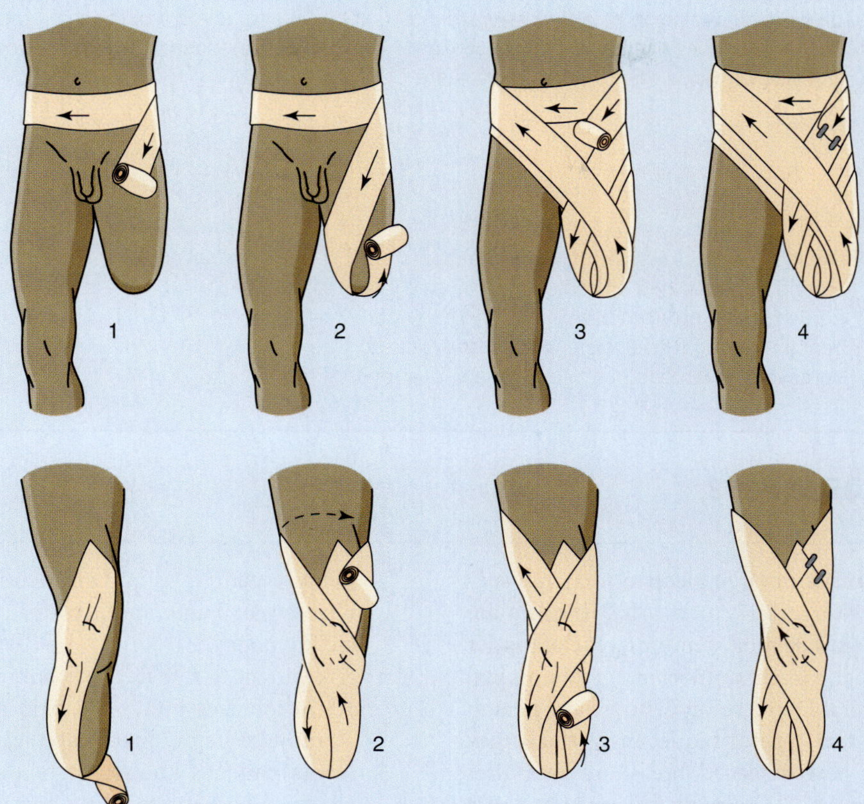

STEP 11b-f *Top,* Correct method for bandaging midthigh amputation stump. Note that bandage must be anchored around patient's waist. *Bottom,* Correct method for bandaging midcalf amputation stump. Note that bandage need not be anchored around the waist. (From Monahan F et al: *Phipps' medical-surgical nursing: health and illness perspectives,* ed 8, St Louis, 2006, Mosby.)

TABLE 26-3   TYPES OF BANDAGE TURNS

TYPE	DESCRIPTION	PURPOSE OR USE
Circular Turns	Bandage turn overlapping previous turn completely	Anchors bandage at first and final turn; covers small part (finger, toe)
Spiral Turns	Bandage ascending body part with each turn overlapping previous one by ½ or ⅔ width of bandage	Covers cylindrical body parts such as wrist or upper arm
Spiral-Reverse Turns	Turn requiring twist (reversal) of bandage halfway through each turn	Covers cone-shaped body parts such as the forearm, thigh, or calf; useful with nonstretching bandages such as gauze or flannel

Continued

TABLE 26-3	TYPES OF BANDAGE TURNS—cont'd	
TYPE	**DESCRIPTION**	**PURPOSE OR USE**
Figure-Eight Turns	Oblique overlapping turns alternately ascending and descending over bandaged part, each turn crossing previous one to form figure eight	Covers joints; applies low-grade pressure for venous return; snug fit provides excellent immobilization
Recurrent Turns	Bandage first secured with two circular turns around proximal end of body part; half turn made perpendicular up from bandage edge; body of bandage brought over distal end of body part to be covered with each turn folded back over on itself	Covers uneven body parts such as head or stump

PROCEDURAL GUIDELINE 26.3
Applying a Binder

Binders are bandages made of large pieces of material specially designed to fit a large body part. Most binders are made of elastic or cotton. The most common type of binder is the abdominal binder, which supports large abdominal incisions that are vulnerable to tension or stress as a person moves or coughs. Another type of binder is for the breast, although sports bras have replaced breast binders after surgery (Michaels, et al., 2011). Front-fastening bras are easiest to apply in the postoperative period.

You apply a binder over or around dressings to support a wound, protect surrounding skin, reduce or prevent edema, and decrease pain, promoting physical activity and respiratory function. It is important to apply a binder correctly and monitor a patient's ability to move comfortably. Misplaced binders have the potential to injure the wound and underlying skin, cause discomfort to patients, and interfere with respirations and mobility.

Delegation and Collaboration

The skill of applying binders can be delegated to nursing assistive personnel (NAP). The nurse instructs the NAP by:
- Explaining how to modify the skill for a specific patient.
- Reviewing what to report back to the nurse (e.g., complaints of numbness, pain, tingling, difficulty breathing, or change in skin color below area of application).

Equipment

- Clean gloves (if drainage present)
- Gauze bandage as needed
- Correct type and size of binder or sports bra
- Closure for cloth binder

Procedural Steps

1. **See Standard Protocol (inside front cover).**
2. Review medical record for order for type and size of binder.
3. Identify patient using two identifiers (e.g., name and birthday or name and account number) according to facility policy.
4. Ask patient to rate level of pain using pain scale of 0 to 10. Administer prescribed pain medication as needed 30 minutes before binder application.
5. Assess patient's knowledge of purpose of binder and whether there is a need for patient or family caregiver to participate in binder application.
6. Apply clean gloves (if drainage present).
7. Inspect skin for actual or potential alterations in skin integrity. Observe for irritation, abrasions, and skin surfaces that rub against one another.
8. Assess patient's ability to breathe deeply, cough effectively, and turn or move independently.
9. Cover any exposed area of an incision or wound with a dressing. Change soiled dressing as needed.
10. *Apply abdominal binder:*
    a. Position patient in supine position with head slightly elevated and knees slightly flexed.
    b. Help patient to roll on side away from you toward raised side rail while firmly supporting abdominal incision and dressing with hands.
    c. Place binder flat on bed, right side up. Fanfold far side of binder toward midline of binder so that patient can roll over with minimal effort.
    d. Instruct patient to roll over folded binder.
    e. Instruct patient next to roll onto back.
    f. Unfold and stretch ends of binder out smoothly on far side of bed. Then stretch out ends on near side of bed.
    g. Adjust binder so that supine patient is centered over binder using symphysis pubis and costal margins as lower and upper landmarks.

PROCEDURAL GUIDELINE 26.3
Applying a Binder—cont'd

h. If patient is very thin, pad bony prominences with gauze bandages.

i. Close binder. Pull one end of binder over center of patient's abdomen. While maintaining tension on that end of binder, pull opposite end of binder over center and secure with Velcro closure tabs or metal fasteners (see illustration).

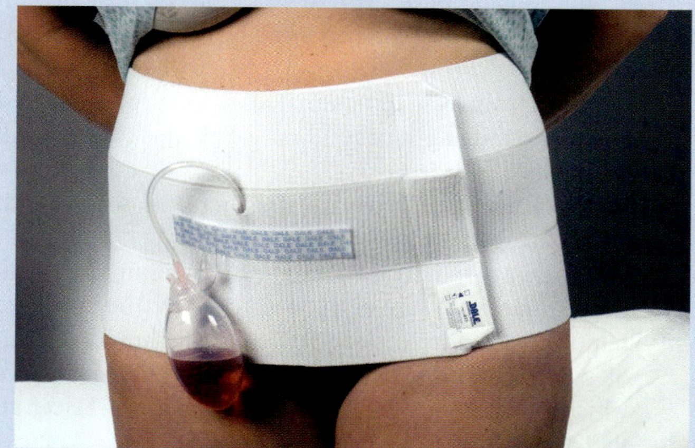

STEP 10i Abdominal binder with Velcro closures. (Courtesy Dale Medical Products, Inc, Plainsville, Massachusetts.)

11. *Apply mastectomy sports bra:*
  a. Protect surgical incision with prescribed dressing.
  b. Slip arms in bra strap openings (same as putting on a blouse) opening to the front.
  c. Fasten bra.
  d. If using a bra with additional support straps or binder, follow manufacturer's instructions in application.

> **SAFE PATIENT ALERT** Recheck patient's ability to breathe deeply and cough effectively.

12. **See Completion Protocol (inside front cover).**
13. Ask patient to rate pain on a scale of 0 to 10. Adjust binder for comfort as needed.
14. Evaluate patient's ability to breathe deeply and cough without discomfort every 4 hours. Report any changes in respiratory status to health care provider.
15. Remove binder and any underlying dressing to evaluate skin and wound characteristics at least every 8 hours.
16. Record type and application of binder, condition of skin, circulation, ease of breathing and coughing, level of comfort, and status of underlying dressing.

CRITICAL THINKING EXERCISES

Case Study

A 15-year-old boy is recovering from surgery following a ruptured appendix. His surgical incision has been left open to heal by secondary intention. His next dressing change is due this morning. In report you learned that the patient observed the steps involved in changing the dressing during the previous dressing change.

1. Before proceeding with the morning dressing change, the nurse should do the following. Select all that apply.
   1. Avoid giving pain medication before the procedure to ensure he is fully awake to participate.
   2. Ask his visiting friend if he would like to stay and watch the dressing change.
   3. Discuss with the patient the condition of his wound before proceeding.
   4. Ask the patient if he would like to do the dressing this time with your guidance.

2. The health care provider has ordered moist-to-dry dressing changes twice a day for the patient using normal saline. Place the following steps in order for the procedure.
   1. Clean the wound with saline-moistened gauze.
   2. Remove the old dressing.
   3. Inspect the appearance and condition of the wound, and measure wound size.
   4. Cover wound with 4 × 4–inch sterile gauze and an ABD.
   5. Loosely pack the wound with saline-moistened gauze.
   6. Blot the wound dry.
   7. Fasten dressing using nonallergenic tape.

3. The nurse gives report on the patient to the NAP. The nurse asks the NAP to assist him with a bath, bed linen change, and getting up in the chair. During today's tasks, what should the NAP be instructed to do? Select all that apply.
   1. Reinforce the dressing if drainage appears.
   2. Notify the nurse if the patient complains of pain.
   3. Report if the patient develops a fever.
   4. Notify the nurse of any bleeding.

Review Questions

1. A hydrocolloid dressing is an adhesive dressing that contains a gel-forming agent. This type of dressing is ideal for which one of the following types of wounds?
   1. Stage I pressure ulcers
   2. Wounds with a large amount of drainage
   3. Wound with dry eschar
   4. Partial-thickness or full-thickness wounds.

2. A patient has a large amount of drainage from a large partial-thickness wound. The previous dressing orders included the use of a hydrocolloid dressing. The patient has developed maceration of the periwound. Which change in choice of dressings should the nurse expect?
   1. Continue the use of the hydrocolloid and apply an absorbent secondary dressing.
   2. Pack the wound and place a transparent dressing.
   3. Pack the wound with gauze and cover with an ABD.
   4. Apply a moisture barrier and then foam dressing with a secondary dressing for support.

3. The nurse caring for a patient with an acute or chronic wound would need to follow which of the following safety guidelines? Select all that apply.
   1. Be aware of any drains in place before removing an old dressing.
   2. Use PPE only if the patient is on isolation.
   3. Know the cause and type of wound the patient has.
   4. Properly dispose of the contaminated dressings.

4. Pain management is an important aspect of caring for a patient with an open wound. Which of the following interventions would you include in a plan of care?
   1. Pack the wound tightly to prevent leakage of drainage on the periwound.
   2. Keep the wound bed as dry as possible.
   3. Medicate the patient for management of pain at least 30 minutes before treatment.
   4. Avoid use of moisture barriers because they can irritate the skin.

5. Moist-to-dry gauze dressings have been traditional treatment options for open wounds for many years. Newer products such as hydrocolloids and hydrogels have replaced moist-to-dry dressing in many cases. Which one of the following characteristics is true of moist-to-dry dressings?
   1. May adhere to healthy tissue
   2. Have the ability to collect exudates and debris
   3. Primarily used to débride a wound bed
   4. Available in many sizes and forms

   A patient had an exploratory laparotomy for removal of abdominal adhesions and an umbilical hernia repair. On postoperative day 2, the patient had a severe coughing episode. During this episode, he experienced a wound dehiscence of the lower third of his incision. The wound opening measures 3.5 cm in length × 2.5 cm in depth (1.4 inch × 1 inch). A small tunneled area approximately 1.5 cm (0.6 inch) in depth appears at the top of the area where the wound dehiscence begins and the incision remains intact. A moderate amount of serosanguineous drainage is present. His dressing change orders include wound packing with hydrogel gauze. (This information applies to questions 6 to 8.)

6. Place the following steps in order for this type of dressing change.
   1. Label dressing with your initials and date dressing changed.
   2. Perform hand hygiene and apply gloves.
   3. Inspect appearance and condition of wound. Measure wound size.
   4. Remove old dressing one layer at a time using a clean gloved hand or forceps.
   5. Partially fill wound bed with hydrogel-impregnated gauze.
   6. Clean from least contaminated to most contaminated area, removing any residual gel in the wound bed; irrigate if needed.
   7. Apply moisture-retentive dressing and secure with nonallergenic tape.

7. The patient is to have an abdominal binder in place at all times. The NAP has been instructed by the nurse to remove the binder only to adjust it if it should slip out of place. The nurse also instructs the NAP to observe which of the following signs and symptoms? Select all that apply.
   1. Difficulty breathing
   2. Skin irritation under the binder
   3. Change in skin color of his lower abdomen
   4. Increased circumference of abdomen.

8. The patient's wife has arrived this morning to observe and learn how to change her husband's dressing. Which of the following statements by the wife would indicate the need to revise your teaching?
   1. "I would dispose of the dressing in the regular trash."
   2. "I would report any signs and symptoms of infection, such as redness, increased drainage, or an odor."
   3. "I should always wash my hands before and after the dressing change."
   4. "I will make sure I have plenty of dressings on hand before I change the dressing."

9. Which of the following is not a characteristic of an ideal dressing?
   1. Maintains physiologic wound environment
   2. Is impermeable to microorganisms
   3. Removes exudate and allows the wound to dry
   4. Is cost-effective

10. The skin of an older-adult patient is fragile, and the patient has a 5-cm (2-inch) skin tear along the lower arm. The skin is still attached. A transparent dressing is covering the wound. Which of the following ways does a nurse remove a transparent dressing covering a skin tear?
    1. Remove old dressing by stretching film in direction parallel to wound
    2. Take edge of dressing and pull off in direction of closed edge of skin tear
    3. Remove transparent film in direction of the open edge of the tear
    4. Place a moist gauze over dressing before removing

REFERENCES

Baranoski S, Ayello E: Wound dressing: an evolving art and science, *Adv Skin Wound Care* 25(2):88, 2012.

Benbow M: Addressing pain in wound care and dressing removal, *Nursing & Residential Care* 13(10):474, 2011.

Bishop S, Walker M, Spivak M: Family presence in the adult burn intensive care unit during dressing changes, *Crit Care Nurse* 33(1):14, 2013.

Denyer J: Reducing pain during the removal of adhesive and adherent products, *Br J Nurs* 20(15):S28, 2011.

Doughty D, Sparks-DeFriese B: Wound healing physiology. In Bryant RA, Nix DP, editors: *Acute and chronic wounds: nursing management*, ed 4, St Louis, 2011, Mosby.

Jones J: Exploring the link between the clinical challenges of wound exudate and infection, *Br J Nurs* P8, 2013.

Jones M: The prevention and management of skin tears, *Nursing & Residential Care* 13(9):418, 2011.

Krazner DL: Wound pain: impact and assessment. In Bryant RA, Nix DP, editors: *Acute and chronic wounds: nursing management*, ed 4, St Louis, 2011, Mosby.

Meaume S, Barrols B, Faucher N: French national wound management survey: choice criteria of dressing, *Br J Nurs* 20(20):S10, 2011.

Michaels J, Coon D, Rubin P: Complications in postbariatric body contouring: postoperative management and treatment, *Plast Reconstr Surg* 127(4):1695, 2011.

Newton H: An introduction to wound healing and dressings, *Br J Healthc Manag* 19(6):270, 2013.

Nilsson S, Hallqvist C, et al: Children's experiences of procedural pain management in conjunction with trauma wound dressings, *J Adv Nurs* 67(7):1449, 2011.

Phillips PL, et al: Biofilms made easy, *Wounds Int* 1(3):1, 2010.

Rolstad BS, Bryant RA, Nix DP: Topical management. In Bryant RA, Nix DP, editors: *Acute and chronic wounds: current management concepts*, ed 4, St Louis, 2012, Mosby.

Siddique K, Mirza S, Housden P: Effectiveness of hydrocolloid dressing in postoperative hip and knee surgery: literature review and our experience, *J Perioper Pract* 21(8):275, 2011.

Stephen-Hayes J, Callaghan R, et al: The assessment and management of skin tears in care homes, *Br J Nurs* 20(11):S12, 2011.

The Joint Commission (TJC): *National Patient Safety Goals*, Oakbrook Terrace, IL, 2014, The Commission. Available at: http://www.jointcommission.org/standards_information/npsgs.aspx.

Wodash A: Wet-to-dry dressings do not provide moist wound healing, *J Am Coll Clin Wound Special* 4(3):63, 2012.

The Wound Healing and Management Node Group: Wet-to-dry saline moistened gauze for wound dressing, *Wound Pract Res* 19(1):48, 2011.

CHAPTER

27

Intravenous and Vascular Access Therapy

Placement of an intravenous (IV) device is one of the most invasive procedures a nurse can perform, putting a patient at risk for complications associated with infusion therapy. Critical thinking is required before initiation of infusion therapy and during the course of treatment. Assessment of a patient's anatomy and physiology of the circulatory system, fluid and electrolyte balance, disease pathophysiology, type and duration of prescribed therapy, allergies, and the patient's response to illness plays a key role in decision making to ensure safe delivery of infusion solutions or medications. The goal of IV therapy is to maintain and prevent fluid and electrolyte imbalances, administer continuous or intermittent medications (e.g., antibiotics and analgesics), and replenish blood volume (Felver, 2013; Phillips, 2014).

Follow the six rights of administering parenteral solutions or medications: *right* drug/solution, *right* dose/concentration, *right* patient, *right* route, *right* date/time, and *right* documentation (Alexander et al., 2014; INS, 2011a). The six *rights* also include knowledge of the correct solution and equipment, how to initiate and regulate an infusion, how to care and maintain the infusion equipment, how to identify and correct any infusion-related complications, and how to discontinue the infusion. To provide infusion therapy safely and correctly, you need astute clinical management and specialized IV therapy skills in addition to your knowledge and professional

accountability. Know and follow these standards, your facility's policy and procedures, and your state or government practice guidelines and standards when providing infusion therapy.

PATIENT-CENTERED CARE

The approach you take can directly affect a patient's response to infusion therapy. Preparing a patient before placing a short-peripheral IV device may help to alleviate fears associated with infusion therapy. Consider any psychological factors related to your patient's previous experience with infusion therapy because these will affect how you place the IV device and the patient's ability to understand the therapy prescribed (Corrigan et al., 2014). Depending on the age of a patient or factors that may affect his or her ability to comprehend, you may need to establish a rapport with a family caregiver.

You can make the experience less traumatic if you appear confident, speak directly to the patient, ensure his or her privacy, and answer questions as directly and honestly as possible. Have a patient use diversional techniques, such as deep breathing, avoiding looking at a catheter during insertion, and focusing on pleasant images or past experiences to lessen anxiety (Corrigan et al., 2014; Phillips, 2014). As a nurse, be aware of the diversity found within health care, including age, gender, race, ethnicity, sexual orientation, and religious beliefs (Corrigan et al., 2014). Such diversity means that you must provide culturally sensitive care. A careful assessment of a patient's beliefs and attitudes about IV therapy and the meaning behind those beliefs helps you to know your patient and be better able to meet his or her physical, psychosocial, spiritual, and cultural needs (Corrigan et al., 2014; Petroulias et al., 2013).

SAFETY

The risk of incurring a needlestick injury or being exposed to a bloodborne pathogen is a safety concern during the insertion of a short-peripheral IV device and when managing infusion therapy. The Needlestick Safety and Prevention Act (OSHA, 2006) requires health care employers to identify and use effective and safer medical devices. In addition, the Infusion Nurses Society (INS) standards recommend that all devices have engineered sharps injury protection mechanisms that are activated before disposal (Hadaway, 2012; INS, 2011b). Most devices have either a self-sheathing mechanism that covers the needle tip when the catheter is placed or a spring action mechanism in which the needle is retracted into a protective housing after the catheter is inserted (Alexander et al., 2014; Hadaway, 2012). It would be impossible to eliminate the need to use short-peripheral IV devices; however, devices with built-in sharps injury protection features can reduce the risk of an accidental needlestick injury. You will become familiar with the safety devices specific to your facility and the correct method to activate the safety mechanisms. Another way to prevent sharps injury is to discard all sharps material in ridged sharps disposal containers (INS, 2011b; O'Grady et al, 2011). Safety issues related to placing and removing the short-peripheral IV device and initiating and completing the setup of the infusion equipment are covered in each skills section.

EVIDENCE-BASED PRACTICE

Infusion Nurses Society (INS): 2011 Infusion nursing standards of practice, *J Infus Nurs* 34(1 Suppl), 2011b.

The Joint Commission: Preventing central line associated bloodstream infections, 2013. http://www.jointcommission.org/assets/1/6/CLABSI_Toolkit_Tool_3-18_CVC_Insertion_Bundles.pdf. Accessed September 11, 2014.

Adhering to evidence-based practices can significantly reduce the risk of local and systemic infusion-related complications. The U.S. Centers for Disease Control and Prevention (CDC), Institute for Health Improvement (IHI), INS, and National Quality Forum (NQF) have demonstrated that the increased risk of infusion-related complications is directly linked to poor infection control practices. These include poor hand hygiene, inadequate site preparation, and inadequate nursing judgment when assessing for the appropriate insertion site and catheter selection. The use of vascular visualization devices (i.e., ultrasound) should be considered as an option for vein identification and selection before placement of short-peripheral and centrally placed catheters (INS, 2011b).

The use of evidence-based care bundles has been shown to decrease the incidence of central line–associated bloodstream infections (CLABSI) in central vascular access devices (CVADs), and these care bundles are now considered best practice with respect to improving patient outcomes. The Joint Commission (2013) is among numerous government and professional organizations such as the INS that support the evidence for bundle components to be considered a standard of care. According to The Joint Commission, the care bundle for CLABSI is a group of evidence-based interventions that result in better outcomes when implemented together than when implemented individually. The Care bundle for CLABSI (TJC, 2013) includes:

- Meticulous hand hygiene
- Maximal barrier precautions (mask, gown, gloves) during central line insertion
- Use of chlorhexidine as a cleaning agent
- Optimal catheter site selection, with avoidance of femoral vein in patients younger than 18 years old
- Daily review of the necessity for a central line with prompt removal of any unnecessary lines

SKILL 27.1 INSERTION OF A SHORT-PERIPHERAL INTRAVENOUS DEVICE

• Nursing Skills Online: Intravenous Fluid Administration Module, Lessons 1 and 2

IV infusions deliver isotonic, hypotonic, or hypertonic fluids through a variety of catheters and access devices either continuously or intermittently to maintain or correct fluid and electrolyte balance. Infusion therapy provides access to the venous system to deliver various medications in emergent and nonemergent situations and to infuse blood or blood products. Reliable venous access for infusion therapy is essential (Felver, 2013).

Successful IV therapy depends on patient preparation, site selection, catheter selection, and catheter insertion. Several

vascular access devices (VADs) are available for use in peripheral veins (Table 27-1). The INS standards of practice recommend using the smallest device and smallest gauge possible to give the prescribed therapy (INS, 2011b). Because potential exposure to bloodborne pathogens is high during insertion and care of IV devices, adherence to asepsis and standard precautions is required (see Chapter 5).

Steel-winged infusion devices (butterfly needles) should be limited to short-term or single-dose IV administration. They are easier to insert but may easily infiltrate. Commonly

TABLE 27-1	**INTRAVENOUS ACCESS DEVICE OPTIONS**	
TYPE	**USE**	**TYPES OF INFUSIONS**
Winged infusion butterfly needle	One-time infusion, IV push administration	Solutions or medications with a pH between 5.0 and 9.0 Osmolarity <600 mOsm/L (INS, 2011b)
Short, over-the-needle catheter (7.5 cm [<3 inches])	Most common, continuous infusion, intermittent infusion, short-term duration (rotate site every 72 hours) (INS, 2011b)	Solutions or medications with a pH between 5.0 and 9.0 Osmolarity <600 mOsm/L (INS, 2011b)
Midline peripheral catheters (7.5-20 cm [3-8 inches])	Continuous and intermittent infusion (1-4 weeks) (INS, 2011b)	Solutions or medications with a pH between 5.0 and 9.0 Osmolarity <600 mOsm/L (INS, 2011b)

IV, Intravenous.

used over-the-needle catheters include (1) a metal stylet to pierce the skin and (2) a catheter made of silicone, polyurethane, polyvinyl chloride, or polytetrafluoroethylene (Teflon) that threads into a vein and remains there for the infusion of fluid. These flexible catheters do not dislodge from veins as easily as stainless steel needles. In choosing a catheter, always select the shortest catheter with the smallest gauge because this ensures proper administration of fluid and minimizes irritation and damage to blood vessel walls.

ASSESSMENT

1. Review accuracy and completeness of health care provider's order for patient name and correct IV solution type, volume, infusion rate, and length of therapy. Check medication and additives for the correct dosage and their compatibility with primary and secondary solutions. *Rationale: Before administering solutions or medications, an order from a licensed independent practitioner is needed (INS, 2011b). Assists in selection of an appropriate access device and early placement of longer term infusion devices, which minimize multiple venipunctures.*

2. Identify patient using two identifiers (e.g., name and birthday or name and account number) according to facility policy. Compare identifiers with information on the patient's MAR or medical record. *Rationale: Ensures correct patient. Complies with The Joint Commission standards and improves patient safety (TJC, 2014).*

3. Assess patient's previous experience and understanding of IV therapy and arm placement preference. *Rationale: Provides patient-centered care by determining level of emotional support and instructions needed (INS, 2011a).*

4. Determine if patient is to undergo any planned surgeries or procedures. *Rationale: Allows you to place an appropriate-size catheter and avoids placement in an area that will interfere with surgeries or procedures.*

5. Assess patient's hand/arm dominance. *Rationale: Ensures that placement does not impair therapy or interfere with activities of daily living or mobility.*

6. Assess for risk factors: child or older adult, presence of heart failure or oliguric renal disease, skin lesions or infection near potential IV site, low platelet count, or anticoagulant use. *Rationale: Conditions pose a risk for fluid overload, affect IV site selection, and determine a patient's risk for bleeding.*

7. Assess for clinical variables that will respond to or be affected by IV fluid administration:
   a. Body weight
   b. Clinical markers of vascular volume:
      (1) Blood pressure (BP) (orthostatic hypotension or hypotension with extracellular fluid volume [ECV] deficit)
      (2) Pulse (rapid, thready with ECV deficit; bounding with ECV excess)
      (3) Fullness of neck veins (flat or collapsing with ECV deficit; full or distended with ECV excess)
      (4) Capillary refill (sluggish with ECV deficit)
      (5) Auscultation of lungs
      (6) Urine output (decreased; dark yellow with ECV deficit)
   c. Clinical markers of interstitial volume:
      (1) Dependent edema—pitting or nonpitting
      (2) Oral mucous membranes (dry between cheek and gum with ECV deficit)
      (3) Skin turgor
   d. Thirst

8. Assess condition of both arms. Palpate veins. *Rationale: Allows for initial selection of appropriate vein to accommodate device and therapy. Avoids veins that are sclerosed or damaged from previous IV therapy or contraindicated for an IV start (mastectomy or dialysis shunt). Consider using an ultrasound device if veins are difficult to locate.*

9. Assess laboratory data. *Rationale: Establishes baseline for evaluating if therapy is effective.*

10. Assess patient's history of allergies, especially to iodine, adhesive, or latex. *Rationale: Equipment used during insertion of VAD may contain substances to which patient is allergic. Use alternatives if patient has allergy.*

11. Assess patient's medical history for chronic illnesses and all prescribed and over-the-counter medications. *Rationale: Reveals background information that might result in adverse effects on patient (e.g., heart failure may require slower infusion rate) or conflict with the prescribed therapy such as drug-drug interactions.*

PLANNING

Expected Outcomes focus on avoiding complications related to IV therapy, minimizing patient discomfort, and establishing a patent route for delivery of therapies.

1. Fluid and electrolyte balance returns to normal, blood volume is replenished, or both.
2. Vital signs are stable.
3. Laboratory values return to within normal limits for patient.
4. Intake and output (I&O) are within normal limits for patient's condition.
5. No signs or symptoms of IV-related complications are observed.
6. IV access is patent, and infusion is delivered at prescribed rate and volume.

Delegation and Collaboration

The skill of inserting a short-peripheral IV access device and monitoring infusion solutions and medications cannot be delegated to nursing assistive personnel (NAP). A nurse directs the NAP to inform the nurse if:

- Patient indicates pain, bleeding, burning, redness, or swelling at IV site.
- The volume of fluid is low in the IV bag or the electronic infusion device (EID) is sounding its alarm.
- An IV dressing becomes wet or loose.

Equipment

- IV start kit, which contains tourniquet, tape, clear occlusive dressing, cleansing agent(s) (2% chlorhexidine and 70% alcohol), and 2 × 2–inch gauze pads
- Appropriate short IV catheter: for continuous fluid infusions, peripheral 22-gauge catheter for adult, 24-gauge for children, and 22- to 24-gauge for older adults and children (INS, 2011b); for short-term therapy or a single dose, steel-winged device (INS, 2011b)
- Clean gloves (latex-free for patient with latex allergy)
- Short extension tubing with fused needleless connector or separate needleless connector (also called *injection cap, IV plug, saline lock, heparin lock, PRN adapter, buff cap, or buffalo cap*).
- Prefilled 5-mL syringe with flush agent (preservative-free normal saline [NS])
- Alcohol pads
- Manufactured catheter stabilization device if available (INS, 2011b)
- IV tubing appropriate for EID
- Prescribed IV solution or medications
- EID and IV pole
- Ultrasound device (optional based on facility's policy and procedure)
- Needle disposal container (sharps container)

IMPLEMENTATION *for* INSERTION OF A SHORT-PERIPHERAL INTRAVENOUS DEVICE

STEPS	RATIONALE
1. **See Standard Protocol (inside front cover).**	
2. Instruct patient about rationale for infusion and procedure for inserting IV.	Promotes patient understanding and adherence.
3. Change patient's gown to more easily removed gown with snaps at shoulder.	
4. Select appropriate-size catheter, and open and prepare sterile packages.	The catheter selected uses the smallest size and shortest length to accommodate prescribed therapy (INS, 2011b).
5. Prepare IV infusion tubing and solution for continuous infusion using sterile technique.	Maintaining the sterility of a closed IV system decreases the risk of bacterial contamination (Corrigan et al., 2014).
a. Check IV solution using the six rights of medication administration. If using bar-code system, scan bar code on patient's wristband and then bar code on IV fluid container. Ensure that prescribed additives such as potassium and vitamins are included on the label. Check solution for leaks, color, clarity, and expiration date. Hang solution on IV pole.	IV solutions are medications and need to be checked carefully to reduce the risk for error. Bar-code systems reduce medication errors by verifying right patient, medication, dose, and time with the electronic medical record (Voshall et al., 2013).
b. Open infusion set, maintaining sterility of both tubing ends. Note: Many EID pumps have special administration sets.	Prevents touch contamination, which prevents microorganisms from entering infusion equipment and bloodstream.

Continued

c. Removing appropriate end caps, attach extension tubing with injection port to distal end of infusion set, maintaining sterility of the connection. Do not touch point of entry of connection. Leave end cap on distal end of extension tubing.

Distal end of extension tubing with injection port attaches to IV catheter hub after venipuncture, providing greater ease of access and ability to change easily between continuous and intermittent IV infusions. Prevents touch contamination.

d. Place roller clamp 2 to 5 cm (1 to 2 inches) below drip chamber, and move roller clamp to "off" position (see illustration).

Close proximity of clamp to drip chamber allows more accurate regulation of flow rate. "Off" position prevents leakage during priming.

e. Remove protective sheath from IV tubing port on plastic IV solution bag (see illustration) or from top of glass bottle. Insert infusion set into fluid bag or bottle by removing protector cap from insertion spike (not touching the spike) and inserting it into opening of IV container (see illustration). *Cleanse rubber stopper on glass-bottled solution with single-use antiseptic, and insert spike into black rubber stopper of IV bottle. Bottle needs vented tubing.*

Provides access for insertion of infusion tubing into the solution using sterile technique. Flat surface on top of a bottled solution may contain contaminants, whereas the port on the plastic bag is recessed.

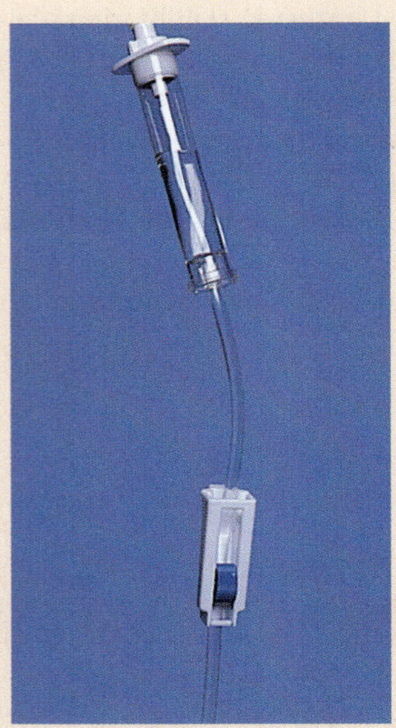

STEP 5d Roller clamp in "off" or closed position.

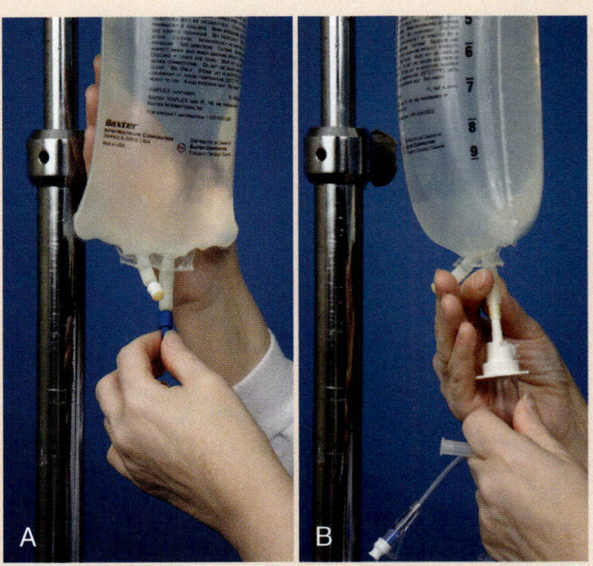

STEP 5e A, Remove protective covering from IV solution tubing port. **B,** Insert tubing spike into IV container.

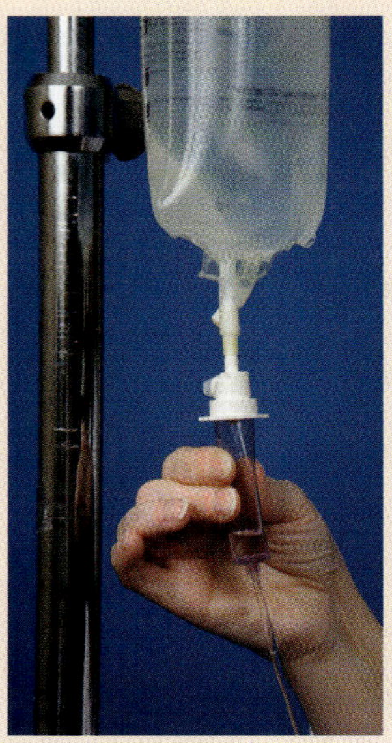

STEP 5f Squeeze drip chamber to fill with fluid.

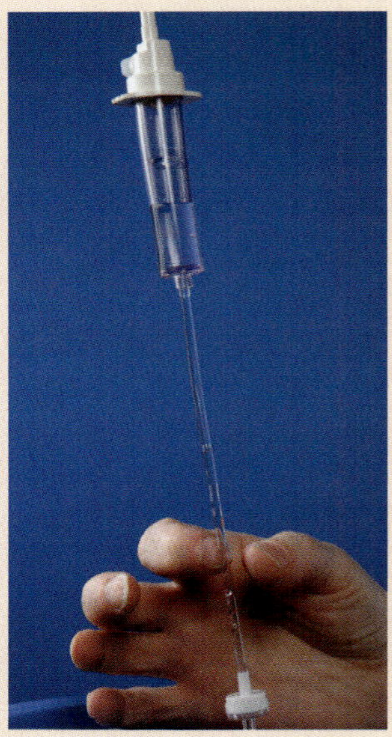

STEP 5g Removing air bubbles from tubing.

f. Prime infusion tubing by filling with IV solution: Compress drip chamber and release; allow it to fill one third to one half full (see illustration).

Ensures tubing is cleared of air and filled with saline before connection with IV catheter.

g. Remove protective cap on end of tubing (you can prime some tubing without removal), and slowly open roller clamp to allow fluid to travel from drip chamber through tubing to needle adapter. Invert Y-connector sites to displace air. Close roller clamp. Ensure tubing is clear of air and air bubbles (see illustration). Remove small air bubbles by firmly tapping IV tubing where bubbles are located. Check entire length of tubing to ensure that all air bubbles are removed. Replace cap protector on end of infusion tubing.

Priming ensures that tubing is clear of air before connecting with VAD. Slow fill of tubing decreases turbulence and chance of bubble formation. Closing clamp prevents continued flow of fluid. Cap on end of tubing maintains system sterility.

h. Insert primed tubing into EID with power off.

Facilitates starting infusion as soon as IV site is ready.

6. *Option:* Prepare an extension set to be used as an extender for standard tubing or prepare a saline lock (capped catheter).

Many facilities use short extension tubing for continuous infusions and stand-alone saline locks (capped catheter) for intermittent infusions. Continuous infusion attaches to the needleless connector on short extension tubing. Saline locks provide IV access for antibiotic infusions.

a. Remove protective cap, and swab injection cap with antiseptic swab. Insert syringe with sterile saline flush, and inject through the cap into the lock or short extension tubing removing all of the air. Keep syringe attached. Maintain sterility and set aside for attaching to catheter hub after successful venipuncture.

Scrubbing the hub decreases incidence of microorganisms (Wright et al., 2013). Removes air from tubing and prevents air from being introduced into vein. Sterile syringe will be used later after IV line is established.

7. Perform hand hygiene and apply clean gloves. Note: Gloves may be left off to locate the vein but must be applied before preparing the site. Apply tourniquet around arm above antecubital fossa or 10 to 15 cm (4 to 6 inches) above proposed insertion site (see illustration). Do not apply too tightly to cause injury or bruising to skin. Verify presence of a radial pulse. Option: Use BP cuff instead of tourniquet. Inflate it to a level just below the patient's normal diastolic pressure (<50 mm Hg).

Tourniquet should be tight enough to impede venous return but not occlude arterial flow. Use of BP cuff reduces trauma to the skin and underlying tissue.

> **SAFE PATIENT CARE** According to the INS (2011b), the use of visualization technologies (ultrasound) aids in vein identification and selection. Use an ultrasound device if veins are difficult to visualize or palpate.

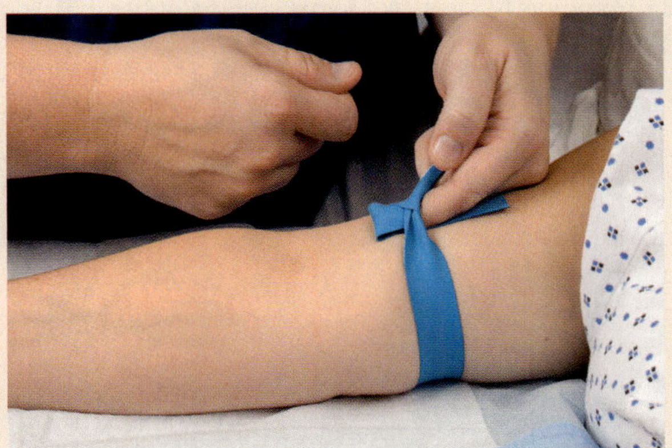

STEP 7 Tourniquet placed on arm for initial vein selection.

Continued

STEPS	RATIONALE

8. Select the vein for device insertion.

a. Veins on the dorsal and ventral surfaces of upper extremities (e.g., cephalic, basilica, and median veins) are preferred in adults. Use most distal site in patient's nondominant arm if possible.

Venipuncture should be performed distal to proximal, which increases availability of other sites for future IV therapy (INS, 2011b).

b. Avoid areas that have already been compromised from previous IV insertions (e.g., areas that are painful, sclerosed, bruised, or inflamed or have a rash).

It would be difficult to assess for any signs or symptoms of complications if an IV device were inserted in an area already compromised.

c. Select a well-dilated vein large enough for device placement (see illustration). Methods to foster venous distention include:

Prevents interruption of venous flow while allowing adequate blood flow around catheter.

(1) Placing extremity in dependent position if possible and stroking from distal to proximal below proposed venipuncture site.

Promotes venous filling.

(2) Applying warmth to extremity for several minutes (e.g., with a warm washcloth).

Increases blood in vein by dilating it.

> **SAFE PATIENT CARE** Choose appropriate dilation method. Vigorous friction and multiple tapping of a vein, especially in older adults, can cause hematoma or venous constriction (INS, 2011b).

d. Choose a site that does not interfere with patient's activities of daily living or planned surgery or procedures.

Maintains patient's mobility as much as possible.

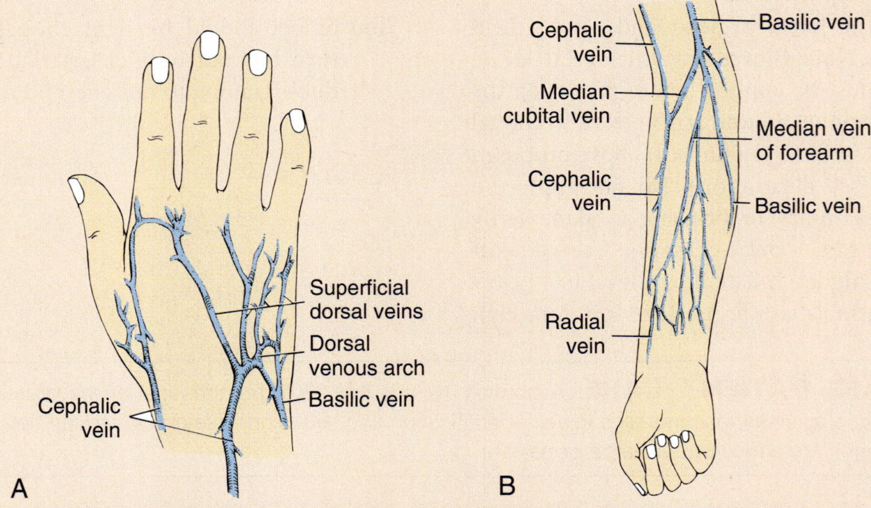

STEP 8c Common IV sites. **A,** Dorsal surface of hand. **B,** Inner arm.

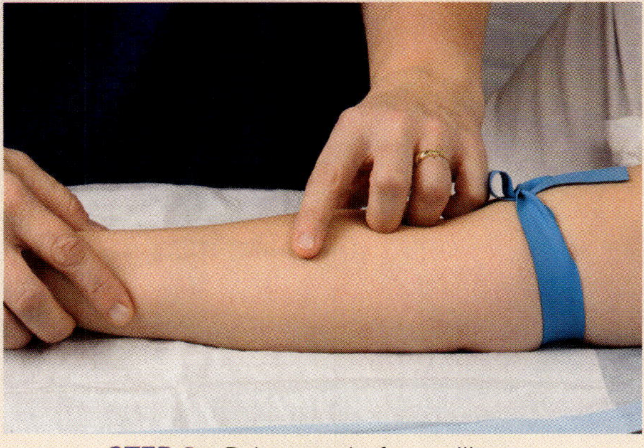

STEP 8e Palpate vein for resilience.

STEPS	RATIONALE

e. With the index finger, palpate the vein by pressing downward and noting a resilient, soft, bouncy feeling as the pressure is released (see illustration). Avoid veins that feel hard.

Use of the same finger causes a development of sensitivity to assess the vein condition better. Hard veins are veins that are sclerosed and have been damaged from previous IV insertions (Corrigan et al., 2014).

f. Avoid sites distal to a previous venipuncture site, veins in the antecubital fossa or inner wrist, sclerosed or hardened cordlike veins, an infiltrated site or phlebotic vessels, bruised areas, and areas of venous valves or bifurcation.

Such sites increase risk of IV-related complications and limit mobility. Veins in antecubital fossa are used for blood draws, placement of midlines, or peripherally inserted central catheter (PICC) lines.

g. Avoid fragile dorsal veins in older adults and vessels in an extremity with compromised circulation (e.g., in cases of mastectomy, dialysis graft, or paralysis).

Venous alterations can increase risk of complications (e.g., infiltration, decreased catheter dwell time).

9. Carefully release tourniquet temporarily. Clip arm hair with scissors if necessary. Do not shave IV site area. Option: You may apply a local anesthetic to site at least 30 minutes before IV start (per facility policy).

Prevents damage to skin and restores blood flow while preparing for venipuncture. Hair impedes venipuncture or adherence of dressing. Shaving causes microabrasions and increases the risk of infection. Local anesthetic reduces discomfort of venipuncture.

10. Apply clean gloves if not done in Step 7. Place adapter end of filled infusion tubing or extension set nearby, keeping it inside its sterile packing.

11. If area for insertion appears to need cleansing, use soap and water first, then dry. Apply chlorhexidine solution using friction in a repeated back-and-forth motion for a minimum of 30 seconds. Prepared area should be in a 5- to 7.5-cm (2- to 3-inch) diameter (see illustration). Allow to air-dry completely between agents if agents are used in combination (chlorhexidine gluconate and alcohol).

Mechanical friction allows penetration of antiseptic into epidermal layer of skin. Drying prevents chemical reactions between agents and allows time for maximum microbicidal activity. Chlorhexidine (2%) has been shown to be an effective agent (INS, 2011b). Touching cleansed area introduces organisms from nurse's hand to site (Corrigan et al., 2014).

12. Reapply tourniquet or BP cuff, and verify presence of radial pulse.

Promotes vein engorgement.

13. Perform venipuncture. Anchor vein below proposed insertion site by placing thumb over vein and pulling skin against direction of insertion 4 to 5 cm (½ to 2 inches) distal to the site (see illustration). Instruct patient to relax hand.

Stabilizing vein for needle insertion prevents vein from rolling. Provides ease for needle insertion for skin puncture and then into vein. Skin becomes taut, decreasing drag on insertion of IV device.

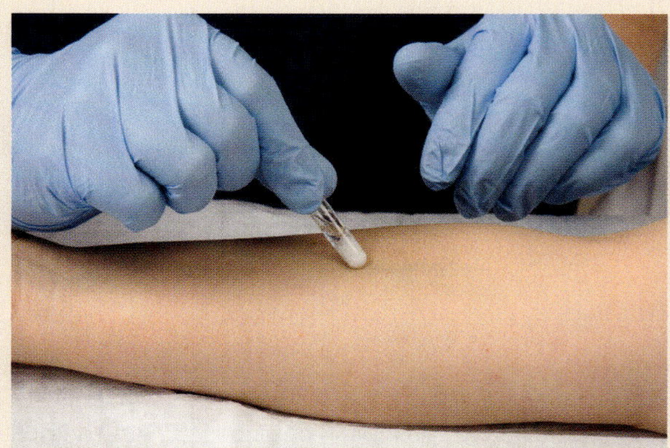

STEP 11 Cleanse site with chlorhexidine.

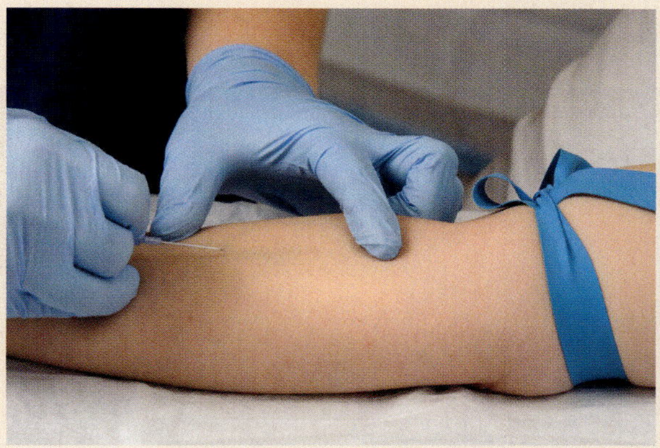

STEP 13 Stabilize vein below insertion site.

Continued

STEPS	RATIONALE

14. Warn patient of a sharp, quick stick. Puncture skin and vein, holding catheter at a 10- to 30-degree angle with bevel in the up position (see illustration).

Superficial veins require a smaller angle; deeper veins require a greater angle. Depth of vein is related to amount of subcutaneous tissue.

15. Observe for a brisk, dark blood return in flashback chamber of catheter, indicating catheter tip is in vein (see illustration A). Lower catheter until almost flush with skin, and slowly advance another 0.6 cm ($\frac{1}{4}$ inch) into vein (see illustration B). Loosen stylet of over-the-needle catheter.

Allows for full penetration of vein wall, placement of catheter in inner lumen of vein, and easy advancement of catheter off stylet.

16. If no blood return is observed or catheter does not advance, venipuncture was unsuccessful; device should be removed, with firm direct pressure applied to insertion site until bleeding stops. Obtain a new catheter and attempt a second time in another location proximal to the previous attempt. Note: No more than two attempts at VAD placement should be made by any one nurse.

Never reinsert the stylet (needle) into the catheter because this may damage the catheter and cause catheter embolism. When the catheter is partially withdrawn through the stylet or reinserted, the damage can range from a small nick in the catheter to complete severing of the distal tip (Corrigan et al., 2014; INS, 2011b). Multiple unsuccessful attempts limit future vascular access and cause patient unnecessary pain (INS, 2011b).

17. Advance catheter off stylet to thread catheter into vein. Continue until catheter hub rests at venipuncture site. *Do not reinsert stylet once it is loosened.* Advance catheter while safety device automatically retracts stylet. (Techniques for retracting stylet vary with different VADs.) Follow manufacturer guidelines for specific safety catheter use. Place stylet directly into sharps container. Continue to hold skin taut.

Reduces risk of introduction of infectious microorganisms along catheter length. Advancing entire stylet into vein may penetrate posterior vein wall, causing a hematoma. Reinsertion of stylet can cause catheter shearing and potential catheter embolization (INS, 2011b).

18. Stabilize catheter with one hand, and release tourniquet with the other.

Restores blood flow to arm.

19. Apply gentle but firm pressure with middle finger of nondominant hand 3 cm ($1\frac{1}{4}$ inch) above insertion site. Keep catheter stable with middle finger.

Obstructs venous flow, minimizing blood loss.

20. Hold catheter firmly and quickly connect Luer-Lok end of either the primed extension tubing/infusion tubing or the prepared saline lock to the catheter.

Stabilizing cannula prevents accidental withdrawal or dislodgment (INS, 2011b). Prompt connection of infusion set maintains patency of vein.

21. Flush VAD. Slowly flush a primed extension set or saline lock with remaining saline from prefilled syringe (see illustration A), or begin a primary infusion by slowly opening slide clamp (see illustration B) or adjusting roller clamp of IV tubing to correct rate. Observe for swelling.

Establishes patent infusion.

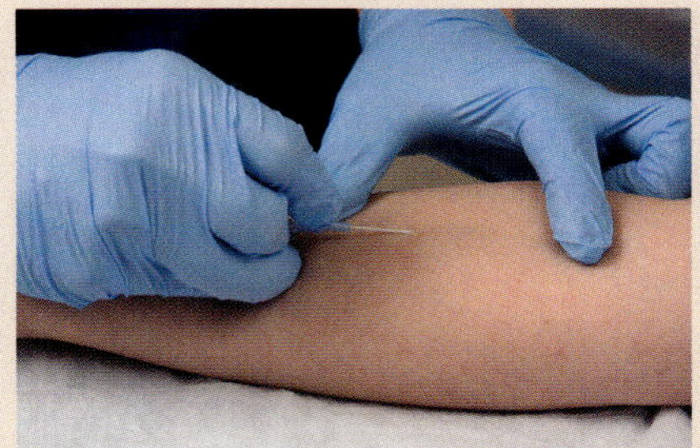

STEP 14 Puncture vein with catheter held at a 10- to 30-degree angle. Catheter enters vein.

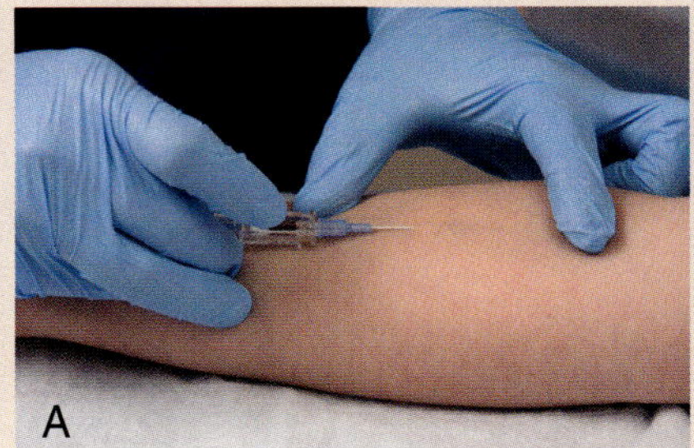

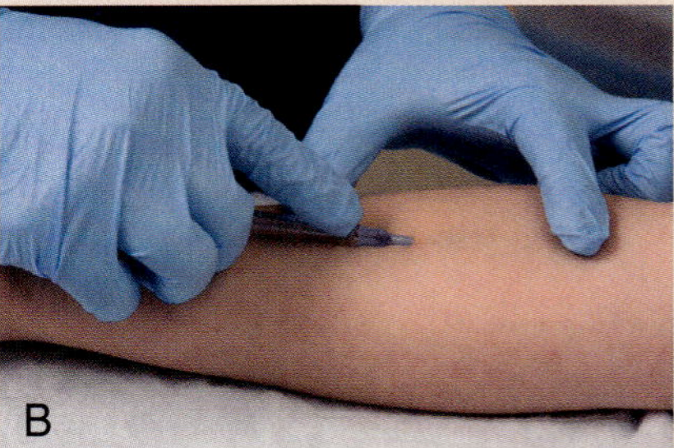

STEP 15 A, Observe for blood return in flashback chamber. **B,** Advance catheter into vein until hub is near insertion site.

STEPS	RATIONALE
22. Remove the syringe from lock. For a continuous primary infusion, be sure tubing is correctly inserted into EID, program it, open roller clamp wide open, and begin infusion at correct rate. If using gravity flow instead of EID, begin infusion by slowly opening roller clamp.	Initiates flow of fluid through IV catheter, preventing clotting of device.
23. Secure IV catheter.	
a. *Sterile transparent dressing:* Secure catheter with nondominant hand while preparing to apply dressing.	Prevents accidental catheter dislodgment.
b. *Manufactured catheter stabilization device* (see illustration): Wipe selected area with single-use skin protectant and allow to dry. Slide device under catheter hub, and center hub over device. Holding catheter in place, peel off half of liner, and press to adhere to skin. Repeat on the other side. Holding catheter in place, pull tab out from center of device to create opening, and insert catheter into slit. This frames the IV site. Cover insertion site with a transparent dressing (see Step 24a).	The stabilization device is a sterile adhesive pad that holds the catheter in place, reduces the risk for infection and needlestick injuries, and improves patient outcomes (INS, 2011b).
c. *Sterile gauze dressing:* Place a narrow, 1.25-cm (½-inch) piece of sterile tape, about 10 cm (4 inches) long over catheter hub. Place tape only on the catheter hub, not over the insertion site (see illustration).	Use sterile tape under a sterile dressing to prevent site contamination. Regular adhesive tape is a potential source of pathogenic bacteria (INS, 2011b). Prevents back-and-forth motion of catheter.
24. Apply sterile dressing over IV site.	
a. *Transparent dressing:*	
(1) Carefully remove adherent backing. Apply one edge of dressing over IV site and gently smooth remaining dressing. Leave connection between IV tubing and catheter hub uncovered (see illustration). Remove outer covering, and smooth dressing gently over site.	Transparent dressing allows continuous inspection of site and surrounding tissue, is more comfortable, and is occlusive to moisture and microorganisms (INS, 2011b). Prevents accidental dislodgment of catheter.

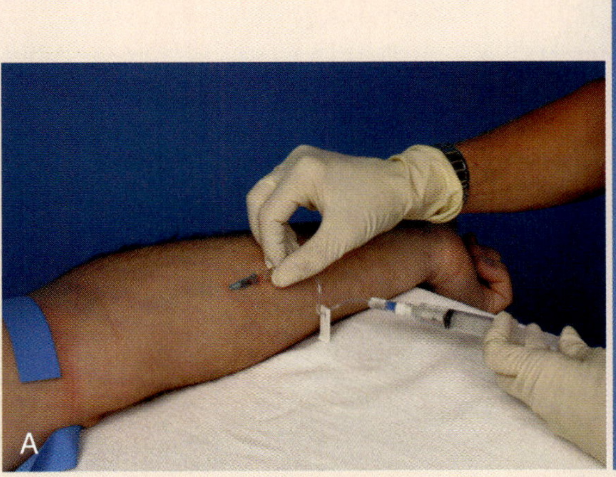
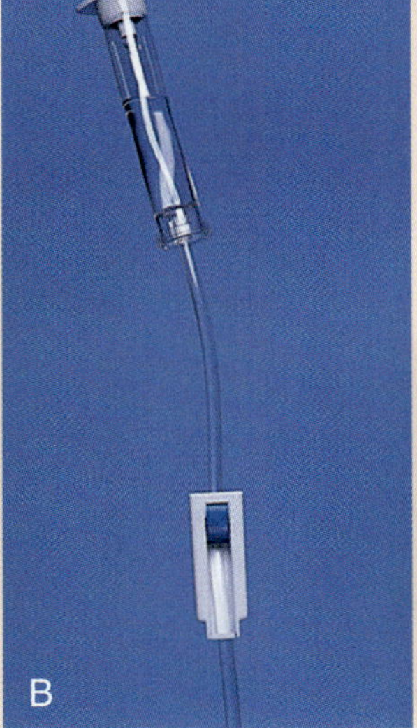

STEP 21 **A,** Flush extension set slowly. **B,** Open roller clamp.

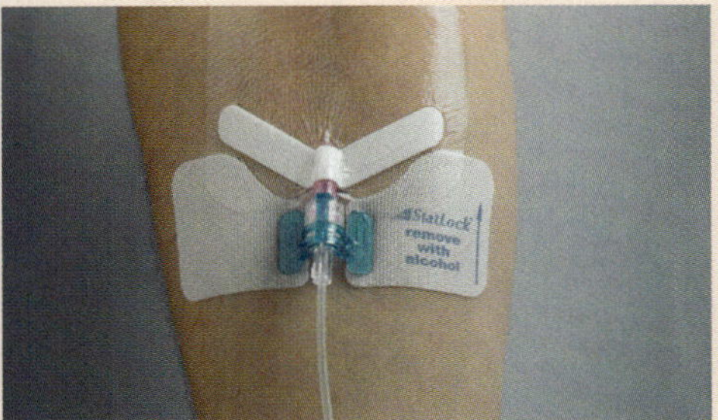

STEP 23b Catheter stabilization device in place. (Courtesy CR Bard Inc.)

Continued

(2) When a stabilization device is not being used, take a 1-inch piece of tape and place it over end of tubing just behind connection point with catheter but not over transparent dressing.

b. *Sterile gauze dressing:*

Optional method of securing IV device if patient is allergic to transparent dressing. However, it is not the preferred method to cover and secure IV device because gauze prevents visualization of the insertion site (INS, 2011b).

(1) Place 2 × 2–inch gauze pad over venipuncture site and catheter hub (see illustration). Secure all edges with tape. Do not cover the connection between IV tubing and catheter hub with the dressing.

25. Loop the continuous infusion or extension set tubing along the outside of the arm and secure with a strip of tape (see illustration).

Initiates flow of fluid through IV catheter, preventing clotting and initiating therapy.

26. Remove and dispose of gloves.

27. Label IV dressing, including date, time, catheter gauge size and length, and your initials (see illustration), and apply to IV dressing being sure not to obscure IV insertion site.

Allows for easy recognition of type of device. Short-peripheral IV devices are not routinely replaced; however, devices placed in an emergent situation should be replaced as soon as possible and not later than 48 hours (Corrigan et al., 2014; INS, 2011b).

28. Show patient how to avoid placing pressure on venipuncture site or dislodging catheter when attempting to reposition in bed or getting out of bed. Discuss signs and symptoms of possible infiltration or phlebitis (e.g., pain, swelling, burning, redness, moisture on dressing) and to report them.

Demonstrates patient understanding of IV therapy (INS, 2011b).

29. Dispose of sheathed stylet and any uncapped sharps in appropriate sharps container as soon as device is secured. Dispose of remaining trash.

Prevents accidental needlestick injury, and transmission of microorganisms is reduced (INS, 2011b).

30. **See Completion Protocol (inside front cover).**

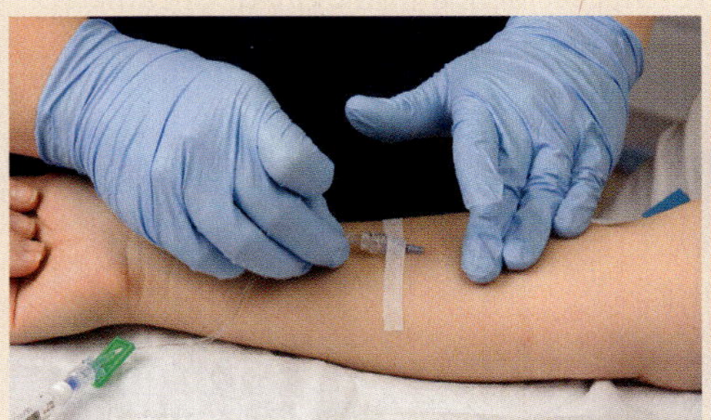

STEP 23c Apply tape over catheter hub.

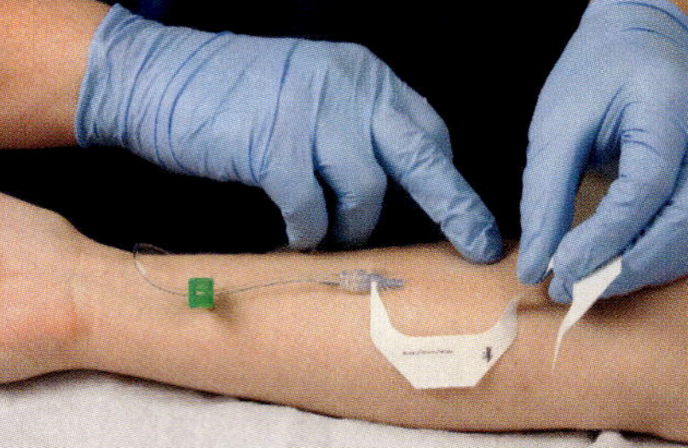

STEP 24a(1) Apply transparent dressing.

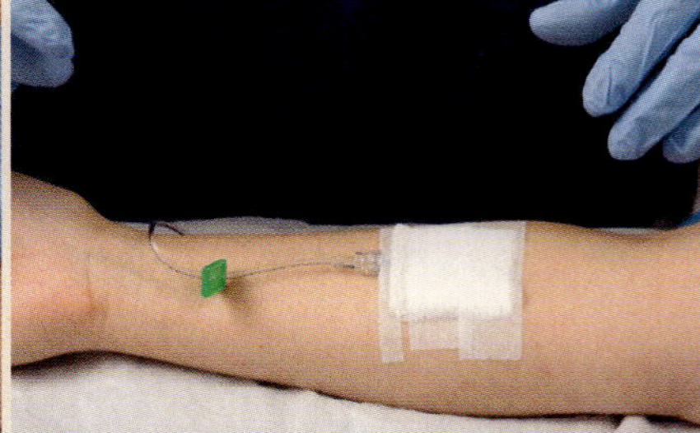

STEP 24b(1) Place 2 × 2–inch gauze over insertion site and catheter hub.

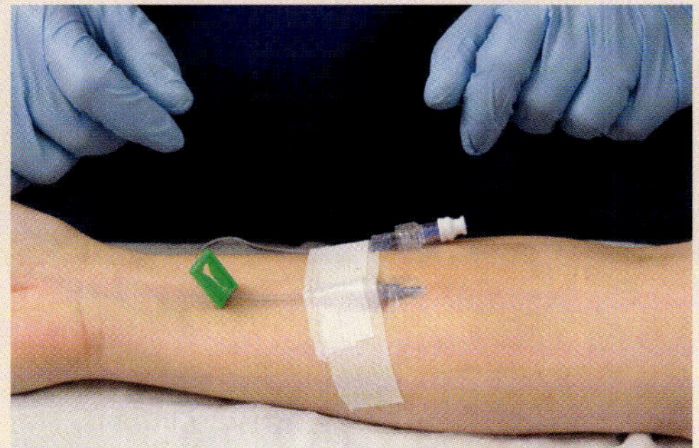

STEP 25 Loop and secure extension set tubing.

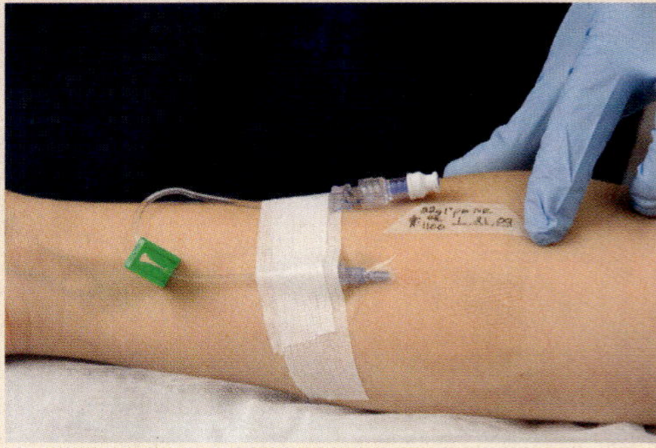

STEP 27 Label IV dressing.

EVALUATION

1. Observe patient every hour and check for:
   a. Patency of IV catheter.
   b. Correct type and amount of IV solution that has infused by comparing time tape or EID record.
   c. The infusion drip rate (if gravity drip) or the rate/volume on EID.
2. Monitor patient's I&O, daily weights as indicated, and evidence that prescribed therapy is working: return of normal fluid volume, resolution of infection, and laboratory values in appropriate range.
3. Inspect patient's IV site and extremity every hour for signs and symptoms of IV-related complications, such as pain, swelling, heat, or redness during the infusion (Tables 27-2 and 27-3).
4. Use *Teach Back:* State to the patient, "I want to make sure that I explained the signs and symptoms to report while having your IV in place. Can you tell me some of the signs and symptoms to report?" Evaluates what the patient is able to explain or demonstrate. Revise your instruction now or develop plan for revised patient teaching to be implemented at an appropriate time if patient is not able to teach back correctly.

Unexpected Outcomes and Related Interventions

1. *Phlebitis:* Patient complains of pain and tenderness at IV site with erythema at site or along path of vein. Insertion site is warm to touch, and rate of infusion may stop.
   a. Stop the infusion and discontinue IV. Reinsert new IV if continued therapy is required. Restart in opposite extremity or proximal to previous site.
   b. Apply moist warm compress over area of phlebitis. Monitor site according to facility policy.
   c. Document degree of phlebitis and nursing interventions per facility policy and procedure (see Table 27-2).
2. *Infiltration:* Patient's rate of infusion slows; insertion site is swollen, cool to touch, pale, and painful.
   a. Stop infusion and discontinue the IV. Reinsert new IV if continued therapy is necessary, preferably in opposite extremity.
   b. Elevate affected extremity.
   c. Monitor previous insertion site per facility protocol until resolution of swelling.
   d. Document degree of infiltration and nursing intervention (see Table 27-3).
3. Infusion is completed before or after appropriate time frame.
   a. Evaluate access device for position and patency; regulate remainder of infusion over prescribed time; assess need for EID.
   b. Assess IV site for need to restart IV infusion at another site.
   c. Continue to monitor hourly for proper rate of infusion.
   d. Monitor with too-rapid infusion for fluid overload. Obtain vital signs, respiratory status, and I&O.
   e. Notify health care provider.
4. IV site infection (redness, induration, temperature change, drainage).
   a. Notify health care provider for appropriate interventions.

Recording and Reporting

- Record number of attempts for insertion; type of solution and additives infusing; rate and method of infusion (e.g., gravity or name of EID); purpose of infusion; insertion

TABLE 27-2	PHLEBITIS SCALE
SCORE	**CLINICAL SIGNS**
0	No symptoms
1	Erythema at access site with or without pain
2	Pain at access site with erythema and/or edema
3	Pain at access site with erythema and/or edema Streak formation Palpable venous cord
4	Pain at access site with erythema and/or edema Streak formation Palpable venous cord >2.5 cm (1 inch) in length Purulent drainage

Data from Infusion Nurses Society (INS): 2011 Infusion nursing standards of practice, *J Infus Nurs* 34(1 Suppl):S65, 2011b.

TABLE 27-3	INFILTRATION SCALE
GRADE	**CLINICAL CRITERIA**
0	No symptoms
1	Skin blanched Edema <2.5 cm (1 inch) in any direction Cool to touch With or without pain
2	Skin blanched Edema 2.5-15 cm (1-6 inches) on skin surface in any direction Cool to touch With or without pain
3	Skin blanched, translucent Gross edema >2.5-15 cm (6 inches) in any direction Cool to touch Mild-to-moderate pain Possible numbness
4	Skin blanched, translucent Skin tight, leaking Skin discolored, bruised, swollen Gross edema >15 cm (6 inches) in any direction Deep pitting tissue edema Circulatory impairment Moderate-to-severe pain Infiltration of any amount of blood product, irritant, or vesicant

From Corrigan A, et al: *Core curriculum for infusion nursing*, ed 4, Philadelphia, 2014, Lippincott Williams & Wilkins.

site by location and vessel; brand, length, and gauge of IV device; patient's response to insertion (e.g., what he or she reports); and when infusion was started. Use facility infusion therapy flow sheet. Always complete entry with full signature and credentials.

- Document your evaluation of patient learning.
- Report any significant information, such as signs or symptoms of IV-related complications (e.g., infiltration, phlebitis, change in flow rate, infection).

Sample Documentation

1400   IV started in left midcephalic vein with 22-gauge 1-inch Insyte catheter × 1 attempt. IV D$_5$ ½ NS infusing at 125 mL/hr. No signs or symptoms of IV-related complications observed. Patient stated, "I hardly felt that at all." Patient able to verbalize back when to report signs and symptoms of complication (e.g., redness, swelling, pain, moist dressing, slowing or stoppage of infusion).

Special Considerations
Pediatric

- In addition to usual venipuncture sites, use the four scalp veins and the dorsum of the foot in infants. Needle selection is based on age: 26- to 24-gauge for neonates; 24- to 22-gauge for children (Corrigan et al., 2014; INS, 2011b).
- Apply latex-free tourniquet or rubber band or use a blood pressure cuff inflated to just below the patient's diastolic BP. In accessing scalp veins, aim the catheter downward, toward the heart, so the flow of infusion can follow venous return (Corrigan et al., 2014; INS, 2011a).

- Maintain skin integrity, especially in neonates. Use adhesives such as tape sparingly, and remove tape gently.
- Stabilization is essential, especially in young children who cannot comprehend the importance of not "playing" with IV device.

Geriatric

- Older adults have less subcutaneous tissue, making veins more prominent. Loss of elasticity makes skin more fragile and prone to skin tears. Anchor catheters carefully to prevent damage to skin. Attempt to insert catheter without the use of a tourniquet if veins are visible. Place tourniquet over clothing to prevent bruising or skin tears. Use of smaller gauge devices is recommended; ideal size is 22- or 24-gauge (Corrigan et al., 2014; INS, 2011a, 2011c).

Home Care

- Ensure the ability and willingness of the patient or family caregiver to administer and monitor IV therapy in the home. Determine if patient or family caregiver has the manual dexterity and cognitive ability to manage the infusion or seek assistance in an emergency (Alexander et al., 2014; Petroulias et al., 2013).
- Ensure that all sharps and equipment contaminated by blood are disposed of in leak-proof, puncture-resistant containers with lids (Clark, 2010).
- Ensure availability of 24-hour assistance with provider of home infusion therapy pharmaceuticals and equipment.

SKILL 27.2   REGULATING INTRAVENOUS INFUSION FLOW RATES

• **Nursing Skills Online: Intravenous Fluid Therapy Management Module, Lesson 2**

Accurate infusion rates in IV therapy are essential to deliver infusion solutions and medications safely (see Chapter 21). Complications associated with IV therapy (e.g., infiltration, phlebitis, clotting of device, or circulatory overload) are reduced or eliminated with a properly regulated IV infusion. Various factors interfere with infusion rates (Table 27-4). Hourly observation of the flow rate and IV system assists in achieving the therapeutic outcome and reducing complications.

Various infusion devices exist for ensuring accurate hourly infusion of IV therapy. An EID maintains correct flow rates and catheter patency and prevents an unexpected bolus of IV fluids. An EID delivers a measured amount of fluid over a period of time (e.g., 100 mL/hr) using positive pressure. Infusion pumps are needed for patients requiring low hourly rates, at risk for volume overload, with impaired renal function, or receiving solutions or medications that require a specific hourly volume. EIDs use an electronic sensor and an alarm that signals if pressure in the system changes and the desired flow rate changes.

Fluids that run by gravity are adjusted through use of a flow control/regulator clamp. In contrast to an electronic

TABLE 27-4	FACTORS THAT ALTER INTRAVENOUS FLOW RATES	
PATIENT FACTORS	**MECHANICAL FACTORS**	
Change in patient position	Height of parenteral container (should be >90 cm [36 inches] above heart)	
Flexion of involved extremity	Positional access device	
Partial or complete occlusion of IV device	Viscosity or temperature of IV solution; occluded air vent	
Venous spasm	Occluded in-line filter	
Vein trauma (phlebitis)	Improperly placed IV devices	
Manipulated by patient or visitor	Crimped administration set tubing; tubing dangling below bed; low battery of an electronic device	

IV, Intravenous.
From Corrigan A, et al: *Core curriculum for infusion nursing*, ed 4, Philadelphia, 2014, Lippincott Williams & Wilkins.

pump, a rate controller can be affected by many mechanical and patient factors.

Health care providers usually order the volume of fluid a patient is to receive within a specific time frame (Felver, 2013). For example, "1 L of D_5NS over 8 hours." You must be able to calculate hourly flow rates to ensure that the prescribed amount of fluid to be infused over the prescribed hours is correct. Assess infusion rates hourly regardless of whether you infuse an infusion by gravity or an EID. The minimal rate used to keep a vein patent is about 10 to 15 mL/hr in an adult and 5 mL/hr in an infant or child. The use of an EID does not absolve you from checking to ensure that the pump is functioning and infusing at the prescribed rate.

Many EIDs have operating and programming capabilities that allow for infusions of single or multiple solutions at different rates. Various detectors and alarms respond to air in IV lines, completion of infusion, high and low pressure, low battery power, occlusion, and the inability to deliver at a preset rate. An anti–free-flow safeguard (preventing bolus infusion in the event of machine malfunction) is a component of an EID. Follow facility and manufacturer's recommendations for selecting infusion pump controls, including infusion volume, rate, alarm settings, or pump malfunction (Alexander et al., 2014; TJC, 2014).

Patients in alternative care settings often have ambulatory infusion pumps. Most pumps weigh less than 2.7 kg (6 pounds) and range from palm to backpack size. They function on battery power, allowing patients freedom to perform normal daily activities. Programming options include automatic rate adjustments, remote site adjustments via a telephone modem, and therapy-specific settings such as patient-controlled analgesia (see manufacturer directions) (Fig. 27-1).

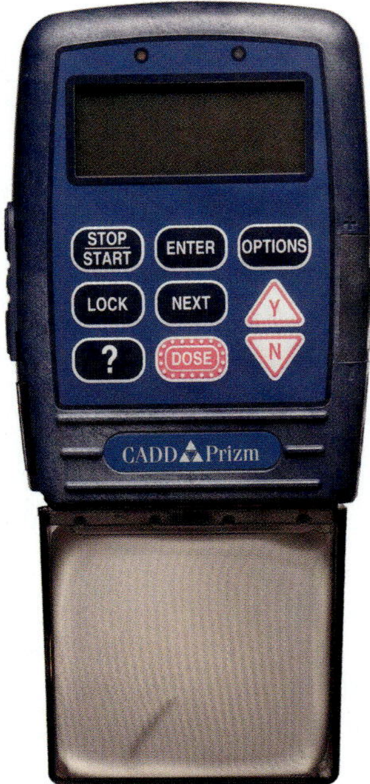

FIG 27-1 Patient-controlled ambulatory infusion pump. (Courtesy Smiths Medical ASD, Inc., St Paul, Minnesota.)

ASSESSMENT

1. Review accuracy and completeness of health care provider's order in patient's medical record for patient's name and correct IV solution: type, volume, additives, rate, and duration of IV fluid order. Apply the six rights of medication administration. *Rationale: Ensures that correct IV fluid is administered (INS, 2011b).*
2. Identify patient using two identifiers (e.g., name and birthday or name and account number) according to facility policy. Compare identifiers with information on the patient's MAR or medical record. *Rationale: Ensures correct patient. Complies with The Joint Commission standards and improves patient safety (TJC, 2014).*
3. Assess patient's experience with having an IV, including knowledge about how positioning of IV site affects flow rate. *Rationale: Determines level of patient instruction or reinforcement needed.*
4. Perform hand hygiene. Apply clean gloves. Inspect existing IV site for swelling and redness, and ask patient if there is tenderness at site when palpated. *Rationale: Signs and symptoms may be early indicators of phlebitis and the need to change IV site (INS, 2011a).*
5. Verify patency by observing infusion flow rate.
6. Identify patient's risk for fluid imbalance (e.g., child; older adult; history of heart, renal, or respiratory disease; electrolyte imbalance). *Rationale: Strict infusion volume control is required (Corrigan et al., 2014).*

PLANNING

Expected Outcomes focus on infusion of prescribed solutions without any adverse effects.
1. Patient receives prescribed volume of solutions or medication over desired time interval.
2. Response to prescribed therapy is achieved (e.g., return to normal fluid and electrolytes, laboratory values within normal limits for patient).
3. No signs or symptoms of IV-related complications develop.

Delegation and Collaboration

The skill of regulating IV flow rates cannot be delegated to nursing assistive personnel (NAP). The nurse directs the NAP to:
- Report patient complaints of burning, bleeding, swelling, or coolness at catheter insertion site.
- Report the EID alarm signals or there is a delayed or sudden emptying of IV bag.
- Report if the fluid container is almost empty.

Equipment
- Watch with a second hand
- Calculator, paper, and pencil/pen
- Label
- IV fluid bag and appropriate infusion tubing
- IV regulating device: EID (optional)

IMPLEMENTATION *for* REGULATING INTRAVENOUS INFUSION FLOW RATES

STEPS	RATIONALE

1. **See Standard Protocol (inside front cover).**
2. Have paper and pencil or calculator ready to calculate rate.
3. Obtain IV solution and appropriate tubing, and know calibration (drop factor) in drops per milliliter (gtt/mL) of infusion set used by facility:

   Use of correct tubing ensures more accurate infusion delivery.

   a. *Macrodrip:* Delivers a rate *greater than* 100 mL/hr. (Drip factor is 10 to 15 gtt/mL; see label on administration set packaging).

   Macrodrip tubing allows for larger infusion volumes.

   b. *Microdrip:* Delivers 60 gtt/mL.

   Used for slow delivery and smaller volumes.

4. Check order to see how long each liter of fluid should infuse. If rate (mL/hr) is not noted, calculate by dividing the volume by hours ordered. For example:

   Provides even infusion of fluid over prescribed hourly rate. A volume of 1 L = 1000 mL.

   a. $\text{Flow rate (mL/hr)} = \dfrac{\text{Total infusion (mL)}}{\text{Hours of infusion}}$

   Example: 1000 mL/8 hr = 125 mL/hr

> **SAFE PATIENT CARE** Health care providers commonly write abbreviated IV orders, such as "D_5W with 20 mEq of KCL 125 mL/hr continuous." This order means that the IV infusion should be maintained at this rate until an order has been written to change the rate or for IV infusion to be discontinued. Clarify with the health care provider if any part of the order is unclear.

5. If KVO (keep vein open) (or TKO [to keep open]) rate is ordered, check order or facility policy regarding the flow rate. KVO often falls in the range of 10 to 15 mL/hr.

   KVO rate prevents catheter clotting, preserving IV access, while infusing a minimal amount of fluid. INS standards (2011a) indicate that KVO orders should contain a specific infusion rate (INS, 2011b).

6. Use one of the following formulas to calculate minute flow rate (drops per minute) based on drop factor of infusion set.

   a. Drop factor × mL/min = Drops/min *or*

   b. mL/hr × drop factor/60 min = Drops/min

   Example: Calculate minute flow rate for a bag 1:1000 mL with 20 mEq KCL at 125 ml/hr:10 gtt/mL:

   10 gtt/mL:

   $$\frac{125}{60} \times \frac{10}{1} = 21\,\text{gtt/min}$$

   15 gtt/mL:

   $$\frac{125}{60} \times \frac{15}{1} = 31\,\text{gtt/min}$$

   60 gtt/mL (microgtt):

   $$\frac{125}{60} \times \frac{60}{1} = 125\,\text{gtt/min}$$

   c. Time-tape the IV bag by securing marked adhesive tape or fluid indicator tape alongside of fluid container. Document each IV fluid bag sequentially, and note type of fluid, patient's name, infusion time, and beginning and expected end of infusion.

   Gives a visual scale to assess progress of infusion hourly. Avoid use of felt-tip pens or permanent markers on plastic bag; these can contaminate IV solutions by permeating the IV bag (INS, 2011b).

STEPS	**RATIONALE**

7. Prepare IV tubing and infusion bag and prime tubing (see Skill 27.1). Be sure roller clamp is turned off. Use tubing compatible with EID if pump is to be used.

Removes air from tubing.

8. *Gravity infusion*

Confirm hourly rate and minute rate. With IV fluid bag hung on pole at a minimum of 90 cm (36 inches) above IV insertion site, slowly open roller clamp and adjust rate to deliver drops per minute. Using a watch, count drops in drip chamber for 1 minute. Then adjust roller clamp to increase or decrease drip rate until you obtain the desired number of drops per minute.

Fluid container height is usually sufficient to overcome venous pressure and other resistance from tubing and catheter (Corrigan et al., 2014; INS, 2011b).

9. *EID (infusion pump or smart pump):*

a. Consult manufacturer directions for setup of the infusion. Insert IV compatible tubing into chamber of control mechanism (see illustration). Roller clamp on IV tubing goes between EID and patient. (Consult manufacturer's instructions for use of pump.)

Pump chamber moves fluid through IV tubing.

b. Secure portion of IV tubing through "air in line" alarm system.

Detects air in tubing, which can enter vascular system, causing an embolus.

c. Close door to control chamber. Turn on EID power and test the alarm, select volume per hour, volume to be infused, and any other information required.

Follow pump instructions. Ensures that correct volume is administered.

d. Open rate-controlling clamp wide open on tubing and press start button.

Keeping control clamp wide open while infusion controller or pump is in use ensures accurate volume of infusion.

e. Monitor infusion on a scheduled frequency to assess patency of system when in alarm mode, and monitor for proper infusion rate and infiltration.

Ensures patient receives proper volume of fluid and ensures any complications are identified early.

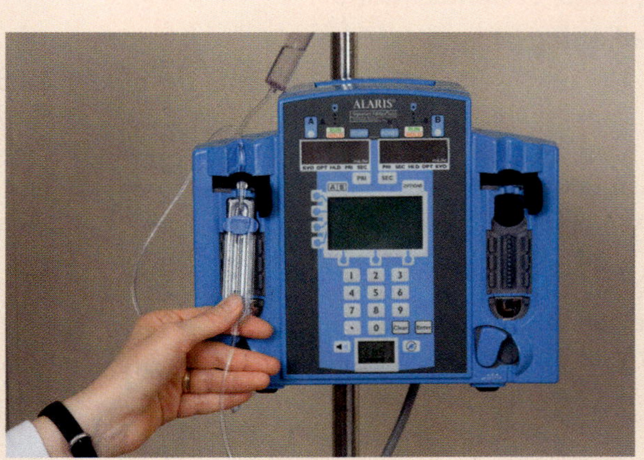

STEP 9a Insert IV tubing into chamber of control mechanism.

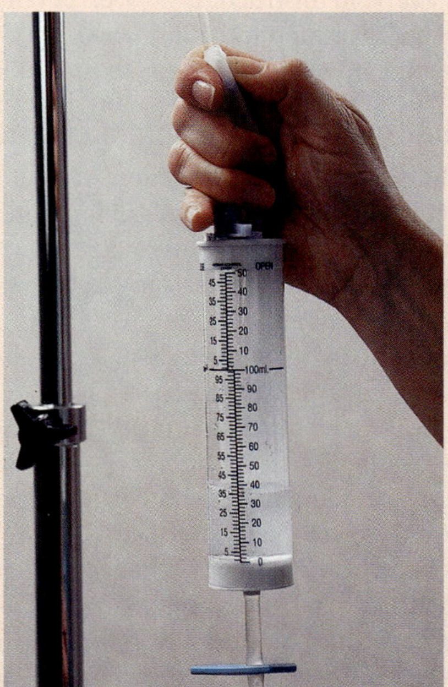

STEP 10b Open regulator clamp to fill volume control device.

Continued

STEPS	RATIONALE
10. Volume-control device:	
a. Place volume control device between IV bag and infusion set using sterile technique.	Delivers small volume but must be refilled as it empties.
b. Fill volume control device with fluid by opening regulator clamp (see illustration). Place 2 hours of fluid allotment in chamber device. Regulate flow rate.	This prevents infusion from running dry if 60 minutes elapse before nurse returns. Should infusion rate accidentally increase, only 2 hours of fluid will infuse.
11. Instruct patient about the following:	
a. To avoid placing hand or arm in a position that will affect flow rate.	Instruction informs patient about how to protect IV site and importance of not altering rate control.
b. To avoid manipulation of rate control clamp.	
c. Purpose and significance of alarms.	
12. See Completion Protocol (inside front cover).	

EVALUATION

1. Monitor IV infusion at least every 1 hour, noting volume of IV fluid infused and rate.
2. Observe patient and monitor his or her response to therapy. Evaluate laboratory values, fluid, and electrolytes.
3. Observe for signs and symptoms of infiltration and phlebitis, for clot in catheter (slowed flow of infusion), kink or knot in infusion tubing, or infusion pump malfunction.
4. Use *Teach Back:* State to the patient, "I want to make sure I have explained how to prevent the infusion from being slowed down or stopping. Can you tell me what not to do so we can be sure the IV runs on time without problems?" Evaluates what the patient is able to explain or demonstrate. Revise your instruction now or develop plan for revised patient teaching to be implemented at an appropriate time if patient is not able to teach back correctly.

Unexpected Outcomes and Related Interventions

1. Sudden infusion of large fluid volume of solution. Patient has symptoms of dyspnea, crackles in lung, and increased urine output, indicating fluid overload.
   a. Temporarily slow infusion rate to 10 gtt/min and notify health care provider.
   b. Place patient in high-Fowler's position; patient may require diuretic medications.
   c. Notify health care provider immediately; new IV orders will be required.
   d. Monitor vital signs and laboratory reports.
2. IV infusion is slower than prescribed.
   a. Assess patient for positional change that might affect rate such as IV catheter or tubing obstruction.
   b. If volume is deficient, consult with health care provider for new prescribed order to provide required volume.
3. IV fluid container empties with subsequent loss of catheter patency.
   a. Discontinue present IV infusion, and start a new IV line in other extremity or proximal to previous insertion site.

Recording and Reporting

- Record type and rate of infusion in milliliters per hour (drops per minute in gravity flow) in patient's medical record and any ordered change in fluid rates. Document use of EID.
- Document your evaluation of patient learning.
- Report at change of shift or break time the rate of infusion and volume left in infusion to nurse in charge or next nurse assigned to care for patient.

Sample Documentation

1400   Complaining of SOB. HOB elevated. Lungs auscultated with inspiratory crackles bilaterally. Health care provider notified. Order noted to decrease IV fluids of D_5NS to 25 mL/hr. IV site left midcephalic without redness, tenderness, or swelling. IV infusion converted to infusion pump at 25 mL/hr. Purpose of fluid restriction and symptoms of pulmonary edema reviewed with patient and wife, who verbalized understanding.

Special Considerations
Pediatric

- Do not use containers exceeding 150 mL in children younger than 2 years old, exceeding 250 mL in children younger than 5 years, or exceeding 500 mL in children younger than 10 years. *Always* use tamper-resistant, volume-controlled EIDs to ensure accurate fluid delivery (Corrigan et al., 2014; Hockenberry, 2013).

Geriatric

- Use an EID with microdrip tubing. Carefully monitor patient's clinical status, laboratory results, vital signs, weight gain or loss, and I&O (Corrigan et al., 2014; INS, 2011a, 2011c).
- Infusing dextrose too rapidly may cause cerebral edema more readily in older patients. NS given to an older patient with impaired renal function can cause hypernatremia (Corrigan et al., 2014).

Home Care

- Ensure that patient or family caregiver is able and willing to operate an ambulatory infusion pump. Assess any physical or visual limitations with ability to connect and disconnect infusion therapy and problem solve pump malfunction (Corrigan et al., 2014; Petroulias et al., 2013).

- A nurse should be in the home during initiation of IV therapy to ensure correct pump settings for solution, rate, time, and alarms.
- Provide telephone numbers for 24-hour service and emergencies with written instructions regarding infusion procedure and pump use.

- **Nursing Skills Online: IV Fluid Therapy Management Module, Lessons 3 and 4**
- **Nursing Skills Online: IV Fluid Administration Module, Lesson 3**

Short-peripheral IV catheters and infusion therapy are often associated with systemic and local complications. Appropriate ongoing management of IV sites prevents or minimizes these complications. The skin insertion site is the most common source of infection for IV catheters; you apply catheter dressings securely and change when loose, wet, or soiled. A transparent dressing or sterile gauze secured with tape is used to cover an IV site (Corrigan et al., 2014; INS, 2011b). You will change a transparent dressing every 7 days or with each catheter site rotation and immediately if integrity of a dressing is compromised (INS, 2011b; O'Grady et al., 2011). Change gauze dressings every 48 hours and immediately if the integrity of a dressing is compromised (O'Grady et al., 2011). When using gauze along with a transparent dressing, it is considered a gauze dressing and changed every 48 hours (Corrigan et al., 2014; O'Grady et al., 2011; INS, 2011b).

Solution and medication containers include plastic bags, plastic bottles, and glass bottles. These containers are changed frequently, depending on the rate of infusion, volume in the container, and stability of the solution or medication (INS, 2011b). The CDC (O'Grady et al., 2011) does not make a recommendation for the hang time of IV solutions or medications, but the INS recommends that each container be changed within 24 hours after the administration set is added (Corrigan et al., 2014; INS, 2011b). Solution and medication containers on ambulatory infusion devices may remain longer than 24 hours if aseptic technique is used, the system remains closed without injection ports or add-on tubing, and the medication is stable for the anticipated infusion time (Corrigan et al., 2014).

It is more efficient to change infusion tubing when hanging a new fluid container. The CDC and INS recommend changing continuous infusion tubing, used for fluids other than lipids, blood, or blood products, no more frequently than every 96 hours but at least every 7 days (O'Grady et al., 2011). Extending a tubing change to every 7 days may be considered when an antiinfective CVAD is being used or if fluids that enhance microbial growth are not administered through the set (INS, 2011b). The INS (2011b) also recommends changing tubing used for intermittent infusion through an injection/access port every 24 hours because both ends of this tubing are handled more frequently than tubing used for continuous infusion.

Placement of a short extension tubing or loop between a catheter hub and injection cap allows you to manipulate the injection cap without moving the catheter. This extension tubing remains attached to the short-peripheral catheter and is changed when the catheter is changed. The fluid pathway and capped ends on all infusion tubing, stopcocks, extension tubing, and injection caps are sterile. Use caution to prevent contamination of these surfaces during changes (INS, 2011b).

You may need to assist patients with many aspects of hygiene (e.g., gown changes, bathing) while patients are receiving IV therapy. *Never* disconnect infusion tubing to change a gown or any article of clothing. Coordinate care so that bathing or hygiene activities are done after discontinuing an IV site and before another venipuncture is performed. If infusion cannot be discontinued, use special "IV gowns" if available.

ASSESSMENT

1. Identify patient using two identifiers (e.g., name and birthday or name and account number) according to facility policy. If changing IV solution containing medication, compare identifiers with information on the patient's MAR or medical record. *Rationale: Ensures correct patient. Complies with The Joint Commission standards and improves patient safety (TJC, 2014).*
2. Determine patient's understanding of the need for continued IV infusion. *Rationale: Determines level of instruction or reinforcement needed.*
3. Perform hand hygiene. Apply clean gloves. Inspect and palpate over dressing covering IV insertion site, note swelling, coolness of skin surrounding site, or tenderness over IV site. In case of transparent dressing in place, observe site for redness or drainage. *Rationale: These symptoms are consistent with phlebitis or infiltration, indicating need to discontinue and replace IV site.*
4. Observe IV system for proper functioning. Verify patency of current IV access site; check for kinks in tubing. Verify IV is running at correct rate. If not, carefully adjust roller clamp to regulated ordered rate or place tubing into EID and reset rate. *Rationale: If IV is not patent, infusion rate cannot be maintained; a new IV access site may be needed.*

> **SAFE PATIENT CARE** Lowering IV container below level of IV site for blood return is an unreliable indicator and can damage the blood vessel.

5. Assessment for changing a short-peripheral IV dressing:
   a. Look at dressing label to determine when the dressing was last changed. *Rationale: Information on label determines status of the site (INS, 2011b).*
   b. Observe present dressing for moisture and occlusiveness. Determine if moisture is caused by leaking from the puncture site or an external source. *Rationale: Change a soiled or wet dressing immediately (O'Grady et al., 2011).*
   c. Monitor body temperature. *Rationale: Increase in body temperature could be a sign of infection at IV site.*

6. Assessment for changing infusion tubing:
   a. Determine when new infusion set is needed (e.g., according to facility policy, after contamination, or after puncture of infusion tubing). *Rationale: Changing of continuous infusion tubing and intermittent infusion tubing at recommended times reduce catheter-related bloodstream infection.*
   b. Observe for occlusions in tubing such as kinking, drug or mineral precipitate, and blood. *Rationale: Infusion of incompatible medications can lead to precipitate formation. Blood may flow retrograde from vein and adhere to tubing. Infusion of viscous blood components may cause adherence to walls of tubing and decrease size of lumen.*

7. Assessment for changing infusion solution:
   a. Review completeness and accuracy of health care provider's order. Check patient's name; type and amount of IV solution, medication, additives, and dose; infusion rate; and length of therapy. Follow six rights of medication administration. *Rationale: The original order is the more reliable source of infusion and medication information. Ensures safe and correct administration of IV therapy. A specific rate must be ordered; KVO is not an appropriate order (INS, 2011b).*
   b. Determine the compatibility of all IV fluids and additives by consulting appropriate literature or the pharmacy. *Rationale: Patency of inside of catheter depends on prevention of chemical interactions. Precipitation can occur because of concentration of drugs in solution and pH changes (INS, 2011a).*

▮ PLANNING

Expected Outcomes focus on reducing risk of IV-related complications, minimizing patient discomfort, reducing risk of overhydration, providing appropriate therapy, and maintaining a patent IV catheter.

1. IV site remains free of signs and symptoms of IV-related complications, including but not limited to infection, redness, swelling, pain, or drainage.
2. Patient's IV catheter and tubing are patent.
3. IV solution and medication infuse at proper rate.

Delegation and Collaboration

The skills of maintaining an IV site cannot be delegated to nursing assistive personnel (NAP). The nurse directs the NAP to:

- Watch for appropriate position of patient to avoid kinking of IV tubing and injury at insertion site.
- Report any leakage that occurs from or around the IV tubing.
- Report observations of changes in patient's temperature, signs and symptoms of IV-related complications such as pain and tenderness, and drainage at IV site.

Equipment
Changing a Short-Peripheral IV Dressing
- Antiseptic swabs (2% chlorhexidine, 70% alcohol, povidone-iodine)
- Skin protectant solution (optional)
- Adhesive remover (optional)
- Clean gloves
- Strips of sterile, precut nonallergic tape (or 36-inch roll of tape)
- Transparent dressing or sterile 2 × 2–inch gauze pads and tape
- Commercially available IV site protector (optional) (Fig. 27-2)
- Manufactured catheter stabilization device if available.

Changing Infusion Tubing
- Clean gloves
- Sterile 2 × 2–inch gauze pads (optional)
- Microdrip or macrodrip infusion tubing or appropriate EID tubing (check manufacturer's requirements)
- 0.22-mcg filter and extension tubing if necessary
- Tubing label
- 5-mL syringe filled with preservative-free NS (check facility policy)
- Antiseptic swabs
- Handheld bar-code scanner if using bar-code system

Changing Infusion Container
- Correct volume and type of solution (with additives if indicated) as ordered by health care provider
- Time tape
- Pen

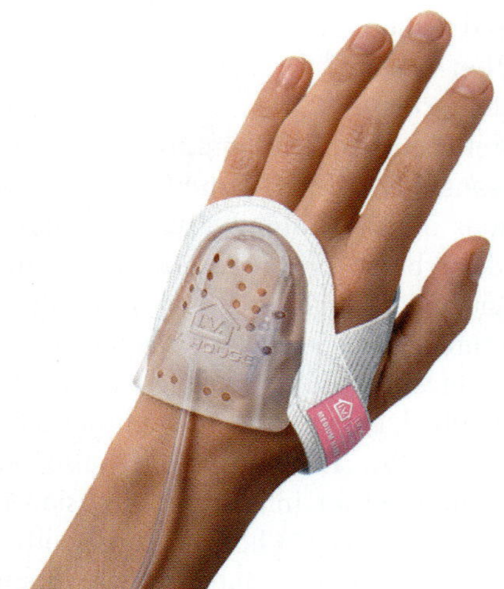

FIG 27-2 Commercially available IV site protector. (Courtesy I.V. House.)

IMPLEMENTATION *for* MAINTENANCE OF AN INTRAVENOUS SITE

STEPS	RATIONALE

1. **See Standard Protocol (inside front cover).**
2. Apply clean gloves.

3. *Changing short-peripheral IV dressing:*

   a. Remove transparent membrane dressing by picking up one corner above IV site and stretch the dressing down laterally while holding catheter hub and tubing with nondominant hand. Repeat for other side (see illustration). Discard dressing in trash container. Leave underlying tape or stabilization device that secures IV in place.

   Or

   Technique minimizes discomfort during removal. Use alcohol swab on transparent dressing next to patient's skin to loosen dressing (if needed).

   b. Remove gauze dressing and tape from old dressing one layer at a time by pulling away from insertion site while holding catheter hub and tubing. Be cautious if IV tubing becomes tangled between two layers of dressing. Leave tape or stabilization device that secures IV in place.

   Prevents accidental catheter displacement.

   c. Observe insertion site for signs and symptoms of phlebitis, infection, or infiltration (see Step 3 under Assessment). If present, discontinue infusion (see Procedural Guideline 27.1).

   Catheter moved during dressing change could accidentally dislodge and puncture blood vessel.

   d. Prepare new strips of sterile adhesive tape as needed and catheter stabilization device. If IV solution is infusing properly, gently remove any tape or stabilization device securing catheter. Using nondominant hand, stabilize hub of catheter with one finger.

   Exposes venipuncture site and prevents accidental displacement of cannula. Adhesive residue decreases ability of new tape to adhere securely to skin.

> **SAFE PATIENT CARE** Keep one finger stabilizing VAD at all times until tape or dressing is applied. If patient is restless or uncooperative, ask another nurse to assist.

   e. While stabilizing VAD, cleanse insertion site using chlorhexidine in a repeated back-and-forth motion with friction for a minimum of 30 seconds. Prepared area should be in a 5-7.5 cm (2- to 3-inch) diameter (see illustration).

   Friction penetrates antiseptic into epidermal layer of skin. Antimicrobial solutions should be allowed to air-dry completely to reduce microbial counts effectively (Corrigan et al., 2014; INS, 2011b).

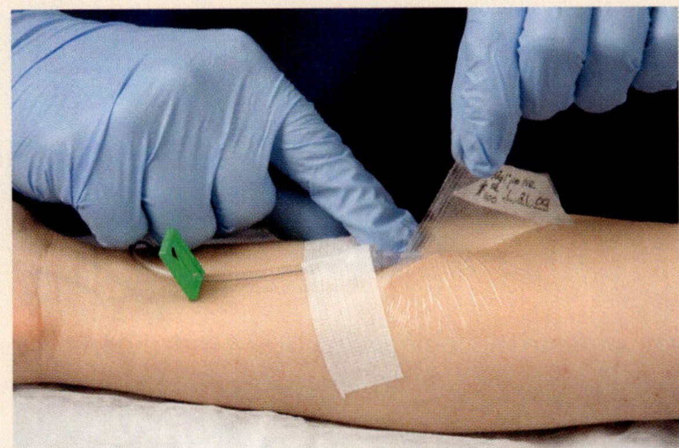

STEP 3a Remove transparent dressing by pulling side laterally.

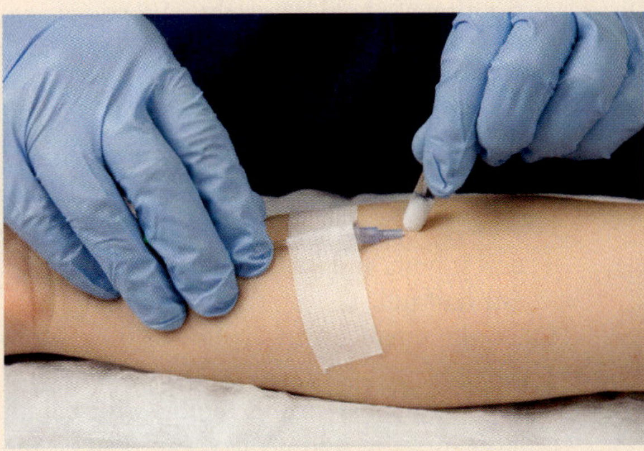

STEP 3e Cleanse insertion site with antiseptic swab.

Continued

STEPS	RATIONALE
f. Option: Apply skin protectant solution to area where you will apply the tape or transparent dressing. Allow to air-dry.	Coats skin with protective solution to maintain skin integrity, prevents irritation from adhesive, and promotes adhesion of dressing.
g. Option: Apply new stabilization device. See Skill 27.1, Step 23.	Prevents accidental catheter dislodgment.
h. Apply sterile dressing over site. (Follow facility policy.)	
(1) Transparent dressing: See Skill 27.1, Step 24a.	Transparent dressing allows for inspection of IV site.
(2) Gauze dressing: See Skill 27.1, Step 24b.	Gauze dressings must be occlusive to prevent introduction of microorganisms at entry site (Alexander et al., 2014).
i. Curl a loop of the infusion tubing along the outside of the arm, and place a piece of tape directly over tubing.	Securing tubing reduces risk of dislodging catheter from accidental pull.
j. Anchor IV tubing with additional pieces of tape if needed. When using transparent dressing, avoid placing tape over dressing.	
k. Label dressing with date and time of insertion, date and time of dressing change, gauge and length of catheter, and your name (initials).	Allows easy recognition of type of device.
4. *Changing infusion tubing:*	
a. Open new infusion set and connect add-on pieces such as filters or extension tubing. Keep protective covering over spike and distal adapter. Secure all connections.	Separation of infusion tubing increases risk of air emboli, hemorrhage, and infection. Protective covers reduce entrance of microorganisms.
b. If catheter hub is not accessible, remove IV dressing (see Step 3a and b). Do not remove tape or stabilization device that secures catheter to skin. Expose catheter hub or end of extension set on existing IV.	Movement of catheter may cause it to dislodge. IV solutions and medications can be administered either by connecting directly to the IV device or through an end cap or extension set.
c. For continuous IV solutions:	
(1) Move roller clamp to "off" position of new tubing.	
(2) Slow rate of infusion on existing IV by regulating roller clamp on old tubing or by turning off EID, removing tubing from pump and decreasing infusion rate.	
(3) Compress and fill drip chamber of old tubing.	Ensures that fluid chamber remains full until new tubing is changed.
(4) Remove old tubing from IV container. Continue to hold it upright until you are ready to connect new tubing. Optional: Tape old drip chamber to IV pole without contaminating spike.	Fluid in drip chamber runs slowly to keep catheter patent.
(5) Place insertion spike of new tubing into old fluid container opening. Hang container on IV pole, compress and release drip chamber on new tubing, and fill drip chamber one third to one half full.	Permits drip chamber to fill and promotes rapid, smooth flow of solution through tubing.
(6) Slowly open roller clamp of new tubing, remove protective cap from adapter (if necessary), and prime tubing with solution. Stop infusion and replace cap. Place capped end of adapter near patient's IV site.	Removes air from tubing and replaces it with fluid. Position equipment for quick, smooth connection of new tubing.
d. For extension set or saline lock:	IV tubing is attached to extension set without disconnecting from the hub of the catheter.

STEPS	RATIONALE
(1) If loop or short extension tubing is needed, use sterile technique to connect the new injection cap to the new loop or tubing.	Prepares extension set for connecting with IV.
(2) Swab injection cap with antiseptic swab. Insert syringe with saline solution, and inject through the injection cap into the loop of the extension tubing.	Scrubbing the hub prevents introduction of microorganisms (Wright et al., 2013).
e. Reestablish infusion:	
(1) Remove manufactured catheter stabilization device from tubing if present. Gently disconnect old tubing or old extension set from IV catheter hub (see illustration *A*). Quickly insert adapter of new tubing or new extension set and saline lock into hub of IV catheter (see illustration *B*).	Allows smooth transition from old to new tubing, minimizing time system is open.

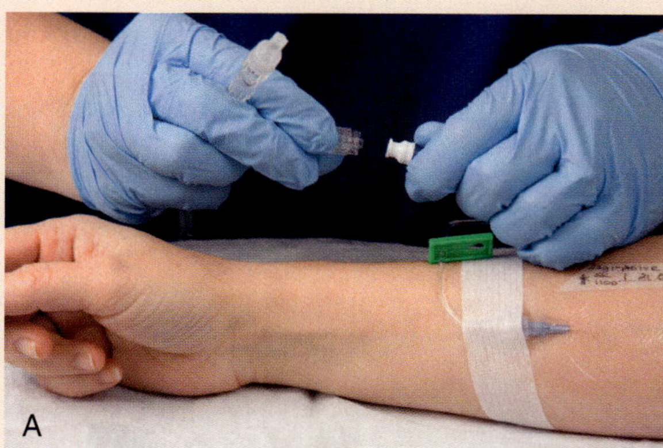
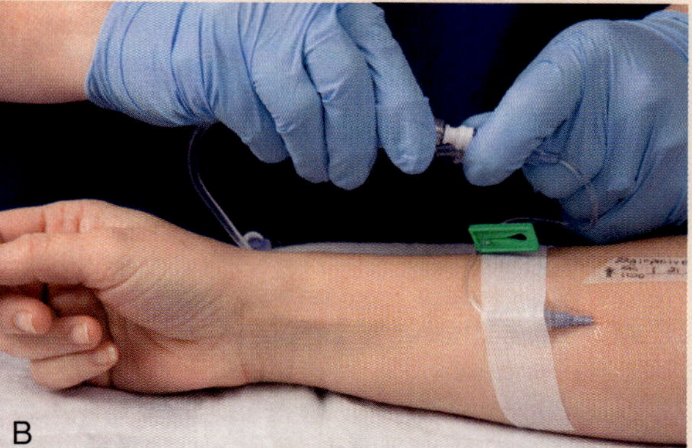

A   B

STEP 4e(1) A, Disconnect old IV tubing. **B,** Luer-Lok adapter of new IV tubing.

STEPS	RATIONALE
(2) For continuous infusion, open roller clamp on new tubing, allowing solution to run rapidly for 30 to 60 seconds and then regulate drip to ordered rate. For EID, rethread tubing into EID, set rate, and start infusion.	Ensures catheter patency and prevents occlusion.
(3) See facility policy. When reestablishing extension set, you will flush tubing and catheter with sterile saline flush.	
f. Apply new manufactured catheter stabilization device if used. Form a loop of tubing and secure it to patient's arm with a strip of tape.	Avoids accidental pulling against IV site and stabilizes the catheter.
g. Attach a piece of tape or a preprinted label with date and time of tubing change onto tubing below the drip chamber.	Provides reference to determine next time for tubing change.
h. Form a loop of tubing and secure it to patient's arm with a strip of tape.	
i. If it was necessary to remove old dressing to access tubing, apply new dressing (see Step 3).	Avoids accidental pulling against site and catheter movement.
5. *Changing IV solution:*	
a. Prepare next solution at least 1 hour before needed. If prepared by pharmacy, ensure that it has been delivered to patient care unit. Ensure that the solution is correct and properly labeled. Allow to warm to room temperature if refrigerated. Follow six rights of drug administration. Verify solution expiration date. Observe for leakage, precipitate, and discoloration.	Ensures no disruption in fluid therapy to patient (Corrigan et al., 2014).

Continued

STEPS	RATIONALE

b. Change solution when about 50 mL fluid remains only in old container or when new type of solution has been ordered. Be sure drip chamber is half full.

Prevents air from entering tubing and vein from clotting from lack of flow. Ensures correct administration of any new solution or change in IV orders.

c. Prepare new IV fluid container. If using plastic bag, remove protective cover from IV tubing port. If using glass bottle, remove metal cap and disk, and cleanse spike insertion site with antiseptic swab.

Permits quick, smooth, and organized change from old to new solution.

d. Close roller clamp to stop flow of existing solution. Remove tubing from EID. Then remove old IV fluid container from IV pole and hold it with tubing port pointing upward.

Prevents solution remaining in drip chamber from emptying while changing IV fluid container. Port held upward prevents IV fluid from spilling.

e. Quickly remove spike from old container end and, without touching tip, insert spike into new container.

Maintains sterility of solution and reduces risk of solution in drip chamber running dry. If spike is contaminated, a new IV tubing set is required.

f. Hang new bag or bottle of solution on IV pole.

g. Check for air in infusion tubing. If bubbles form, they can be removed by closing the roller clamp, stretching the tubing downward, and tapping the tubing with the finger (the bubbles rise in the tubing to the drip chamber).

Infusion of air in tubing can result in air embolus, which can be fatal to patient.

h. Ensure that drip chamber is one third to one half full. If drip chamber is too full, pinch off tubing below it, invert the container, squeeze the drip chamber, hang the container, and release the tubing (see illustration).

If chamber is completely filled, you cannot observe drip rate.

i. Regulate flow to prescribed rate or set up EID per manufacturer's instructions.

j. Place time label on side of container and label with time hung, time of completion, and appropriate interval. If using plastic bags, mark only on the label and not the container.

Do not use permanent marker to write on bag because it could leach into bag and contaminate fluid (Corrigan et al., 2014).

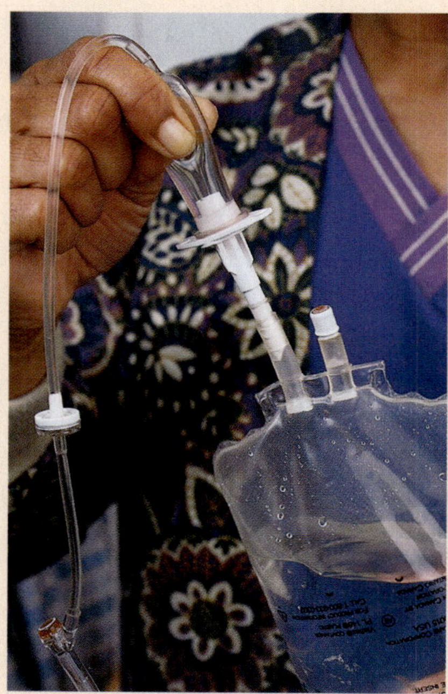

STEP 5h Remove excess fluid from the drip chamber.

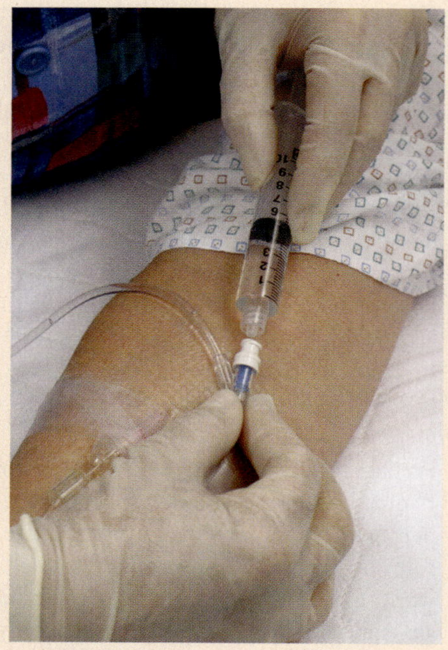

STEP 6e Flush injection port slowly.

STEPS	RATIONALE
6. *Discontinuing IV solutions or medications:*	
a. Move roller clamp on infusion tubing to the "off" position.	Prevents spillage of fluid.
b. Remove any clasping devices and disconnect medication delivery tubing from injection port or end cap of main IV.	If the tubing spike, connector end, fluid pathway, or solution container is contaminated, a new tubing set or solution container is required.
c. Cover end of IV medication tubing with a sterile cap or cover as required.	Infusion tubing can be reused with next ordered medication.
d. Swab injection port or end cap on main IV tubing with antiseptic swab.	Scrubbing the hub prevents introduction of microorganisms (Wright et al., 2013).
e. For intermittent medication piggybacked into a continuous infusion (see Chapter 23), attach 5-mL saline-filled syringe to injection port and flush the line gently (see illustration). Regulate fluid flow of continuous infusion as ordered.	Saline flush prevents incompatible medications from contacting the infusion tubing. There is no way to know how much pressure is exerted inside catheter lumen. A 5-mL or 10-mL syringe generates less pressure than a 3-mL syringe. Do not force irrigation against resistance.
f. For intermittent medications through an end cap or extension set, attach saline-filled 5-mL needleless syringe to injection port and flush catheter gently or attach heparin flush solution–filled needleless syringe to injection port and flush gently if necessary per facility policy. Do not force flushing of solution.	Flushing with saline instills any remaining medication in tubing. Volume of flush depends on lumen size, catheter length, and medication infused (Corrigan et al., 2014). Size of syringe used for flushing should be in accordance with manufacturer's guidelines. The smaller the syringe, the higher the pressure exerted (INS, 2011b). If resistance is met, assess for mechanical causes such as closed clamps or kinked tubing. Forcing the flush may cause catheter to fracture within the vein.
7. See Completion Protocol (inside front cover).	

▌EVALUATION

1. Observe intactness and patency of IV system and flow rate after changing dressing, tubing, or solution container and after administering IV medications.
2. Inspect condition of IV site for signs and symptoms of IV-related complications. Palpate for skin temperature, edema, and tenderness.
3. Monitor patient's body temperature.
4. Observe patient and monitor for signs of fluid volume excess or deficit to determine response to new IV solution.
5. Monitor laboratory values.

Unexpected Outcomes and Related Interventions

1. IV catheter is infiltrated; phlebitis is present; or site is red, edematous, or painful or has presence of exudate.
   a. Stop infusion and discontinue IV (see Procedural Guideline 27.1).
   b. Notify health care provider to evaluate patient for source of infection; antibiotic therapy may be prescribed.
   c. Culture of cannula may be ordered; confirm before removal of IV device.
   d. Restart new IV infusion in other extremity if continued therapy is required. Follow facility policy for complication management.
2. Decreased or absent flow of IV fluid indicated by a slowed or obstructed flow.
   a. Open roller clamp and slide clamps, and recalibrate drip rate. Check for kinks in tubing, and reposition patient's arm.
   b. Evaluate any pain or discomfort at the site for infiltration or temporary venous spasm.
3. Flow rate is incorrect; patient receives too little or too much fluid.
   a. Regulate to correct rate.
   b. Determine and correct the cause of incorrect flow rate (e.g., change in patient position, change in catheter position, kinked tubing).
   c. Use EID when accurate flow rate is critical.
   d. Notify health care provider if patient received less than or greater than 100 to 200 mL as prescribed (follow facility policy).

Recording and Reporting

- Record time short-peripheral dressing was changed, reason for dressing change, type of dressing material used, patency of system, and observation of venipuncture site.
- Record tubing or solution change, type of infusion solution, volume of container, and rate of infusion on IV flow sheet or medical record.
- Record time of discontinuing solution or IV medication; tubing or catheter flush with type, volume, and concentration of flush solution; and the IV site condition.

- Report to charge nurse or oncoming nurse dressing change, any significant information about IV site or system, and time medication or IV solution was discontinued.

Sample Documentation

0700   IV dressing over left metacarpal site became wet during shower; new transparent dressing applied; insertion site clear without redness, swelling. Patient denies tenderness. D_5NS infusing at 125 mL/hr via gravity. Patient states, "It does not hurt at all."

1125   Rocephin infusion complete; line flushed with 5 mL NS. D_5NS continues infusing at 125 mL/hr via gravity. IV site without signs and symptoms of complications. Patient able to verbalize what to report to nurse (e.g., redness, pain, swelling, decrease or stoppage of infusion).

Special Considerations
Pediatric

- Use commercially available IV site protectors to cover and protect the IV site in young active children. Ensure that identification band is visible and nonrestricting (INS, 2011b).

Geriatric

- Infiltration may go unnoticed because of the decreased elasticity of the skin and loose skin folds. Because of decreased tactile sensation, a large amount of fluid may infiltrate before patient experiences pain (Alexander et al., 2014; INS, 2011a).
- Phlebitis may develop without pain but with significant inflammation resulting from the decreased sensitivity of the nerve endings of the skin.

Home Care

- Have family caregiver demonstrate hand hygiene and aseptic technique for changing IV site dressing. If the catheter comes out, instruct caregiver to apply gauze pressure dressing and notify home care facility nurse.
- Teach patient to keep site dry during bath (preferred) or shower by wrapping in plastic bag and taping occlusively. Ensure EID or ambulatory infusion pump safety during hygiene activity.
- Discuss the signs and symptoms of possible IV-related complications (Corrigan et al., 2014).

PROCEDURAL GUIDELINE 27.1
Discontinuing a Short-Peripheral Intravenous Device

You discontinue a short-peripheral vascular access device (VAD) when the prescribed length of therapy is completed or a complication occurs (e.g., phlebitis, infiltration, or catheter occlusion). Removal of a short-peripheral catheter or winged needle should be based on assessment of patient's condition, access site, skin and vein integrity, length and type of prescribed therapy, integrity and patency of device, and condition of dressing (Gorski et al., 2012; INS 2011b). You will remove and then restart an IV (if ordered) every 72 hours to reduce chance of infection (INS, 2011b). If a catheter-related bloodstream infection is suspected, consult with the health care provider to determine if culturing the catheter after removal is needed (INS, 2011b) (see facility policy). Use infection control guidelines when discontinuing a peripheral VAD.

Delegation and Collaboration

The skill of discontinuing a short-peripheral VAD cannot be delegated to nursing assistive personnel (NAP). The nurse directs the NAP to:

- Watch for and report immediately any bleeding at the site after the catheter has been removed.

Equipment

- Clean gloves
- Sterile 2 × 2–inch or 4 × 4–inch gauze sponge
- Antiseptic swab
- Tape

Procedural Steps

1. Review health care provider's order for discontinuation of IV therapy.
2. Identify patient using two identifiers (e.g., name and birthday or name and account number) according to facility policy.
3. **See Standard Protocol (inside front cover).**
4. Observe existing site for signs and symptoms of complications (e.g., infection, infiltration, phlebitis).
5. Explain procedure to patient, describing sensation (burning) the patient may feel and the need to hold affected extremity still.
6. Turn IV tubing roller clamp to "off" position or turn EID off and turn roller clamp to "off" position.
7. Apply clean gloves. Remove IV site dressing or stabilizing IV device. Remove any tape securing catheter.
8. With dry gauze held above site, apply light pressure above where the tip of IV catheter would be and withdraw the catheter, using a slow, steady movement, keeping the hub parallel to the skin (see illustration).
9. Apply pressure to the site for 2 to 3 minutes until bleeding stops, using a dry, sterile gauze pad. Secure with tape. Note: Apply pressure for 5 to 10 minutes if patient is on anticoagulants.
10. Inspect catheter for intactness, noting tip integrity and length.

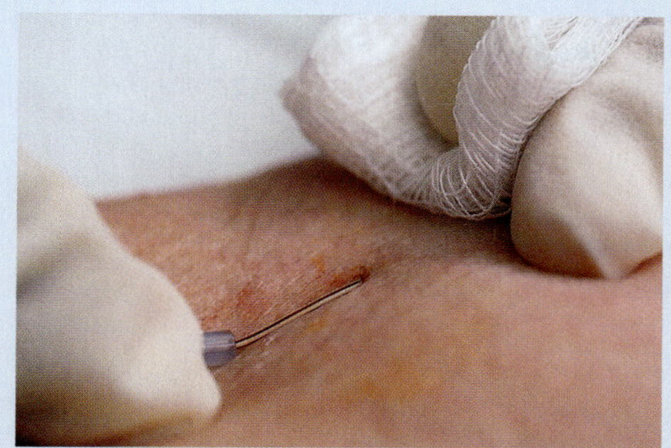

STEP 8 IV catheter is removed slowly, keeping catheter parallel to vein.

11. Apply clean folded gauze dressing over insertion site and secure with tape.
12. Instruct patient to report any redness, pain, drainage, or swelling that may occur after catheter removal.
13. **See Completion Protocol (inside front cover).**
14. Record removal of VAD and condition of site in nurse's notes or IV flow sheet.

SKILL 27.4 MANAGING CENTRAL VASCULAR ACCESS DEVICES

The need for safe and convenient long-term IV therapy led to the development of central vascular access devices (CVADs). Physicians or credentialed advanced practice nurses place these devices into the central vascular system. A CVAD differs from a short-peripheral or midline catheter with respect to the location of the catheter tip. The tip of a central venous catheter lies in the lower third of the superior vena cava (SVC) near the junction of the right atrium (Fig. 27-3) (INS, 2011b). The catheter tip of a central venous catheter in the femoral region typically lies in the inferior vena cava (IVC) above the level of the diaphragm (INS, 2011b). CVADs are categorized as short-term or long-term, with various types within each category (Table 27-5).

Many factors are considered when placing a CVAD, such as pH and osmolarity of the IV solution or medication (pH <5 or >9, osmolarity >600 mOsm/L), duration of therapy (>7 days), poor condition of peripheral veins, and diagnosis or disease processes (cancer, pain management). A nurse's role is to assist the health care provider in placing a CVAD, maintain the device, administer solutions and medications, and assess for signs and symptoms of complications (Alexander et al., 2014; INS, 2011b).

The nurse needs to be aware of the similarities and differences of each device. Characteristics of the devices affect care and maintenance of each CVAD as well as the type of patient education. Both types of devices are made of similar material, such as silicone or polyurethane, and can be coated with heparin, antibiotics, or chlorhexidine (Alexander et al., 2014). Tip configuration is either open-ended or valve-ended. In an open-ended device (e.g., Hickman or Broviac), the catheter tip is open like a "straw." Open-ended devices carry a higher degree of complications, such as hemorrhage, air embolism, and occlusion from fibrin or clots (Alexander et al., 2014). A valve-tipped device (e.g., Groshong) has a tip configured with a three-way pressure-activated valve, or the hub of the device has a pressure-activated valve (e.g., PAS V). Fewer complications occur with valve-tipped devices.

CVADs have single or multiple lumens. The choice of how many lumens are necessary depends on a patient's condition and prescribed therapy. Patients requiring numerous infusions and perhaps blood sampling will have a multilumen device that allows for administration of solutions and medications at the same time without disrupting therapy. Additionally, multiple lumens allow for administration of incompatible solutions or medications at the same time. You access a CVAD to administer medications or blood therapy through the hub of the device located on the end of each external lumen.

An implanted venous port is a CVAD that has a reservoir placed in a pocket under the skin with the catheter inserted into a major vessel (e.g., subclavian). The CVAD has no external lumen and hub. Instead, you access an implanted venous port through the septum of the reservoir. Medications and fluids are administered via a special 90-degree angle noncoring needle. It is inserted through the skin into the septum's self-sealing injection port. A port may not be used for several days between infusions. To keep a port patent, it is necessary to flush monthly at a minimum with 3 to 5 mL heparin (100 units/mL) (INS, 2011b).

Primary complications associated with CVADs are usually related to infection. A local infection can develop around a catheter insertion site. A more serious infection of the bloodstream, a CLABSI, often causes a prolonged hospital stay and increased cost and risk of mortality (CDC, 2014; IHI, n.d.; O'Grady et al., 2011). According to NQF, CLABSI is included in a list of Serious Reportable Events, and a set of evidence-based interventions is recommended for its prevention (see Evidenced-Based Practice earlier) (NQF, 2013). The

SHORT-TERM DEVICES	LONG-TERM DEVICES
Nontunneled percutaneous	**External tunneled (Hickman, Broviac)**
• Length of dwell: Days to several weeks • Insertion sites: Subclavian, external/internal jugular and femoral vein • Insertion technique: Not surgically placed, done at bedside using sterile technique, direct puncture into intended vein without passing through subcutaneous tissue • Held in place: With sutures or manufactured securement device	• Length of dwell: Considered permanent • Insertion sites: Chest region through the subclavian or jugular vein • Insertion technique: Surgery required, tunneling of the proximal end subcutaneously from the insertion site and bringing it out through the skin at an exit site (Fig. 27-5) • Held in place: By Dacron cuff coated in antimicrobial solution. Scar tissue forms around cuff in about 2-3 weeks fixing the catheter in place
PICCs (Fig. 27-4)	**Implanted venous ports**
• Length of dwell: Months or up to 1 year as long as there is evidence of IV-related complications (see manufacturer's recommendations) • Insertion sites: Antecubital fossa or upper arm (basilic or cephalic vein) and advanced until catheter tip reaches SVC • Insertion technique: Not surgically placed, done at bedside using sterile technique, in home setting or in radiology setting • Held in place: With sutures or manufactured securement device	• Length of dwell: Considered permanent • Insertion sites: Chest, abdomen, or inner aspect of forearm • Insertion techniques: Requires surgery, catheter is placed via subclavian or jugular vein and attached to a reservoir located within a subcutaneous pocket (Fig. 27-6) • Held in place: Within reservoir pocket and accessed using a noncoring needle (Fig. 27-7)

IV, Intravenous; *PICCs,* peripherally inserted central catheters; *SVC,* superior vena cava.

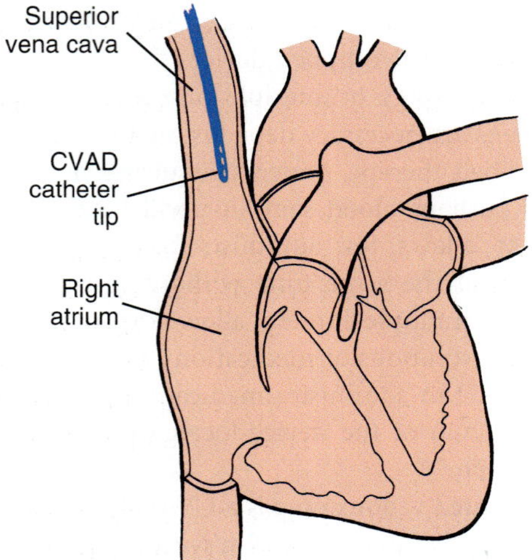

FIG 27-3 CVAD tip placement in SVC.

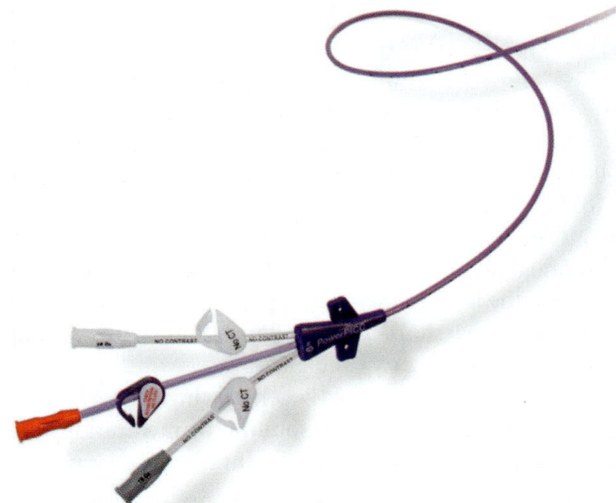

FIG 27-4 PICC line.

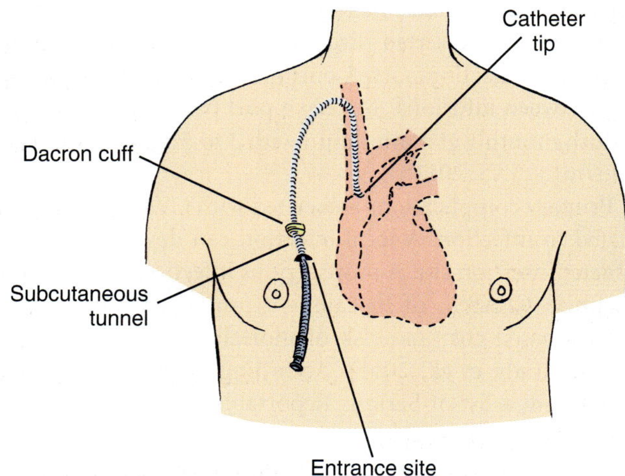

FIG 27-5 Tunneled catheter in place threaded to SVC.

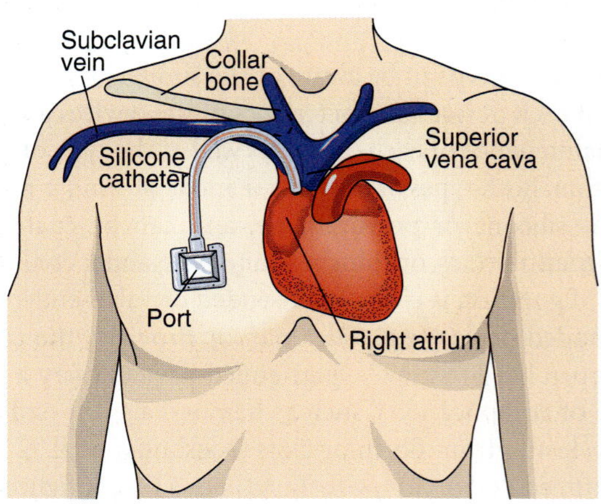

FIG 27-6 Implanted port and catheter.

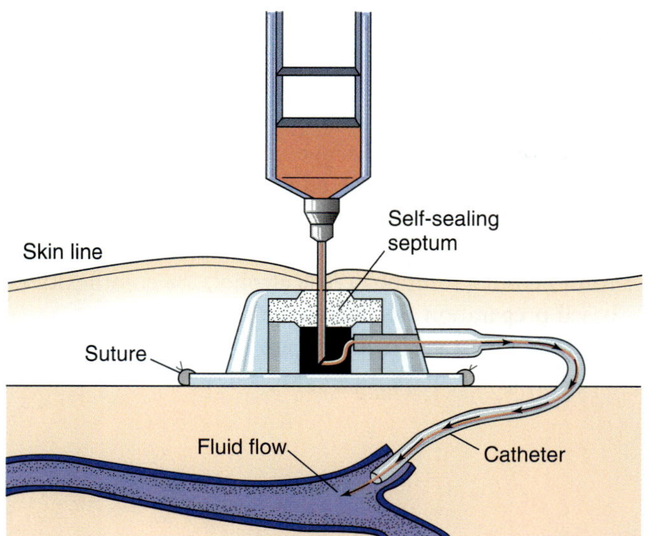

FIG 27-7 Cross section of implanted port accessed with noncoring needle.

set of interventions, or care bundle, is incorporated into this skill. Patients with CVADs require health education and teaching about infection prevention practices and skin care.

ASSESSMENT

1. Review medical record and assess appearance of device to determine its type. Review manufacturer's directions concerning catheter maintenance. *Rationale: Care and management depend on type and size of catheter or port, number of lumens, and purpose of therapy.*
2. Review medical record for evidence of final catheter tip location. *Rationale: CVADs should have final tip placement in the SVC or IVC verified by x-ray for safe administration of medication or solutions having pH and osmolarity within recommended parameters (INS, 2011b).*
3. Determine if any lumens require flushing or if insertion site needs dressing change by referring to medical record, nurses' notes, facility policies, and manufacturer's recommendations. *Rationale: Provides guidelines for maintaining catheter patency and prevention of infection.*
4. Identify patient using two identifiers (e.g., name and birthday or name and account number) according to facility policy. *Rationale: Ensures correct patient. Complies with The Joint Commission standards and improves patient safety (TJC, 2014).*
5. Perform hand hygiene. Apply clean gloves. Assess for proper functioning of existing CVAD before any therapy, note the integrity of catheter or reservoir, and review nurses notes for indication of any difficulty aspirating blood. *Rationale: Determines if CVAD is functioning without complications (INS, 2011b).*
6. Assess patient's reaction to CVAD and knowledge of purpose, care, and maintenance. For long-term use, ask patient or family caregiver to discuss steps in care and perform procedure (e.g., catheter site care or dressing change). *Rationale: Determines patient's level of understanding. Provides opportunity to educate patient or family caregiver for home care of CVAD (Petroulias et al., 2013).*
7. Assess patient's understanding of any procedures to be performed (e.g., insertion of device, dressing change, or discontinuation of CVAD). *Rationale: Promotes patient cooperation with procedure.*
8. Assess patient for allergy to iodine, lidocaine, latex, or medications in parenteral nutrition (PN) solution. *Rationale: Medications, solutions used during catheter maintenance, and use of gloves may cause serious allergic response.*

PLANNING

Expected Outcomes focus on prevention of CVAD-related complications; uninterrupted infusion of fluids, medications, blood products, or PN; and patient and family caregiver understanding of the purpose of CVAD therapy and ability to perform catheter care (if required for home therapy).

1. Catheter tip remains placed in desired location.
2. CVAD is free of clotting, local inflammation at insertion site, phlebitis, CLABSI, venous thrombosis, infiltration or extravasation (medication leaks into tissues around site), air embolus, or catheter migration.
3. Medications, fluids, blood products, and PN infuse as prescribed.
4. Patient and family caregiver perform dressing changes and site care as needed.

Delegation and Collaboration

The skills of inserting, maintaining, and administering therapies through a CVAD cannot be delegated to nursing assistive personnel (NAP). The nurse directs the NAP to:

- Watch for bleeding or swelling at or around CVAD insertion site; shortness of breath; damp, loosened, or soiled dressing; patient complains of pain; fever or catheter becomes dislodged.
- Report above-listed complications immediately.
- Report when volume of fluid infusing is low in the bag or EID alarm is sounding.

Equipment
Site Care and Dressing Change

- CVAD dressing change kit, which includes (Fig. 27-8) sterile gloves, mask, antimicrobial swabs (2% chlorhexidine, alcohol [see facility policy]), transparent dressing (transparent semipermeable membrane), gauze pads, tape measure, sterile tape, label
- Catheter stabilization device (if not sutured) for PICC or nontunneled catheters
- Needleless injection cap for each lumen

Changing the Injection Cap

- Clean gloves
- Antimicrobial swabs (2% chlorhexidine, 70% alcohol [see facility policy])
- Needleless injection cap
- 10-mL syringe with 10 mL NS flush 0.9% NS solution

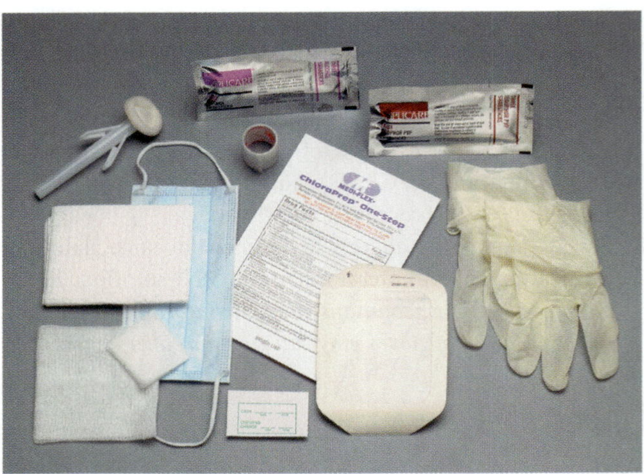

FIG 27-8 CVAD dressing change kit.

Flushing a Positive Pressure Device
- Clean gloves
- Alcohol swabs
- Positive pressure injection cap
- 10-mL prefilled saline syringe

Discontinuation of Nontunneled Catheter or PICC
- CVAD dressing change kit
- Tape
- Antimicrobial solutions (70% alcohol, 2% chlorhexidine-based preparation [see facility policy])
- Suture removal kit (if sutures are in place)
- Goggles, gown, mask, clean gloves

IMPLEMENTATION *for* MANAGING CENTRAL VASCULAR ACCESS DEVICES

STEPS	RATIONALE
1. See Standard Protocol (inside front cover).	

> **SAFE PATIENT CARE** Meticulous hand hygiene is a component of CLABSI prevention care bundles.

STEPS	RATIONALE
2. *Site care and dressing change:*	
a. Position patient in a comfortable position with head slightly elevated and turned away from insertion site, or in the case of a PICC or midline device, have arm extended.	Provides easy access to CVAD insertion site.
b. Apply mask. Gown is optional (see facility policy).	Prevents spread of airborne microorganisms over CVAD insertion site.
c. Apply clean gloves. Remove old dressing by lifting and removing transparent dressing or tape and gauze in direction of catheter insertion while stabilizing catheter with other hand. Discard in biohazard container.	Stabilizes catheter as you remove dressing. Allows for visualization of insertion site.
d. Inspect catheter insertion site and surrounding skin, noting color and presence of swelling. Palpate for tenderness. Per facility policy, midline and PICC devices may require external catheter and midarm circumference measurements above insertion site. Compare with previous measurements. If sutures used to stabilize catheter have become loosened or are no longer intact, an alternative stabilization measure should be considered.	Insertion site requires regular inspection for signs of complications (INS, 2011b). Measurement of external catheter is completed to determine if device has migrated externally. Midarm circumference determines if upper arm has increased in size, which could indicate venous thrombus or postinsertion phlebitis (INS, 2011b).
e. Remove and discard clean gloves, and perform hand hygiene.	Hand hygiene is one component of decreasing CLABSIs (IHI, n.d.; NQF, 2013).
f. Open central line dressing change kit using sterile technique and **apply sterile gloves.** If mechanical securement device is in use, disengage CVAD from housing and remove stabilization device with alcohol.	Sterile technique prevents transmission of microorganisms. Alcohol loosens adhesive backing to prevent damage to skin during removal.

> **SAFE PATIENT CARE** Use of chlorhexidine skin antisepsis as a cleansing agent is a component of CLABSI prevention care bundles.

STEPS	RATIONALE

g. Cleanse site:

   (1) Using chlorhexidine swab, apply with friction using repeated back-and-forth motions vertically and horizontally for at least 30 seconds; allow to dry completely.

   Allowing antiseptic solutions to air-dry completely reduces microbial counts (INS, 2011b).

   (2) Povidone-iodine may be used (see facility policy).

h. Apply skin protectant to entire area around insertion site. Allow to dry completely so skin is not tacky.

   Skin protectant is used to protect irritated or fragile skin from dressing. It must be used if mechanical stabilization devices are being used.

i. Option: Use chlorhexidine-impregnated dressing for short-term CVADs in patients older than 2 months of age if the CLABSI rate is not decreasing despite adherence to basic prevention measures (CDC, 2014).

j. Apply new catheter stabilization device per manufacturer's instructions if catheter is not sutured in place (see illustration in Skill 27.1, Step 23b).

   Provides catheter stability to minimize dislodgment.

k. Apply sterile transparent semipermeable dressing or gauze dressing over insertion site (see Skill 27.1).

   Transparent dressing allows for clear visualization of catheter insertion site between dressing changes.

l. Apply label with date, time, and your initials.

   Provides information about when dressing change was completed.

3. *Change injection cap:*

a. Perform hand hygiene.

   Meticulous hand hygiene is a component of CLABSI prevention care bundles.

b. 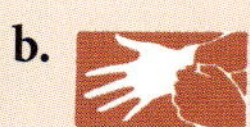 Apply clean gloves. Determine if injection caps should be changed.

   Caps usually are changed when removed for IV fluid administration, if integrity is compromised, after blood specimen sampling, or if they have been accessed beyond manufacturer's directions.

c. Prepare new injection cap:

   (1) Remove cap from package and cleanse septum with alcohol using friction.

   Scrubbing the hub prevents incidence of microorganisms (Wright et al., 2013).

   (2) Keep protective cap on tip of injection cap.

   Maintains sterility.

   (3) Prime injection cap by flushing with 0.9% NS through cap until fluid is seen in protective cap. Keep syringe attached.

   Removes air from system.

d. Clamp catheter lumens one at a time by using slide or squeeze clamp.

   Prevents air from entering system when opened.

e. Remove old injection caps using aseptic technique.

   Routinely changing injection cap decreases catheter infections.

f. Cleanse catheter hub with antiseptic swab. Allow to dry and then connect new injection cap on catheter hub.

   Allowing antiseptic solutions to air-dry completely effectively reduces microbial counts (INS, 2011b; Wright et al., 2013).

g. Flush catheter with 10-mL syringe of 0.9% sodium chloride or attach new IV tubing and begin infusion.

   Prevents clot formation in catheter lumen.

4. *Flush positive-pressure device:*

a. Perform hand hygiene.

   Meticulous hand hygiene is a component of CLABSI prevention care bundles.

b. Apply clean gloves. Prepare a new positive pressure device by attaching prefilled saline syringe. Prime through device and leave syringe attached.

   Maintains sterility of device.

Continued

STEPS	RATIONALE

   c. Vigorously cleanse the cap-catheter junction of the CVAD with alcohol swab for 5 to 10 seconds and allow to dry.

Ensures microbial action of antiseptic (Corrigan et al., 2014; Wright et al., 2013).

   d. Clamp catheter. Remove old needleless cap and discard in proper container.

Prevents loss of blood through catheter.

   e. Connect positive pressure device, unclamp catheter, and flush through with saline as ordered. Do not add extension tubing, which negates positive pressure action of valve.

Establishes catheter patency.

   f. Do *not* reclamp catheter.

Reclamping negates positive pressure action of valve.

> **SAFE PATIENT CARE** Daily review of line necessity with prompt removal of unnecessary lines is a component of CLABSI prevention care bundles.

5. Discontinue nontunneled catheter or PICC.

   a. Perform hand hygiene.

Meticulous hand hygiene is a component of care bundles.

   b. If solutions or medications are to be continued, prepare to convert them to a short-peripheral IV infusion device before CVAD discontinuation.

Prevents interruption of ordered solutions or medications. Prevents fluid loss during CVAD removal.

   c. Apply clean gloves. Apply mask, goggles, and gown (optional) (see facility policy), and remove old transparent dressing (see Skill 27.3, Step 3a). Discard in appropriate receptacle. Inspect insertion site and surrounding area for any signs or symptoms of IV-related complications.

Evaluates baseline condition of catheter site.

   d. Remove gloves, and perform hand hygiene.

Ensures that sterility is maintained while preparing equipment needed for removal of device.

   e. Apply clean gloves. Cleanse CVAD insertion site using combination antiseptic or chlorhexidine swabs (check facility protocol). With chlorhexidine, use a back-and-forth motion vertically and horizontally for at least 30 seconds; allow to dry completely.

Removes microorganisms from skin surrounding insertion site. Allowing antiseptic solutions to air-dry completely reduces microbial count effectively (INS, 2011b). Reduces incidence of CLABSI (IHI, n.d.; NQF, 2013).

   f. *If* mechanical securement device is present, disengage catheter from housing and remove sticky adhesive padding on skin using alcohol swab. Make sure to hold catheter securely so that it does not come out. Discard sticky adhesive padding.

Disengaging catheter from securement device and holding securely ensures that catheter will not come out until you are ready to remove it appropriately. Alcohol loosens sticky backing, preventing skin tears during removal.

   g. *If* sutures are present, remove clean gloves and **apply sterile gloves.** With nondominant hand, grasp suture with forceps. Using dominant hand, carefully cut suture with sterile scissors; avoid damaging skin or catheter. Lift suture out and discard. Continue until all sutures are removed (see facility policy).

Prevents accidental damage to catheter, causing a portion to break off in the arm or chest. Technique prevents pulling contaminated end of suture through patient's skin. Suture removal may require special training by facility.

   h. Using nondominant hand, apply sterile 4 × 4–inch gauze with antimicrobial ointment at insertion site. **Instruct patient to take a deep breath and hold it as you withdraw catheter.**

Ointment on sterile gauze provides a seal over insertion site after catheter is removed, preventing air from entering insertion site. Valsalva maneuver reduces risk of air embolism by decreasing negative pressure in respiratory system (Alexander et al., 2014; INS, 2011b).

   i. With dominant hand, remove catheter in a smooth, continuous motion an inch at a time. Note any resistance while removing catheter. Inspect catheter for intactness as you withdraw it. Keeping fingers near insertion site, immediately apply pressure with the sterile 4 × 4–inch gauze with ointment and hold until bleeding stops.

Gentle removal of catheter prevents stretching and breaking. Damaged catheters may break off and leave a piece in patient's body. Direct pressure reduces risk for bleeding and hematoma formation (Corrigan et al., 2014).

STEPS	RATIONALE
j. Apply sterile transparent dressing directly over sterile 4 × 4–inch gauze with ointment. Date, time, and initial dressing. Change every 24 hours until healed or per facility protocol.	Identifies date of catheter removal and need for dressing change.
k. Per facility protocol, measure length of catheter removed and inspect for integrity. Dispose of in biohazard container. *If catheter was removed for suspected bloodstream infection, place in appropriate specimen container according to facility protocol.*	Ensures that entire catheter has been removed. Compare with initial catheter insertion measurement (INS, 2011a, 2011b).
l. Discard items visibly contaminated with blood in biohazard container.	Prevents transmission of bloodborne pathogens.
6. See Completion Protocol (inside front cover).	

EVALUATION

1. Routinely assess patient's vital signs, noting changes symptomatic of infection (e.g., fever, chills, tachycardia, flushed skin). Monitor laboratory values for white blood cell count.
2. Observe and palpate catheter insertion site for erythema, warmth, tenderness, edema, or drainage.
3. If mechanical securement device is in place, assess that catheter is intact and has not migrated externally, or assess that sutures are intact. For tunneled devices, assess that Dacron cuff is not visible.
4. Inspect condition of catheter and connection tubing for leaks or tears; secure connections, kinks or obstructions, or cracked hubs.
5. Evaluate for signs of clot formation in catheter: difficulty flushing, sluggish infusion, and absent or sluggish blood return.
6. Use *Teach Back:* State to the patient, "We covered a lot today about your CVAD (or PICC line) and I want to make sure that I explained things clearly. So let's review what we discussed. Can you name at least three symptoms or problems to report to your home health nurse when you get home?" Evaluates what the patient is able to explain or demonstrate. Revise your instruction now or develop plan for revised patient teaching to be implemented at an appropriate time if patient is not able to teach back correctly.

UNEXPECTED OUTCOMES

1. *Catheter damage or breakage:* CVAD leaks during flushing or administration of solutions or medications. Insertion site appears wet or damp under transparent dressing or dressing is not occlusive.
   a. Stop infusion of solution or medication (if applicable).
   b. Clamp catheter with nonserrated clamp near insertion site.
   c. Place sterile gauze over break or hole, and have catheter removed or repaired.
2. *Occlusion—venous thrombus:* Difficulty or inability to flush device, aspirate blood return, or administer solutions or medications; enlarged neck veins; increase in midarm circumference (PICC).
   a. Stop infusion of solution or medication.
   b. Obtain order for radiograph film to confirm tip placement.
   c. Administer thrombolytics if ordered.
   d. Remove or assist with removal of device per facility protocol.
3. *Infection at site (exit site, tunnel, port pocket) or suspected CLABSI:* Drainage, tenderness, erythema at insertion site, elevated temperature.
   a. Obtain blood cultures: one set from CVAD and one set from peripheral venipuncture (if ordered) (see Chapter 8).
   b. Administer antibiotic therapy as ordered.
   c. Remove or assist with removal of device.
4. *Catheter migration:* PICC external catheter is longer than previously noted. Dacron cuff is exposed on chest wall with tunneled devices.
   a. Stop infusion of medications or solutions.
   b. Obtain chest radiograph film to verify that tip is placed in SVC or IVC. Physician or advanced practice nurse may reposition tip under fluoroscopy.
   c. Remove or assist with removal of device.
5. *Air emboli:* New onset of shortness of breath or dyspnea, hypotension, and tachycardia.
   a. Close off open end of catheter immediately.
   b. Place patient in Trendelenburg's position on left side.
   c. Remove or assist with removal of device as ordered.

Recording and Reporting

- Record in nursing notes type of CVAD, number of lumens, location and appearance of site; condition and type of dressing, procedure performed, and any signs and symptoms of complications.

- Document your evaluation of patient learning.
- Report any unexpected outcomes (e.g., signs and symptoms of complications), interventions, and patient's response to treatment to health care provider.

Sample Documentation

0800   Right upper extremity double-lumen PICC line dressing changed. New mechanical securement device applied. Insertion site and surrounding area without signs or symptoms of IV-related complications observed. Both lumens with positive brisk blood return and flush without resistance. Midarm circumference measures 32 cm (13 inches) at 10 cm (4 inches) above insertion site, and external catheter measures 1 cm ($\frac{1}{2}$ inch), both measurements unchanged from last dressing changes. Patient states, "I will let you know if I notice any redness or swelling or if I have pain where the catheter comes out."

Special Considerations

Pediatric

- Do not use chlorhexidine gluconate in infants younger than 2 months of age (INS, 2011b).
- CVADs are available in smaller diameters and shorter lengths for children and infants (Corrigan et al., 2014).
- Take care to secure infant catheters in a manner that does not allow them to twist. Small-diameter catheters are fragile, and twisting them will cause them to tear.

- Amount and dosage of flush solution (heparin/saline) varies with age and size. Record volume of blood draws on intake and output record.

Geriatric

- Some older adults have difficulty with lying flat in bed, and a modification of the totally supine position during CVAD insertion or removal is often necessary.
- PICC insertion may provide an alternative route of administration and reduce the risk of complications associated with subclavian or jugular insertion.

Home Care

- Initiate early referral for discharge planning to social service, counselor, or home care coordinator for assessment of resources (Petroulias et al., 2013).
- Provide patient with written list of providers for supplies and equipment.
- Instruct patient or family caregiver in flushing technique, site care and dressing change, and emergency interventions (Corrigan et al., 2014).
- Instruct patient and family caregiver in adaptations of hospital procedures that they can make at home (e.g., good hand hygiene instead of sterile gloves).
- Assess home environment, and determine suitable area for dressing changes, avoiding areas where contaminants are potential hazards.
- Provide appropriate information about home disposal of soiled dressings and equipment (see Chapter 31).

SKILL 27.5   ADMINISTRATION OF PARENTERAL NUTRITION

PN is a specialized form of nutritional support in which nutrients are given intravenously through a CVAD by an infusion pump to patients with significant gastrointestinal (GI) dysfunction. PN is composed of amino acids, glucose, and lipid as energy sources with the addition of various electrolytes, minerals, and trace elements as a means to provide complete or partial nutritional supplementation (Alexander et al., 2014; Phillips, 2014). The base solution of PN is a dextrose solution ranging from 5% to 70% dextrose. In some situations, fat emulsion is added directly to a PN solution rather than being administered separately. When the fat emulsion is added to the PN solution, it is referred to as a 3:1 solution or total nutrition admixture solution. A 3:1 mixture allows for lipid infusion over 24 hours, decreasing risk of hypertriglyceridemia from rapid infusion. If a patient has fluid restrictions such as with heart failure, PN allows for the appropriate nutritional support without the addition of fluid. Because of the high osmolarity of total PN (total nutrition admixture) (>600 mOsm/L), a solution is administered through a CVAD and not peripherally because of the increased risk of complications such as phlebitis (Corrigan et al., 2014; INS, 2011b). With the lower dextrose and amino acid concentration of partial PN (<600 mOsm/L), this type of solution is given through a peripheral IV device, but it may also be administered via CVAD.

Several complications are associated with PN, the most frequent being catheter-related bloodstream infection. PN has also been associated with liver disease, particularly in patients with multiple bloodstream infections, severe GI disease, and longer PN duration (Worthington and Gilbert, 2012). There is a risk of allergic reaction to PN, although the risk is low.

PN regimens are individually designed for patients with the formulas prescribed by the health care provider (in consultation with a dietitian) and are reviewed daily, with special consideration given to each patient's fluid, electrolyte, and nitrogen balance. Nurses collaborate with health care providers and members of the nutritional support team in administering PN and monitoring a patient's nutritional status, blood glucose levels, and signs or symptoms of catheter-related complications. Indications for short-term PN are seen in patients requiring preoperative bowel rest and in patients whose GI tracts are unusable for more than 4 to 5 days. Long-term indications include, but are not limited, to a nonfunctional GI tract seen with massive bowel resection, GI surgery, or massive GI bleed or trauma to abdomen, head, or neck. The skill of infusing PN requires you to know the composition and indications thoroughly and to follow the policy and procedure of your facility.

ASSESSMENT

1. Review medical record for indications of and risks for protein/calorie malnutrition: weight loss from baseline or ideal body weight, muscle atrophy or weakness, failure to wean from a ventilator, edema, lethargy, chronic illness, and NPO for more than 6 days. Confer with the health care provider and nutritional support team. *Rationale: Indications for use of PN (Corrigan et al., 2014).*

2. Assess patient's medical history for electrolyte levels and renal, cardiac, and hepatic function. Assess for history of allergies. *Rationale: Factors influenced by PN include elements to which patient may be allergic.*

3. Consult with health care provider and nutritional support team on calculation of calorie, protein, and fluid requirements for patient. *Rationale: Provides multidisciplinary plan for patient's nutritional support and goals for therapy (Corrigan et al., 2014).*

4. Perform hand hygiene. Apply clean gloves. Assess for type and status of venous access device. Note signs and symptoms of IV-related complications: tenderness, inflammation, edema, and drainage or inability to flush or aspirate blood return. *Rationale: Ensures correct device is in place (based on formula concentration). Identifies early signs of catheter-related complications, which contraindicate infusion of PN and may indicate need to establish a new IV site (Worthington and Gilbert, 2012).*

5. Assess baseline vital signs, auscultate lung sounds, and measure weight and I&O. *Rationale: Provides baseline for monitoring patient's response to infusion of PN.*

6. Assess laboratory test results for serum albumin, total protein, transferrin, prealbumin, and triglycerides, and check blood glucose by fingerstick. *Rationale: Provides baseline for measuring patient's nutritional status and tolerance to PN.*

7. Verify health care provider's order for nutrients, vitamins, minerals, trace elements, electrolytes, and added medication and flow rate. Check for compatibility of added medications. *Rationale: Health care provider must order PN. Pharmacies that prepare PN will check for medication compatibility.*

8. Assess patient's understanding of need for PN and any risks associated with therapy. *Rationale: Determines level of instruction required.*

PLANNING

Expected Outcomes focus on achieving adequate nutrition and fluid volume, preventing complications related to PN therapy, and promoting patient understanding of therapy.

1. Patient's ideal weight gain is usually 1 to 3 pounds (0.5 to 1.5 kg) per week.

2. Serum glucose levels are less than 150 mg/dL or maintained between 80 and 110 mg/dL. (Check health care provider's order for desired glucose level and other laboratory parameters.)

3. Venous access device is patent and free of signs or symptoms of IV-related complications.

4. Patient is able to describe purpose of PN and symptoms representing complications to report to nurse.

Delegation and Collaboration

Administration of PN cannot be delegated to nursing assistive personnel (NAP). The nurse directs the NAP to:

- Measure urinary output and patient's weight per facility protocol.
- Report when the pump alarms, catheter dressings are wet, temperature is elevated, or patient has any complaints such as shortness of breath, headache, weakness, feeling shaky, or discomfort or bleeding at IV site.
- Report vital signs outside of normal range to nurse.
- Perform fingerstick blood glucose monitoring as directed and report abnormal findings.

Equipment

- PN solution (IV)
- EID
- IV infusion tubing with Luer-Lok tip
- Appropriate IV filter (0.22 micron for dextrose/amino acids that do not contain lipids; 1.2 micron for 3:1 solution) (INS, 2011b)
- 5- to 10-mL syringe with sterile saline flush
- Bedside blood glucose monitoring kit
- Adhesive tape or tubing label
- Alcohol swabs
- Clean gloves
- Medication administration record (MAR) or computer printout

IMPLEMENTATION *for* ADMINISTRATION OF PARENTERAL NUTRITION

STEPS	RATIONALE
1. **See Standard Protocol (inside front cover).**	
2. When obtaining bag of PN in medication room, check label on PN bag with health care provider's order on MAR or computer printout and patient's name. Also check any additives, and note solution expiration date. Prepare solution at least 30 minutes to 1 hour before needed by removing from refrigerator.	Prevents medication error. *This is first check for accuracy.* Solution should be at room temperature for administration (INS, 2011b). Preparation prevents delay of infusion.

Continued

STEPS	RATIONALE

3. Inspect 2:1 PN solution for particulate matter. Inspect 3:1 solution for a cream layer or separation of fat into a layer.

Presence of particulate matter or fat emulsion separation requires that solution be discarded.

4. Before leaving medication room, check IV solution a second time using the six rights of medication administration. Check label on PN bag against MAR or computer printout.

This is second check for accuracy.

5. At the bedside, identify patient using two identifiers (e.g., name and birthday or name and account number) according to facility policy. Compare identifiers with information on the patient's MAR or medical record. If using bar-code system, scan bar code on patient's wristband and bar code on PN fluid container.

Ensures correct patient. Complies with The Joint Commission standards and improves patient safety (TJC, 2014). *This is the third check for accuracy.*

6. Apply clean gloves. Perform hand hygiene. Attach appropriate IV filter to IV tubing. Prime tubing with PN solution, making sure that no air bubbles remain; turn off the flow with the roller clamp (see Skill 27.1).

Maintains sterility of solution. Air introduced into central circulation can result in air embolus, a fatal IV complication.

> **SAFE PATIENT CARE** *If* patient has CVAD, meticulous hand hygiene is a component of CLABSI prevention care bundles.

7. Wipe end port of CVAD with alcohol, allow to air-dry, and then attach syringe of 0.9% NS solution to needleless port; aspirate for blood return, then flush with saline per facility policy.

Scrubbing the hub decreases microorganisms (Wright, 2013). Determines patency of IV device before infusing PN.

8. Remove syringe. Connect Luer-Lok end of PN IV tubing to end port of CVAD; for multilumen lines, label tubing used for PN.

Ensures that tubing is securely connected to IV line. Dedicated line should be used for multilumen devices. Labeling of high-risk catheters prevents connection with inappropriate tube or catheter (TJC, 2014).

9. Place IV tubing into EID. Open roller clamp. Set and regulate flow rate on pump as ordered (see illustration).

Flow rates are ordered to meet patient's metabolic and electrolyte needs. Maintaining rates prevents electrolyte imbalances.

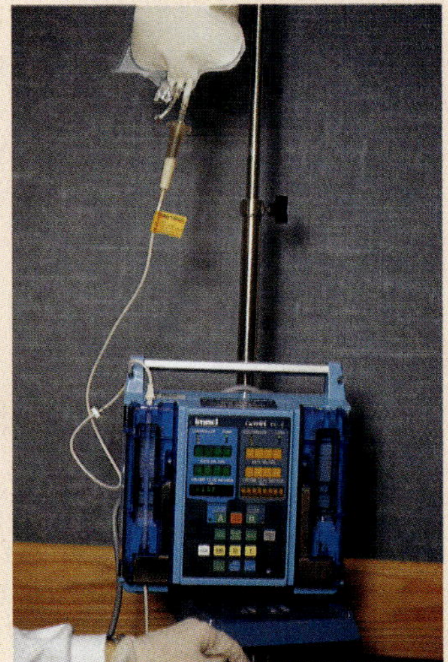

STEP 9 Place PN IV tubing into EID.

a. *Continuous infusion (optional):* Flow rate is immediately set at ordered rate and given over a 24-hour period.

Ensures that blood glucose levels are maintained to prevent hypoglycemia or hyperglycemia (Corrigan et al., 2014).

STEPS	RATIONALE

b. *Cycle infusion (optional):* Flow rate is initiated at about 40 to 60 mL/hr, and rate is gradually increased until patient's nutritional needs are met. Before completion of the infusion, the rate is decreased at about the same amount of milliliters per hour until PN has completed. This infusion is generally given over a shorter time frame (12 to 18 hours).

Infusion rates are gradually increased and decreased to prevent hypoglycemia or hyperglycemia (Corrigan et al., 2014).

10. Infuse all IV medications or blood through an alternative IV site or multilumen devices. Do not obtain blood samples or central venous pressure readings through same lumen or port used for PN.

Prevents drug incompatibility and IV device occlusion (Corrigan et al., 2014).

11. Do not interrupt a PN infusion (e.g., during showers, transport, blood transfusion).

Prevents development of catheter-related bacteremia (Corrigan et al., 2014; Worthington and Gilbert, 2012).

12. PN containing dextrose and amino acids alone or with fat emulsion added as a 3:1 formulation shall have a hang time not to exceed 24 hours. Fat emulsions alone shall have a hang time not to exceed 12 hours.

Prevents bacterial infection and deterioration of emulsion (INS, 2011b).

13. Change IV administration sets for PN every 24 hours and immediately on suspected contamination (see Skill 27.3).

Reduces transmission of infection (INS, 2011b).

14. **See Completion Protocol (inside front cover).**

EVALUATION

1. Monitor flow rate according to facility policy and procedure. If infusion is not running on time (ahead or behind of prescribed order), do not attempt to catch up because this could cause a hypoglycemic or hyperglycemic reaction and fluid overload.
2. Inspect IV site routinely for signs and symptoms of swelling, inflammation, drainage, warmth, tenderness, or edema.
3. Measure blood glucose levels as ordered (see Chapter 8), and check other laboratory values as ordered by health care provider or nutrition support team.
4. Measure weights daily or as ordered.
5. Monitor I&O and assess for signs of fluid retention: palpate skin of extremities and auscultate lung sounds, which could indicate fluid retention.
6. Monitor for signs of systemic infection such as fever, elevated white blood cell count, or malaise.
7. Use *Teach Back:* State to the patient, "We covered a lot today about your administration of PN and I want to make sure that I explained things clearly, so let's review what we discussed. What signs and symptoms should you report to your health care team immediately?" Evaluate what the patient is able to explain or demonstrate. Revise your instruction now or develop plan for revised patient teaching to be implemented at an appropriate time if patient is not able to teach back correctly.

Unexpected Outcomes and Related Interventions

1. Patient develops signs and symptoms of hypoglycemia or hyperglycemia or has blood glucose level lower or greater than target set by health care provider.
   a. Gradually adjust concentration of glucose in PN solution per orders.
   b. Administer insulin, if ordered, to maintain proper blood glucose levels.
2. Infusion stops flowing or flows at rate slower than ordered.
   a. Check patency of IV device and attempt to flush.
   b. Infuse a thrombolytic agent, if ordered (see facility policy).
   c. Prepare for line removal if occlusion remains.
3. Patient experiences weight gain greater than $\frac{1}{2}$ kg/day (1 pound), taut skin turgor is present, and crackles are auscultated over lung fields.
   a. Notify health care provider and obtain orders to reduce infusion rate.
   b. Anticipate need to administer diuretics.
4. Development of fever, chills, malaise, and elevated white blood cell count, indicating systemic infection.
   a. Notify health care provider and discuss possibility of obtaining wound cultures from insertion site and blood culture from peripheral site.
   b. Systemic antibiotic therapy may be initiated or IV device removed or both.

5. Solution is unavailable or unable to be infused because of particulate matter, leakage of bag, or separation of fat emulsion.

  a. Obtain and infuse 10% dextrose in water solution at same flow rate that PN was infusing to prevent sudden decrease in blood glucose level.

  b. Evaluate for signs and symptoms of hypoglycemia (e.g., weakness, confusion) and report to health care provider.

  c. Monitor blood glucose levels and report to health care provider.

Recording and Reporting

- Document assessment of physical condition, bedside blood glucose values, condition of IV site, and IV solution infusing on applicable flow sheet.
- Document I&O and weights on graphic sheets per facility policy and procedure.
- Document your evaluation of patient learning.
- Report to health care provider deviation from baseline assessment or laboratory parameters and signs or symptoms of dehydration, fluid overload, and signs or symptoms of local or systemic IV-related complications.

Sample Documentation

0800   PN solution initiated through proximal lumen of nontunneled triple-lumen subclavian IV. Infusing at rate of 150 mL/hr via EID. Laboratory results reported to health care provider with no new changes to formula. Complete chemistry panel to be obtained in AM. Current weight maintained at 58 kg for last week. IV site without signs or symptoms of related complications observed. Patient states, "I don't feel as shaky as I did last week."

Special Considerations
Pediatric

- Partial PN is suggested for nonstressed infants for a brief course of maintenance therapy when full growth and development is not the primary goal (Corrigan et al., 2014).

Geriatric

- Some older adults have impaired ability to manage higher fluid volumes or are at risk for an increased incidence of hypoglycemia (INS, 2011c).

Home Care

- Patients requiring long-term PN benefit from referral to a home nutrition therapy team.
- Patient and family caregiver need to learn to perform catheter site care, dressing changes, and techniques for adding and removing PN solutions.
- Some patients receive PN at night during sleep (cycle therapy) to allow freedom to leave home or work during the day.
- Teach patient and family caregiver to monitor patient's weights, calorie count, I&O, and serum glucose levels (Worthington and Gilbert, 2012).

SKILL 27.6   TRANSFUSION OF BLOOD PRODUCTS

The transfusion of blood and blood components restores and maintains quality of life for patients with hematological disorders, cancer, injury, or surgical intervention. Caring for patients receiving blood or blood components is a nursing responsibility. However, you should never view the transfusion of blood products as routine; overlooking a minor detail is dangerous and life-threatening to a patient (Alexander et al., 2014; AABB, 2014a; Phillips, 2014).

Transfusion of blood and blood products is closely regulated and monitored. Standards of operations for all blood bank centers are set by the American Association of Blood Banks (AABB, 2014b, OSHA, the U.S. Food and Drug Administration (FDA), and the American Red Cross. These standards include the collection of donor blood, distribution of the product, and standards for transfusion. Before any transfusion, always verify specific facility policy regarding procedural requirements.

Blood and blood component therapies treat and restore hemodynamic homeostasis or provide treatment for diseases related to coagulation deficiencies (Clark, 2011). A written health care provider's order to transfuse should always include which component to transfuse and the duration of the transfusion. A single unit of whole blood or blood components should be infused within a 4-hour period (INS, 2011a). If more than one blood product is to be given, the sequence or order of transfusion should be specified. Any additional medications such as an antihistamine (given when the history shows previous allergic response), antipyretics (given when the history shows previous febrile nonhemolytic response), diuretics (given when the history shows potential for heart failure), or other special treatment of the components should also be included in a written transfusion order.

Three blood typing systems, ABO, Rh, and most recently HLA typing (e.g., single donor), are used to ensure that transfusion products match a recipient's blood as closely as possible (Table 27-6). Before transfusion in nonemergent situations, always verify a patient's blood type and Rh to be sure it is compatible with the donor transfusion (see facility policy for procedure).

There is increasing public awareness of the possible transmission of infectious diseases through transfusion of blood products. The risk of a blood recipient developing an infectious disease is lower than ever before because of improved testing of donor blood. However, viral, bacterial, and parasitic diseases can still be transmitted through blood. Screening of blood donors is an important first step to identify people with a medical history, behavior, or events that put them at risk of transmissible disease (Alexander et al., 2014; Clark, 2011). Be prepared to inform your patients thoroughly about the options, benefits, and risks of transfusion and reassure them

TABLE 27-6   ABO SYSTEM

PATIENT'S BLOOD TYPE	RED BLOOD CELLS ANTIGEN	TRANSFUSION WITH TYPE A	TRANSFUSION WITH TYPE B	TRANSFUSION WITH TYPE AB	TRANSFUSION WITH TYPE O	TRANSFUSION OPTIONS
A(+)	A	Yes	No	No	Yes	A+, A–, O+, O–
A(–)	A	Yes	No	No	Yes	A–, O–
B(+)	B	No	Yes	No	Yes	B+, B–, O+, O–
B(–)	B	No	Yes	No	Yes	B–, O–
AB(+)	AB	Yes	Yes	Yes	Yes	A+, A–, B+, B–, O+, O–, universal recipient
AB(–)	AB	Yes	Yes	Yes	Yes	A–, B–, O–
O(+)	None	No	No	No	Yes	O+, O–
O(–)	None	No	No	No	Yes	O–, universal donor

From Corrigan A, et al: *Core curriculum for infusion nursing*, ed 4, Philadelphia, 2014, Lippincott Williams & Wilkins.

that every effort is taken to ensure a safe blood supply and transfusion. Patients should know that there is never a completely risk-free transfusion.

One avenue for preventing the transmission of infectious diseases during blood transfusion is the use of autologous blood (e.g., a patient's own blood). Autologous transfusions can be done in several ways; however, the most frequent method is preoperative collection from a patient. AABB standards establish the process for determining patient eligibility and collecting, testing, and labeling the blood product unit. Before transfusion, ABO and Rh typing of the patient are performed. Autologous units must be used before units from the general blood supply. Identification and verification processes and methods of administration for autologous units are the same as those used for other units of blood (AABB, 2014b). This method is not without risk because human error still exists in collection and storing of the blood.

ASSESSMENT

1. Verify health care provider's order for specific blood or blood product with appropriate date, time to begin transfusion, duration, and any pretransfusion or post-transfusion medications to be given. *Rationale: Correct identification of ordered blood product is the first step to ensure safe administration (AABB, 2014b; Alexander et al., 2014).*

2. Review medical record for patient's baseline laboratory values (e.g., hematocrit, hemoglobin, platelet count) and transfusion history, including known allergies and previous transfusion reaction. Verify that type and cross-match have been completed within 72 hours of transfusion and that patient consent for transfusion is completed. *Rationale: Baseline provides means to evaluate response to transfusion. Record review identifies patient's prior response to blood or blood product transfusion (including a reaction), which allows you to anticipate and be prepared to intervene rapidly.*

3. Know the indications or reasons for a transfusion (e.g., low hematocrit secondary to postoperative bleeding).

Rationale: Allows you to anticipate patient's response to therapy (Clark, 2011).

4. Identify patient using two identifiers (e.g., name and birthday or name and account number) according to facility policy. Compare identifiers with information on the patient's MAR or medical record. *Rationale: Ensures correct patient. Complies with The Joint Commission standards and improves patient safety (TJC, 2014).*

5. Perform hand hygiene. Apply clean gloves. Verify that IV catheter is patent and site is without signs or symptoms of IV-related complications, such as infiltration or phlebitis. In adults, use a 14- to 24-gauge catheter; in neonates or children, use a 22- to 24-gauge device; 1.9-Fr is the smallest CVAD that can be used (INS, 2011b). *Rationale: Catheters used for blood transfusion must be patent and large enough to accommodate the appropriate flow rate but not large enough to damage the vein. The major concern is completing the transfusion within the recommended 4-hour time frame. If a smaller gauge catheter is used, consider requesting split blood units to ensure timely administration (INS, 2011b).*

6. Obtain and record pretransfusion baseline vital signs and review hourly urine output for last 24 hours. If patient is febrile (temperature >100° F [37.8° C]), notify health care provider prescribing the transfusion (follow facility policy). *Rationale: This provides a comparison to detect change in patient's condition during transfusion.*

7. Assess patient's level of comfort and understanding of the procedure and rationale. *Rationale: Clarifying patient's need for and associated benefits of therapy may alleviate some of the patient's anxiety.*

PLANNING

Expected Outcomes focus on safe, complication-free transfusion therapy, including restoration of normal hemodynamics and improvement in clinical condition.

1. Patient's systolic blood pressure improves, urine output is 0.5 to 1 mL/kg/hr, and cardiac output returns to baseline.

2. Patient's laboratory values reflect improvement in targeted areas; factor levels are within therapeutic range for patient; improved coagulation function.
3. Patient verbalizes understanding of rationale for therapy.

Delegation and Collaboration

Skills of initiating and monitoring blood therapy cannot be delegated to nursing assistive personnel (NAP). The nurse directs the NAP about:

- Frequency of vital sign monitoring needed (after stabilization determined by nurse).
- What to observe for, such as complaints of shortness of breath, sudden back pain, hives, or chills or signs or symptoms of IV site complications such as swelling, pain, or redness and to report immediately to RN.
- Obtaining blood components from blood bank (check facility policy).
- Report when volume of blood is low in the blood bag.

Equipment

- Y-type blood administration set with standard filter and macrodrip drop factor (Note: Depending on blood product, special tubing and filters may be necessary)

- Prescribed blood product
- IV 250-mL bag 0.9% NaCl (NS) IV solution
- 5- to 10-mL syringe containing NS
- Clean gloves
- Tape
- Antiseptic wipes or swabs (chlorhexidine preferred)
- Vital sign equipment: thermometer, blood pressure cuff, stethoscope, and pulse oximeter
- Signed transfusion consent

Optional Equipment

- Rapid infusion pump
- EID (verify that infusion pump can be used to deliver blood or blood products)
- Option: Leukocyte-depleting filter (Note: Facility may irradiate blood products within its blood bank facility)
- Blood warmer (used mainly when large-volume or rapid transfusion is needed)
- Pressure bag (used for rapid infusion in acute blood loss)

IMPLEMENTATION *for* TRANSFUSION OF BLOOD PRODUCTS

STEPS	RATIONALE
1. **See Standard Protocol (inside front cover).**	
2. Obtain blood bag from laboratory following facility protocol (see illustration). Blood transfusions must be initiated within 30 minutes after release from laboratory, blood bank, or controlled environment.	Facilities differ as to personnel who can release a blood bag from a blood bank, but they always require two witnesses and some form of patient identification. Usually only one unit is released at a time (INS, 2011a).

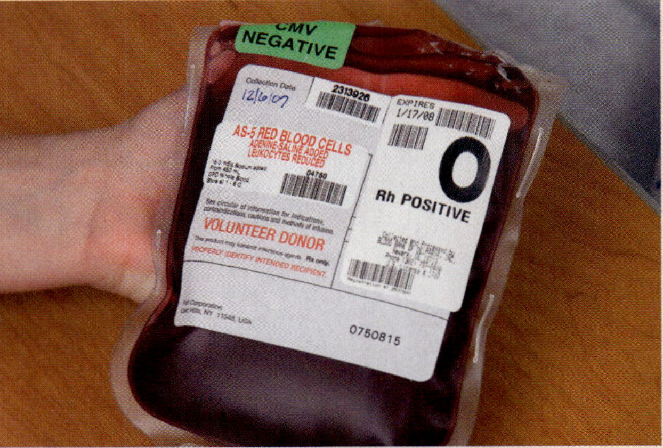

STEP 2 Blood bag with label.

3. Check appearance of blood product for signs of contamination (e.g., bubbles, clumping or clots, purplish color, and presence of leaks).	Determines integrity of bag. Air bubbles, clots, or discoloration indicate bacterial contamination or inadequate anticoagulation of components and are contraindications for transfusion (AABB, 2014b).
4. Verbally compare and correctly verify patient, blood product, and blood and Rh type with another person considered qualified by your facility (e.g., registered nurse or licensed practical nurse) before initiating transfusion (see illustrations). Check the following:	Ensures that patient receives correct blood or blood product (Clark, 2011). Most hemolytic transfusion errors are caused by clerical errors (Alexander et al., 2014).

STEPS	RATIONALE

a. Reconfirm patient identity.

b. Transfusion record number and patient's identification number must match.

c. Patient's name is correct on all documents. Check identification number and date of birth on identification band and patient record.

d. Check unit number on blood bag with blood bank slip to ensure that they are a match.

e. Blood type matches on transfusion record and blood bag. Verify that component received from blood bank is same component that health care provider ordered.

f. Check that patient's blood type and Rh type are compatible with donor blood type and Rh type.

g. Check expiration date and time on unit of blood.

Prevents accidental administration of wrong component.

Prevents transfusion reaction.

Expired blood should never be used because the cell components deteriorate and may contain excess citrate ions.

> **SAFE PATIENT CARE** When discrepancy is noted during verification process, do not administer blood or blood product. Notify blood bank and appropriate personal per facility policy.

5. Have patient void or empty urinary drainage collection container.

If transfusion reaction occurs, urine specimen obtained must be recent and preferably taken after transfusion is initiated to assess for presence of red blood cells from a hemolytic reaction.

6. Review purpose of the transfusion and ask patient (or visiting family member) to report immediately any signs and symptoms (during or after transfusion), including chills, low back pain, shortness of breath, nausea, excessive perspiration, rash, itching, or a vague sense of uneasiness.

Once transfusion reaction occurs, staff must respond immediately with treatment (Clark, 2011; Phillips, 2014).

7. Perform hand hygiene and apply clean gloves. Reinspect blood product for signs of leakage or unusual appearance.

Verifies quality of blood product. If signs of contamination are present, return blood product to laboratory.

8. Open Y-tubing blood administration set for single unit. Use multiset if multiple units transfused. Set all clamps to "off" position.

"Y"-tubing facilitates maintenance of IV access with NS in case patient will need more than 1 unit of blood.

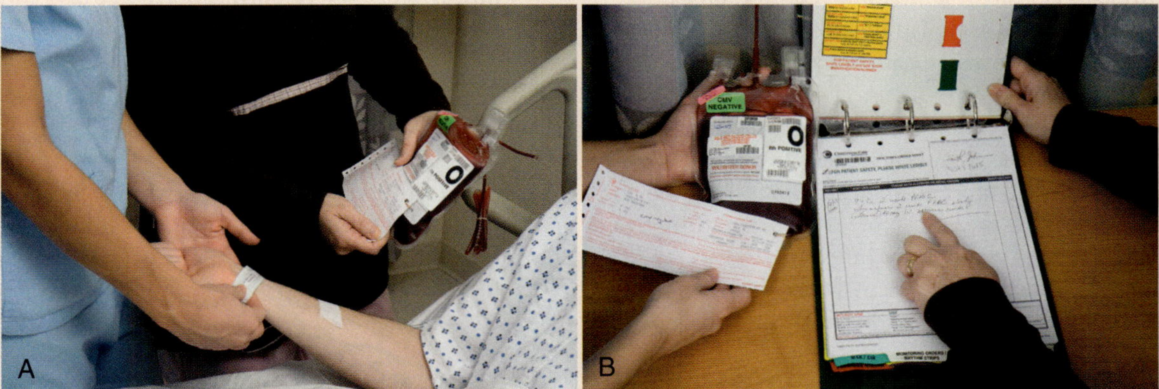

STEP 4 A, Checking patient identification, comparing information with arm band. **B,** Two clinicians verifying identification of patient and blood product.

Continued

9. Use aseptic technique and spike bag of 0.9% NS with one of Y-tubing spikes. Hang bag on pole and prime tubing, completely filling filter chamber with saline. Close lower clamp. Maintain clamp on blood product side of Y-tubing in the "off" position.

Eliminates air in tubing. IV is ready to be connected to patient's VAD. If filter is not completely primed with NS, transfusion will slow because of collection of debris in partially primed filter.

10. Open common tubing clamp to finish priming tubing to distal end of tubing connector. Close when tubing is filled with saline. All three tubing clamps should now be closed. Keep sterile cap on connector.

Prevents blood from entering NS bag.

11. Prepare blood component for administration. Gently invert bag two to three times, back and forth. Remove protective covering from access port on blood bag. Spike blood component bag with other Y-tubing connector located next to NS 0.9% tubing (see illustration). Close NS clamp above filter and open clamp above filter to blood product; prime Y-tubing with blood. Blood will flow into drip chamber.

Gentle agitation suspends red blood cells in anticoagulant. Tubing is primed with blood unit and ready for transfusion into patient.

SAFE PATIENT CARE Only use NS solution to administer blood. Do not piggyback other solutions or medications with blood (AABB, 2014b; INS, 2011b).

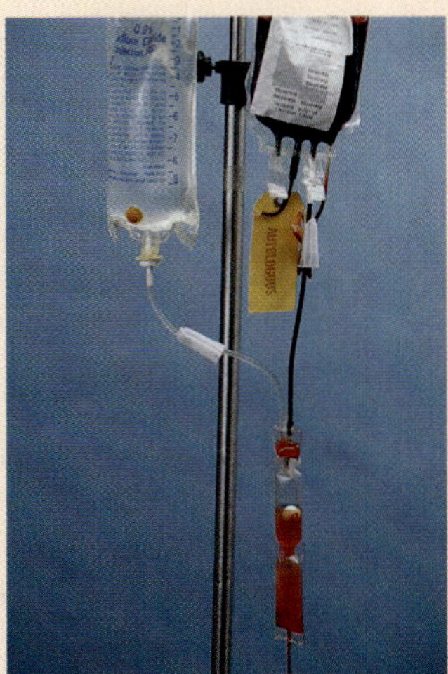

STEP 11 Unit of blood connected to Y-tubing setup.

12. Turn off any existing IV infusion and disconnect tubing from catheter hub. Keep tubing end sterile with sterile cap. Maintaining asepsis, attach the primed blood administration tubing to patient's VAD by first cleansing catheter hub with antiseptic swab. Then quickly connect NS-primed blood administration tubing directly to patient's IV site. Option: Connect to newly placed IV catheter.

Scrubbing the hub prevents incidence of microorganisms (Wright, 2013). Once blood or blood product begins to infuse, no other IV medications will be administered through the same IV line or device.

13. Open lower clamp and regulate blood infusion to allow only 2 mL/min (or 20 gtt/min using a macrodrip 10 gtt/mL) to infuse in the initial 15 minutes. Remain with patient for the first 15 minutes of the transfusion. Remove and discard gloves. Perform hand hygiene.

Most transfusion reactions occur within the first 5 to 15 minutes. Infusing a small amount of blood component initially minimizes the amount of incompatible blood to which patient is exposed, minimizing the severity of a reaction.

14. Obtain vital signs at 5 minutes, 15 minutes, and every 30 minutes until 1 hour after transfusion (AABB, 2014b) or per facility policy after that.

Change from baseline vital signs may indicate transfusion reaction.

STEPS	RATIONALE
15. If there is no transfusion reaction, regulate rate according to health care provider's orders, and infuse the remaining volume of blood as ordered (packed red blood cells [PRBCs] infused over 2 hours; whole blood infused over 3 to 4 hours). For other blood products such as IV immunoglobulin or factor replacement, follow facility recommendations.	Reduces risk of fluid volume excess while restoring vascular volume. Patient's condition and health care provider's orders dictate rate of blood infusion. If patient is at risk for fluid overload, blood bank can split units (Alexander et al., 2014).

> **SAFE PATIENT CARE** *Do not let a unit of blood hang for more than 4 hours because of danger of bacterial growth.* Change administration sets and add-on filters at completion of each unit or at end of 4 hours, whichever comes first (INS, 2011b). *Never* store blood in facility refrigerator.

STEPS	RATIONALE
16. After blood has infused, close roller clamp above filter to blood, open NS, and infuse until blood administration tubing is completely clear. Restart primary IV fluids as ordered only after assessing IV site for patency and signs and symptoms of IV-related complications. Discard blood bag according to facility policy.	NS infusion clears IV catheter of blood product. If transfusing more than 1 unit of blood or blood products, maintain 0.9% NS via blood administration set at prescribed rate until second unit is started.
17. **See Completion Protocol (inside front cover).**	

EVALUATION

1. Observe for any changes in vital signs and any sign of transfusion reaction such as chills, flushing, itching, hives, dyspnea, or tachycardia during transfusion.
2. Monitor I&O and laboratory values after transfusion. In a hematologically stable adult, 1 unit of PRBCs should increase the hemoglobin by 1 g/100 mL and the hematocrit by 3%. A unit of platelet concentrate prepared from a single unit of whole blood should increase a patient's platelet count by 5000 to 10,000/mL (INS, 2011b).
3. Monitor IV site for signs and symptoms of phlebitis or infiltration each time vital signs are taken.
4. Use *Teach Back:* State to the patient, "I want to make sure I explained the purpose of your blood transfusion and symptoms to report back to me. Can you name two symptoms to report?" Evaluates what the patient is able to explain or demonstrate. Revise your instruction now or develop plan for revised patient teaching to be implemented at an appropriate time if patient is not able to teach back correctly.

Unexpected Outcomes and Related Interventions

1. Patient displays signs and symptoms of transfusion reaction.
   a. Stop the transfusion. Stay with patient and *notify* the health care provider.
   b. Connect a new NS infusion solution to the IV access site to prevent any subsequent blood from infusing from original blood tubing. Keep vein open with slow infusion at 10 to 12 gtt/min to ensure patency and maintain venous access for medication or to resume transfusion.
   c. Monitor vital signs per facility policy.
   d. Send entire blood setup back to blood bank (per facility policy).
2. Rate of infusion slows in the absence of infiltration.
   a. Verify patency of IV catheter and that all clamps are open.
   b. Ensure that blood bag is elevated to proper height and filter is completely primed.
   c. Gently flush IV line with NS or use a pressure bag or EID that permits blood transfusion.
3. Patient experiences pain, swelling, or redness at IV site.
   a. Stop transfusion and discontinue IV infusion and catheter.
   b. Reinsert a new IV catheter in another site proximal to the old site or opposite arm.
4. Fluid overload occurs or patient exhibits difficulty breathing or has crackles on auscultation.
   a. Slow or stop transfusion, elevate head of the bed, and notify health care provider.
   b. Administer prescribed diuretics, analgesics, or oxygen as prescribed.
   c. Continue frequent assessments, and closely monitor vital signs and I&O.

Recording and Reporting

- Record pretransfusion medications, vital signs, and location and condition of the IV site.
- Record the type and volume of blood component; blood type or Rh; blood unit, donor, and recipient identification; compatibility; and expiration date according to facility policy.
- Record volume of NS and blood component infused.
- Record vital signs before, during, and after transfusion.

- Report signs and symptoms of a transfusion reaction immediately.
- Document your evaluation of patient learning.

Sample Documentation

0900   Early AM CBC noted. Health care provider aware of Hct 22. Type and cross-match drawn with two witnesses per phlebotomy.

1330   Voided 320 mL clear, amber urine. 20-gauge 1-inch Insyte inserted into L midcephalic × 1 attempt. Patient stated, "Only hurt a little." NS 0.9% initiated at 25 mL/hr. 1 unit PRBCs started at 40 mL/hr; vital signs: Temp 98.9° F, Pulse 80, Resp 20, BP 140/78. Patient verbalized understanding of transfusion and to report any feeling of SOB, back pain, headache, or chills. Transfusion assessment and vital sign record initiated per policy.

Special Considerations
Pediatric

- Pediatric blood units are prepared in special units (aliquots) and usually equal half the volume of a conventional adult unit (Corrigan et al., 2014).
- Administer 5% to 10% of total transfusion volume the first 15 minutes of transfusion, then if no adverse effects, increase administration rate to 2 to 5 mL/kg/hr (Corrigan et al., 2014).
- Usual dose of PRBCs is 10 to 15 mL/kg (Corrigan et al., 2014).

Geriatric

- Older adults may have compromised cardiac, renal, and respiratory systems. Adjust flow rate if patient cannot tolerate prescribed flow rate. Flow rate should be 1 mL/kg/hr in patient at risk for circulatory overload.
- Vigilance in monitoring an access site during transfusion is vital in an older adult who may be less sensitive to the symptoms of infiltration and the generalized symptoms of a transfusion reaction (INS, 2011c).

Home Care

- Patients who have had prior transfusion reactions, acute angina, or heart failure are not considered good candidates for home transfusion.
- Nursing personnel must be present for the entire transfusion process and for 30 to 60 minutes after transfusion.
- Whole blood must not be administered in the home.
- Blood and blood products must be transported in a container with appropriate coolant. Verify and record the temperature at the time of delivery.
- Post-transfusion instructions must be given in writing, and the patient or family caregiver must be provided with names and phone numbers of individuals available to be called in the event of a delayed problem (e.g., unexplained fever, malaise, jaundice). Complications may occur days to weeks after transfusion.
- The container, empty bags, and tubing should be returned to the home care facility on completion of the transfusion.

CRITICAL THINKING EXERCISES

Case Study

A 62-year-old woman is 4 days postoperative following a left total knee replacement. She has been receiving IV fluids of D_5 ½ NS solution at 83 mL/hr via an EID. She has a 22-gauge 1-inch Insyte IV device in her left midcephalic vein. When getting report, the nurse finds out the patient has been complaining of nausea and is unable to eat. Her blood work reveals she is mildly dehydrated, but her vital signs are stable. The patient is to continue her IV fluids for 2 more days on recommendation of her surgeon. Her IV site shows no signs or symptoms of IV-related complications and had been restarted yesterday.

1. The patient is due for her next bag of IV fluids. Place the steps to change the IV bag in the correct order.
   1. Remove spike from old IV bag.
   2. Label new IV bag with date, time, and time of completion.
   3. Close roller clamp on old IV tubing.
   4. Check for air in tubing.
   5. Regulate flow rate.
   6. Insert spike into new IV bag and fill tubing.
   7. Remove new IV bag from refrigerator at least 1 hour before hang time.

2. The patient rings her call bell 30 minutes after a new 1-L bag of IV fluids is hung. On entering the patient's room, the nurse notices that her IV bag is ¾ empty and she is complaining of shortness of breath and is dyspneic. The nurse's assessment reveals bilateral crackles in lung bases, tachycardia, and increased urinary output. What should the nurse suspect is happening?
   1. Fluid volume deficit
   2. Fluid volume overload
   3. Obstructed IV catheter
   4. Air emboli

3. True or false. Administration of the patient's IV fluids cannot be delegated to the NAP.

Review Questions

1. Which set of symptoms is indicative of phlebitis?
   1. Tenderness, pitting edema, dyspnea, cough
   2. Chest pain, cyanosis, hypotension, weak pulse
   3. Headache, nausea, diarrhea, chills
   4. Pain, erythema, swelling

2. A patient is receiving a blood transfusion of PRBCs after a total hip replacement. The nurse checks the patient's vital signs 30 minutes after beginning the transfusion and finds an oral temperature of 101° F, pulse of 100 beats/min, and respiratory rate of 20. What is the nurse's first priority?
   1. Notify the health care provider.
   2. Stop the transfusion and begin the NS infusion.
   3. Notify the blood bank immediately.
   4. Wait 30 minutes and repeat the vital signs.
   5. Administer acetaminophen (Tylenol) 650 mg by mouth.

3. Considerations for selecting a peripheral IV catheter for a patient include which of the following?
   1. Selecting the longest catheter with a larger gauge
   2. Selecting the longest catheter with the smallest gauge
   3. Selecting the shortest catheter with a larger gauge
   4. Selecting the shortest catheter with the smallest gauge

4. What is the correct anatomical tip location for a PICC line?
   1. Right ventricle
   2. Midaxillary
   3. Antecubital fossa
   4. SVC

5. A patient returning from surgery has an order for 1000 mL D_5NS to infuse at 100 mL/hr. If the drop factor on the patient's infusion tubing is 10 gtt/mL, what is the correct infusion rate?
   1. 34 gtt/min
   2. 10 gtt/min
   3. 60 gtt/min
   4. 17 gtt/min

6. True or false. Partial PN can be administered only through a CVAD.

7. Which of the following is a key component in the central line care bundles?
   1. Chlorhexidine skin antisepsis
   2. Soap and water skin antisepsis
   3. Alcohol skin preparation
   4. Hydrogen peroxide skin preparation

8. Which solution should the nurse use to prime the Y administration blood set?
   1. 0.45% sodium chloride (½ NS)
   2. Dextrose 5% in 0.45% sodium chloride (D_5 ½ NS)
   3. 0.9% sodium chloride (NS solution)
   4. Dextrose 5% in 0.9% sodium chloride (D_5 NS)

9. Place the steps for changing a dressing over a short-peripheral IV device in correct order.
   1. Cleanse insertion site with antiseptic swab.
   2. After removing tape anchoring catheter, remove transparent membrane dressing.
   3. Apply new transparent semipermeable membrane (TSM).
   4. Observe site for signs and symptoms of IV device–related complications.
   5. Label dressing with date, time, catheter gauge size, and initials.

10. Which of the following is an acceptable way to verify patient identification before administering an IV fluid or medications?
    1. Check arm band against MAR
    2. Ask a second RN to verify
    3. Scan bar code on wrist band
    4. Delegate NAP to identify patient

REFERENCES

Alexander M, et al: *Core curriculum for infusion nursing*, ed 4, Philadelphia, 2014, Lippincott Williams & Wilkins.

American Association of Blood Banks (AABB): *Technical manual*, ed 18, Bethesda, MD, 2014a, AABB.

American Association of Blood Banks (AABB): *Standards for blood banks and transfusion services*, ed 29, Bethesda, MD, 2014b, AABB.

Centers for Disease Control and Infection (CDC): *Central line-associated bloodstream infection (CLABSI) event*, 2014, http://www.cdc.gov/nhsn/pdfs/pscmanual/4psc_clabscurrent.pdf. Accessed April 9, 2014.

Clark C: Recent effects and available technologies for safety in delivery of blood products, *J Infus Nurs* 34(1):23, 2011.

Clark P: Emergence of infection control surveillance in alternate health care setting, *J Infus Nurs* 33(6):363, 2010.

Corrigan A, et al: *Core curriculum for infusion nursing*, ed 4, Philadelphia, 2014, Lippincott Williams & Wilkins.

Felver L: Fluid and electrolyte balance. In Giddens JF, editor: *Concepts for nursing practice*, St Louis, 2013, Mosby.

Gorski L, et al: Recommendations for frequency of assessment of short peripheral IV catheter sites, *J Infus Nurs* 35(5):290, 2012.

Hadaway L: Needle stick injuries, short peripheral IV devices, *J Infus Nurs* 35(3):164, 2012.

Hockenberry MJ: *Essentials of pediatric nursing*, ed 9, St Louis, 2013, Mosby.

Infusion Nurses Society (INS): *Policy and procedures for infusion nursing*, ed 4, Norwood, MA, 2011a, Infusion Nurses Society.

Infusion Nurses Society (INS): 2011 Infusion nursing standards of practice, *J Infus Nurs* 34(1 Suppl):S65, 2011b.

Infusion Nurses Society (INS): *Policy and procedures for infusion nursing of the older adult*, ed 2, Norwood, MA, 2011c, Infusion Nurses Society.

Institute for Healthcare Improvement (IHI): *Implement the IHI central line bundle*, n.d. http://www.ihi.org/knowledge/Pages/Changes/ImplementtheCentralLineBundle.aspx. Accessed April 5, 2014.

National Quality Forum (NQF): *Prevention of central line associated blood stream infections*, 2013, http://www.qualityforum.org/ProjectMeasures.aspx?projectID=73701. Accessed September 12, 2014.

Occupational Safety and Health Administration (OSHA): *Occupational exposure to blood borne pathogens, needle stick, and other sharps injuries: final rule, CFR 29, part 1910 (Fed Reg 66:5317, Jan 18, 2001)*, 2006, https://www.osha.gov/pls/oshaweb/owadisp.show_document?p_table=FEDERAL_REGISTER&p_id=16265. Accessed April 5, 2014.

O'Grady N, et al: Healthcare infection control practices advisory committee: guidelines for the prevention of intravascular catheter-related infections, *Am J Infect Control* 39(4 Suppl 1):S1, 2011.

Petroulias P, Groesbect L, Wilson FL: Providing culturally competent care in home infusion nursing, *J Infus Nurs* 36(2):108, 2013.

Phillips L: *Manual of IV therapeutics: evidence based practice for infusion therapy*, ed 6, Philadelphia, 2014, FA Davis.

The Joint Commission: *Preventing central line associated bloodstream infections*, 2013, http://www.jointcommission.org/assets/1/6/CLABSI_Toolkit_Tool_3-18_CVC_Insertion_Bundles.pdf. Accessed September 11, 2014.

The Joint Commission (TJC): *National Patient Safety Goals*, Oakbrook Terrace, IL, 2014, The Commission. Available at: http://www.jointcommission.org/standards_information/npsgs.aspx.

Voshall B, et al: Barcode medication administration workarounds: A systematic review and implications for nurse executives, *JONA* 43(10):530, 2013.

Worthington P, Gilbert K: Parenteral nutrition risk, complications and management, *J Infus Nurs* 35(1):52, 2012.

Wright MO, et al: Continuous passive disinfection of catheter hubs prevents contamination and bloodstream infection, *Am J Infect Control* 41(1):33, 2013.

Preoperative and Postoperative Care

Surgery is both psychologically and physiologically stressful for patients. A patient has little control over the situation or the outcome, resulting in feelings of anxiety, fear, and powerlessness. The goal of preoperative nursing care is to reduce stress and place patients in the best conditions possible to undergo surgery.

During preoperative preparation, the nursing role focuses on physical, psychological, sociocultural, and spiritual preparation; validates existing information; reinforces preoperative teaching; reviews discharge information; and provides nursing care to complete preparation for the surgical experience (ASPAN, 2014). A nurse thoroughly assesses a patient's condition and collects and reviews relevant laboratory and diagnostic data. In addition, a nurse teaches a patient and family caregiver what to expect, and prepares the patient physically and psychologically for surgery.

The care of postoperative patients can be divided into three phases: immediate postanesthesia phase, early recovery phase, and convalescent phase. The immediate postanesthesia phase extends from the time a patient leaves the operating room (OR) to the time of transfer from the postanesthesia care unit (PACU) to the nursing unit. This phase requires 2 or more hours and frequent assessments for complications. Patients having surgery in ambulatory outpatient surgery centers have the same recovery needs as patients having surgery in a hospital. The early recovery phase includes several days after surgery followed by a convalescent phase of several additional days or weeks at home for the continued healing process. Patients with chronic medical condition, such as chronic respiratory disease or diabetes mellitus may require a longer convalescent phase.

PATIENT-CENTERED CARE

Often a patient is unsure of what to expect and has concerns about the amount of pain, possible complications, and length of recovery after surgery. Newer technologies such as laser and laparoscopy are less invasive and decrease the need for prolonged hospitalization or inpatient admission. Because many patients return home the same day, it is a challenge to meet patients' and families educational needs. Family caregivers may be unsure about their role in a patient's care and recovery. During both the preoperative and the postoperative periods, nurses need to continually educate patients and families about the normal healing process and how to optimize recovery, while also making them aware of signs and symptoms of surgical site infections (SSIs) (TJC, 2014). Ambulatory outpatient surgeries and shorter hospitalizations lower costs and decrease the risk of health care–associated infections.

Patients must be asked about their cultural practices and religious beliefs that may alter their family caregiver's acceptance of necessary education and procedures. For example, it is helpful to assess patient preference for pain medication before and after surgery. In addition, some religious practices may include receiving sacraments immediately before surgery and wearing religious medals or undergarments until just before surgery. Some cultural practices may prohibit cutting hair or include wearing a turban over long hair. Communicating all information pertaining to specific patient findings, practices, and beliefs to all members of the health care team is important and ensures each patient receives comprehensive and holistic care.

SAFETY

Physically preparing patients to undergo surgery and anesthesia involves important skills, including a thorough preoperative assessment. Regardless of the setting, the preoperative assessment forms the basis for a plan of care for a patient during and after surgery. Safety measures such as verifying correct patient, correct procedure and surgical site, signed consent, and relevant documentation (e.g., history and physical examination, nursing assessment, and preanesthesia assessment) and ensuring the availability of required blood products, implants, devices, or special equipment for the procedure are critical preparation steps. The timing and duration of antibiotic administration and proper surgical site preparation are critical in preventing SSIs. Other physical preparation procedures focus on minimizing the risks involved with surgery and anesthesia, while optimizing the patient's condition. The surgical site must be marked before surgery to allow staff to identify clearly the intended site for the procedure. A time-out must be performed immediately before starting the procedure and skin incision to ensure right patient and right site. This is the Universal Protocol (TJC, 2014). Glycemic control and normothermia restoration in the immediate postoperative period are also important care goals in specific surgical populations that help reduce the risk of SSIs (IHI, 2014).

Patient assessment in the immediate postoperative recovery phase emphasizes the *ABCs*—*A*, airway; *B*, breathing; and *C*, circulation. Postoperative patients are still under sedation and can easily become hypoxic. Nurses routinely monitor oxygen saturation levels and provide supplemental oxygen for as long as needed. Assess the wound size, location, and depth, all of which influence the type and amount of drainage. It is important to know what type of drainage to expect from the dressing, tubes, and catheters. You must implement prophylactic venous thromboembolism measures. Patients who are overweight or obese have increased risk of postoperative complications such as obstructive sleep apnea (OSA). Patients with OSA have a greater incidence of airway management problems in the PACU and postoperative pulmonary complications. Longer lengths of stay and unanticipated postoperative admission to the intensive care unit are common.

EVIDENCE-BASED PRACTICE

Institute for Healthcare Improvement (IHI): Surgical infection prevention, 2014, http://www.ihi.org/Engage/ Memberships/MentorHospitalRegistry/Pages/Infection PreventionSSI.aspx. Accessed September 15, 2014.

Magill SS, et al: Prevalence of healthcare-associated infections in acute care hospitals in Jacksonville, Florida, *Infect Control Hosp Epidemiol* 33(3):283, 2012.

Schwulst SJ, Mazuski JE: Surgical prophylaxis and other complication avoidance care bundles, *Surg Clin North Am* 92(2):285, 2012.

Spivey J: Infection prevention: 2013 criteria for reporting surgical site infections, *OR Nurse2013* 7(4):13, 2013.

Wound infections are among the most common surgical complications and occur in 2% to 5% of all surgical procedures. These infections are identified as SSIs and represent one quarter of all nosocomial infections. SSI adds to the morbidity in terms of hospital stay, pain, need for additional interventions, and cost (Schwulst and Mazuski, 2012).

The estimated 500,000 SSIs that occur annually in the United States represent the second most common infection among surgical patients, prolong hospitalization by 7 to 10 days, and increase the risk of death 2 to 11 times higher than patients without SSIs (IHI, 2014; Spivey, 2013).

The U.S. Centers for Disease Control and Prevention (CDC) has developed criteria that define SSI as infection related to an operative procedure that occurs at or near the surgical incision within 30 days of the procedure or within 90 days if prosthetic material is implanted at surgery (Magill et al., 2012). The impact on morbidity, mortality, and cost of care has resulted in SSI reduction being identified as a top national priority by the U.S. Department of Health and Human Services Action Plan to Prevent Healthcare-Associated Infections. Most SSIs are largely preventable, and evidence-based strategies have been available for more than 10 years and implemented in many hospitals. The current evidence-based strategies of the SSI bundle include:

- Antibiotics within 1 hour before the incision (2 hours for vancomycin or fluoroquinolone)
- Prophylactic antibiotics consistent with recommendations
- Discontinue prophylactic antibiotics within 24 hours of surgery end time (48 hours for cardiac procedures)
- Discontinue urinary catheters within 24 hours of surgery (preferably in PACU or by the morning of day 1 after surgery)
- Appropriate hair removal
- Appropriate surgical site skin antisepsis
- Proper hand scrub before surgery
- Hand hygiene before and after touching the patient or before and after clean or aseptic procedures by members of the surgical team who have not scrubbed
- Control of blood glucose levels in diabetic patients who are having cardiac surgery

SKILL 28.1   PREOPERATIVE ASSESSMENT

To identify risks and plan for care during and after surgery, a thorough preoperative nursing assessment of a patient's physiological and psychological condition documents baseline data for future comparisons to determine the effect of instruction and whether complications develop during the perioperative period. Many health care facilities have a designated department devoted to completing thorough preoperative screening and testing. Laboratory tests, electrocardiograms (ECGs), chest x-ray films, and other tests are often obtained in these facilities 1 to 2 weeks in advance of the scheduled surgical procedure. Perioperative staff performs a thorough assessment and reviews the test results to identify any potential abnormalities that may need further evaluation and treatment before surgery. The nurse assesses patients again 1 to 2 hours before the scheduled time of surgery to ensure that there are no changes to their medical condition. Advanced planning allows time for nurses to follow up on any unexpected outcomes. Before beginning this assessment, establish a trusting relationship with the patient. It is not unusual for the patient to remember and report at this time facts that were not previously told to the surgeon. Provide the patient privacy and a location free of interruption to encourage open communication. A preprocedure checklist is initiated, beginning with the decision to perform a procedure, maintained with ongoing data collection and assessment, and verified immediately before moving the patient to the procedure room (TJC, 2014). Typically an assessment is completed by the surgeon, anesthetist, or nurse, and a consent form is signed. Current test results should be available, as well as notices of any special considerations during the procedure, such as a need for blood products or special equipment.

PLANNING

Expected Outcomes focus on obtaining accurate information and identifying risk factors related to the intended surgery.

1. Patient can state which surgical procedure is being performed and the risks and benefits of surgery.
2. Patient provides appropriate preoperative information required to establish a plan of care.
3. Patient remains alert and appropriately responsive to nurse's assessment questions.

Delegation and Collaboration

The skill of preoperative assessment cannot be delegated to nursing assistive personnel (NAP). Each state has its own delegation rules. The following is an example of delegation (ASPAN, 2014):

- Obtain vital signs and weight and height measurements.

Equipment

- Stethoscope
- Blood pressure monitoring equipment
- Pulse oximetry
- Thermometer
- Watch or clock with a second hand
- Method to measure height and weight
- Access to laboratory, ECG, x-ray films, and other diagnostic equipment as needed
- Preprocedure checklist
- Preoperative assessment form

IMPLEMENTATION *for* PREOPERATIVE ASSESSMENT

STEPS	RATIONALE
1. **See Standard Protocol (inside front cover).**	
2. Identify patient using two identifiers (e.g., name and birthday or name and account number) according to facility policy.	Ensures correct patient. Complies with The Joint Commission standards and improves patient safety (TJC, 2014).
3. Determine if patient has any communication impairment (e.g., blindness, hearing loss), is able to read and understand English, and is mentally competent. For example, give patient an informational brochure and have him or her explain a portion of the contents.	Patient may not fully comprehend a diagnosis, understand proposed treatment, or effectively consider alternatives that are presented without effective communication.
4. Assess patient's understanding of the intended surgery and anesthesia. Ask patient to offer a description rather than asking a simple yes or no question (e.g., "Do you understand your surgery?"). Have patient describe in his or her own words. Ask about expectations of patient and family caregiver of surgery and care. Include questions concerning fears, cultural practices, and religious beliefs if applicable.	Patients may have misconceptions and incomplete knowledge. Asking about fears, cultural practices, and religious beliefs allows you to anticipate priorities of patient and family caregiver and adapt your plan so that you can give appropriate instruction and support.

Continued

STEPS	RATIONALE
5. Ask if patient has an advance directive (see Chapter 30).	Advance directives protect patient's rights by communicating a patient's treatment preferences if he or she is unable to communicate.
6. Collect nursing history and identify surgical risk factors:	Allows for anticipation of possible complications and planning for interventions to reduce risks. Allergies, to medications or latex, can be life-threatening.

SAFE PATIENT CARE If patient is having emergency surgery, focus on assessment of primary body system affected.

STEPS	RATIONALE
a. Condition leading to surgery.	Allows you to anticipate postoperative needs and complications.
b. Chronic illnesses and associated risks (e.g., hypertension—bleeding and stroke; OSA—postoperative respiratory depression and arrest; asthma—impaired ventilation; hiatal hernia—aspiration; diabetes mellitus—poor wound healing; methicillin-resistant *Staphylococcus aureus*—impaired wound healing and sepsis).	Some chronic conditions increase the risk of complications from surgery and anesthesia.
c. Last menstrual period (for female patients in childbearing years).	Anesthetic agents and other medications could injure the fetus.
d. Previous hospitalizations.	Determines if patient is familiar with hospital procedures.
e. Full medication history, including prescription, over-the-counter (OTC), and herbal remedies and date and time of last doses.	Patient may not report OTC medications and herbal remedies unless specifically asked. All may interact with anesthetic agents or other medications given during surgery. Patient may be instructed to take any routine blood pressure, cardiac, or seizure medications. Changes in dosages of oral diabetic agents or insulin may be ordered.
f. Previous experience with surgery and anesthesia; have patient clarify if any undesirable outcomes occurred.	Information assists in preventing recurrent problems with the planned surgery.
g. Family history of complications from surgery or anesthesia.	A family history of reactions to anesthetic agents may indicate a familial condition such as malignant hyperthermia, which is life-threatening.
h. Allergies to medications, food, or tape, including specific questions about natural rubber latex. Ask patients if they have had any problem with medication or anything placed on their skin.	Reactions to latex can be life-threatening, and prevention in sensitized patients requires specific precautions. Often patients with latex allergies are scheduled as the first case of the day. In addition, many patients do not understand that rubber and latex are the same. Using both words helps obtain accurate information.
i. Physical impairment.	Physical impairments may cause limited mobility and situations that could lead to problems with positioning and risk for pressure ulcer formation. Communicate this information to the OR nurse because these patients may need special positioning or OR bed surfaces.
j. Prostheses and implants (e.g., implantable medication delivery pump, dentures, hearing aid, pacemaker, internal defibrillator, hip prosthesis).	These devices could become damaged or malfunction from electrical equipment used during surgery. Report this information to the OR nurse.
k. Smoking, alcohol, and drug use.	Increases risk of intraoperative and postoperative complications.
l. Occupation.	Anticipates how postoperative restrictions affect patient's return to work.
7. Obtain patient's weight, height, and vital signs (see Chapters 6 and 7).	Height and weight are used to calculate drug dosages. Vital signs provide a baseline for postoperative comparison.

STEPS	RATIONALE
8. Assess patient's respiratory status, including auscultation of lungs, adventitious sounds, character and rate of respirations, oxygen saturation, ability to breathe lying flat, use of oxygen or continuous positive airway pressure (CPAP) at home, and chest x-ray film report.	Poor respiratory condition can affect patient's response to general anesthesia. Use of CPAP may indicate that patient has OSA, a condition that poses risks after surgery.
9. Auscultate heart sounds, and evaluate patient's circulatory status, including apical pulse, ECG report, and peripheral pulses (see Chapter 7, Skill 7.4).	Circulation may be a factor in positioning patient on the OR table.
10. Assess for patient's risk for postoperative thrombus formation (e.g., older adults, immobilized patients, patients with personal or family history of blood clots, use of birth control pills, hormones). Ask patient about any leg pain. Observe calves for swelling, warmth, and redness; observe calves for symmetry; and palpate pedal pulses.	Circulation slows after general anesthesia, increasing the tendency for blood clot formation. Immobilization during the surgical procedure promotes venous stasis. Manipulation and positioning can cause accidental trauma to leg veins.

> **SAFE PATIENT CARE** Homans' sign is not always present when a DVT exists. If you suspect a thrombus, notify the surgeon and refrain from manipulating the extremity any further. Surgery will usually need to be postponed. Antiembolism stockings or pneumatic compression cuffs may be ordered for patients at risk for thrombus formation (Chapter 16).

STEPS	RATIONALE
11. Complete gastrointestinal assessment; identify the time of patient's last intake of food or drink (see Chapter 7, Skill 7.5).	With patient under general anesthesia, the esophageal sphincter relaxes and the stomach contents can be aspirated.
12. Complete neurological assessment, determine patient's neurological status including level of consciousness (LOC), and note neurological deficits (see Chapter 7, Skill 7.7).	Patient's neurological status affects attentiveness to instruction. Offers important baseline for postoperative evaluation.
13. Evaluate patient's musculoskeletal system, including range of motion (ROM) of joints (see Chapter 7, Skill 7.7).	If ROM is limited, extra care is needed to prevent injury related to positioning in surgery.
14. Examine patient's skin; identify any breaks in skin integrity, and determine level of hydration (see Chapter 7, Skill 7.1). Pay particular attention to area of body on which patient will be positioned.	If skin is thin, broken, or bruised, extra padding is needed in surgery. Hydration may affect skin integrity.
15. Evaluate patient's emotional status, including level of anxiety, coping ability, and family caregiver support. Assess the potential for abuse.	If patient has high level of anxiety or fear, consultation with a social worker, pastoral care, or advanced practice nurse might be useful.
16. Review results of laboratory tests, including complete blood count, electrolytes, urinalysis, and other diagnostic tests.	Laboratory work provides an assessment of major body systems.
17. **See Completion Protocol (inside front cover).**	

EVALUATION

1. Determine if patient information is complete so that plan of care can be established. Validate unclear information with family caregiver.
2. Evaluate patient's ability to cooperate (e.g., makes eye contact, answers appropriately).
3. Use **Teach Back:** State to the patient, "I want to be sure I explained what you need to know about your intended surgery and anesthesia. Can you tell me why you are having surgery?" Evaluates what the patient is able to explain or demonstrate. Revise your instruction now or develop plan for revised patient teaching to be implemented at an appropriate time if patient is not able to teach back correctly.

Unexpected Outcomes and Related Interventions

1. Patient does not understand what surgery will be performed.
   a. Notify the surgeon.

2. The patient reports a condition that is a risk factor for surgery or after surgery such as hiatal hernia, pregnancy, family history of complications with anesthesia, cold or upper respiratory infection, recent chest pain, or obstructive sleep apnea (OSA).
   a. Notify the surgeon and anesthesia provider.
3. Patient has been taking anticoagulants.
   a. Notify the surgeon.
4. Patient reports an allergy to latex.
   a. Remove all supplies containing latex from patient's room.
   b. Post a latex precautions sign on the door or stretcher.
   c. Notify surgeon, anesthesia provider, and OR nurse.
5. Appropriate laboratory tests were not ordered or completed.
   a. Notify surgeon and anesthesia provider and make arrangements for tests to be completed.
6. Chest x-ray film report, ECG, or laboratory tests show abnormal findings.
   a. Notify surgeon and anesthesia provider.

Recording and Reporting

- Document findings on the preoperative portion of the nurses' detailed preoperative notes or other designated facility form.

- Report abnormal laboratory values or other concerns to the surgeon or anesthesiologist.
- Document your evaluation of patient learning.

Sample Documentation

0830   Nursing history completed. Patient states that after knee surgery last year she "vomited for 6 hours." Anesthesiologist notified of patient history of vomiting after surgery.

Special Considerations
Pediatric

- Consider a child's developmental level when performing preoperative preparation (e.g., use films, books, tours, toys, and games to demonstrate preoperative procedures) (Hockenberry and Wilson, 2013).
- Take the developmental level of the child into consideration during the preoperative assessment.

Geriatric

- Age-related changes may result in diminished short-term memory. Additional assessment and teaching may be necessary.
- An older adult may have some limitation in ROM. If this limitation is significant, notify the OR nurse so that surgical position can be modified.

SKILL 28.2 PREOPERATIVE TEACHING

With shortened hospital lengths of stay and growth in ambulatory surgical procedures, there is a greater demand for patient preparation and support. Patient education must go beyond simply providing information because patients and families must assume more preoperative and postoperative responsibilities (Johansson et al., 2010). Preoperative patient teaching involves assisting a patient to understand and prepare mentally for the surgical experience. Effective education focuses on each patient's individual needs and leads to empowered patients who have sufficient knowledge that meets their needs, expectations, or preferences.

In the past, patients received preoperative teaching the day or evening before surgery, when patients were most anxious. Health care cost reduction practices now have most patients entering the hospital or ambulatory care center the morning of surgery. Preoperative teaching is not effective at this time because of patient anxiety and stress related to surgical preparation (Stannard and Krenzischek, 2012). Many health care agencies now provide outpatient education programs to prepare patients and their family caregivers for a specific surgery. For example, patients who require a total knee replacement will go to preoperative preparation classes with other patients requiring the same surgery. Effective preoperative teaching increases patient satisfaction, promotes psychological well-being, and may decrease complications leading to an increased length of stay (Lewis et al., 2014). Plan your teaching based on the preoperative assessment. Make every attempt to ensure the patient's privacy. Select the best

learning method for the patient. In many settings, videotape and written materials are available to assist you. Whenever possible, have the family caregivers responsible for the patient's care after surgery present. Later the family caregivers serve as coaches and assist the patient in performing exercises. Plan to have the patient demonstrate expected postoperative skills to allow for practice and facilitate understanding.

Patients and their families are often anxious about impending surgery, which hinders learning. Speak in a clear, slow voice to reduce the patient's anxiety and promote understanding. You may need extra time for teaching and reinforcement to ensure patient understanding. After surgery, high anxiety can lead to negative psychological and physiological outcomes. Preoperative information about expected perioperative sensations decreases the distress associated with surgery. By teaching and setting expectations before surgery (pain level, average length of surgery), the patient and the nurse can make a significant contribution to success in the postoperative recovery phase.

ASSESSMENT

1. Identify patient using two identifiers (e.g., name and birthday or name and account number) according to facility policy. *Rationale: Ensures correct patient. Complies with The Joint Commission standards and improves patient safety (TJC, 2014).*

2. Ask about patient's previous experiences with surgery and anesthesia. *Rationale: This allows you to individualize teaching and address specific patient concerns.*

3. Determine if patient and family caregiver understand the surgery. *Rationale: This information determines if correction of misunderstanding is necessary.*

4. Identify patient's cognitive level, language, and culture. *Rationale: These factors may alter patient's ability to understand the meaning of surgery and can affect the postoperative healing course if there are mixed messages or misunderstanding.*

5. Assess patient's risk for postoperative respiratory complications. Identify underlying lung conditions. Determine patient's ability to perform deep breathing and coughing and inspiratory spirometer activity. *Rationale: General anesthesia predisposes patient to respiratory problems. The presence of underlying respiratory conditions or patient's inability to perform postoperative respiratory exercises increases patient's risk for pulmonary complications.*

6. Assess patient's anxiety related to surgery. *Rationale: Directs you to provide additional emotional support and indicates patient's readiness to learn.*

7. Assess family caregiver's willingness to learn and support patient following surgery. *Rationale: Family caregiver's presence after surgery can be a potential motivating factor for patient recovery. In addition, the caregiver can coach patient through postoperative exercise and observe for any postoperative problems.*

8. Assess patient's medical orders. *Rationale: Preoperative and postoperative orders often require adaptations in the way a patient performs exercises.*

PLANNING

Expected Outcomes focus on reducing the anxiety level of patient and family caregivers and having patient demonstrate understanding of key information and specific skills necessary to prevent complications.

1. Patient demonstrates eye contact and asks and answers questions appropriately.

2. Patient correctly performs splinting, turning and sitting, breathing exercises, and leg exercises.

3. Family caregivers identify the location of the waiting room and time frame when they can expect a status on their family member.

4. Family caregivers verbalize ability to help prepare patient at home preoperatively.

5. Family caregivers provide emotional support for patient before surgery.

Delegation and Collaboration

The skills of preoperative teaching cannot be delegated to nursing assistive personnel (NAP). NAP can reinforce and assist patients in performing postoperative exercises. The nurse instructs the NAP about:

- Any precautions or safety issues unique to the patient (e.g., fall precautions, bleeding precautions, weight-bearing issues, dietary concerns).
- Informing the nurse of any identified concerns (e.g., patient is unable to perform the exercises correctly).

Equipment

- Stretcher or bed
- Pillow
- Incentive spirometer
- Preoperative education flow sheet
- PEP device
- Stethoscope

IMPLEMENTATION *for* PREOPERATIVE TEACHING

STEPS	RATIONALE
1. **See Standard Protocol (inside front cover).**	
2. Inform patient and family caregiver of date, time, and location of surgery; anticipated length of surgery; additional time in the postanesthesia recovery area; and where to wait.	Accurate information helps reduce the stress associated with surgery.
3. Answer questions patient and family caregiver ask.	Responding to patient and family caregiver questions helps to decrease anxiety and demonstrates your concern for them.
4. Instruct patient on preoperative bowel or skin preparations as needed. Check facility policy regarding number of preoperative showers and agent to be used for each shower (2% chlorhexidine gluconate is used most often). Following each preoperative shower, the skin should be rinsed thoroughly and dried with a fresh, clean, dry towel; and patient should don clean clothing.	Proper skin preparation is a critical element in preventing SSIs. Rinsing the skin removes residual antiseptic preparation that may cause skin irritation. After use, towels contain microorganisms that can grow in the presence of moisture. Using a fresh towel after each shower and donning clean clothing minimizes the risk of reintroducing microorganisms to clean skin (AORN, 2013; Graling and Vasaly, 2013).

Continued

STEPS	RATIONALE
5. Instruct patient on extent and purpose of food and fluid restrictions for period specified before surgery (e.g., no oral intake for 2 hours before surgery; no meat or fried foods 8 hours before surgery, unless otherwise specified by surgeon or anesthesiologist) (ASA, 2011).	During general anesthesia, muscles relax, and gastric contents can reflux into esophagus, leading to aspiration. Anesthetic eliminates patient's ability to gag.
6. Describe perioperative routines (e.g., time-out, site marking, intravenous [IV] therapy, urinary catheterization, enema, hair clipping or removal, laboratory tests, transport to OR).	Allows patient to anticipate and recognize routine procedures, reducing anxiety.
7. Describe planned effect of preoperative medications.	Provides information about what to expect, decreasing anxiety.
8. Review which routine medications patients need to discontinue before surgery.	Some medications are discontinued before surgery to minimize effects that can cause surgical risks. For example, anticoagulants may increase bleeding and are usually discontinued several days before surgery. Insulin dosages are usually adjusted because of the reduced intake of food before surgery.
9. Describe perioperative sensations (e.g., blood pressure cuff tightening, ECG leads, cool room, and beep of monitor).	Misconceptions and concerns about anesthesia have been ranked high among preoperative patients.
10. Describe pain-control methods to be used postoperatively. Many patients have a patient-controlled analgesia (PCA) pump (see Chapter 13).	Patients are fearful of postoperative pain. Explaining pain-management techniques reduces this fear. Establish what pain is acceptable, knowing that they will not be pain-free, but their pain will be managed.
11. Describe what patient will experience after surgery (e.g., where patient will be on awakening, frequent vital signs, turning, catheters, drains, tubes, alternating pressure from sequential compression device).	Provides a concrete description of what patient can expect after surgery so that patient is prepared.
12. Teach turning.	
a. Instruct patient on turning and sitting up (especially suited for abdominal and thoracic surgery):	
(1) Turn onto right side: Instruct patient to flex knees while lying supine and move toward left side of bed.	Promotes circulation and ventilation.
(2) Have patient splint incision with right arm and pillow; keep right leg straight and flex left knee up; and grab right side rail with left hand, pull toward right, and roll onto right side. Reverse process to turn to left side.	Supports incision and decreases discomfort while turning.
(3) Instruct patient to turn every 2 hours from side to side while awake.	Reduces risk of vascular, pulmonary, and pressure ulcer complications.
(4) Sit up on right side of bed: Elevate head of bed and have patient turn onto right side. While lying on right side, patient pushes on mattress with left arm and swings feet over edge of bed with nurse's assistance. To sit up on left side of bed, reverse this process.	Sitting position lowers diaphragm to permit fuller lung expansion.
13. Teach coughing, deep breathing, and incentive spirometry (see Step 14):	Patient may be unable or reluctant to deep breathe because of weakness or pain, resulting in secretions remaining in the base of the lungs. Collection of secretions increases the risk of pulmonary atelectasis and pneumonia.

STEPS	**RATIONALE**

a. Assist patient to high-Fowler's position in bed with knees flexed or sitting on side of bed or chair in upright position.

Sitting position facilitates diaphragmatic expansion.

b. Instruct patient to place palms of hands across from each other lightly along the lower border of the rib cage or upper abdomen (see illustration).

This allows patient to feel the rise and fall of the abdomen during deep breathing (Lewis et al., 2014).

c. Have patient take slow, deep breaths, inhaling through nose. Explain that patient will feel normal downward movement of diaphragm during inspiration. Demonstrate as needed.

Helps to prevent hyperventilation or panting. Slow deep breath allows for more complete lung expansion.

d. Have patient avoid using chest and shoulder muscles while inhaling.

Increases unnecessary energy expenditure and does not promote full lung expansion.

e. Have patient take slow, deep breath; hold for count of 3 seconds; and slowly exhale through mouth as if blowing out a candle (pursed lips).

Resistance during exhalation helps to prevent alveolar collapse.

f. Have patient repeat breathing exercise three to five times.

Repetition reinforces learning.

g. Have patient take two slow, deep breaths, inhaling through nose and exhaling through pursed lips.

Deep breaths expand lungs fully so air moves behind mucus to facilitate coughing.

h. Have patient inhale deeply a third time and hold breath to count of 3. Cough fully for two to three consecutive coughs without inhaling between coughs.

Deep breathing moves up secretions in the respiratory tract to stimulate the cough reflex without voluntary effort on the part of patient (Lewis et al., 2014).

i. Caution patient against just clearing throat.

Clearing throat does not remove mucus from deeper airways.

j. Have patient practice several times. Instruct patient to perform turning, coughing, and deep breathing every 2 hours. Have family caregiver coach patient to exercise.

Ensures mastery of technique. Frequent pulmonary exercises and movement decrease risk of postoperative pneumonia (Lewis et al., 2014).

14. Teach use of an incentive spirometer (see illustration):

Provides visual aid of respiratory effort. Encourages deep breathing to loosen secretions in lung bases.

a. Position in sitting or reclining position.

Facilitates diaphragm lowering and lung expansion.

b. Instruct patient to exhale completely and place mouthpiece so that lips completely cover it and inhale slowly, maintaining constant flow through unit.

Promotes complete inflation of lungs and minimizes atelectasis.

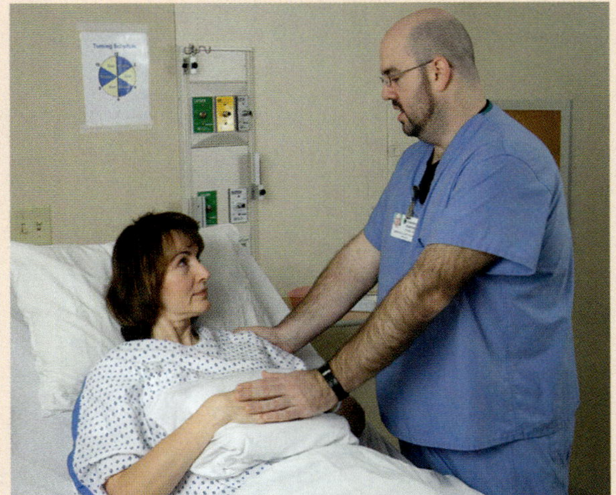

STEP 13b Deep-breathing exercise—placement of hands on upper abdomen during inhalation.

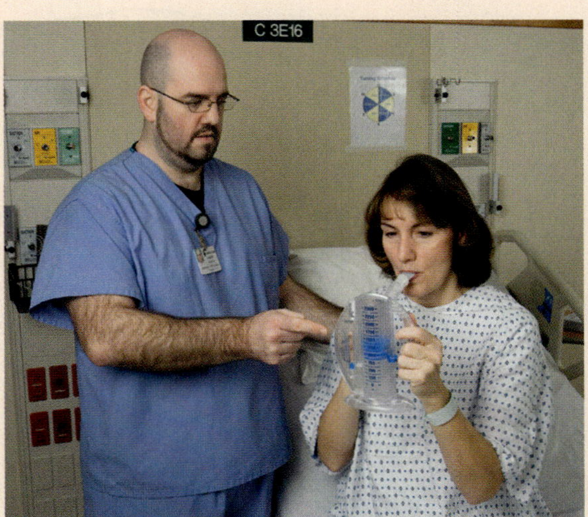

STEP 14 Patient demonstrates incentive spirometry.

Continued

STEPS	RATIONALE
c. After maximum inspiration, patient should hold breath for 2 to 3 seconds and exhale slowly.	Promotes alveolar inflation.
d. Set marker on spirometer at maximum inspiration point to establish postoperative target.	Establishes measure of normal maximum breath for patient. Provides outcome measure to determine postoperative return to preoperative volumes.
e. Instruct patient to breathe normally for a short period and repeat process 10 times every hour while awake.	Prevents hyperventilation and fatigue.
15. Teach positive expiratory pressure therapy and "huff" coughing:	
a. Set positive expiratory pressure device for setting ordered.	Higher settings require more effort.
b. Instruct patient to assume semi-Fowler's or high-Fowler's position, and place nose clip on patient's nose (see illustration).	Promotes optimum lung expansion and expectoration of mucus.
c. Have patient place lips around mouthpiece. Instruct patient to take a full breath and then exhale 2 or 3 times longer than inhalation. Repeat pattern for 10 to 20 breaths.	Ensures that patient does all breathing through mouth. Ensures that patient uses the device properly.
d. Remove device from mouth and have patient take a slow, deep breath and hold for 3 seconds.	Promotes lung expansion before coughing.
e. Instruct patient to exhale in quick, short, forced "huffs."	"Huff" coughing, or forced expiratory technique, promotes bronchial hygiene by increasing expectoration of secretions.
16. Teach leg exercises:	
a. Instruct and encourage patient in leg exercises to be performed every 1 to 2 hours while awake: ankle rotation, dorsiflexion and plantar flexion, leg extension and flexion, and straight leg raises.	Leg exercises facilitate venous return from the lower extremities and reduce the risk of circulatory complications such as venous thrombus.
b. Position patient supine.	
c. Instruct patient to rotate each ankle in a complete circle and draw imaginary circles with the big toe 5 times (see illustration).	Promotes joint mobility.

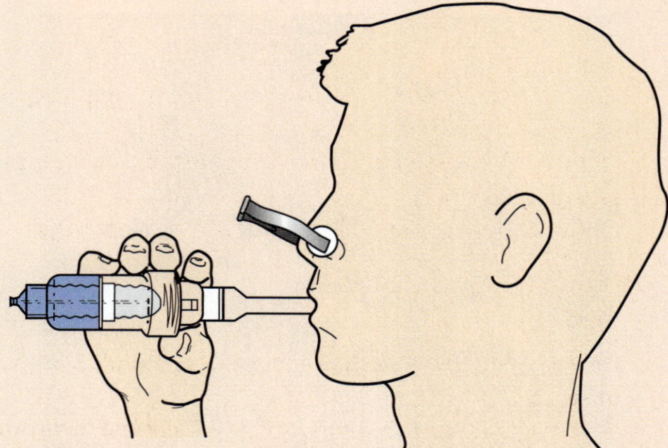

STEP 15b Diagram of use of positive expiratory pressure device.

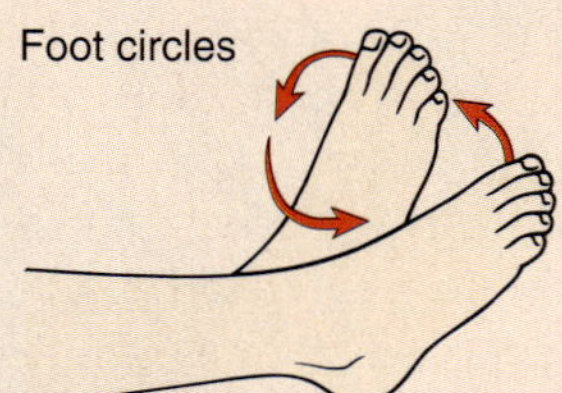

STEP 16c Foot circles. (From Lewis S et al: *Medical-surgical nursing: assessment and management of clinical problems,* ed 9, St Louis, 2014, Mosby.)

STEPS	RATIONALE

d. Alternate dorsiflexion and plantar flexion while instructing patient to feel calf muscles tighten and relax. Repeat 5 times (see illustration).

Helps maintain joint mobility and promote venous return to prevent thrombus formation.

e. Instruct patient to alternate flexing and extending knees one leg at a time. Repeat 5 times (see illustration).

Maintains knee joint mobility and contracts muscles of upper leg.

f. Instruct patient to alternate raising legs straight up from bed surface. Leg should be kept straight. Repeat 5 times (see illustration).

Causes quadriceps muscle contraction and relaxation that helps promote venous return (Lewis et al., 2014).

g. Instruct patient to perform these four leg exercises 10 to 12 times every 1 to 2 hours while awake.

Leg exercises stimulate circulation, which prevents venous stasis to help prevent formation of deep vein thrombosis (DVT) (Lewis et al., 2014).

17. Verify that patient's expectations of surgery are realistic. Correct expectations as needed.

Can prevent postoperative anxiety or anger.

18. Reinforce therapeutic coping strategies. If ineffective, encourage alternatives.

Therapeutic coping strategies promote postoperative compliance and recovery.

19. **See Completion Protocol (inside front cover).**

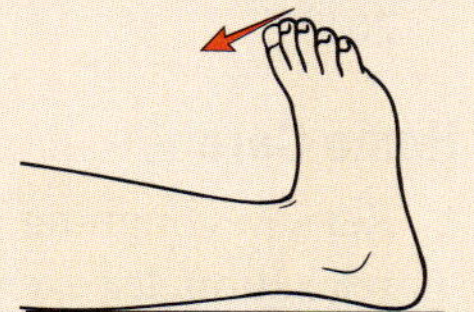
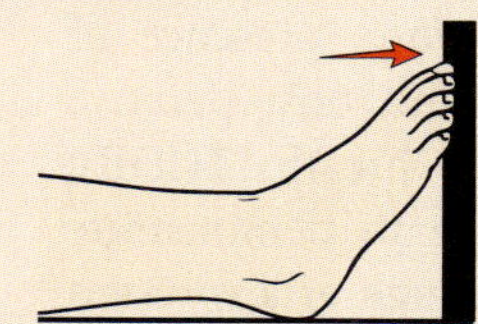

STEP 16d Alternate dorsiflexion and plantar flexion. (From Lewis S et al: *Medical-surgical nursing: assessment and management of clinical problems,* ed 9, St Louis, 2014, Mosby.)

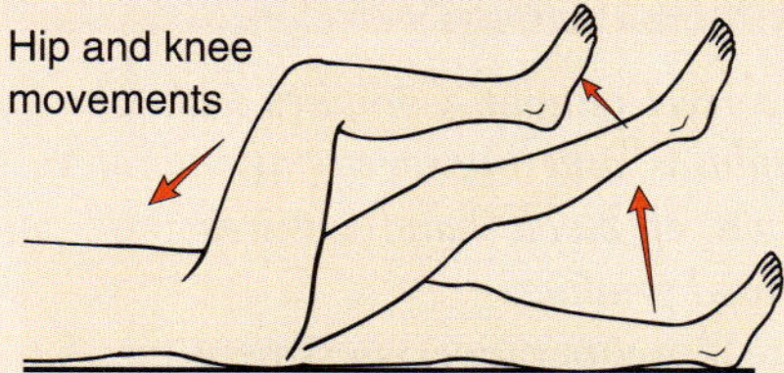

STEP 16e Hip and knee movements. (From Lewis S et al: *Medical-surgical nursing: assessment and management of clinical problems,* ed 9, St Louis, 2014, Mosby.)

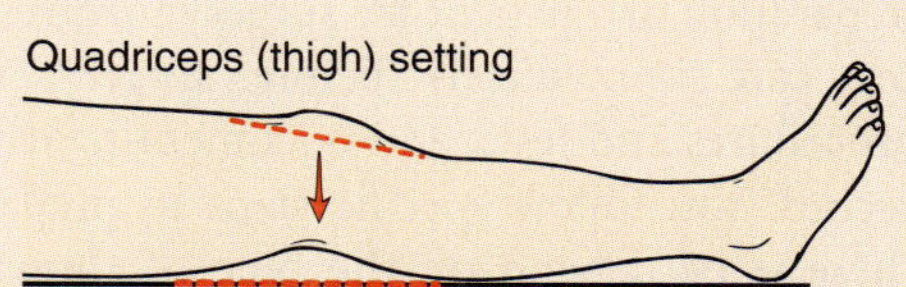

STEP 16f Quadriceps (thigh) setting. (From Lewis S et al: *Medical-surgical nursing: assessment and management of clinical problems,* ed 9, St Louis, 2014, Mosby.)

EVALUATION

1. Ask patient to repeat key information (e.g., rationale for withholding medications, food, and fluids). Use **Teach Back:** State to the patient, "I want to be sure I explained what you need to know about getting ready for surgery. Can you tell me which medications you should not take before surgery?" Evaluates what the patient is able to explain or demonstrate. Revise your instruction now or develop plan for revised patient teaching to be implemented at an appropriate time if patient is not able to teach back correctly.

2. Observe patient demonstrating splinting, turning and sitting, deep breathing, and leg exercises.

3. Ask family caregiver to identify location of the waiting room and validate if correct.

4. Ask family caregiver if he or she is able to help prepare patient at home before surgery.

5. Observe the level of emotional support family caregiver provides patient.

6. Observe patient and family caregiver coping strategies.

Unexpected Outcomes and Related Interventions

1. Patient identifies an incorrect procedure, site, date, or time of surgery.
   a. Provide the correct information verbally and in writing for patient and family caregiver.

2. Patient questions the importance of not drinking the morning of surgery.
   a. Explain that under anesthesia the fluid can come up from the stomach and go into the lungs.

3. Patient incorrectly performs breathing exercises.
   a. Explain and demonstrate correct breathing technique.
   b. Explain the importance of postoperative breathing.
   c. Instruct patient to repeat demonstration.
4. Family caregiver verbalizes anxiety about helping patient at home before surgery.
   a. Explain that these feelings are normal.
   b. Provide written instructions and a telephone number for contact if there are further questions.
5. Family caregiver indicates that he or she is unable to care for patient at home after surgery.
   a. Contact health care provider and discuss the alternative of a home health care referral.

Recording and Reporting

- Record preoperative teaching on the preoperative education flow sheet or designated facility form.
- Document your evaluation of patient learning.

Sample Documentation

0940   Instructed on continued need to be NPO; routine events to expect in OR and recovery room; presence of oxygen; IV fluid; postoperative drains; and postoperative activities, including turn, cough, and deep breath (TCDB); use of IS; and leg exercises. Patient able to demonstrate breathing and leg exercises correctly. Daughter expressed willingness to care for her mother at home after surgery.

Special Considerations

Pediatric

- Use an age-appropriate level of communication, and provide simple explanations using familiar terms.
- The use of pictures, models, equipment, and play rather than verbal explanations increases learning in preschool and school-age children.

Geriatric

- Age-related changes in the central nervous system may diminish short-term memory. Additional time and reinforcement may be necessary for older adults to learn and comprehend information (Spry and Goodman, 2013). The greater the number of different exposures to new material, the higher the probability that the material will be learned.
- Reinforce teaching with verbal explanations, audiovisual resources, pamphlets, and demonstrations. Consider sight and hearing deficits when providing both written and verbal instructions (Spry and Goodman, 2013).

Home Care

- Review coughing, deep breathing, abdominal splinting, relaxation, leg exercises, and ambulation before admission to hospital or surgical clinic and after discharge.

SKILL 28.3   PHYSICAL PREPARATION FOR SURGERY

Physical preparation of a patient for surgery involves providing nursing care immediately before surgery, verifying required procedures and tests, and documenting care in the patient's record. You follow specific steps to prepare every patient. These steps depend on the type of surgery being performed and the risks involved. For example, you use compression stockings, intermittent compression devices (ICDs), and the venous foot pump for adult patients undergoing surgery that will last several hours and require a long period of immobilization afterward. You provide a bowel preparation, administering an enema, laxative, or cathartic (this may be done at home by patients admitted the morning of surgery) for abdominal surgery on or near the intestine. You may need to clip hair near the incision site. Always check the surgeon's orders to determine what procedures are needed for the surgical patient. Regardless of the type of surgery, the goal of physical preparation is to place the patient in the best condition possible to minimize the risks of the planned surgery.

ASSESSMENT

1. Identify patient using two identifiers (e.g., name and birthday or name and account number) according to facility policy. Ask patient to state name. Apply identification bracelet if all information is correct. Apply blood band if applicable and used by the facility. *Rationale:*

Ensures correct patient. Complies with The Joint Commission standards and improves patient safety (TJC, 2014). Application of blood band ensures that patient receives correct blood product.

2. Complete a preoperative assessment (see Skill 28.1).

PLANNING

Expected Outcomes   focus on the proper physical preparation of the patient for surgery.

- Patient cooperates during preparatory measures (e.g., starting an IV line, undergoing an enema).
- Patient can state the surgical procedure being performed.
- Patient able to discuss remaining concerns about surgery.

Delegation and Collaboration

The skill of coordinating the patient's preparation for surgery cannot be delegated to nursing assistive personnel (NAP). However, the NAP may administer an enema or a douche; obtain vital signs in stable patients; apply antiembolism stockings; and assist patients in removing clothing, jewelry, and prostheses. The nurse instructs the NAP about:

- Using basic infection control practices and proper precautions when preparing a patient for surgery.
- Observing and using precautions if the patient has an IV catheter in place.

Equipment

Note: Equipment varies by procedure ordered.
- Vital sign equipment: Stethoscope, BP cuff, thermometer, pulse oximeter
- Oxygen equipment as ordered
- Suction equipment as ordered
- Hospital gown
- IV solution and equipment (see Chapter 27)
- Skin cleansing solution
- Compression (antiembolism) stockings
- ICD
- Venous foot pump
- Urinary catheterization kit (see Chapter 18)
- Preoperative checklist
- Medications (e.g., sedative)

IMPLEMENTATION *for* PHYSICAL PREPARATION FOR SURGERY

STEPS	RATIONALE
1. **See Standard Protocol (inside front cover).**	
2. Assist patient with putting on hospital gown and removing personal items. Patients are often anxious before surgery. Before any procedure, decrease anxiety by explaining how equipment or preparation will feel (e.g., cold, tight) before touching patient.	
3. Instruct patient to remove makeup, nail polish, hairpins, and jewelry.	During and after surgery, anesthesiologist and nurse must assess the skin and nails to determine tissue perfusion. (In some settings, patients are allowed to have a ring taped and remove polish from only one nail.)
4. Ensure that money and valuables have been locked up or given to a family caregiver.	Patient may not return to same location after surgery. Prevents valuables from being misplaced or lost.
5. Ensure that patient has followed appropriate fluid and food restrictions per surgeon or anesthesiologist order (see Skill 28.2).	Extent and type of restriction vary by facility and health care provider. Under general anesthesia, the sphincters in the stomach relax, and contents can reflux into the esophagus and trachea.
6. Verify presence of allergies and ensure that allergy/sensitivity band or other safety arm bands are present.	Alerts surgeons and health care team to potential allergies, risk of falls, etc.
7. Verify that patient has followed instructions about omission or ingestion of medications as instructed.	Missed or inaccurate dosage could precipitate complications.
8. Verify that a bowel preparation (e.g., laxative, cathartic, enema) has been completed, by patient or family caregiver at home, if ordered.	Proper bowel evacuation needed for surgery to be performed.

> **SAFE PATIENT CARE** In some situations, additional enemas and/or cathartics are ordered. Emptying the bowel is necessary for bowel surgery and to decrease the risk of postoperative ileus. Enemas are used when surgery is near the lower intestine.

STEPS	RATIONALE
9. Ensure that a medical history and physical examination results are in patient's record.	Establishes database for future comparison.
10. Verify that surgical consent, anesthesia consent, and consent for blood transfusion are complete. The name of procedure; name of surgeon; date; name of person authorized to obtain surgical consent; signature of surgeon (or authorized person) obtaining consent, anesthesia provider delivering anesthesia, and witness (often the nurse); and the patient's signature all should be present.	Ensures patient's agreement to undergo intended procedure. In most settings, the surgeon obtains the consent, and the nurse verifies that it is complete and consistent with patient's understanding (refer to facility policy).
11. Ensure that necessary laboratory work, ECG, and chest x-ray film studies are completed and results are on the chart.	Diagnostic test results may indicate a medical problem and provide data for postoperative comparison.

Continued

STEPS	RATIONALE
12. Verify that blood type and cross-match are completed if ordered by the surgeon and that blood transfusions are available as needed.	In many cases, surgery cannot begin without availability of blood units.
13. Ask if patient has an advance directive. If so, place it in patient's record.	Document conveys patient's wishes if life-support measures are necessary.
14. Assess and record patient's heart rate, blood pressure, respiratory rate, oxygen saturation, and temperature.	Provides baseline for patient's preoperative status.
15. Instruct patient to void.	Prevents risk of bladder distention or rupture during surgery.
16. Start an IV line; refer to unit standards or surgeon's orders (see Chapter 27).	IV provides access for fluids and medications administered in OR.
17. Administer preoperative medications as ordered (e.g., preoperative antibiotics, prophylactic agents).	Preoperative medications are used for various reasons and should be administered as ordered for maximum effectiveness.
18. Apply compression stockings (see Chapter 16, Procedural Guideline 16.2).	Compression stockings promote circulation during periods of immobilization, reducing the risk of an embolism.
19. Apply ICD if ordered (see illustrations and Procedural Guideline 16.2). Note: ICDs may or may not be used in combination with compression stockings. Verify order.	ICDs push blood from the superficial veins into the deep veins, decreasing venous stasis.

> **SAFE PATIENT CARE** ICDs do not provide effective DVT prophylaxis if the device is not applied correctly or if the patient does not wear the device continuously except during bathing, skin assessment, and ambulation. ICDs are *not* to be worn when a patient has an active DVT because of risk of pulmonary embolism.

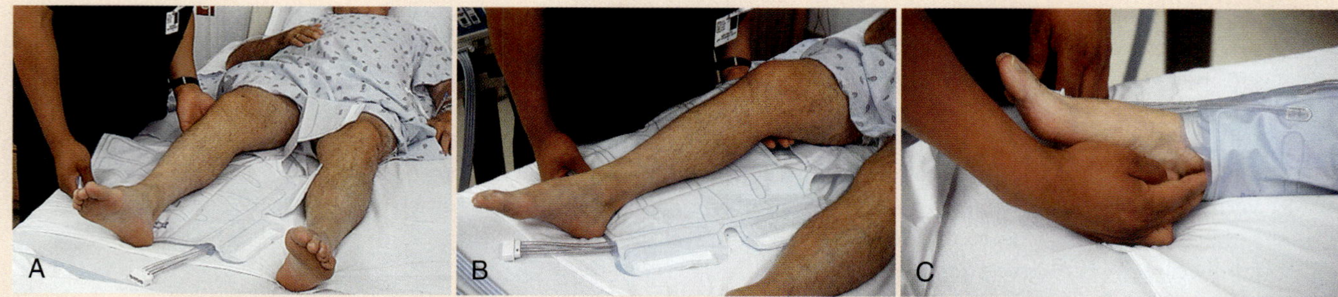

STEP 19 **A,** Correct leg position on inner lining. **B,** Position back of patient's knee with popliteal opening. **C,** Check fit of ICD sleeve.

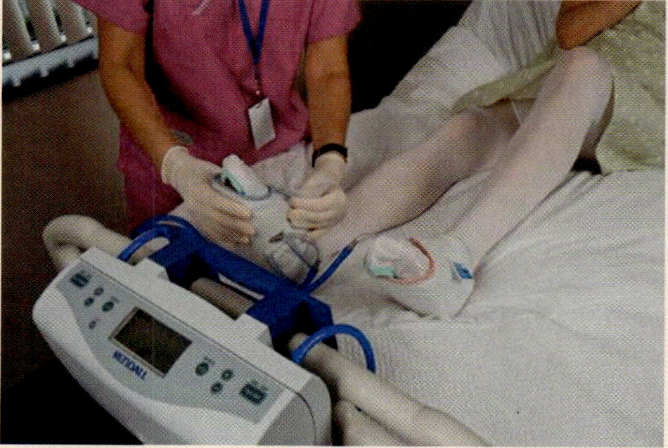

STEP 20 Venous plexus foot pump with bedside controls. (Courtesy Tyco Healthcare Group LP.)

STEPS	RATIONALE
20. Cleanse and prepare the surgical site if ordered.	Cleansing with an antimicrobial soap decreases bacterial flora on the skin.
21. Insert a urinary catheter if ordered (see Chapter 18). Note: There are times when the urinary catheter is placed in the OR.	Maintains bladder decompression and provides for monitoring output during surgery.
22. Allow the patient to wear eyeglasses or hearing aid as long as possible before surgery so that patient is able to sign consents and read materials. Remove contact lenses, eyeglasses, hairpieces, and dentures just before surgery (see checklist completed preoperatively noting that all items are removed before proceeding to OR).	These aids facilitate patient cooperation by ensuring that patient has clear vision and maximal auditory perception throughout the preoperative phase.
23. Place cap over patient's head and hair.	The cap contains the hair and minimizes OR contamination during surgery. Plastic or reflective caps reduce heat loss during surgery.
24. Assist patient onto stretcher for transport to OR.	Some ambulatory surgery patients walk to OR.
25. **See Completion Protocol (inside front cover).**	

EVALUATION

1. Observe patient's level of cooperation during preparation.
2. Ask patient to identify any concerns about surgery.

Unexpected Outcomes and Related Interventions

1. Patient reports having eaten breakfast or drinking fluids.
   a. Notify surgeon and anesthesia provider.
2. Patient refuses to go to surgery until contacting a family caregiver.
   a. Notify surgeon.
   b. Assist patient with contacting family caregiver.
3. Consent is incomplete or incorrect.
   a. Notify surgeon and anesthesia provider.
4. Patient did not follow instructions regarding medications at home.
   a. Notify surgeon and anesthesia provider.
5. Patient has a reaction to a preoperative medication.
   a. Discontinue medication.
   b. Treat the reaction per facility policy.
   c. Notify surgeon.

Recording and Reporting

- Document preoperative physical preparation on preoperative checklist.

Sample Documentation

0850   Verified patient has been NPO since midnight. Dentures, yellow wedding band, and wallet given to patient's wife. Fleets enema given with results of large amount soft brown stool. Compression stockings applied. Patient stated he did not take his bedtime dose of 30 units of Lantus insulin. Bedside blood sugar 110. Surgeon notified. 20 units of Lantus insulin administered subcutaneously per order. IV of $D_5\frac{1}{2}$ normal saline started in right hand per order. Voided and taken to OR by stretcher per transporter.

Special Considerations
Pediatric

- Give the child as many choices related to procedures as possible.
- Keep parent-child separation to the minimum time possible. When a parent cannot be present, it is important to leave a favorite possession with the child.

Geriatric

- Because of cognitive, sensory, or physical impairments, it may take an older patient increased time to dress for surgery and complete needed physical preparation.

SKILL 28.4 PROVIDING IMMEDIATE ANESTHESIA RECOVERY IN THE POSTANESTHESIA CARE UNIT

The first phase of postoperative care takes place during the immediate recovery period. This phase extends from the time the patient leaves the OR to the time he or she is stabilized in the PACU, meets discharge criteria, and is transferred to the nursing unit. Table 28-1 provides an overview of expected monitoring following anesthesia.

TABLE 28-1 POSTANESTHESIA MONITORING

CONDITION	INTERVENTIONS
Airway	
Mechanical obstruction: Decreased LOC and muscle relaxants, resulting in flaccid muscles and tongue blocking airway	Hyperextend neck; pull mandible forward; use nasal or oral airway; encourage deep breathing.
Retained thick secretions: Irritation from anesthesia; anticholinergic medications; history of smoking	Suction; encourage coughing.
Laryngospasm: Stridor from excessive secretions or airway irritation	Encourage to relax and breathe through the mouth. If extreme, it may require positive-pressure ventilation with oxygen, small dose of muscle relaxant (ordered by anesthesiologist), and intubation.
Laryngeal edema: Allergic reaction, irritation from ET tube, fluid overload	Administer humidified oxygen, antihistamines, steroids, sedatives; in some cases, perform reintubation.
Bronchospasm: Preexisting asthma, anesthetic irritation (expiratory wheeze)	Administer bronchodilators as ordered.
Aspiration: Vomiting from hypotension, accumulated gastric secretions and delayed gastric emptying, pain, fear, position changes	Position on side; suction airway; administer antiemetic as ordered.
Breathing: Hypoventilation/Hypoxemia	
CNS depression: Anesthesia, analgesics, muscle relaxants (respiratory rate shallow)	Encourage to cough and deep breathe; use mechanical ventilator; administer narcotic antagonist and muscle relaxant reversal agent.
Mechanical restriction: Obesity, pain, tight cast or dressings, abdominal distention	Reposition; give analgesic; loosen cast or dressings; implement measures to reduce gastric distention (e.g., NG intubation, NG suction).
Circulation	
Hypovolemia: Blood loss, dehydration	Administer IV fluids or blood replacement.
Hypotension: Anesthesia/drug effects, vasodilation (possibly from spinal anesthesia); narcotics	Elevate legs; give oxygen, IV fluids, or blood replacement; administer vasopressors; monitor I&O, stimulation, hemoglobin, and hematocrit.
Cardiac failure: Preexisting cardiac disease; circulatory overload; excessive/too-rapid fluid replacement	Provide digitalization and diuretics; monitor ECG.
Cardiac arrhythmias: Hypoxemia; MI; hypothermia; imbalance of potassium, calcium, magnesium	Provide IV fluid replacement; monitor ECG and urine output; identify and treat cause.
Hypertension: Pain; distended bladder; preexisting hypertension; vasopressor drugs	Compare with preoperative baseline; identify and determine cause.
Compartment syndrome: Pressure from edema causing enough compression to obstruct arterial and venous circulation resulting in ischemia, permanent numbness, loss of function; forearm and lower leg most common sites	Obtain compartment pressures to diagnose, and elevate extremity no higher than heart level; remove or loosen bandage or cast to relieve compression; if left untreated, amputation may be required. Do not apply ice.

CNS, Central nervous system; *ECG,* electrocardiogram; *ET,* endotracheal; *I&O,* intake and output; *IV,* intravenous; *LOC,* level of consciousness; *MI,* myocardial infarction; *NG,* nasogastric.

The first 1 to 2 hours are the most critical for assessing the aftereffects of anesthesia, including airway clearance, cardiovascular complications, temperature control, and neurological function. A patient's condition can change rapidly; assessments must be timely, knowledgeable, and accurate. You need to be aware of the common complications and problems associated with specific types of anesthesia (Table 28-2). Quick judgment regarding the most appropriate interventions is essential. A patient is usually ready for discharge to the general unit when specific standardized criteria are met. The Aldrete score is one of several scoring systems for assessment (Table 28-3). It uses parameters of activity, respiration, circulation, consciousness, and oxygen saturation. A score of 8 or less indicates additional monitoring is required. A score of 10 indicates full recovery of the patient.

Recovery from ambulatory surgery requires the same assessments. However, the depth of general anesthesia may be less because the surgery is less involved and of shorter duration. Some patients have only IV conscious sedation, and intensive monitoring is required for a shorter time period. As soon as the patient is stable and alert, give instructions for

TABLE 28-2	FOCUSED ASSESSMENT OF PATIENT PROBLEMS RELATED TO ANESTHESIA TYPE
ANESTHESIA TYPE	**FOCUSED ASSESSMENT**
General	Hypotension; changes in heart rate or rhythm; lowered body temperature; respiratory depression; emergence delirium in the form of shivering, trembling, confusion, or hallucinations
Spinal	Headache, hypotension, decreased cardiac output, cyanosis, difficulty breathing
Local	Skin rash; allergic reaction with edema of the face, lips, mouth, or throat; restlessness; bradycardia; hypotension; ischemic necrosis at injection site
Conscious sedation	Respiratory depression, bradycardia, hypotension, nausea and vomiting
Epidural	Cyanosis, breathing difficulties, decreased heart rate, irregular heart rate, pale skin color, nausea and vomiting

Data from Lilley LL, Rainforth Collins S, Snyder J: *Pharmacology and the nursing process*, ed 7, St Louis, 2014, Mosby; and Rothrock JC: *Alexander's care of the patient in surgery*, ed 15, St Louis, 2014, Mosby.

TABLE 28-3	ALDRETE SCORE FOR POSTANESTHESIA MONITORING	
		SCORE
Activity (moving voluntarily on command)	4 extremities	2
	2 extremities	1
	0 extremities	0
Respiration	Able to deep breathe and cough freely	2
	Dyspnea, shallow or limited breathing	1
	Apneic	0
Circulation	BP + 20 mm Hg of presedation level	2
	BP + 20-50 mm Hg of presedation level	1
	BP + 50 mm Hg of presedation level	0
Consciousness	Fully awake	2
	Arousable on having name called	1
	Not responding	0
Color	Normal	2
	Pale, dusky, blotchy, jaundiced, or other change	1
	Cyanotic	0

BP, Blood pressure.
From American Society of PeriAnesthesia Nurses (ASPAN): *2012-2014 perianesthesia nursing standards, practice recommendations and interpretive statements*, Cherry Hill, NJ, 2014, ASPAN; Phillips NM, et al: Post-anaesthetic discharge scoring criteria: key findings from a systematic review. *Int Evid Based Healthc* 11(4):275–284, 2013.

home care to the patient and caregiver, including demonstrations and written instructions.

ASSESSMENT

1. On patient's arrival in PACU, identify patient using two identifiers (e.g., name and birthday or name and account number) according to facility policy. *Rationale: A patient hand-off identification protocol ensures patient safety and continuity of care. Ensures correct patient. Complies with The Joint Commission standards and improves patient safety (TJC, 2014).*
2. Obtain hand-off report from circulating nurse and anesthesia provider and a review of patient's surgery course, physiological status, and baseline data. Rationale: Information helps you assess for potential problems, identify changes in condition, and plan appropriate nursing interventions for patient in PACU.
3. Review patient's preexisting conditions during operative procedure, including baseline and intraoperative vital signs; oxygen saturation; blood volume or fluid loss; fluid replacement; type of anesthesia; type of airway and size; and extent of surgical wound, including presence of surgical drains. Rationale: Determines patient's general status and allows you to anticipate the need for special equipment, nursing care, and activities in PACU.

4. Consider the effects of patient's type of surgery, anesthesia, and restrictions to movement. Rationale: Information influences type of assessments you initiate, type of complications for which you observe, and specific nursing interventions.

PLANNING

Expected Outcomes focus on early detection of complications from surgery or anesthesia and adequate pain control by the time of transfer (usually 1 to 2 hours).
- Patient's airway remains clear; respirations are deep, regular, and within normal limits by the time of transfer. Oxygen saturation remains greater than 95%.
- Patient's blood pressure, pulse, and temperature remain within previous baseline or normal expected range by the time of transfer.
- Dressings are clean, dry, and intact by discharge from recovery.
- Intake and output (I&O) is within expected parameters by discharge from recovery.

- Patient reports relief of discomfort after analgesia or other pain-relief measures by the time of transfer from immediate recovery area (usually 1 to 2 hours).
- Patient's postoperative assessments are within expected normal postoperative parameters.

Delegation and Collaboration

The skill of initiating immediate anesthesia recovery of a patient cannot be delegated to nursing assistive personnel (NAP). The NAP may provide basic comfort and hygiene measures. The nurse instructs the NAP by:

- Explaining any restrictions for how to provide comfort measures (e.g., repositioning, turning, applying warming blanket).
- Offering instruction in providing needed supplies.
- **NOTE:** NAP may be allowed to do more in ambulatory surgery recovery, such as provide initial PO liquids.

Equipment

- Stethoscope, sphygmomanometer, pulse oximeter, cardiac monitor, thermometer
- Oxygen equipment such as mask, oxygen regulator and tubing, and positive-pressure delivery system
- Suction equipment
- Dressing supplies
- Warmed blanket or active rewarming device
- Emergency equipment
- Emergency medications

IMPLEMENTATION *for* PROVIDING IMMEDIATE ANESTHESIA RECOVERY IN THE POSTANESTHESIA CARE UNIT

STEPS	RATIONALE
1. **See Standard Protocol (inside front cover).**	
2. As patient enters PACU on stretcher, immediately attach oxygen tubing to regulator and check IV flow rates.	Inhaled oxygen promotes tissue oxygenation during recovery from anesthesia. IV fluids maintain circulatory volume and provide route for emergency drugs.
3. Connect or secure drainage tubes to intermittent suction, depending on drain and order.	Drainage tubes must remain patent to prevent pressure within wound cavity.
4. Attach monitoring devices (e.g., blood pressure cuff, pulse oximeter, ECG, arterial lines).	Provides continual assessment and monitoring of physiological parameters.
5. Compare vital signs, ECG, and pulse oximetry with patient's preoperative baseline. Continue assessing vital signs and other parameters at least every 5 to 15 minutes until stable.	May show respiratory depression, cardiac irregularity, hypotension, or hypothermia.
6. Maintain airway after general anesthesia:	
a. If patient is supine, elevate head of bed slightly, pull jaw forward, or turn head to side unless contraindicated. Initially patient may need to be reminded to breathe.	Maintains open airway by keeping tongue out of the way while patient has decreased LOC.

> **SAFE PATIENT CARE** Always stay with a sedated patient until respirations are well established. Patients with an artificial airway may gag and vomit, become restless, or stop breathing.

STEPS	RATIONALE
b. Suction artificial airway and oral cavity with Yankauer suction tip if secretions accumulate (see Chapter 14). Encourage patient to spit out oral airway as gag reflex returns.	Indicates that patient is able to maintain patent airway independently.
7. Call patient by name in normal tone of voice. If there is no response, attempt to arouse patient by touching or gently moving a body part. Explain that surgery is over and patient is in the recovery area.	Determines patient's LOC and ability to follow commands. Assists patient in being oriented to place.
8. Encourage patient to cough and deep breathe every 15 minutes (see Skill 28.2).	Promotes lung expansion, elimination of inhalation anesthetic, and expectoration of mucus secretions.
9. Inspect color of nail beds and skin. Palpate for skin temperature.	Indicators of peripheral tissue perfusion.

STEPS	RATIONALE
10. Assess closely for any potential cardiovascular and pulmonary complications of general anesthesia (see Table 28-1) Monitor laboratory findings.	Postoperative patients who are sedated often become hypoxic.
11. If patient had general anesthesia: As patient arouses, introduce yourself and orient him or her to surroundings.	
12. Monitor sensory, circulatory, and neurological responses after spinal or epidural anesthesia:	
a. Monitor for hypotension, bradycardia, and nausea and vomiting.	Blockage of sympathetic nervous system results in vasodilation of major vessels and systemic hypotension.
b. Maintain adequate IV infusion.	Maintains blood pressure by increasing fluid volume and fills temporarily expanded vascular space.
c. Keep patient supine or with head slightly elevated and maintain position.	Minimizes risk of post–spinal anesthesia headache from leakage of spinal fluid at injection site, with increased pressures caused by elevation of upper body. Headache is more common with spinal than epidural anesthesia. Headache occurs less frequently with use of smaller gauge spinal needles (Lewis et al., 2014).
d. Observe patients in PACU until they regain movement in extremities.	Patients fear permanent loss of function.
e. Assess respiratory status, level of spinal sensation, and mobility in lower extremities. Drowsiness will be apparent after IV sedation. The level of anesthesia depends on the location of sensation change. Have patient close eyes and use an alcohol wipe to test sensation along sensory dermatomes. Have patient identify if warm or cold. *If patient had spinal anesthesia:* Remind him or her that loss of extremity sensation and movement is normal and will return in several hours.	Spinal block is set within 20 minutes of onset. However, if level of anesthesia moves above sixth thoracic vertebra (T6), respiratory muscles are affected. Patients often feel short of breath and may require mechanical ventilation if respiratory muscles are severely affected.
13. Monitor source of intake and output:	
a. Observe dressing and drains for any evidence of bright red blood.	Dressing maintains hemostasis and absorbs drainage. First dressing changes usually occur 24 hours after surgery and are done by the surgeon unless otherwise ordered.
b. Inform surgeon of unexpected bloody drainage and reinforce dressing as indicated. Apply direct pressure. Also look underneath patient for any pooling of bloody drainage. Monitor for decreased blood pressure and increased pulse.	Hemorrhage from a surgical wound is most likely within first few hours, indicating inadequate hemostasis during surgery. As dressing becomes saturated, blood often oozes down patient's side and collects underneath patient.
c. Inspect condition and contents of any drainage tubes and collecting devices. Note character and volume of drainage.	Determines patency of drainage tube and extent of wound drainage.
d. Observe amount, color, and appearance of urine from indwelling Foley catheter (if present).	Urine output of less than 30 mL/hr is a sign of decreased renal perfusion or altered renal function.
e. If nasogastric (NG) tube is present, assess drainage. If not draining, check placement and irrigate if necessary with normal saline (see Chapter 19).	Maintains patency of tube to ensure gastric decompression. Expected drainage is dark or pale, yellow, or green and 100 to 200 mL/hr. Bloody drainage occurs after some surgeries.
f. Monitor IV fluid rates. Observe IV site for signs of infiltration (see Chapter 27).	Provides adequate hydration and circulatory function.
14. Promote comfort:	
a. Provide mouth care by placing moistened washcloth to lips, swabbing oral mucosa with dampened swab, or applying petrolatum to lips.	Mouth is dry from NPO status and preoperative anticholinergics such as atropine.

Continued

STEPS	RATIONALE
b. Provide a warm blanket or active rewarming therapy to promote warmth and minimize shivering.	General anesthesia impairs thermoregulation, the OR environment is cold, and exposure of the body cavity results in internal heat loss. Shivering increases oxygen consumption, predisposes patient to arrhythmias and hypertension, impairs platelet function, alters drug metabolism, impairs wound healing, and increases hospitalization costs because of cumulative adverse outcomes (ASPAN, 2014).
c. Assist with position changes and provide supportive pillows.	Improves ventilation and circulation.
15. Continue monitoring pain as patient awakens and until transfer to surgical unit or discharge, including quality, severity, and location (see Chapter 13). Do not assume that all postoperative pain is incisional pain.	Pain is often not directly related to the surgical procedure (e.g., chest pain [myocardial infarction or pulmonary embolism] or muscle pain [trauma from positioning]). Referred pain (in shoulder) often occurs after a laparoscopy. Systematic assessment of pain helps patients achieve functional status.
16. Provide pain medication as ordered and when vital signs have stabilized.	Promotes patient comfort.
17. Explain patient's condition to patient and inform of plans for transfer to nursing unit or discharge.	Decreases anxiety that can interfere with recovery process.
18. When patient's condition stabilizes (see Table 28-3), contact anesthesiologist to approve transfer to nursing unit or release to home.	A surgeon is responsible for authorizing transfer or discharge.

19. Before discharge to home from the ambulatory surgery unit, provide verbal and written instructions about:
  a. Signs and symptoms of possible complications.
  b. Not driving for 24 hours.
  c. Avoiding important legal decisions for 24 hours.
  d. Surgical site care.
  e. Activity restrictions.
  f. Pain control.
  g. Dietary modifications or restrictions.
  h. Medications as prescribed.
  i. Plan for follow-up visit.
  j. Reasons to call surgeon and number to call.
	Patients and home care providers must be aware of potential complications and follow-up care.

20. See Completion Protocol (inside front cover).	

EVALUATION

1. Observe respirations: rate, depth, and rhythm. Auscultate breath sounds. Monitor pulse oximetry.
2. Compare all blood pressure, pulse, and temperature readings with patient's baseline and expected normal values.
3. Inspect surgical wound and dressings for drainage. Be sure to assess for wound drainage under the patient.
4. Measure I&O. Urine output should be at least 30 to 50 mL/hr.
5. Auscultate bowel sounds and ask if patient has passed flatus.
6. Ask patient to rate pain on a scale of 0 to 10, and determine location and characteristics.
7. Complete system-specific physical assessments as appropriate according to patient's unique type of surgery (e.g., craniotomy—neurological assessment; neck surgery—airway status; vascular surgery—circulation and bleeding; orthopedic surgery—neurovascular status and immobility or positioning).

Unexpected Outcomes and Related Interventions

1. Patient exhibits respiratory depression (pulse oximetry <95%, respiratory rate <10 breaths per minute or shallow).
   a. Promptly report to surgeon.
   b. Administer oxygen as ordered by nasal cannula. Give patients with chronic obstructive pulmonary disease (COPD) 2 L/min or less of oxygen.
   c. Encourage deep breathing every 5 to 15 minutes.
   d. Position to promote chest expansion (on side or semi-Fowler's).

e. Administer prescribed medications (e.g., epinephrine, muscle relaxant, narcotic reversal agent).

2. Patient exhibits respiratory obstruction (e.g., abnormal lung sounds, snoring, stridor or crowing sounds, wheezing).
   a. Reposition head and jaw to open airway.
   b. Administer oxygen at 6 to 10 L/min by mask as ordered.
   c. Encourage to cough and deep breathe.
   d. Suction if needed.
   e. Notify anesthesiologist if unresponsive to interventions; may need to be reintubated if severe.

3. Patient exhibits signs of hypovolemia related to internal or incisional hemorrhage.
   a. Elevate patient's legs enough to maintain a downward slope toward the trunk of the body. Do not lower the head past the flat position because this position increases respiratory effort and potentially decreases cerebral perfusion.
   b. Promptly report patient's present status to surgeon.
   c. Administer oxygen at 6 to 10 L/min by mask per order.
   d. Increase rate of IV fluid or administer blood products as ordered.
   e. Monitor blood pressure and pulse every 5 to 15 minutes.
   f. Apply pressure dressings as follows per order:
      (1) *Abdominal dressing:* Cover bleeding area with several thicknesses of gauze compresses, and place tape 7 to 10 cm (3 to 4 inches) beyond width of dressing with firm, even pressure on both sides close to bleeding source. Maintain pressure as you tape entire dressing to maximize pressure at source of bleeding.
      (2) *Dressing on extremity:* Apply rolled gauze, pressing gauze compress over bleeding site. Do not continue tape around entire extremity.
      (3) *Dressing in neck region:* Cover with several thicknesses of gauze and place tape 7 to 10 cm (3 to 4 inches) beyond width of dressing. Apply with pressure, but do not occlude carotid artery or airway. Assess every 5 to 15 minutes for carotid pulse and evidence of airway obstruction.
   g. Patient remains NPO because it is often necessary to return to surgery for control of bleeding.

4. Patient complains of severe incisional pain.
   a. Administer analgesics, then reassess and provide analgesia before the pain is severe.
   b. Pain sometimes lowers blood pressure; analgesia may restore vital signs to normal. Monitor vital signs carefully.
   c. For patients with PCA, be sure that patient is using device correctly. Warn family caregiver not to manipulate the PCA.
   d. Orthopedic surgery: The earliest symptom of compartment syndrome in an extremity is pain unrelieved by analgesics. Other symptoms include numbness,

tingling, pallor, coolness, and absent peripheral pulses. The surgeon *must* be notified. Do not elevate extremity above the level of the heart because this increases venous pressure. Application of ice is contraindicated because vasoconstriction will occur (Lewis et al., 2014).

5. Patient has hypothermia (temperature <36°C [96.8°F]). Shivering increases oxygen consumption, predisposes patient to arrhythmias and hypertension, impairs platelet function and wound healing, and alters drug metabolism. This problem is seen more in infants and children because of immature thermoregulation centers.
   a. Use warm blankets, socks, head coverings, or active rewarming device.
   b. Monitor temperature and patient's thermal comfort level every 30 minutes until normal temperature is reached.

Recording and Reporting

- Document in progress notes patient's arrival time at PACU; include vital signs and other physical parameters, LOC, and pain severity. Also include condition of dressings and tubes, character of drainage, and all nursing measures initiated.
- Record vital signs and I&O on appropriate flow sheets.
- Report any abnormal assessment findings and signs of complications to surgeon.

Sample Documentation

1000   Received from OR via stretcher. Alert and oriented ×3. Oxygen administered at 3 L/min per nasal cannula. Abdominal dressing saturated with bright red blood, and pad under patient saturated, 12-cm × 20-cm area. Dressing reinforced with pressure dressing. IV in left forearm infusing with lactated Ringer's at 150 mL/hr. Surgeon notified of excessive drainage and immediate interventions. Vital signs: BP 110/60, HR 98, R 22, SpO_2 96%. Remains NPO. Warm blanket applied.

Special Considerations
Pediatric

- Maintenance of body temperature in infants and children after surgery is a priority because of their immature temperature-control mechanisms.
- Infants and children normally have higher metabolic rates and differences in physiological makeup than adults, resulting in greater oxygen, fluid, and calorie needs.

Geriatric

- The ability of older adults to tolerate surgery depends on the extent of physiological changes that have occurred with aging, the presence of any chronic diseases, and the duration of the surgical procedure.
- When communicating with older adults, be aware of any auditory, visual, or cognitive impairment that may be present.

Home Care

- Teach ambulatory surgery patient and primary caregiver about any postoperative exercises, home modifications, or activity limitations.

- If patient is discharged with dressing changes, suggest that bedroom or bathroom is usually ideal for procedure.
- Assess need for a home health care referral.

SKILL 28.5 PROVIDING EARLY POSTOPERATIVE AND CONVALESCENT PHASE RECOVERY

Careful monitoring and comfort measures are essential during the early postoperative recovery period, which extends from the time a patient is discharged from the PACU to the time he or she is discharged from the hospital. Patients who have outpatient surgery undergo convalescence at home. Individualize your nursing care depending on the type of surgery, preexisting medical conditions, the risk or development of complications, and the rate of recovery. Teaching promotes the patient's independence, educates the patient about any limitations, and provides resources needed for the patient to achieve an optimal state of wellness.

The convalescent phase lasts for several days or weeks after discharge. During this phase, it is important to promote the patient's independence and active participation in care. The patient must have adequate nutrition and hydration to enhance healing. Make sure that patient's goals are realistic. It is also important that the patient and family caregiver (if available) have the required supplies and support services at home to promote healing. Some patients require a home health nurse.

ASSESSMENT

1. Obtain phone report from nurse in PACU. *Rationale: A preliminary report allows you to prepare hospital room with necessary supplies and equipment for patient's special needs.*
2. Assist with transfer to unit and obtain hand-off report. Review chart to identify type of surgery, preoperative medical risks, and baseline vital signs. *Rationale: Provides baseline to detect any change in patient's condition.*
3. Review surgeon's postoperative orders. *Rationale: Provides continuity of postoperative orders and maintains ongoing progress through the patient's convalescent phase.*

PLANNING

Expected Outcomes focus on preventing complications, maintaining adequate pain control for recovery activities, and promoting patient's self-care postoperatively.
- Patient's breath sounds remain clear bilaterally.
- Patient's vital signs remain within normal limits consistent with preoperative baseline.
- Patient describes pain as less than 4 on a scale of 0 to 10 while engaged in moderate activity by discharge.

- Fluid balance is evident by I&O records.
- Normal bowel sounds are present after bowel surgery or general anesthesia within 48 to 72 hours after surgery.
- Incision wound edges are well approximated; no drainage is noted.
- Patient or family caregiver describes plans for coping with stress of surgery.
- Patient or family caregiver describes evidence of complications that should be reported to surgeon by discharge.
- Patient or family caregiver describes or demonstrates incision care, dietary modifications, activity restriction, and plans for follow-up visit.

Delegation and Collaboration

The skill of providing early postoperative and convalescent phase recovery cannot be delegated to nursing assistive personnel (NAP). NAP may obtain vital signs (if patient is stable), apply nasal cannula or oxygen mask, and provide hygiene or repositioning for comfort. The nurse instructs the NAP by:
- Explaining how often to take vital signs.
- Reviewing specific safety concerns and what to observe and report back to the nurse.
- Explaining any precautions that affect how to provide basic hygiene and comfort measures.

Equipment

- Postoperative bed (recliner for day surgery recovery)
- Stethoscope, sphygmomanometer, thermometer
- IV fluid poles and infusion pumps as needed
- Emesis basin
- Washcloth and towel
- Waterproof pads
- Equipment for oral hygiene
- Pillows
- Facial tissue
- Oxygen equipment and mask
- Suction equipment (to suction airway)
- Dressing supplies
- Intermittent suction (to connect to NG or wound drainage tubes)
- Orthopedic appliances (if needed)
- Clean gloves
- Personal protective equipment as indicated

STEPS	RATIONALE
1. See Standard Protocol (inside front cover).	

Early Recovery Initial Postoperative Care

STEPS	RATIONALE
2. If patient is being transported by stretcher, prepare for transfer with bed in high position (level with the stretcher), with sheet folded to side and room for a stretcher to be placed beside bed easily (see Chapter 15).	Arrangement of equipment facilitates safety and smooth transfer process.
3. Assist transport staff to move patient from stretcher to bed (see Chapter 15). Identify patient using two identifiers (e.g., name and birthday or name and account number) according to facility policy.	Ensures correct patient. Complies with The Joint Commission standards and improves patient safety (TJC, 2014).
4. Attach any existing oxygen tubing, position IV fluids, verify IV flow rate settings on infusion pump, and check drainage tubes (e.g., Foley catheter or wound drainage).	Maintains patency of IV and integrity of drainage tubing.
5. Maintain airway. If patient remains sleepy or lethargic, keep head extended and support in side-lying position (see Chapter 14, Skill 14.2).	Minimizes chances of aspiration and obstruction of airway with tongue.
6. Conduct an initial assessment of LOC and vital signs, and compare findings with vital signs in recovery area and patient's baseline values. Continue monitoring as ordered.	Patient's status may change during transfer. Movement of patient and pain level influence stability of vital signs.
7. Encourage coughing, deep breathing, and incentive spirometry (see Skill 28.2) to prevent atelectasis.	Anesthesia, medications, and intubation irritate airways, resulting in secretions and atelectasis. Coughing expands chest, aerates lungs, and mobilizes secretions.
8. If NG tube is present, check placement and irrigate (see Chapter 19, Skill 19.3). Connect to proper drainage device. Connect all other drainage tubes to appropriate suction or collection device. Secure to prevent tension on tubing.	Transfer and movement may dislodge tubes, which would interfere with drainage.
9. Assess patient's surgical dressing for appearance, presence, and character of drainage. Unless contraindicated by surgeon, outline drainage along the edges with a pen and reassess in 1 hour for change. If no dressing is present, inspect condition of wound (see Chapter 24).	Hemorrhage is most likely to occur on the day of surgery. Dressing should be clean, dry, and intact.
10. Palpate abdomen for bladder distention or use bladder ultrasound when available. If Foley catheter is present, check placement. Ensure that it is draining freely and properly secured. Patient may have continuous bladder irrigations or suprapubic catheter (see Chapter 18).	Anesthesia often contributes to urinary retention. Urinary stasis increases the risk for urinary tract infection.
11. If no urinary drainage system is present, explain that voiding within 8 hours after surgery is expected. Male patients may void successfully if allowed to stand.	After spinal or epidural anesthesia, risk for urinary retention is increased. Other risks for urinary retention include male sex, age older than 50 years, previous history of pelvic surgery or voiding problems, and concurrent neurological diseases (Baldini et al., 2009). Patients may not feel the urge to void. If patient is unable to void and bladder is distended, catheterization is required.
12. Measure all sources of fluid I&O (including estimated blood loss during surgery).	Altered fluid and electrolyte balance is a potential complication of major surgery.
13. Describe the purpose of equipment and frequent observations to patient and significant others.	Unfamiliar sights (e.g., equipment, patient's appearance) are often anxiety-provoking.

Continued

STEPS	RATIONALE
14. Position patient for comfort, maintaining correct body alignment. Avoid tension on surgical wound site.	Reduces stress on suture line. Helps patient relax and promotes comfort.
15. Place call light within reach and raise side rails (one of two or three of four). Instruct patient to call for assistance to get out of bed.	Promotes patient's safety as effects of anesthesia continue to diminish. Raising all side rails may be considered a physical restraint.
16. Assess patient's level of pain on an age-appropriate pain scale. Assess the last time analgesic was given. PCA may be used for pain control (see Chapter 13). Medicate patient as ordered either around-the-clock or prn as ordered during the first 24 to 48 hours. Explain to patient how you plan to control pain; review orders of what is prescribed and frequency.	Determines level of discomfort. Adequate pain control is needed to permit patient to participate with breathing exercises, coughing, and ambulation.

Continued Postoperative Care

STEPS	RATIONALE
17. Assess vital signs at least every 4 hours or as ordered.	Temperature greater than 38°C (100.4°F) in the first 48 hours may indicate atelectasis, the normal inflammatory response, or dehydration. Temperature greater than 37.7°C (99.86°F) on the third day or after often indicates wound infection, pneumonia, or phlebitis (Lewis et al., 2014). Altered blood pressure or pulse is associated with cardiovascular complications (see Table 28-1).
18. Provide oral care at least every 2 hours as needed. If permitted, offer ice chips.	Medication such as an anticholinergic given before surgery makes mouth dry. Oral care and ice chips promote comfort.
19. Encourage patient to turn, cough, deep breathe, and use incentive spirometer at least every 2 hours (see Skill 28.2).	Promotes adequate ventilation and minimizes hypoventilation and atelectasis. Especially necessary for patients with a history of smoking, pneumonia, or COPD or patients who are confined to bed rest.
20. Promote ambulation and activity as ordered. Assess vital signs before and after activity to assess tolerance. Patients often are encouraged to be up in a chair the evening of surgery or the next morning and progress to walking in room or hallway.	Ambulation is the most significant nursing intervention to prevent postoperative complications. Mobility promotes circulation, lung expansion, and peristalsis. Postural hypotension is caused by sudden position changes.
21. Progress from clear liquids to regular diet as tolerated if nausea and vomiting do not occur.	Nausea and vomiting are associated with anesthesia and surgery. IV fluids are usually discontinued when oral intake is tolerated. Some patients must be NPO for several days until bowel sounds are heard.
22. Include patient and family caregiver in decision making; answer questions as they arise.	Promotes patient's sense of control and independence and improves self-esteem.
23. Provide opportunity for patients who must adjust to a change in body appearance or function to verbalize feelings.	Radical surgery, amputation, or inoperable cancer often results in anxiety and depression. The grief response to loss of a body organ is common and should be expected.

Convalescent Phase

STEPS	RATIONALE
24. Assess patient's home environment for safety, cleanliness, and availability of assistance for patient.	Provides information about patient's need for home care. Verifies patient's and caregiver's level of knowledge and any additional teaching needs for discharge. Assists in promoting uncomplicated discharge and patient's independence and participation in care.
25. Keep patient and family caregiver informed of progress made toward recovery. Explain the time expected to reach a level of maximal recovery. Provide answers to individual patient questions or concerns.	Decreases anxiety and helps patient know what to anticipate during the convalescent period.
26. **See Completion Protocol (inside front cover).**	

EVALUATION

1. Auscultate breath sounds bilaterally.
2. Obtain vital signs.
3. Ask patient to describe pain on a scale of 0 to 10 after moderate activity.
4. Evaluate I&O records. Assess time of patient's first postoperative urination.
5. Auscultate bowel sounds.
6. Inspect incision (wound edges well approximated, no drainage noted).
7. Use *Teach Back:* State to the patient, "I want to be sure I explained what you need to know about your postoperative activity level. Can you tell me how you will increase your activity level during the first week at home?" Evaluates what the patient is able to explain or demonstrate. Revise your instruction now or develop plan for revised patient teaching to be implemented at an appropriate time if patient is not able to teach back correctly.
8. Ask patient or family caregiver to indicate symptoms of complications that should be reported to the surgeon by discharge.
9. Have patient or family caregiver describe incision care with teach back, dietary modifications or restrictions, activity restrictions, and plans for follow-up visit.

Unexpected Outcomes and Related Interventions

1. Vital signs are above or below patient's baseline or expected range. Initially this could be related to anesthesia effects, pain, hypovolemic shock, airway obstruction, fluid and electrolyte imbalance, or hypothermia.
   a. Identify contributing factors.
   b. Notify surgeon.
2. Bowel sounds are absent or decreased. Patient experiences nausea and vomiting. Patient is unable to pass flatus, and abdomen is hard and distended. Paralytic ileus is a common complication after bowel surgery. Intestinal motility may return slowly.
   a. Report to surgeon.
   b. Insert NG tube as ordered (see Chapter 19).

Recording and Reporting

- Document patient's arrival at nursing unit; describe vital signs, assessment findings, and all nursing measures initiated in progress note. Document every 4 hours or more frequently as patient's condition warrants.
- Record vital signs and I&O on appropriate flow sheet.
- Report any abnormal assessment findings and signs of complications to surgeon.
- Document your evaluation of patient learning.

Sample Documentation

Third postoperative day after abdominal surgery

1800   Vomited 300 mL dark green mucus. Abdomen firm and distended. No bowel sounds heard. Not passing flatus. Rates pain at 7 (scale 0 to 10). Morphine sulfate 10 mg IV. Instructed not to eat or drink anything.

1910   Vomited 200 mL dark green material and C/O being "very nauseated." Abdominal pain now rated at 6 (scale 0 to 10). Surgeon notified. NG tube inserted and connected to low intermittent suction as ordered with return of 400 mL dark green material within 15 minutes. Phenergan 5 mg given intramuscularly for nausea.

1950   Resting comfortably. Denies nausea. Pain now rated at 4 (scale 0 to 10). NG tube draining 200 mL of dark green drainage.

Special Considerations
Pediatric

- Assessment of a child's perceptions of the surgical experience enforces positive experiences and clarifies misconceptions. Drawing and storytelling are effective methods that allow children to share their thoughts and feelings (Hockenberry and Wilson, 2013).
- Use appropriate pain assessment tools to determine child's pain level.

Geriatric

- Older adults often experience a longer and more difficult postoperative recovery. Assess carefully for the development of postoperative complications.
- Assess for postoperative delirium and changes in mental status along with potential causes.
- Postoperative pain tends to be undertreated in older adults. Some patients fear "becoming addicted" or minimize pain because they are stoic. Assess for pain and encourage use of nonpharmacological measures such as relaxation and imagery along with pain medications (Lewis et al., 2014).

Home Care

- Teach patient and family caregiver about postoperative exercises, home modifications, activity limitations, wound dressing care, medications, and nutritional needs.
- If patient is discharged with dressing changes, the bedroom or bathroom is usually ideal for the procedure. Have patient and family caregiver perform return demonstration of dressing change.
- Make referral to home health services if patient and family caregiver will have difficulty providing the expected level of care needed.

CRITICAL THINKING EXERCISES

Case Study

A 39-year-old man arrived for a same-day-surgery admission to have arthroscopic surgery on his left knee. He is scheduled to have spinal anesthesia with light sedation. He is a runner, does not smoke, drinks one or two beers daily, and has a negative health history.

1. At which points in the procedural planning and actual procedure should The Joint Commission Universal Protocol for preoperative verification of correct person, correct site, and correct procedure occur for this patient? Select all that apply.
   1. At the time the procedure was scheduled
   2. At the time of preadmission testing and assessment
   3. At the time of admission or entry into the facility for the procedure
   4. Before the patient leaves the preprocedure area or enters the procedure room
   5. Any time the responsibility of care of the patient is transferred to another member of the procedural care team

2. Which of the following elements are required on the patient's procedural checklist? Select all that apply.
   1. Assessment (surgeon, nursing, anesthesia)
   2. Signed consent form
   3. Family caregiver contact information
   4. Any required blood products, implants, or special equipment for the procedure
   5. Test results

Review Questions

1. Which of the following is true about the immediate post-anesthesia phase?
   1. Includes several days after surgery
   2. Extends from the time the patient leaves the operating room (OR) to the time of transfer from the postanesthesia care unit (PACU) to the nursing unit
   3. Includes several additional days or weeks at home for the continued healing process
   4. Begins as the patient enters the operating room

2. A new patient for admission has arrived, and the surgical unit is very busy. Which of the following activities is not delegated to the NAP?
   1. Vital sign collection
   2. Preoperative teaching
   3. Placement of antiembolism stockings
   4. Assisting patient with deep-breathing exercises

3. The nurse's role in informed consent includes which of the following?
   1. Informing the patient of the prognosis if patient refuses surgery
   2. Explaining the risks, benefits, and alternatives of the planned surgery
   3. Verifying the patient's understanding of the surgical procedure and ensuring the patient's signature is complete on the consent form
   4. Asking the patient for consent for the planned surgery

4. A nurse is responsible for properly instructing patients on breathing exercises before surgery. Place the following steps for deep breathing and coughing in the correct order.
   a. Have patient place palms of hands across from each other along the lower rib cage or upper abdomen.
   b. Have patient take slow, deep breath; hold for count of 3 seconds; and exhale.
   c. Have patient sit in high-Fowler's position with knees bent.
   d. Have patient take slow, deep breaths, inhaling through nose.
   e. Have patient repeat breathing exercise three to five times.
   1. a, c, b, d, e
   2. c, a, d, b, e
   3. b, c, a, d, e
   4. c, b, a, d, e

5. Which assessment findings in a patient in the PACU need to be reported to the surgeon? Select all that apply.
   1. Respiratory rate less than 10 per minute with shallow breathing
   2. Bright red wound drainage saturating dressing
   3. Pain rating of 3 on a scale of 0 to 10
   4. Scattered crackles in posterior lung bases

6. The nurse is checking a patient into the room on the surgical unit after abdominal surgery. There is a 1.5-cm (½-inch) diameter spot of serosanguineous drainage on the dressing. What action should the nurse take at this time?
   1. Notify the surgeon of bleeding from the wound
   2. Note the amount of drainage on the dressing and continue to monitor
   3. Remove the dressing to check for bleeding from the suture line
   4. Apply gentle pressure to the site for 5 minutes

7. Which position is used to minimize the chance of aspiration in a patient who is lethargic after general anesthesia?
   1. High-Fowler's
   2. Semi-Fowler's
   3. Side-lying
   4. Supine

8. A local anesthetic may cause which of the following side effects?
   1. Hypertension
   2. Vasodilation
   3. Cyanosis
   4. Skin rash

9. With stable patients, what preoperative skills can be delegated to nursing assistive personnel (NAP)?
   1. Vital signs
   2. Education for use of incentive spirometer
   3. Preoperative assessments
   4. Nothing can be delegated to the NAP

10. A postoperative patient is dehydrated and has symptoms of blood loss, including hypotension. The nurse can expect to implement which interventions?
    1. Administer antibiotics and epinephrine
    2. Continue to monitor vital signs only
    3. Double the intravenous fluid rate
    4. Administer intravenous fluids and possible blood products

REFERENCES

American Society of Anesthesiologists (ASA) Committee: Practice guidelines for preoperative fasting and the use of pharmacologic agents to reduce the risk of pulmonary aspiration: application to healthy patients undergoing elective procedures: an updated report by the American Society of Anesthesiologists Committee on Standards and Practice Parameters, *Anesthesiology* 114(3):495, 2011.

American Society of PeriAnesthesia Nurses (ASPAN): *2012-2014 perianesthesia nursing standards, practice recommendations and interpretive statements*, Cherry Hill, NJ, 2014, ASPAN.

Association of PeriOperative Registered Nurses (AORN): *Perioperative standards and recommended practices*, Denver, CO, 2013, AORN.

Baldini G, et al: Postoperative urinary retention, *Anesthesiology* 110(5):1139, 2009.

Graling PR, Vasaly FW: Effectiveness of 2% CHG cloth bathing for reducing surgical site infections, *AORN J* 97(5):547, 2013.

Hockenberry MJ, Wilson D: *Wong's essentials of pediatric nursing*, ed 9, St Louis, 2013, Mosby.

Institute for Healthcare Improvement (IHI): *Surgical Infection Prevention*, 2014. http://www.ihi.org/explore/SSI/Pages/default.aspx.

Johansson K, Katajisto J, Salanterä S: Pre-admission education in surgical rheumatology nursing: towards greater patient empowerment, *J Clin Nurs* 19(21–22):2980, 2010.

Lewis S, et al: *Medical-surgical nursing: assessment and management of clinical problems*, ed 9, St Louis, 2014, Mosby.

Lilley LL, Rainforth Collins S, Snyder J: *Pharmacology and the nursing process*, ed 7, St Louis, 2014, Mosby.

Phillips NM, et al: Post-anaesthetic discharge scoring criteria: key findings from a systematic review, *Int Evid Based Healthc* 11(4):275, 2013.

Rothrock JC: *Alexander's care of the patient in surgery*, ed 15, St Louis, 2014, Mosby.

Spry C, Goodman T: *Essentials of perioperative nursing*, ed 4, Gaithersburg, MD, 2013, Aspen.

Stannard D, Krenzischek D: *PeriAnesthesia nursing care: a bedside guide for safe recovery*, Sudbury, MA, 2012, Jones & Bartlett Learning.

The Joint Commission (TJC): *National Patient Safety Goals*, Oakbrook Terrace, IL, 2014, The Commission. http://www.jointcommission.org/standards_information/npsgs.aspx. Accessed September 17, 2014.

Emergency Measures for Life Support in the Hospital Setting

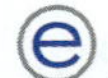 **EVOLVE WEBSITE/EVOLVE RESOURCES LIST**

http://evolve.elsevier.com/Perry/nursinginterventions
Audio Glossary • Checklists • Review Questions

Cardiac arrest is the cessation of circulating blood flow that greatly reduces oxygen transport and perfusion of body cells and tissue. The condition is life threatening. All patients receive cardiopulmonary resuscitation (CPR) in the event of a cardiopulmonary arrest unless otherwise indicated, such as a patient having an advance directive for final health care or a "do not resuscitate" status.

PATIENT-CENTERED CARE

Nurses have a unique relationship with their patients, and because of the associated high level of trust, nurses are the ideal facilitators for the initiation of advance directives. As a nurse, you have the opportunity to assist patients and their families in making informed decisions about end-of-life care. Advance directives offer valuable information about a patient's decisions regarding resuscitation efforts. Although advance directives are often addressed before or during a patient's hospital admission, you play an important role in encouraging patients and families to discuss this issue and determine the patient's wishes regarding life-support interventions. You also have the opportunity to assist in completion of the patient's advance directive document. Often an advance directive document can minimize disagreements among family members when a patient is physically or mentally unable to make decisions.

SAFETY

Certain types of lethal arrhythmias can be quickly converted back to a regular heart rhythm if electricity is applied to a patient early in cardiac arrest. The treatment for ventricular fibrillation (V Fib; VF) or ventricular tachycardia (V Tach; VT) without a pulse requires an externally applied electrical shock called defibrillation to a patient's chest. For every minute of delay of the first shock, the chances of survival are reduced by 10% (Meaney et al., 2013). The American Heart Association (AHA) Get With The Guidelines-Resuscitation (2014) registry has set the goal for hospitals to deliver the first electrical shock to patients in ventricular fibrillation in less than 2 minutes. When electrical energy is used during an emergency, good skin contact between the pad and patient's chest is essential to avoid the release of live electricity into the environment. Clear communication to all others in the room is essential at the time of defibrillation so that everyone is aware and does not touch the patient or the bed at the time of the shock.

Rapid Response Teams composed of a critical care nurse, a physician or an advanced practice nurse, and respiratory therapists are present in many hospitals (Jones et al., 2011). The goal of a Rapid Response Team is to intervene in the care of patients with unexpected clinical deterioration. Many clinicians believe that one key component of improving outcomes involves earlier detection of clinical compromise

(Jones et al., 2011). Automated computer systems that analyze vital signs, laboratory results, and physical assessments can be used to trigger Rapid Response Teams. The effects of these early warning systems are still being investigated.

Finally, proper hand position when performing chest compressions ensures effective perfusion, while minimizing internal injury to a patient. A mask with a one-way valve provides a filter between the patient and the rescuer during artificial ventilations. This mask provides a safety barrier for both the staff performing mouth-to-mask ventilations and the patient.

EVIDENCE-BASED PRACTICE

Jones D, DeVita M, Bellomo R: Rapid-response teams, *N Engl J Med* 365(2):139, 2011.

Meaney P, et al: Cardiopulmonary resuscitation quality: [corrected] improving cardiac resuscitation inside and outside the hospital: a consensus statement from the American Heart Association, *Circulation* 128(4):417, 2013.

Every 5 years, the AHA reviews all the resuscitation studies to provide the latest recommendations for basic, adult, pediatric, and neonatal life support. The last year these recommendations were updated was 2010. The previous 2010 AHA CPR guidelines focus on methods to ensure high-quality chest compressions. Future updates are expected in 2015.

Since 2010, other studies have focused on issues concerning the quality of CPR and earlier interventions to prevent arrest (Meaney et al., 2013). Research demonstrated that early, high-quality CPR and early defibrillation are the primary components influencing survival. Metrics such as end-tidal carbon dioxide (CO_2) and arterial pressures (when available) provide valuable feedback to the chest compressor and the provider of ventilations.

The goal of high-quality CPR is to maintain end-tidal CO_2 greater than 20. This feedback plus recommended team level logistics to switch chest compressors every 2 minutes help improve performance of high-quality CPR. There are four additional critical components of high-quality CPR. A list of what needs to be performed from highest to lowest priority follows:

- Minimize interruptions in chest compressions.
- Provide compressions at adequate depth and rate.
- Avoid leaning between compressions.
- Avoid excessive ventilation.

SKILL 29.1   INSERTING AN OROPHARYNGEAL AIRWAY

An oropharyngeal airway is a semicircular-shaped, minimally flexible, curved piece of hard plastic (Fig. 29-1). When inserted, it extends from just outside the lips, over the tongue, and to the pharynx (Fig. 29-2). Oral airways allow you to suction through a central core or along the side of the airway, facilitate resuscitation, and maintain airway patency in an unconscious patient.

The oral airway is sized for adults and children, varying in length and width (Table 29-1). Choose the size of an oral airway on the basis of a patient's age and the width and length of the patient's mouth. Size is correct if the end of the curve reaches the angle of the jaw when the flange is held parallel to the front teeth with the airway against the patient's cheek.

ASSESSMENT

1. Identify need to insert oral airway. Signs and symptoms include upper airway "gurgling" with respiratory cycle, absent cough or gag reflex, increased oral secretions or

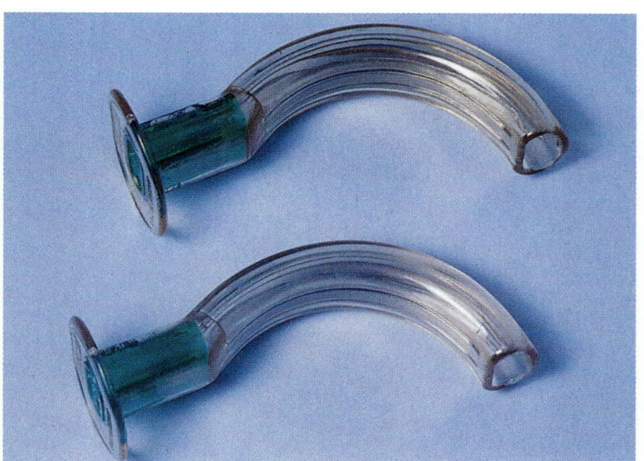

FIG 29-1 Oral airways.

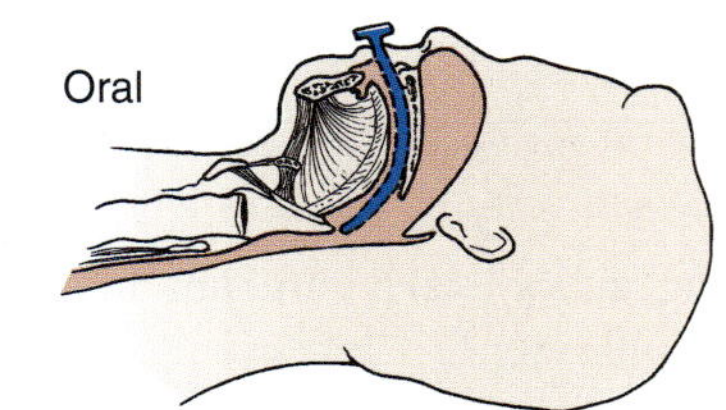

FIG 29-2 Placement of oral airway.

TABLE 29-1	ORAL AIRWAY GUIDELINES FOR SIZE BY AGE		
SIZE	**AGE**	**SIZE**	**AGE**
000	Premature neonates	3	6-18 yr
00	Newborn	4	Adult medium
0	Newborn to 1 yr	5	Adult large
1	1-2 yr	6	Adult extra large
2	2-6 yr		

excretions, excessive drooling, grinding teeth, biting of oral tracheal or gastric tubes, labored respirations, and increased respiratory rate. *Rationale: These conditions place patients at risk for obstruction of upper airway.*

SAFE PATIENT CARE Use oral airways only for unresponsive patients without an active gag reflex. Placement of an oral airway may stimulate vomiting and possible aspiration or cause laryngospasm if inserted in a semiconscious patient.

SAFE PATIENT CARE Never insert an oropharyngeal airway in a patient with recent oral trauma, oral surgery, or loose teeth.

---

2. Determine factors that may be contributing to upper airway obstruction, such as age (children have a proportionally larger tongue), loss of consciousness, seizure disorder, neuromuscular disease affecting swallowing, or facial trauma. *Rationale: Identifying risk factors for airway obstructions allows you to accurately assess the need for an oral airway.*
3. In postoperative patients awakening from anesthesia, assess for presence of cough or gag reflex; gently place tongue blade on back of patient's tongue. *Rationale: Action elicits a cough or gag reflex if one is present, which demonstrates patient's ability to manage oral secretions.*
4. Before attempting an oral airway, ensure that patient does not have dentures in place. *Rationale: An oral airway can dislodge loose fitting dentures and cause worsening airway obstruction.*

PLANNING

Expected Outcomes focus on the improvement in airway patency and respiratory status.
1. Patient's rate of respirations is normal, removal of secretions is easier, lack of gurgling noise in throat.
2. Patient is not able to grind teeth or bite endotracheal or other tubes.
3. Patient's tongue does not relax back into pharynx and obstruct airway.

Delegation and Collaboration

The skill of inserting an oropharyngeal airway cannot be delegated to nursing assistive personnel (NAP). Respiratory therapists have the training to insert an oral airway on delegation. The nurse instructs the NAP to:
• Report immediately to the nurse any signs of airway distress, vomiting, or change in level of consciousness.

Equipment
• Appropriate-size oral airway (see Table 29-1)
• Clean gloves
• Gown if needed
• Tissues or washcloths
• Suction equipment if indicated
• Nonallergic tape
• Face shield if indicated
• Tongue blade
• Stethoscope

IMPLEMENTATION *for* INSERTING AN OROPHARYNGEAL AIRWAY

STEPS	RATIONALE
1. **See Standard Protocol (inside front cover).**	
2. Position unconscious patient; semi-Fowler's position is preferred.	Provides easy access to oral cavity.
3. Apply clean gloves and face shield (when possible).	Reduces transmission of microorganisms.
4. Use padded tongue blade whenever possible if you need to open patient's mouth.	Provides access to oral cavity.

SAFE PATIENT CARE Do not use your fingers to try to open airway, there is the risk of patient biting you.

---

5. Insert oral airway:	When inserting airway, take care not to push patient's tongue into pharynx.

STEPS	RATIONALE

a. Hold oral airway with curved end up and insert distal end until airway reaches back of throat; then turn airway over 180 degrees and follow natural curve of tongue. *Option:* Hold airway sideways and insert halfway; rotate airway 90 degrees while gliding it over natural curvature of tongue. Make sure outer flange is just outside patient's lips.

Provides patent airway and prevents displacement of patient's tongue into posterior oropharynx. Secure airway temporarily with tape on upper and lower flange. May need to insert an endotracheal (ET) airway as soon as possible.

6. Suction secretions as needed.
7. Reassess patient's respiratory status; auscultate lungs.
8. Clean patient's face with soft tissue or washcloth.
9. Administer frequent oral hygiene such as oral swabbing and tooth brushing.

Removes secretions; maintains patent airway.
Verifies respiratory status and patent airway.
Promotes hygiene.
Increases patient comfort and removes debris. Provides moisture to oral mucosal tissues. Prevents bacterial translocation into the lungs and pneumonia.

10. Oral airway needs to be removed, cleaned, and reinserted routinely in patients with copious amount of oral mucus secretions (see facility policy).
11. **See Completion Protocol (inside front cover).**

Reduces risk of aspiration.

EVALUATION

1. Observe patient's respiratory status, and compare respiratory assessments before and after insertion of oral airway.
2. Determine that airway is patent, that patient does not occlude airway by biting tubes, and that patient's tongue does not obstruct airway.

Unexpected Outcomes and Related Interventions

1. Patient pushes airway out of place or out of mouth.
   a. If patient regains consciousness and is gagging, place in lateral recumbent (rescue) position and suction.
   b. Determine patient's continued need for oral airway.
2. Airway obstruction is not relieved.
   a. Obtain immediate assistance.
   b. Reinsert airway.

Recording and Reporting

- Record and report assessment findings while inserting oral airway; size of oral airway; placement; any other procedures performed at same time, especially positioning, secretions obtained, patient's tolerance of procedure.

Sample Documentation

1000 Unresponsive, airway secretions increasing, upper airway gurgling auscultated. Gag reflex absent. Size 4 oropharyngeal airway inserted without trauma. Airway suctioned for yellow airway secretions. Bilateral lung sounds; no adventitious sounds.

Special Considerations
Pediatric

- Oral airways are seldom used in treatment of airway obstruction in children and infants. A child's airway is narrow; thus oral airways are often more occlusive than beneficial (Berg et al., 2010b).
- For infants and small children, sliding oral airway along side of mouth rather than with tip up is recommended because the soft palate is easily injured.

SKILL 29.2 USING AN AUTOMATED EXTERNAL DEFIBRILLATOR

An automated external defibrillator (AED) incorporates a heart rhythm analysis system. It eliminates the need for training in rhythm interpretation and makes early defibrillation practical. The device is attached to a patient's chest via two adhesive pads with conductive gel. An AED can be a stand-alone box (Fig. 29-3) with a very simple three-step function, or it can be incorporated into a manual defibrillator. In most hospitals, the pads used for the stand-alone box are the same as the pads used for the manual defibrillators. On pad application, the AED automatically analyzes a patient's cardiac rhythm to determine if it is a shockable rhythm (i.e., ventricular tachycardia or ventricular fibrillation). If a shock is advised, the device automatically charges and gives the user audible and visible prompts to press the shock button.

ASSESSMENT

1. Establish patient's unresponsiveness and call for help. *Rationale: Assists in determining if the patient is unresponsive rather than asleep, intoxicated, hearing impaired, or postseizure (postictal).*

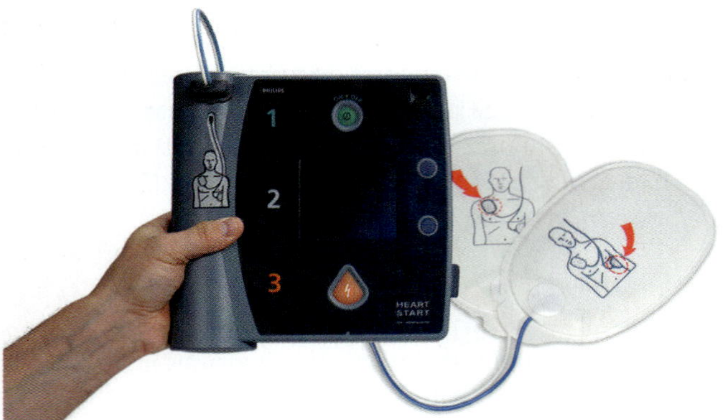

FIG 29-3 AED device. (Courtesy Philips Medical Systems.)

2. Establish absence of respirations and lack of circulation within 10 seconds: no palpable pulse, no respirations, no movement. *Rationale: Indicates need for emergency measures, including AED.*

> **SAFE PATIENT CARE** An AED should be applied only to a patient who is unconscious, not breathing, and pulseless.

PLANNING

Expected Outcomes focus on restoring cardiac rhythm, pulse rate, and respirations.
1. Patient's cardiac rhythm is converted back to a stable rhythm.
2. Patient regains pulse and respirations.

Delegation and Collaboration
Basic life support (BLS) certification provides hands-on training with an AED for laypersons, nursing assistive personnel, and licensed health care professionals. Most hospitals using AEDs have given the authority to use an AED to all CPR-certified personnel, including nursing assistive personnel. Refer to specific facility policies for use of the AED.

Equipment
- AED
- Pair of AED adhesive pads

IMPLEMENTATION *for* USING AN AUTOMATED EXTERNAL DEFIBRILLATOR

STEPS	RATIONALE
1. Assess patient for unresponsiveness, no breathing, pulselessness, and no movement within 10 seconds.	Rapid response ensures ongoing resuscitation support.
2. Activate code team in accordance with facility policy and procedure. (In community setting have someone call 9-1-1.)	First available person to bring resuscitation cart and AED.
3. Start chest compressions and continue until AED is attached, turned on, and verbal prompt advises you, "do *not* touch the patient."	To minimize the interruption time of chest compressions, continue CPR while AED is being applied and turned on.
4. Place AED next to the patient near the chest or head and turn on the power (see illustration).	Turning on the power begins the verbal prompts to guide you through the next steps.

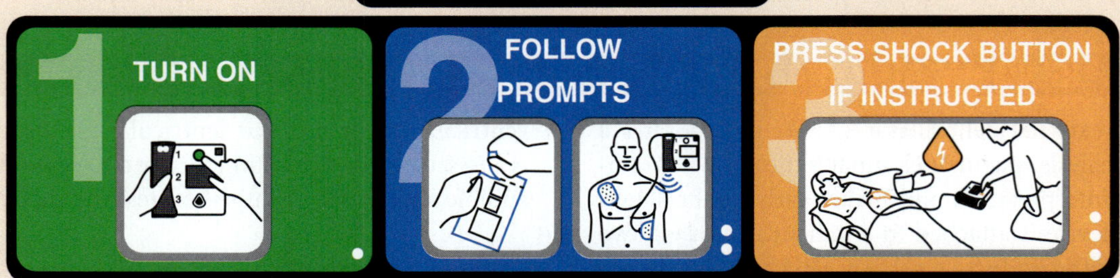

STEP 4 Power panel with AED prompts. (Courtesy Philips Medical Systems.)

> **SAFE PATIENT CARE** If the AED is available immediately, attach it to patient as soon as possible. The faster defibrillation is delivered, the better the survival rate (Berg et al., 2010a).

STEPS	RATIONALE

5. Attach device. Place first AED pad on upper right sternal border directly below the clavicle. Place second AED pad lateral to left nipple with the top of the pad a few inches below the axilla (see illustration). Ensure that cables are connected to AED. Do not attach pads to a wet surface, over a medication patch, or over a pacemaker or implanted defibrillator.

Alternative pad placement of AED pads is not recommended. The fastest application technique is the one mentioned. If AED pads are placed as directed, patient's heart rhythm is analyzed in lead II. Patients with large amounts of chest hair may require shaving to obtain adequate pad contact. Wet surfaces, implanted defibrillators, and medication patches reduce the effectiveness of the defibrillation attempt and result in complications.

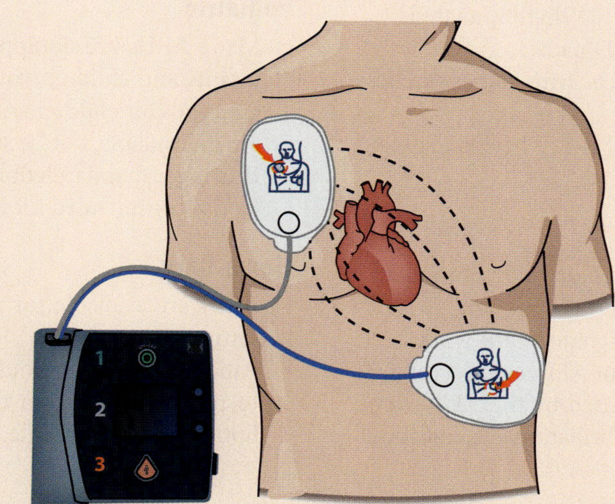

STEP 5 Placement of AED pads with device next to patient.

6. Do *not* touch the patient when AED prompts you. Direct rescuers and bystanders to avoid touching the patient by announcing "Clear!" Allow AED to analyze the rhythm. Some devices require that an analysis button be pressed. The AED takes approximately 5 to 15 seconds to analyze the rhythm.

Each brand of AED is different; familiarity with the model is important. Not touching the patient when directed prevents artifact errors, avoids all movement during analysis, and prevents shock from being delivered to bystanders.

7. Before pressing the shock button, announce loudly "Clear!" to clear the victim. Perform a visual check to ensure that no one is in contact with victim.

Clearing patient ensures safety for individuals involved in rescue efforts.

8. Immediately begin chest compression after the shock and continue for 2 minutes with a ratio of 30:2 (30 compressions and 2 breaths). Do NOT remove the pads.

Continues cardiac perfusion.

9. Deliver two breaths using mouth-to-mouth with barrier device or mouth-to-mask device or bag-mask device. Watch for chest rise and fall. Deliver 10 to 12 breaths/min

Mouth to mouth without a barrier in a health care setting is not recommended because of risk for microbial contamination

10. After 2 minutes of CPR, AED prompts you not to touch patient and resumes analysis of patient's rhythm. This cycle continues until patient regains a pulse or the health care provider determines death.

EVALUATION

1. Inspect pad adhesion to chest wall. If pads are not in good contact with chest wall, remove them and apply a new set. Attach new set of pads to AED.
2. Monitor vital signs and continue resuscitative efforts until patient regains pulse or health care provider determines death.

Unexpected Outcomes and Related Interventions

1. Patient's heart rhythm does not convert into a stable rhythm with pulse after defibrillation.
   a. Observe pad contact with patient's chest wall.
   b. Do not touch patient during AED rhythm analysis.
2. Patient's skin has burns under AED pads.
   a. Observe that AED pad contacts with patient's chest wall.
   b. Ensure that patient's chest wall is dry before applying pads.

Recording and Reporting

- Immediately report arrest via facility-wide communication system, indicating exact location of victim.
- Record in nurses' notes or on designated CPR worksheet: onset of arrest, time and number of AED shocks (you will not know the exact energy level used by the AED), time and energy level of manual defibrillations, medications given, procedures performed, cardiac rhythm, use of CPR, and patient's response.

Sample Documentation

0900   Patient found unresponsive on floor of room; code team activated. No palpable pulse or observable respirations. CPR initiated at 0901.

0903   AED attached and pads placed on patient's chest, 1 shock delivered, CPR resumed immediately after shock.

0905   Second shock applied; no palpable pulse and CPR continued. Code team arrived.

Special Considerations
Pediatric

- Many AEDs are equipped to deliver energy suitable for infants and children younger than 8 years old using specific pads for children. Adult pads can be used if child pads are unavailable, but be sure not to overlap or cut the pads. If using a manual defibrillator, energy setting of 2 to 4 J/kg is recommended for infants (Haskell and Atkins, 2010).

Home Care

- AEDs are available for use in the community and home setting.
- Patient and family should keep emergency numbers taped to phone or program them into speed dial function on both home and mobile phones. Stress the use of 911.

SKILL 29.3   CODE MANAGEMENT

This skill includes the initial response and management of a patient in cardiopulmonary arrest. All who respond to cardiopulmonary arrests should arrive well trained in a simple, easy-to-remember approach. The advanced cardiac life support (ACLS) provider course teaches the primary and secondary survey approach to arrest situations. With each step, the responder performs an assessment and then, if the assessment indicates, a management intervention. Initially a code is managed by the first responder performing the basic skills of CPR, which includes the primary survey of *C* (circulation), *A* (airway), *B* (breathing), *D* (early defibrillation). This survey continues until the code team arrives. CPR is initiated and maintained by the first responders until the code team arrives. As soon as possible, determine the patient's cardiac rhythm and, if appropriate, defibrillate the patient with a manual defibrillator or an AED (see Skill 29-2).

The initial process also includes the notification of the hospital resuscitation team or code team. Most of the code team members have been trained in the ACLS guidelines and the performance of the secondary survey: *C* (rhythm analysis of cardiac rhythm), *A* (airway intubation), *B* (confirmation of airway and ventilation), and *D* (differential diagnosis of the cause). Both surveys must be reassessed continually and managed as appropriate throughout the code situation.

The hospital code team may include a physician, intensive care nurse, respiratory therapist, anesthesiologist, and pharmacist. A representative from pastoral care is often available to be with the family.

CPR certification is required of most nursing students or for entry into the nursing program. As a result, CPR is not covered in detail in this chapter. Table 29-2 summarizes health care provider guidelines for CPR.

ASSESSMENT

1. Determine if patient is unconscious by shaking patient and shouting, "Are you OK?" Assess patient's unresponsiveness. *Rationale: Confirms that patient is unconscious rather than asleep, intoxicated, or hearing impaired. Substance abuse, hypoglycemia, ketoacidosis, and shock can also cause unconsciousness.*

SAFE PATIENT CARE If an unconscious patient has adequate respirations and pulse, remain with him or her until further assistance is present. Place victim in a modified lateral recovery position (Fig. 29-4) if patient is not injured. Continue to determine presence of respirations and pulse throughout because a respiratory or cardiopulmonary arrest is still possible. Lateral recovery position helps to avoid airway blockage by the tongue and aspiration of oral fluids.

TABLE 29-2 HEALTH CARE PROVIDER GUIDELINES FOR ADULT, CHILD, AND INFANT CPR TECHNIQUES

TECHNIQUE	ADULT	CHILD (1-8 YEARS OLD)	INFANT (<1 YEAR; DOES NOT INCLUDE NEWBORNS)
Chest compressions: Push hard and fast to allow complete recoil	Begin compressions if no pulse Lower half of sternum, between nipples Heel of one hand, other hand on top 3.75-5 cm (1½-2 inches) in depth One or two rescuers: 30 compressions, 2 breaths (30:2) Continue until AED is available and ready to analyze rhythm	Begin compressions if no pulse or pulse <60/min Lower half of sternum, between nipples Heel of one hand or as for adults At least $\frac{1}{3}$ depth of chest One rescuer: 30 compressions, 2 breaths (30:2) Two rescuers: 15 compressions, 2 breaths (15:2)	Begin compressions if no pulse or pulse <60/min Just below nipple line (lower half of sternum) Two fingers, two thumb (encircling hands) At least $\frac{1}{3}$ depth of chest One rescuer: 30 compressions, 2 breaths (30:2) Two rescuers: 15 compressions, 2 breaths (15:2)
Defibrillation using AED	Use adult pads Provide 5 cycles of CPR before shock if response time is >4-5 minutes and arrest was not witnessed; otherwise AED should be applied as soon as available and shock as soon as advised; resume compressions immediately after shock	Use child pads whenever possible; if none, use adult pads, but do not overlap them; do not cut pads Apply AED as soon as available and shock as soon as advised	Use child pads whenever possible; if none, use adult pads, but do not overlap them; do not cut pads Apply AED as soon as available and shock as soon as advised
Airway	Head tilt–chin lift (HCP: Suspected trauma, use jaw thrust)	Head tilt–chin lift (HCP: Suspected trauma, use jaw thrust)	Head tilt–chin lift (HCP: Suspected trauma, use jaw thrust)
HCP: Rescue breathing with mouth-to-mask or bag-mask without chest compressions	10-12 breaths/min (approximate) 1 breath every 5-6 seconds	12-20 breaths/min (approximate) 1 breath every 3 seconds	12-20 breaths/min (approximate) 1 breath every 3 seconds
HCP: Rescue breaths for CPR with advanced airway (ET tube/tracheotomy)	8-10 breaths/min (approximate) 1 breath every 6-8 seconds	8-10 breaths/min (approximate) 1 breath every 6-8 seconds	8-10 breaths/min (approximate) 1 breath every 6-8 seconds
Foreign body airway obstruction	Abdominal thrusts	Abdominal thrusts	Back slaps and chest thrusts

AED, Automated external defibrillator; *CPR,* cardiopulmonary resuscitation; *ET,* endotracheal; *HCP,* health care provider.
Data from Berg RA et al: Part 5: adult basic life support: 2010 American Heart Association Guidelines for Cardiopulmonary Resuscitation and Emergency Cardiovascular Care, *Circulation* 122(Suppl 3):S685, 2010a; and Berg RA et al: Part 13: pediatric basic life support: 2010 American Heart Association Guidelines for Cardiopulmonary Resuscitation and Emergency Cardiovascular Care, *Circulation* 122(Suppl 3):S862, 2010b.

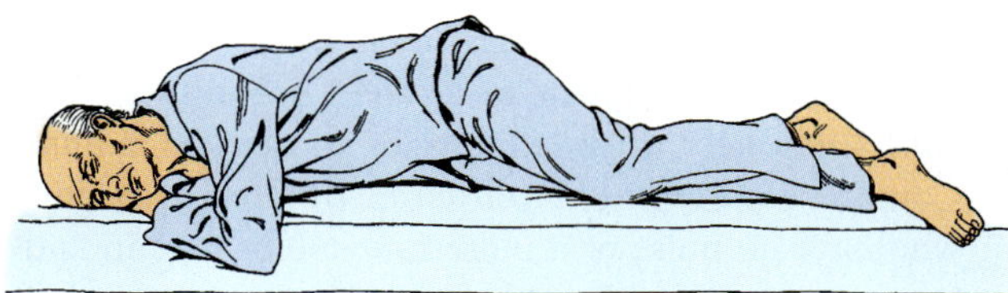

FIG 29-4 Recovery position.

2. Activate the hospital's code team or emergency medical services (EMS). Tell co-workers to bring AED and crash cart to bedside. *Rationale: Many adult victims are in ventricular fibrillation and need defibrillation and medications as soon as possible. Early access to emergency cardiac care systems improves patient outcomes (Meaney et al., 2013).*

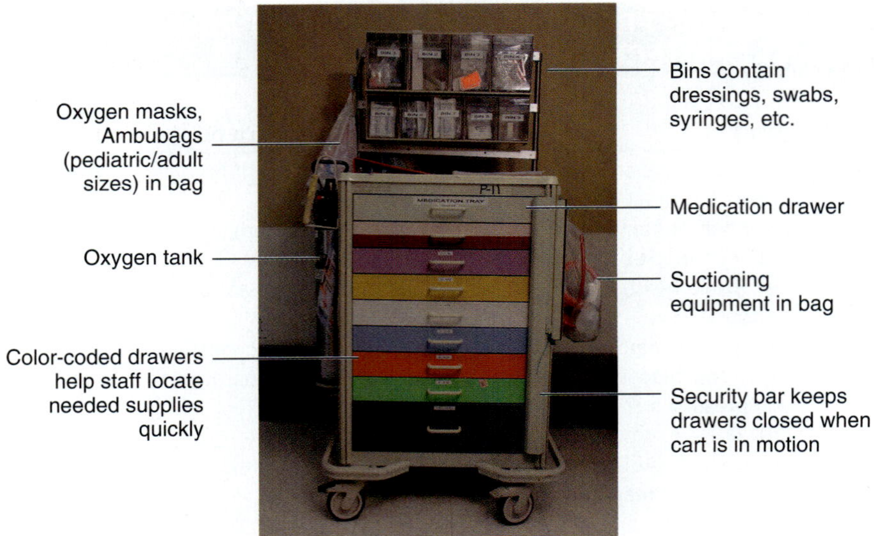

FIG 29-5 Emergency resuscitation cart.

PLANNING

Expected Outcomes focus on the restoration of cardiac and pulmonary function before irreversible organ damage occurs.
1. Patient regains pulse and respirations or is assisted with a ventilator as long as a pulse exists.
2. No complications occur from the resuscitation.
3. Health care provider may terminate CPR and pronounce death.

Delegation and Collaboration
The skill of code management cannot be delegated to nursing assistive personnel (NAP). However, NAP who are certified in BLS techniques can perform the basic skills of CPR. Most NAP are certified in BLS and may use an AED. However, manual defibrillation is usually reserved for licensed personnel who have ACLS certification. All other skills in the code situation are directed by the code team leader and performed by nurses, respiratory therapists, and other health care professionals.

Equipment
Code cart (Fig. 29-5): Most adult code carts have the following equipment:

- Clean and sterile gloves, gown, protective eyewear
- Oxygen source
- Bag mask
- Oral airways
- Laryngoscope, handle, and straight and curved laryngoscope blades
- ET tube, various sizes (6- to 8-Fr)
- End-tidal CO_2 detector or monitor
- Tape
- Backboard
- AED or manual defibrillator
- Intravascular needles (14- to 22-gauge)
- Central vascular access kit
- Intravenous (IV) tubing, fluids (9% normal saline, D_5W)
- Syringes
- Laboratory specimen tubes
- Arterial blood gas kit
- Emergency medications
- ACLS guidelines or algorithms
- Suction machine and suction equipment if not with crash cart

IMPLEMENTATION *for* CODE MANAGEMENT

STEPS	RATIONALE
Primary Survey: C (Circulation) 1. Check carotid pulse on adult or child; use brachial pulse on an infant. Check if victim is unresponsive and not breathing or only gasping. If no definite pulse within 10 seconds, begin chest compressions.	Carotid pulse is present when other peripheral pulses are not palpable. Because the neck of an infant is short, the carotid pulse is difficult to locate. Compressions are contraindicated when a pulse is present in adults. Compressions are to be started in children or infants who have no pulse or a pulse rate <60 beats/min and are unresponsive and not breathing.

STEPS	**RATIONALE**

2. Place victim on a hard surface such as floor, ground, or backboard. Victim must be flat. If necessary, logroll victim to flat, supine position using spine precautions.

Facilitates external compression of heart. Heart is compressed between sternum and spinal vertebrae, which must be on a hard, flat surface.

Primary Survey: A (Airway)

3. Open airway: Determine if patient has spontaneous respirations. Tongue is common cause of blocked airway.

Determines if patient has spontaneous respirations.

   a. Apply clean gloves and face shield.

Reduces transmission of microorganisms.

   b. Open airway: Head tilt–chin lift (no trauma) (see illustration) *or*

   c. Jaw thrust (spinal cord trauma suspected) (see illustration).

Suspect a spinal cord injury with any type of trauma. Jaw thrust maneuver prevents head extension and neck movement and further paralysis or spinal cord injury.

> **SAFE PATIENT CARE** If neck trauma is known or suspected, a cervical brace should be applied as soon as possible to maintain cervical spine stability.

Primary Survey: B (Breathing)

4. Attempt to ventilate patient with slow breaths, using one of these methods:

Slow breaths deliver air at a low pressure to reduce the risk of gastric distention.

   a. Mouth-to-mouth using barrier device.

Forms airtight seal and prevents air from escaping through nose.

   b. Mouth-to-mask using a pocket mask (see illustration).

Provides secure seal and permits use of supplemental oxygen.

   c. Bag-mask ventilation (see illustration).

Give breaths with enough force to make chest rise.

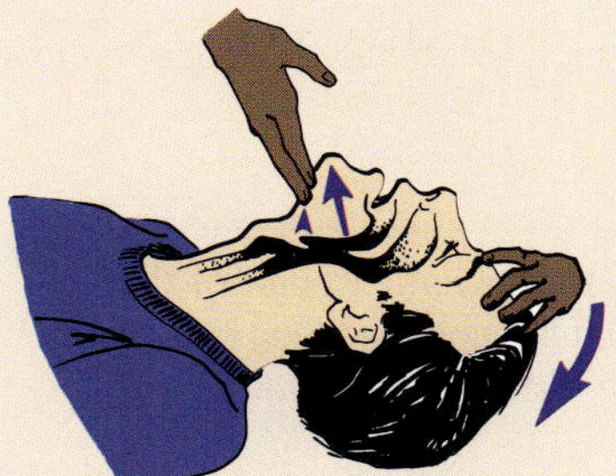

STEP 3b Head tilt–chin lift.

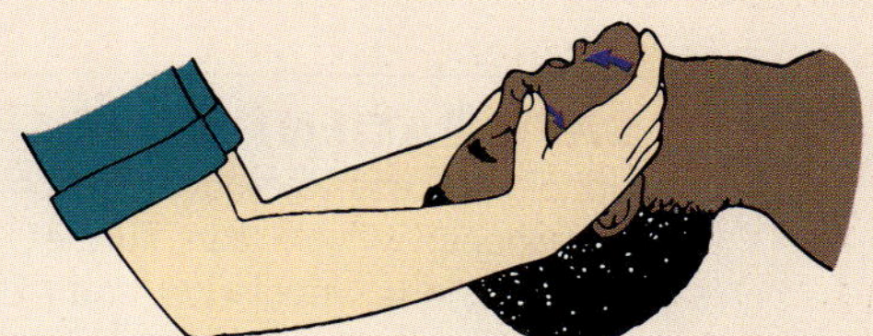

STEP 3c Jaw thrust without head tilt.

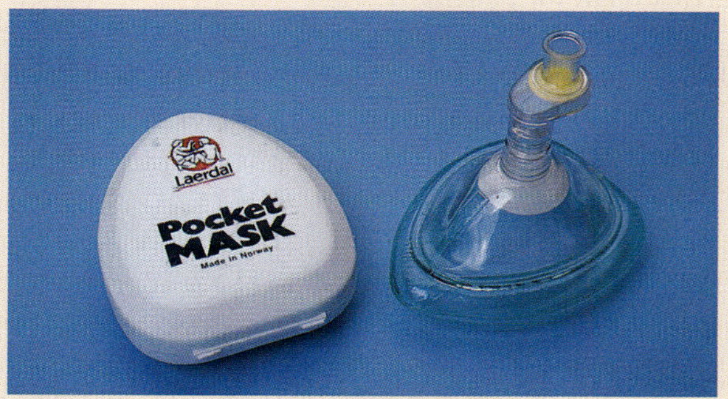

STEP 4b Pocket mask.

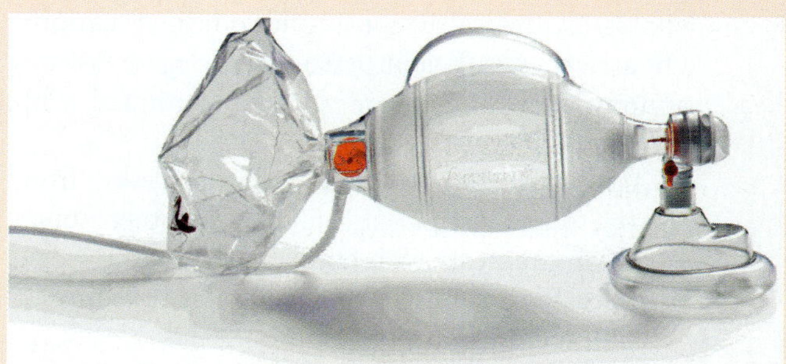

STEP 4c Bag mask. (Courtesy AMBU, United States.)

Continued

STEPS	RATIONALE

5. If readily available, insert oral airway (see Skill 29.1).

Maintains tone on anterior floor of mouth and prevents obstruction of posterior airway by tongue.

6. Suction secretions if necessary or turn victim's head to one side unless trauma is suspected.

Suctioning prevents airway obstruction. Turning patient's head to one side allows gravity to drain any secretions, decreasing risk of aspiration.

Primary Survey: D (Defibrillation)

7. If pulse is absent and AED is available, apply AED immediately as appropriate.

Most successful defibrillation rates occur when AED is applied and used within 3 minutes after collapse. Survival rates decline when defibrillation is delayed.

  a. After one shock, resume CPR for 5 cycles and then begin rhythm analysis and shock sequence again.

One shock followed by chest compressions for 5 cycles provides sufficient blood movement and improved perfusion before another set of shocks is delivered.

8. If pulse is absent and an AED is unavailable, immediately initiate chest compressions:

  a. Assume correct hand position and compression ratio for patient (see illustration).

Specific hand position, compression depth, and ratio are different for adult, child, and infant to avoid injury to heart, lung, or liver.

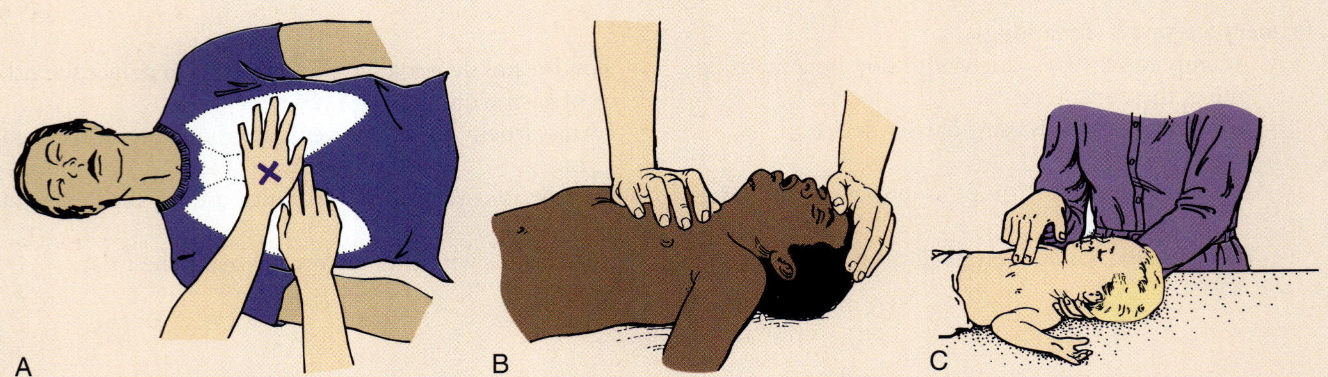

STEP 8a **A,** Proper hand position for an adult. **B,** Proper hand position for a child. **C,** Proper hand position for an infant.

> **SAFE PATIENT CARE** Ensure that fingers are off ribs and lowermost part of the xiphoid process to reduce chance of rib fractures that could result in punctured lung or liver lacerations, which can further compromise cardiopulmonary status. Continue chest compressions, ventilation, and AED use.

Secondary Survey: Implementation

1. Give code leader brief verbal report on events performed before arrival of code team (i.e., code, vital signs, medical diagnosis, and code intervention).

This information is critical in selection of appropriate treatment for patient.

2. On arrival of sufficient personnel, delegate tasks as appropriate (while core group continues with resuscitation efforts):

Delegation of duties is essential to meet all needs of patient and his or her family in a timely manner.

  a. Assist victim's roommate or visitors away from code scene. Assign pastoral care or other nurses to communicate with family.

  b. Delegate someone to remove excess furniture or equipment from room.

  c. Have someone bring patient's chart to bedside or be able to access patient's electronic medical record.

Clarifies patient's present medical condition, code status, and presence of any allergies.

STEPS	**RATIONALE**

d. Assign a nurse as recorder to document events of code.

Documents events of code and medications and treatments administered.

e. Assign another nurse to get medications and supplies from code cart and hand them off to code team members. The bedside nurse is involved in tasks such as medication administration, vital signs, and assisting with procedures.

Provides code personnel with appropriate medication and equipment in a timely manner.

Secondary Survey: C (Analysis of Cardiac Rhythm)

3. Attach manual defibrillator/monitor to patient using electrocardiogram electrodes, quick-look paddles with gel pads, or "hands-off" defibrillation pads. Visualize cardiac rhythm.

Cardiac rhythm monitor devices provide immediate rhythm display for visual analysis without disruption of rescue breathing and chest compression.

4. If cardiac rhythm is "shockable," continue CPR until command is verbalized to clear the patient:

It is important to minimize interruptions in CPR. Pad application, intubation, and ventilations all can be performed during CPR. Interruptions must be kept to a minimum and must not exceed 30 seconds.

a. Turn on defibrillator and select proper energy level following facility policy and equipment directions.

Energy is delivered in prescribed doses. For VT and VF, the maximum energy level should be selected. For most manual biphasic devices, deliver a maximum of 200 J; monophasic devices deliver a maximum of 360 J.

b. Most defibrillators use "hands-off pads" that are applied to patient's chest and directly connected to the manual defibrillator.

Decreases thoracic impedance and helps minimize burns to patient's skin (Berg et al., 2010a).

c. Place pads on the patient's chest wall in the same position as AED pads.

Pictures of proper pad placement on the patient's chest are visible on most pads.

d. Verify that no one is in physical contact with patient, bed, or any item contacting patient during defibrillation. A warning must be called out before initiating the charge. Announce "Clear!"

Prevents accidental delivery of shock or injury to personnel.

5. Establish IV access with large-bore needle (14- to 22-gauge) and begin infusion of 0.9% normal saline. If unable to obtain peripheral IV access, physician may order placement of central venous access.

Provides route for rapid drug administration and access for blood samples and fluid administration. Normal saline is isotonic.

6. Assist with procedures as needed.

Much of the equipment needed for special procedures during a code is on the code cart. Knowledge of code cart contents and their location is essential to provide personnel with appropriate equipment without delay.

7. Continue CPR until rescuer is relieved, victim regains spontaneous pulse and respiration, rescuer is exhausted and unable to perform CPR correctly, or physician discontinues. To maintain CPR quality, switch chest compressors every 2 minutes or every five cycles.

Artificial cardiopulmonary function is maintained. Interruption of CPR is planned and organized. Interruptions occur seamlessly during changing of CPR personnel, defibrillation, and intubation. Interruptions must be kept to a minimum and must not exceed 10 seconds (Berg et al., 2010a).

Secondary Survey: A (Intubate Airway)

8. If respirations are absent, assist code team with endotracheal (ET) intubation:

Intubation provides patent airway and improves pulmonary ventilation. A laryngeal mask airway or esophageal-tracheal Combitube can also be used to provide advanced airway support.

a. Have laryngoscope blade, laryngoscope handle, curved and straight blades, and ET tubes available. Ensure that light source on laryngoscope is functional.

Functional laryngeal light facilitates visualization of vocal cords and placement of ET tube into trachea.

Continued

STEPS	RATIONALE
Secondary Survey: B (Confirmation of Airway and Ventilation)	
9. Assist in confirmation of ET tube placement or advanced airway support by auscultating lungs for bilateral breath sounds. CO_2 detector or esophageal detector devices are used as secondary methods to confirm correct airway placement.	Auscultation of lungs and exhaled CO_2 monitoring or esophageal detector device further verifies correct airway placement and adequacy of ventilation and gas exchange.
10. Ventilate using a bag on intubation.	Bag provides ventilation through ET tube.
Secondary Survey: D (Differential Diagnosis)	
11. Assist health care provider in obtaining laboratory and diagnostic studies. Placement of advanced airway and central venous lines needs to be confirmed after arrest via x-ray.	Helps in determining cause of the arrest. X-ray confirms correct placement of devices.
12. **See Completion Protocol (inside front cover).**	

EVALUATION

1. Reassess primary and secondary survey CABDs throughout code event.
2. Palpate carotid pulse at least every 2 minutes after first minute of CPR.
3. Observe for spontaneous return of pulse or respirations.
4. Observe that interruptions in CPR are minimized.

Unexpected Outcomes and Related Interventions

1. Patient experiences skeletal injury such as fractured ribs or sternum or internal organ injury such as lacerated lung or liver.
   a. Obtain appropriate diagnostic tests to document fractures.
   b. Assess patient's postarrest breathing and chest wall asymmetry.
   c. Observe for hemoptysis or gastrointestinal bleeding.
   d. Observe for distended abdomen.
2. Resuscitation efforts are unsuccessful.
   a. Contact chaplain services, social worker, or other family support systems.
   b. Provide privacy for patient's family to begin grieving process (see Chapter 30).
   c. Complete postmortem care on patient per facility policy. Some states might also require notification of local organ donor services and the medical examiner before any postmortem care.

Recording and Reporting

- Record on a designated CPR worksheet or electronic medical record. The following should be documented to give the timeline of events in this order: time of patient discovery, time of first chest compression, time of first shock (if delivered), time of first assisted ventilations. Other documentation should include number of AED shocks (you need to know the device-specific energy level delivered by the AED), time and energy level of manual defibrillations, medications given, procedures performed, cardiac rhythm strips, use of CPR, and patient's response. Most hospitals use a form designed specifically for in-hospital arrests.
- Immediately report arrest, indicating exact location of victim. In hospital setting, follow facility policy for alerting the code team. In community setting, activate emergency response system.

Sample Documentation

1030   Telemetry service called with report of patient in V Tach. Immediately went to room to discover patient unconscious, not breathing, and pulseless. CPR started. AED applied. Advised shock, shock delivered × 1. CPR restarted immediately and continued for 2 minutes. Pulse palpable. BP 76/50. Dopamine IV 320 mcg/min started. Patient intubated. Transferred to ICU with physician and ICU nurse.

Special Considerations
Pediatric

- Infants and children experience respiratory arrest more frequently than full cardiopulmonary arrest.

Geriatric

- Older adults, especially older adults with osteoporosis, are at greater risk for rib fractures.
- Remove loose-fitting dentures to avoid airway obstruction during CPR and airway insertions. Leave properly fitting dentures in place because they assist in ensuring a tight seal during artificial ventilation.

CRITICAL THINKING EXERCISES

Case Study

An 84-year-old woman with a long history of heart failure and renal disease was admitted to a hospital's cardiology unit with pulmonary edema. A telemetry monitor was attached to the patient while diuretics were administered. The nurse receives a call from centralized telemetry 2 hours after the last IV diuretic was administered stating that the patient is in V Fib. The nurse has a NAP to assist with patient care.

1. What is the first thing the nurse should do on receiving this phone call?
   1. Tell the nurse manager.
   2. Establish patient's unresponsiveness and call for help.
   3. Activate code team in accordance with facility policy.
   4. Prepare or draw laboratory specimens from the patient.
2. Place the following interventions in correct sequence on entering this patient's room.
   a. Check responsiveness.
   b. Begin 30 chest compressions.
   c. Provide 2 breaths.
   d. Attach the AED
   e. Check for pulse.
   1. e, b, c, a, d
   2. a, e, b, d, c
   3. b, c, e, d, a
   4. a, e, b, c, d
3. The nurse instructs the NAP to use the AED if the patient becomes unresponsive and pulseless. Is this an appropriate delegation? Support your answer.
   1. Yes
   2. No

Review Questions

1. After one shock from the AED, the nurse should do which of the following first?
   1. Palpate the carotid pulse
   2. Immediately begin chest compressions
   3. Perform a rhythm analysis
   4. Place patient in the recovery position
2. Name the preferred technique to open the airway when there is no suspected trauma.
   1. Head tilt–chin lift
   2. Jaw thrust
   3. Lateral-lying position
   4. All of the above
3. What is the ideal time goal from victim discovery to first defibrillation for in-hospital patients?
   1. 3 minutes or less
   2. 5 minutes or less
   3. 7 minutes or less
   4. 10 minutes or less

4. Identify a possible unexpected outcome when performing chest compressions.
   1. Return of spontaneous pulse
   2. Possible skin burns
   3. Lacerated lung or liver
   4. Intubated airway
5. Which of the following statements about an oral airway is true?
   1. It eliminates the need to position the head of an unconscious patient.
   2. It eliminates the possibility of an upper airway obstruction.
   3. It is of no value after an ET tube is inserted.
   4. It may stimulate vomiting in a semiconscious patient.
6. During a cardiac arrest, an endotracheal tube is inserted. How many breaths per minute should be delivered to the patient via the bag?
   1. 8 to 10
   2. 4 to 6
   3. 20 to 24
   4. 18 to 20
7. Which of the following statements regarding quality chest compressions is true?
   1. Adults require chest compression depth of 1 inch.
   2. After each shock, the pulse should be checked before beginning chest compressions.
   3. Chest compressions-to-ventilation rate ratio should be 30:2.
   4. Adult CPR can be performed using one hand.
8. Which of the following is of the highest priority in performing high-quality CPR?
   1. Provide compressions at adequate depth and rate
   2. Minimize interruptions in chest compressions
   3. Avoid excessive ventilation
   4. Avoid leaning between compressions
9. When measuring CPR quality, which of the following provides feedback information to the chest compressor?
   1. Central venous pressure
   2. Pulse oximetry
   3. End-tidal CO_2
   4. Body temperature
10. Which of the following are the only two interventions shown to improve survival in cardiac arrest?
    1. Advanced airway and central line placement
    2. Artificial ventilation and early CPR
    3. Early IV medications and defibrillation
    4. Early CPR and early defibrillation

REFERENCES

American Heart Association (AHA): *Get with the guidelines—resuscitation recognition criteria*, 2014. http://www.heart.org/HEARTORG/HealthcareResearch/GetWithTheGuidelines/GetWithTheGuidelines-Resuscitation/Get-With-The-Guidelines-Resuscitation-Recognition-Criteria_UCM_433238_Article.jsp. Accessed September 15, 2014.

Berg RA, et al: Part 5: adult basic life support: 2010 American Heart Association Guidelines for Cardiopulmonary Resuscitation and Emergency Cardiovascular Care, *Circulation* 122(Suppl 3):S685, 2010a.

Berg RA, et al: Part 13: pediatric basic life support: 2010 American Heart Association Guidelines for Cardiopulmonary Resuscitation and Emergency Cardiovascular Care, *Circulation* 122(Suppl 3):S862, 2010b.

Haskell SE, Atkins DL: Defibrillation in children, *J Emerg Trauma Shock* 3(3):261, 2010.

Jones D, DeVita M, Bellomo R: Rapid-response teams, *N Engl J Med* 365(2):139, 2011.

Meaney P, et al: Cardiopulmonary resuscitation quality: [corrected] improving cardiac resuscitation inside and outside the hospital: a consensus statement from the American Heart Association, *Circulation* 128(4):417, 2013.

CHAPTER

30

Palliative Care

 **EVOLVE WEBSITE/EVOLVE RESOURCES LIST**

http://evolve.elsevier.com/Perry/nursinginterventions
Audio Glossary • Checklists • Review Questions

Nurses play a vital role in helping patients with chronic, life-limiting illnesses maintain the best possible quality of life (QOL) by providing expert palliative care and helping patients reach peaceful deaths at the end of life. The goal of palliative care is to prevent and relieve the suffering of patients and family caregivers facing serious, life-limiting illness by early identification, diagnosis, and treatment of pain and other physical, psychological, and spiritual symptoms (Lynch et al., 2011). Patients of all ages with any diagnosis can receive symptom management with palliative care throughout the duration of their illness, even as they seek treatment and curative interventions. As a patient's condition changes, the goals of care may shift away from curing an illness to care completely focused on symptom management and maintaining the highest possible QOL. Ideally, patients who receive palliative care would move seamlessly into hospice care when they no longer benefit from curative treatments (Fig. 30-1).

Patients, family members, and health care professionals sometimes resist palliative care because of a lack of understanding about its benefits or the mistaken belief that palliative care is used only at the end of life (Matsuyama et al., 2011; Melvin, 2010). You can offer care alternatives and meaningful education when you understand the similarities and differences between palliative and hospice care (Box 30-1). Because end of life care is an excellent example of palliative care, the skills in this chapter focus on nursing care at the end of life.

PATIENT-CENTERED CARE

Patient-centered care lies at the heart of palliative care and hospice nursing. Each person will die in his or her own way, influenced by culture, religion, ethnicity, availability of financial resources, belief systems, and key relationships. As the plan of care shifts toward patient comfort and QOL, less emphasis is placed on following medical regimens. Listen carefully to patients' and family members' descriptions of their needs and wishes, and set nursing care priorities accordingly. Think creatively about how to help patients live as well as possible as they approach the end of life. For example, you might extend visiting hours in a hospital setting to meet the needs of a family to be together as a loved one dies. When you provide palliative care, you should develop the ability to understand, acknowledge, and be present with people experiencing intense and changing emotional reactions to their situation. Compassion and attentiveness are conveyed in many ways, including the therapeutic use of touch (Fig. 30-2), active listening, or silently sitting with a patient (Andrus, 2010).

Spiritual concerns arise in situations of serious illness and impending death. All patients, including individuals who do not practice a particular religion, have spiritual strengths, needs, and practices. The terms *spirituality* and *religion* are often used interchangeably and for many people are closely related. However, there are important differences in these terms. Religion refers to a person's specific beliefs and

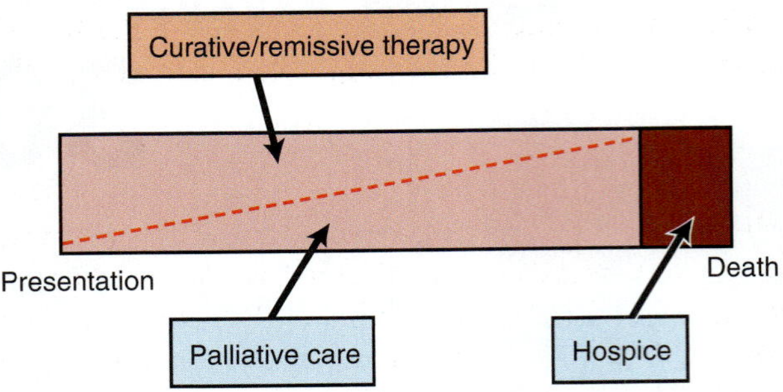

FIG 30-1 Palliative care and hospice. (From Emanuel L et al: The education in palliative and end of life care [EPEC] curriculum: The EPEC Project, 2003, Northwestern University Feinberg School of Medicine.)

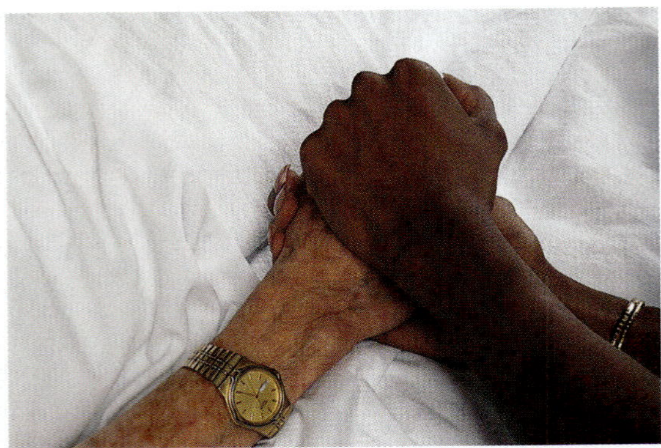

FIG 30-2 Touch can communicate caring and compassion.

behaviors associated with a religious tradition. Spirituality refers to a dynamic dimension of human life, expressed in a person's search for meaning and hope. Spirituality also includes the way people connect with their deeper selves, other people, their communities, nature, and what they consider to be a Higher Being or Holy Other (Edwards et al., 2010; Milligan, 2011). Explore a patient's spirituality by organizing a patient-centered nursing assessment focused on four conceptual areas: meaning, hope, community, and a sense of the Holy Other (Box 30-2).

Cultural sensitivity is crucial in providing patient-centered care at the end of life. A patient's culturally influenced health care beliefs and practices, communication patterns, and family structures affect the dying process (Bullock, 2011; Fiorelli and Jenkins, 2012). To provide appropriate care, look beyond your own cultural assumptions and preconceived ideas and focus on the needs of the patient and family and their specific cultural practices. Be especially aware of religious diversity in end-of-life care (Box 30-3). People with the same religion have varying beliefs or practices and may adhere more or less strictly to their beliefs.

A patient-centered care approach allows patients to communicate their preferences clearly for end of life care. An advance directive provides a patient with a mechanism to make personal values and wishes known and guide others in making care decisions when the patient can no longer participate (e.g., overwhelming illness, unconsciousness, or sedating drugs). Advance directives are written documents such as living wills or durable powers of attorney for health care, which designate a patient-appointed representative. In a living will, patients express their wishes concerning the use

---

BOX 30-1   SIMILARITIES AND DIFFERENCES BETWEEN PALLIATIVE AND HOSPICE CARE

Similarities
- Prioritize for quality of life and relief from pain and other distressing symptoms.
- Integrate physical, psychological, social, and spiritual dimensions into plan of care.
- Affirm life and regard dying as a normal process.
- Involve the patient and family members as active participants in all decisions and care.
- Rely on the expertise of an interdisciplinary team for planning and implementing care.
- Appropriate for all patients, regardless of diagnosis, age, or setting.

Differences
- Palliative care is used in varying extent at any time during an illness. Hospice care is designed exclusively for patients near the end of life.
- Palliative care is often used in conjunction with curative interventions, whereas patients who receive hospice care can no longer pursue curative care.
- Palliative care helps people living with chronic illness over an extended period of time rather than the shorter time frame (approximately 6 to 12 months) designated for hospice.

BOX 30-2   ASSESSING THE SPIRITUAL DIMENSION

Meaning
- What gives your life meaning and purpose in your current situation?
- What are your goals? What do you still want to achieve?
- What do you live for now?

Hope
- What do you hope for right now?
- How have your hopes changed?
- What gives you hope during difficult times?

Community
- Who are the people most important to you?
- Who gives you comfort in difficult times?
- Are you able to participate in community activities (i.e., church, family, friends)?

Sense of Holy Other or God
- What is God like for you? What is your concept of that which is larger than yourself?
- Is religion or God significant to you? If yes, describe how.
- What religious practices or spiritual rituals are meaningful to you?

of extraordinary medical procedures, artificial nutrition and fluids, comfort measures, life-support interventions, or other care preferences. Because laws relating to advance directives vary from state to state, know the state laws in which you practice. Facilities usually have policies and sample forms for advance directives to help patients and families in their deliberations. Patients should give copies of completed advance directives to their health care providers and responsible family members and request that their advance directives be placed in their medical record. If a patient expresses his or her wish to forego cardiopulmonary resuscitation (CPR) in an advance directive, a health care provider must also write a "do not resuscitate" (DNR) order in the medical chart. Because discussions about care decisions are very sensitive and emotional for patients and families, provide a quiet setting for conversation and participate when your involvement is appropriate. Recognize that cultural, ethnic, and religious values influence the likelihood that a patient will complete an advance directive (Zager and Yancy, 2011).

End of life care poses many challenging ethical questions, including a patient's right to have assisted dying, use of artificial food and hydration, pain management, or the appropriate use of technology. To ensure that you are providing patient-centered care in ethical deliberations, listen carefully and nonjudgmentally to concerns of patients and family caregivers (Clabots, 2012). Patients, family caregivers, and members of the interdisciplinary team determine the best course of action by having meaningful conversations together.

SAFETY

Patients who are seriously ill experience decreased muscle strength and limited endurance. However, they may prefer to get out of bed for meals or to walk to the bathroom as long as possible. Guard against falls by having patients use appropriate assistive devices for walking. Remain with patients until they are safely seated or lying down. Patients at the end of life also lose the ability to chew and swallow safely (D'Arcy, 2012). Place a patient who wants to eat or drink in an upright position and offer small bites of food or sips of water slowly to avoid aspiration (see Chapter 12). Be sure that the call bell system is available at all times, and consider calls as a high priority.

In some facilities, patients who do not want to be resuscitated (DNR) wear a wrist bracelet that alerts care providers that they should not start CPR when the patient's heart or breathing stops. Identify a patient with DNR status by using two identifiers (i.e., name and birthday or name and account number, according to facility policy). Compare identifiers with information on the patient's identification bracelet. Placing a DNR bracelet on the wrong patient may lead to unintentional death or the resuscitation of a patient against

---

<table>
<tr><td colspan="2" style="background:green;color:white">BOX 30-3   SOME RELIGIOUS PRACTICES RELATED TO DEATH AND DYING</td></tr>
<tr><td>

Judaism

Persons dying may want to hear prayers and scripture at the time of death. After death, there should be minimal handling of the body by non-Jews. A family member may stay with the body until burial. Close the eyes after death. It is customary for burial to occur within 24 hours except on the Sabbath. Families participate in a mourning period during which grief is expressed openly and in keeping with ritual. Because life is valued as a gift of God, all efforts to continue life are supported, even when it appears that there is no hope, especially in Orthodox Judaism. In some, but not all, types of Judaism, cremation, autopsy, and embalming are avoided.

Christianity

Christians believe in life after death and eternal life. Some may request rituals of confession, laying on of hands, anointing the sick, baptism, or Holy Communion. Prayer and reading from the Bible may be appropriate. There may be a period of viewing the body or a wake before burial, and funerals or memorial services are common. Cremation, autopsy, and embalming are usually permitted.

Islam

Muslims believe in eternal life and the will of God (Allah). Patients may wish to face Mecca (the East) as they are dying. Cleanliness and modesty are very important. Regular prayer five times a day should continue as long as possible. Loved ones usually remain with the dying person 24 hours a day.

</td><td>

Non-Muslims should wear gloves when touching the body. Cover the body with a plain sheet until a person of Muslim faith can give the ritual bath and wrap the body in a white cloth. Burial is usually in a Muslim cemetery within 24 hours. Autopsy is usually forbidden, but organ donation is becoming more acceptable.

Hinduism

Hindus believe in one supreme deity and in lesser gods with powers and interests in specific areas of life. Core beliefs include community connectedness, reincarnation, and karma (how one has lived in this world affects how one might return in the next one). Patients may want the presence of a Brahmin priest who may chant prayers. Only the family should touch the body after death, and they are responsible for washing and preparing it. Cremation is traditional, but autopsy and organ donation are not commonly practiced.

Buddhism

In Buddhism, the state of the mind at the time of death is relevant in the person's rebirth into a new life. The goal of life and death is to reach the eternal state of nirvana, or inner peace and happiness. A patient may want to remain conscious to be able to meditate or contemplate the dying process. Allow for a peaceful environment at the time of death, and notify a Buddhist priest. Time from death to burial varies from 3 to 7 days. Mourners wear white to the funeral. Cremation and autopsy are usually allowed.

</td></tr>
</table>

Adapted from Sherman D: Culture and spirituality as domains of quality palliative care. In Matzo M, Sherman D, editors: *Palliative care nursing: quality care to the end of life*, ed 3, New York, 2010, Springer, p 26.

his or her wishes. Use the same patient identification methods before sending a body to the morgue. Improper identification of a body may lead to a serious miscommunication with family members.

After a death, the nurse communicates to others who will care for the patient's body (e.g., transporters, morgue attendants, and funeral home employees) of potential infection risks. The bodies of patients that pose a high infectious risk should be carefully marked, and the body should be prepared after death to avoid leakage of infectious body fluids.

EVIDENCE-BASED PRACTICE

Epiphaniou E, et al: Adjusting to the caregiving role: the importance of coping and support, *Int J Palliat Nurs* 18(11):541, 2012.

Stajduhar K, Funk L, Outcalt L: Family caregiver learning—how family caregivers learn to provide care at the end of life: a qualitative secondary analysis of four datasets, *Palliat Med* 27(7):657, 2013.

Family dynamics significantly influence the QOL for most patients with serious, life-limiting illness. Family caregivers assume an increasing role as direct care providers at the end of life. Additionally, you enhance your ability to care for patients when you understand the families' preferences and lived experiences better. Qualitative studies involving interviews with family caregivers of patients at the end of life revealed two areas of importance: timely, meaningful communication and support of family values and preferences (Epiphaniou et al., 2012; Stajduhar et al., 2013).

- Help family caregivers optimize their existing coping strategies by providing emotional support and understanding, characterized by conveying respect and dignity.
- Communicate with family caregivers at regular intervals, keep family members updated, and provide guided teaching sessions related to practical information on the physical and emotional aspects of caregiving.

- Family caregivers appreciate having a quiet, private environment during the dying process. Work to create peaceful environments, especially in busy hospital settings.
- Allow time for family caregivers to share their caregiving experiences and identify their learning needs.

NURSES' SELF-CARE: ADDRESSING COMPASSION FATIGUE

To nurture your capacity to remain empathically engaged with patients and family members, you must also care for yourself physically, spiritually, and emotionally. Nurses who are routinely involved in care of seriously ill and dying patients are positively affected and changed by their intimate experiences with patients and families (Sinclair, 2011). However, over time and after many losses, you may feel overwhelmed or struggle with feelings of distress or sadness. Sharing in others' grief, sadness, helplessness, and loss can lead to compassion fatigue (Showalter, 2010). Compassion fatigue leaves you feeling tired, depressed, angry, "stressed out," and eventually apathetic and leads to an inability to relate well to people in your care (Boertje, 2013; Warden, 2012).

To prevent or manage compassion fatigue, talk about your feelings and experiences with a trusted friend or peer. Identify ways in which you can work with others to address workplace barriers to effective self-care. Sometimes a debriefing after a particularly long or difficult death helps you feel support and gain perspective. Regularly practice stress management techniques such as relaxation exercise when feeling stressed, physical exercise, nutritious eating patterns, humor, hobbies, and adequate sleep. Strengthen yourself spiritually with meditation, prayer, or consultation with a spiritual care provider (Thornton, 2010). It may help to attend the funeral of a patient with whom you shared special bonds. You might also gain insight by reflecting on your own personal beliefs and feelings about death and loss.

SKILL 30.1 SUPPORTING PATIENTS AND FAMILIES IN GRIEF

In end of life situations, patients and family members experience intense feelings such as anxiety, sadness, regret, or relief. They ask questions of spiritual significance about the meaning of life, pain, suffering, and loss of personal power and control. In short, they experience grief, an intense emotional and behavioral response to perceived and actual losses. Grief experiences often begin before a patient dies. Survivors grieve as they anticipate a loss and continue to feel the grief after the patient dies. Most people gradually move through their grief and learn to adjust to life without their loved one. You will journey with patients and family members in their grief and provide emotional and spiritual support.

ASSESSMENT

1. Limit your initial grief assessment to concerns most important to the patient and family. Expand the assessment through observation, and explore concerns as they arise. *Rationale: Discussing emotional and spiritual concerns may arouse uncomfortable feelings, anxiety, or uncertainty. Refrain from probing issues before people are ready to talk about them.*
2. Discuss spiritual and emotional concerns at an appropriate time in a quiet place and in an unrushed manner. *Rationale: People participate when timing and location feel appropriate for them.*

3. Observe for physical symptoms and behaviors that might be related to grief. *Rationale: Grief might cause insomnia, change in appetite, isolation, angry outbursts, anxiety, or frequent crying. In nonverbal patients, restlessness may indicate emotional distress.*

4. Listen for statements that might indicate spiritual distress, such as: "I haven't accomplished what I wanted to in life"; "I must have done something wrong to deserve this." *Rationale: Spiritual matters are expressed in religious or nonreligious language and should be recognized for their spiritual significance.*

5. Identify barriers to expression of feelings. *Rationale: Lack of privacy, pain, stress, distrust, or fatigue may create barriers to self-expression.*

6. Gather information about the person's usual coping style, relationship to the deceased, and the nature of the loss. *Rationale: A person's familiar coping patterns are of more use near the end of life than trying new strategies or strategies designed by others.*

7. Identify spiritual and religious needs, resources, and strengths. *Rationale: Acts of forgiveness, reconciliation, blessing, and community often help.*

8. Ask patient or family members if they would like to meet with a priest, rabbi, pastor, or the facility's spiritual care provider to obtain a full spiritual assessment. *Rationale:*

Patients and family members may benefit from professionals' assessment skills.

PLANNING

Expected Outcomes focus on providing emotional and spiritual support for patients and family members in the grief process.

1. Patient and family members share feelings and grief responses related to perceived and actual losses.
2. Patient and family members identify sources of strength and hope.
3. Patient and family members express satisfaction with emotional and spiritual aspects of palliative and end of life care.

Delegation and Collaboration

The skill of psychosocial and spiritual care cannot be delegated to nursing assistive personnel (NAP). The nurse instructs the NAP to:

- Watch for specific changes in patient's affect or interaction, maintaining a respectful, quiet demeanor when interacting with patient and family members.
- Report notable changes in patient's affect or statements indicating distress or suffering.

IMPLEMENTATION *for* SUPPORTING PATIENTS AND FAMILIES IN GRIEF

STEPS	RATIONALE
1. **See Standard Protocol (inside front cover).**	
2. Provide emotional support for grieving patients and family members.	
a. Use active listening, therapeutic communication skills, and quiet presence to help people feel and express their grief. Validate that grief feelings are normal.	Listening to patients and family members without interruption or trying to fix things validates their feelings (Sandor, 2012).
b. Allow sufficient time for patients and family members to have conversations when they are ready.	Patients and family members may be in different phases of grief or have unresolved conflicts (Newson, 2012).
c. Respect individual differences in willingness to share concerns. Be alert for opportunities to have discussions when patient is ready.	Some people share feelings more than others. As a trusting relationship develops, people may share what they have been working on privately (Wittenberg-Lyles et al., 2010).
d. Explore realistic goals and offer practical help to address immediate problems. Do not focus on long-term problems that cannot be solved at the time.	Goal setting gives patients and family members a sense of control and achievement even in limited circumstances.
3. Promote emotional well-being.	
a. Talk with patients and family members about fears, stressors, anxieties, and care options. Assure them that they will not be abandoned.	Patients feel valued and respected when they are included in discussions. Many patients fear being alone or abandoned.
b. Consult interdisciplinary team for help with emotional, spiritual, or psychological issues.	Creative team approaches enhance care. Patients and family members may benefit from professional consultation.

Continued

STEPS	RATIONALE
c. Administer prescribed antianxiety medication for significant depression or anxiety.	Although sadness is normal with significant loss, severe anxiety or depression decreases QOL (Handsaker et al.,, 2012).

4. Promote spiritual well-being.
   a. Facilitate prayer, meditation, or reading a patient's spiritual texts.
   b. Consult with spiritual care team.
	Spiritual activities sustain patients' hope and help them find peace and reconciliation (Milligan, 2011).
	A spiritual care professional can design individualized interventions.

c. Use therapeutic presence and active listening. Provide information and answer questions in an honest, helpful manner. **d.** Honor cultural and religious beliefs and rituals. People without a religious affiliation may have rituals for remembering and honoring their loved one.	Allowing patients to talk about their feelings and providing assistance and information promotes hope and sense of community (Revier et al., 2012). Religious and cultural beliefs provide opportunity for closure, community support, and belief that the dying process conformed to one's own valued customs and behaviors (Sherman, 2010).
5. Assist patient and family members in advance planning and involve them in care decisions. Identify who will manage the patient's affairs and make funeral plans.	Being involved in planning minimizes fear and loss of control in decision making and increases the sense of having one's death supported and honored.
6. See Completion Protocol (inside front cover).	

EVALUATION

1. Evaluate degree of relief from grief and emotional and spiritual symptoms.
2. Monitor effectiveness of decision making related to important concerns.
3. Observe quality of interactions among patient, family members, and caregivers.
4. Evaluate patient's and family members' satisfaction with emotional and spiritual support.

Unexpected Outcomes and Related Interventions

1. Patient continues to have emotional symptoms and spiritual distress.
   a. Collaborate with interdisciplinary team to develop new strategies. Make referrals as needed.
   b. Talk with patient and family members about what actions they believe may be helpful.
2. Patient and family members experience ethical conflicts or disagreements in decision making.
   a. Clarify patient's wishes or consult patient advance directives.
   b. Use active listening to identify and clarify the issues affecting decision making.

Recording and Reporting

- Record in nurses' notes interventions for psychological and spiritual grief responses, including patient response; patient and family preferences; family presence and involvement; and evidence of unresolved issues and concerns.
- Report when a patient or family member requests therapeutic intervention from social worker, counselor, or spiritual care provider.

Sample Documentation

1500 Patient stated that she wanted to talk more openly with family members about her impending death and wants to make decisions about her funeral and disposition of her possessions. Requested that a conversation with her pastor and family members be arranged for tomorrow afternoon. Patient states she knows this will be difficult but believes that decisions must be made.

Special Considerations
Pediatric

- Encourage parents to share information about their child's coping style and the degree of openness with which death is addressed in the family.
- Decisions to end treatment can be very difficult when children are involved.
- Many children know they are dying and are able to have age-appropriate conversations about their feelings and fears.

Geriatric

- Older adults have experienced multiple losses in their lives, which may affect their reactions to subsequent losses and their grief response.
- Do not assume that older adults accept or have addressed their feelings about death.
- Older adults may have fewer relatives and friends available to offer support.

Home Care

- Family members need support and role modeling for talking about emotional, relational, and spiritual issues.

• Family members may have ambivalent feelings about having a loved one die at home. Encourage them to express their concerns.

• Family members need respite care to meet caregiving demands and to attend to their own grief and responses to loss.

SKILL 30.2 SYMPTOM MANAGEMENT AT END OF LIFE

Palliative care at the end of life involves caring for the whole person—body, mind, and spirit. Do not underestimate the importance of attending to a patient's physical needs. Patients and family members identify relief from pain and other troublesome physical symptoms as a high priority in end of life care. Their grief and response to loss are based in part on memories of their loved one's care and whether or not it was free from suffering (Dosser and Kennedy, 2012). Lessen the fear and uncertainty often associated with the dying process by helping patients and family members understand and anticipate the common physical changes associated with impending death (Table 30-1).

ASSESSMENT

1. During assessment, do not impose judgment on a patient's reports of pain and discomfort. *Rationale: A symptom is what a patient says it is, not what the nurse says it is. Patients with persistent pain or other symptoms often exhibit behaviors different from patients experiencing symptoms of acute onset.*
2. Assess each symptom for onset, precipitating factors, quality, severity, and anything that has helped to relieve symptoms in the past (see Chapter 13). In nonverbal patients, look for facial grimacing and restlessness or changes in breathing as indicators of distress, and validate with family members. *Rationale: A full assessment determines the level of distress for planning patient-specific interventions.*
3. Involve family members in symptom assessment. *Rationale: Patients near the end of life may be unable to self-report. Family members who know patient behavior patterns provide valuable assessment information.*

PLANNING

Expected Outcomes focus on promoting comfort, autonomy, family involvement, and dignity throughout the dying experience.

1. Patient demonstrates relief from pain and other physical symptoms.
2. Patient and family members participate in end of life care decisions as desired.
3. Patient and family members are involved in care, based on their abilities and preferences (Fig. 30-3).
4. Patient and family members express satisfaction with all aspects of palliative care.

TABLE 30-1	PHYSICAL CHANGES COMMONLY ASSOCIATED WITH IMPENDING DEATH
SIGNS AND SYMPTOMS	**INTERVENTIONS**
Coolness and color changes in extremities	Use slippers or socks; cover person with light blankets, not tucked tightly over toes.
Increased periods of sleeping and unresponsiveness	Sit with patient, perhaps holding a hand and talking quietly; speak to patient even though there may be a lack of response.
Bowel or bladder incontinence	Change bedding as appropriate, use bed pads, and give frequent skin care. An indwelling urinary catheter may be indicated because of patient fatigue or skin breakdown.
Congestion and increased secretions	Explain that noisy breathing is not uncomfortable for patient. Elevate head of bed; turn the head to drain secretions. Avoid suctioning.
Restlessness or disorientation	Speak calmly. Gently massage hands or feet. Play soothing music and lower lights.
Decreased intake of food or fluids	Do not force patient to eat or drink. Offer ice chips, popsicles, or sips of fluid. Apply lip balm and give oral care.
Decreased urine output	Consider advocating for the removal of indwelling urinary catheters. Change bed pads as needed.
Altered breathing patterns (apnea, labored, and irregular breathing)	Elevate the head, hold a hand, and use quiet voice tones. Administer prescribed anxiolytics and opioids for pain and apprehension. Explain common changes in breathing patterns at end of life to decrease concerns.

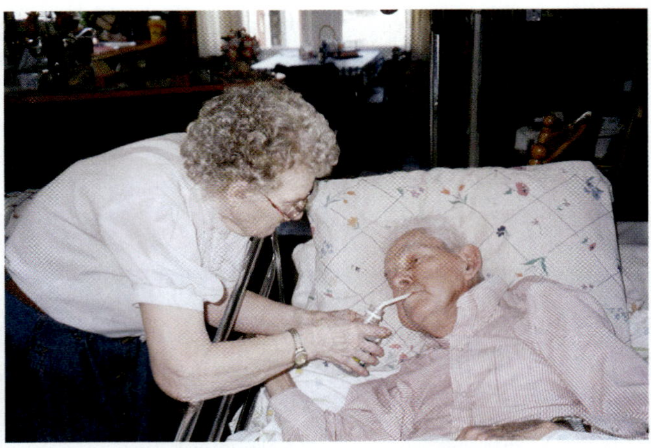

FIG 30-3 Encourage family involvement in care.

Delegation and Collaboration

Providing physical care activities for patients receiving palliative care may be delegated to nursing assistive personnel (NAP). The nurse instructs the NAP to:

- Watch for specific signs of patient discomfort or loss of skin integrity and to use gentle touch and quiet tone of voice.
- Report unrelieved patient discomfort and patient preferences for comfort measures or positioning.

Equipment

- Personal care items most preferred by patient
- Comfort and hygiene products
- Clean gloves

IMPLEMENTATION *for* SYMPTOM MANAGEMENT AT THE END OF LIFE

STEPS	RATIONALE
1. **See Standard Protocol (inside front cover).**	
2. Promote pain relief (see Chapter 13).	
a. Administer prescribed analgesics around the clock (ATC), and give extra doses for breakthrough pain.	ATC dosing is the most effective method for maintaining adequate pain control. Using breakthrough doses minimizes pain episodes without overmedicating (Paice, 2010).
b. Collaborate with health care provider to consider use of adjuvant pain medications (e.g., antidepressants and anticonvulsants for neuropathic pain and antiinflammatory drugs for bone pain).	Adjuvant medications can enhance opioid effectiveness or treat pain not relieved by opioids (Paice, 2010).
c. Advocate for the most effective, least invasive route for analgesic administration.	The best route is based on patient's level of consciousness, gastrointestinal and circulatory status, type of medication, and ease of delivery.
d. Monitor effectiveness of medication regimen and adverse side effects at regular intervals.	Patients often need larger opioid doses as disease progresses, drug tolerance builds, and symptoms increase. Pain medication doses may have to be decreased when liver and kidney function declines. Treating symptoms before they worsen ensures more consistent pain relief (D'Arcy, 2012).
e. Monitor for constipation, sedation (usually transitory), nausea, vomiting, or dry mouth.	These are side effects of opioids and sedatives. Excessive sedation may require decrease in opioid dose.
f. Use nonpharmacological methods of pain control (e.g., relaxation, repositioning, heat or cold, massage, diversion).	Enhance the effectiveness of pain medication and allow patients to participate in their symptom management (Mariano, 2010).
3. Provide regular skin care and take action to prevent pressure ulcers (see Chapter 25).	
a. Reposition at least every 2 hours, more often or less depending on patient comfort. Use pressure-reducing devices.	Skin integrity is compromised by immobility, poor nutrition, and weight loss. Immobility and prolonged pressure on an area cause pain, skin breakdown, and stiffness.
b. Apply alcohol-free lotion as needed and desired to hands, feet, or back.	Local massage may increase patient comfort.

> **SAFE PATIENT CARE** Do not massage any reddened area on patient's skin. Massaging causes breaks in the surface of the skin capillaries and increases risk of skin breakdown.

STEPS	RATIONALE

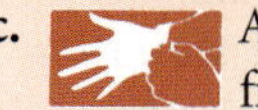 **c.** Apply clean gloves. Cleanse perineal area frequently if incontinent.

Promotes skin integrity and patient dignity and well-being.

4. Provide nutrition and hydration; adjust to changing patterns at end of life.

  a. Offer patient preferred food and liquids as tolerated, slowly, and in small amounts at patient-determined times.

Anorexia and difficulty swallowing are common at end of life. Patients are more likely to enjoy eating favorite foods (D'Arcy, 2012).

  b. Apply clean gloves. Provide oral care q2h or as requested: offer frequent sips of water; use soft toothbrush to brush teeth and oral cavity gently; rinse mouth with diluted salt water after eating and at bedtime (usually three to four times daily).

Oral care reduces oral bacteria, mouth odor, and bad taste. A clean mouth gives a sense of well-being.

  c. Avoid offering foods with strong odors.

Strong smells can intensify nausea.

  d. Allow patient to decide what and when to eat or drink. Accept patient's refusal of food or liquids.

Gradual dehydration may be a natural way for the body to decrease distressing symptoms, such as congestion, excess secretions, shortness of breath, vomiting, and edema (D'Arcy, 2012).

  e. Inform family members about normal decrease in appetite at end of life. Help family shift hope focus and find other ways to help.

Talking about the issue reduces family distress. Offering food and fluid symbolizes life, love, and nurturing. No longer sharing meals can be a difficult adjustment.

5. Assist with changing elimination patterns.

  a. Administer prescribed stool softeners and laxatives, especially with use of opioid analgesia.

Opioid analgesia, inactivity, and decreased fluid intake contribute to constipation (Lentz and McMillan, 2010).

  b. Apply clean gloves. Use bedside commode as long as possible.

The natural position for defecation promotes elimination and maintains patient autonomy (Kyle, 2010).

6. Promote comfort with breathing patterns.

  a. Keep head of bed elevated.

The diaphragm can move more easily in sitting position than when lying flat.

  b. Increase air movement with fans or open windows.

Airflow stimulates trigeminal nerve in the cheek, which inhibits feelings of dyspnea. Use of oxygen is not routine at end of life (Freeman, 2013).

  c. Use actions that conserve energy, and balance periods of rest and activity.

Reducing activity decreases patient oxygen use and minimizes shortness of breath.

  d. Offer prescribed oral, intravenous, or inhaled opioids for severe dyspnea and benzodiazepines for anxiety.

Medications decrease anxiety and may alter perception of breathlessness.

  e. Decrease anxiety related to shortness of breath by massage therapy, relaxation therapy, and listening to music.

Feelings of suffocation are very distressing and frightening. Use multiple methods for symptom relief (Freeman, 2013).

  f. Address family caregivers' distress with noisy breathing ("death rattle") at end of life. Educate family that patient cannot clear throat and is not choking or uncomfortable. Try elevating head of bed, side positioning, or use of anticholinergic drugs. Suctioning is rarely indicated for noisy breathing.

Noise is caused by secretions at back of throat rattling with breath airflow and relaxed tongue. Offering support and education help relieve family caregivers' distress, even though few interventions work consistently well. Anticholinergic drugs can be used but have side effects. Suctioning increases discomfort and does not help (Twomey and Dowling, 2013).

7. See Completion Protocol (inside front cover).

EVALUATION

1. Perform frequent ongoing evaluation of symptom relief before and after each intervention.
2. Observe level of patient's and family members' participation and comfort in giving care.
3. Ask patient and family members to describe their satisfaction with and knowledge of symptom management interventions.

Unexpected Outcomes and Related Interventions

1. Pain or other symptoms are not well managed with prescribed treatment plan.
   a. Collaborate with interdisciplinary team for alternative medications or adjuvant therapies.
   b. Talk with patient and family members about what they believe may be helpful.
   c. Consider emotional or spiritual issues that may interfere with symptom management.
2. Family members are not present or participating in care.
   a. Determine cause of nonparticipation. Consider cultural influences on participation. Provide information to increase family members' comfort with care interventions.
   b. Maintain a nonjudgmental attitude and support patient and family coping styles and relationships.

Recording and Reporting

- Record in nurses' notes interventions for pain and symptom management, including patient response; changes in physical, mental, emotional, or spiritual status; patient and family preferences; family presence and involvement; evidence of unresolved issues and concerns with physical care or patient symptoms.
- Report when a previously alert patient becomes unresponsive.

Sample Documentation

1500 Patient less responsive to verbal stimuli with occasional periods of restlessness. No oral intake this shift. Mouth care provided every 2 hours. Unable to rate pain. Hospital pastor and grandchildren visiting. Family members tearful and verbalize awareness that death is near. A daughter wishes to remain with patient until the time of death.

Special Considerations
Pediatric

- Treat family and child as one unit. Encourage parents to stay with child and participate in care as much as desired or possible.
- Consider child's age and developmental level in care planning, symptom management, and sibling support (Crozier and Hancock, 2012).

Geriatric

- Older patients may have more than one disease process and multiple physical symptoms and medications.
- Drug metabolism changes with increased age, requiring careful monitoring to determine proper dose.
- Older adults may experience pain, respiratory distress, and confusion at end of life, but evidence suggests less than optimal symptom management in elderly patients (Derby, O'Mahony, and Tickoo, 2010).

Home Care

- Primary family caregivers need ongoing teaching and support.
- Educate family caregivers about symptom management approaches and when to seek help.
- Volunteers may be needed to give family members respite time.

SKILL 30.3 CARE OF THE BODY AFTER DEATH

After a patient dies, the designated health care provider, often a physician or nurse practitioner, certifies the death and records the time and actions taken at the time of death in the medical record. The health care provider may request permission from the family for an autopsy or postmortem examination, although this is less likely with an anticipated death or when the cause of death is known. An autopsy consent form must be signed by the appropriate family member and the health care provider. Autopsies normally do not delay burial. You are responsible for providing respectful, thorough care of the body after death. Some family members wish to view the body immediately after death, or they may wish to help with preparing the body. Give family members ample time to say good-bye before transferring the body to the morgue or funeral home. Consider that some family members may have to travel from distant locations.

ASSESSMENT

1. Identify patient using two identifiers (e.g., name and birthday or name and account number) according to facility policy. Compare identifiers with information on patient's identification bracelet. Leave identification (tag) in place on the body as directed by facility policy. *Rationale: Ensures correct patient. Complies with The Joint Commission standards and improves patient safety (TJC, 2014). Ensures proper identification of body in morgue, autopsy room, and funeral home.*
2. Assess for presence of family members or significant others, and determine whether they have been informed of patient's death. Determine who is responsible for any legal matters after death. *Rationale: Assists in coordinating facility-based procedures for care after death.*

3. Assess family members' grief response. *Rationale: Determines level of support and guidance needed.*
4. Determine if patient is an organ and tissue donor. Federal law mandates that family members be given a chance to authorize organ and tissue donation. Call organ and tissue request and procurement team (consult facility policy). *Rationale: Trained requestors usually approach families for donation and manage care of the body for successful organ retrieval. Successful recovery of organs and tissues depends on skillful and timely requests.*
5. Assess patient's religious preference and cultural heritage. *Rationale: Religious or cultural preferences for body preparation may require changes in routine procedures.*
6. Determine if autopsy is ordered. *Rationale: The removal of tubes, drains, catheters, and lines may be altered or prohibited with an autopsy. Consult facility guidelines.*
7. Assess the general condition of the body. Note presence of dressing, tubes, and medical equipment. *Rationale: Validates tissue damage and type of postmortem care required.*

▌PLANNING

Expected Outcomes focus on preventing injury to the body and facilitating grieving of family and friends.
1. Survivors are able to grieve in a manner consistent with religious, cultural, and personal values.
2. Patient's body is prepared in a respectful manner consistent with cultural and religious practices and with family involvement if desired.

3. Patient's body is free of new skin damage and optimally prepared for the mortuary.

Delegation and Collaboration

The skill of providing emotional and supportive care at the time of death cannot be delegated to nursing assistive personnel (NAP). NAP can provide physical care. The nurse instructs the NAP to:
- Follow specific religious, cultural, or physical measures needed for postmortem care of the body.
- Prepare the room for family to view the body, if desired.
- Report specific family needs promptly.

Equipment
- Clean gloves, gown, and other protective clothing for caregivers
- Clean gown or disposable gown for body (consult facility policy)
- Washbasin, washcloth, warm water, and bath towel
- Absorbent pads
- Plastic bag for hazardous waste disposal
- Body bag or shroud kit (consult facility policy)
- Paper tape and gauze dressing
- Bag or receptacle for patient's clothing and other items to be returned to family
- Envelope for valuables
- Identification tags as specified by facility policy

IMPLEMENTATION *for* CARE OF THE BODY AFTER DEATH

STEPS	RATIONALE
1. **See Standard Protocol (inside front cover).**	
2. Place pillow under head or slightly elevate head of bed.	Decreases pooling of blood and discoloration of the face while you make other preparations.
3. Consult facility policy for guidelines if tissue, or organ, or body donation or an autopsy has been requested.	Retrieval of tissues (e.g., corneas, skin) and an autopsy require special body preparation.
4. Determine if the patient had an infectious disease and proceed by following infection control guidelines and universal precautions.	Withdrawal of lines or tubes may cause oozing of blood or release of body fluids that can be source of infection to others who will handle the body.
5. Discuss routine postmortem care with family members. Ask if they wish to participate or give instructions concerning their cultural or religious practices. Offer support from spiritual care provider in facility.	Including the family facilitates culturally sensitive patient-centered care. Family members may welcome the presence of a spiritual care professional.
6. Ensure as much environmental privacy as possible before beginning postmortem care.	Providing private space gives family a respectful place for rituals, body preparation, and grief expressions.
7. Do not rush. Proceed at a pace that honors family's cultural, spiritual, and personal preferences and expectations.	A rushed pace may seem disrespectful and increases family distress. Allow time for reflection and saying good-bye.
8. Apply protective clothing and clean gloves before beginning physical care.	Be consistent with universal precautions to avoid spread of infection. Some cultural practices prohibit direct touch of body by nonfamily members.

Continued

STEPS	RATIONALE
9. Remove indwelling catheters, tubes, tape, and airways (check facility policy). Disconnect and cap off (no need to remove) intravenous lines. ***Leave all devices in place if autopsy is requested or required.***	Creates a normal, nonmedical appearance for family at time of viewing the body.
10. Remove soiled dressings (except in cases of known infection) and replace with clean gauze dressings using paper tape. Cover puncture wounds with a small dressing.	Helps to control odors caused by microorganisms and creates more acceptable appearance. Paper tape minimizes skin trauma.
11. If the person wore dentures, clean and insert them. If the mouth fails to close, place a rolled-up towel under chin. If dentures do not stay securely in mouth, place in denture cup and transport with body to mortuary.	It is easiest to insert dentures immediately after death. Dentures maintain natural facial expression if body is to be viewed.
12. Close the eyes by gently holding them shut for short time. Some cultures prefer eyes to remain open.	Closed eyes present a more natural appearance in death for many people.
13. Wash body parts soiled by blood, urine, feces, or other drainage with warm water. Place an absorbent pad under patient's perineal area.	Bathing prepares the body for viewing and reduces odors. Relaxation of sphincter muscles at death releases urine or feces.
14. Place a clean gown on patient. Facility policy may require replacement with disposable gown after viewing.	Dressing the patient's body creates a natural, modest, and dignified state for viewing.
15. Brush and comb patient's hair. Remove clips, hairpins, or rubber bands. Respect any preferences or prohibitions before shaving male facial hair. Shaving is forbidden in some religions, or the person may have worn a beard.	Patient should appear well-groomed. Objects can damage or discolor face and scalp. Shaving can sometimes leave facial discoloration.
16. Remove all jewelry. Give personal belongings to designated family member. Exception: If family requests that wedding band be left in place, place a small strip of tape around patient's finger over the ring.	Prevents loss of patient's valuables.
17. Place a sheet or light blanket over the body with only the head and upper shoulders exposed. Remove medical equipment from room. Provide soft lighting and offer chairs. Determine if family prefers to be alone or have a nurse with them during viewing.	Covering the body maintains patient's dignity and respect and limits body exposure. People viewing body are provided with a peaceful, comfortable environment.
18. After body has been viewed, remove hospital linen. Send body to morgue clothed, per facility policy. Place body in body bag with extremities at side and cover with shroud in accordance with facility policy.	Respect is conveyed by not exposing patient's body after death. Tying wrists together can discolor and damage skin on a visible part of the body.
19. Before transport to the morgue, place identification on *outside* of body bag (see facility policy). Identify the patient using two identifiers (i.e., name and birthday or name and account number, according to facility policy). Compare identifiers with information on patient's identification bracelet. Place isolation tag on body bag if applicable.	Ensures proper identification of body and alerts transporters and morgue personnel of potential infectious hazard.
20. Arrange transportation of body to morgue or mortuary.	A body should be kept in a cooled morgue to delay tissue decomposition.
21. Respond to family questions or concerns. Review with family members who they might want to notify of the death. Confirm name of funeral home.	After a death, grieving people may have difficulty remembering details and may appreciate guidance.
22. See Completion Protocol (inside front cover).	

EVALUATION

1. Observe family and significant others' responses to the loss.
2. Ask family members if they believe they received emotional and spiritual support and respect for their cultural or religious practices after the death.
3. Note appearance and condition of patient's skin during preparation of the body.

Unexpected Outcomes and Related Interventions

1. Grieving survivors become immobilized by grief and have difficulty functioning.
   a. Stay calm and unhurried. Allow time for questions and expressions of grief.
   b. Offer spiritual or psychological consultation from interdisciplinary team.
2. Lacerations, bruises, or abrasions are noted on deceased's skin surfaces.
   a. Cleanse areas thoroughly before family viewing.
   b. Inform family of any notable bruises or lacerations that they may see.
   c. Document any new skin tears or breakdown.

Recording and Reporting

- Record in nurses' notes the date and time of death as determined by designated health care professional. Include the time professional notified, name of professional pronouncing death, completion of postmortem care, identification and disposition of body, information provided to significant others, whether autopsy consent (if needed) was signed, and how valuables and personal belongings were handled and who received them. Secure signatures as required by facility policy.
- Report any marks, bruises, or wounds on body before death or observed during care of body.

Sample Documentation

0245   Pronounced dead by health care provider. Wife and daughter present at time of death and assisted with preparation of the body. Family pastor was present, offering support. Two bruises on left forearm, both approximately 1 cm (0.4 inch) in diameter. Funeral home notified of death. Glasses and clothes sent with body to morgue with transport personnel. White-colored metal ring left in place at wife's request, taped to left hand ring finger.

Special Considerations
Pediatric

- Parents need opportunity to hold their deceased child and help with body preparation.
- If parents agree, assess siblings' developmental level and readiness to view their brother's or sister's body.
- In cases of neonatal deaths or stillbirths, many parents appreciate having a picture or lock of hair from their child as a remembrance.

Geriatric

- Some geriatric patients have a limited support group. The nurse may be the person who stays with the patient in the final stages of life.
- For older adults who live in an extended care facility, the residents and staff are often regarded as family members and should be notified of the patient's death.

Home Care

- Many people choose to die at home with hospice care.
- Family caregivers need ongoing education on end of life care, signs of impending death, who to call for help with symptom control, what to do and who to call at the time of death, and how to arrange for transportation of the body.

CRITICAL THINKING EXERCISES

Case Study

A retired schoolteacher with advanced heart failure, has been admitted to the hospital four times in the past year and feels weaker after each hospitalization. He no longer believes that his medical treatments are effective for managing his disease. He is now in the hospital again, and he asks the nurse what he should do if he no longer wants to be admitted to the hospital. His wife says that she is afraid to take care of her husband at home alone.

1. Which of the following responses would be best at this time?
   1. "It sounds like both of you have concerns about what lies ahead."
   2. "It would be very difficult to take care of your husband alone at home. The hospital is the best place for patients who have serious illness."
   3. "Have you talked this over with your doctor? She might be able to tell you more about your medical condition."
   4. "Has anybody talked to you about being admitted into hospice care?"

2. The patient's wife has more questions for you after they received a visit from a nurse specializing in palliative care. Which of the following approaches would be best to further the conversation at this time?
   1. Encourage them to think more positively about possible new medical therapy.
   2. Avoid the discussion because it has to do with medical, not nursing, issues.
   3. Initiate a discussion about advance directives with the patient, family, and health care team.
   4. Ask both of them what they each believe the goals of care should be.
3. The nursing assistive personnel reports that the couple is having an angry discussion, and the patient is crying. What delegation decision should you make, given this information?

Review Questions

1. A patient tells the nurse that she was given information about preparing an advance directive when she entered the hospital. She asks the nurse to explain how advance directives work. Which of the following explanations is accurate?
   1. "Advance directives have to be written documents."
   2. "You can indicate in an advance directive what kind of care you want and do not want if you are unable to speak for yourself."
   3. "Be sure to store your advance directive in a safe deposit box."
   4. "Advance directives are the same across the country."
2. A patient has just entered home hospice care. Which of the following nursing interventions would be best to ensure that the patient will receive patient-centered care?
   1. Talk to the patient and her family caregivers to understand their usual daily routine better
   2. Provide the patient and her family caregivers with a diet that will help her sustain her muscle mass and energy
   3. Ensure that the patient has completed an advance directive
   4. Explain the purposes of all of her medications
3. You are providing postmortem care. Which action should be the highest priority?
   1. Locating the patient's clothing
   2. Transporting the body to the morgue quickly to prevent body decomposition
   3. Providing culturally and religiously sensitive care in body preparation
   4. Providing all postmortem care to protect the family from having to see the body

4. A patient receiving home hospice care wants to get out of bed for meals. What would be your best response to the patient's request, considering patient-centered care and patient safety?
   1. "Maybe you could get up only on special occasions."
   2. "Your muscle strength will decrease as illness progresses. It will be very risky for you to try to walk to the dining room."
   3. "Why don't you let your family bring food into the bedroom to eat with you?"
   4. "Let's talk about how we can work together to help you get safely to the dining room."
5. A nurse begins to prepare the body of a deceased patient for family viewing and transport to the morgue. Place the following actions in proper sequence, beginning with what the nurse should do first.
   a. Wash body parts soiled by blood, urine, feces, or other drainage.
   b. Slightly elevate the head of the bed.
   c. Place a clean gown on the patient.
   d. Apply gloves, gown, or protective barriers as applicable.
   e. Apply fresh dressings to open wounds.
   f. Ask family members if they want to be involved in final preparation of the body.
      1. d, f, a, e, c, b
      2. b, f, d, e, a, c
      3. d, a, f, e, b, c
      4. f, a, d, e, c, b
6. A self-care goal to avoid developing compassion fatigue would include:
   1. Maintain life balance, and reflect on the meaning of your work
   2. Learn not to take loss so seriously
   3. Realize that you are responsible for everything that happens on the job
   4. Admit that you are not well suited to care for grieving patients and families
7. You suggest that a patient receive a palliative care consultation for symptom management related to anxiety and increasing pain. A family member asks the nurse if this means the patient is dying and is now "in hospice." What should the nurse tell the patient about the care she is receiving? Select all that apply.
   1. Hospice (end of life care) and palliative care are the same thing.
   2. Palliative care is for any patient, any time, any disease, in any setting.
   3. Palliative care strategies are primarily designed to treat the patient's illness.
   4. Palliative care interventions relieve the symptoms of illness and treatment.

8. Which of the following activities would be most consistent with what family caregivers of patients at the end of life report as a helpful nursing behavior?
   1. Leave the family alone as much as possible for private conversations
   2. Avoid difficult conversations or questions that may upset a family member
   3. Provide timely, guided instruction on matters of concern to the family caregiver
   4. Teach new coping skills for managing the acute period of grief

9. Which of the following would be the best first response to a family member who states that he believes it is wrong not to encourage patients at the end of life to eat?
   1. Suggest that the family member consult with a spiritual care provider for advice
   2. Recommend that the family member discuss the matter with the health care provider
   3. Ask the family member why he thinks that way
   4. Seek further clarification of the family member's point of view

10. Which of the following descriptions of spiritual care at the end of life is most accurate?
    1. Spiritual and religious concerns are the same thing.
    2. Spiritual concerns can be described in religious or nonreligious terms.
    3. A priest, pastor, or rabbi can best address spiritual concerns.
    4. Spiritual matters are personal, and they do not include interpersonal matters.

REFERENCES

Andrus V: Therapeutic presence: bringing comfort to our patients, *Beginnings* 30(4):18, 2010.

Boertje J: Tired of caring? You may have compassion fatigue, *Am Nurs Today* 8(7):16, 2013.

Bullock K: The influence of culture on end of life decision making, *J Soc Work End Life Palliat Care* 7(1):83, 2011.

Clabots S: Strategies to help initiate and maintain the end of life discussion with patients and family members, *Medsurg Nurs* 21(4):197, 2012.

Crozier F, Hancock L: Pediatric palliative care: beyond the end of life, *Pediatr Nurs* 38(4):198, 2012.

D'Arcy Y: Managing end of life symptoms, *Am Nurs Today* 7(7):22, 2012.

Derby S, O'Mahony S, Tickoo R: Elderly patients. In Ferrell B, Coyle N, editors: *Textbook of palliative nursing*, ed 3, New York, 2010, Oxford University Press, p 713.

Dosser I, Kennedy C: Family carers' experiences of support at the end of life: carers' and health professionals' views, *Int J Palliat Nurs* 18(10):491, 2012.

Edwards A, et al: The understanding of spirituality and the potential role of spiritual care in end of life and palliative care: a meta-study of qualitative research, *Palliat Med* 24(8):753, 2010.

Fiorelli R, Jenkins W: Cultural competency in grief and loss, *Beginnings* 32(3):11, 2012.

Freeman B: CARES: an acronym organized tool for the care of the dying, *J Hosp Palliat Nurs* 15(3):147, 2013.

Handsaker S, Dempsey L, Fabby C: Identifying and treating depression at the end of life and among the bereaved, *Int J Palliat Nurs* 18(2):91, 2012.

Kyle B: Bowel and bladder care at the end of life, *Br J Nurs* 19(7):408, 2010.

Lentz J, McMillan S: The impact of opioid induced constipation on patients near the end of life: perspectives of patients, family caregivers and nurses, *J Hosp Palliat Nurs* 12(1):29, 2010.

Lynch M, et al: Palliative care nursing: defining the discipline? *J Hosp Palliat Nurs* 13(2):106, 2011.

Mariano C: Holistic integrative therapies in palliative care. In Matzo M, Sherman D, editors: *Palliative care nursing: quality care to the end of life*, ed 3, New York, 2010, Springer, p 39.

Matsuyama R, et al: Will patients want hospice or palliative care if they do not know what it is? *J Hosp Palliat Nurs* 13(1):41, 2011.

Melvin C: Patients and families' misperceptions about hospice and palliative care: listen as they speak, *J Hosp Palliat Nurs* 12(2):107, 2010.

Milligan S: Addressing the spiritual care needs of people near the end of life, *Nurs Stand* 26(4):47, 2011.

Newson P: The elephant in the room: communication at the end of life, *Nurs Res Care* 14(2):96, 2012.

Paice J: Pain at the end of life. In Ferrell B, Coyle N, editors: *Textbook of palliative nursing*, ed 3, New York, 2010, Oxford University Press, p 161.

Revier S, Meiers S, Herth K: The lived experience of hope in family caregivers caring for a terminally ill loved one, *J Hosp Palliat Nurs* 14(6):438, 2012.

Sandor MK: Becoming a catalyst for conscious change at end of life, *Beginnings* 32(3):15, 2012.

Sherman D: Culture and spirituality as domains of quality palliative care. In Matzo M, Sherman D, editors: *Palliative care nursing: quality care to the end of life*, ed 3, New York, 2010, Springer, p 26.

Showalter S: Compassion fatigue: what is it? Why does it matter? Recognizing the symptoms, acknowledging the impact, developing the tools to prevent compassion fatigue, and strengthen the professional already suffering from the effects, *Am J Hosp Palliat Med* 27(4):239, 2010.

Sinclair S: Impact of death and dying on the personal lives and practices of palliative and hospice care professionals, *Can Med Assoc J* 183(2):180, 2011.

The Joint Commission (TJC): *National Patient Safety Goals*, Oakbrook Terrace, IL, 2014, The Commission. Available at:

http://www.jointcommission.org/standards_information/npsgs.aspx.

Thornton L: Coping with stress holistically, *Beginnings* 30(1):16, 2010.

Twomey S, Dowling M: Management of death rattle at end of life, *Br J Nurs* 22(2):81, 2013.

Warden A: Keeping your compassion, *Am Nurs Today* 7(3):54, 2012.

Wittenberg-Lyles E, Goldsmith J, Ragan S: The COMFORT initiative: palliative nursing and the centrality of communication, *J Hosp Palliat Nurs* 12(5):282, 2010.

Zager BS, Yancy M: A call to improve practice concerning cultural sensitivity and advance directives: a review of the literature, *Worldviews Evid Based Nurs* 4(4):202, 2011.

In the home setting, the recipient of care is commonly referred to as the *client* rather than *patient*. Clients and family caregivers need instruction so that they are prepared to assume self-care in the home and to be able to function safely in their environment. Home care instruction begins at the time of admission to a health care facility and often includes multiple topics, including health care promotion (e.g., exercise or diet), coping with impaired function (e.g., making adaptive changes in the home), and restoration of health (e.g., learning how to take medicines or perform exercises). It is common for a family caregiver to be a partner in any education effort. Instruction should continue in the home setting, where you can help clients attain healthy behaviors, access available education programs or resources in the community, and learn how to adjust to any health-related restrictions so that they can be safe in the home.

CLIENT-CENTERED CARE

Home care clients include older adults, individuals with a chronic illness, disabled adults and children, and individuals who have experienced an acute illness or injury. A nurse takes a holistic approach to care of clients by considering physiological, mental, emotional, social, spiritual, and environmental aspects that influence individuals and their communities (Edlin and Golanty, 2010). This approach is critical for clients to be willing to change their behavior when change is required. A nurse delivers care in a culturally sensitive manner by showing understanding and respect for a client's beliefs and learning needs (Cohen, 2014).

Home care is part of the continuum of care. Nurses are instrumental in helping clients to achieve their maximum functional ability and adjust to changes when back in their home. Older adults can be at greater risk for environmental hazards and mistreatment as they age. The nurse works with clients in the home and encourages them to share the responsibility for maintaining a healthy lifestyle (Touhy and Jett, 2012). An in-depth client-centered assessment is needed to provide relevant and appropriate education and intervention.

SAFETY

The Joint Commission (TJC, 2014) identified five goals related to client safety in home care, focusing on problems in safety and how to solve them. These goals focus on:
- Identifying clients correctly—following procedure to ensure clients receive the correct medications
- Using medicines safely—ensuring a client has one up-to-date medication list and understands his or her medications
- Preventing infection—using hand hygiene
- Preventing clients from falling—recognizing fall risks and implementing preventive strategies
- Identifying client safety risks—identifying specifically risks associated with oxygen therapy

Home safety modifications affect all people living in a home. A nurse must include the client and family caregiver in all discussions. Be prepared to discuss concerns about the number of modifications required, costs of modifications, and change in home decor. Accident prevention begins with making timely and adequate home repairs; however, it may also be necessary to modify the home to make it more accessible for the client. The goal is to provide an environment in which the client or the family caregiver can provide care safely and effectively.

EVIDENCE-BASED PRACTICE

Abusalem SK, Coty MB: Home health nurses coping with practice care errors, *J Res Nurs* 18(4):336, 2013.

Sears N, et al: The incidence of adverse events among home care patients, *Int J Qual Health Care* 25(1):16, 2013.

A study showed that 13.2% of clients receiving home care experience adverse events, and approximately one third of those events were considered preventable (Sears et al., 2013). Nurses in home care strive to deliver safe and effective care to their clients. Much research has been published related to how adverse care effects clients; however, a survey of 192 home care nurses sought to examine the effect of practice errors on the nurses themselves (Abusalem and Coty, 2013). Four different scales were used to assess the nurses' coping mechanisms and emotional responses to practice errors. Most nurses felt they were supported by their facility when practice errors occur; however, the nurses identified areas lacking within their facilities to prevent similar errors from occurring again:

- A focus on problem solving within home care facilities
- A need for ongoing dialogue in home care facilities
- Continued education for nurses in all practice settings to address safety concerns
- Encouragement to seek appropriate solutions to prevent injury to clients.

SKILL 31.1   HOME ENVIRONMENT SAFETY

The home environment should be a place in which individuals feel healthy, comfortable, and safe. Older adults are at risk for threats to safety as a result of physiological changes associated with aging. For example, a hearing loss prevents a client from hearing a smoke alarm, whereas a cognitive deficit affects a person's ability to organize or store medications properly.

Fall prevention is a critical component of home care safety. Falls can occur at any age. Older adults are at high risk; however, younger adults who have experienced an illness may be at risk as a result of medication effects or alterations in balance and lower extremity strength. After a fall, an adult may experience physical injury and psychological trauma (Meiner, 2011). When a fall occurs, it is important to assess the consequences of the fall as well as the client's fear of falling to develop an appropriate plan of care and prevention.

Prevention of unintentional injury and violence is a goal of *Healthy People 2020* (HHS, 2014). Included in this topic area is a focus on the emerging issue of elder maltreatment and the effects of the environment on risk for injury and violence. It is important for a nurse working in a home setting to focus on specific motor and cognitive developmental needs of clients in the home setting, while also considering the impact of individual, family, social, and community influences. Assessing for the potential for injury for each client, the nurse identifies areas of risk and designs interventions to eliminate or reduce threats to the client's safety.

┃ASSESSMENT

1. Assess for presence of sensory, motor, cognitive, or other physical changes or deficits (see Chapter 7). *Rationale: These factors increase client's risk of injury, and assessment aids in determining client's actual or potential limitations that create safety risks.*

2. Assess for adaptations necessary in the home on the basis of client's physical and mental status. *Rationale: The nature of physical and cognitive limitations determines the type of adjustments to be made in the home. Home health care services can assist family caregivers of clients in their home in later stages of dementia (Meiner, 2011).*

3. Assess client's attitudes about returning home and following health care provider recommendations. Determine client's perceived benefit of action, perceived barrier to action, interpersonal influences such as family and peers, and commitment to a plan of action. *Rationale: Clients may feel unprepared or think they lack the knowledge needed to transition to home (Barnason et al., 2012).*

4. Consult other health care team members (e.g., social worker, physical therapist) about client needs in the home. *Rationale: Members of all health care disciplines collaborate to determine client's needs and functional abilities (Meiner, 2011).*

5. Assess developmental stage of client. *Rationale: Safety needs of clients vary based on their developmental age.*

6. Assess client's history of falls in the past. If client has fallen at home, use the mnemonic SPLATT to assess the client. *Rationale: Previous falls often indicate an increased risk for falling or a client's fear of falling. Assessing prior falls helps identify factors that contribute to or prevent future falls. SPLATT test allows patient to explain symptoms in own words and helps to clarify circumstances surrounding a fall (Meiner, 2011).*
   - **S**ymptoms at time of fall
   - **P**revious fall
   - **L**ocation of fall
   - **A**ctivity at time of fall
   - **T**ime of fall
   - **T**rauma after fall

7. Assess family caregiver's knowledge of client's condition and willingness and ability to provide support. *Rationale: Family caregiver needs to understand client's risks for injury and how to provide assistance that will reduce risks.*

PLANNING

Expected Outcomes focus on identifying risk factors and providing a safe home environment.

1. Client or family caregiver identifies safety risks in the home.
2. Client or family caregiver identifies community resources available and how to initiate contact.
3. Client does not experience injury in the home.

Delegation and Collaboration

The skill of risk assessment and accident prevention cannot be delegated to nursing assistive personnel (NAP). The nurse may need to consult with a physical therapist or an occupational therapist to conduct a thorough home safety assessment and determine appropriate adaptations needed based on client's physical or cognitive limitations.

Equipment

- Home safety checklist

IMPLEMENTATION *for* HOME ENVIRONMENT SAFETY

STEPS	RATIONALE
1. **See Standard Protocol (inside front cover).**	
2. Involve client and family caregiver as active participants in a home safety assessment using a checklist (Table 31-1).	Active participation enhances learning and empowers making decisions about care.
3. General safety in the home:	
a. Ensure that there is a direct light source in areas where patient reads, cooks, uses tools, performs hobby activities, prepares medication, etc.	Older adults or patients with diabetes mellitus are at risk for visual changes due to cataracts, macular degeneration, glaucoma, or diabetic retinopathy (Touhy and Jett, 2012).

> **SAFE PATIENT CARE** Avoid fluorescent lighting, which may cause excessive glare.

b. With client and family caregiver, identify ways to make home environment safe; post emergency phone numbers near all telephones.	A safe environment helps maintain or improve level of independence and function.
c. If client is an older adult who is alone frequently, suggest use of a home monitoring system (HMS) and set a schedule for client to "check in" with family, neighbors, or friends.	HMS technologies support and enable safe independent living. Checking in with others at regular times communicates that client is safe at home (Meiner, 2011).
d. Reduce the number of different pain and sleep medications the client uses if possible (consult with health care provider and pharmacist).	Prevents oversedation and enhances ability of client to make safe decisions.
e. Offer client and family caregiver appropriate information about community health care resources.	The goal is to keep client in the home for as long as it is safe and desirable. When deciding about the need for care outside the home, the role of the nurse is to support client and family caregiver and provide information about available options (Meiner, 2011).
f. Instruct client and family caregiver to have HVAC (heating, ventilation, and air-conditioning) system inspected annually.	Improper venting prevents escape of carbon monoxide.
g. Instruct patient and family caregiver to have carbon monoxide detector installed in the home and to verify battery and proper functioning annually.	Carbon monoxide system alarm will sound if carbon monoxide reaches unsafe levels (Meiner, 2011).

Continued

4. Electrical safety:

a. Verify that major electrical appliances are grounded and that there are no overloaded plugs or sockets (see illustration). Examine plugs, cords, and switch plates for signs of damage.

Reduces risk of electrical shock and fire (ESFi, 2014).

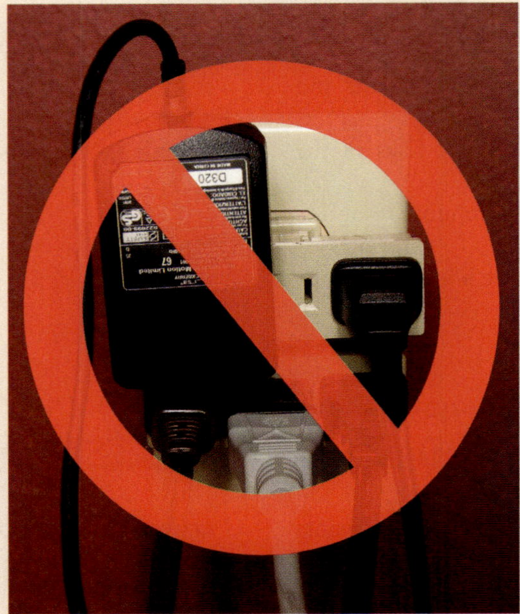

STEP 4a Overloaded electrical socket.

b. If small children or confused clients are in the house, cover unused outlets with safety plugs.

Prevents electrical shock.

c. Check fuse box accessibility and wattage of light bulbs.

Correct wattage lessens risk of fire.

5. Fire safety and burn prevention:

a. Have smoke detectors installed near each bedroom and other areas according to building codes in patient's community.

Provides early warning in the presence of smoke or fire and alerts the family in a timely manner.

b. Instruct client to keep thermostat on hot water heater below 120°F (49°C).

Prevents scalding burns from hot water (Meiner, 2011).

c. Encourage client not to smoke; offer access to smoking cessation classes. If he or she smokes, educate client not to smoke while tired or in bed.

Smoking and secondhand smoke are health hazards; falling asleep while smoking is associated with preventable deaths and injuries (Meiner, 2011).

d. Instruct clients, especially those with small children in the home, about stove safety (e.g., turn pot handles inward, away from edge of stove; install stove knob protectors and a stove lock).

Safe stove use helps prevent burns (Hockenberry and Wilson, 2013).

e. Instruct client on safe usage of portable space heaters. Electrical space heaters are only unvented heaters safe to use in the home (Energy.Gov, 2013):

Prevents accidental fire.

(1) Do not use extension cords with space heaters unless absolutely necessary.

(2) Plug heater directly into a wall outlet. If an extension cord is necessary, use the shortest possible heavy-duty cord of 14-gauge wire or larger. Always check and follow any manufacturer's instructions about use of extension cords.

(3) Buy a unit with a tip-over safety switch, which automatically shuts off the heater if the unit is tipped over.

f. Discuss emergency exit plan with client.

Assists in rapid evacuation of home.

STEPS	RATIONALE
6. Fall prevention:	
a. Schedule diuretics early in the day and space antihypertensives and antiarrhythmics at different times to minimize side effects.	Appropriate diuretic schedule minimizes interruption in sleep and trips to the bathroom at night. Antihypertensives and antiarrhythmics often cause hypotension and dizziness, increasing risk of falls (Touhy and Jett, 2012).
b. Consider changing the physical environment to reduce predisposition to falls: remove clutter, remove tripping hazards on the floor, install proper lighting, and install safety grab bars in the bathroom.	Modifying the home environment is effective in preventing falls (Meiner, 2011).
c. Have client visit eye care professional if vision is blurred.	Blurred vision contributes to falls.
d. Inspect client's shoes. Teach client to wear shoes with thin, firm soles and moderate traction, especially if he or she has a shuffling gait. Velcro-type fasteners are helpful on shoes.	Better stability and proprioception are provided by shoes that have a thin, firm sole with moderate traction. Footwear with thicker soles (e.g., sneakers) can result in tripping if the client has a shuffling gait.
e. Refer client to physical or occupational therapist for rehabilitative or therapeutic exercise or adaptive devices if indicated.	Tailored exercise programs and assist devices help decrease the risk of falls.
f. Teach client and family caregiver about risks for falling and specific plan for reducing falls in the home.	Clients who understand their fall risk and how to adapt are less fearful of falling.
7. Firearm safety:	
a. Teach client about dangers associated with keeping guns in the home.	Firearms are associated with higher rates of suicide (Meiner, 2011).
b. Teach client to install trigger locks on any guns and store them unloaded in a locked cabinet. Have client store ammunition in a secured area separate from the guns. Store keys in a place inaccessible to children.	Restricting access to firearms decreases the risk of injury or death for children by firearms (Hepp et al., 2012).
8. **See Completion Protocol (inside front cover).**	

EVALUATION

1. Ask client or family caregiver to identify safety risks present in the home and steps recommended to minimize risks for injury
2. Ask client or family caregiver to identify resources available for a particular problem and how to initiate contact with that resource.
3. Ask client or family caregiver if anyone has experienced an injury in the home.
4. Have client keep a fall diary if he or she falls or almost falls at home. (**Note:** Any fall with injury should be reported to a health care provider immediately.) Organize diary so that client enters date and time of each fall, activity at time of fall, and any related symptoms or injury. If family caregiver witnesses fall, he or she should make an entry. Instruct client to share diary with all health care providers.
5. Use **Teach Back:** State to the client, "I want to be sure I explained clearly the ways you can make the kitchen safer. Can you tell me what you could do to reduce hazards in the kitchen?" Evaluates what the client is able to explain or demonstrate. Revise your instruction now or develop plan for revised client teaching to be implemented at an appropriate time if client is not able to teach back appropriately.

Unexpected Outcomes and Related Interventions

1. Client is unable to identify safety risks.
   a. Consider using different teaching approach.
   b. Reinforce information about preventing and removing potential hazards from home environment.
2. Client or family caregiver does not make changes to reduce risks in home.
   a. Assess the concerns or views of client or family caregiver about making changes; make changes client will accept.
   b. Assess client's finances.
3. Client or family caregiver is unaware of community resources.
   a. Provide informational brochures and contact information for resources.
4. Client or family caregiver reports that an injury has occurred in the home.

TABLE 31-1   HOME SAFETY CHECKLIST

SAFETY CRITERIA	YES	NO
Front and Back Entrances		
1. Walkways and steps are smooth and well lighted. Sturdy handrail is on both sides of stairs to entrance.	____	____
2. If client lives in an apartment or assisted living facility, elevators are in working order.	____	____
3. Nonskid strips/safety treads or bright paint is used on outdoor steps. All steps have the same rise and depth (standard: 7-inch rise and 11-inch depth).	____	____
4. A shelf or bench is kept by front and back doors to place grocery bags or packages if needed.	____	____
5. Doormats are in good condition.	____	____
Kitchen		
1. Client wears clothes with short or close-fitting sleeves when cooking.	____	____
2. Stove control dials are easy to see and use, and stovetop and oven are clean and grease-free.	____	____
3. A working refrigerator is present.	____	____
4. Items in kitchen cabinets and shelves are easy to reach; expiration dates on food items are appropriate.	____	____
5. Lighting over sink, stove, and work areas is bright.	____	____
6. Client stays in kitchen while cooking.	____	____
7. Fire extinguisher is functional, available, and easy to handle and use.	____	____
Floors		
1. All carpeting and mats are secure. Skid backing is present under area rugs, or throw rugs are removed.	____	____
2. Walkways are free of clutter.	____	____
Bathrooms		
1. Door lock can be unlocked from both sides.	____	____
2. Tub or shower has nonskid mats or abrasive strips. Floor mats have nonskid backing.	____	____
3. Tub or shower has at least one grab bar kept free of towels or other items.	____	____
4. Shower has a stable stool or chair and handheld sprayer.	____	____
5. Cold and hot water faucets are clearly marked and functional, and temperature on water heater is 120°F (49°C) or lower.	____	____
6. An automatic nightlight is present and functional.	____	____
Bedroom		
1. Client can turn on light without having to get out of bed in the dark. Lighting is adequate for clear vision.	____	____
2. Furniture is arranged to provide clear path from bed to bathroom.	____	____
3. Phone with large-print emergency numbers is within easy reach of bed.	____	____
4. Alarm systems are available. There are listening devices for invalid clients.	____	____
Living Room/Family Room		
1. Light can be turned on without having to walk into dark room.	____	____
2. Lamp, extension, or phone cords are kept out of traffic ways.	____	____
3. Furniture is arranged so it can be walked around easily, and walking paths are free of clutter.	____	____
Fire Safety		
1. Sufficient numbers of working smoke detectors are in appropriate locations.	____	____
2. Emergency exit plans are in place in case of fire.	____	____
3. Family has determined a meeting place outside the house.	____	____
4. Portable space heaters have a UL mark and are placed on flat, level surfaces 3 feet away from flammable items.	____	____
5. Furnace area is free of things that can catch on fire.	____	____
6. Furnace and chimney are checked annually by a qualified professional. Wood fireplaces are cleaned regularly of ash and soot.	____	____
7. Emergency numbers for police, fire, and poison control are posted near phone.	____	____
8. Fire extinguisher is functional, available, and easy to handle and use.	____	____

TABLE 31-1	HOME SAFETY CHECKLIST—cont'd		
SAFETY CRITERIA		YES	NO
Electrical Safety			
1. Electrical cords are in good condition and not frayed, spliced, or cracked.		____	____
2. Electrical cords are kept away from water.		____	____
3. Extension cord/outlet extenders have built-in circuit breaker or fuse; outlets are not overloaded.		____	____
4. Wall outlets and switches have cover plates.		____	____
5. Light bulbs are of correct wattage for each fixture.		____	____
6. Fuse box is easily accessible and clearly labeled.		____	____
7. Lamp switches are easy to turn on to avoid burns from hot light bulbs.		____	____
Carbon Monoxide Prevention			
1. Furnace flues are checked regularly for patency.		____	____
2. Battery operated carbon monoxide detector is in home. Battery is checked regularly each spring and fall.		____	____

Modified from Meiner SE: *Gerontologic nursing*, ed 4, St Louis, 2011, Mosby.

   a. Notify health care provider immediately if injury involves a fall, loss of consciousness, or other serious injury.

   b. Determine cause and extent of injury. Suggest further modifications that can be made in the home to prevent future injuries.

Recording and Reporting

- Record assessment of physical and cognitive status, home barriers or risks, recommended interventions, instruction provided, and response of client or family caregiver, and changes client makes to home environment.
- Document your evaluation of client learning.
- Report any physical or cognitive changes not previously identified and remaining barriers in the home environment.

Sample Documentation

0900   Safety checklist completed with client and daughter. Daughter states will remove throw rugs and have handrails installed in bathroom. Referred client to physical therapy for selection of ambulation assistive device.

Special Considerations

Pediatric

- Ensuring the safety of children in the home is based on child's developmental level. Instruct families to use safety devices as applicable (Hockenberry and Wilson, 2013).
- Suggest that parents get down on the floor to look at the environment from child's view to identify dangers present in the home (Hockenberry and Wilson, 2013).

- Children imitate and copy what they see and hear. Instruct parents that practicing safety teaches safety (Hockenberry and Wilson, 2013).
- Teach families car safety based on child's age, developmental level, and size. Place children in appropriate restraint system; if the car has airbags, children younger than 12 years of age need to ride in the back seat or as defined by state law.

Geriatric

- Physiological and mental status changes (e.g., slower reaction time, reduced pain and temperature perception, reduced visual acuity) place older adults at risk for injury.
- Older adults are usually more aware of potential dangers when they are in a familiar setting.
- Frail older adults should not ride in the passenger side of the car if the car has airbags. Teach them to sit in the back seat or at least 10 inches away from the airbag.

Home Care

- Make changes in client's home environment to keep him or her as independent as possible.
- Before making changes to a client's home, know his or her financial resources. Let client be the final decision maker in the types of changes to be made whenever possible. Consider client's physical strengths and remaining functional abilities, not just the disabilities.
- Educate family caregivers about the importance of preserving client autonomy.

SKILL 31.2   HOME SAFETY FOR CLIENTS WITH COGNITIVE DEFICITS

Clients with cognitive impairments and their family caregivers need assistance in making the adaptations needed to preserve the client's ability to function safely within the home. To be safe, a person needs to be able to perform routine activities of daily living (ADLs) and instrumental activities of daily living (IADLs) (e.g., check writing, buying groceries) and make sound decisions. When there are cognitive limitations, a person's independence is threatened. Family caregivers often do not understand changes in cognition and function and need help to determine whether a client is competent to remain at home safely.

It is a myth that all older adults experience cognitive dysfunctions; however, older adults are more likely to develop them. In addition to mental status and cognitive changes, many older adults experience depression. Depression often results from social isolation (e.g., the older adult is homebound and has few visitors). An accurate assessment includes mental and physical health, social and economic status, functional status, and the environment (Touhy and Jett, 2012). Some mental processes may be intact (e.g., orientation to name, time, and place), while other processes are compromised (e.g., short-term memory of life events).

Many clients who have dementia experience wandering. Wandering refers to moving about without having a definite place to go or a purpose. It is characterized by a repeated, prolonged, and sometimes compulsive need to walk, with or without an aim. Clients who wander can leave their home and walk endlessly until found by a family caregiver or local police. Family caregivers need to learn how to make the home safe to discourage wandering and prevent clients from leaving the home unattended.

ASSESSMENT

1. Assess client over several short periods and be ready to adapt assessment if client has sensory disabilities. *Rationale: Improves likelihood of gathering relevant data (Touhy and Jett, 2012).*
2. Listen carefully to client in a quiet, well-lit space, without interruptions or distractions. Speak slowly, clearly, and in a normal tone of voice. *Rationale: Providing an optimal environment ensures accurate assessment of client's cognitive and mental status.*
3. Ask client to describe own level of health and ability to provide self-care skills. Ask family caregiver to confirm description. Also assess for risky behaviors (e.g., medication nonadherence, unsupervised use of stove). *Rationale: Question requires client to describe abilities and health challenges. Family caregivers are able to provide helpful insight, especially about risky behaviors. Minimizing risky behaviors is essential in making the environment safe.*
4. Ask how client manages home responsibilities and manages medications or other health care. Ask family caregiver to confirm description. *Rationale: Allows you to assess short-term memory, judgment, and problem solving. Family caregivers provide helpful insight.*
5. If you suspect cognitive or mental status change, complete Mini-Mental State Examination (MMSE) or other depression scales as requested. *Rationale: Reliable scales provide a reliable measure for baseline and subsequent changes in patients' mental status or level of depression.*
5. If you suspect that client is wandering or at risk for wandering, observe and assess for the following characteristics and behaviors. Consult with family caregiver. *Rationale: Clients who exhibit these behaviors or have these characteristics are more prone to wandering (Alzheimer's Association, 2012):*
   - Higher level of cognitive impairment
   - Difficulty sleeping
   - Active lifestyle before becoming cognitively impaired
   - Use of psychotropic medications
   - Pacing or walking that cannot be redirected easily
   - Getting lost in familiar places
   - Client explains he or she is searching for "missing" people or places
6. Determine if client has a family caregiver or friend who helps with self-care or home management responsibilities. *Rationale: Determines availability of potential resources for client.*
7. Assess competency of family caregiver and his or her perception of ability to care for client safely in the home. *Rationale: Caring for family caregiver and ensuring that family caregiver can care for client competently are essential in providing a safe environment for client.*

PLANNING

Expected Outcomes focus on adaptation of the home environment and promoting client's ability to perform ADLs and IADLs safely.
1. Client is able to complete home management responsibilities (specify) within existing limitations.
2. Family caregiver verbalizes recognition that cognitive impairment may be progressive; uses adaptations in the home that help client perform home management activities as needed.
3. Client does not wander alone from the home.

Delegation and Collaboration

The skill of adapting the home setting for clients with cognitive deficits cannot be delegated to nursing assistive personnel (NAP). The nurse instructs the NAP to:
- Observe for and report any changes in client mood, memory, and ability to maintain the home.

Equipment
- Mini-mental state examination (MMSE)
- Calendar
- Paper for making lists
- Bulletin board or poster board (optional)
- Motion detector (optional)

IMPLEMENTATION *for* HOME SAFETY FOR CLIENTS WITH COGNITIVE DEFICITS

STEPS	RATIONALE
1. **See Standard Protocol (inside front cover).**	
2. If client has difficulty remembering when to perform self-care routines, create a list or post reminder notes written in large print in a noticeable place. Suggest use of a wristwatch with an alarm to signal time of scheduled activity and use of a medication organization container to help with medication administration.	Memory function in older adults tends to be preserved for relevant, well-known material (Meiner, 2011). Lists and other reminders help client remember and complete required tasks. Large print is helpful when client has limited eyesight.
3. If necessary to take, schedule medications that cause confusion or drowsiness at bedtime.	Maintains mental status during the day at the maximum level possible.
4. Instruct family caregiver to focus on client's abilities rather than disabilities. Encourage allowing client to make decisions when possible.	Retains client's autonomy and sense of self-worth.
5. When client has difficulty completing tasks with multiple steps, reduce number of steps or simplify task.	Prevents frustration and forgetting one or more steps that lead to not finishing task.
6. Help client and family caregiver develop a schedule for routine ADLs such as eating, bathing, and exercise.	Consistency creates a sense of security and keeps client oriented to ADLs. Activity reduces agitation.
7. Have family caregiver set up activities so that client can complete them (e.g., lay out clothes to wear for the day, place food for meals out on the counter).	Helps client complete tasks even though unable to plan and perform all the steps.
8. Instruct family caregiver to use simple and direct communication with calm and relaxed approach. Use eye contact and touch. Speak in simple words and short sentences.	Facilitates effective communication and reduces anxiety.
9. Place clocks, calendars, and personal mementos throughout rooms within the home.	Maintaining familiar surroundings maximizes cognitive function.
10. Enhance the environment with addition of tactile boards or three-dimensional art.	
11. If client wanders, follow these interventions (Alzheimer's Association, 2012):	
a. Provide a safe place (e.g., large room in den free of obstacles) for client to wander.	Reduces risk of client leaving residence.
b. Provide clues (e.g., signs) to guide client to a desired location.	Reduces aimless wandering.
c. Recommend that family caregiver install door locks or electronic guards.	Reduces chance of wandering out of home.
d. Address the cause of wandering (e.g., provide food if hungry) and eliminate or lessen stressors (e.g., pain).	Reduces causes of wandering.
12. Have family caregiver routinely remind client of who he or she is and what the next step will be.	Improves client's responses to activities and environment (Meiner, 2011).
13. Facilitate regular naps or rest periods.	Fatigue adds to mental status changes.
14. Encourage and support frequent visits by family and friends. Encourage use of humor and reminiscing about favorite stories.	Prevents boredom and reduces restlessness.
15. **See Completion Protocol (inside front cover).**	

EVALUATION

1. Ask client to review the home management activities completed that day and previous day.
2. Use ***Teach Back:*** State to the family caregiver, "We talked about ways to keep your mother independent. I want to be sure I explained the options clearly. Tell me two ways to help your mom stay active and involved." Evaluates what the family caregiver is able to explain or demonstrate. Revise your instruction now or develop plan for revised family caregiver teaching to be implemented at an appropriate time if family caregiver is not able to teach back appropriately.

Unexpected Outcomes and Related Interventions

1. Client is unable to complete daily activities as planned.
   a. Review what occurred and identify barriers.
   b. Identify strategies for maintaining adequate support and overcoming barriers.
2. Family caregiver is unable to carry out techniques that improve orientation and ability of client to complete activities.
   a. Offer reinstruction for family caregiver. Reassess family caregiver's knowledge of client's progressive condition.
   b. Reassess family caregiver's ability to provide necessary support. Consider other living arrangements or support services if indicated.

Recording and Reporting

- Record cognitive abilities and mental status, recommended interventions, and responses of client and family caregiver.
- Document your evaluation of family caregiver learning.
- Report significant decline in cognitive or mental status to health care provider.

Sample Documentation

2100   Oriented to person only. States is "waiting for breakfast." Reoriented by having client identify location. Reoriented client to look outside to see that it is dark and telling her that it will soon be bedtime. Sister reports that client has wandered less since offering more frequent meals and planning naps.

Special Considerations
Pediatric

- Children with cognitive impairments often are unaware of dangers normally present during play and daily activities. Adult supervision is critical.

Geriatric

- Many clients experience progressive loss of function, requiring continuous adaptations and adjustments. If client becomes unable to complete any ADLs or experiences major behavioral changes (e.g., excessive wandering), you may need to help family caregiver determine need for alternative living arrangements.
- Refer family caregivers to resources for safety and communication tips, such as the Alzheimer's Association.

SKILL 31.3 **MEDICATION AND MEDICAL DEVICE SAFETY**

Clients with chronic disease frequently take multiple medications. The effects of treatment, progression of disease, and physical and cognitive changes that can occur if a client is elderly all affect the ability to take medications safely. You need to provide interventions that allow clients to store and prepare medications correctly, understand and follow their medication schedule, administer medications correctly, and dispose of unused or expired medications properly. It is frequently necessary to teach family caregivers how to perform medication preparation and administration.

The use of medical devices in the home places clients and their family caregivers at risk for injury. Medical devices include syringes, blood glucose monitoring equipment, dressings, and intravenous devices. Clients need to know how to store and handle medical devices properly and dispose of medical waste properly to prevent infection. Clients with special needs because of acute sensory or neurological impairment, chronic illnesses, and physical limitations may have difficulty manipulating medical devices and handling medications. In some cases, a family caregiver or other caregiver must learn to provide this care (Fig. 31-1).

ASSESSMENT

1. Assess client's visual, cognitive, musculoskeletal (ability to open and manipulate devices), and neurological function; level of consciousness or sedation; vision; hearing; literacy

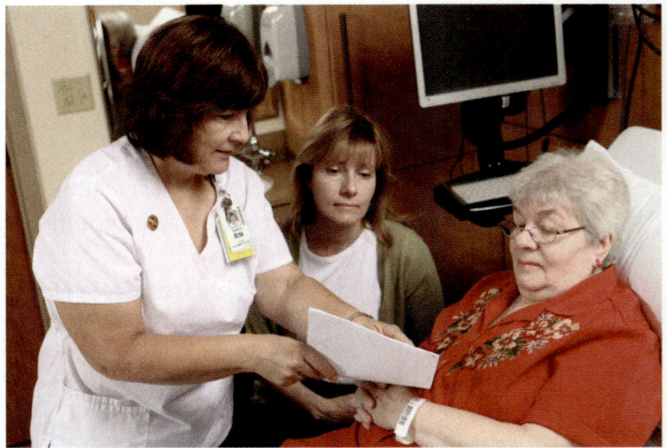

FIG 31-1 A family caregiver or other caregiver often needs to learn about prescribed medications.

level; and willingness to learn. *Rationale: Helps to identify instructional approaches and appropriate assistive devices needed.*

2. Assess client's and family caregivers' knowledge of medication regimen and compare with actual regimen. Also assess length of time client has been receiving each drug. *Rationale: Determines complexity of medication regimen and client's familiarity with each drug.*

3. Assess client's beliefs, previous experiences, and attitudes about medication therapy. *Rationale: Client-centered approach to selecting interventions might enhance client's adherence.*

4. Identify where medications are stored and the type of storage containers used. If patient uses glucose monitoring device, also locate where the monitor, lancets, and glucose strips are stored. *Rationale: Determines safe use and storage of medications and related supplies.*

5. Assess resources for obtaining medications when needed. *Rationale: Lack of resources interferes with self-medication at home.*

6. Assess family caregiver's ability and willingness to assist client. *Rationale: Determines extent to involve family caregiver in instruction.*

PLANNING

Expected Outcomes focus on client's ability to manage medications and medical devices safely.

1. Client states purpose of each medication, common side effects, and when to notify health care provider about problems.

2. Client is able to read each medication label and explain when each drug is to be taken.

3. Client or family caregiver prepares and administers prescribed medications independently.

4. Client or family caregiver stores medications and medical devices properly and disposes of medical wastes safely.

Delegation and Collaboration

The skill of medication and medical device safety cannot be delegated to nursing assistive personnel (NAP). The nurse instructs the NAP to:

- Observe for and report unsafe behaviors, improper disposal of sharps and contaminated supplies, and use of infection control practices.

Equipment

- Written instructions or charts
- Medications
- Pill organizer for daily or weekly medication preparation
- Measuring devices (e.g., medicine cup, teaspoon, syringe) if needed
- Colored marking pens
- Labels
- Assistive device (e.g., syringe magnifier) or medical device (e.g., blood glucose monitor)
- Puncture-resistant sharps container or hard plastic bottle (e.g., laundry detergent or fabric softener bottle) with cap

IMPLEMENTATION *for* MEDICATION AND MEDICAL DEVICE SAFETY

STEPS	RATIONALE
1. **See Standard Protocol (inside front cover).**	
2. Educate client and family caregiver about prescribed medications and over-the-counter medications that are scheduled and taken prn, including:	Education enhances adherence with medication therapy and reduces errors in medication self-administration.
a. Purpose of medications and their expected effects.	
b. How medications work and affect the body.	
c. Dosage schedules and rationale.	
d. Common side effects and what to do to relieve side effects.	
e. What to do if a dose is missed.	
f. When to call the health care provider.	
3. Suggest use of appropriate devices to help client take medications as scheduled:	Helps client decrease medication administration errors.
a. Provide a large-print chart for client or family caregiver to list each medication (see illustration).	Provides resource to check medication doses and frequencies.
b. Use pill organizers that are set up daily or weekly to separate pills into slots for each day of the week and appropriate time of day (see illustration).	Assists client in adhering to correct dosage schedule.
c. Set an alarm on clock or cell phone to alert client to medication administration time.	

Continued

STEPS	RATIONALE
4. Educate client and family caregiver about the principles of safe medication administration and the recommended modifications for safe administration.	Medication prescriptions specify frequency, dosage, and special instructions (e.g., take before meals).
a. Take prescribed medication only as prescribed and by the person for whom it was prescribed.	It is unsafe for anyone to take medications prescribed for another person.
b. Do not take expired medications.	Medication may be toxic or no longer effective.
c. Keep medications in original containers and ensure that label is clear and legible. Have pharmacy provide large-print or braille labels if needed.	Putting several different kinds of medications in the same container is unsafe because client can mix up dosages or schedules of administration. Large print makes label reading easier.
d. Finish prescribed medications and, if ordered, get refills before container is empty.	It is unsafe for client to keep some medication when symptoms are gone, planning to use it later. It is essential to order refills so there is no interruption in medication routine.

HOME CARE MEDICINE FORM

Allergic to/describe reaction:	Allergic to/describe reaction:

List all prescription and over-the-counter (non-prescription) medicines such as vitamins, aspirin, Tylenol, and herbals (ex: ginseng, gingko biloba).
Include prescription medicines taken only as needed, (eg. Dulcolax, Zyrtec)

Start date	Name of medicine/ ordered by?	What is it for? How is it working?	How much (dose)	When to take	Date stopped

1. Take this form with you to ALL doctor visits and ALL medical testing (lab, x-ray, MRI, CT, etc).

Update the form as changes are made to the person's medicines. If a medicine is stopped, draw a line through it and record the date it was stopped.

STEP 3a Medication schedule chart for home use.

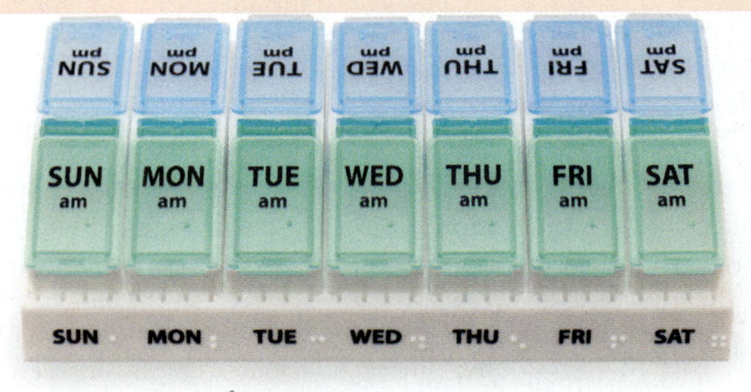

STEP 3b Pill organizers.

STEPS	RATIONALE

e. Have pharmacist put medications in a container that client can open easily if manual dexterity is limited.

Childproof containers may be difficult to open if client has limited mobility of fingers or hands.

f. Follow specific disposal instructions on prescription drug labeling or patient information that accompanies the medicine. Do not flush medicines down a sink or toilet unless drug information specifically instructs to do so. Take advantage of a community take-back program. If there is no take-back program, remove drugs from their original containers and mix them with an undesirable substance, such as used coffee grounds or cat litter (FDA, 2014).

Safe drug disposable protects adults, children, and pets in the home from injury.

> **SAFE PATIENT CARE** Identify a safe place for storage of medication to reduce risk of accidental ingestion by children.

5. Instruct client or family caregiver about safe use and disposal of medical devices and supplies:

Prevents injuries from contaminated supplies (FDA, 2013).

a. Instruct how to use medical device, using diagrams, written information, and other resources (e.g., Internet), and validate competence via return demonstration.

Clear written information, diagrams, and other resources enhance client learning and allow reinforcement of information.

b. Instruct on proper storage, cleaning, and care of medical device.

Ensures that device will continue to work safely and accurately.

c. Instruct to place used needles, syringes, lancets, or other sharp objects in sharps container or hard plastic soda bottle or laundry detergent bottle with screw-on or tightly secured cap. FDA-cleared sharps disposal containers are also available through pharmacies, medical supply companies, and online (FDA, 2013).

Reduces transmission of microorganisms and prevents exposure to body fluids (FDA, 2013).

d. Instruct to put soiled dressings, disposable sheets, and medical gloves in securely fastened plastic bag before being placed in garbage can.

Ensures safe disposal of medical supplies (EPA, 2012).

6. **See Completion Protocol (inside front cover).**

EVALUATION

1. Ask client or family caregiver to state purpose of each medication, common side effects, and when to notify health care provider about problems associated with medications.

2. Ask client to explain when each medication is to be taken.

3. Observe client or family caregiver preparing and administering medications and using medical devices independently.

4. Complete a pill count at specific intervals.

5. Use *Teach Back:* State to the family caregiver, "During my last visit we talked about how to throw away expired medicines and used syringes. I want to be sure I explained the options clearly. Tell me what you remember discussing." Evaluates what the family caregiver is able to explain or demonstrate. Revise your instruction now or develop plan for revised family caregiver teaching to be implemented at an appropriate time if family caregiver is not able to teach back appropriately.

Unexpected Outcomes and Related Interventions

1. Client or family caregiver makes errors in preparing medications or is unable to recall information.
  a. Try alternative approaches (e.g., written instruction or pictures).
  b. Repeat and reinforce important information. Give positive feedback for accurate recall of information.
  c. Provide repeated supervised practice until client is able to self-administer medications safely.

2. Client's self-care deficits prevent safe self-medicating.
  a. Consider need for alternative living arrangements.

3. Excess or insufficient pills are found in pill container during pill count.

a. Reevaluate use of dosage reminders.

b. Establish monitoring system until client is able to self-medicate accurately.

4. Medications and medical devices and supplies are not stored or disposed of in a secure or appropriate location.

a. Identify barriers and appropriate alternatives.

b. Explain risks posed when supplies and devices are not handled safely.

Recording and Reporting

- Record all instructions given, including details of medication administration and use of medical devices.
- Document your evaluation of client or family caregiver learning.
- Report client's inability to adhere to medication safety plan to health care provider.

Sample Documentation

0900 Instructed on self-administration of digoxin. Client states purpose of medication, common side effects, and when to notify health care provider about medication-related concerns. Able to read each label and state when drug is to be taken. Demonstrated how to take pulse correctly.

Special Considerations

Pediatric

- Keep all medications, medical supplies, and equipment safely out of reach of children. Children are curious and put things in their mouth; risk is high for accidental poisoning (CDC, 2011).
- Tell family caregivers not to refer to medications as treats; this could add to risk of child overdosing by mistaking medicine for candy (CDC, 2011).

Geriatric

- Capacity for learning new information remains as adults age (in the absence of dementia). Additional time is needed to accomplish learning; allow adequate time and number of teaching sessions to support successful learning.
- Keep medications locked in a secure place for clients with cognitive impairment.
- The assistance of a home health nurse or trained family caregiver is often needed to fill weekly pillbox containers.

CRITICAL THINKING QUESTIONS

Case Study

A 4-year-old girl with a history of diabetes mellitus was recently discharged from the hospital after an acute hypoglycemic event. The home health nurse arrives to find her mother smoking a cigarette while cooking fried eggs as the 4-year-old plays nearby.

1. The home care nurse instructs the mother in ways to make the home environment safer. Her instructions include which of the following safety measures? Select all that apply.
   1. Turn pot handles to face inward when cooking on stovetop
   2. Install a stove lock
   3. Set hot water heater above 120°F (49°C)
   4. Offer smoking cessation classes
2. The nurse evaluates the mother's ability to care for her daughter's needs related to being a diabetic. Which of the following actions by the mother would the nurse identify as a need for further education? Select all that apply.
   1. The mother disposes of the used syringe in an empty plastic soda bottle
   2. The daughter's insulin bottle is being stored on the child's bedroom dresser
   3. Testing supplies are mailed to the family from a private company
   4. The mother tells her daughter that the insulin is a "treat" for being a good patient
3. Medication adherence is particularly important for a diabetic to be able to manage blood glucose levels. List two areas to assess with this mother to determine the likelihood of her ability to administer insulin as ordered to her daughter.

Review Questions

1. Home care instruction begins at the time of admission to a health care facility. Which of the following topics are appropriate to discuss with a client preparing to go home after surgery? Select all that apply.
   1. Health care promotion
   2. Coping with impaired function
   3. The medical history of family caregiver
   4. Measures to restore health
2. An elderly client with a recent history of three falls has moved in with his daughter and has started keeping a fall diary. When the nurse visits, she asks to see the diary; however, the daughter becomes angry and tells the nurse that her father feels this information should be kept private. How should the nurse respond to the daughter?
   1. Call the Center for Aging and report the daughter for bullying
   2. Explain to the daughter why this information is helpful in planning care
   3. Request that the daughter leave the home so the nurse can meet with the client alone
   4. Agree with the daughter and begin to write a private diary on the client instead
3. The nurse instructs the daughter who is the family caregiver of a client at risk for wandering to follow which of the following safety measures? Select all that apply.
   1. Provide signs in the home to guide the client
   2. Remove locks from doors
   3. Allow wandering in a safe place
   4. Use restraints to discourage wandering

4. The home care nurse visits an 83-year-old woman who has multiple health problems. The client takes eight different medicines. Which of the following measures would help prevent a medication administration error? Select all that apply.
   1. Have client get a refill before a medicine container is empty
   2. Have pharmacist place pills in an easy-to-open container
   3. Dispense pills into a pill organizer for a full week
   4. Do not take expired medications

5. In helping an older adult manage his or her medications safely, the nurse performs which of the following actions? Select all that apply.
   1. Provides large-print medication chart in home
   2. Disposes of used needles in a plastic bag
   3. Reviews safe storage techniques for medications
   4. Has pharmacist put medication in container that client cannot easily open

6. A home care nurse visits a client who has an ulcer on his lower leg. The client's wife performs the dressing change for the nurse. The nurse knows that the wife is able to dispose of medical supplies correctly by which of the following actions?
   1. Does not wear gloves because they would offend her husband
   2. Places sharp objects in a trash bag
   3. Discards disposable sheet in trash bag
   4. Places the soiled bandages in a securely fastened plastic bag

7. During a visit with a family with two children, ages 10 and 15 years, the home care nurse observes that a gun is lying on a table in the living room. What is the best response the nurse can make to this observation?
   1. Engage the father in conversation about how he uses the gun
   2. Encourage the father to move the gun to a nightstand in his bedroom
   3. Advise the father to install trigger locks and store the gun in a locked cabinet
   4. Suggest that he teach his children how to use the gun by practicing in their backyard

8. The home care nurse is assessing a Hispanic male client who is obese and was recently diagnosed with diabetes. The nurse is practicing in a culturally sensitive manner as evidenced by which of the following actions?
   1. Provide the client with a low-fat, low-carbohydrate cookbook
   2. Listen to the client explain his holiday meal traditions
   3. Enroll the client at a local gym in aerobic step classes
   4. Support the client in continuing his usual dietary practices

9. An elderly client uses a cane to walk. The home care nurse is concerned about risk for falls. Which of the following actions could the nurse take to prevent a fall?
   1. Discourage use of the cane
   2. Encourage client to wear shoes with thick soles
   3. Advise client to remove area rugs from home
   4. Schedule diuretic medications in late evening

10. An 82-year-old man who lives with his son recently sustained a fractured elbow when he fell at home. His son tells the home care nurse that he is concerned because his father is afraid to be at home alone now and the son travels often for business. How should the nurse respond to the son's concerns?
    1. Tell the son not to worry because the father has to get used to being alone
    2. Explain to the son that the father's fear is a normal reaction to falling
    3. Assist the son to find a new job so he can stay at home with his father
    4. Begin organizing the placement of the father in a skilled care facility

REFERENCES

Alzheimer's Association: *Preparing for and preventing wandering,* 2012, http://www.alz.org/national/documents/topicsheetwandering.pdf. Accessed September 5, 2013.

Barnason S, et al: Patient recovery and transitions after hospitalization for acute cardiac events: an integrative review, *J Cardiovasc Nurs* 27(2):175, 2012.

Centers for Disease Control and Prevention (CDC): *Put your medicines up and away and out of sight,* 2011, http://www.cdc.gov/features/medicationstorage/. Accessed September 5, 2013.

Cohen R: *Cultural competence in holistic nursing: a core value of practice,* 2014, http://www.ahna.org/Resources/Publications/eNewsletter/CulturalCompetence/tabid/9789/Default.aspx. Accessed October 2014.

Edlin G, Golanty E: *Health and wellness,* ed 10, Sudbury, MA, 2010, Jones & Bartlett.

Electrical Safety Foundation International (ESFi): *How to conduct a basic home electrical safety check,* 2014, http://esfi.org/index.cfm/cd/FAP/cdid/11246/pid/10272. Accessed February 25, 2014.

Energy.Gov: *Portable heaters,* 2013, http://energy.gov/energysaver/articles/portable-heaters. Accessed October 2014.

Hepp U, et al: Methods of suicide used by children and adolescents, *Eur Child Adolesc Psychiatry* 21(2):67, 2012.

Hockenberry MJ, Wilson D: *Wong's essentials of pediatric nursing,* ed 9, St Louis, 2013, Mosby.

Meiner SE: *Gerontologic nursing,* ed 4, St Louis, 2011, Mosby.

Sears N, et al: The incidence of adverse events among home care patients, *Int J Qual Health Care* 25(1):16, 2013.

The Joint Commission (TJC): *National Patient Safety Goals,* Oakbrook Terrace, IL, 2014, The Commission. Available at: http://www.jointcommission.org/standards_information/npsgs.aspx. Accessed October 2014.

Touhy TA, Jett K: *Ebersole and Hess' toward healthy aging: human needs and nursing response,* ed 8, St Louis, 2012, Mosby.

US Department of Health and Human Services (HHS): *Healthy People 2020 topics and objectives,* 2014, http://healthypeople.gov/2020/topicsobjectives2020/default.aspx. Accessed February 25, 2014.

US Environmental Protection Agency (EPA): *Medical waste, 2012,* http://epa.gov/wastes/nonhaz/industrial/medical/. Accessed November 2014.

US Food and Drug Administration (FDA): *Sharps disposal containers,* 2013, http://www.fda.gov/MedicalDevices/ProductsandMedicalProcedures/HomeHealthandConsumer/ConsumerProducts/Sharps/ucm263236.htm. Accessed September 5, 2013.

US Food and Drug Administration (FDA): *How to dispose of unused medicines,* 2014, http://www.fda.gov/forconsumers/consumerupdates/ucm101653.htm. Accessed October 2014.

Answer Key to End-of-Chapter Exercises

CHAPTER 1

Case Study

1. Does the use of the teach-back method (I) compared with a standard teaching handout (C) improve demonstration of safe insulin injections (O) by patients with diabetes (P)?
2. An outcome would be patients' ability to demonstrate safe insulin injection on themselves with needle safety principles. The nurses could measure this by the number of times patients successfully inject insulin, recording if patients prepare the correct subcutaneous site with alcohol, safely and accurately draw up the insulin, inject insulin at a 45-degree angle, inject insulin slowly and completely, and dispose of the needle in a sharps container. Each factor could be recorded, comparing the rates of success between the patients with the verbal handout training and the patients who received the teach-back method.

Review Questions

1. **3, 5, 2, 4, 6, 1.**
2. **3. Rationale:** Evidence review and critique determine if the evidence is strong enough eventually to apply in practice.
3. **3. Rationale:** The nurses seek scientific information about local anesthesia as an opportunity to build knowledge about a new procedure.
4. **1, 3. Rationale:** Background questions are broad and less focused than a foreground or PICO question; they often lead to too many articles to read on diverse topics not relevant to the PICO question.
5. **1. Rationale:** A descriptive study describes phenomena, in this case nurses' perceptions of communication during handoffs. It usually involves analysis of surveys, interviews, observation, or questionnaires.
6. **2, 3. Rationale:** Randomized trials are experimental studies involving a control and experimental (intervention) group. Both the control and the intervention groups are measured by the same outcomes to determine if the intervention was more effective than the control.
7. **1. Rationale:** The literature review summarizes available literature on the researcher's topic of interest. A good review explains why the author decided to study or report on a topic, usually because of a gap in the literature.
8. **P:** Medical inpatients; **I:** Hourly rounds; **C:** Standard observations; **O:** Fall incidence or rate.
9. **4. Rationale:** Question 4 has the primary components of an identified patient population (P), the intervention thought to be worthwhile (I), and a desired outcome (O). The question also has a comparison intervention. Questions 1 and 2 have no outcome. Question 3 has no population or area of interest.
10. **2, 3 Rationale:** Resources for implementation of an EVP change include staff from all disciplines (as appropriate) and administrative support and costs of the implementation. Accuracy of the device is not a resource but a clinical factor that should be addressed in your literature review supporting use of the device. Patient satisfaction could be an outcome measure that you choose to include in the pilot.

CHAPTER 2

Case Study

1. **2. Rationale:** This is an example of an ineffective and nontherapeutic communication technique and is likely to result in increased agitation and frustration in the patient.
2. **3, 4. Rationale:** The patient's daughter is avoiding participating in the decision-making process regarding placement for her mother. She needs to get involved.
3. **2. Rationale:** The nurse can delegate to the NAP to reorient the patient to person, place, and time.

Review Questions

1. **1. Rationale:** This statement is empathetic and acknowledges the patient's feelings.
2. **4. Rationale:** Nonverbal communication is very powerful; however, the nurse must validate that the message perceived is the intended message.

3. **1. Rationale:** Touch can be a therapeutic nonverbal communication technique, but it should not be used with suspicious patients. It may be perceived as an invasion of personal space and may heighten the level of suspiciousness.
4. 1, 2, 4, and 6 are examples of therapeutic techniques.
5. **3. Rationale:** Facial expressions communicate emotions and are the most important source of nonverbal communication.
6. **1, 4. Rationale:** These nursing statements are examples of a nontherapeutic communication block of belittling feelings. Belittling feelings occur when the nurse misjudges the degree of the patient's discomfort, and a lack of empathy and understanding may be conveyed.
7. **2, 4. Rationale:** Asking "why" questions is nontherapeutic and sets up a feeling of defensiveness in the patient. Information may be obtained by asking questions using other words such as "how," "where," "what," and "when." It is not therapeutic to challenge patients, demanding proof from them.
8. **4. Rationale:** Many factors may adversely affect patient outcomes; all of the factors listed have the potential to have a negative effect on patients.
9. **3. Rationale:** Maintaining personal space, encouraging safe coping behaviors, and using silence all are therapeutic techniques. The use of touch is discouraged with angry patients because it may escalate the situation.
10. **3. Rationale:** The patient needs to agree with the discharge plan for it to be successful.

CHAPTER 3

Case Study

1. **1, 2. Rationale:** A hip fracture is an adverse event and deviates from the standard of care. The fall is documented in the medical record and incident report. Personal notes of incidents should not be maintained. The other two answers are inappropriate.
2. **4. Rationale:** SBAR is a framework to communicate the situation, background, assessment, and recommendation to other members of the health care team. SOAP, PIE, and DAR are methods to record data in the medical record.
3. **3. Rationale:** Obtaining vital signs when a patient is stable may be delegated to the NAP. A nurse cannot delegate assessments to the NAP. Teaching and evaluation of responses to teaching are the nurse's responsibilities.

Review Questions

1. **3. Rationale:** Nurses document only factual and objective information in the medical record and not opinions or assumptions.
2. **4. Rationale:** The nurse quotes what the patient states if it is relevant and appropriate to nursing care.
3. **2, 5. Rationale:** Administration of any treatments is documented as soon as possible after administration. A pain assessment occurs before the intervention of pain medication. The other activities are part of routine charting

either periodically during the shift or at the end of the shift.
4. **3. Rationale:** Charting by exception (CBE) is a method of recording that aims to eliminate redundancy and make documentation of routine care more concise. The emphasis is on recording abnormal findings and trends in clinical care.
5. **3. Rationale:** Do not leave patient information on the monitor where others can view. Never share user passwords and keep your own password private. Dispose of patient data in official disposable units. Nurses must use the EHR as needs arise.
6. **1. Rationale:** Descriptive and objective information that is factual is recorded in the medical record. Using vague terms such as *good* and *bad* may be interpreted differently by care providers and should be avoided.
7. **3. Rationale:** Nurses must legally and ethically keep patient information confidential. Without the patient's permission, data cannot be shared with family. Patients have the right to access their medical record. Only health care providers directly involved in a specific patient's care have legitimate access to the medical record.
8. **3. Rationale:** 8:45 PM is 2045 in military time. 0845 is equivalent to 8:45 AM, 1845 is equivalent to 6:45 PM, and 1945 is equivalent to 7:45 PM.
9. **3. Rationale:** DAR (*Data*, *Action*, and patient *Response*) is used in focus charting. Other formats include SOAP (*Subjective* data, *Objective* data, *Assessment* or *Analysis*, and *Plan*), SOAPE (SOAP plus *Evaluation*), and PIE (*Problem*, *Intervention*, and *Evaluation*).
10. **4. Rationale:** Documentation is accurate, concise, and objective, reflecting the patient's status.

CHAPTER 4

Case Study

1. **3. Rationale:** Using the acronym RACE, the first step is to rescue a patient from immediate injury, followed by activation of the alarm, containing the fire, and patient evacuation.
2. **1. Rationale:** The order of steps for containing a fire include (1) closing all doors and windows, (2) turning off oxygen and electrical equipment, and (3) placing wet towels along base of doors.

Review Questions

1. **3. Rationale:** If a person receives an electrical shock, immediately turn off power to electrical source and then assess for presence of a pulse.
2. **2, 4, 5. Rationale:** The nurse should assess any previous fall using the acronym SPLATT: *Symptoms* at time of fall, *Previous* fall, *Location* of fall, *Activity* at time of fall, *Time* of fall, and *Trauma* after fall. It is important to assess medications and medical conditions to determine a patient's fall risks but not as the information relates to a previous fall.
3. **3. Rationale:** The first step is to position the patient safely, guiding the patient to the floor. This step is

followed by calling for help, suctioning the mouth as needed, and observing the sequence and timing of the seizure. It is not appropriate in this case to insert an oral airway, unless at end of seizure the patient has difficulty breathing.

4. Correct sequence is 3, 2, 4, 1.

5. **1, 2, 3, 4. Rationale:** All of these interventions are important for a patient in restraints. Without ROM exercises, the patient may experience rapid deconditioning. Restraints can restrict circulation and lead to skin breakdown. These assessments must be made at least every 2 hours. Toileting and hydration are basic human needs that a restrained person cannot provide for himself. All of these interventions also show respect for the patient.

6. **3. Rationale:** A facility must support a "culture of safety" in which a safety concern can be voiced by anyone without fear. Responses 1 and 2 are ways to measure and reinforce competency training. Response 4 is an example of a nurse being accountable for following organizational policies.

7. **1, 2, 3. Rationale:** Planned activities such as walks or other activities can decrease wandering. Keeping the patient near the nurses' station where her activities can be watched more closely is also helpful.

8. **2. Rationale:** The one evidence-based intervention among the choices is a standard vision assessment. Restraints do not prevent falls. Diversional activities and the RAWS are designed to reduce the use of restraints, not to prevent falls.

9. **2, 3, 4, 1. Rationale:** Follow the acronym RACE—*R*escue, *A*ctivate alarm, *C*ontain fire, *E*vacuate patient.

10. **3, 4. Rationale:** QSEN skills for safety competency include demonstrating effective use of strategies such as evidence-based assessment guidelines to reduce the risk of harm to patients. In addition, communicating to staff members any observations related to errors such as a fall occurrence is essential. Reliance on memory is not a safety competency, nor is the use of a new technology without first receiving proper training.

CHAPTER 5

Case Study

1. Airborne precautions
2. N95 or P100 mask
3. The nurse can delegate basic care to the NAP; however, the selection of the mask is based on patient assessment and implementation of isolation precautions, which are in the scope of professional nursing practice and cannot be delegated.

Review Questions

1. **2. Rationale:** Small droplets cannot be transmitted when there is a barrier such as a hand or tissue in place. This barrier reduces the risk of transmission of infection.

2. **3, 4, 2, 6, 5, 1, 7. Rationale:** This sequence ensures that the risk of contaminating any other surfaces or health care personnel is reduced.

3. **2, 4, 5. Rationale:** The condition described in option 1 happened outside of the hospital, and option 3 describes testing for an infection, not the acquisition of that infection. All other answers describe conditions acquired in a hospital setting.

4. **4. Rationale:** Gloves protect health care personnel from contamination with body fluids, which is a method of blocking the portal of exit from the patient.

5. **1. Rationale:** A dressing serves as a source of a reservoir for microorganisms. Changing dressings reduces the risk of bacterial growth.

6. **1, 2, 5. Rationale:** Nos. 1, 2, and 5 all require sterile technique because of the high risk of bacterial entrance into sterile body cavities through the urethra, trachea, or central nervous system.

7. **1. Rationale:** The second glove was picked up incorrectly, causing the first glove to be contaminated. The nurse should have picked up the second glove under the cuff because the right hand already had a sterile glove in place.

8. **2. Rationale:** To maintain a sterile field, objects must be maintained and handled above the waist. All other choices are appropriate to maintaining a sterile field while opening a sterile pack.

9. **2. Rationale:** Individuals who have frequent exposure to latex have a higher risk of developing a latex allergy.

10. **1. Rationale:** The first flap in a sterile field is opened away from, not toward, the nurse.

CHAPTER 6

Case Study

1. **4. Rationale:** If patient is unable to keep the mouth closed, the nurse should select another site.

2. **2, 3, 5. Rationale:** Insufficient information is available to notify the health care provider. The nurse cannot assume that the patient has not taken her medications. A complete vascular assessment is not indicated until blood pressure measurements are verified. Lower extremity blood pressure measurements are not needed in this situation. The correct blood pressure cuff should be used for the initial measurement. The measurements should be verified and compared with baseline before taking any action.

3. **4. Rationale:** Cough and complaints of dyspnea indicate the potential for respiratory compromise in this patient. The patient's right hand is compromised, and capillary refill is likely to be increased. Values of 95% and greater are normal. Oximeter pulse rate is not always accurate.

Review Questions

1. **2. Rationale:** Acute pain increases heart rate and respiratory rate. Pain causes vasoconstriction, which increases blood pressure. There is no effect on temperature.

2. **1. Rationale:** The difference between right arm and left arm blood pressure is of concern and needs to be reconfirmed. The temperature should be reconfirmed, but this is not as critical as the blood pressure. The pulse is acceptable and does not require an apical rate. A focused respiratory assessment is not indicated at this time.

3. **3. Rationale:** The blood pressure and heart rate are acceptable for a patient with a fever. The respiratory rate reflects complications of pneumonia, and interventions are needed.

4. **3. Rationale:** The associated symptoms of hypertension (e.g., headache, flushing) support the blood pressure measurements, making repeating the blood pressure values unnecessary. Although the social worker should be contacted, the physician needs to be notified to treat the hypertension.

5. **2. Rationale:** The student is displaying symptoms of an infection. A full set of vital signs is needed, but an elevated temperature is the most likely abnormality the school nurse will find.

6. **2. Rationale:** Cheyne-Stokes is a pattern of apnea and hyperventilation. The respiratory rate of 12 was counted with the apneic phase.

7. **1. Rationale:** Choices 2 and 3 create a false low blood pressure. The gown would not alter the blood pressure measurement.

8. **4. Rationale:** Decreased pulse strength on the affected side may indicate vascular compromise.

9. **1, 2, 3, 5, 6. Rationale:** An increased temperature may result in vasodilation and lower blood pressure. The remaining factors can potentially increase blood pressure.

10. **4, 1, 3, 2.**

CHAPTER 7

Case Study

1. Focused assessments would include skin, cardiovascular, peripheral neurovascular, respiratory, abdominal and perineal, and intake and output (I&O) assessments. Key elements of each system are as follows: (a) skin—condition of the skin at the IV site (b) cardiovascular—blood pressure; heart rate; inspection, palpation, and auscultation of the heart; (c) peripheral neurovascular—inspection and palpation of extremities; checking peripheral pulses; edema, skin color, and temperature; capillary refill; sensation and movement; (d) respiratory—checking rate and depth of respirations, chest excursion, and lung sounds; (e) abdominal—checking size and shape of abdomen, palpation of bladder, assessing bowel sounds, assessing condition of dressing; (f) I&O—intake, output (Foley, Jackson-Pratt drain).

2. Respiratory. Unilateral leg swelling around the calf could indicate deep venous thrombosis, so the respiratory system should be assessed because of the possibility of the complication of pulmonary embolism.

3. You must listen for 5 minutes over each quadrant before deciding that bowel sounds are absent. It is common for bowel sounds to be hypoactive for 24 hours or more after abdominal surgery.

Review Questions

1. **1, 5, 7. Rationale:** The general survey includes assessment of vital signs, height and weight, general behavior, posture, and appearance.

2. **3. Rationale:** A lesion colored blue-black or with variegated, nonuniform pigmentation or variations or multiple colors (tan, black) with areas of pink, white, gray, blue, or red may indicate a melanoma.

3. **4. Rationale:** Crackles sound like crushing cellophane; rhonchi sound like blowing air through fluid with a straw.

4. **4. Rationale:** S_1 and S_2 are normal components of the cardiac cycle and an expected physical assessment finding.

5. Auscultation. Auscultation follows inspection because of the risk for causing increased bowel sounds that could be interpreted as an abnormal finding.

6. **3. Rationale:** The dorsum of the hand is most sensitive to temperature variations.

7. **1 and 2. Rationale:** In a normal get-up-and-go test, a patient does not use the arms to sit up from a chair or to sit back down. Muscle strength graded as 1 indicates minimal strength.

8. Total 352 mL intake (3 ounces apple juice = 90 mL; $\frac{1}{4}$ carton milk = 63 mL; 6 ounces soda = 180 mL; and 8 ounces ice [$\frac{1}{2}$ volume] = 120 mL).

9. The fourth to seventh day of the menstrual cycle or right after the cycle ends. The breasts are least likely to be tender at this time.

10. **2, 3, 5, 6. Rationale:** Frequency, loudness, quality, and duration are all the characteristics that can be heard through auscultation.

CHAPTER 8

Case Study

1. **4. (2, 4, 1, 5, 3). Rationale:** Performing the procedure using appropriate steps minimizes contamination of the specimen, increases efficiency, and allows timely delivery to the laboratory.

2. **3. Rationale:** This response indicates the daughter's understanding that a culture is for identification of the pathogenic microorganism, and sensitivity identifies medications that are active against the microorganism.

Review Questions

1. **1. Rationale:** The forearm is an appropriate alternate site, especially if blood sugar values are not changing. The patient is having a routine check. Applying pressure to the puncture site might cause an abnormal reading because of the changes of cellular metabolism. Warm water increases blood flow to the area but does not address the patient's discomfort. Placing the lancet firmly against the skin is not likely to reduce pain in fingers.

2. **4. Rationale:** The median cubital vein is easier to puncture and less likely to rupture. The basilic and cephalic veins of the lower arm and hand are preferred for administering IV fluids. The antecubital vein is often less visible.

3. **1. Rationale:** Diets rich in red meats and peroxidase-rich vegetables (turnips, horseradish, artichokes, mushrooms, radishes, broccoli, bean sprouts, cauliflower, oranges, bananas, cantaloupes, and grapes) may affect results (Pagana and Pagana, 2013).

4. **3. Rationale:** A repeat wound specimen is necessary to identify the pathogenic organism correctly. Antibiotic therapy begins after results from the specimen are obtained. Monitoring a patient is not indicated as a result of specimen contamination. Water would cause drying of the wound.

5. **1. Rationale:** Assessing the patient's understanding would allow reinforcement of the information and determine what action the nurse may need to take to ensure that all urine is collected for 24 hours. All urine needs to be collected for a full 24-hour period; not including urine results in an inaccurate report. Restarting the procedure is necessary, but the nurse must first determine the patient's ability to collect the specimen. Drinking water would be helpful for voiding but would not influence the patient's ability to collect the specimen.

6. **2. Rationale:** Do not attempt throat cultures if you suspect acute epiglottitis because trauma from swabbing might cause an increase in edema and resulting occlusion of the airway (Hockenberry and Wilson, 2013). It is important to collect a throat culture before mealtime or at least 1 hour after eating or drinking to lessen the chance of inducing vomiting and risk for aspiration. Assess the patient's understanding of the purpose of the procedure and the patient's ability to cooperate. You may need assistance to obtain throat cultures from confused, combative, or unconscious patients.

7. **1, 4. Rationale:** These are the only correct steps for this procedure. Leaning the head forward increases difficulty entering the mouth and decreases visualization of the oral cavity. Rinsing the mouth before collection of a specimen would decrease flora. You swab the tonsillar area, not the uvula. Blowing the nose does not affect a throat culture.

8. **1, 3, 4. Rationale:** The patient's blood sugar remains uncontrolled. To control his diabetes it is important for him to understand the need to be consistent and to follow his personal regimen for blood sugar monitoring.

9. **3. Rationale:** The absence of the radial pulse indicates absence of arterial blood flow, which can cause injury to the patient. Blood returns to the arterial system immediately, and in 60 seconds flow is normal.

10. **1, 2, 5, 6. Rationale:** Option 3 is incorrect; the head of the penis is wiped in a circular motion, not back and forth. Option 4 is incorrect; the amount of urine needed is 30 to 60 mL.

CHAPTER 9

Case Study

1. **2, and 4. Rationale:** Cardiac catheterization poses a risk for blood loss and complications that require immediate cardiac surgery. Baseline assessment should include the patient's hemoglobin and hematocrit (CBC). The PT and PTT provide a baseline to determine if the patient is at risk for postprocedure bleeding. BUN, creatinine, and urine specific gravity are used to assess the patient's dehydration status further. Patients who are dehydrated, have diabetes, or have renal failure are at risk for impaired excretion of the contrast dye. Because the liver is responsible for the metabolism of most drugs, liver function should be assessed preoperatively.

2. **2. Rationale:** Patients who have not given informed consent must wait until the health care provider fully explains the procedure. Sedatives impair decision making, and informed consent is obtained first. Laboratory values may determine if the health care provider proceeds with the procedure or delays the procedure for other treatment, but they do not affect consent process.

Review Questions

1. **1, 2 and 4. Rationale:** Catheter site pain, loss of distal pulses, and pooling of blood under the patient can be caused by arterial bleeding from the arterial site. Anxiety, backache, and increased heart rate can be signs of internal bleeding and must be evaluated.

2. **1. Rationale:** The patient with renal failure is not able to filter out the toxins from the contrast medium and may be nephrotoxic. The patient with one kidney may have complete renal function in the remaining kidney.

3. **1. Rationale:** "Apply topical anesthetic to the bone marrow aspiration site 10 minutes before the procedure is scheduled to begin" is not a nursing intervention and requires a health care provider's order.

4. **4, 5, 3, 1, 2 is the correct order.**

5. **1. Rationale:** Assisting to help maintain the patient's side-lying position is the only appropriate option. Options 2 and 3 deal with assessment; assessment is always the responsibility of the nurse. Preparing a site and a sterile tray is also a nursing responsibility.

6. **3. Rationale:** When fluid is removed from the abdominal cavity, the abdominal girth decreases. Removing abdominal ascetic fluid allows the lungs to expand further to meet oxygen needs. As this occurs, the respiratory rate declines.

7. **1, 3 and 4. Rationale:** The patient is assisted into left side-lying position before the procedure. The patient is instructed not to drive or operate machinery for 24 hours after any sedation procedure. Bowel preparation occurs 36 to 24 hours before the procedure to ensure an empty colon.

8. **1, 2, 3, 4, 5, and 6. Rationale:** 1, 2, 5, and 6 are necessary evaluation measures to compare with baseline data to determine if the patient's condition worsens. The patient's status is unstable or likely to become unstable requiring emergency resuscitative procedures (Rapid Response Team) and oxygen. Obtaining vital signs are part of the NAP's responsibility; delegating this to the NAP at this time, after obtaining a baseline set of vital signs, frees the nurse to assess and treat the patient.

9. **1. Rationale:** Symptoms of shallow and reduced respirations, tachycardia, and difficulty to arouse indicate oversedation.

10. **3. Rationale:** Naloxone (Narcan) is the reversal agent for opioids. Midazolam is the benzodiazepine and would lead to additional sedation. Flumazenil is the reversal

agent for benzodiazepines. Morphine is an opioid that would result in additional sedation.

CHAPTER 10

Case Study

1. **2. Rationale:** It is important to ask about patient preferences before beginning a procedure so that you know what supplies to gather. Perform hand hygiene and don gloves before removing dentures. After upper and lower dentures are removed, hold dentures over an emesis basin or lined sink to protect them in the event they are dropped while brushing the dentures. Storing dentures would be the last step.
2. **2. Rationale:** The patient becomes short of breath with any exertion. It would be best at this time to give a partial bath. A complete bath requires more time and movement. A tub bath and shower require more exertion and would be inappropriate at this time.

Review Questions

1. **1, 3, 5, 7. Rationale:** To be safe, the bed must be elevated to working height. Tuck in the top sheet and spread at the foot of the bed and then make a modified mitered corner. To save steps, apply all bottom linen on one side of bed before moving to opposite side. Horizontal toe pleats are made on all beds. Gloves do not need to be worn except if linen is soiled with drainage. Soiled linen should be placed in linen bag, not on the floor. Top covers need to be fanfolded to the end of the bed when the procedure is complete.
2. **3. Rationale:** Follow the principle of cleansing from least contaminated area to most contaminated area. Leaving a foreskin retracted results in tightening of the foreskin around the shaft of the penis, which can lead to permanent urethral damage. Cleansing the perineum should proceed from the least to most contaminated area, in this case, from "front to back" or perineum to rectum. A patient with a Foley catheter needs more frequent perineal care because of the increased risk of infection.
3. **4. Rationale:** The patient is less likely to aspirate in the side-lying position because fluid would most likely pool in the mouth, where it can be suctioned. Options 1, 2, and 3 place the patient at risk for aspiration.
4. **4. Rationale:** Although bath bags are easy to use, are quick, and promote comfort, the patient was concerned about not using a basin. Option 4 addresses that concern. Bath basins may be a reservoir and a way that harmful bacteria can spread.
5. **3. Rationale:** Washing from distal to proximal promotes venous return to the right side of the heart. It does not enhance comfort, prevent skin irritation, or reduce swelling.
6. **1, 3. Rationale:** Using the razor at 45 degrees and shaving in the direction of hair growth facilitates shaving of facial hair. A warm, moist washcloth is used, and short downward strokes are recommended.

7. **1. Rationale:** Eyes are first, using plain water without soap. Bathing then proceeds from top (face) to bottom so that the most contaminated areas are last.
8. **4. Rationale:** Patients with diabetes have poor circulation. Cutting nails could cause trauma, impaired skin integrity, and infection. Always use nail clippers to trim nails straight across; clipping nails to fit the contour of the fingers could result in ingrown nails. Use an emery board to shape nails after being trimmed.
9. **1. Rationale:** Before shaving a patient, the nurse should ask what his preference is and take into consideration his cultural and spiritual beliefs. Some religions do not allow cutting or shaving hair.
10. **4. Rationale:** All are signs and symptoms of a VTE. Other signs and symptoms include redness, warmth, and tenderness.

CHAPTER 11

Case Study

1. **2. Rationale:** Apply clean gloves when drainage is present. Turn off the aid volume before it prevents feedback (whistling) during removal. Grasping the device prevents accidentally dropping the aid. The brush supplied with the aid is used to dislodge any wax that is transferred from the ear canal to the aid. Wash the ear canal to remove any drainage or wax. Storing the aid in its storage case further reduces the risk of damage to the aid.
2. **1, 3. Rationale:** Options 1 and 3 are safety concerns. The batteries are very toxic to children and pets when swallowed, and the child would need to be seen by a health care professional. The aids are small and present a choking hazard to the child. Option 2 teaches the patient to have his grandchildren face him to increase his hearing clarity when the children are speaking but is not related to child safety. Option 4 offers the patient a way to show the children about the aid to address some of their curiosity.

Review Questions

1. **1. Rationale:** Ear irrigations are contraindicated when a foreign matter such as a vegetable is present. Potentially the foreign object could absorb the solution and expand in the ear canal.
2. **2. Rationale:** This position straightens the ear canal and facilitates entrance of the irrigant.
3. **2. Rationale:** Holding the syringe correctly directs the irrigant into the ear canal without occluding the canal and damaging the internal ear structures.
4. **4. Rationale:** Some disposable contact lenses are intended to be cleaned and reused. There is increased risk for infection with any contact lens use.
5. **4. Rationale:** The nurse needs more information about the pain and any other related symptoms, such as drainage, odor, or fever. The assessment is needed to gather further information on which treatment can be recommended.
6. **1. Rationale:** This is an urgent situation. The priority of care is to determine the level of injury and prevent

further damage. The nurse must quickly assess the injured eye; determine the level of pain, which might indicate the need for pain relief; and prepare to irrigate the eye to flush out any remaining chemical and reduce further damage to the eye. Although teaching eye safety is important and needs to occur before discharge, it is not an immediate nursing action. The fact that the patient's wife ran water over the eyes to remove the chemical before coming to the emergency department was good; however, this action has no relevance to the nurse's immediate actions.

7. 3. **Rationale:** Eye care practices include providing artificial tears or moisturizers to lubricate and hydrate the eye. These artificial tears wash debris from the eye, moisten the cornea, and prevent microorganisms from adhering to the cornea.

8. 4. **Rationale:** It is the nurse's responsibility to assess the patient's eyes further before contacting the patient's health care provider. The NAP was instructed to notify the nurse for further assessment if drainage, redness, or irritation was present when performing eye care.

9. 2. **Rationale:** Before any interventions are undertaken, the nurse must first assess the patient's ear for signs of irritation, including any presence of infection. From there, the nurse can determine what needs to be done. This follows the sequence of the nursing process to assess first before implementing. Teaching the patient how to reposition his hearing aids if they are uncomfortable would be appropriate based on the assessment findings. Reducing the volume of the hearing aid in the ear not causing a problem is inappropriate.

10. 2. **Rationale:** The patient will be unable to care for her contact lenses immediately after surgery. No signs or symptoms have been presented to justify any of the other choices.

CHAPTER 12

Case Study

1. 2. **Rationale:** The nurse would expect a pH of 6.0 because of the continuous tube feeding in the small bowel. A pH of 4.0 would be expected for gastric secretions, and a pH of 2.0 would be expected if feedings were not being administered and the tube was in the stomach. A pH of 8.0 would suggest that the tube is in tracheobronchial tree.

2. 4. **Rationale:** Sterile water is indicated for irrigation when a patient is immunocompromised. Sterile water is not necessary for routine irrigation, and pH values of gastric aspiration do not influence selection of irrigation fluid. Extended-release medications should not be crushed.

Review Questions

1. 1, 3. **Rationale:** A wet voice and coughing on food are two common signs of dysphagia that are predictive for the risk of aspiration. The patient may have difficulty smiling if there is facial nerve paralysis after stroke. The ability to smile has not been associated with dysphagia.

Aversion to food and change in taste are not predictors of aspiration.

2. 3. **Rationale:** Placing a patient upright at a 90-degree angle reduces the incidence of gastric reflux. Providing oral hygiene reduces the number of bacteria in the saliva that could be aspirated. Pulse oximetry may reveal oxygen desaturation in patients who have aspirated. Adding thickener to liquids reduces risk of aspiration.

3. 1. **Rationale:** The correct technique requires the nurse to check tube placement first and then irrigate. The procedure is done every 4 hours.

4. 1, 3, 4. **Rationale:** Unexpected outcomes of a tube feeding include aspiration, the retention of large residual volumes of 250 mL or more, and clogging of a tube indicated by the inability to irrigate. Diarrhea, not constipation, is a symptom of tube-feeding intolerance. The ulcer on the naris is an unexpected outcome resulting from improper tube care, not the feeding.

5. 1, 3. **Rationale:** Always wash hands before touching food, and keep the refrigerator at 4.4°C (40°F). Discourage drinking unpasteurized milk, which might contain bacteria. Never use leftovers past 2 days.

6. 4. **Rationale:** A patient unable to chew is able to have a clear-liquid, full-liquid, or pureed diet. A full-liquid diet is indicated if the patient cannot tolerate solid foods. However, a pureed diet provides the most nutrients of the three and is indicated when the patient's GI function is normal. Mechanical and high-fiber diets require chewing.

7. 2. **Rationale:** High-fiber foods such as fresh uncooked fruits and steamed vegetables are useful in relieving constipation. Just because the patient has dentures does not mean that he is unable to chew; a pureed diet would be inappropriate. There is no indication for a fat-modified diet, and a low-residue diet is low in fiber content.

8. 2. **Rationale:** When a patient is forced to remain supine, place the patient in reverse Trendelenburg's position when administering a tube feeding.

9. 4. **Rationale:** The head of bed should be elevated at all times during tube feeding administration unless there is a contraindication, such as physiologic instability or spine injury. Tube feedings should be paused just before medication administration. Frequent pausing can lead to a decrease in caloric intake. The closed system should be changed every 24 to 48 hours. Medications should be mixed individually in 60 to 120 mL of water, depending on the patient's fluid volume status.

10. e, f, d, a, c, g, b.

CHAPTER 13

Case Study

1. This patient would benefit from a nonpharmacological approach because she has incomplete pain relief with NSAIDs, she would benefit from not taking an NSAID because she is an older adult, and she has expressed anxiety about her pain relief method.

2. When a patient reports pain intensity greater than desired after using nonpharmacological pain therapies, the nurse should try alternative nonpharmacological pain relief measures, ask the patient and family members what other options might be helpful, and consult with the patient's health care provider about the type of analgesic being used and other analgesic options.

Review Questions

1. 1, 2, 3. **Rationale:** Minority patients are at high risk for poor pain outcomes because of their difficulty in explaining and reporting.
2. 4. **Rationale:** Nonselective NSAIDs such as ibuprofen must be given with caution after other treatments have been tried. NSAIDs are given in the lowest dose possible and for the shortest time. Nonopioids such as acetaminophen are a first-line treatment against acute and persistent pain. Opioids such as morphine are safe to use in elderly patients. Dilantin is an example of a coanalgesic that can be given safely.
3. The correct order is 4, 1, 2, 5, 3, 6. **Rationale:** *P* stands for precipitating or palliative factors, *Q* stands for quality of pain, *R* stands for region or location of pain, *S* stands for severity or acuity of pain, *T* stands for timing, and *U* stands for the patient ("you") in "how does pain affect U."
4. 2. **Rationale:** Give analgesics at least 30 minutes before a nonpharmacological measure. All other measures are appropriate.
5. The correct order is 3, 1, 4, 2. **Rationale:** *S* stands for situation, *B* stands for background, *A* stands for assessment, and *R* stands for recommendation.
6. 2. **Rationale:** Relaxation should be first taught when a patient is not in acute discomfort or severe pain and is able to concentrate. It often takes several coaching sessions before patients effectively reduce pain. Relaxation techniques have few side effects and can be used with a variety of pain conditions.
7. 2. **Rationale:** Morphine is an opioid that works on higher centers of the brain and spinal cord to modify moderate to severe pain perception. In contrast to NSAIDs, it has no antiinflammatory properties. Nonopioids such as acetaminophen relieve mild pain by acting peripherally on nerves and centrally on the brain. Many adjuvants are more effective than opioids for neuropathic pain.
8. 1. **Rationale:** An analgesic should be given as soon as the patient perceives pain.
9. 3. **Rationale:** Teenagers usually are comfortable with technology; at this developmental stage the autonomy of being able to determine when to take their pain medication is very satisfying and reassuring.
10. 2. **Rationale:** A person with sleep apnea already has periods of decreased oxygenation due to episodes in which they briefly stop breathing while asleep (apnea). Obesity often causes partial obstruction of the trachea, especially when the pharynx is relaxed during sleep. These patients need frequent pain and sedation assessment. When they receive prn medications, the nurse will assess pain and sedation with each injection of analgesia.

CHAPTER 14

Case Study

1. 1, 3, 4. **Rationale:** The nurse initially observes the patient throughout the respiratory cycle. It is also important to obtain vital signs in this patient because these data give the nurse information about the overall status of the patient. Auscultation provides information about lung expansion, but this area cannot be assessed if the patient is lying flat. The chest tube should not show bubbling within the chambers; this indicates an air leak and needs to be evaluated.
2. 2. **Rationale:** The change in the assessment means that the patient is becoming hypoxic. A health care provider needs to be notified. The NAP is not qualified to stay with this patient. The nasal cannula delivers a maximum of 40% oxygen; the partial rebreathing mask must be set at a minimum of 8 L.
3. 1 and 4. **Rationale:** The nurse should assess for the location of the leak by clamping the chest tube with two rubber-shod or toothless clamps close to the chest wall. If bubbling stops, an air leak is inside the patient's thorax or at the chest insertion site. If bubbling continues with the clamps near the chest wall, the nurse should gradually move one clamp at a time down the drainage tubing away from the patient and toward the suction control chamber. When the bubbling stops, the leak is in a section of tubing or the connection between the clamps. If the tube becomes kinked, tidaling will stop, but bubbling will not be noted unless there is a breach in a connection of the system. The nurse should never disconnect the tubing unless hemostats are in place when changing the drainage system; research states that this should be completed quickly so as not to cause a tension pneumothorax.

Review Questions

1. 3. **Rationale:** Although assessing the level of consciousness of this patient is appropriate, it is not directly related to the primary assessment needs of the ETT. The student and nurse need to understand the differences in assessment for the neurologic versus the respiratory system.
2. 2, 3. **Rationale:** Tracheostomy care and suctioning can be delegated to NAP if the tracheostomy is well established and not for an acutely ill patient. The NAP can attach a nasal cannula if the nurse previously adjusted oxygen flow rate and assessed the patient. Suctioning for any patient with an ETT cannot be delegated to NAP.
3. 2, 3. **Rationale:** When caring for an intubated patient, nurses are encouraged to use positive verbal and nonverbal communication with direct eye contact and questions that require only "yes" or "no" responses. Alphabet charts, pen and paper, slates or chalkboards, and magnetic pen boards are some common communication tools. Intubated patients do not have a hearing loss; speaking loudly does not help communication and may frustrate the

patient even more. Families can speak to the patient, but the patient still needs a mechanism with which to reply. Families are not responsible for explaining the plan of care.

4. 4. **Rationale:** Smoking is not permitted in health care facilities, and because oxygen is combustible, open flames must be kept at least 10 feet away.

5. 2, 3, 6. **Rationale:** Toothbrushes should be used every 12 hours to provide oral care for ventilated patients. Toothettes are inadequate to clean dental plaque, but they may be used between brushing for moistening mucosa. The cuff pressure should be no more than 30 cm H_2O and needs to be assessed every 2 hours to prevent microaspirations or oral secretions. Although increasing mobility in this population is challenging, interventions such as repositioning, sitting, or standing at the bedside or ambulation have decreased the risk of VAP.

6. 1, 2, 3. **Rationale:** Alcohol may cause pain if the tops of the ears are excoriated and causes drying of the tissue. The best intervention is application of foam padding to the tops of the ears.

7. 3. **Rationale:** The patient needs to understand that OSA will not go away in a few weeks and that the CPAP machine will not provide adequate oxygenation and depth of sleeping needed in a couple of hours. Many patients may complain of feeling suffocated by the mask, but this feeling passes with continued use.

8. 4. **Rationale:** This sequence prompted correct PEFR measures. See Procedural Guideline 14.1.

9. 2. **Rationale:** The nurse needs to document the color, amount, and consistency of the sputum produced after CPT is complete. This information indicates for other health care providers the effectiveness of the treatment and the continued need for the treatment.

10. 4. **Rationale:** Promotes safe suction procedure. See Skill 14.4.

CHAPTER 15

Case Study

1. 1, 3, 5. **Rationale:** The patient is in pain most likely related to his lacerations and fractures. Pain management is a priority at this time. To transfer the patient safely, three nurses are necessary because of the patient's weight. In addition, explaining to him the purpose of the CT scan helps elicit his cooperation. This patient is most likely fearful of movement because of his pain and uncertainty of his condition. Two nurses are insufficient for the transfer. The nurse may inform the patient that it is the health care provider's orders, but the patient has the right to refuse treatment.

2. Logrolling. **Rationale:** The patient maintains proper alignment by moving all body parts at the same time, preventing tension or twisting of the spinal column.

3. 3. **Rationale:** Caution must be taken to prevent tension or twisting of the spinal column. The nurse must be present to supervise and assist in the transfer of the patient.

Review Questions

1. 1, 2, 3, 4. **Rationale:** It is important to perform a thorough assessment of the patient before attempting to transfer; this will prevent injury to the nurse and patient. A 24-hour calorie count would not be needed to determine the safest transfer technique.

2. 3. **Rationale:** Holding objects away from the body improves leverage. To prevent injury, do not keep the knees in a locked position or bend at the waist to pick up objects. Maintain a wide base of support to improve stability.

3. 1. **Rationale:** A mechanical transfer device would be appropriate because of the weight of this patient to prevent injury to the nurse and patient. Even though the patient is cooperative and has agreed to assist, the potential for injury is present.

4. 2. **Rationale:** The move from a supine to a vertical position redistributes about 500 mL of blood. Immobile patients may have decreased ability for the autonomic nervous system to equalize blood supply, resulting in orthostatic hypotension; this increases a patient's risk of fainting or falling during transfer.

5. 2. **Rationale:** Because of the patient's weight and limited ability to bear weight, a bariatric transfer aid provides the best and safest technique to transfer this patient. A friction-reducing device is used when transferring a patient from a bed to stretcher. A three-person carry is inappropriate and not recommended any longer. Option 4 is incorrect because of the patient's weight and limited weight bearing.

6. 2. **Rationale:** Logrolling and moving the patient as a unit prevents twisting and damage to the unstable spinal cord. The step-by-step method causes twisting and bending of the spine, resulting in further damage. The patient should remain non–weight-bearing to prevent further damage to the injured spine. Option 4 is incorrect because there is risk of twisting and bending the spine during transfer.

7. 1. **Rationale:** The patient may be refusing to move because his pain is not under control. Options 2, 3, and 4 are important assessment data once the patient has agreed to transfer.

8. 4. **Rationale:** Allowing the patient to dangle his or her feet at the side of the bed for a few minutes allows the nurse to determine if the patient is experiencing symptoms of orthostatic hypotension such as dizziness. Place the transfer belt around the patient's waist after the patient is in a sitting position. The under-axilla method may cause injury to the patient and places undue stress on the patient's axilla area. Offer the patient his or her glasses after positioning in a chair to prevent damage to eyeglasses.

9. 4. **Rationale:** A slide board is the most appropriate method to transfer this patient because the patient is unable to assist. If a caregiver must lift more than 35 pounds, there is a risk of injury. Body mechanics alone are insufficient. A slide board is the most appropriate method.

10. **7, 1, 4, 3, 2, 5, 6. Rationale:** This sequence first positions the bed and wheelchair at equal height, with the wheelchair appropriately angled to the bed. The safety features of the wheelchair are used, and the patient is safely transferred to the wheelchair.

CHAPTER 16

Case Study

1. **1, 2. Rationale:** Use of the device on the patient's strong side provides more support; a dry surface prevents slipping and falls. A patient should walk while wearing firm shoes with nonslip sole. The elbow should remain flexed when using a cane.
2. **3, 4. Rationale:** Space activities to avoid exhaustion. Rest is needed between activities such as bathing and ambulation. Sitting on the side of the bed and dangling helps resolve any dizziness resulting from orthostatic hypotension. The patient should stand straight while walking. An opioid could result in dizziness.
3. **3. Rationale:** The skill of teaching the use of the assistive device cannot be delegated to the NAP. The nurse is responsible for teaching. The NAP can assist the patient to walk with a device.

Review Questions

1. **2. Rationale:** Walking does not cost the older adults anything, and it is a safe means of exercise. A local fitness club and purchase of exercise equipment would be costly. A readers' club is an excellent social activity but does not involve exercise.
2. **1. Rationale:** The four-point gait provides the most support and improves balance.
3. **1, 3, 4. Rationale:** Pallor, nausea, and dizziness all are signs of orthostatic hypotension. Bradycardia is incorrect; tachycardia is actually a symptom. Irritability is not a classic sign of the condition.
4. **3. Rationale:** Raising the arm above the head achieves 180-degree abduction.
5. **1, 2, 3. Rationale:** Identifying methods to increase activity, such as increased range-of-motion exercises during daily hygiene routines, encourages routine exercise. Determining what activities are available and an appropriate age-group for exercise increase a person's likelihood of participating in exercise and increases socialization. A referral to a psychologist is inappropriate that this time.
6. **3. Rationale:** NAP can make sure that the patient's environment is free from potential threats to patient safety, such as spills or clutter.
7. **2. Rationale:** The success of a skin graft could be compromised by the application of elastic stockings to the site.
8. **2, 4, 3, 1. Rationale:** By providing a wide base of support first, the patient is able to balance.
9. **1, 2, 3, 4. Rationale:** The nurse must consider the unique characteristics of her unit and unique needs of her patients, such as overall physical health and conditions.

In addition, the literature supports that patients be involved in the individual plans so that their preferences are taken into consideration.

10. **4. Rationale:** This is ROM for the hips that the patient can perform while lying on her back. The exercise can take some stress and pressure off the patient's hips.

CHAPTER 17

Case Study

1. **2. Rationale:** Any sharp edges of a cast should be covered with tape or moleskin to prevent skin damage to adjacent tissues. A plaster cast needs to breathe and should not be covered completely for any length of time. In addition, a fiberglass cast can sustain exposure to water without losing structural integrity, but a plaster cast will begin to crumble.
2. **2. Rationale:** The health care provider may need to bivalve the cast by cutting it in two lengthwise along each side. A heating pad would increase swelling. There is concern of compartment syndrome and altered neurovascular status. In addition, the wadding underneath is cut to relieve pressure.
3. **2. Rationale:** The first step involves appropriate positioning. Before using the saw, it is important to explain to the patient what to expect from it to prevent anxiety and fear. Inspecting the skin determines if the skin is intact and can be washed. An enzyme wash assists in dissolving dead skin, and gentle manipulation of tissue prevents damaging delicate skin.

Review Questions

1. **2, 4. Rationale:** The boot should fit snugly to prevent slipping and ensure the traction pull but not be so tight that it leads to pressure on the tissues under the boot. Shaving is unnecessary and may create micronicks that could become inflamed under the traction apparatus. The heel should sit properly in the boot without the need for padding. Padding can cause pressure to the heel. Adding weight slowly and gently avoids involuntary muscle spasms and pain. Neurovascular status should be assessed distal to the traction, primarily in the foot.
2. **3. Rationale:** A fiberglass cast sets up and is dry in 14 to 20 minutes, so it is not necessary to prevent indentations, and the cast does not remain damp after that time period. A plaster of Paris cast takes much longer to dry and is susceptible to indentation and dampness, and assistance is needed in the drying process.
3. **1, 2, 3, 5, 7. Rationale:** The symptoms indicate swelling of the tissues under the cast. Elevating the cast to promote venous return and decrease edema may relieve the symptoms. More frequent neurovascular checks are needed because swelling could increase. Checking for the degree of tightness will reflect any change. The health care provider must be notified Analgesics do not relieve edema and could mask increasing symptoms. Lowering the cast or applying heat increases the edema.
4. **2. Rationale:** The brace should be inspected for anything that could damage the skin. A cotton T-shirt should be

worn beneath the brace to protect the skin. Metal joints should be cleaned only with pipe cleaners and oiled weekly. Plastic parts would be damaged by ammonia and should be wiped with a damp cloth and dried thoroughly.

5. 4. **Rationale:** Erythema (redness), warmth, or purulent drainage from the pin site indicates infection. It is normal to expect a small amount of crusting from the serous (clear) drainage from pin sites. An ashen skin color may indicate circulatory problems but not an infection.

6. 2. **Rationale:** The pull of traction should be in a straight line, with the rope going over a pulley at a 90-degree angle. Weights can be moved so that they hang freely for the traction force to be engaged. It is not within the scope of nursing to determine the amount of weight to be applied to traction or to manipulate traction pins. Pins should be stationary and not move. The nurse would not adjust a pin but would notify the health care provider of any pin that moved.

7. 3. **Rationale:** Proper alignment of the injured limb ensures proper pull of the traction. Patients can use an overhead trapeze to move in bed without disrupting the pull of the traction. Weights are never removed from skeletal traction because removal may damage the callus forming at the ends of the broken bones and delay healing. If weights are not hanging freely at the end of the bed, the pull of the traction is affected.

8. 1. **Rationale:** Itching is expected but can be managed with medication. Scratching of any sort can lead to skin infection.

9. 2. **Rationale:** The patient is receiving pain medication, and the assessment indicates muscle spasms. The nurse does not release the traction because it is in place to reduce muscle spasm.

10. 3, 2, 4, 1, 5. **Rationale:** These are the steps in placing a sling in an emergency or temporary situation to ensure the arm is aligned and the sling is secured so that skin at the back of the neck does not become irritated.

CHAPTER 18

Case Study

1. 3. **Rationale:** Advancing the catheter to the bifurcation avoids inflating the catheter balloon in the prostatic urethra causing trauma and pain. Catheter balloons are never inflated with saline or inflated quickly. Securing the catheter drainage tubing to the bedsheets increases the risk for accidental pulling or tension on the catheter. The advancement of the catheter until urine flows and then inserting $\frac{1}{4}$ inch more is not acceptable practice for male patients.

2. 1. **Rationale:** Emptying the drainage bag when $\frac{1}{2}$ full helps prevent unnecessary pulling and traction on the catheter, preventing trauma to the urinary meatus, urethra, and bladder neck. Washing the catheter helps prevent CAUTI, not trauma. Not replacing the foreskin after catheter insertion and care causes pain and discomfort for the patient

and causes dangerous swelling of the penis, trauma not directly caused by the catheter. Attaching the bag to a movable object increases the risk for trauma.

3. 1 and 3. **Rationale:** Securement of the male catheter to the abdomen reduces traction on the urethra and prevents urethral injury. Securing the catheter to the upper leg not the lower leg reduces the risk of urethral erosion, CAUTI, or accidental catheter removal. Attachment of the securement device above or below bifurcation per manufacturer's direction prevents occlusion of the catheter. Catheter traction should always be avoided to minimize risk for urethral trauma.

Review Questions

1. 1 and 2. **Rationale:** Evidenced-based interventions shown to decrease the risk for CAUTI include ensuring that there is a free flow of urine in the catheter to the bag and keeping the catheter bag below the level of the bladder. The urinary meatus should be cleansed with soap and water. The system should remain closed as much as possible, so it would not be appropriate to change the urinary drainage bag daily or to irrigate the catheter daily.

2. 3. **Rationale:** The recommended size for a routine indwelling catheter is 14 to 16 Fr with a 10-mL balloon. Larger catheters and balloons have been associated with increased complications, such as trauma, leakage, and discomfort.

3. 4, 5, 2, 3, 6, 1, 7.

4. 2, 3. **Rationale:** By allowing the balloon to drain by gravity, the development of creases or ridges in the balloon may be avoided minimizing trauma to the urethra during withdrawal. All patients who have a catheter removed should have their voiding monitored. The best way to do this is with a voiding record or bladder diary. The size syringe used to deflate the balloon is dictated by the size of the balloon. In an adult patient, balloon sizes are either 10 mL or 30 mL. Catheters should be pulled out slowly and smoothly. There is no evidence to support clamping catheters before removal.

5. 1. **Rationale:** The most appropriate initial action would be to determine if there is anything that is interfering with the free flow of urine from the catheter, such as kinked drainage tubing. Fluids should not be encouraged if the catheter is blocked. If the catheter is occluded, it needs to be removed and another reinserted. The health care provider needs to be notified, but the first action is to ensure the catheter is patent.

6. 3. **Rationale:** Hygiene minimizes skin irritation. There needs to be 2.5 to 5 cm (1 to 2 inches) of space between tip of the glans penis and the end of the catheter. Excess space may cause pooling of urine causing excessive exposure to urine. Shaving the pubic area increases the risk for skin irritation. The condom should be secure but not tight. Application of adhesive tape is contraindicated because it could interfere with circulation increasing risk for necrosis of the penis.

7. 1, 3, 4. **Rationale:** A new suprapubic catheter insertion site is a surgical incision and should be treated similarly

to other incisions, including sterile dressing change and inspection of the site for signs of infection. To minimize trauma and increase comfort, the catheter should be anchored to the abdomen. Wiping the catheter toward the skin violates principles of asepsis. Tension to the catheter should be avoided in all circumstances so as to minimize discomfort and potential for damage to the bladder wall.

8. 2 and 4. **Rationale:** If the catheter is in the vagina, leave it there as a landmark indicating where not to insert, and insert another sterile catheter. A catheter needs to be inserted about 2 to 3 inches into a female for the tip to enter the bladder. Pulling the catheter back and reinserting is poor technique that increases the risk for CAUTI. It is not necessary to start over in this case unless it is in the vagina.

9. 3. **Rationale:** To assess bladder function adequately after a catheter is removed, voiding frequency and amount should be monitored. Unless contraindicated, fluids should be encouraged. To promote normal micturition, patients should be placed in as normal a posture for voiding as possible. Suprapubic tenderness and pain are possible indicators of urinary retention or UTI.

10. 3. **Rationale:** All options help prevent CAUTI; only option 3 prevents unnecessary traction on the catheter. Pulling on the catheter is a cause of discomfort for the patient and can damage the urethra and bladder neck.

CHAPTER 19

Case Study

1. 2. **Rationale:** Nasal trauma can cause a deviated septum, which makes passing the NG tube difficult. Assess patency of each naris to determine if a deviation is present before tube insertion. If the deviation is noted, placement of the tube through that naris is contraindicated; use the other naris.

2. 3. **Rationale:** The color and pH of the aspirate are consistent with acidic gastric secretions. All other aspirates have a pH greater than 5.0 and likely come from the esophagus, duodenum, or pleural fluid.

3. 3. **Rationale:** The injection of air through the Salem Sump pigtail ensures that the air vent stays patent.

Review Questions

1. 3. **Rationale:** Breathing slowly helps the patient relax. Lowering the container slows the instillation of the enema solution, which eases cramping. If the patient continues to cramp, the enema solution will be evacuated too soon, altering the effectiveness of the enema.

2. 2. **Rationale:** The oil retention enema is absorbed into the fecal mass, softening it for easier evacuation.

3. 2, 4, 5. **Rationale:** Functional constipation results from multiple causes, such as reduced fluid intake to soften the stool, a lack of fiber in the diet to add bulk to the stool, and ignoring the urge to have a bowel movement.

4. 1. **Rationale:** Reflex bradycardia occurs from the manipulation of the sacral branch of the vagus nerve. The vagus

nerve is a parasympathetic nerve that when stimulated decreases heart rate.

5. 2. **Rationale:** This is the approximate distance from naris to stomach so that the tip of the tube enters the patient's stomach.

6. 1. **Rationale:** Over time, the NG tube may rest along the stomach wall or is no longer patent because of abdominal secretions. Irrigation of the tube gently moves the tube away from the stomach lining and facilitates patency. When the tube is patent, drainage of abdominal secretions occurs, and abdominal distention, discomfort, and nausea are relieved. If irrigation is unsuccessful, the nurse should contact the health care provider.

7. 5, 6, 4, 1, 3, 2. **Rationale:** Following the proper sequence of inserting any type of NG tube is essential for correct placement to prevent harm or possibly death (especially in the case of feeding tubes).

8. 3, 5. **Rationale:** The patient's symptoms suggest the NG tube is not properly decompressing the stomach. Irrigation of the NG tube with saline ensures tube patency for proper drainage. Checking if the suction is functioning properly at an intermittent setting ensures proper drainage if the tube is clear.

9. 1, 2, 3. **Rationale:** The National Pressure Ulcer Advisory Panel recommends strategies for reducing pressure ulcers from medical device insertion, as follows: Choose the correct-size medical device to fit the individual; remove or move the device daily to assess the skin; avoid placement of the device over a site of prior or existing pressure ulceration.

10. 3. **Rationale:** The patient's report of diarrhea, nausea, and vomiting are symptoms of fecal impaction. The diarrheal stool is likely leaking around the impacted stool.

CHAPTER 20

Case Study

1. 1. **Rationale:** The stoma should be red and moist and protruding above the skin level. Stents would be present in a urostomy, not an ileostomy.

2. 3. **Rationale:** The pouch is not *emptied* on a schedule but when it is $\frac{1}{3}$ to $\frac{1}{2}$ full. If the pouch is too full, it is difficult to easily empty. *Changing* the pouch should be done on a schedule to avoid unexpected leakage. The frequency of change should be every 3 to 7 days.

3. 4. **Rationale:** Ideally, the ostomy nurse can begin teaching with the first pouch change. If there is not an ostomy nurse present, the nurse should assess the stoma and the peristomal skin and begin teaching the patient self-care.

Review Questions

1. 3. **Rationale:** After removal of the colon, the bowel movement will never be formed but will have a thin or thick liquid consistency.

2. 3. **Rationale:** Site marking before surgery helps to ensure that the patient will have a well-placed stoma that is easy

to see and is not in an abdominal crease or fold. This will make care of the ostomy easier and a reliable pouching system easier to achieve.

3. 1. **Rationale:** Catheterizing the stoma is the best way to avoid contamination of the specimen.

4. 2, 5, 4, 1, 6, 3. **Rationale:** These steps permit correct disposal of the used pouch and efficient steps to control urinary output from the urostomy while cleansing the peristomal skin and keeping it dry. This facilitates application of a new, secure pouching system.

5. 1, 6, 7. **Rationale:** The pouch should be emptied when it is too full and changed on a schedule that meets the patient's needs and provides a reliable seal on the pouch. Self-care is expected, unless there are limitations posed by disability unrelated to the ostomy. Peristomal skin should be intact and free of pain or itching. Pouches are waterproof and disposable.

6. 4. **Rationale:** Postoperative edema and abdominal distention may be present for 4 to 6 weeks after surgery. During this time, the stoma may change size, but when swelling and distention are resolved, the stoma usually does not change size significantly unless other complications develop.

7. 3. **Rationale:** Family support is more important to adjustment to the body image change and the ability to have a good quality of life than the other factors.

8. 2. **Rationale:** It is normal to be distressed when there is a body image change, and a process of grieving occurs. Allowing the patient to express these feelings is helpful to the patient.

9. 4. **Rationale:** A piece of the ileum is used to make a conduit for urine to be excreted. A nephrostomy is an opening directly in the kidney, and an ileostomy and ascending colostomy are fecal stomas.

10. 2. **Rationale:** Fasting or inducing constipation encourages unhealthy habits. A larger pouch will be heavy and may loosen or be visible under clothing. Irrigation is an appropriate way to regulate a colostomy in patients motivated to do it.

CHAPTER 21

Case Study

1. The nurse should explain that a diuretic is prescribed to help the patient eliminate excess fluid. Failure to take the diuretic may lead to fluid retention and increased lung congestion and peripheral edema, which will increase stress on his heart.

2. 1, 2, 4. **Rationale:** Belief in the ineffectiveness of a medication, unpleasant side effects, cognitive changes, and lack of financial resources contribute to nonadherence. Age alone is not a contributor to nonadherence.

Review Questions

1. 1, 2, 3. **Rationale:** Distraction, the nurse's workload, and a medication being unavailable all contribute to medication errors. A computer code ensures security to the medication system.

2. 3. **Rationale:** Medication should be given 1 hour before physical therapy for peak effectiveness to minimize discomfort during the treatment.

3. 3. **Rationale:** The medication order lacks the route of administration and possible start time.

4. 3, 2. **Rationale:** A stool softener is not a time-critical medication and can be given 1 to 2 hours before or after the time it is ordered to be given.

5. 2. **Rationale:** The nurse needs to clarify medication orders that do not follow safe medication order guidelines.

6. 4. **Rationale:** 1 tbsp = 15 mL (see Table 21-4).

7. 4. **Rationale:**

$$\text{Tablets} = \frac{1\,\text{tablet}}{250\,\text{mg}} \times \frac{500\,\text{mg}}{1} \times \frac{500}{250} = 2\,\text{tablets}$$

8. 2. **Rationale:** The rest of the patients are stable; treating the pain in this situation is the priority.

9. 1, 2, 4. **Rationale:** Never crush, cut, or split a chemotherapy drug. All other precautions should be taken with chemotherapy.

10. 1, 2. **Rationale:** Larger print and a dispensing system can ensure safe medication administration to an older adult. Large-print pamphlets are also available.

CHAPTER 22

Case Study

1. 4. **Rationale:** A cream should be spread evenly over the skin surface, using long, even strokes that follow the direction of hair growth to ensure proper absorption.

2. The patient should measure her blood pressure just before taking the medication to obtain a baseline blood pressure and measure the blood pressure again 30 to 60 minutes after taking the medication to determine response to the medication.

Review Questions

1. 2. **Rationale:** Reading the labels a second time reduces errors and ensures that the nurse is preparing the correct medication.

2. 4. **Rationale:** Syringes for oral dosing are adapted for accurate administration of medication to pediatric patients. They do not have a syringe or needle cap and cannot be accidentally administered as a parenteral medication.

3. 3. **Rationale:** The pharmacist is a good resource. There may be other preparations of the extended-release medication or other medication options. Extended-release tablets are never split or crushed because this would change the dose distribution when the medication is administered. Do not encourage patients to swallow any medication they state they have difficulty swallowing because this could cause the patient to choke.

4. 2. **Rationale:** The current recommendation is to request that the pharmacy split and repackage the medication. This ensures a noncontaminated accurate method to

split the medication and ensures that the second half of the medication is used for the next dose. The nurse should split the medication if there is no other option.

5. 1, 3, 4, 5. **Rationale:** Option 2 is incorrect. The mouthpiece should not be inserted beyond the raised lip on the mouthpiece. Option 6 is also incorrect. When taking two medications prescribed at the same time, the patient should wait 2 to 5 minutes before taking the second medication.

6. 2, 1, 5, 3, 4. **Rationale:** This is the correct order for safe administration of ophthalmic ointment.

7. 4. **Rationale:** It is important to remove any medication residue before applying a new patch to ensure a consistent dosage delivery. When giving a transdermal patch, always rotate the application site. A patient should never cut a patch in half because there is no way to determine dosage. If the patient becomes oversedated, the health care provider should be notified. Always remove a patch before applying the next dose.

8. 3. **Rationale:** Rectal suppositories are contraindicated in patients with rectal surgery or active rectal bleeding. A suppository can be given for hemorrhoids; however, extra lubricant is helpful for insertion. A suppository is often used for treatment of fever. The presence of diarrhea is often an indication for a suppository and does not contraindicate use in this situation.

9. 1, 2, 3. **Rationale:** Option 4 is incorrect. A DPI is breath activated; there is no need to coordinate puffs with inhalation.

10. 2. **Rationale:** A 5-year-old child receives an ear medication the same way as an adult receives it. The nurse straightens the ear canal by pulling the pinna upward and outward.

CHAPTER 23

Case Study

1. The nurse needs to know the following: drug classification, desired effect, and nursing implications related to heparin therapy and the safe medication dose, which must be compared with the order before administration. The nurse needs to calculate how many milliliters to draw from the vial and if a filter needle is required.

2. The nurse needs to know the patient's current diet and use of over-the-counter (OTC) supplements, herbal supplements, and other prescribed medications to ensure that there is no increased risk of bleeding; if anything is affecting blood flow to subcutaneous tissues of the abdomen; and any related laboratory findings of the partial thromboplastin time.

3. The preferred site would be the abdomen for better absorption. The main difference between a vial and an ampule for dose preparation is that a vial does not require injection of air into the vial.

Review Questions

1. 1, 3, 4. **Rationale:** The nurse needs to know the compatibility of existing IV fluids before administering any

medication via IV bolus, pain level is assessed on a scale of 0 to 10, and the patency of the IV site must be established. The rate is per minute, not per hour.

2. 4. **Rationale:** Medication is drawn from the vial first to prevent contamination of the vial with medication from the ampule.

3. 2. **Rationale:** An induration of greater than 10 mm in a healthy individual indicates tuberculosis exposure and requires follow-up.

4. 1. **Rationale:** These symptoms indicate paresthesia and should not be present after an IM injection.

5. 1, b; 2, c; 3, a.

6. 4. **Rationale:** This is an appropriate size needle for administering a subcutaneous medication.

7. 2. **Rationale:** The nurse should calculate how much medication will be used for the injection while considering the route; this should be done before the diluent and powder are mixed.

8. 1. **Rationale:** Stop the infusion. The IV line is infiltrated, and the site needs to be changed.

9. 1. **Rationale:** Assessing the IV site is the nursing priority; medication cannot be given into a problem IV site.

10. 3, 7, 1, 6, 4, 5, 2. **Rationale:** These are the correct steps for administering ID injection.

CHAPTER 24

Case Study

1. 1, 2, 4. **Rationale:** These are important descriptors that provide information about the wound. Over time, the results of a wound assessment help identify how well the wound is healing. Information about the hemoglobin and hematocrit does not provide wound assessment information.

2. 2, 4. **Rationale:** The objective of using wound irrigation on this wound is to help clean any necrotic tissue in the wound base and to ensure that the base of the wound is clean. Using a 19-gauge angiocatheter with a 35-mL syringe provides the necessary amount of pressure to clean the wound. Leaving the gauze in the wound does not give the nurse a clear view of the wound and does not allow the irrigation to reach the wound tissue. Administering warm wound irrigant may harm the wound tissue. The container of wound irrigant should not be placed near the wound because this would contaminate the container and could cause an excessive amount of irrigant to be used (because there is less control when holding a full container over a wound).

3. 2. **Rationale:** The patient's wound contained drainage and was opened by the surgeon and left open to heal by secondary intention; this allows the wound to fill in from the bottom up. A wound healing by primary intention would have the wound edges approximated.

Review Questions

1. 1, 2, 4, 5. **Rationale:** The dimensions including the depth and presence of undermining are two important

measurements along with width and depth that help to determine wound-healing progress. The estimate of the wound-healing progress is not an objective assessment parameter because the time to healing depends on many factors that cannot be predicted. The color of the tissue in the wound also gives an assessment of movement toward healing as well as information needed to choose a wound treatment. A wound filled with granulation tissue will move toward healing; a wound with yellow or brown tissue will need a wound treatment to clean the tissue and support the growth of granulation tissue. The condition of the periwound skin provides data on the appropriateness of the wound treatment; if the surrounding tissue is red, this can indicate inflammation from the wound or the dressing type.

2. 1, 2. **Rationale:** The first intervention would be to check to see if the drainage is coming from around the tube rather than through it, as indicated by an increased amount of drainage on the gauze pad. Next, the nurse should call the surgeon. It is not advisable to wait 8 hours before any intervention because you know that this patient had 100 mL of drainage only 8 hours ago; the drain could be plugged. Jackson-Pratt drains are not irrigated routinely.

3. 3. **Rationale:** The collection bulb should be below the insertion site to facilitate drainage. To prevent pulling of the tube at the insertion site, pin the bulb to the patient's gown. Never allow the bulb to become full because it becomes heavy as it pulls on the insertion site, and a full bulb prevents further drainage collection. Never do anything to prevent drainage, and the insertion site should remain dry and clean with no lubrication to the site.

4. 2. **Rationale:** Start by explaining to patient what will happen. After applying gloves to protect patient's incision, determine if the healing ridge is present; if not, do not proceed. Remove staples and apply Steri-Strips.

5. 2. **Rationale:** The recommended amount of pressure to be used in NPWT is −75 to −125 mm Hg. Using more negative pressure can cause harm to the wound and pain to the patient.

6. 1, 3, 4. **Rationale:** Use pieces of the adhesive drape over the areas where air is leaking. The leak causes a break in the seal, and the suction is no longer effective. Patching maintains the airtight seal. Clip hair in the area that adhesive drape will be located before application if the facility policy allows. Hair can interfere with the seal of the adhesive drape. Do not use adhesive remover because this can leave a residue, preventing a good seal. Many adhesive removers leave a film on the skin that is greasy and does not allow the adhesive drape to make a good seal. Patching the leaking area with gauze does not work because the gauze does not allow an airtight seal. If soap is used on the periwound area, it must be rinsed off thoroughly to obtain an adequate seal.

7. 2. **Rationale:** The Steri-Strips provide support to the wound by distributing tension across the wound.

8. 2. **Rationale:** The deepest part of the wound should be measured to determine the depth because this identifies the area that needs the highest degree of healing. Only one measurement is required, and this would be the deepest because this area would likely take the longest to heal.

9. 1. **Rationale:** Wounds heal in an orderly fashion to clean the wound, stop bleeding, build new tissue and allow the healed tissue to gain strength.

10. 2. **Rationale:** The Jackson-Pratt drain has the smallest capacity of the drains listed.

CHAPTER 25

Case Study

1. 2, 3. **Rationale:** Moisture barrier ointment is applied to areas that will be in contact with the stool. A thick layer prevents the liquid stool from contacting the skin. If the amount of fecal incontinence is high and the consistency is watery to slightly pasty, the use of a fecal incontinence collector can keep the stool from contacting the skin. Talcum powder absorbs moisture and holds the moisture to the skin and should not be used in areas of fecal incontinence. The use of towels under the patient is not indicated because the towels remain moist and may damage the patient's skin.

2. 2. **Rationale:** The location of the skin breakdown is around the anus, and the etiology is likely fecal incontinence. Staging should be used only for pressure ulcers, and this skin breakdown is not from pressure.

3. 2, 3, 4. **Rationale:** Options 2, 3, and 4 are activities that are safely delegated to NAP and assist in reducing the patient's pressure ulcer risk. Option 1 requires nursing assessment; this is the role of the registered nurse. The NAP can report specifics to the registered nurse, such as increased redness in perianal region. However, it is the registered nurse's role to fully assess the patient's skin.

Review Questions

1. 1, 2. **Rationale:** The patient with the surgical wound most likely has an infection that delays wound healing because the inflammatory phase of wound healing is prolonged. A steroid such as cortisol also delays the inflammatory phase of wound healing. Vitamin C and a moist dressing are factors that promote wound healing.

2. 2, 4. **Rationale:** The patient is at risk for device-related pressure ulcers at the mouth or lips because of the endotracheal tube location. All patients have the risk of pressure ulcers over bony prominences, but the risk is greater posteriorly in this patient because of her weight and difficulty turning. The pillows remove the risk of heel ulcers, and the IV site is not subject to pressure. There is no tube exiting the patient's nose.

3. 2. **Rationale:** A moist saline gauze dressing provides a moist environment to the wound and wicks away excessive drainage, facilitating healing.

4. 2. **Rationale:** A hydrocolloid dressing interacts with the moist wound base and forms a gel over the wound to support moist wound healing.

5. 3. **Rationale:** Explain the purpose of the dressing change to the patient before application. Position him in a way that provides easy access to wound for cleansing. After cleansing the wound, select a dressing that extends at least 2.5 cm [1 inch] beyond the wound edge, and remove the paper backing. The dressing adheres best if gently pressed to the skin.

6. 2. **Rationale:** All four patients have some risk factors for developing a pressure ulcer. However, the 45-year-old patient has more factors, three, placing him at risk: lack of sensory perception, limited mobility, and friction and shear with movement.

7. 3. **Rationale:** The category of frictional shear should be added.

8. 2, 3, 4. **Rationale:** Dehydration can become a problem because the air circulating around the patient is warm. Moving a patient out of an air fluidized bed can be difficult because of the high bed edges and the fact that the patient is submerged into the bed. The air fluidized bed is large and very heavy making it difficult to transport.

9. 1, 3, 4, 5. **Rationale:** Unrelieved shear and friction can cause harm to the wound and prevent wound healing. A lack of calories can slow down the development of healthy granulation and epidermal tissue. Lack of psychosocial support also has been shown to have a negative effect on healing.

10. 2. **Rationale:** Obese tissue is poorly vascularized, slowing down the delivery of nutrients to the healing wound.

CHAPTER 26

Case Study

1. 3, 4. **Rationale:** Patients react differently to body image alterations. It is necessary to assess the patient's comfort level with viewing the wound and in participating with the dressing change. This may take time. Provide updates on the progress of wound healing with each dressing change.

2. 2, 1, 6, 3, 5, 4, 7. **Rationale:** The proper order of changing the dressing prevents contamination of supplies and the wound and decreases the risk of infection.

3. 2, 3, 4. **Rationale:** A moist-to-dry dressing change may sometimes be delegated to the NAP, especially if it is a chronic wound. The nurse should instruct the NAP if he or she can change or reinforce the dressing and what signs and symptoms to report to the nurse. In this scenario, the nurse did not delegate the dressing change.

Review Questions

1. 4, 2, 6, 3, 5, 7, 1. **Rationale:** The proper order of changing the dressing prevents contamination of supplies and the wound and decreases the risk of infection. Some gel-type dressings can leave a residual film in the wound bed, which requires irrigation.

2. 1, 2, 3. **Rationale:** Binders support a wound, protect surrounding tissue, and decrease pain. A binder that is too tight can impede breathing and cause damage to underlying tissue. You would not expect a sign of increased abdominal circumference.

3. 1. **Rationale:** The steps involved in the teach-back method require confirmation of patient and caregiver learning. If the caregiver says she is going to dispose of the dressing in the regular trash, further instruction is needed. All other statements are appropriate.

4. 4. **Rationale:** A hydrocolloid dressing is indicated for a low to moderately exuding wound. Thinner versions are generally used on wounds that are dry or that have low levels of exudate. The hydrophilic gel facilitates autolytic débridement, which is ideal for exudate but not dry eschar. The dressings are not designed to absorb large amounts of drainage.

5. 4. **Rationale:** Wounds with large amounts of drainage require a dressing that can absorb the exudate while protecting the periwound from maceration. In this case, a foam dressing would be an appropriate choice following a treatment plan to address the macerated periwound.

6. 1, 3, 4. **Rationale:** Universal precautions and PPE should be used whenever the risk of splashing of bodily fluids is present, regardless of whether or not the patient has a known infection. Knowing the cause and type of wound, including the presence of drains, enables the nurse to ensure the proper treatment plan is followed. Proper disposal of contaminated dressings prevents the spread of microorganisms.

7. 3. **Rationale:** Wound pain can severely affect the patient's physical and psychological well-being. A mutual goal for patient and nurse is to ensure the pain is minimized and controlled during the dressing change. All other options are likely to increase the patient's pain.

8. 1, 2, 3. **Rationale:** The drying of the dressing in a wound bed may cause the dressing to adhere to healthy surrounding tissue. Removal of the dressing can cause injury if the dressing is not moistened before removal, unless the intention is to débride the wound.

9. 3. **Rationale:** A dressing should remove exudate, but it is important not to dry out the wound. Tissue growth occurs in a warm moist environment.

10. 3. **Rationale:** The correct way to remove a transparent dressing is to remove the film in the direction of the open edge of the tear so that additional skin is not torn.

CHAPTER 27

Case Study

1. 7, 3, 1, 6, 4, 5, 2. **Rationale:** IV fluids must be removed from the refrigerator before infusion. Closing roller clamp of old IV tubing prevents fluid from leaking from tubing. Removing spike from old IV tubing maintains sterility and prevents tubing from running dry. Inserting new spike into new IV bag ensures no break in therapy and maintains sterility. Air in tubing can cause emboli and be fatal to the patient. Regulating flow rate ensures that correct rate of fluid is given. Labeling bag provides for accuracy

when assessing right patient and right medication and ensures that fluid is running on time.

2. 2. **Rationale:** The infusion of ¾ of the volume of a 1-L bag would place the patient at risk for fluid overload, which is reflected in the assessment findings.

3. True. **Rationale:** Administration of prescribed IV solutions and medications is not a task the NAP can provide.

Review Questions

1. 4. **Rationale:** Signs and symptoms of phlebitis do not include respiratory, cardiac, or GI presentations, but they do include the local symptoms of erythema and pain.

2. 2. **Rationale:** If a transfusion reaction is suspected based on vital sign changes or complaints of itching or the presence of hives, the priority nursing intervention is to *stop* the blood transfusion but maintain IV access.

3. 4. **Rationale:** Based on INS standards of practice, the smallest device and smallest gauge possible to give the prescribed therapy should be used.

4. 4. **Rationale:** According to the INS, optimal tip placement for a central line is the SVC. A PICC is placed in the arm via the antecubital fossa or upper arm and advanced to the SVC.

5. 4. **Rationale:** The correct answer is derived from the following calculation:

6. False. **Rationale:** Partial PN can be administered through either a peripheral device or a central vascular device because the osmolarity is less than 600 mOsm/L. Total PN must be given through a central device because the osmolarity is greater than 600 mOsm/L.

7. 1. **Rationale:** Current evidence states chlorhexidine skin antisepsis has been proven to reduce the risk of CLABSI when used as a skin preparation.

8. 3. **Rationale:** NS is the only IV solution that should be used with blood because of its isotonic quality. Dextrose solutions can cause hemolysis of RBCs.

9. 2, 4, 1, 3, 5. **Rationale:** After removing tape and dressing, observe the site for signs and symptoms of IV device–related complications. Cleanse site with an antiseptic swab to remove any surface microorganisms before applying a new dressing. Apply a new transparent membrane dressing to the site to prevent any microorganisms from entering the insertion site. Label the site with date, time, catheter gauge, and your initials for identification as to when device was placed and size placed.

10. 3. **Rationale:** The only correct way to identify a patient is to use two identifiers and compare with the MAR. Comparing the patient's arm band with the MAR is not two identifiers. Asking another nurse to verify a patient is not acceptable; likewise, delegating to the NAP to verify the patient is unacceptable. Use of a bar code is an appropriate and acceptable way to identify a patient before fluid administration.

CHAPTER 28

Case Study

1. 4, 5. **Rationale:** Identification of the correct patient, surgical site, and procedure occurs immediately before moving to the procedure area, and a time-out is performed before starting the procedure. This verification is also done during any patient hand-off.

2. 1, 2, 4, 5. **Rationale:** Although family caregiver contact information is important, it is not a requirement for the procedural checklist.

Review Questions

1. 2. **Rationale:** The three phases include the immediate postanesthesia recovery, early recovery, and convalescent phase. The immediate postanesthesia phase extends from the time the patient leaves the operating room (OR) to the time of transfer from the postanesthesia care unit (PACU) to the nursing unit. This phase requires 2 or more hours and frequent assessments for complications. Patients having surgery in ambulatory outpatient surgery centers have the same recovery needs as patients having surgery in a hospital. The early recovery phase includes several days after surgery followed by a convalescent recovery phase of several additional days or weeks at home for the continued healing process.

2. 2. **Rationale:** Patient education is not a skill that can be delegated to the NAP.

3. 3. **Rationale:** The surgeon is ultimately responsible for obtaining informed consent. The nurse should verify the patient's understanding and ensure that the patient's signature is complete before signing the consent form as a witness.

4. 2. **Rationale:** It is important for the patient to be in the correct position to allow for increased lung expansion.

5. 1, 2. **Rationale:** The surgeon should be notified immediately to evaluate bleeding source and possible respiratory depression.

6. 2. **Rationale:** Small amounts of drainage are normal. Marking the amount allows the nurse to evaluate progression of drainage.

7. 3. **Rationale:** The side-lying position minimizes the chances of aspiration and obstruction of the airway with the tongue.

8. 4. **Rationale:** One of the side effects of a local anesthetic can be a skin rash. Its vasoconstrictive property slows the rate of absorption of the anesthetic agent. Hypotension and bradycardia are other possible side effects.

9. 1. **Rationale:** The NAP may obtain preoperative vital signs on stable patients with direction from the registered nurse.

10. 4. **Rationale:** Fluid resuscitation and blood products are needed to increase circulating blood volume.

CHAPTER 29

Case Study

1. 2. **Rationale:** Patient assessment is the first step to verify patient unresponsiveness before any additional therapy for a lethal arrhythmia. The nurse must always assess the patient's condition.

2. 2. **Rationale:** The patient's responsiveness and pulse need to be assessed before chest compressions can begin or AED

application. Begin chest compressions, and once the AED is prepared, attach the AED. Immediately after the first shock or advised no shock, provide 2 ventilations and resume 30:2 CPR.

3. 1. **Rationale:** An NAP who is certified in basic life support techniques may use an AED. Prompt use of an AED by correctly trained personnel increases the chance that the patient's heart will return to normal rhythm and the patient will remain stable until the rapid response team can arrive at the bedside.

Review Questions

1. 2. **Rationale:** According to the American Heart Association 2010 CPR guidelines, begin CPR immediately after the shock to provide immediate perfusion to the heart after shock.
2. 1. **Rationale:** Head tilt–chin lift provides the best technique to open an airway with no suspected trauma.
3. 1. **Rationale:** The patient has a better chance of survival if the first shock is delivered in less than 3 minutes inside a hospital. The chance of survival decreases by 10% for every minute of delay.
4. 3. **Rationale:** In performing chest compressions, fractured ribs may lacerate the liver or puncture the lung.
5. 4. **Rationale:** An oral airway should be inserted only in unconscious patients because of the risk of vomiting.
6. 1. **Rationale:** When an advanced airway is in place, breaths should be delivered at a rate of 8 to 10 per minute to avoid hyperventilation.
7. 3. **Rationale:** To provide more continuous perfusion to the body, chest compressions-to-ventilation rate ratio should be 30 : 2.
8. 2. **Rationale:** Interruption in chest compressions is an interruption in blood flow. Coronary and cerebral blood flow are essential to survival.
9. 3. **Rationale:** End-tidal CO_2 can be used as a measurement of perfusion during CPR. The goal of high-quality CPR is to maintain end-tidal CO_2 greater than 20.
10. 4. **Rationale:** Research has repeatedly shown that basic life support measures of early, quality CPR and early defibrillation improve survival.

CHAPTER 30

Case Study

1. 1. **Rationale:** The nurse recognizes that this couple is having a difficult time making health care decisions. It is important to help them talk about their feelings and fears. Although the nurse may at some point offer alternatives and expand the discussion to include other members of the health care team, at this time the husband and wife would most benefit by being able to talk about their feelings.
2. 4. **Rationale:** After people have been able to express their emotional responses to a situation, and after they have more information, it is helpful to discuss their goals. It is rarely helpful to avoid difficult discussions or shift the conversation to medical management.

3. A nurse should not delegate the responsibility for conflict management or discussions of goals of care to a nursing assistant. These delicate conversations are best managed by a health care provider skilled in psychosocial assessment and interventions. The nurse would instruct the nursing assistant to continue to report communication needs.

Review Questions

1. 2. **Rationale:** An advance directive can be a written document, or a person can appoint a durable power of attorney for health care to make decisions when the patient is no longer able. A person preparing an advance directive should share it with his or her health care providers and family members and place it in his or her medical record. An advance directive provides an opportunity for a person to ask for certain care interventions (effective pain management) or refuse other interventions (artificial food or water), although some states have differing policies regarding the use of advance directives.
2. 1. **Rationale:** In hospice care, priority is given to meeting the needs of the patient and family caregivers and addressing the issues most important to them. The nurse can help the patient make the best care decisions when he or she understands the patient's usual preferred life routines. Although patient education can be very helpful in hospice care, the first activities are geared at understanding patient preferences.
3. 3. **Rationale:** End of life experiences are highly individual. A meaningful, peaceful death is characterized by abiding by religious and cultural norms and expectations of the patient and family. There are times with facility routines may have to be changed to accommodate concerns of the patient and family.
4. 4. **Rationale:** Patient-centered care and safety are important considerations. The nurse should work to maintain both values by collaborating with patients and family caregivers to identify creative, workable ways to mean meaningful patient goals.
5. 2. **Rationale:** It is best to elevate the head of the bed as soon as possible after death to prevent pooling of blood in the face and discoloration. Before beginning body preparations, ask if family members would like to participate. Put on gloves and other protective barriers as needed and proceed from dirty to clean tasks, replacing soaked dressings, bathing, and placing the patient in a clean gown.
6. 1. **Rationale:** Compassion fatigue can best be avoided when caregivers engage in effective self-care strategies and maintain life balance. Acknowledge the importance of your work, but do not assume you are personally responsible for all outcomes. Realize that loss is painful. Your desire to continue to care for people in situations of grief and loss contributes to being an empathic caregiver.
7. 2, 4. **Rationale:** Patients of any age or diagnosis can receive palliative care in any setting. Options 1 and 4

apply to hospice care, a form of palliative care for people who likely have 6 to 12 months or less to live. Option 3 refers to palliative care in the home setting. Palliative care occurs in all health care settings.

8. 3. **Rationale:** Interviews with family caregivers indicate that they appreciate timely, guided instruction when they have questions or concerns. They also appreciate communication and the presence of professional caregivers. Support existing coping skills at this time.

9. 4. **Rationale:** The nurse first should listen nonjudgmentally to the family member and gather more information. Sometimes a clarification helps the person deliberate. Talking also helps validate the person's concerns. People rarely know why they believe what they do, but those beliefs are important to them. The nurse might report the family member's concern, with the added information, to the health care team.

10. 2. **Rationale:** Religious and spiritual concerns overlap for many people, but they are different concepts. Spiritual matters can be expressed in religious or nonreligious terms and involve human dimensions of community, hope, meaning, and a sense of the Holy Other.

CHAPTER 31

Case Study

1. 1, 2, 4. **Rationale:** Pot handles should be turned inward. Hot water heaters should be set below 120°F (49°C). A stove lock is a good safety measure to prevent burns of small children. Smoking is a risk factor for burns; encourage the mother to stop smoking by offering access to classes.

2. 2, 4. **Rationale:** All medication should be stored out of reach of children. Medication should not be referred to as a "treat" to children because it presents a risk that the child would attempt to take more of the medication and potentially overdose.

3. Assess if the mother demonstrates risky behavior (has she missed a dose of insulin or does she ever give it at unscheduled times). Assess what attitudes, beliefs, or previous experience she has in giving or taking medications.

Review Questions

1. 1, 2, 4. **Rationale:** Home instruction is needed to help clients be able to attain healthy behaviors in the home, which includes health promotion, coping with any health-related restrictions, and learning ways to restore their health. Learning the medical history of a family caregiver is private and confidential information. It should be considered only if the family caregiver offers assistance in the home and is willing to share such information.

2. 2. **Rationale:** The daughter and client need to be instructed about the benefits of sharing the diary with health care providers. Information must be documented by the client or family member; however, the health care team can use this information to assess for concerns and plan care.

3. 1, 3. **Rationale:** Signs give clues to guide clients to desired locations. Allowing wandering in a safe place reduces the risk of the client leaving home. Locks and electronic alarms are necessary to reduce wandering. Restraints are inappropriate and increase client's agitation.

4. 3. **Rationale:** A pill dispenser helps a client self-administer medications as scheduled. The other three options are important for medication safety but do not directly affect administration.

5. 1, 3. **Rationale:** Charts help a client be organized in taking medications safely. Storage techniques are important to review because different medications are stored in different ways. Never place needles in a plastic bag. Always keep a medication in an easy-to-open container to make it easier for clients with dexterity problems to self-administer.

6. 4. **Rationale:** Gloves should be worn if there is a risk of contacting medical waste. Sharp objects or disposable sheets are never placed in trash bags. Place sharps in hard plastic containers and disposable sheets in separate plastic bags placed in trash.

7. 3. **Rationale:** Firearms are the second leading cause of death in 10- to 24-year-olds. Guns need to be secured and kept in a locked cabinet to avoid injury.

8. 2. **Rationale:** The obese client will need to make dietary changes relative to his weight and diagnosis of diabetes. The culturally sensitive nurse begins helping this client by first listening to his food traditions and not assuming she can choose lifestyle and diet changes for the client without consulting with him.

9. 3. **Rationale:** Area rugs are trip hazards. A cane is an appropriate assistive device when fitted correctly, and shoes should have thin soles with traction. Diuretics are better scheduled early in the day to avoid the client getting up in the middle of the night to use the bathroom, which increases risk of falls.

10. 2. **Rationale:** Older adults experience physical injury from falls and may have psychological trauma. It is normal for the father to have some fear of falling again; the nurse can explain this to the son and offer assistance to deal with this fear.

Abbreviations and Equivalents

ABBREVIATIONS FOR CONVERSION USING HOUSEHOLD MEASURES

1 drop (gtt) = 1 minim
1 teaspoon (1 tsp) = 5 mL
3 tsp = 1 tablespoon (tbsp)
1 cup = 8 oz
16 oz = 1 pound (lb)

STANDARD EQUIVALENTS, ABBREVIATIONS, AND CONVERSIONS

1000 mg = 1 g
1000 mL = 1 liter (L)
2.2 lb = 1 kilogram (kg) = 1000 g
1 tsp = 5 mL
1 dr = 4 mL
mEq: milliequivalent
mcg: microgram

SYMBOLS

/ Per
≤ Equal to or less than
≥ Equal to or more than
≅ Approximately equal to
+/−, ± Plus or minus
♂ Male
♀ Female
1° Primary; first degree
2° Secondary; second degree
3° Tertiary; third degree
↑ Up; increase
↓ Down; decrease

ABBREVIATIONS

$\bar{a}$: before
abd: abdomen
ABGs: arterial blood gases

ac: before meals
ad lib: as desired
ADH: antidiuretic hormone
ADLs: activities of daily living
AFB: acid-fast bacillus (related to tuberculosis)
AIDS: acquired immunodeficiency syndrome
ALL: acute lymphoblastic leukemia
AMB: ambulatory
AP (and lateral chest): anterior and posterior
ASA: aspirin
ASHD: arteriosclerotic heart disease
ax: axillary
BE: barium enema
bid: twice a day
BM: bowel movement
BP: blood pressure
BPH: benign prostatic hypertrophy
BR: bed rest
BRP: bathroom privileges
BSE: breast self-examination
BSI: body substance isolation
BUN: blood urea nitrogen
bx: biopsy
$\bar{c}$: with
C&S: culture and sensitivity
CA: cancer
CABG: coronary artery bypass graft
CAD: coronary artery disease
cap: capsule
CBC: complete blood count
CBI: continuous bladder irrigation
CBR: complete bed rest
CC: chief complaint
CDC: Centers for Disease Control and Prevention
CHF: congestive heart failure
Cl: chloride
CN: cranial nerve
CNS: central nervous system
c/o: complains of
CO_2: carbon dioxide
COPD: chronic obstructive pulmonary disease

CPM: continuous passive motion
CPR: cardiopulmonary resuscitation
CSF: cerebrospinal fluid
CT: computed tomography
CVA: cerebrovascular accident (stroke)
CVP: central venous pressure
D5NS, D5NS: 5% dextrose in 0.9% (normal) saline
DAT: diet as tolerated
DM: diabetes mellitus
DNR: do not resuscitate
DSD: dry sterile dressing
DTR: deep tendon reflex
DVT: deep venous thrombosis
dx: diagnosis
EC: enteric coated
ECG, EKG: electrocardiogram
elix: elixir
ER: extended release
ESR: erythrocyte sedimentation rate
ESRD: end-stage renal disease
ET: enterostomal therapist
FUO: fever of unknown origin
fx: fracture
g: gram
GI: gastrointestinal
gtt: drops
GU: genitourinary
Hb, Hgb: hemoglobin
HBV: hepatitis B virus
HCO_3^-: bicarbonate
Hct: hematocrit
HCV: hepatitis C virus
HEPA: high-efficiency air
HIV: human immunodeficiency virus
h/o: history of
HOB: head of bed
HR: heart rate
hs: at bedtime
HTN: hypertension
I&O: intake and output
ICP: intracranial pressure
ICU: intensive care unit
IDDM: insulin-dependent diabetes mellitus
IM: intramuscular
IPPB: intermittent positive-pressure breathing
IV: intravenous
JVD: jugular vein distention
K: potassium
KUB: kidney, ureter, bladder
KVO: keep vein open (run IV very slowly)
LLQ: left lower quadrant
LMP: last menstrual period
LOC: level of consciousness
LR: lactated Ringer's solution lytes: electrolytes
MAP: mean arterial pressure
MCHC: mean corpuscular hemoglobin concentration
MCV: mean corpuscular volume

MI: myocardial infarction
N: nitrogen
Na: sodium
NaCl: sodium chloride
neg: negative
NG: nasogastric
NPO: nothing by mouth
NS: normal saline
NSAIDs: nonsteroidal antiinflammatory drugs
O_2: oxygen
OOB: out of bed
OR: operating room
OT: occupational therapy
OTC: over-the-counter (medicine available without prescription)
P: pulse
PACU: postanesthesia care unit
pc: after meals
PCA: patient-controlled analgesia
PE: pulmonary embolism
PID: pelvic inflammatory disease
PMH: past medical history
PMI: point of maximal impulse
PO: by mouth
postop: after surgery
preop: before surgery
prn: as needed
pt: patient
PT: physical therapy
PT: prothrombin time
PTT: partial thromboplastin time
PVD: peripheral vascular disease
q: each
q_h (fill in the number of hours), e.g. q3h: every 3 hours
qs: sufficient quantity
R: respirations
RA: rheumatoid arthritis
RBC: red blood cells
R/O: rule out (eliminate possibility of a condition)
ROM: range of motion
ROS: review of systems
r/t: related to
RUQ: right upper quadrant
Rx: treatment
s̄: without
sl (SL): sublingual
SOB: shortness of breath
sp gr: specific gravity
SR: sustained release
STAT: immediately
STD: sexually transmitted disease
supp: suppository
susp: suspension
sx: symptoms, signs
T: temperature
T&C: type and crossmatch
Tab: tablet

TB: tuberculosis
TCDB: turn, cough, deep breathe
tid: three times a day
TPN: total parenteral nutrition
TPR: temperature, pulse, respirations
TURP: transurethral resection of prostate
UA: urinalysis
up ad: up as desired
URI: upper respiratory infection

US: ultrasound
UTI: urinary tract infection
VS: vital signs
VTBI: volume to be infused
WBC: white blood cell
WC: wheelchair
WNL: within normal limits
wt: weight

OFFICIAL "DO NOT USE" LIST*

DO NOT USE	POTENTIAL PROBLEM	USE INSTEAD
U (unit)	Mistaken for "0" (zero), the number "4" (four), or "cc"	Write "unit"
IU (International Unit)	Mistaken for IV (intravenous) or the number 10 (ten)	Write "International Unit"
Q.D., QD, q.d., qd (daily)	Mistaken for each other	Write "daily"
Q.O.D, QOD, q.o.d., qod (every other day)	Period after the Q mistaken for "I" and the "O" mistaken for "I"	Write "every other day"
Trailing zero (X.0 mg)†	Decimal point is missing	Write X mg
Lack of leading zero (.X mg)		Write 0.X mg
MS	Can mean morphine sulphate or magnesium sulphate	Write "morphine sulphate"
MSO$_4$ and MgSO$_4$	Confused for one another	Write "magnesium sulphate"

Official "Do Not Use" List, Joint Commission on Accreditation of Healthcare Organizations, February 2012; www.jointcommission.org, accessed December 5, 2014.

*Applies to all orders and all medication-related documentation that is handwritten (including free-text computer entry) or on preprinted forms.

†**Exception**: A "trailing zero" may be used only where required to demonstrate the level of precision of the value being reported such as for laboratory results, imaging studies that report size of lesions, or catheter/tube sizes. It may not be used in medication orders or other medical-related documentation.

ADDITIONAL ABBREVIATIONS, ACRONYMS, AND SYMBOLS (FOR POSSIBLE FUTURE INCLUSION IN THE OFFICIAL "DO NOT USE" LIST)

DO NOT USE	POTENTIAL PROBLEM	USE INSTEAD
> (greater than)	Misinterpreted as the number "7" (seven) or the letter "L"	Write "greater than"
< (less than)	Confused for one another	Write "less than"
Abbreviations for drug names	Misinterpreted due to similar abbreviations for multiple drugs	Write drugs names in full
Apothecary units	Unfamiliar to many practitioners Confused with metric units	Write drugs names in full
@	Mistaken for the number "2" (two)	Write "at"
cc	Mistaken for U (units) when written poorly	Write "mL" or "milliliters"
μg	Mistaken for mg (milligrams), resulting in one thousand-fold overdose	Write "mcg" or "micrograms"

Official "Do Not Use" List, Joint Commission on Accreditation of Heathcare Organizations, February 2012; www.jointcommission.org, accessed December 15, 2014.

INDEX OF SKILLS